Thieme

Ear Surgery Illustrated

A Comprehensive Atlas of Otologic Microsurgical Techniques

Robert K. Jackler, MD
Sewall Professor and Chair
Department of Otolaryngology–Head and Neck Surgery
Professor of Neurosurgery and Surgery
Stanford University School of Medicine
Stanford, California

Illustrations by
Christine Gralapp, MA, CMI, FAMI
Medical and Scientific Illustrator
Fairfax, California

1,105 illustrations

Thieme
New York • Stuttgart • Delhi • Rio de Janeiro

Library of Congress Cataloging-in-Publication Data

Names: Jackler, Robert K., author. | Complemented by (work): Jackler, Robert K. Atlas of skull base surgery and neurotology.
Title: Ear surgery illustrated : a comprehensive atlas of otologic microsurgical techniques / Robert K. Jackler ; illustrations by Christine Gralapp.
Description: New York : Thieme, [2019] | A companion volume to Atlas of skull
base surgery and neurotology / Robert K. Jackler. 2nd ed. c2009. | Includes bibliographical references and index.
Identifiers: LCCN 2018061416| ISBN 9781684201105 (hardcover : alk. paper) |
ISBN 9781684201112 (e-book)
Subjects: | MESH: Ear—surgery | Microsurgery—methods | Otologic Surgical Procedures—methods | Ear Diseases—surgery | Atlas
Classification: LCC RD529 | NLM WV 17 | DDC 617.5/1400222—dc23
LC record available at https://lccn.loc.gov/2018061416

Important note: Medicine is an ever-changing science undergoing continual development. Research and clinical experience are continually expanding our knowledge, in particular our knowledge of proper treatment and drug therapy. Insofar as this book mentions any dosage or application, readers may rest assured that the authors, editors, and publishers have made every effort to ensure that such references are in accordance with **the state of knowledge at the time of production of the book.**

Nevertheless, this does not involve, imply, or express any guarantee or responsibility on the part of the publishers in respect to any dosage instructions and forms of applications stated in the book. **Every user is requested to examine carefully** the manufacturers' leaflets accompanying each drug and to check, if necessary in consultation with a physician or specialist, whether the dosage schedules mentioned therein or the contraindications stated by the manufacturers differ from the statements made in the present book. Such examination is particularly important with drugs that are either rarely used or have been newly released on the market. Every dosage schedule or every form of application used is entirely at the user's own risk and responsibility. The authors and publishers request every user to report to the publishers any discrepancies or inaccuracies noticed. If errors in this work are found after publication, errata will be posted at www.thieme.com on the product description page.

Some of the product names, patents, and registered designs referred to in this book are in fact registered trademarks or proprietary names even though specific reference to this fact is not always made in the text. Therefore, the appearance of a name without designation as proprietary is not to be construed as a representation by the publisher that it is in the public domain.

Thieme Publishers New York
333 Seventh Avenue, New York, NY 10001 USA
+1 800 782 3488, customerservice@thieme.com

Thieme Publishers Stuttgart
Rüdigerstrasse 14, 70469 Stuttgart, Germany
+49 [0]711 8931 421, customerservice@thieme.de

Thieme Publishers Delhi
A-12, Second Floor, Sector-2, Noida-201301
Uttar Pradesh, India
+91 120 45 566 00, customerservice@thieme.in

Thieme Revinter Publicações Ltda.
Rua do Matoso, 170 – Tijuca
Rio de Janeiro RJ 20270-135 - Brasil
+55 21 2563-9702
www.thiemerevinter.com.br

Cover design: Thieme Publishing Group
Typesetting by DiTech Process Solutions

Printed in the United States of America by King Printing Co., Inc. 5 4 3 2 1

ISBN 978-1-68420-110-5

Also available as an e-book:
eISBN 978-1-68420-111-2

FSC
www.fsc.org
100%
Paper from well-managed forests
FSC® C103101

Dedicated to Laurie, whose creativity is my inspiration and whose companionship I treasure.

Contents

Foreword

How do surgeons learn their craft? Fundamental to mastering surgery is acquiring a thorough knowledge of anatomy in order to build a three-dimensional vision of a surgical space. This construct is accomplished through the study of any number of anatomic descriptions, diagrams, photographs, models, and dissections. Classically, the student begins by sitting down with a text and reading a description of the local anatomy. This process requires a transformation of the written word into a mental image. Alternatively, the aspiring surgeon may listen to a lecture, which, like reading the written word, requires assimilation of information into a mental image. The surgical atlas helps eliminate the risk of generating a potentially erroneous mental image and, ultimately, makes all those interested in learning otologic surgery "visual learners." Learning through a variety of sources, however, is an iterative process in which the modalities of information can transfer synergistically to accelerate the process of understanding.

Dr. Robert K. Jackler has a unique ability to make complex anatomy accessible through highlighting key landmarks, and further, by defining crucial relationships and concepts. Christine Gralapp, his collaborator and a gifted medical illustrator, transforms these tenets into the actual illustrations we see. This great teaching duo is prolific, producing seemingly countless images that are clear, relevant, and widely utilized. Their depictions have educated an entire generation of otologists and skull base surgeons. No other team or body of work can compare.

We, the authors of this Foreword, are each grateful beneficiaries of the expertise of Dr. Jackler and Ms. Gralapp. Through the years, we, like many others, have used illustrations they created in our presentations and teaching endeavors. The two of us are thrilled that this comprehensive work of otologic surgery is now available. Undoubtedly, Ear Surgery Illustrated, like their previous work, will provide foundational knowledge for current and future generations of surgeons.

Finally, Dr. Jackler has always recognized that a complete surgeon requires a profound understanding of anatomy, but that anatomical knowledge is but one of the abilities the competent surgeon must possess. As a mentor to medical students, residents, fellows, and faculty, Dr. Jackler has demonstrated, through example, that thoughtful planning, respect for the patient's wishes, and the surgical wisdom that comes with considering what should be done for any given patient, will result in the highest level of care. We are indebted to him for his contributions.

Colin L.W. Driscoll, MD
Professor and Chair
Department of Otolaryngology
Mayo Clinic
Rochester, Minnesota

Samuel H. Selesnick, MD, FACS
Professor and Vice Chairman of Otolaryngology and Neurological Surgery
Weill Cornell Medical College
New York, New York
Past President, American Otological Society
Past President, American Neurotology Society

Preface

This book is the product of a collaboration between a surgeon (Robert K. Jackler) and a medical illustrator (Christine Gralapp) that has spanned a period over three decades and produced thousands of original color illustrations. Earlier, we produced a number of illustrated volumes (list below). This book is a companion volume to our *Atlas of Skull Base Surgery and Neurotology* (1st edition 1996, current 2nd edition 2009). This earlier work was intended for neurotologists and neurosurgeons and is thematically focused upon tumors of the posterior and middle cranial fossae and of the skull base. Over the last decade, we have turned our attention to ear microsurgery with the goal of creating an operative resource for otologists and otolaryngologists who care for patients with surgical ear disease. The concept of this book is to provide guidance on the stepwise technical maneuvers required in safe and effective otological microsurgery. The scope is intended to comprehensively cover all of the major surgical disorders involving the temporal bone. Although the great majority of the illustrations herein are new, selected portions of special relevance to otology are reproduced from our earlier atlas.

Today in the 21st century, artistic illustration retains its important role in in both anatomical and surgical education. The emphasis of this book is upon the illustrations with text limited to a concise description of operative techniques—the concept is to let the illustrations speak for themselves. While operative videos and still photography make important contributions to surgical education, illustrations have distinct advantages. Most importantly, drawings can be simplified to highlight key technical points which are the conceptual and intellectual underpinnings of safe and effective surgery. The temporal bone is an anatomical jewel box with highly complex and convoluted three dimensional relationships between critical structures. Operative photos tend to have excessive detail and can be difficult to decipher even for experienced surgeons. Operative videos can be highly valuable, especially if carefully edited and well narrated, but can be time consuming for the learner and are laborious to edit. Illustration, by use of exaggerated color and highlighting, elimination of extraneous detail, and emphasis upon the most surgically relevant structures, enables communication of much useful anatomical and technical information in just a handful of images. While anatomically accurate illustrations can provide the intellectual framework for surgical technique, they are no substitute for actual surgical experience which is essential for true mastery.

It should be pointed out that there is no singular "right way" to perform otologic microsurgery. Considerable variation in methods and styles exist between regions, among surgeons even within a region, as well as among surgeons with differing training backgrounds. While an effort was made to include a spectrum of different approaches rather than merely those preferred by the author, we recognize that while our book is comprehensive it is certainly not exhaustive, and numerous alternative techniques exist in addition to those illustrated.

I affirm that I and Christine Gralapp retain the copyright for all of the illustrations that appear in this book. We encourage use of our illustrations for educational purposes, but written permission should be sought from Dr. Jackler and Ms. Gralapp before their publication or commercial use.

Robert K. Jackler, MD

Jackler RK. Atlas of Skull Base Surgery and Neurotology. 1st edition Mosby. St. Louis 1996, 2nd edition. Thieme. New York. 2009.

Jackler RK, Brackmann DE. Neurotology. Mosby. St Louis. 1994. 2nd edition Elsevier/Mosby. Philadelphia. 2005.

Jackler RK, Driscoll CLW. Tumors of the Ear and Temporal Bone. Lippincott, Williams & Wilkins. Philadelphia. 2000.

Acknowledgments

My thanks go to the generations of otolaryngology residents and neurotology fellows, both at Stanford University and the University of California San Francisco, whose eagerness to learn coupled with keen intelligence and innate curiosity helped to guide me in understanding what was most important in breaking down operative procedures into their most essential steps and stages.

My gratitude to Dr. Jennifer Alyono for her proofreading and editorial suggestions. And my special gratitude goes to medical illustrator Christine Gralapp, who with consummate artistic skill transformed thousands of my crude pencil drawings into beautiful drawings infused with color and dimensionality.

Contributors

Jennifer Alyono, MD
Assistant Professor
Department of Otolaryngology–Head and Neck Surgery
Division of Otology & Neurotology
Stanford University School of Medicine
Stanford, California
(Cochlear Implants, Mastoid Obliteration)

Nikolas H. Blevins, MD
Larry and Sharon Malcolmson Professor of Otolaryngology–Head and Neck Surgery
Chief, Division of Otology & Neurotology
Medical Director, Stanford Cochlear Implant Center
Stanford University School of Medicine
Stanford, California
(Cochlear Implants, Mastoid Obliteration, Transfacial Recess)

Kay W. Chang, MD
Professor of Otolaryngology–Head and Neck Surgery and Pediatrics
Stanford University School of Medicine
Division of Pediatric Otolaryngology
Lucile Packard Children's Hospital at Stanford
Stanford, California
(Atresia, Microtia)

Peter H. Hwang, MD
Professor of Otolaryngology–Head and Neck Surgery
Vice Chair of Clinical Affairs
Chief, Division of Rhinology
Stanford University School of Medicine
Stanford, California
(Transphenoidal Approach to Petrous Apex)

Robert K. Jackler, MD
Sewall Professor and Chair
Department of Otolaryngology–Head and Neck Surgery
Professor of Neurosurgery and Surgery
Stanford University School of Medicine
Stanford, California

Jennifer Y. Lee, MD
Clinical Assistant Professor
Department of Otolaryngology–Head and Neck Surgery
Division of Comprehensive Otolaryngology
Stanford University School of Medicine
Stanford, California
(Eustachian Tuboplasty)

Sam P. Most, MD
Professor
Chief, Division of Facial Plastic and Reconstructive Surgery
Department of Otolaryngology–Head and Neck Surgery
Stanford University School of Medicine
Stanford, California
(Otoplasty)

Jon-Paul Pepper, MD
Assistant Professor
Division of Facial Plastic and Reconstructive Surgery
Stanford University School of Medicine
Stanford, California
(Hypoglossal/Trigeminal Facial Anastomoses, Gracilis Microvascular facial reanimation)

Mai Thy Truong, MD
Clinical Associate Professor
Division of Pediatric Otolaryngology
Department of Otolaryngology–Head and Neck Surgery
Stanford University School of Medicine
Lucile Packard Children's Hospital at Stanford
Stanford, California
(Microtia, Pre-auricular cyst, Atresia)

Yona Vaisbuch, MD
Clinical Instructor
Division of Otology & Neurotology
Department of Otolaryngology–Head and Neck Surgery
Stanford University School of Medicine
Stanford, California
(Ergonomics, Butterfly Tympanoplasty)

1 Surgical Anatomy of the Ear

Robert K. Jackler

1.1 Introduction to Surgical Anatomy of the Ear

A rigorous understanding of anatomy underlies safe and effective ear microsurgery. Traditionally, anatomical dissection of temporal bones was the primary educational means of being introduced to the complex and convoluted relationships of the ear and its related structures. With the increasing difficulty in obtaining anatomical material coupled with the expense of maintaining temporal bone labs, which tend to occupy the most lightly used space in academic departments, imaging-based anatomical tools are likely to gradually supplant dissection as the dominant educational method. Conventional CT and MRI images are a valuable means of learning temporal bone anatomy. With experience, mastery of relationships in the axial, coronal, and sagittal planes can translate into a fused three-dimensional awareness. While the two-dimensionality of the illustrations in this atlas may be considered a limitation, their use of enhanced color and highlighting of surgically relevant structures while eliminating the extraneous efficiently conveys much useful anatomical and surgical information. Although not yet a mature technology at the time of publication, it seems clear that the future of ear microsurgical training lies in virtual three-dimensional simulation using haptically reinforced, computer-generated microsurgical tools.

Further Reading

1. Andersen SAW, Cayé-Thomasen P, Sørensen MS. Mastoidectomy performance assessment of virtual simulation training using final-product analysis. Laryngoscope 2015;125(2):431–435 PubMed
2. Awad Z, Tornari C, Ahmed S, Tolley NS. Construct validity of cadaveric temporal bones for training and assessment in mastoidectomy. Laryngoscope 2015;125(10):2376–2381 PubMed
3. Chan S, Li P, Locketz G, Salisbury K, Blevins NH. High-fidelity haptic and visual rendering for patient-specific simulation of temporal bone surgery. Comput Assist Surg (Abingdon) 2016;21(1):85–101 PubMed
4. Cheattle AH. The Surgical Anatomy of the Temporal Bone. London: J&A Churchill Ltd; 1907
5. Donaldson JA, Duckert LG, Lambert PM, Rubel EW. Surgical Anatomy of the Temporal Bone. 4th ed. New York, NY: Raven Press; 1992
6. Gulya AJ. Anatomy of the Temporal Bone with Surgical Implications, 3rd ed. New York, NY: Informa Healthcare USA; 2007
7. Locketz GD, Lui JT, Chan S, et al. Anatomy-specific virtual reality simulation in temporal bone dissection: perceived utility and impact on surgeon confidence. Otolaryngol Head Neck Surg 2017;156(6):1142–1149 PubMed
8. Lustig LR, Jackler RK, Mandelcorn R. The history of otology through its eponyms I: anatomy. Am J Otol 1998;19(3):371–389 PubMed
9. Piromchai P, Wijewickrema S, Smeds H, Kennedy G, O'Leary S. Correlations of external landmarks with internal structures of the temporal bone. Otol Neurotol 2015;36(8):1366–1373 PubMed
10. Sanna M, Russo A, Taibah A, Piras G, Tang W. The Temporal Bone: Anatomical Dissection and Surgical Approaches. New York, NY: Thieme; 2018

1.2 Temporal Bone

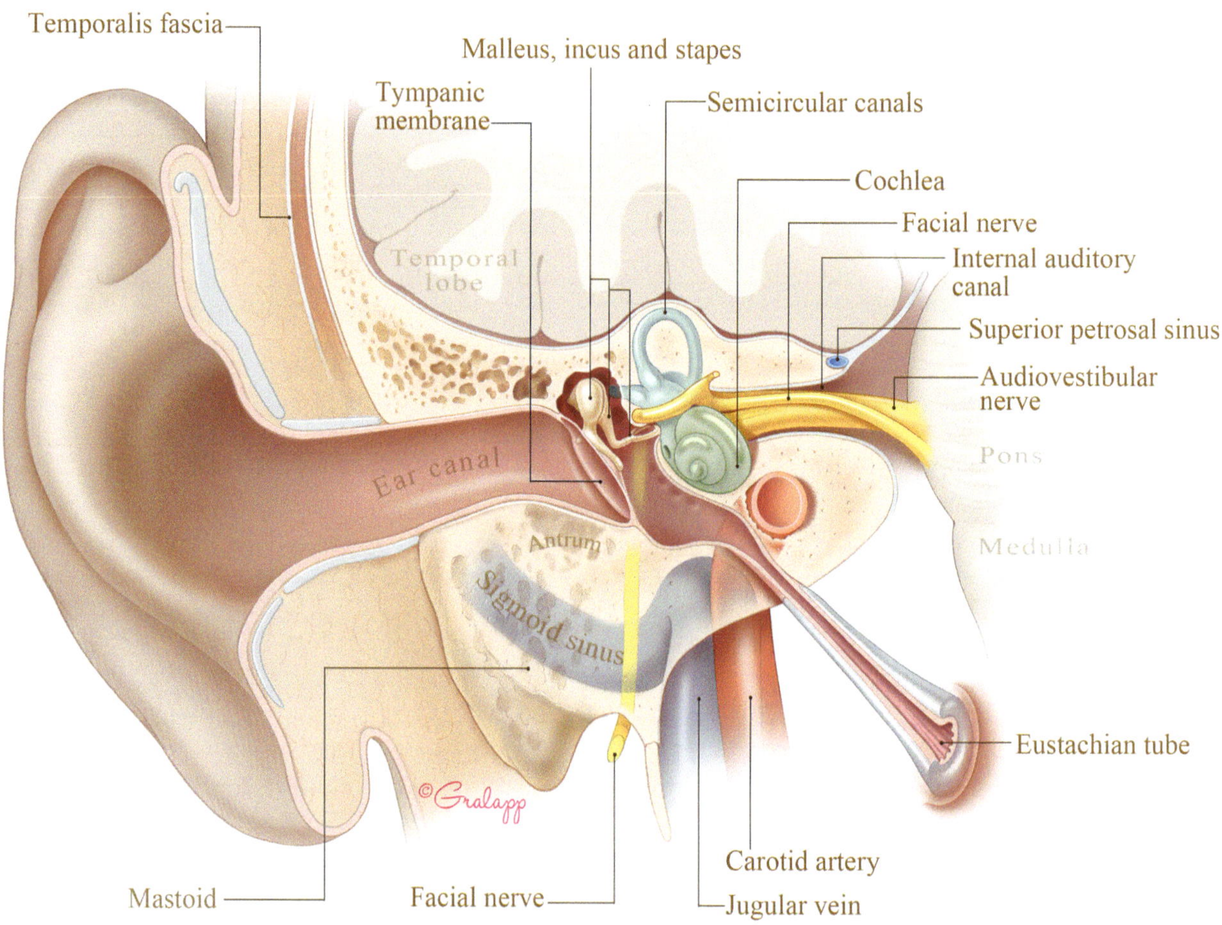

Fig. 1.1 Coronal perspective of the anatomy of the ear which is the illustration used on the cover of this Atlas. This drawing was an effort to modernize the classical coronal depiction of the ear created in 1939 by the eminent medical illustrator Max Brödel. Compressing three dimensional structures into a proportionally correct illustration with accurate anatomical relationships, yet simplified enough to convey an overall perspective, took many iterations over the course of an entire year. For the story of the centuries-long effort to illustrate overall ear anatomy, please see the following study on the subject: Jackler RK, Gralapp CL, Mudry A. Revisiting Max Brödel's classic coronal illustration of the ear. *Otol Neurotol* 2014;35:555–560.

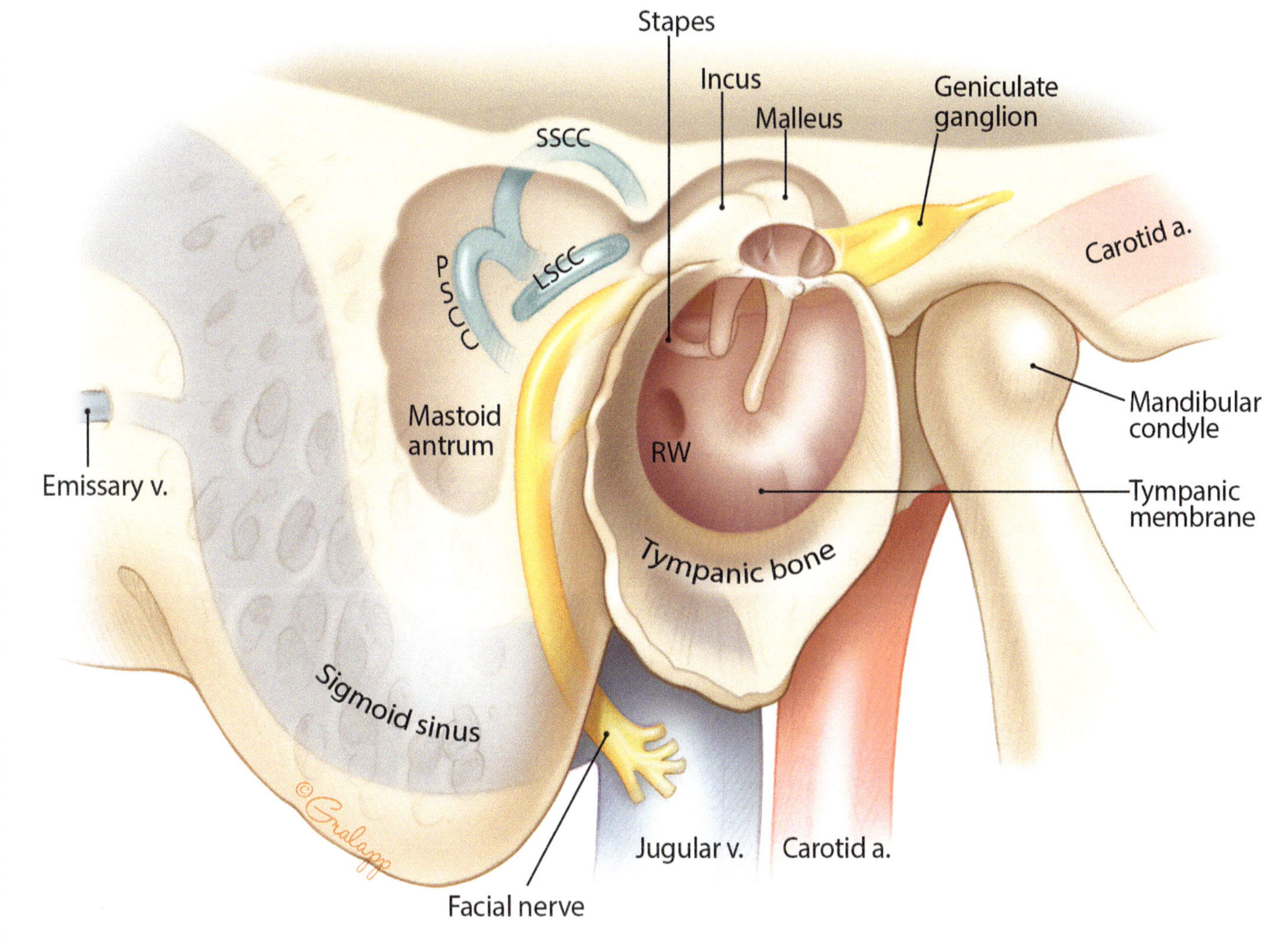

Fig. 1.2 Lateral perspective of the anatomy of the ear. LSCC, lateral semicircular canal; PSCC, posterior semicircular canal; RW, round window; SSCC, superior semicircular canal.

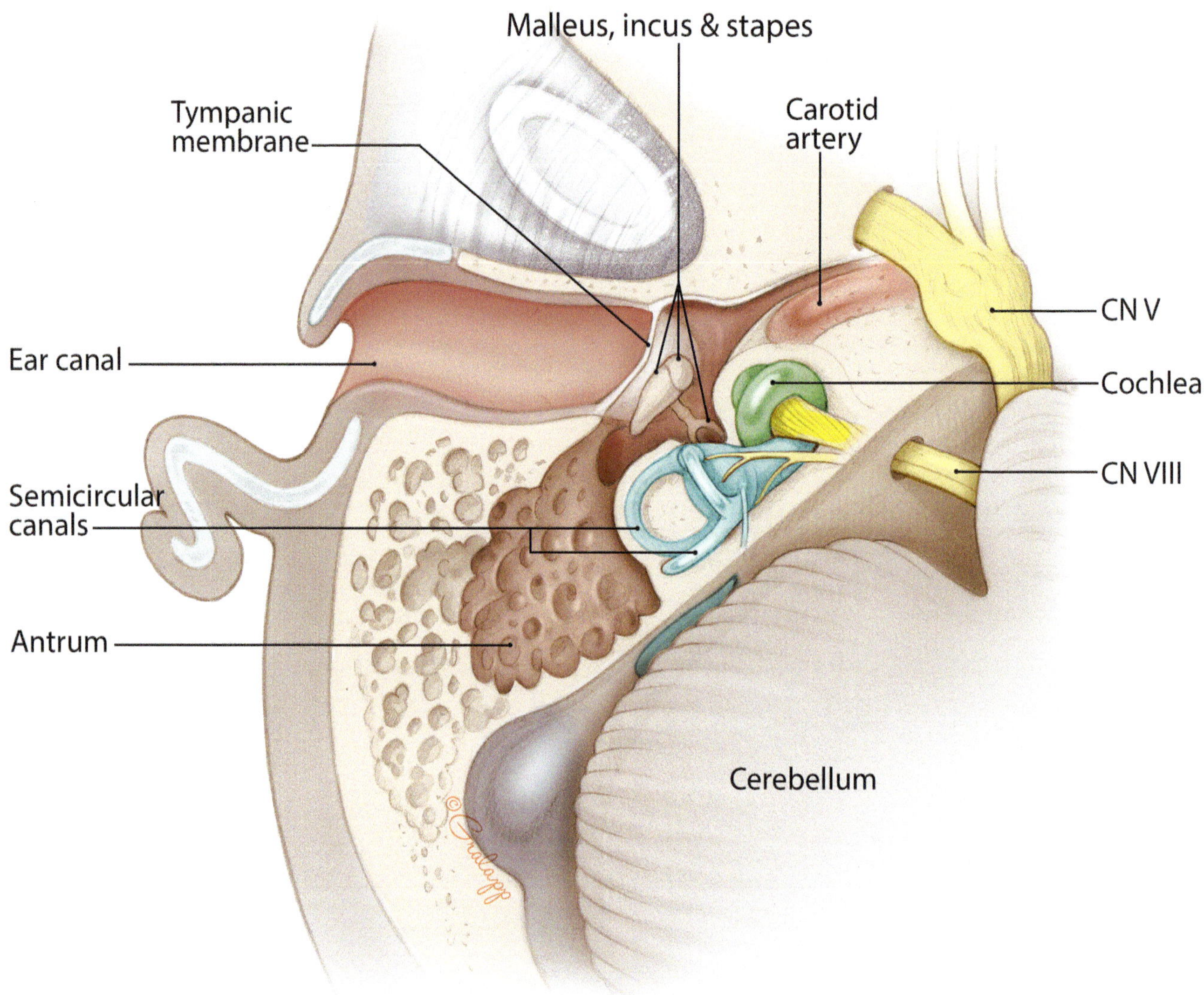

Fig. 1.3 Axial perspective of the anatomy of the ear.

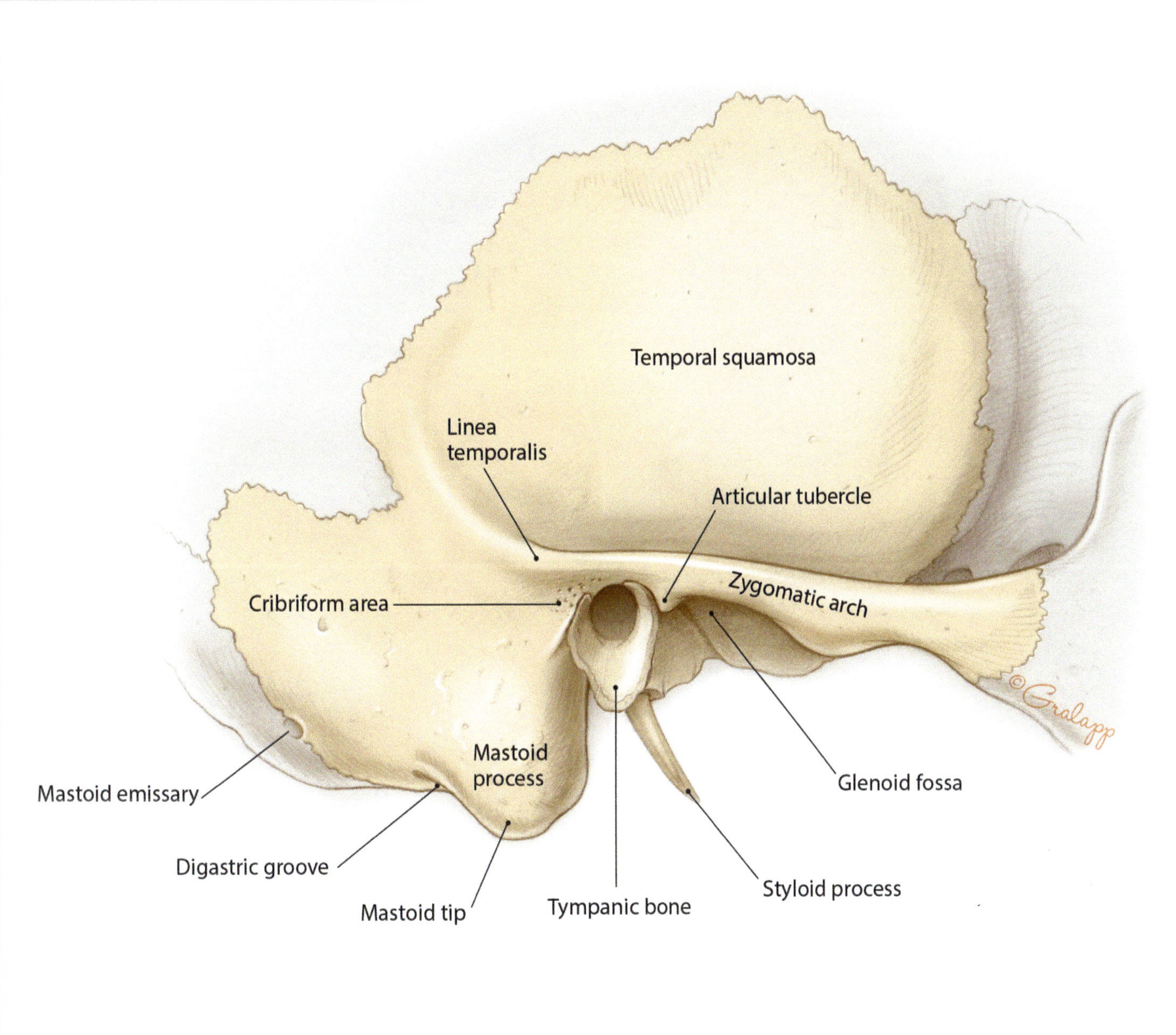

Fig. 1.4 Surface anatomy of the temporal bone.

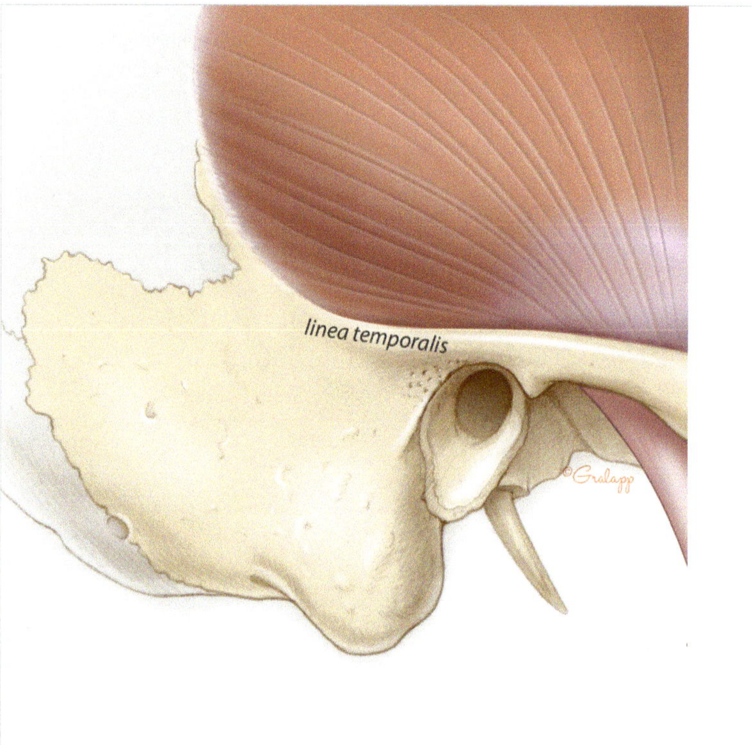

Fig. 1.5 The relationship between the temporalis muscle and the linea temporalis.

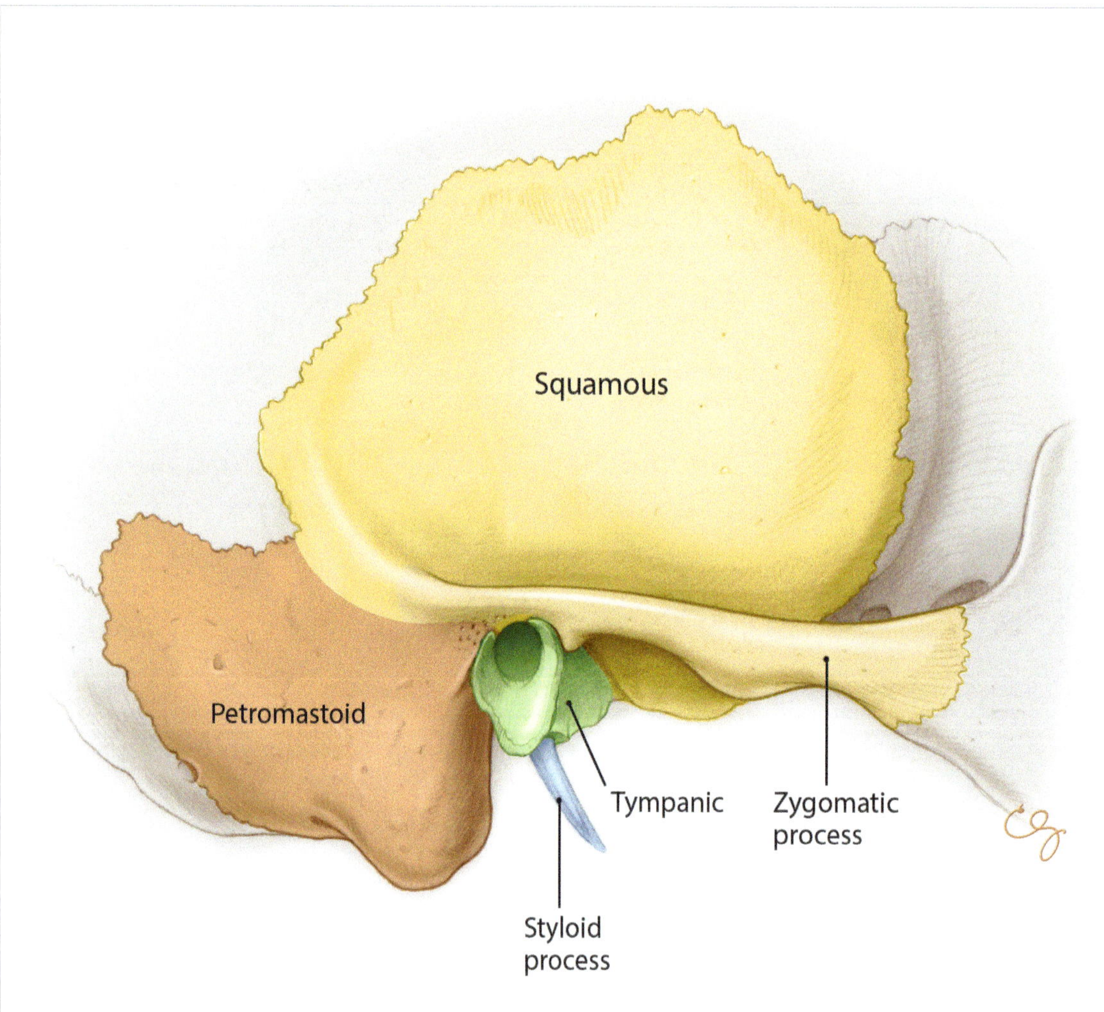

Fig. 1.6 The four osseous components of the temporal bone from lateral perspective.

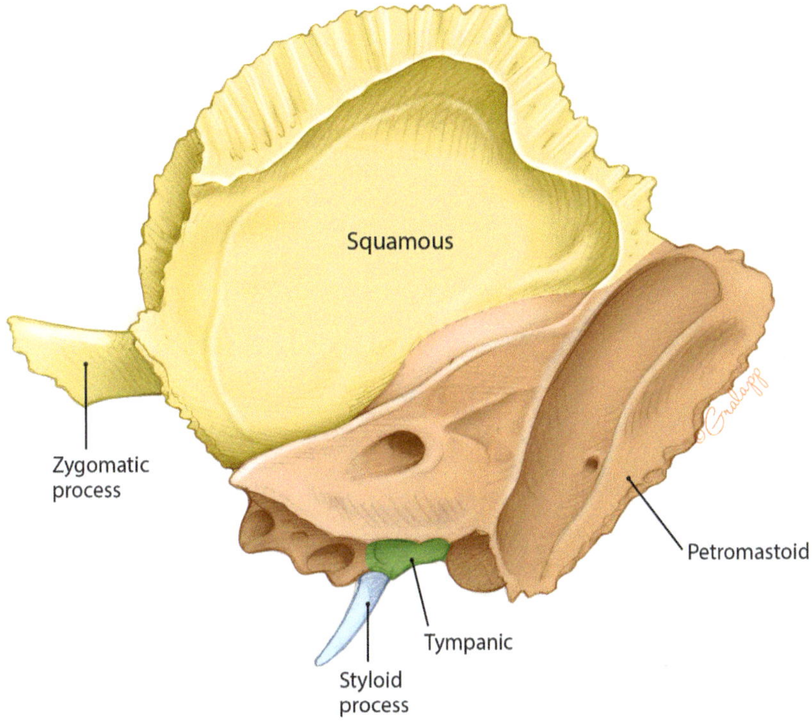

Fig. 1.7 The four osseous components of the temporal bone from medial perspective.

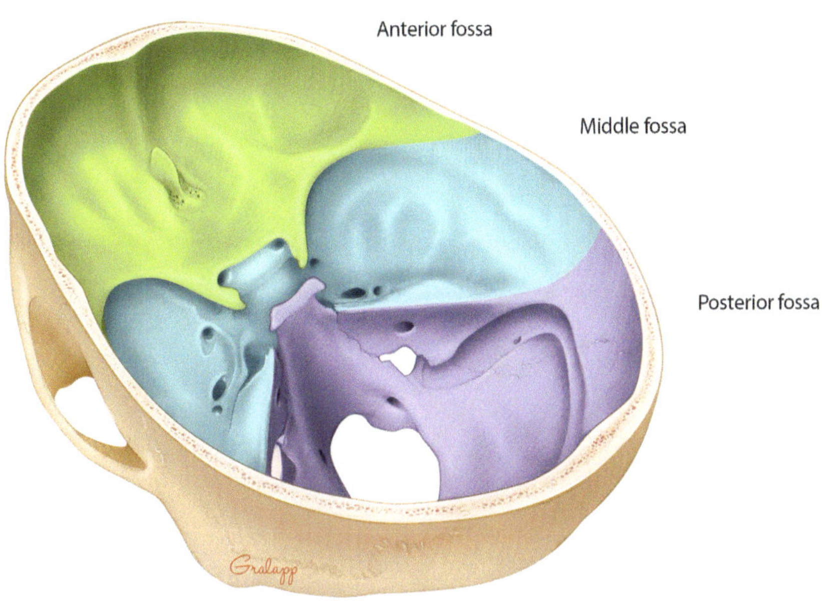

Fig. 1.8 The three fossae of the skull base. The petrous pyramid containing the ear structures separates the middle fossa from the posterior fossa.

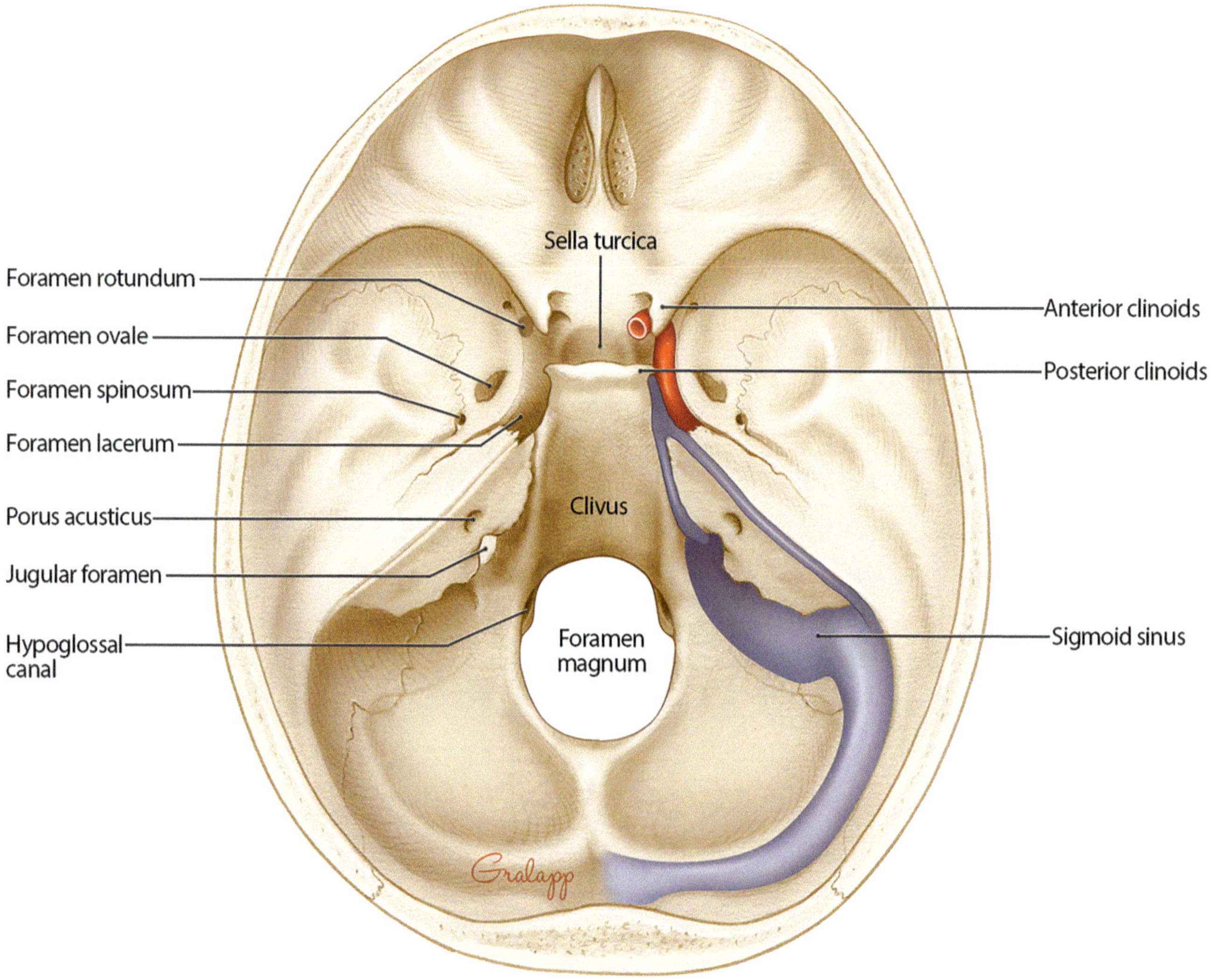

Fig. 1.9 The cranial base as seen from above.

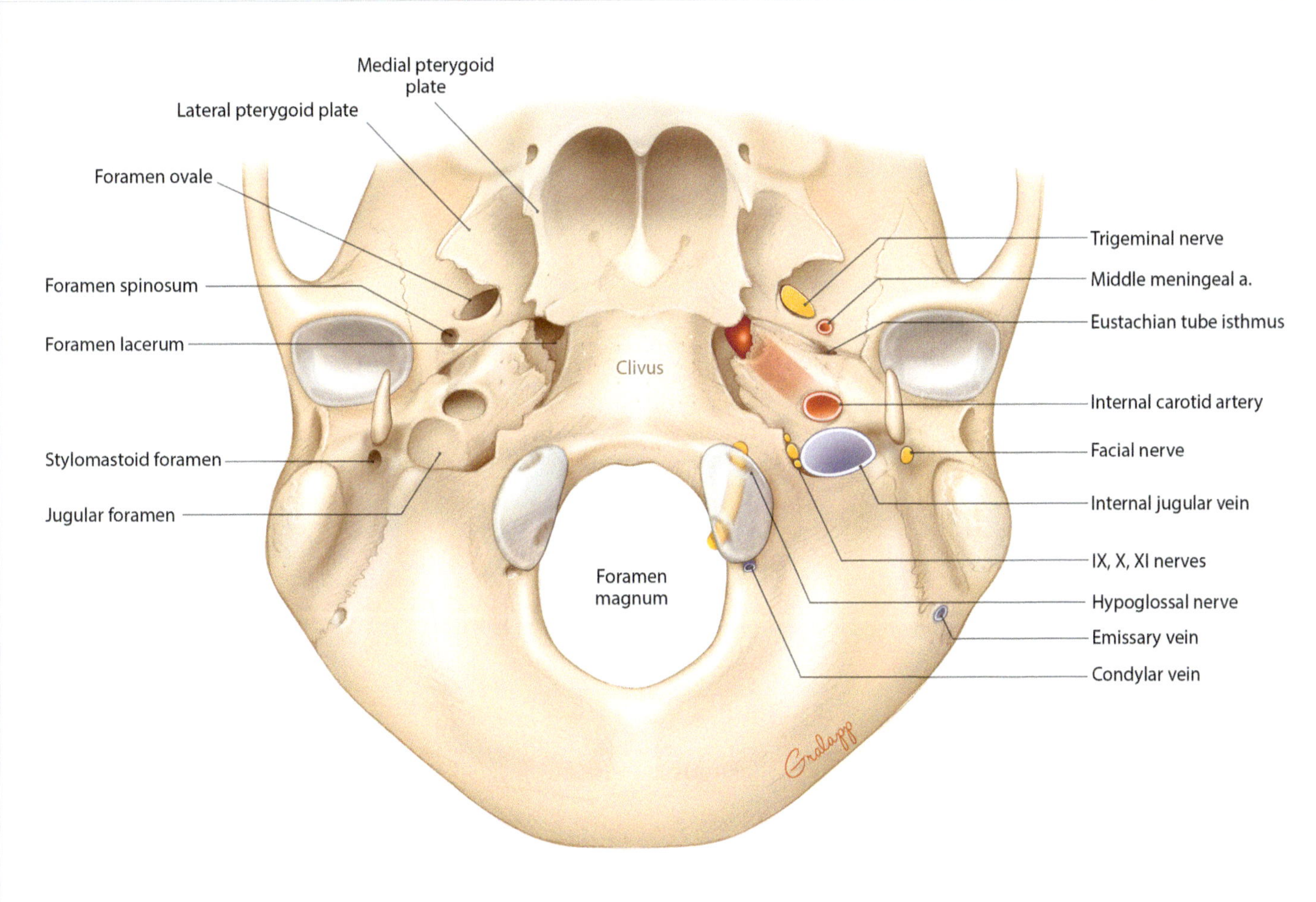

Fig. 1.10 The cranial base as seen from below.

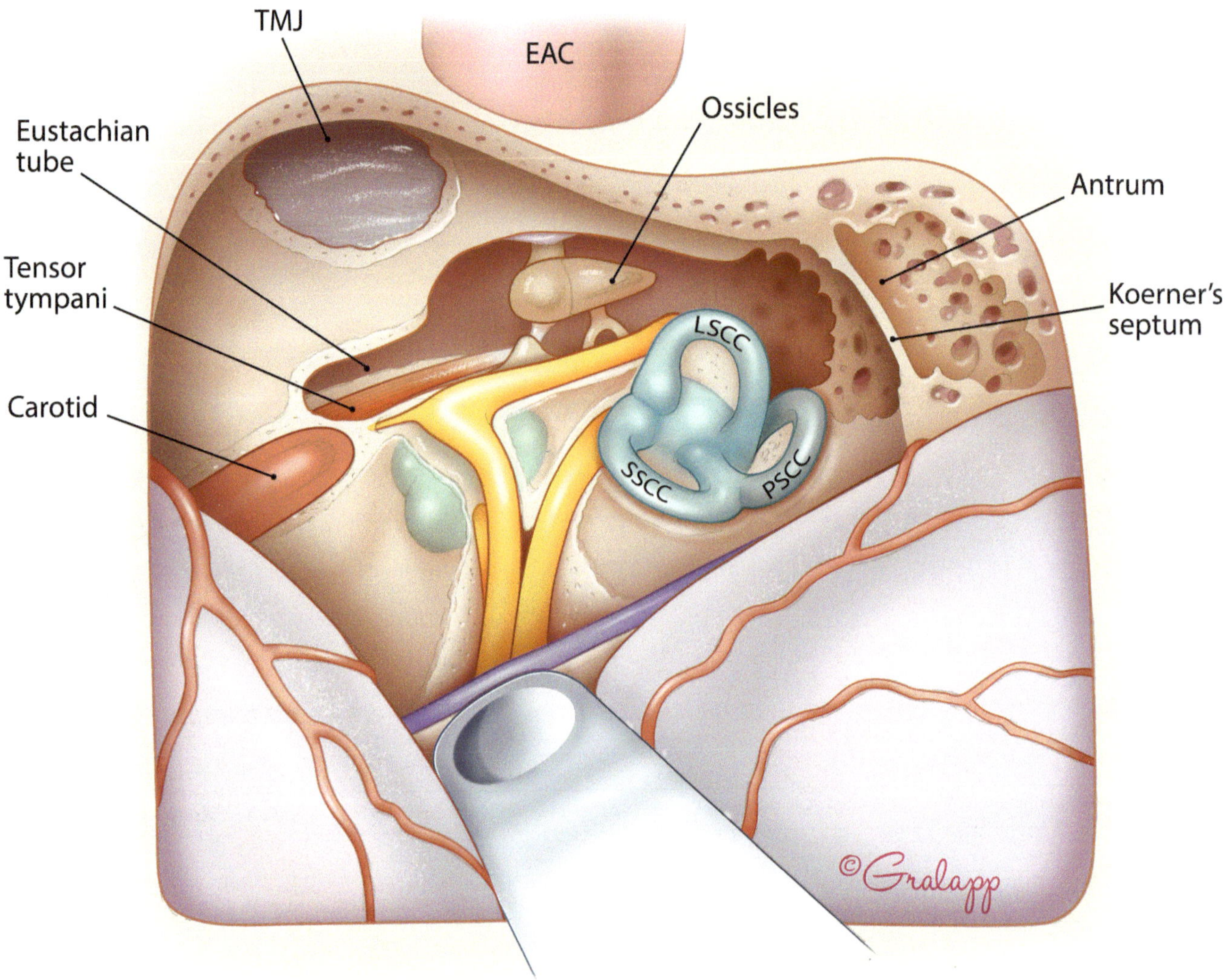

Fig. 1.11 Anatomical dissection of the temporal floor peering from above via the middle fossa approach. EAC, external auditory canal; LSCC, lateral semicircular canal; PSCC, posterior semicircular canal; TMJ, temporomandibular joint; SSCC, superior semicircular canal.

1.3 External Ear

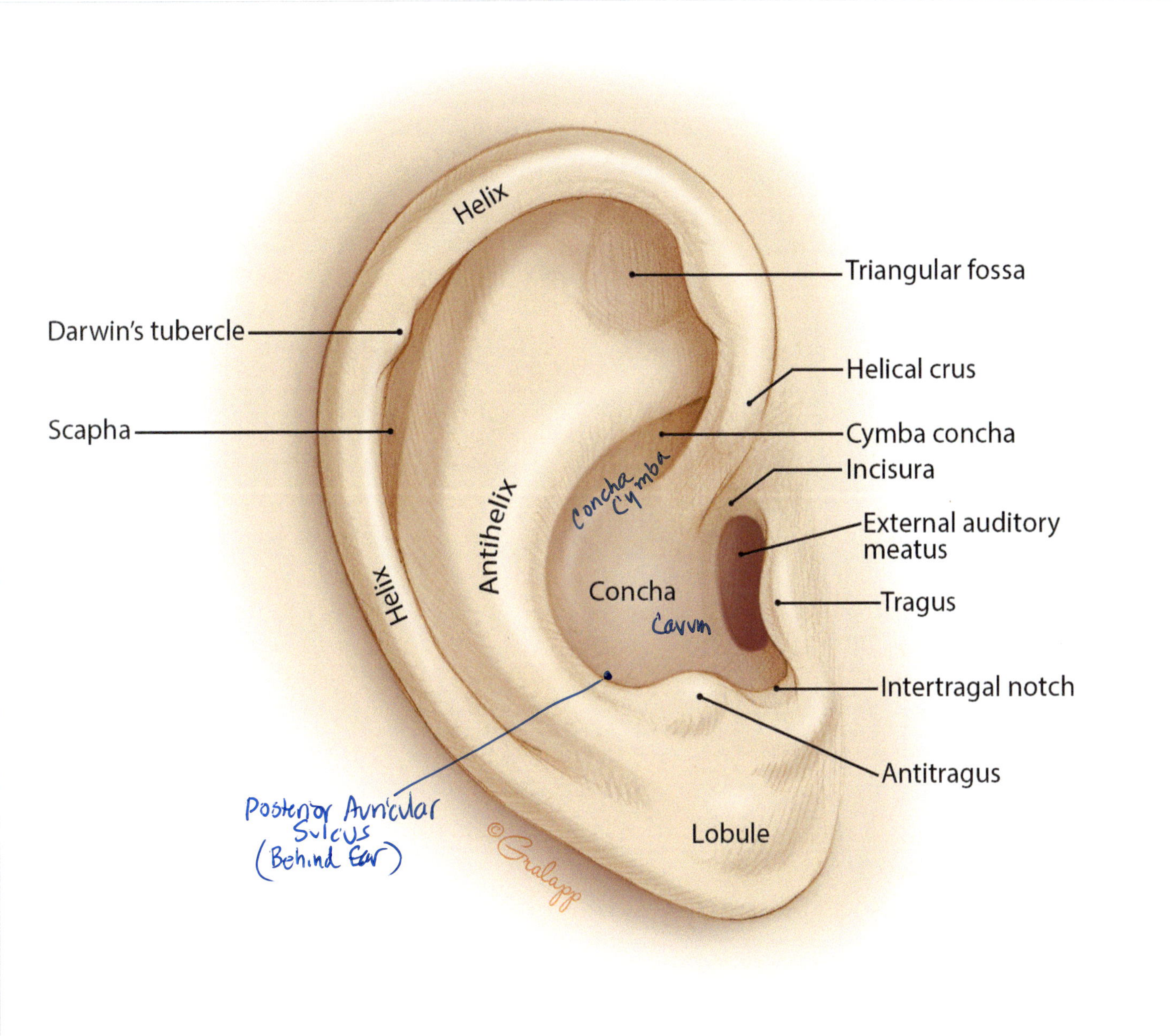

Fig. 1.12 Anatomy of the pinna (auricle).

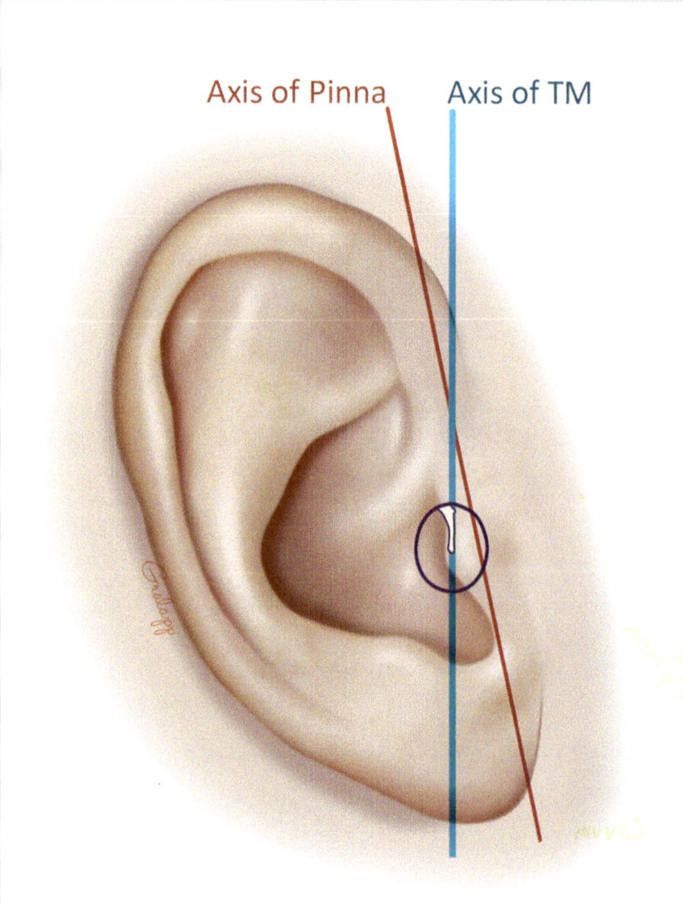

Fig. 1.13 The pinna is tilted posteriorly from the axis of the malleus. Understanding this is important to patient positioning during surgery.

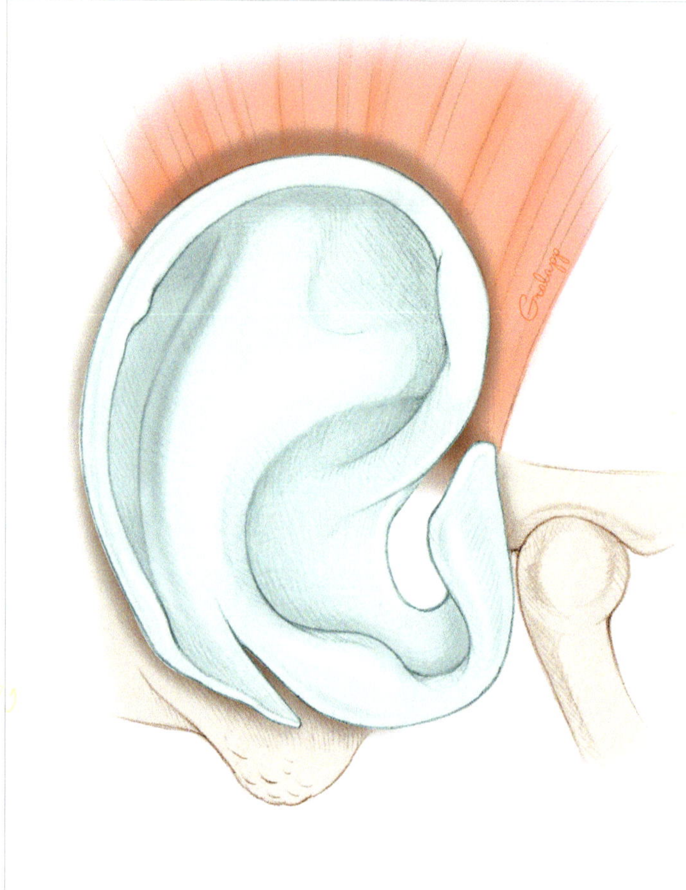

Fig. 1.14 Cartilage skeleton of the auricle. Note the incisura between the crus of the helix and the tragus. This is the location of an endaural incision.

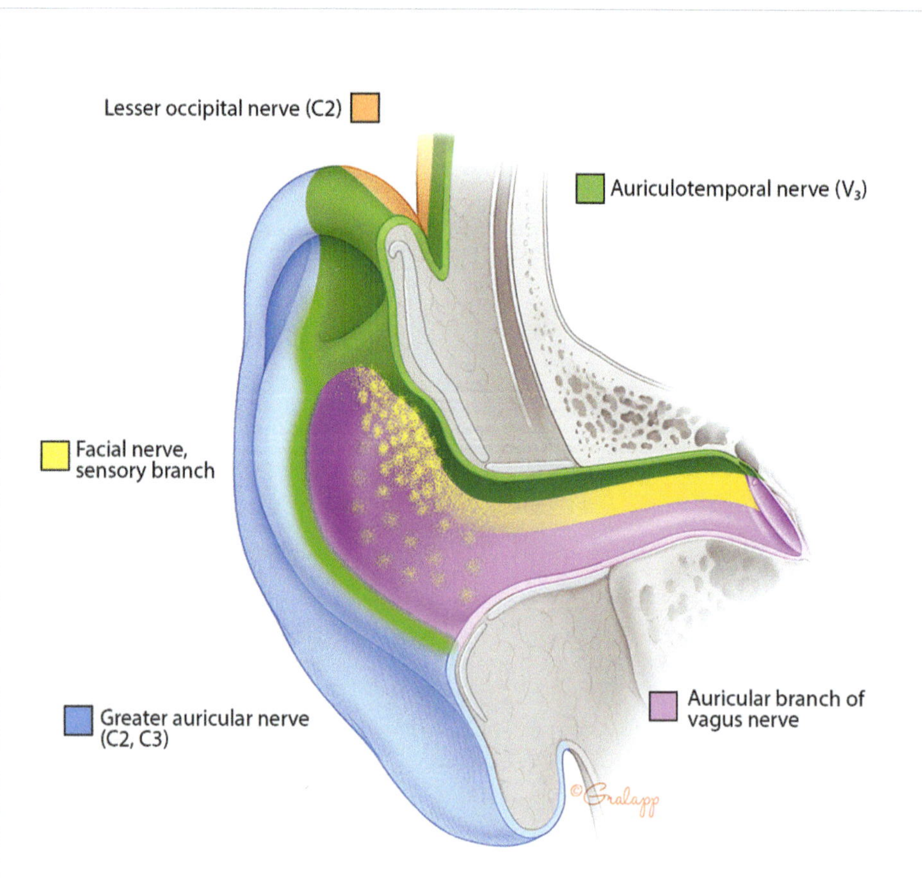

Fig. 1.15 Sensory innervation of the pinna and external auditory canal.

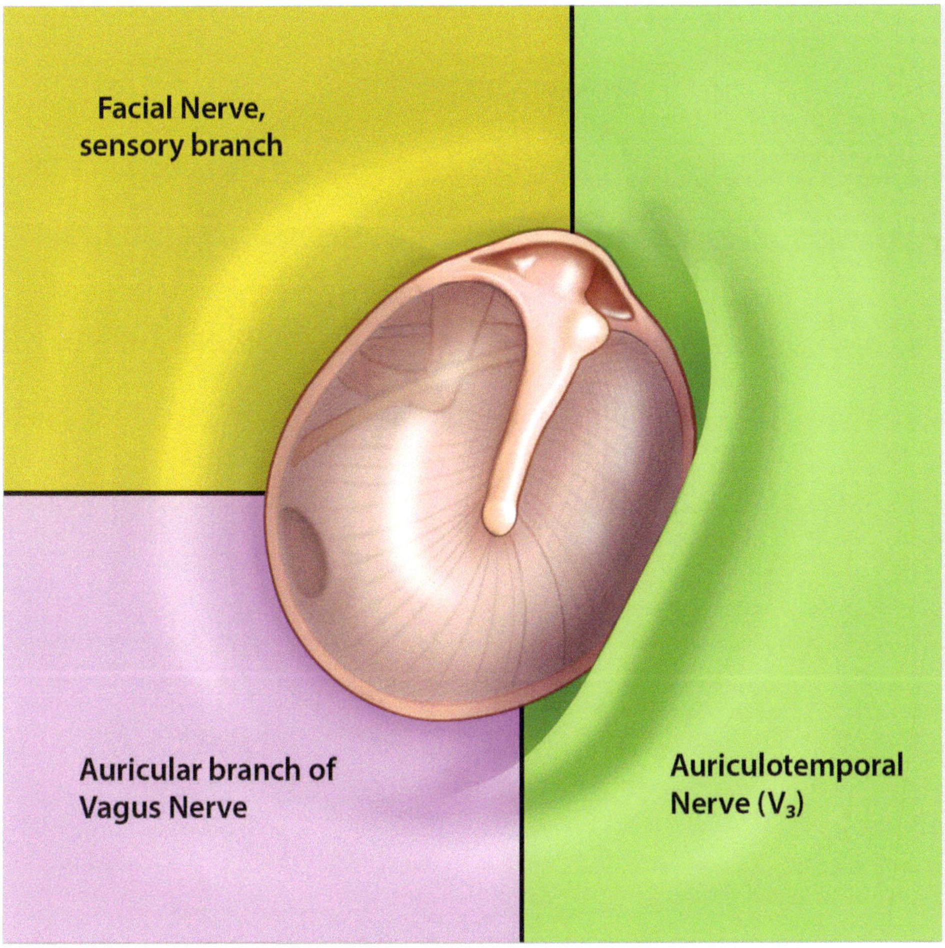

Fig. 1.16 Sensory innervation of the external auditory canal.

1.4 Middle Ear and Mastoid

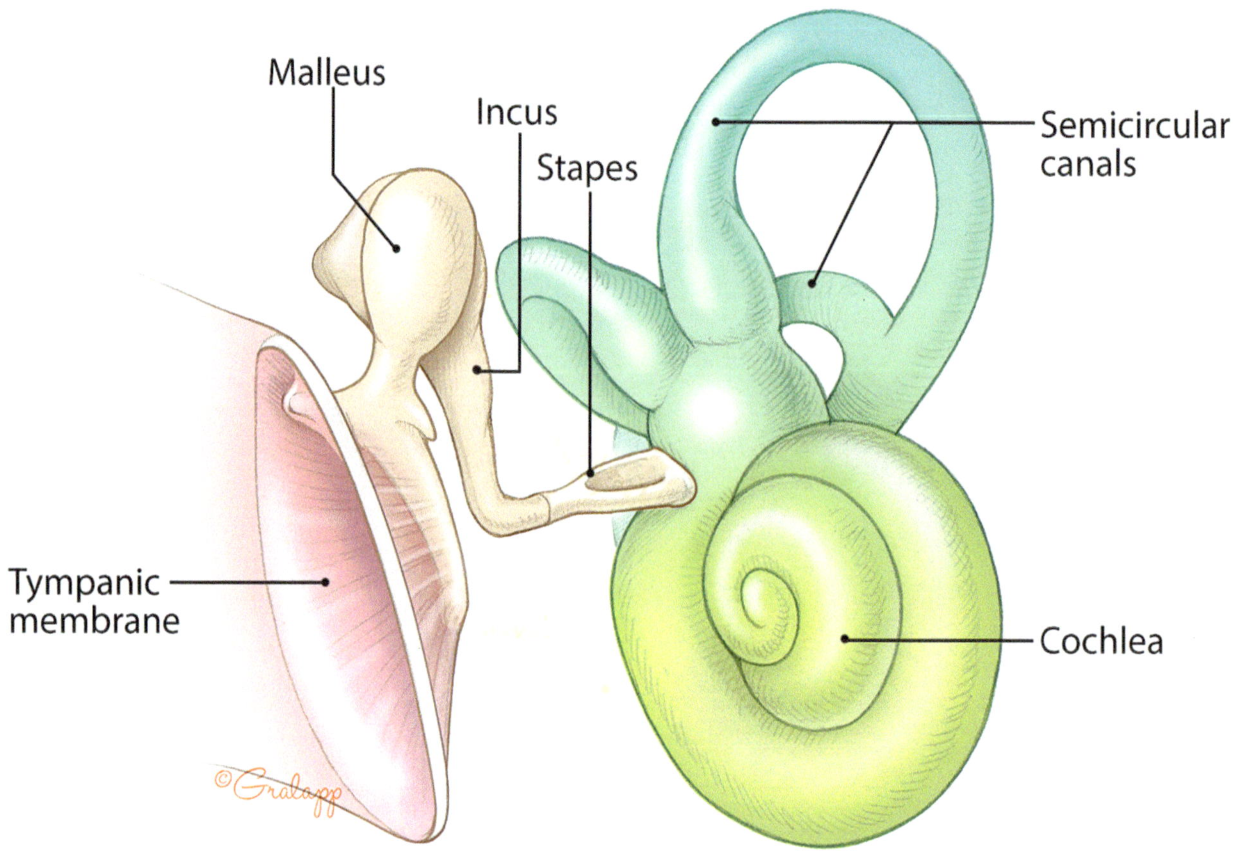

Fig. 1.17 Anatomy of the middle and inner ear.

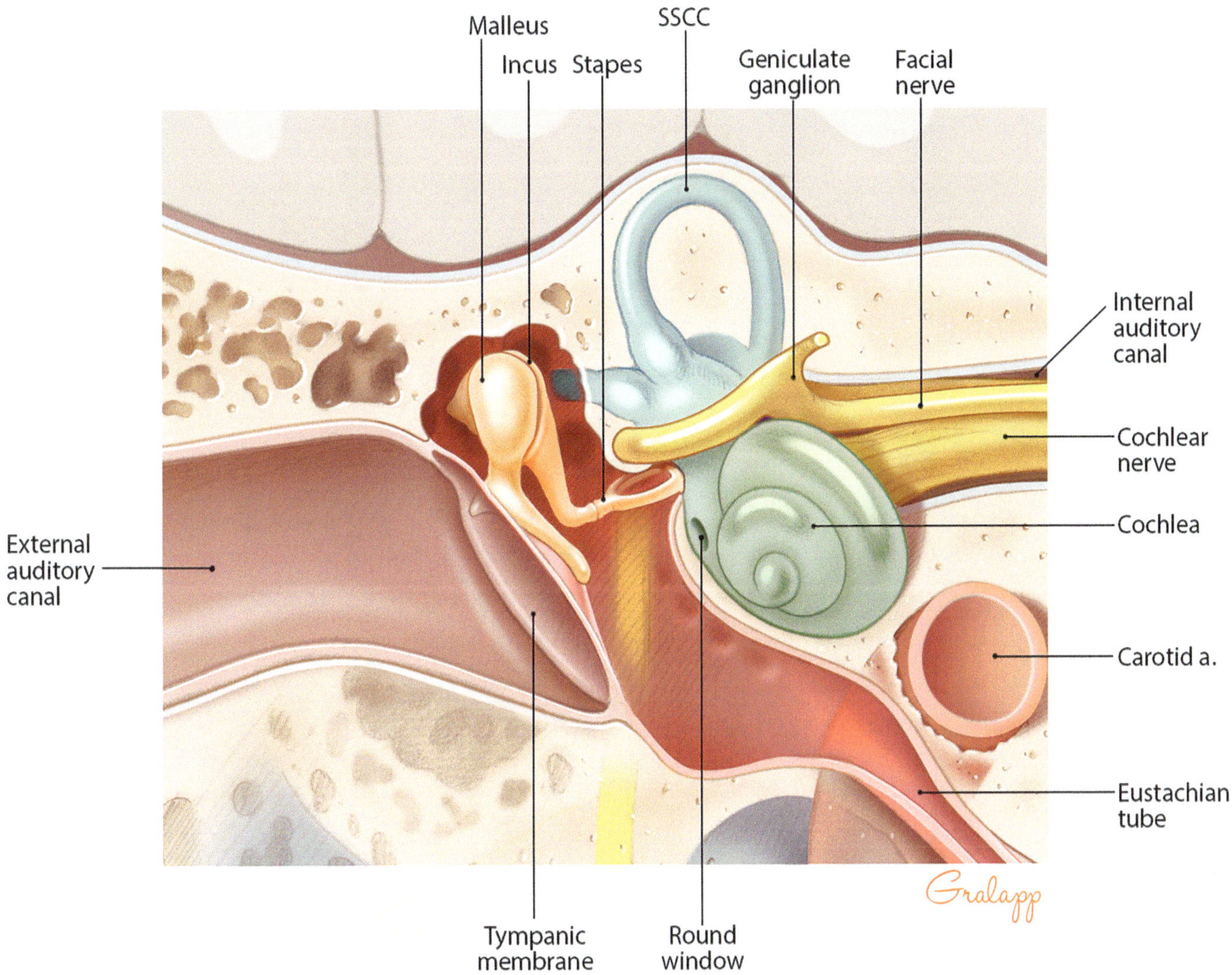

Fig. 1.18 Relationships of the middle ear: coronal aspect.

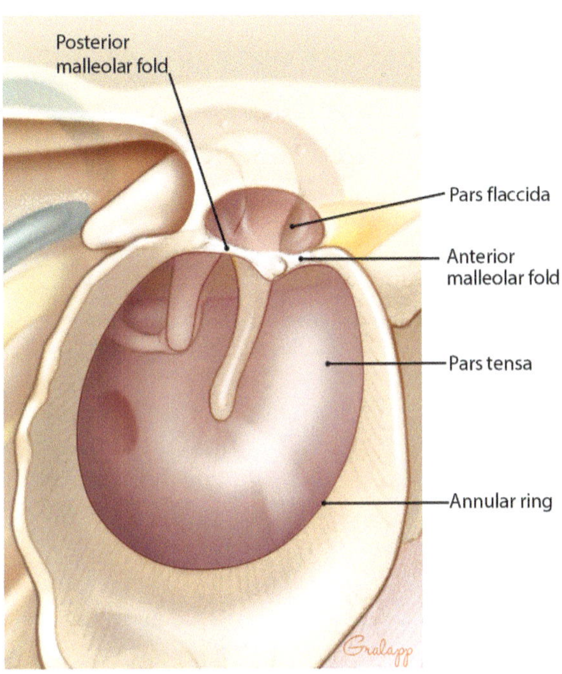

Fig. 1.19 The tympanic membrane and ossicles.

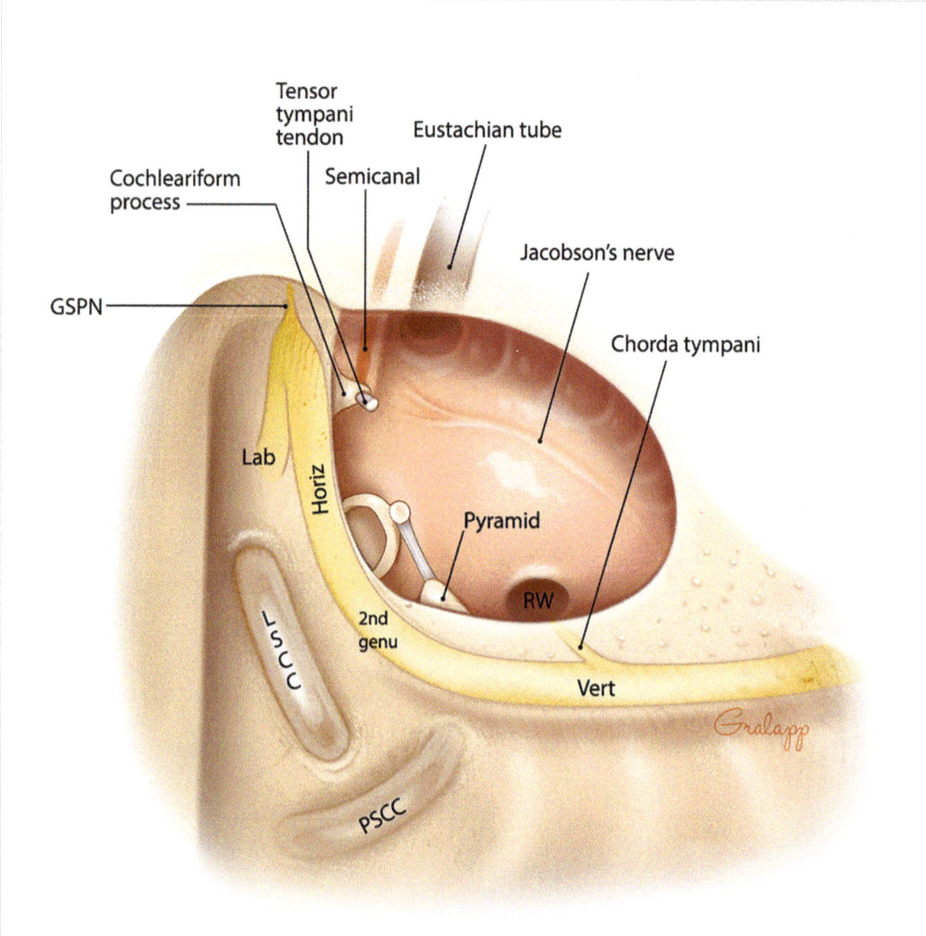

Fig. 1.20 The medial wall of the middle ear and mastoid. Components of the facial nerve: GSPN, greater superficial petrosal nerve; Lab, labyrinthine segment; Horiz, horizontal or tympanic segment; Vert, vertical or mastoid segment; LSCC, lateral semicircular canal; PSCC, posterior semicircular canal.

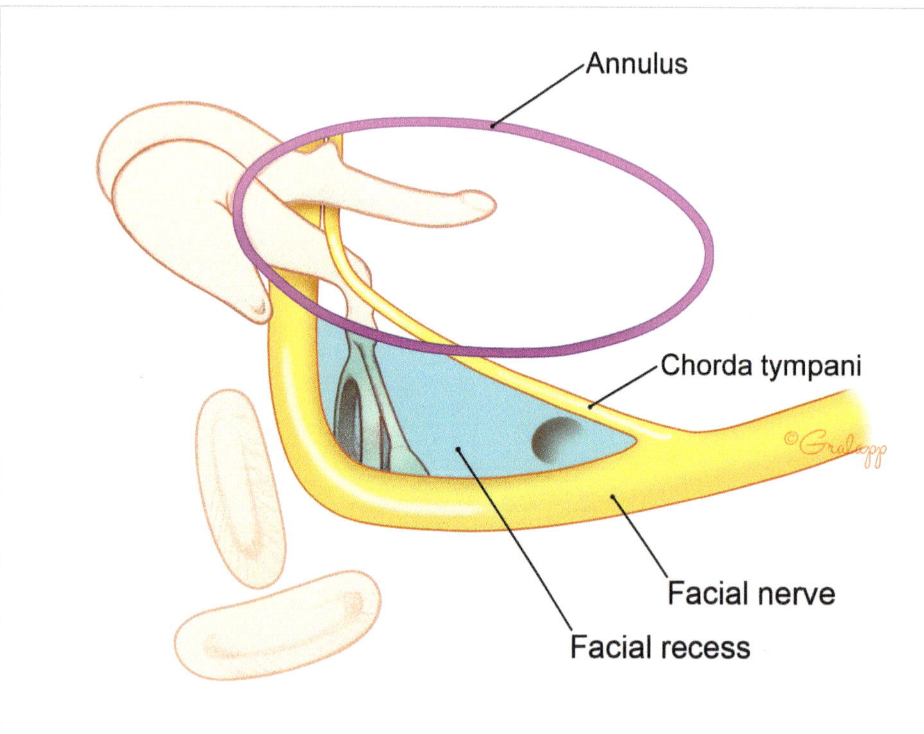

Fig. 1.21 Facial recess (blue): surgical path to middle ear via the mastoid.

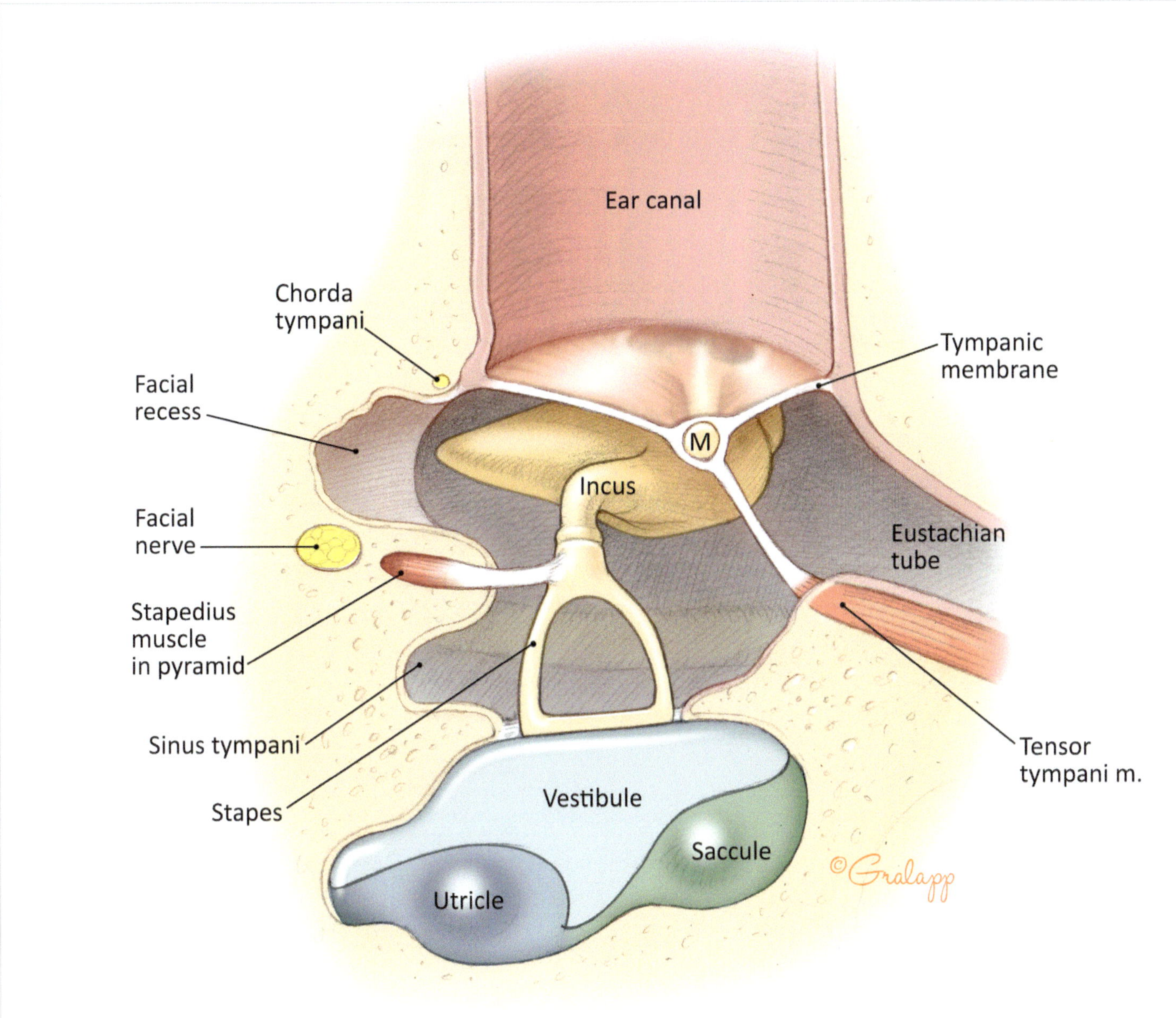

Fig. 1.22 Middle ear and inner ear vestibule from inferior perspective. The facial recess and sinus tympani are important in chronic ear surgery.

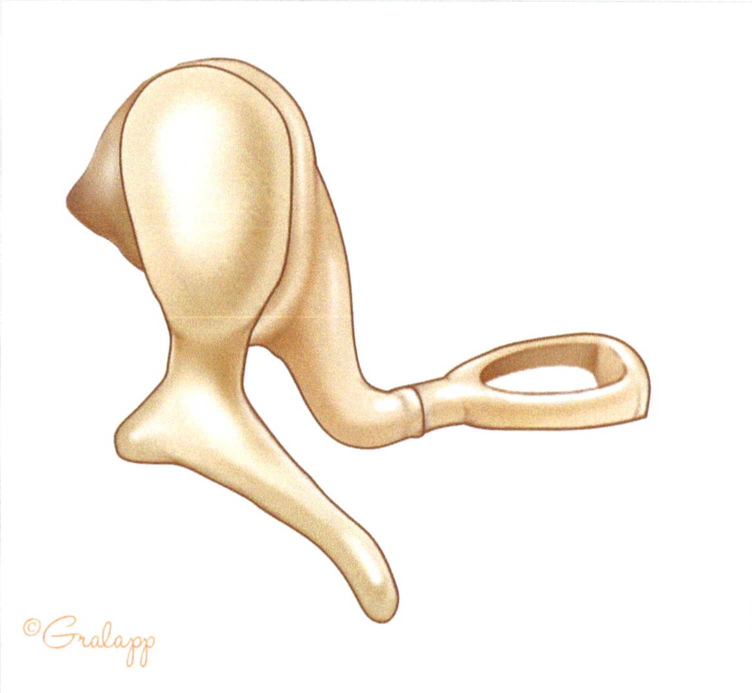

Fig. 1.23 The ossicular chain and its articulations.

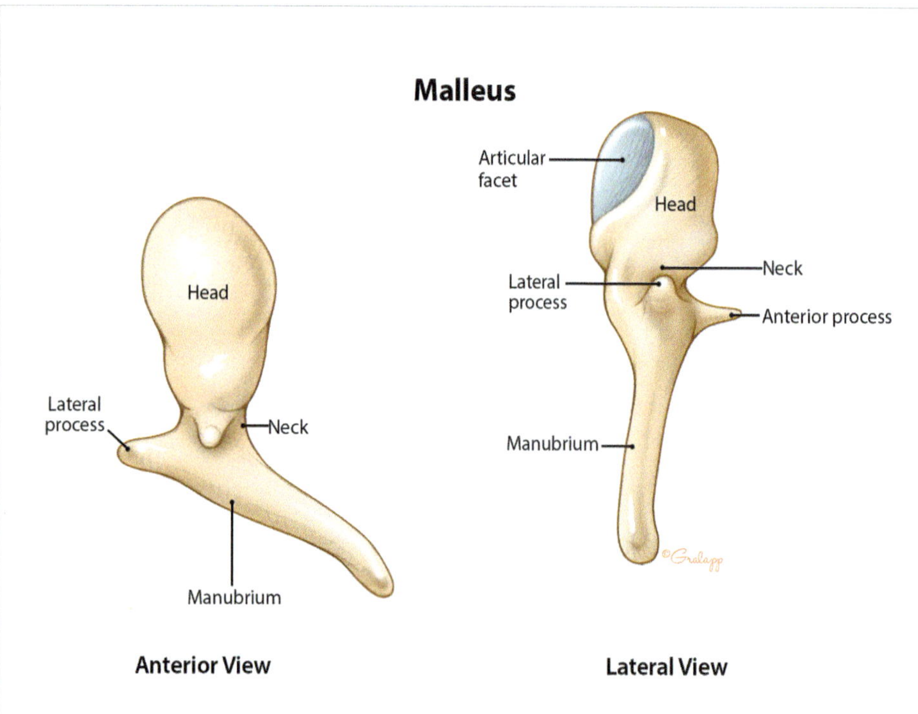

Fig. 1.24 Anatomy of the malleus.

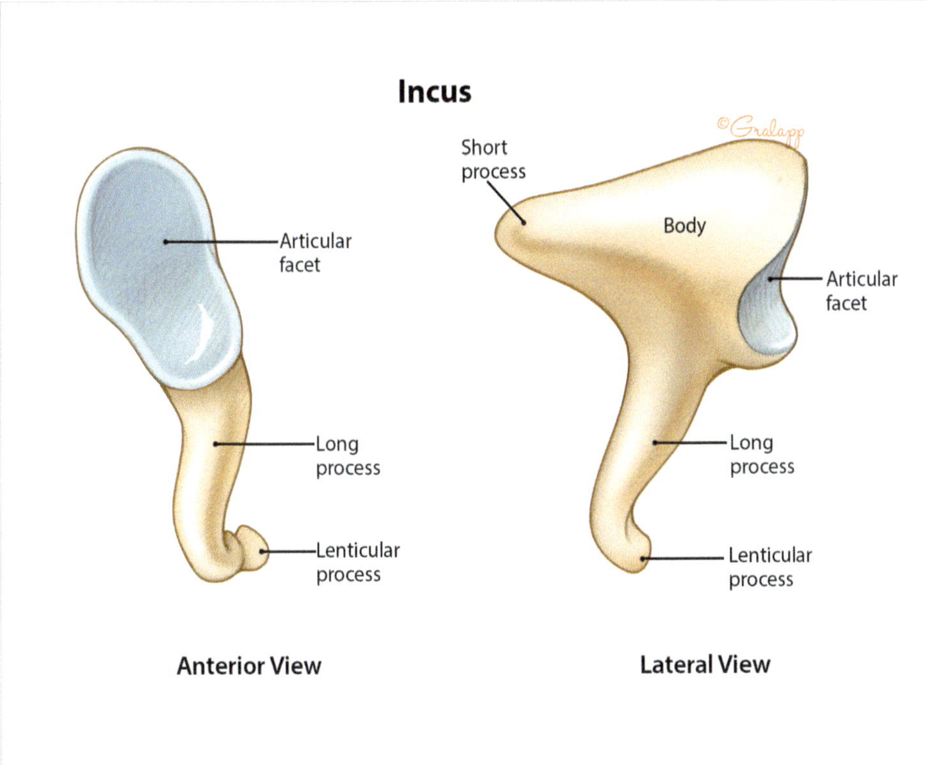

Fig. 1.25 Anatomy of the incus.

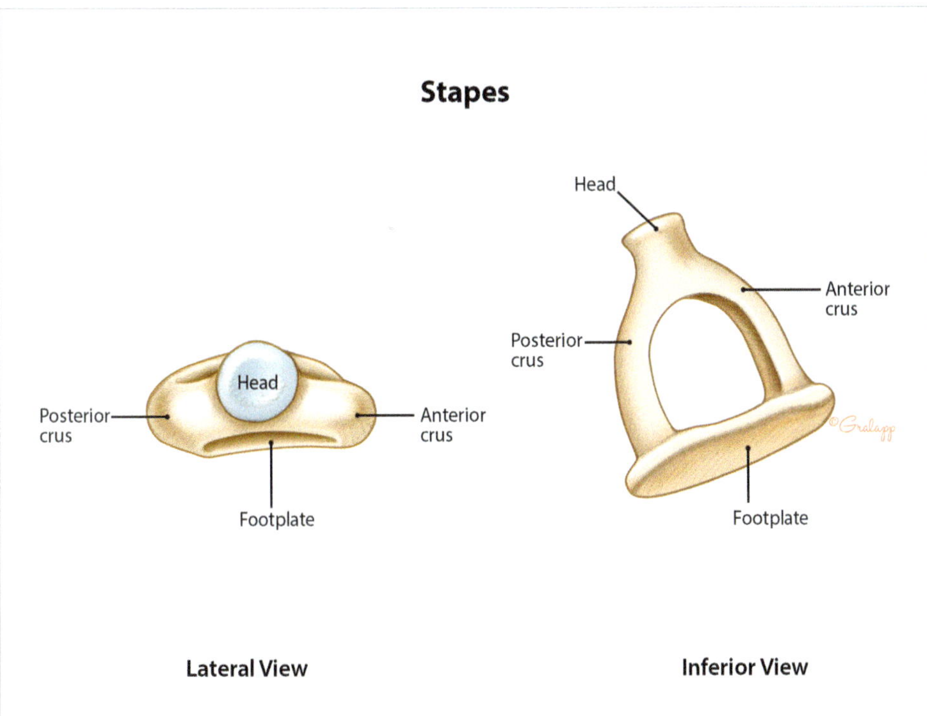

Fig. 1.26 Anatomy of the stapes. The head of the stapes is also known as the capitulum.

1.5 Eustachian Tube

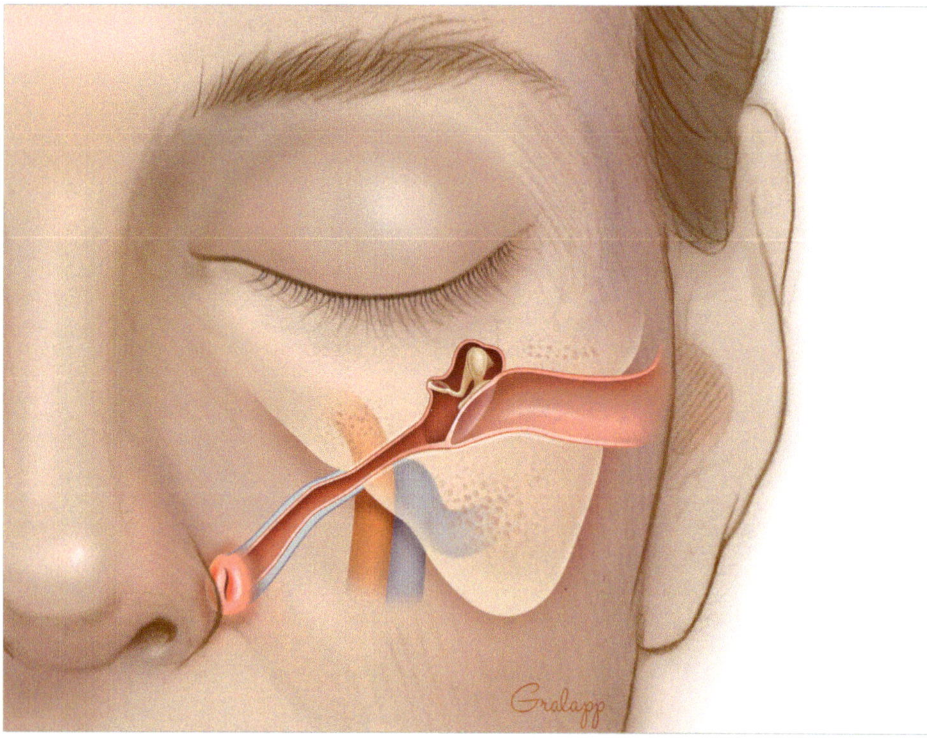

Fig. 1.27 Anatomy of the Eustachian tube.

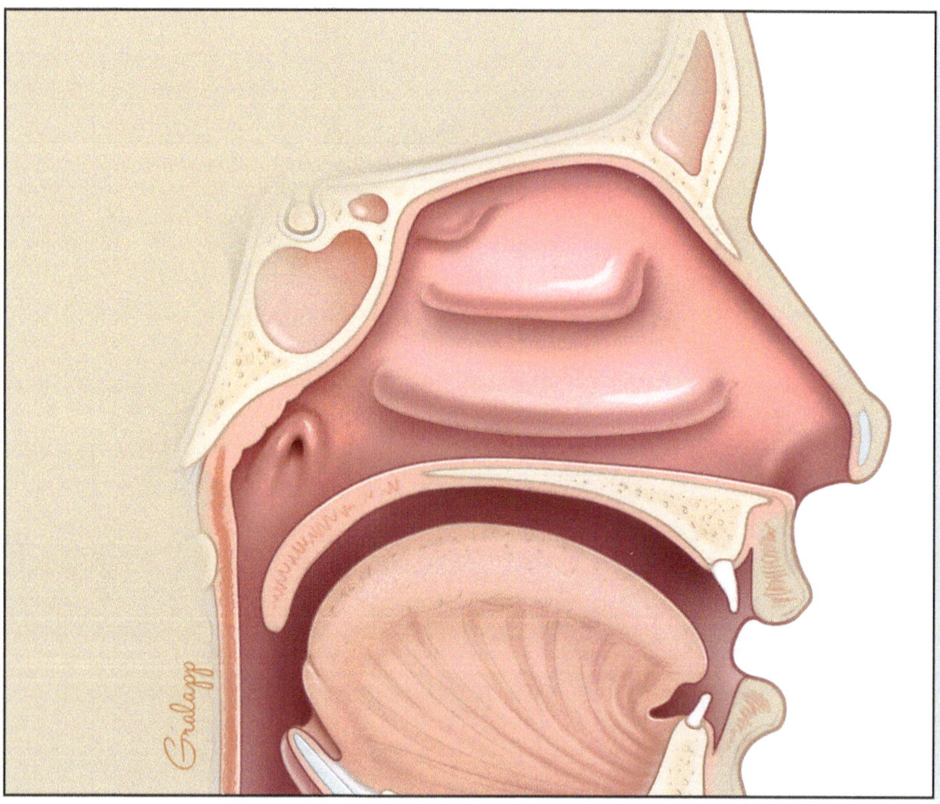

Fig. 1.28 Nasopharyngeal orifice of the anatomy of the Eustachian tube.

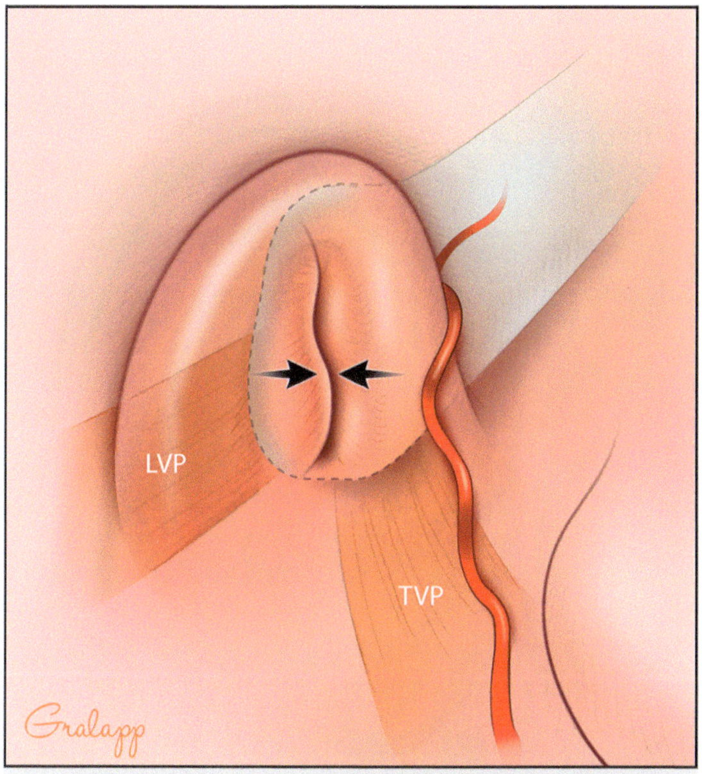

Fig. 1.29 Eustachian tube closed. LVP, levator veli palatini; TVP, tensor veli palatini.

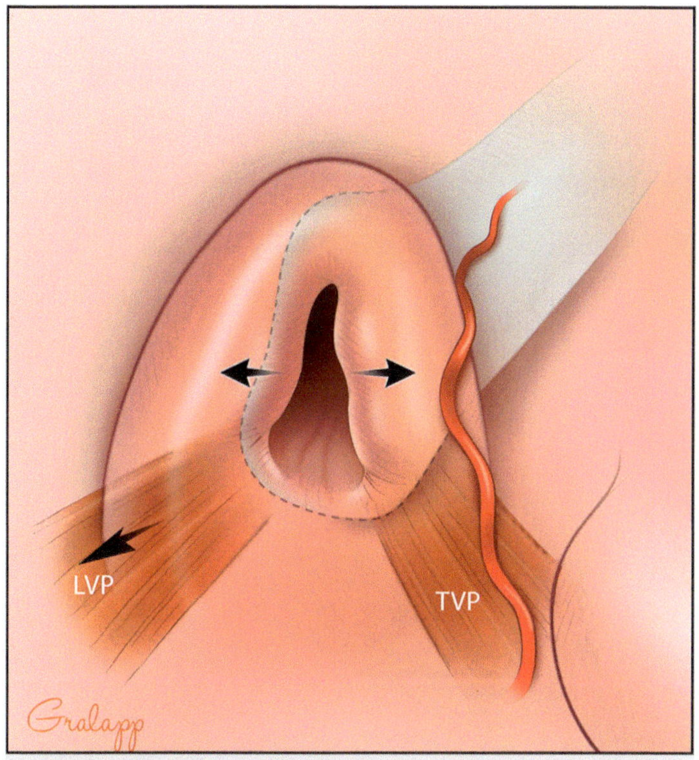

Fig. 1.30 Eustachian tube opening mechanism driven by the tensor and levator muscles.

1.6 Auditory System

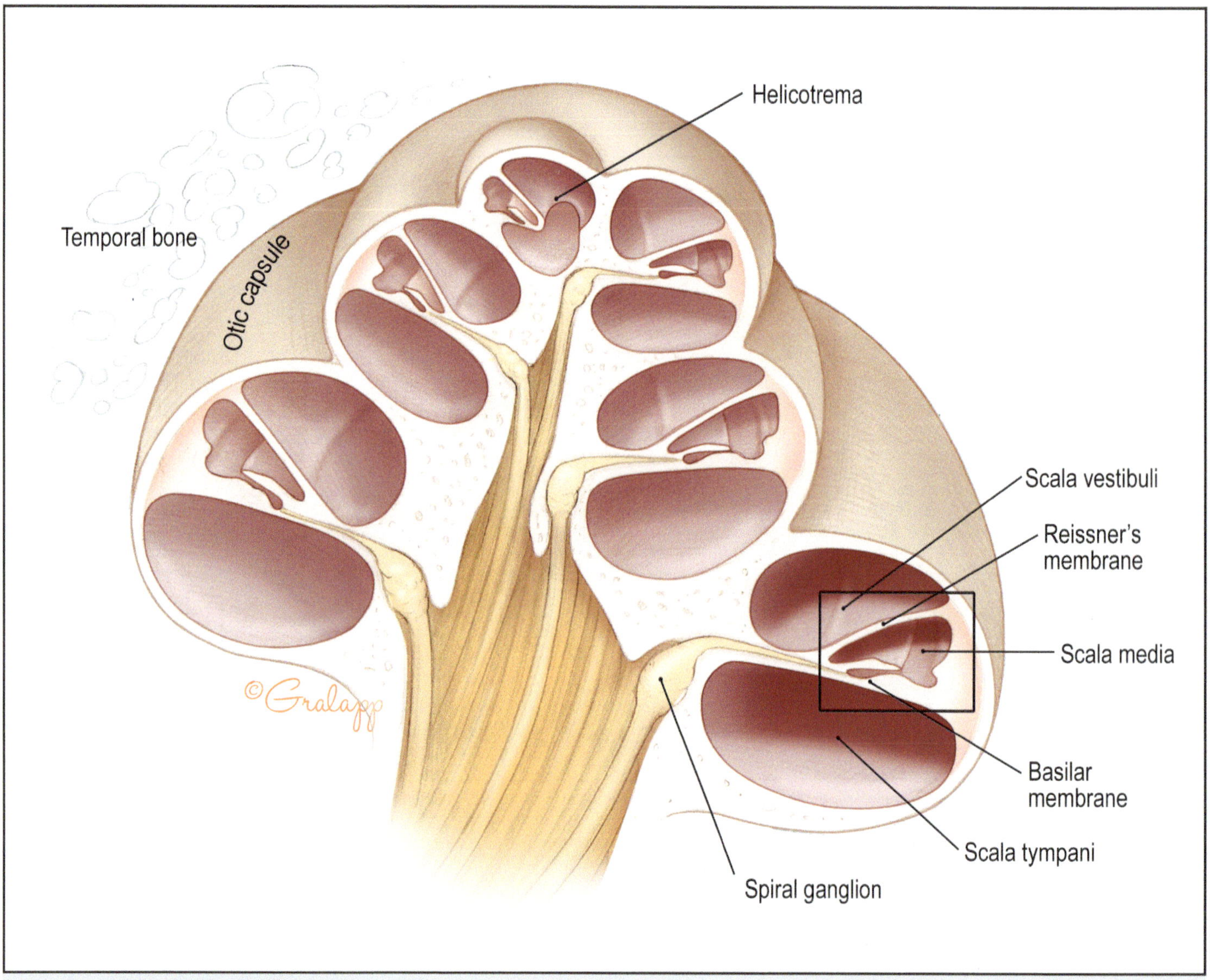

Fig. 1.31 Cochlea in mid-modiolar section.

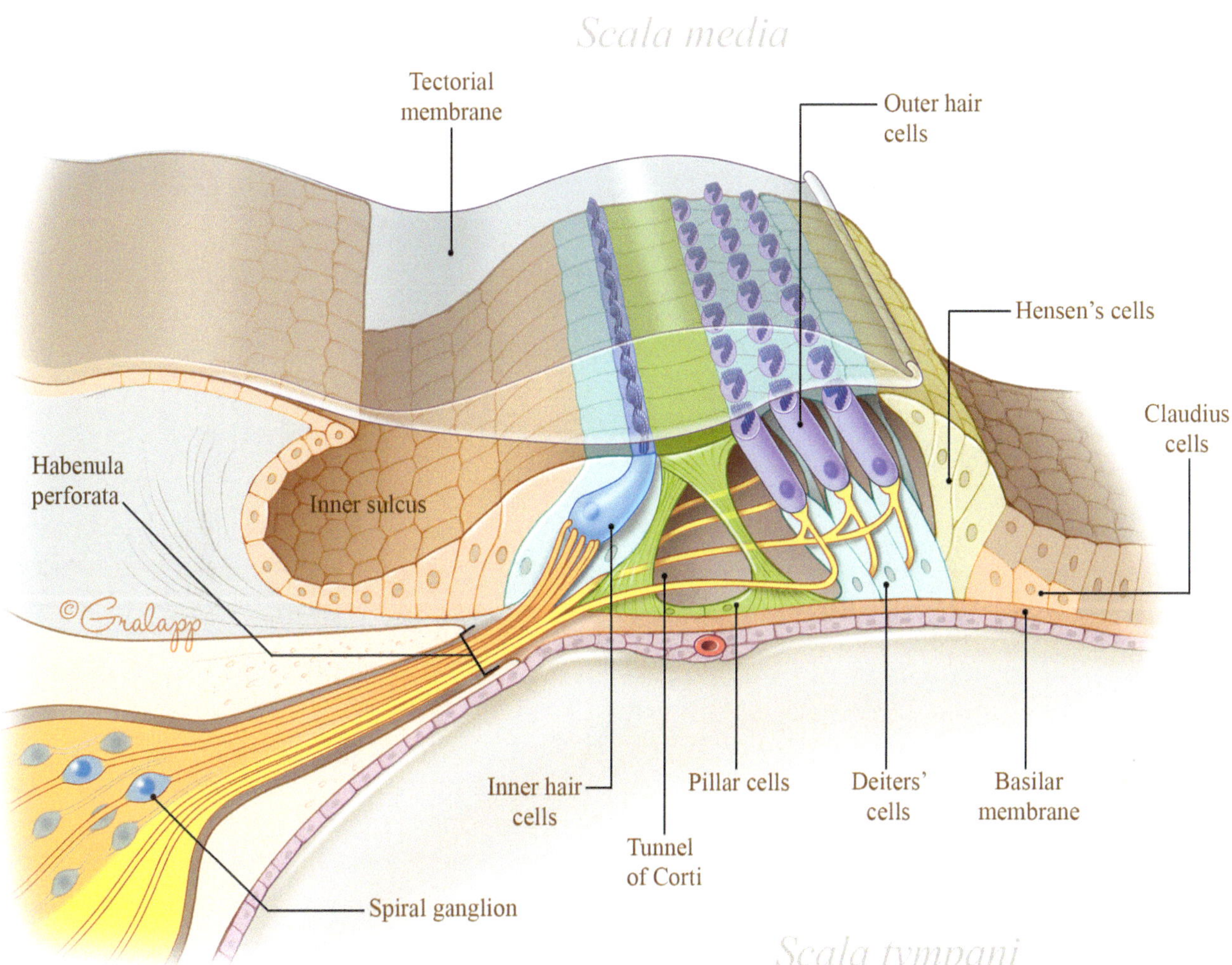

Fig. 1.32 Organ of Corti.

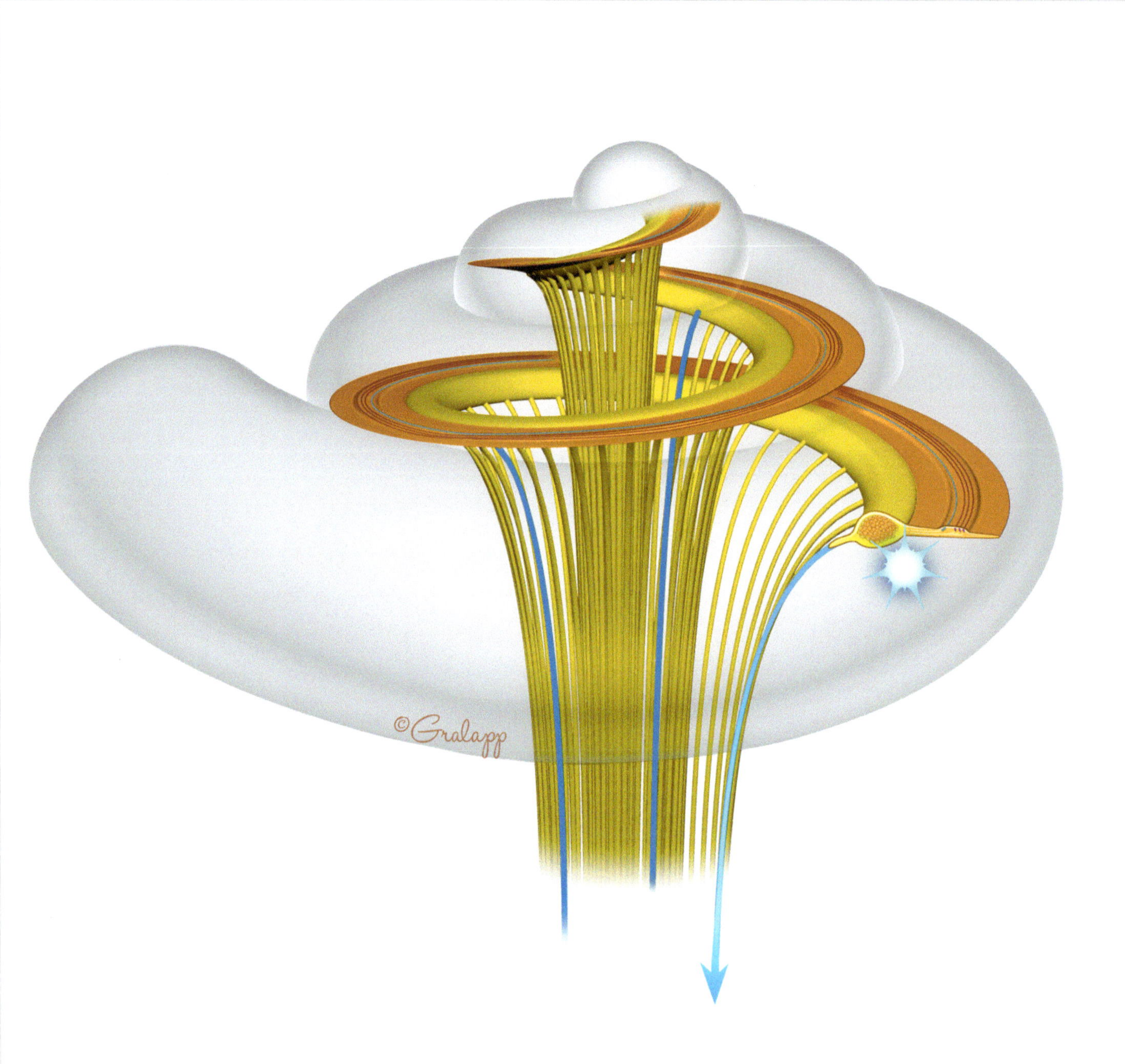

Fig. 1.33 Spiral ganglia (star) and the auditory nerve fibers.

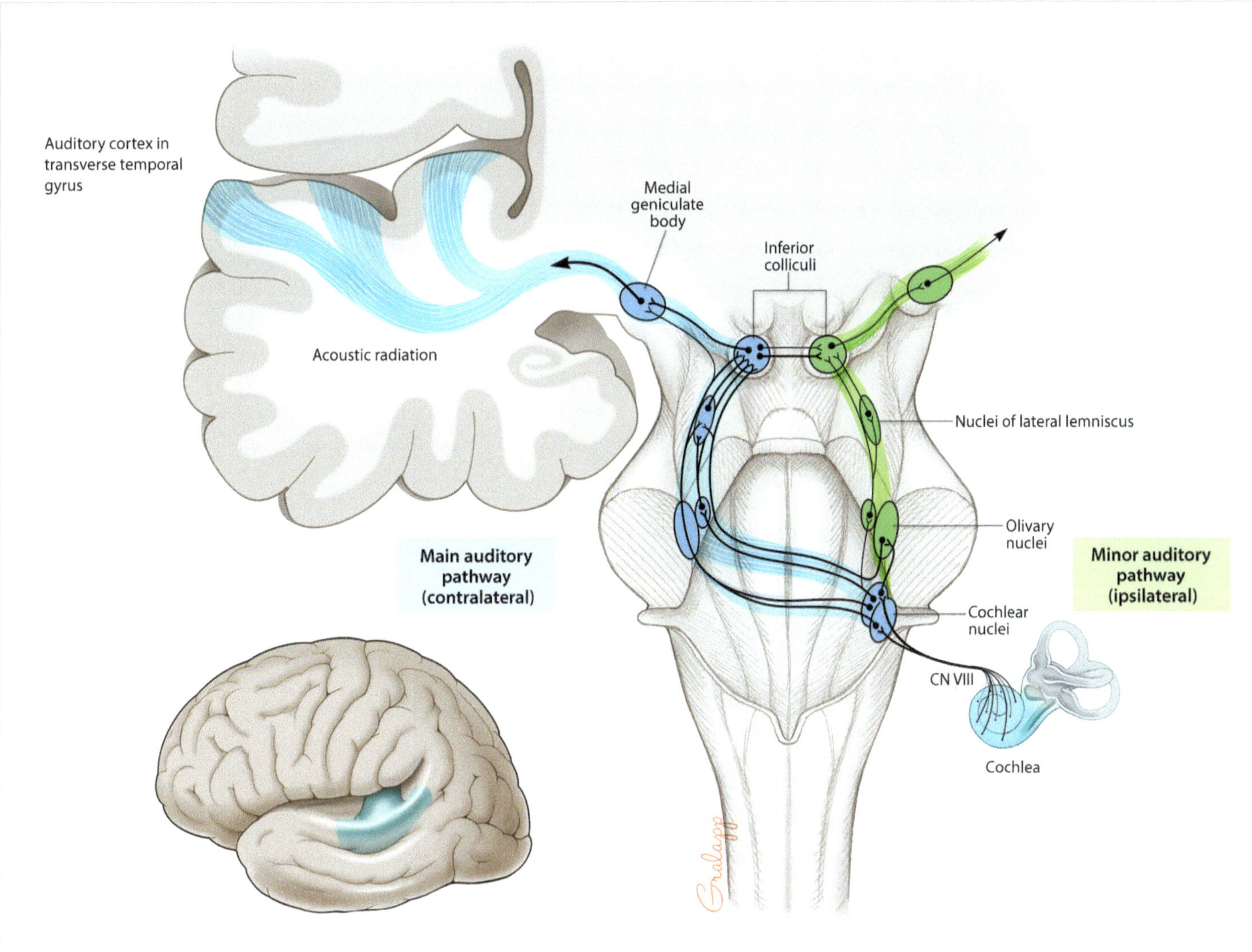

Fig. 1.34 Central auditory pathways.

1.7 Vestibular System

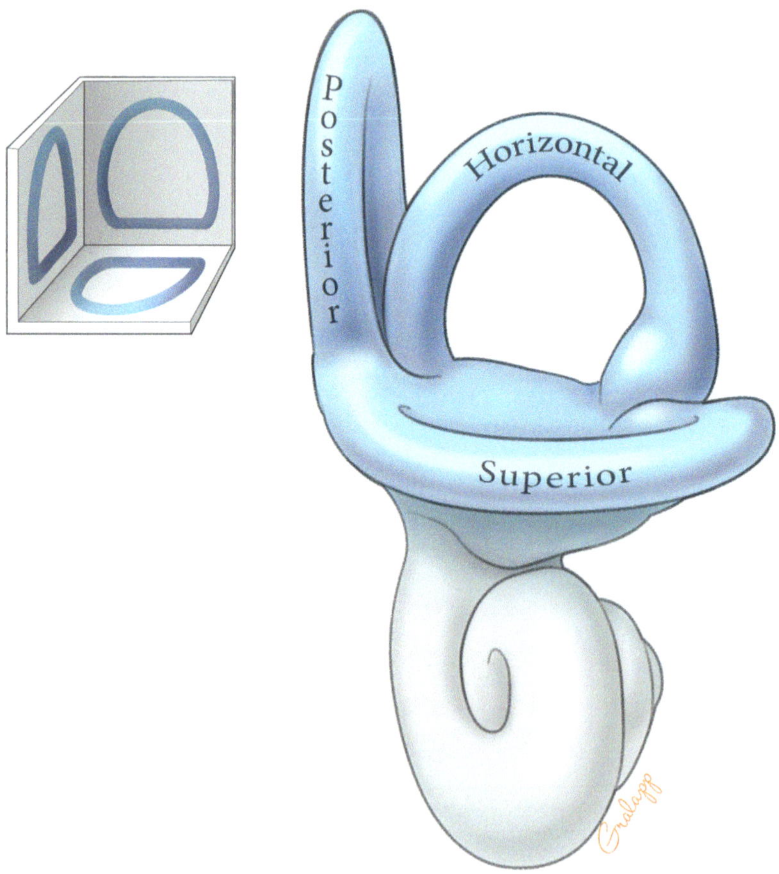

Fig. 1.35 The three semicircular canals, which sense angular accelerations in the three dimensions, are mutually perpendicular.

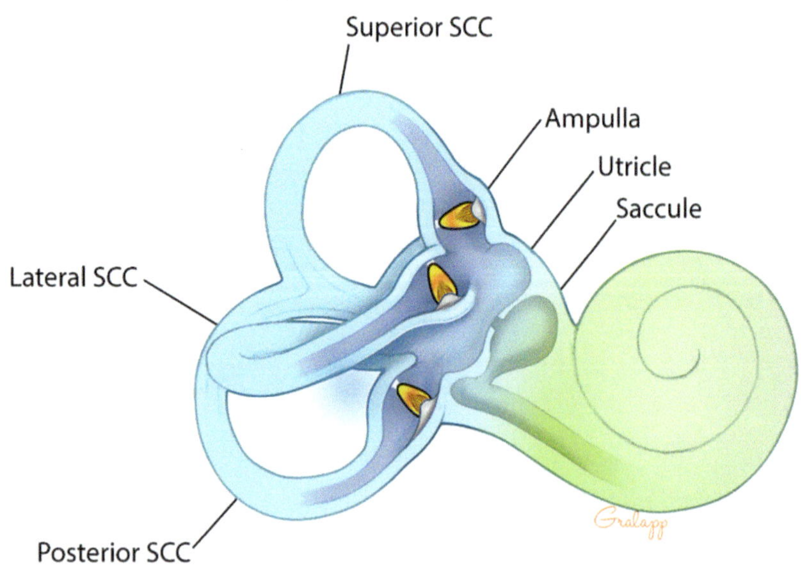

Fig. 1.36 Cupula (orange) in the ampulla of each semicircular canal.

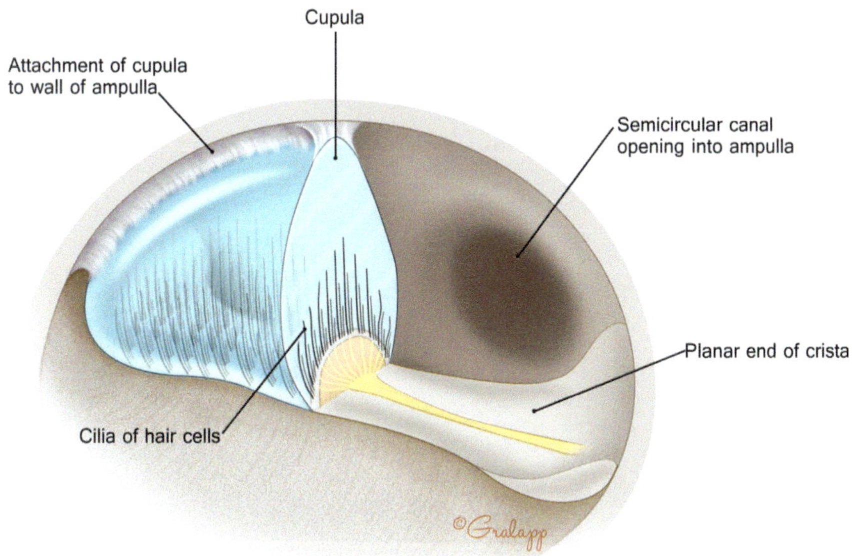

Fig. 1.37 Semicircular canal ampulla.

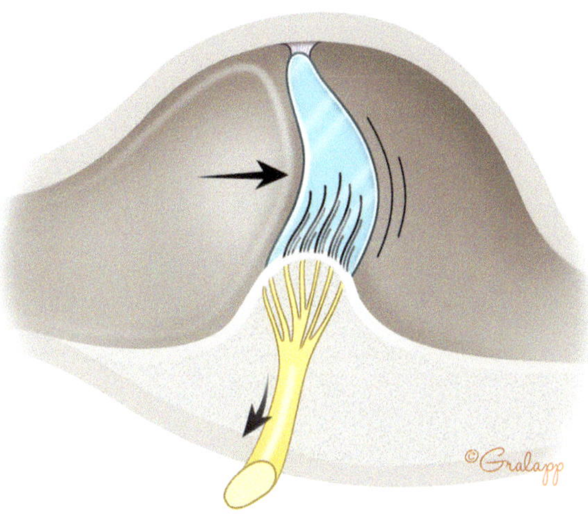

Fig. 1.38 Cupula bowing with endolymph motion.

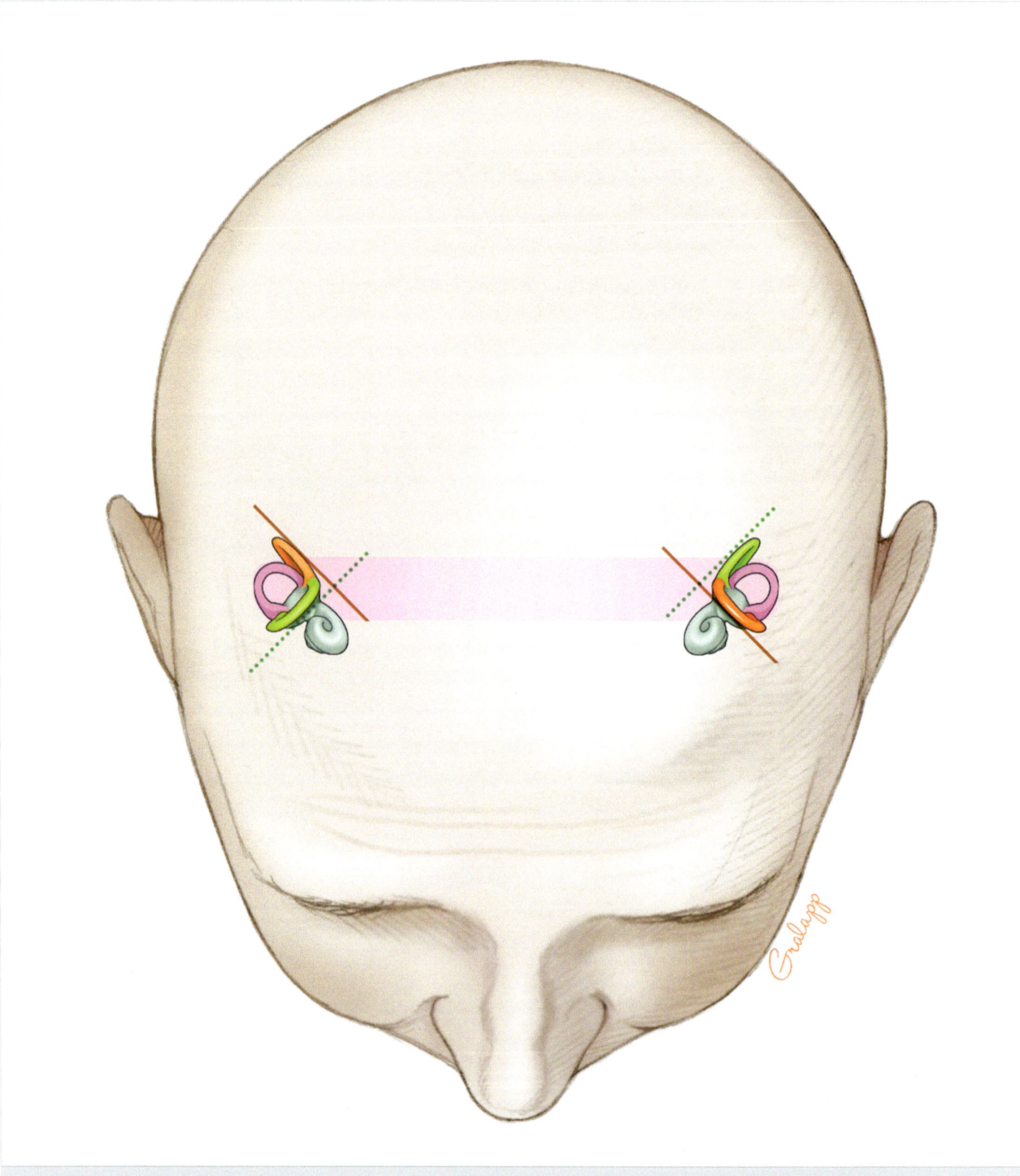

Fig. 1.39 Both lateral semicircular canals are coplanar. Each posterior semicircular canal is coplanar with the opposite superior canal.

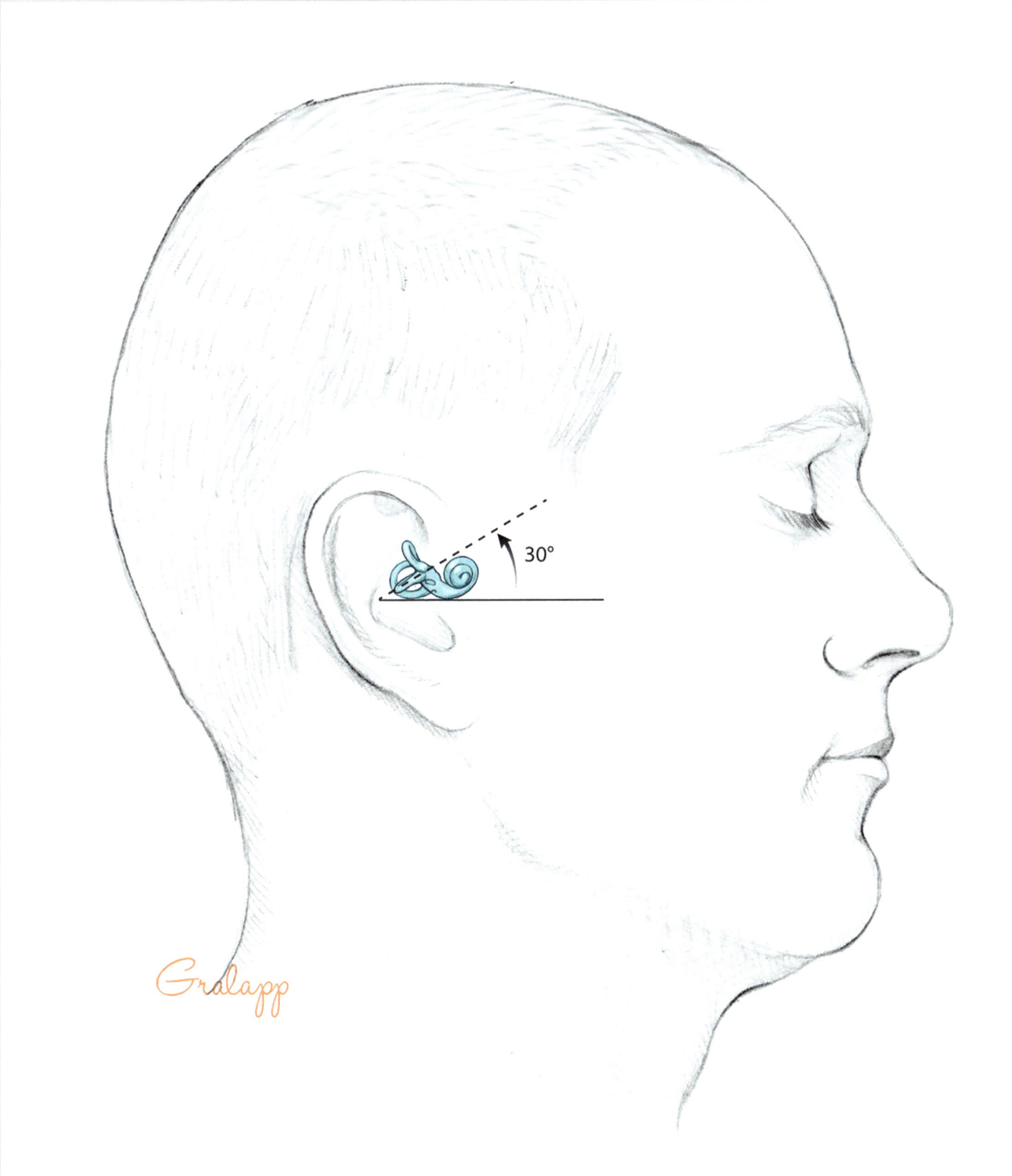

Fig. 1.40 The lateral semicircular canal is tilted upward by 30 degrees.

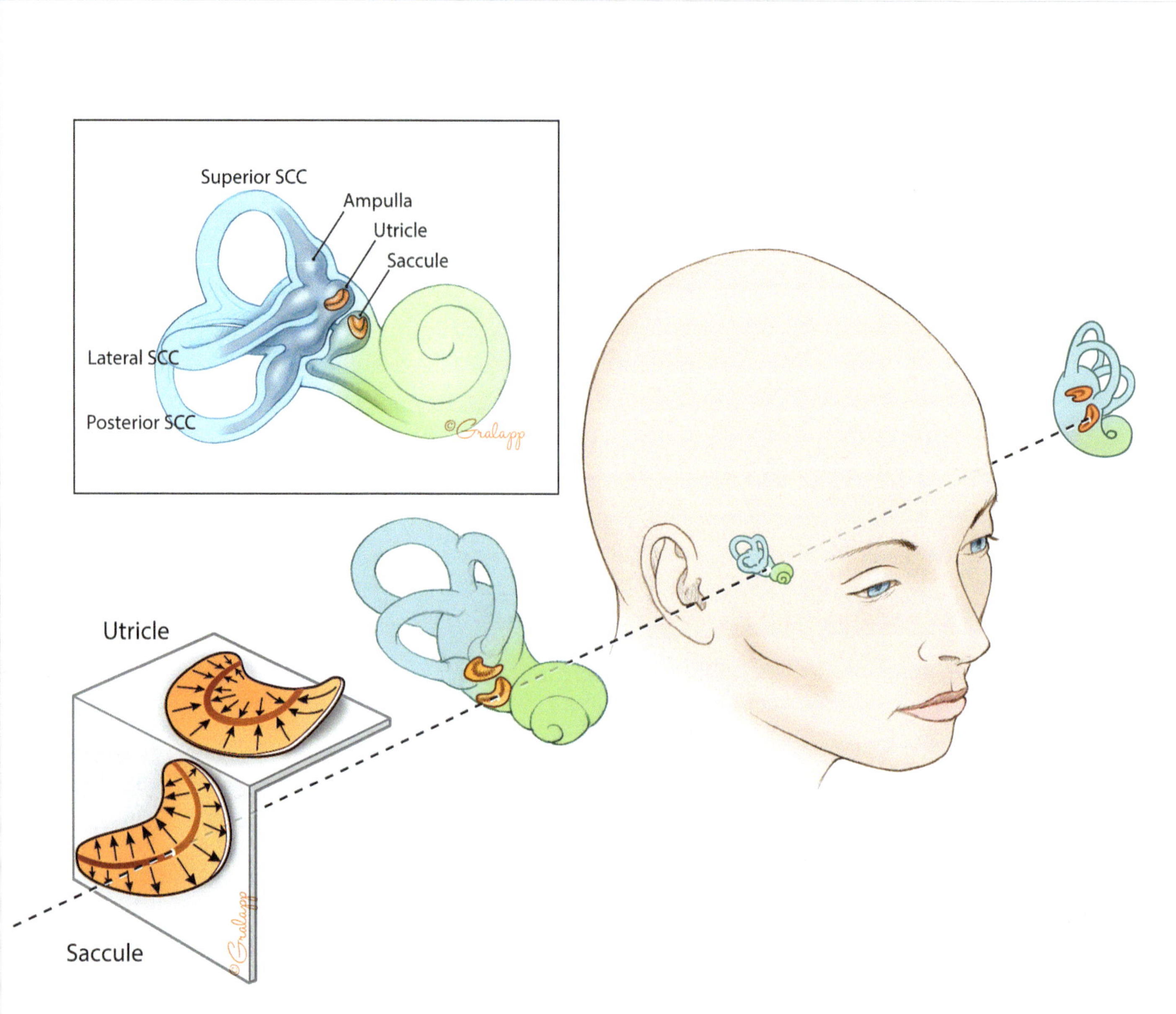

Fig. 1.41 Otolithic organs, the saccule and the utricle, are mutually perpendicular and sense linear accelerations in the horizontal and vertical planes.

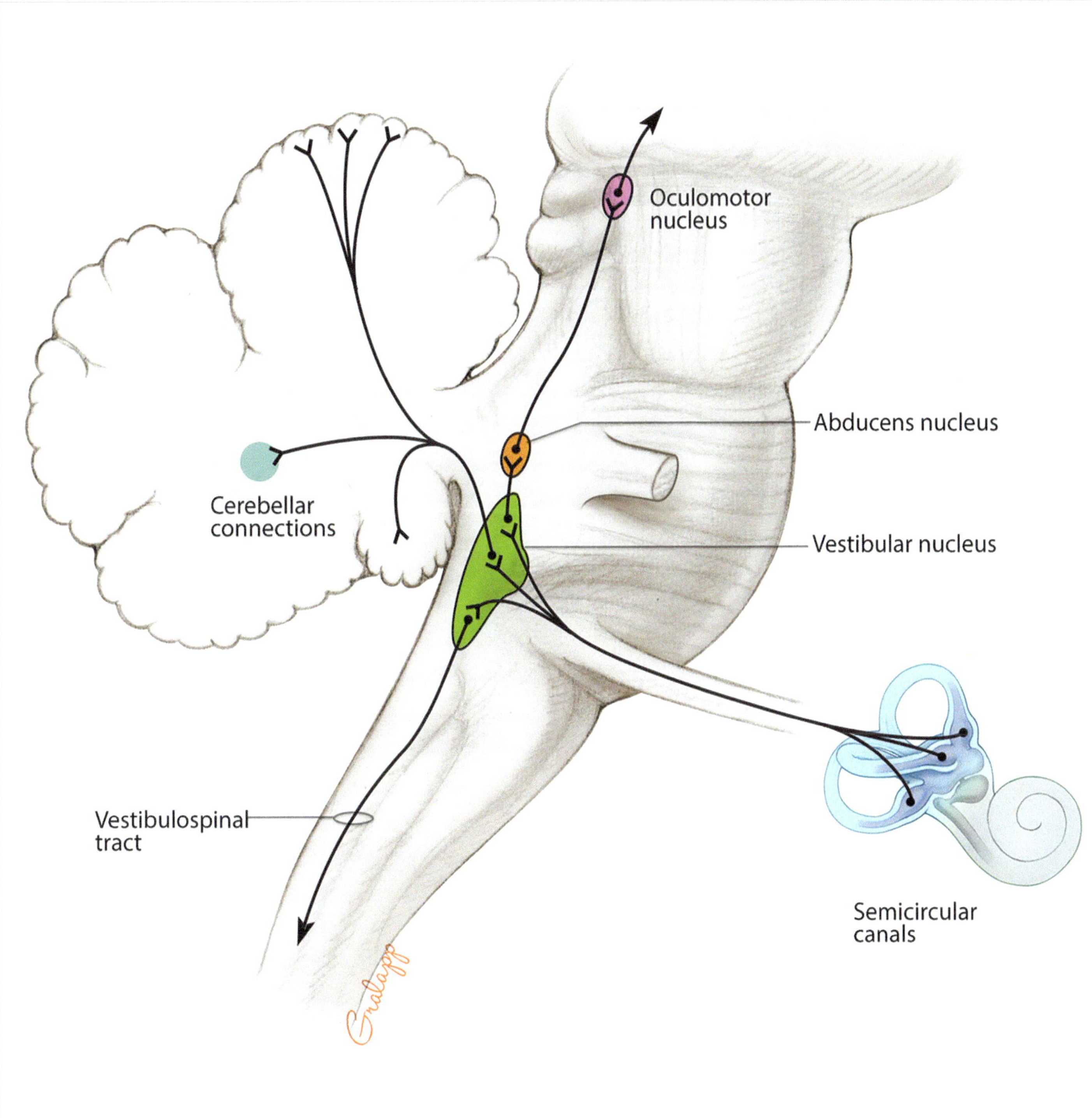

Fig. 1.42 The central vestibular system in sagittal view showing connections to the cerebellum and both oculomotor (eye control) and spinal tract (postural control).

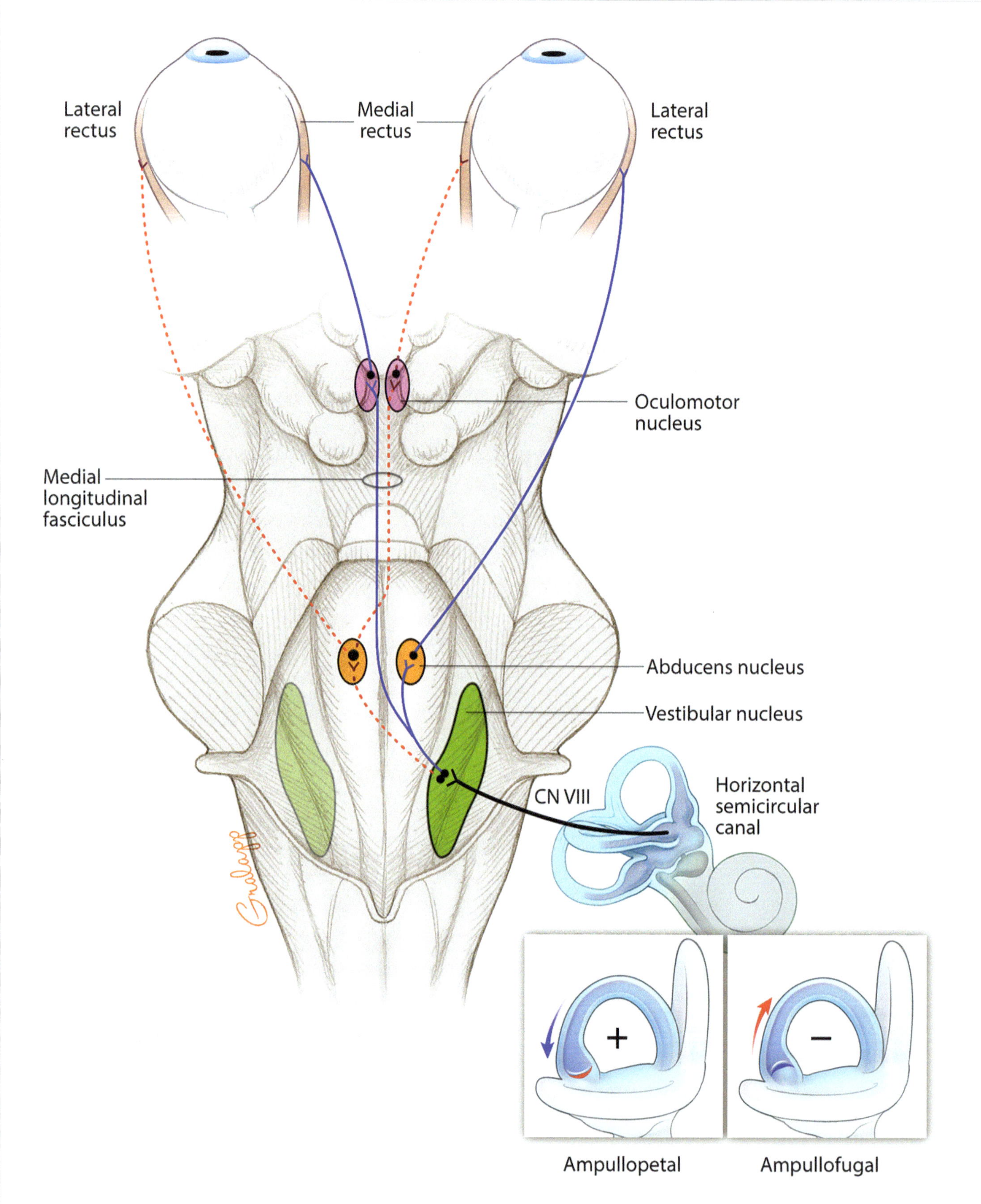

Fig. 1.43 Central vestibular system illustrating connections involved in the oculomotor reflex.

1.8 Internal Auditory Canal and Cerebellopontine Angle

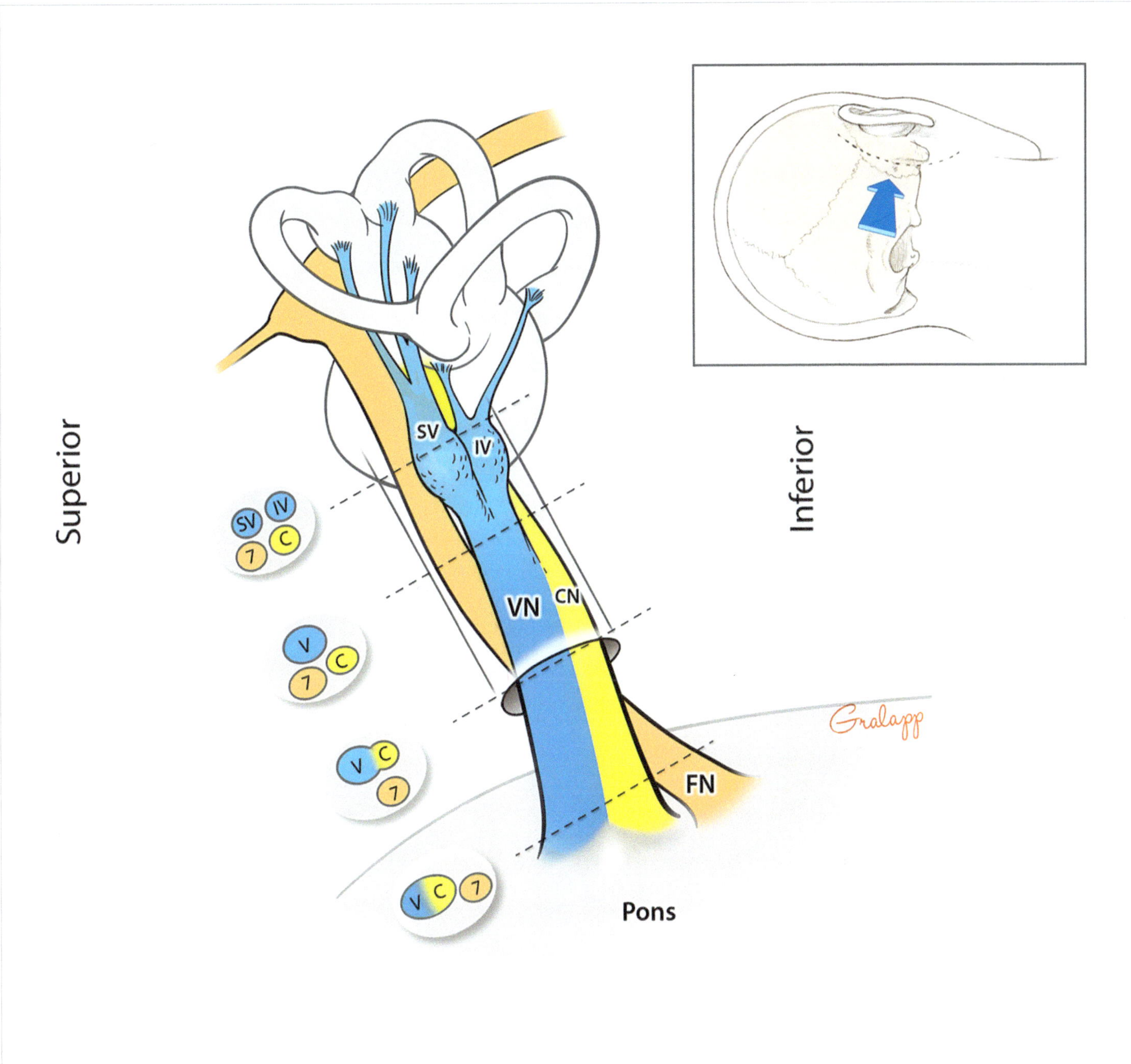

Fig. 1.44 Anatomy of the nerves traversing the internal auditory canal as seen from a retrosigmoid craniotomy perspective. Note the 90-degree rotation of the vestibular and cochlear nerve components of the eighth nerve between inner ear and brainstem entry. C, cochlear nerve; CN, cochlear nerve; IV, inferior vestibular nerve; VN, vestibular nerve; SV, superior vestibular nerve; 7, facial nerve.

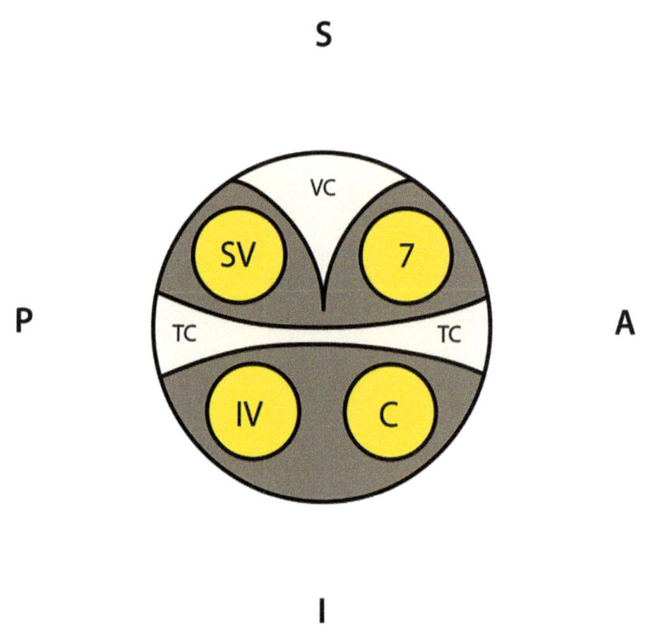

Fig. 1.45 At the lateral extremity of the IAC the relationships of the superior vestibular (SV), inferior vestibular (IV), facial (7), and cochlear (C) nerves are highly predictable. In this location, the canal is completely divided in the horizontal plane by the transverse crest (TC) and its upper compartment is partitioned by a vertical bony crest (VC) also known as Bill's bar (after William F. House, MD). A, anterior; I, inferior; P, posterior; S, superior.

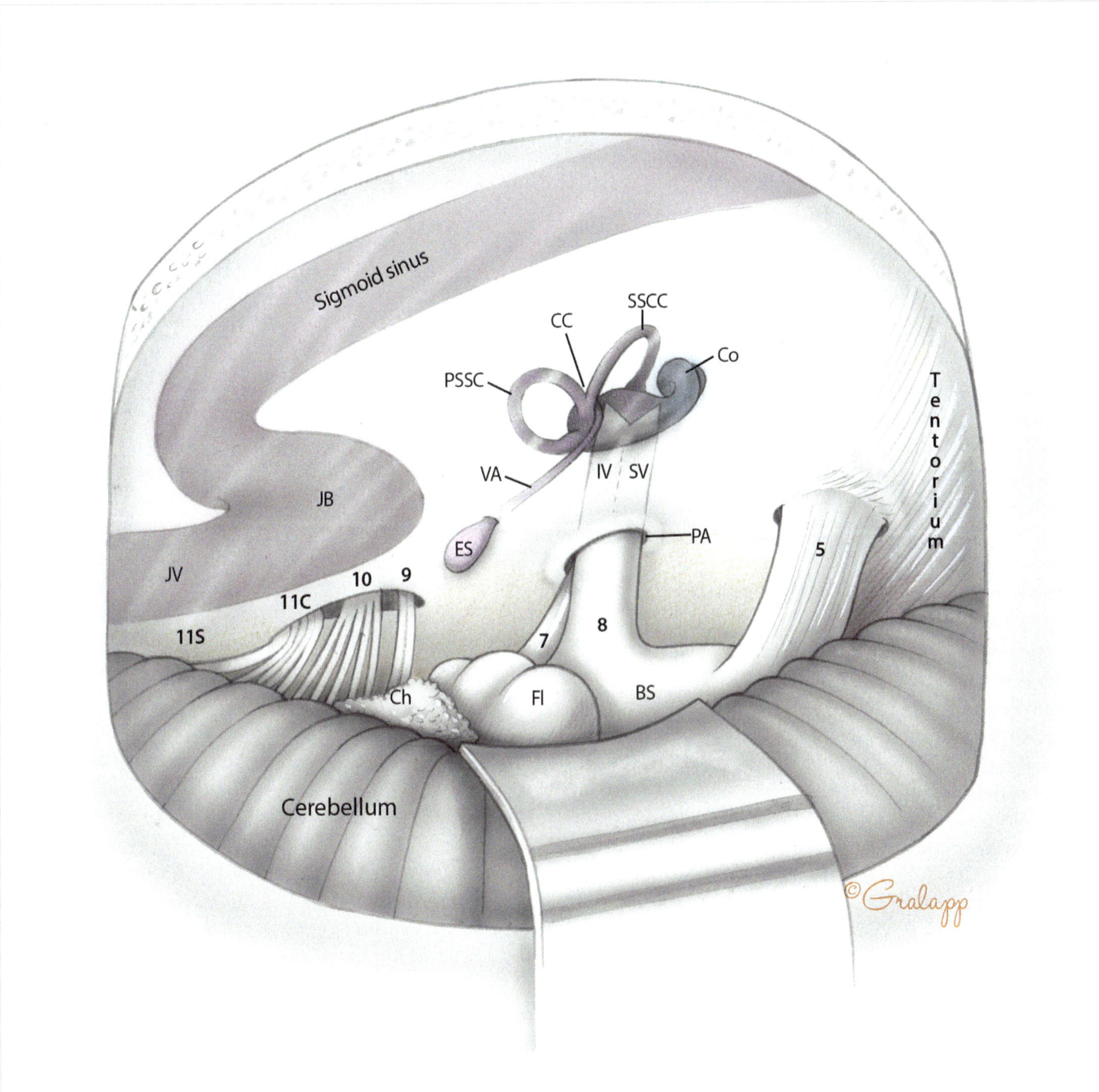

Fig. 1.46 Anatomical relationships of the cerebellopontine as seen through a retrosigmoid posterior fossa craniotomy. JV, jugular vein; JB, jugular bulb; SS, sigmoid sinus; 11 s, spinal component of the accessory nerve; 11c, cranial component of the accessory nerve; 10, vagus nerve; 9, glossopharyngeal nerve; Ch, choroid plexus emanating from the lateral recess to the fourth ventricle; Fl, flocculus; BS, brainstem surface (pons); 7, facial nerve; 8, audiovestibular nerve; 5, trigeminal nerve; PA, porus acusticus; IV, inferior vestibular nerve; SV, superior vestibular nerve; ES, endolymphatic sac; VA, vestibular aqueduct; PSSC, posterior semicircular canal; CC, common crus; SSCC, superior semicircular canal; Co, cochlea.

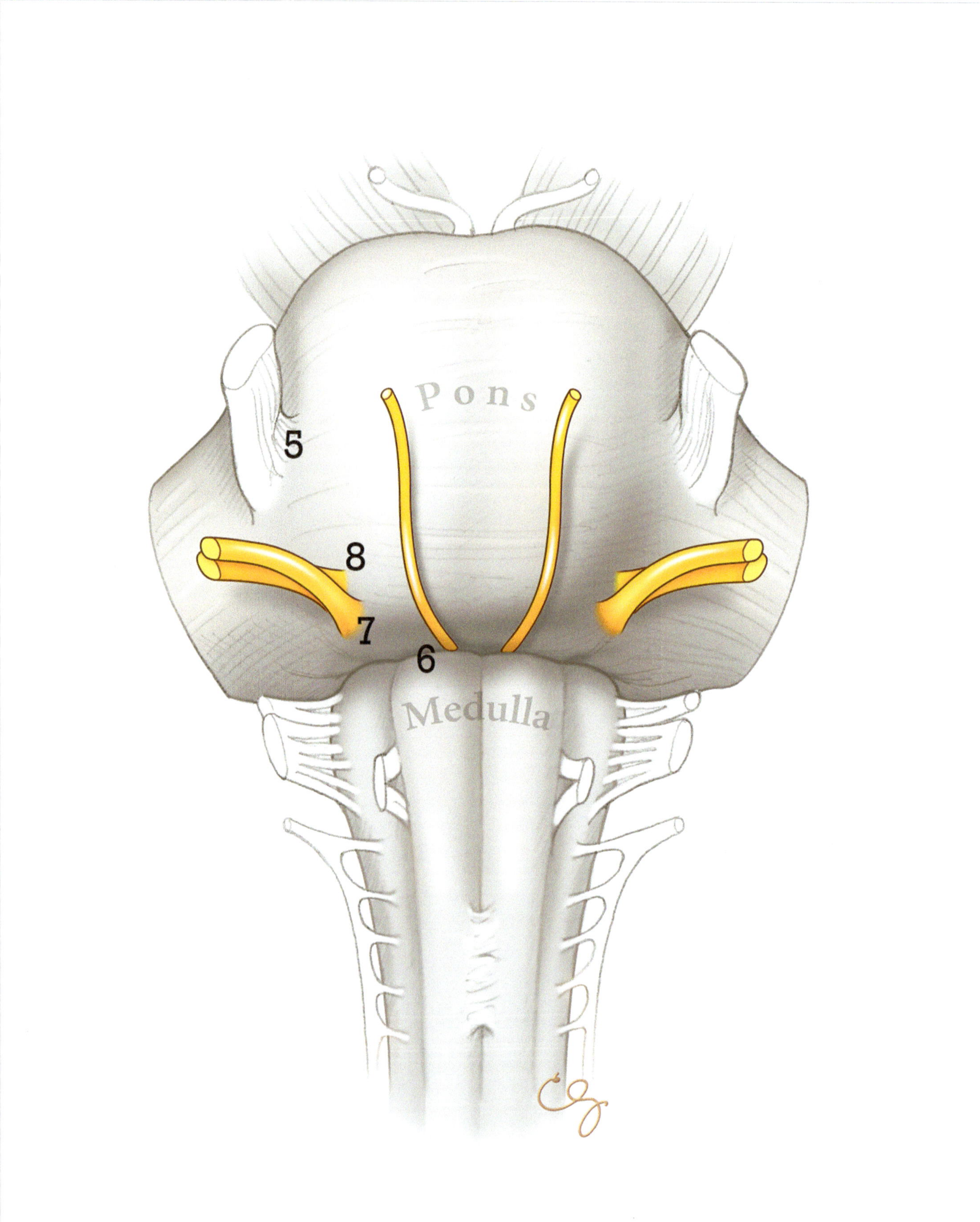

Fig. 1.47 Ventral perspective of the brainstem depicting the root entries and proximal course of cranial nerve entries of V to VIII. Note the seventh nerve enters inferior to the eighth. Most previous illustrations contain errors in the depiction of these anatomical details. (Used with permission from Corrales CE, Jackler RK, Mudry A. Perpetuation of errors in illustrations of cranial nerve anatomy. *J Neurosurg* 2016;28:1–7.)

1.9 Ear Tumors

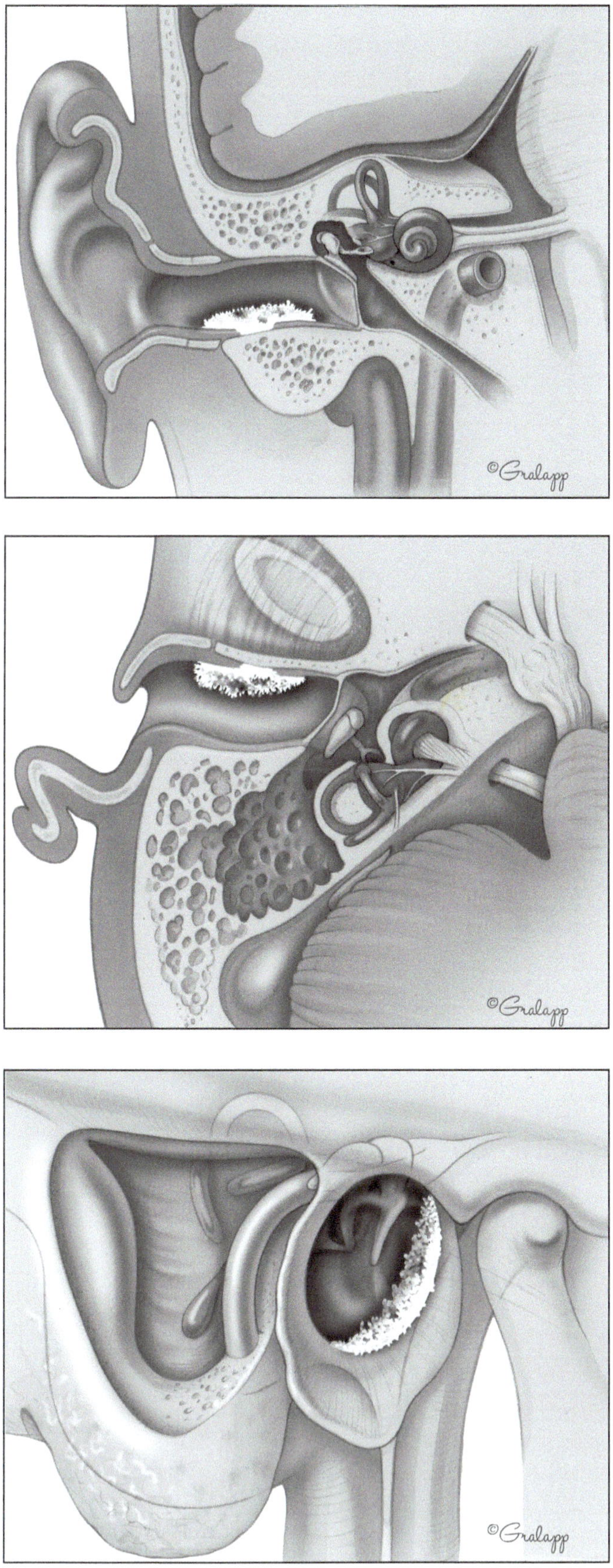

Fig. 1.48 An early squamous cell carcinoma of the ear canal involving the anterior and inferior aspects of the canal. The lesion is still superficial.

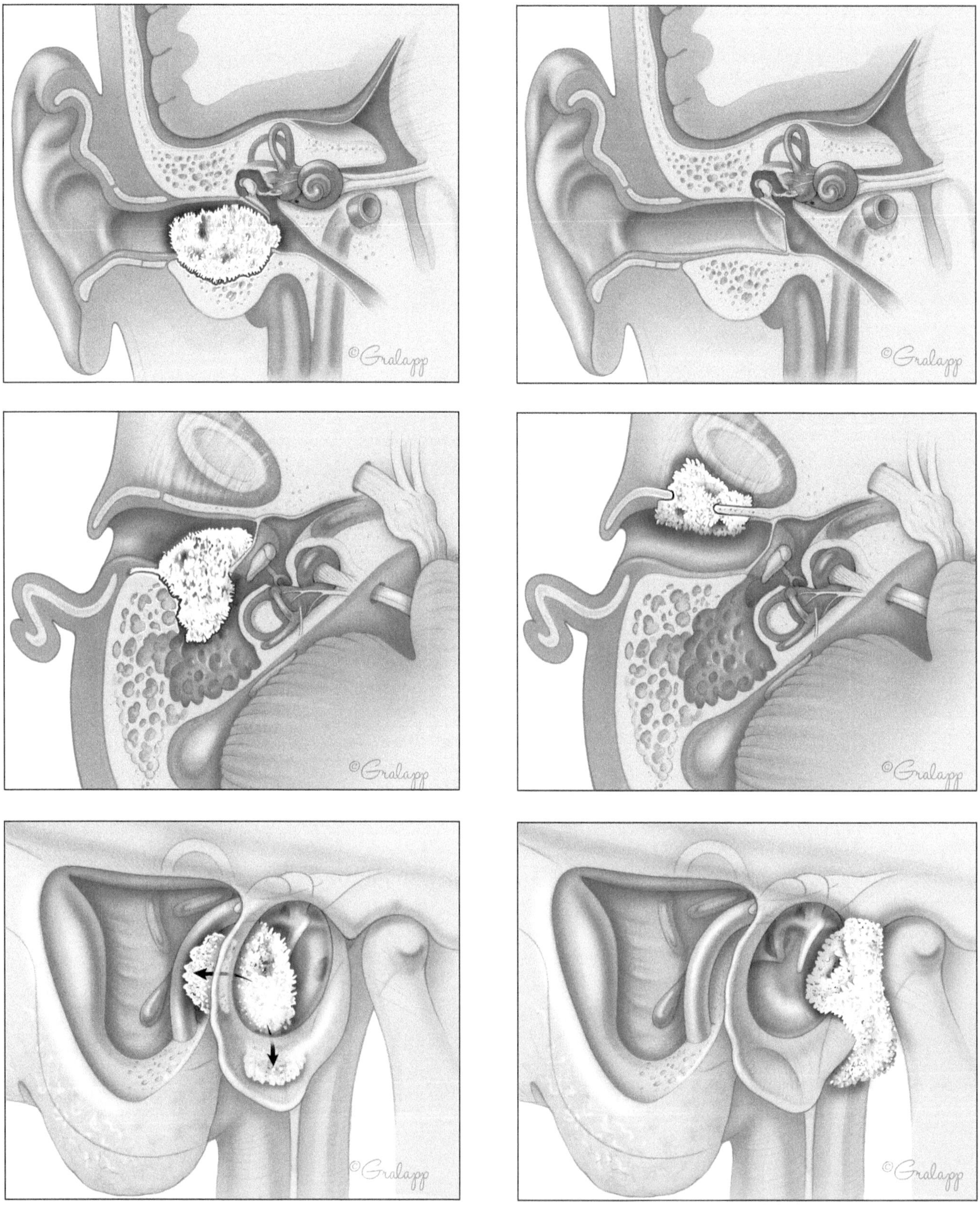

Fig. 1.49 Moderate-size squamous cell carcinoma of the ear canal involving the inferior and posterior aspects of the canal (*left*). Note the breaching of posterior aspect of the canal into the mastoid. In addition, the floor of the canal is eroded and the tympanic membrane is penetrated. Moderate-size squamous cell carcinoma of the ear canal with an anterior invasion pattern (*right*). Note the involvement of the condylar fossa and the tendency for invasion anteriorly and inferiorly along the base of skull.

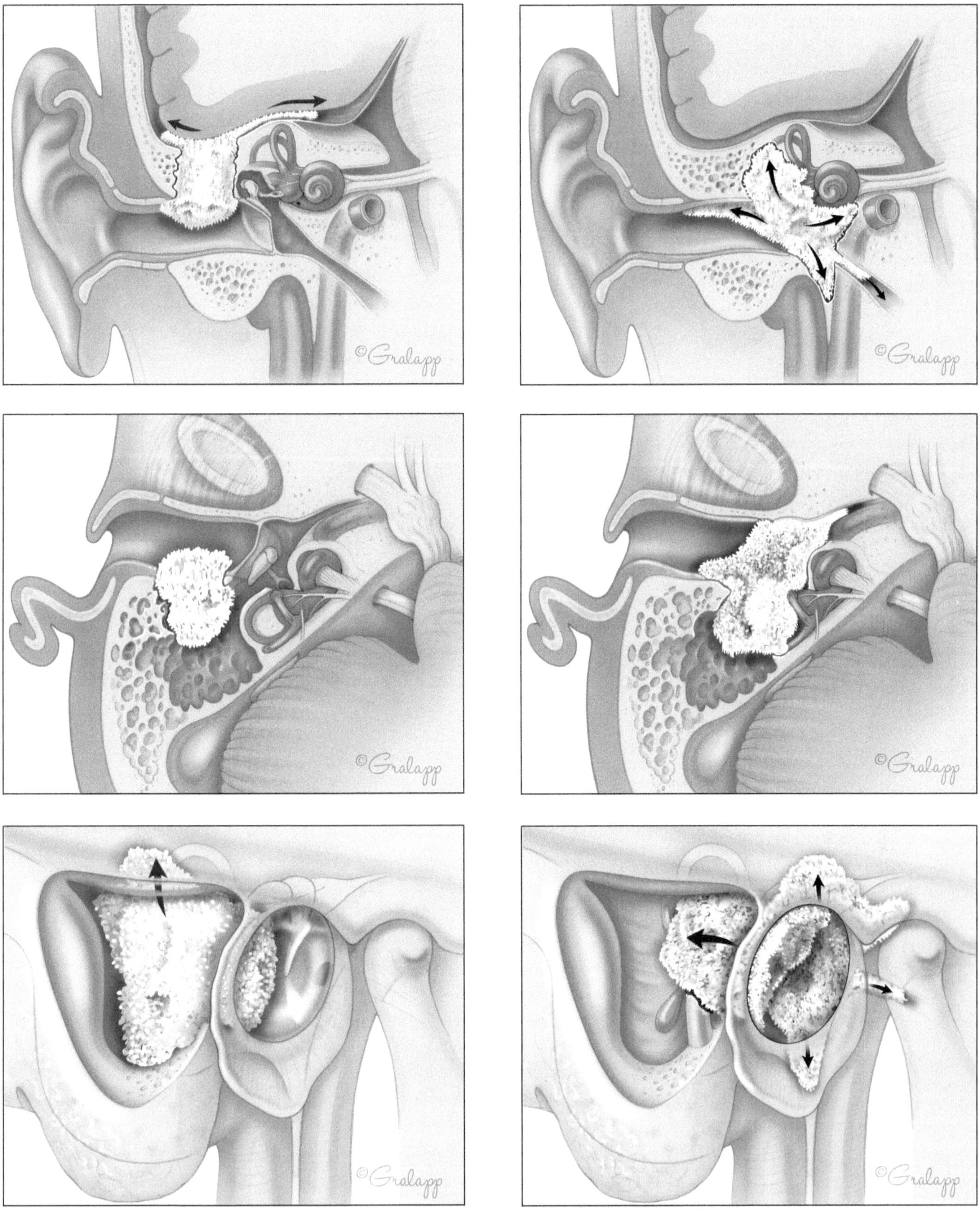

Fig. 1.50 Advanced squamous cell carcinoma of the ear canal with invasion of the middle cranial fossa via the tegmen mastoideum (*left*). Note the tendency for spread along the dural surface. Advanced squamous cell carcinoma of the ear canal with medial invasion through the middle ear into the otic capsule (*right*). Spread into the protympanum and along the Eustachian tube brings the tumor into approximation with the intrapetrous carotid artery.

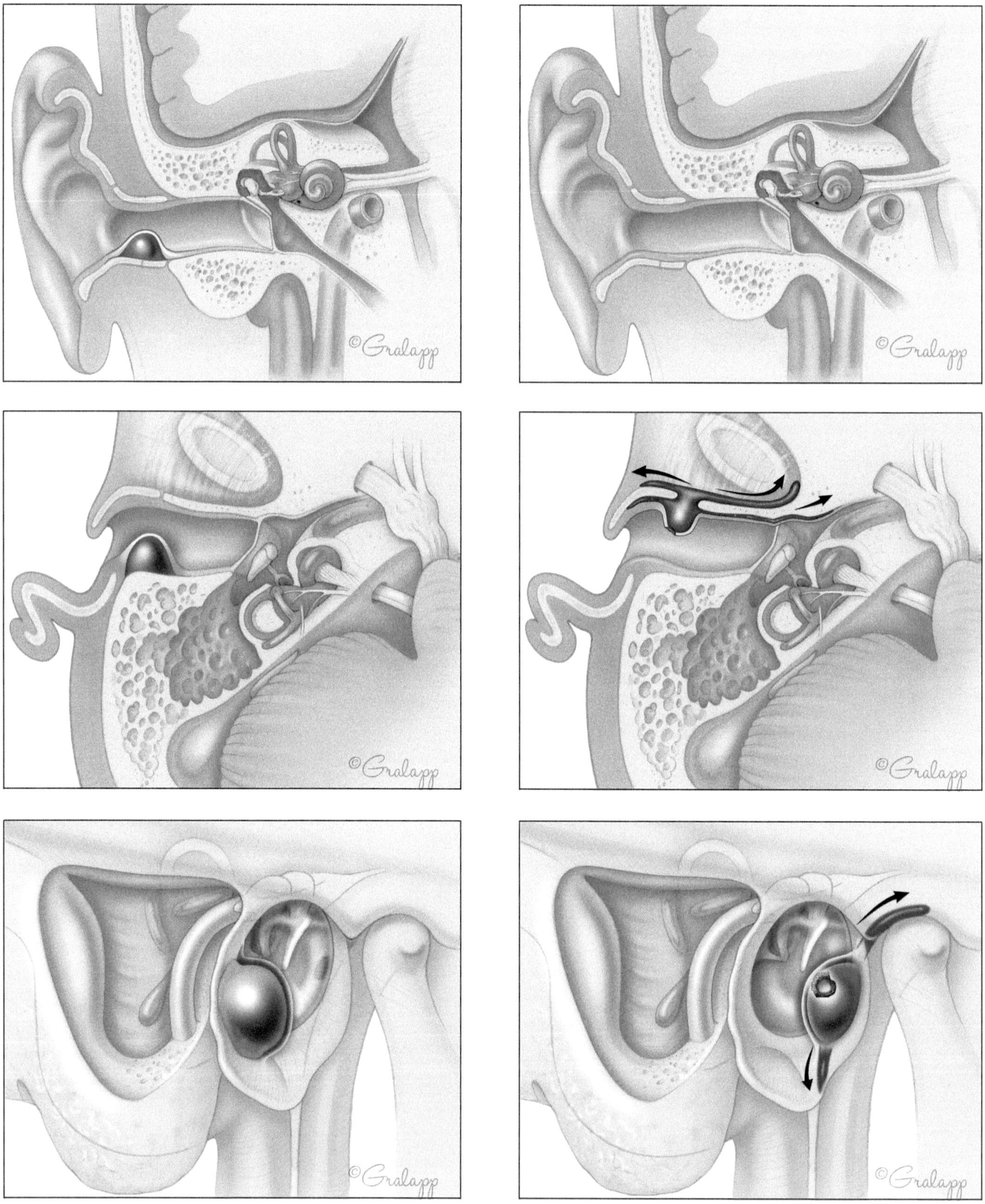

Fig. 1.51 Adenoma of the ear canal. Note the geometric regularity of the lesion and its minimal influence on underlying bone (*left*). Adenocystic carcinoma of the ear canal. Note the widespread subperiosteal spread in the ear canal and the extensive skull base involvement for a relatively modest size primary lesion (*right*). A neurotrophic growth pattern, particularly along the intratemporal course of the facial nerve, may develop.

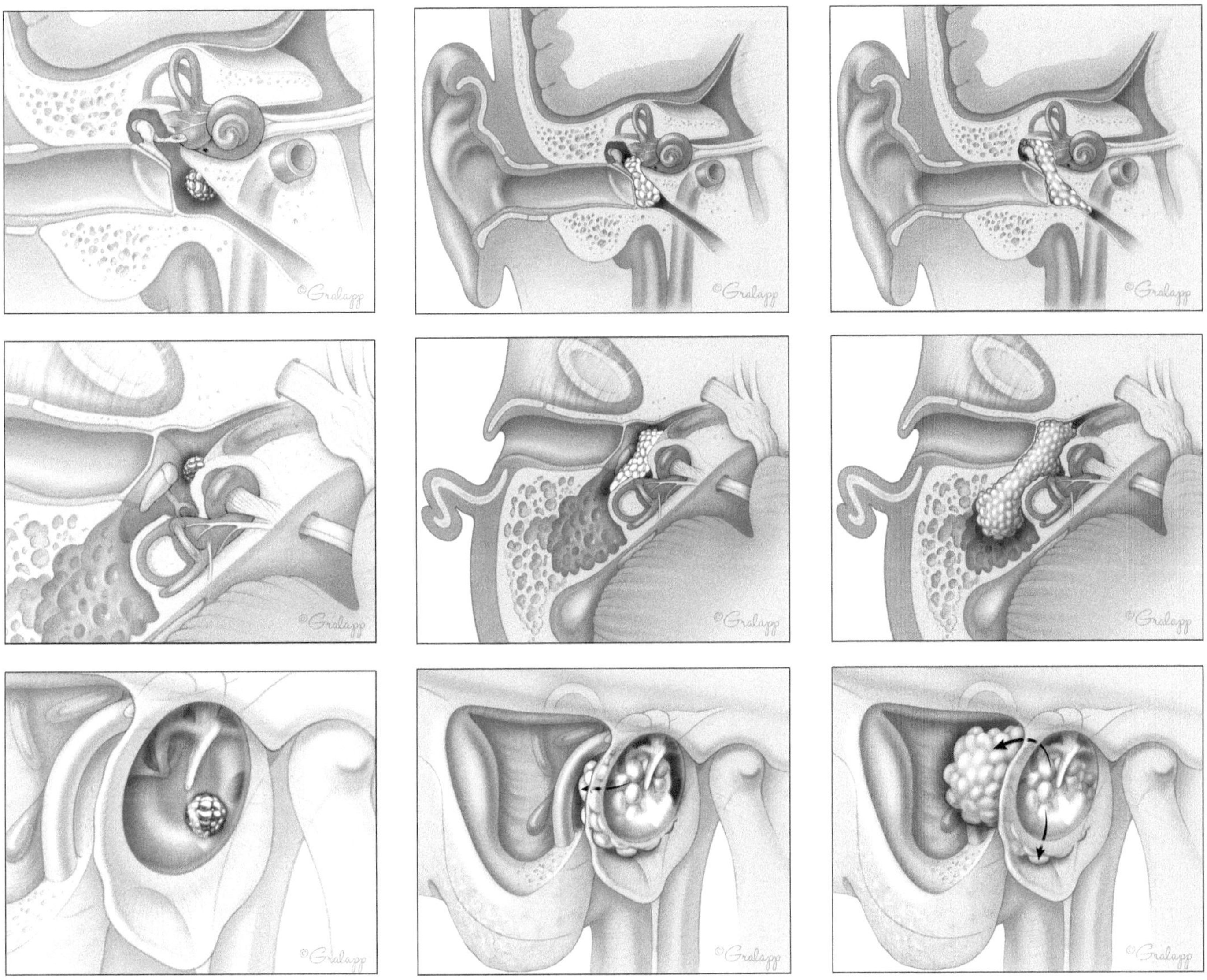

Fig. 1.52 Small glomus tympanicum tumor arising from the anterior–inferior aspect of the promontory (*left*). Glomus tympanicum tumor with growth into the hypotympanum, posterior tympanic spaces (sinus tympani and facial recess), and oval window region with engulfment of the stapes (*center*). Extensive glomus tympanicum tumor with involvement of the entire middle ear cleft and spread via the aditus-ad-antrum to the mastoid (*right*).

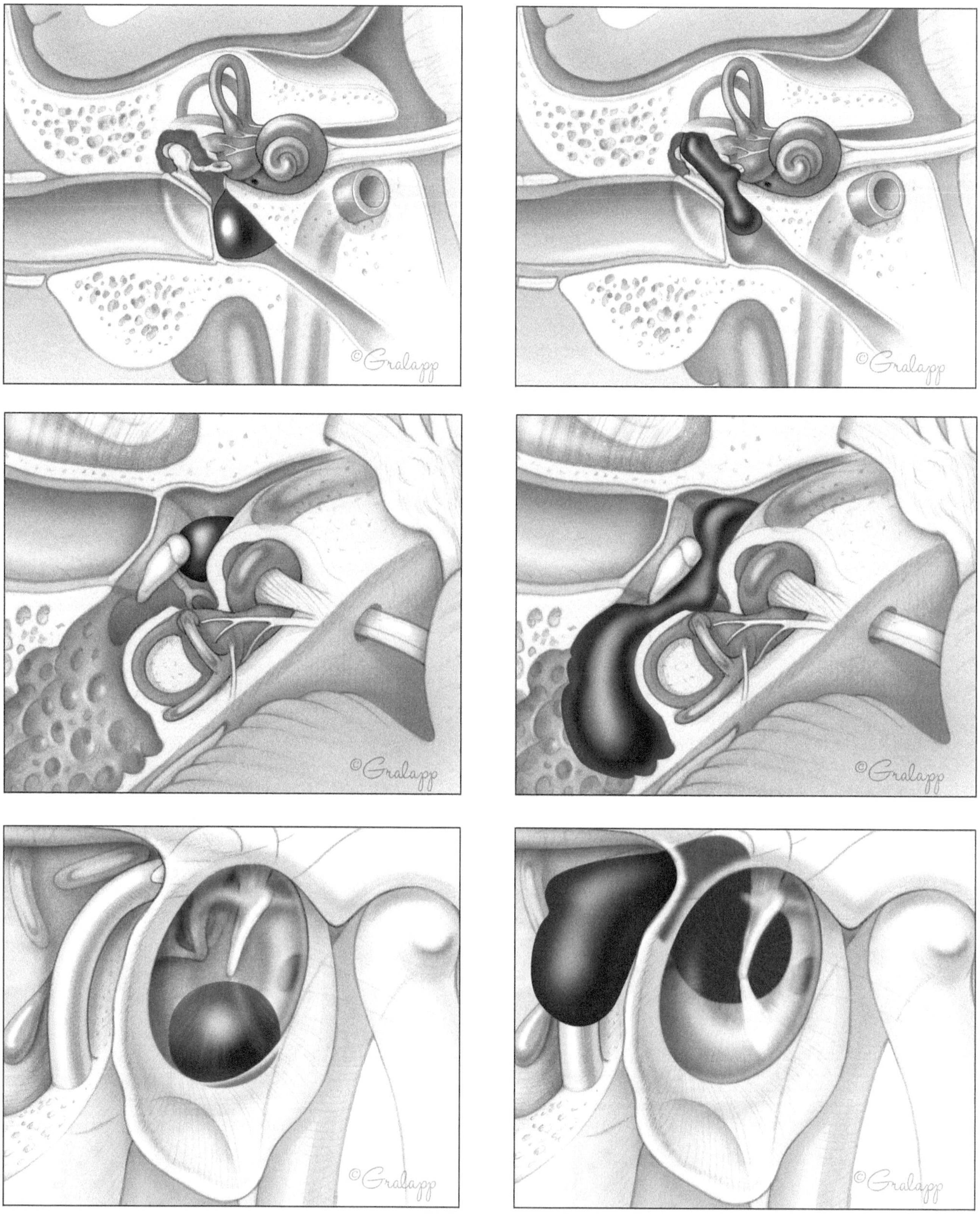

Fig. 1.53 Adenoma arising from the mucosal surface of the middle ear (*left*). Most tympanomastoid adenomas are neuroendocrine tumors (carcinoids). These lesions usually have a smooth, geometrically regular shape with a broad base against the mucosal surface of origin. (*Right*) Extensive mucosal adenoma of the middle ear and mastoid: note the spread along preformed pneumatic pathways and the absence of osseous erosion.

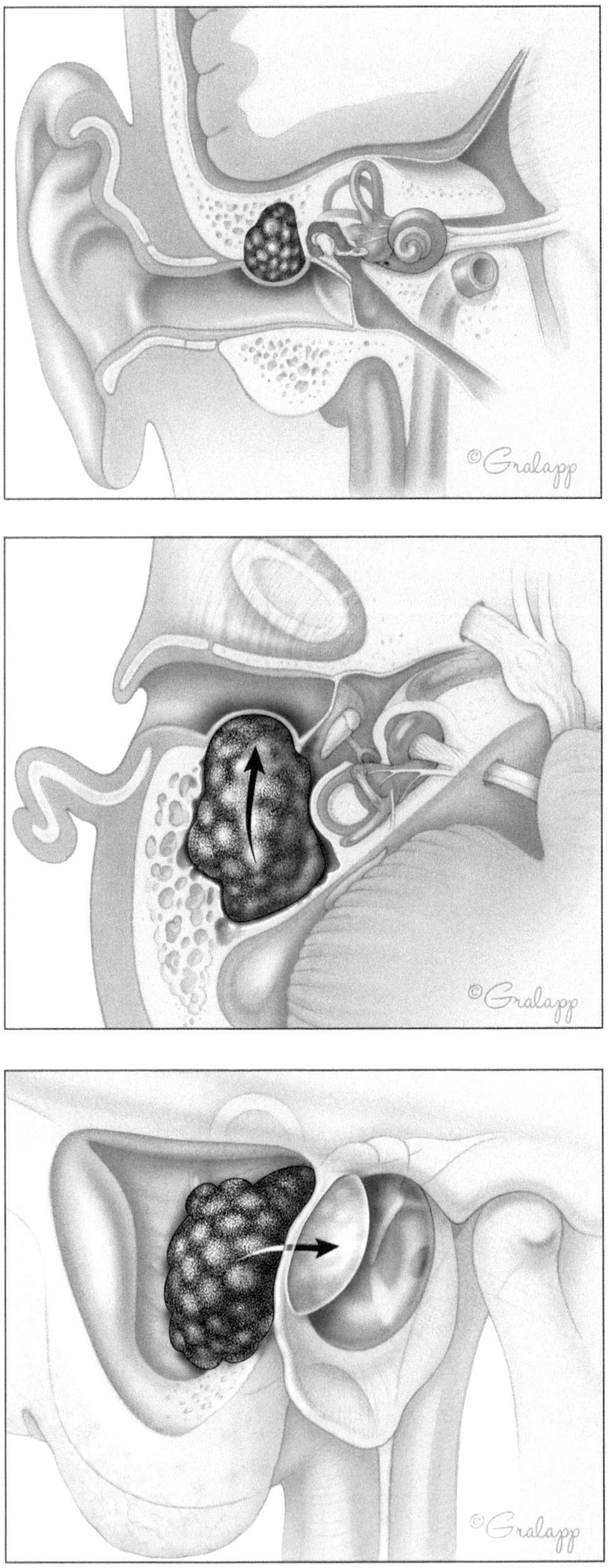

Fig. 1.54 Eosinophilic granuloma of the mastoid. These tumors may erode from the mastoid into the ear canal simulating the clinical presentation of suppurative mastoiditis.

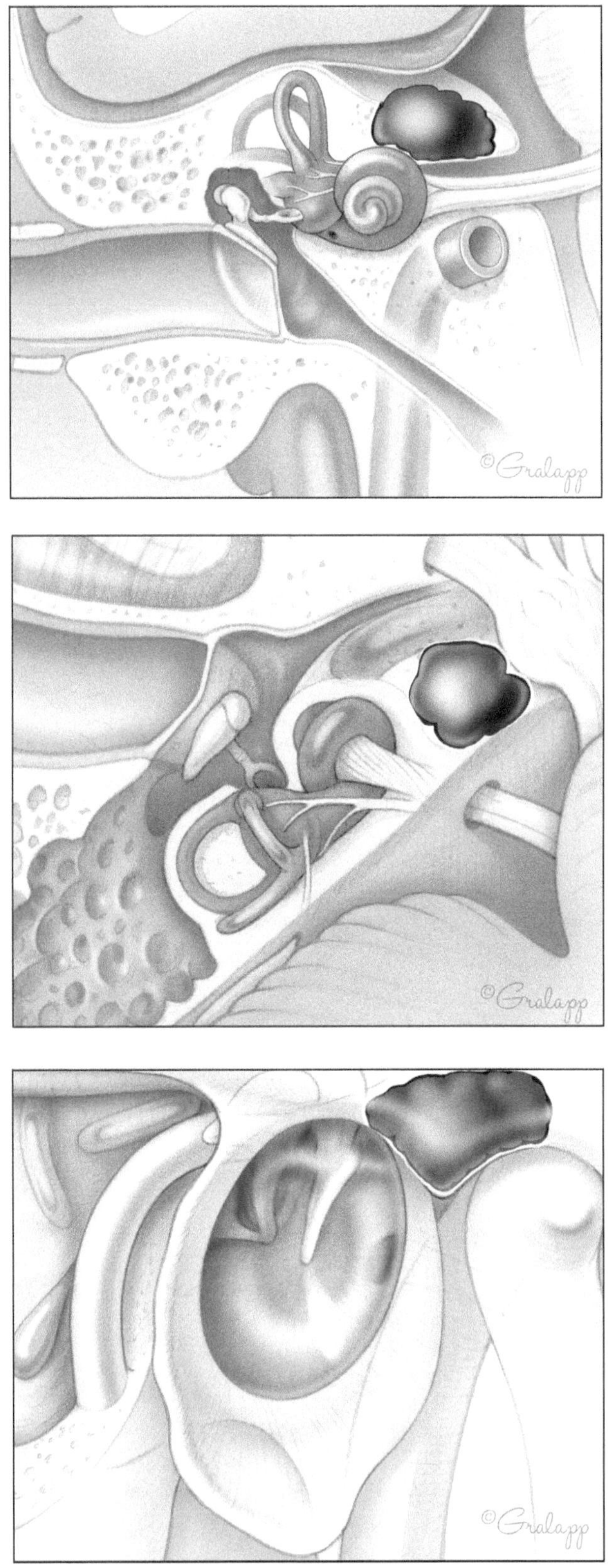

Fig. 1.55 Metastasis to the petrous apex. The marrow space of the petrous apex is the most frequent location for metastases within the temporal bone (e.g., breast, lung, and prostate cancers).

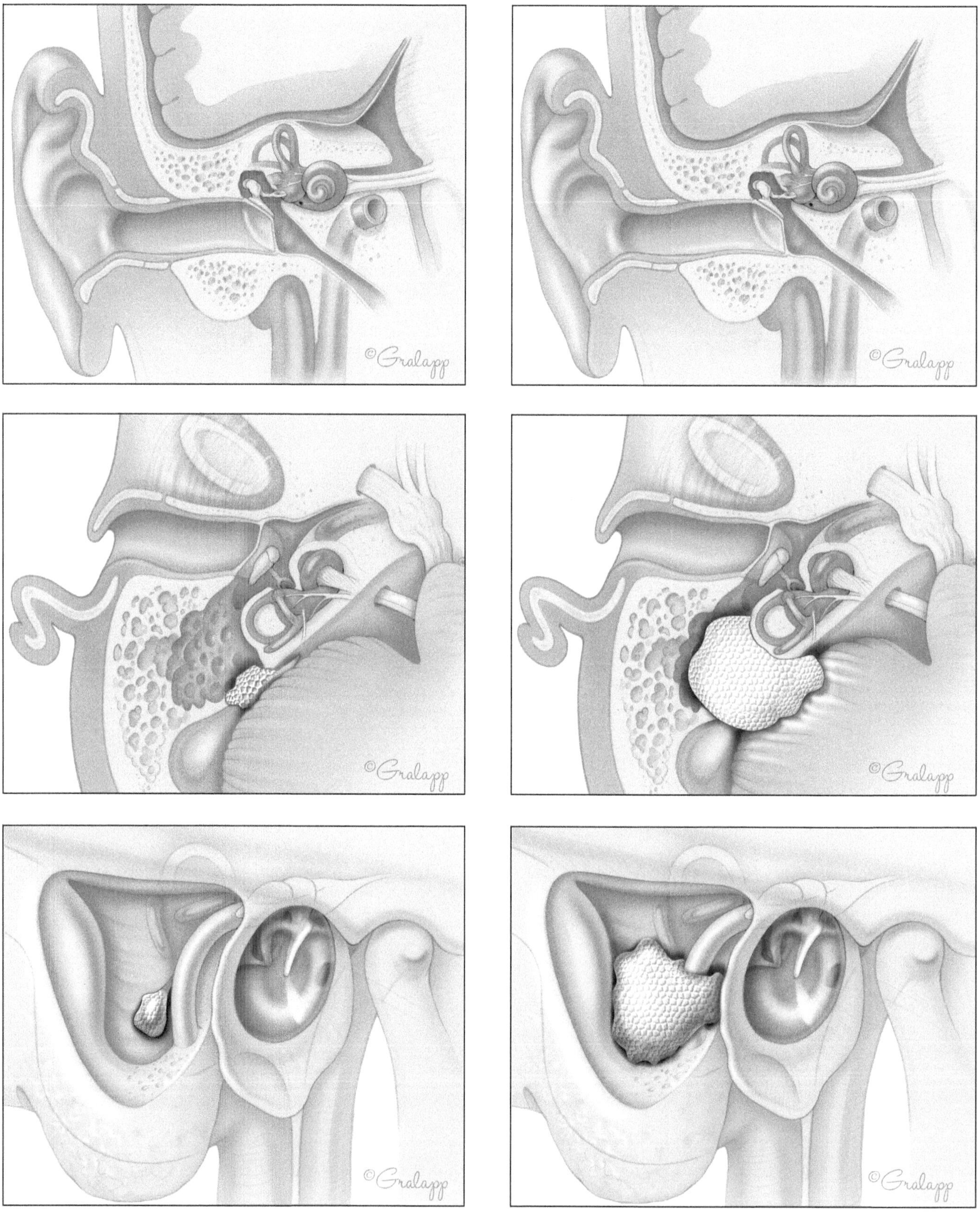

Fig. 1.56 An early papillary adenomatous lesion arising from the rugose portion of the endolymphatic sac (*left*). These tumors may grow laterally into the mastoid, posteriorly into the posterior cranial fossa, or along the vestibular aqueduct to the inner ear. (*Right*) An advanced endolymphatic sac tumor with extensive mastoid involvement, erosion of the semicircular canals, and spread into the posterior cranial fossa and indentation of the cerebellum. In von Hippel–Lindau syndrome, patients may have bilateral endolymphatic sac tumors.

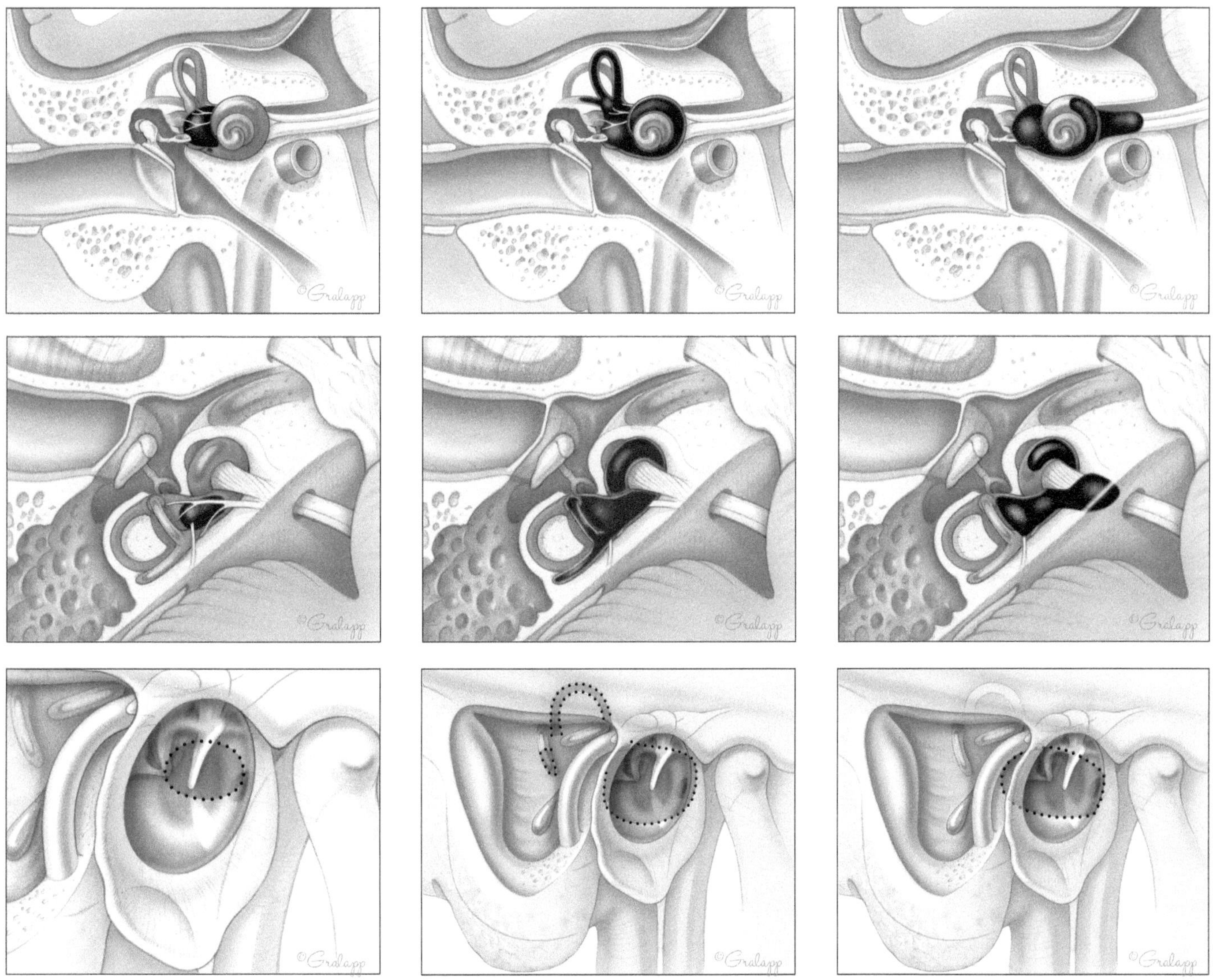

Fig. 1.57 Intralabyrinthine schwannoma of the vestibule spanning from the oval to round windows (a veritable "vestibular schwannoma") (*left*). (*Center*) An inner ear schwannoma with involvement of the posterior and superior semicircular canals lumens as well as the base turn of the cochlea. (*Right*) A schwannoma involving both the inner ear (vestibule and cochlea) and the fundus of the internal auditory canal. Most commonly, this represents a vestibular nerve tumor (acoustic neuroma) which has penetrated through the lateral terminus of canal.

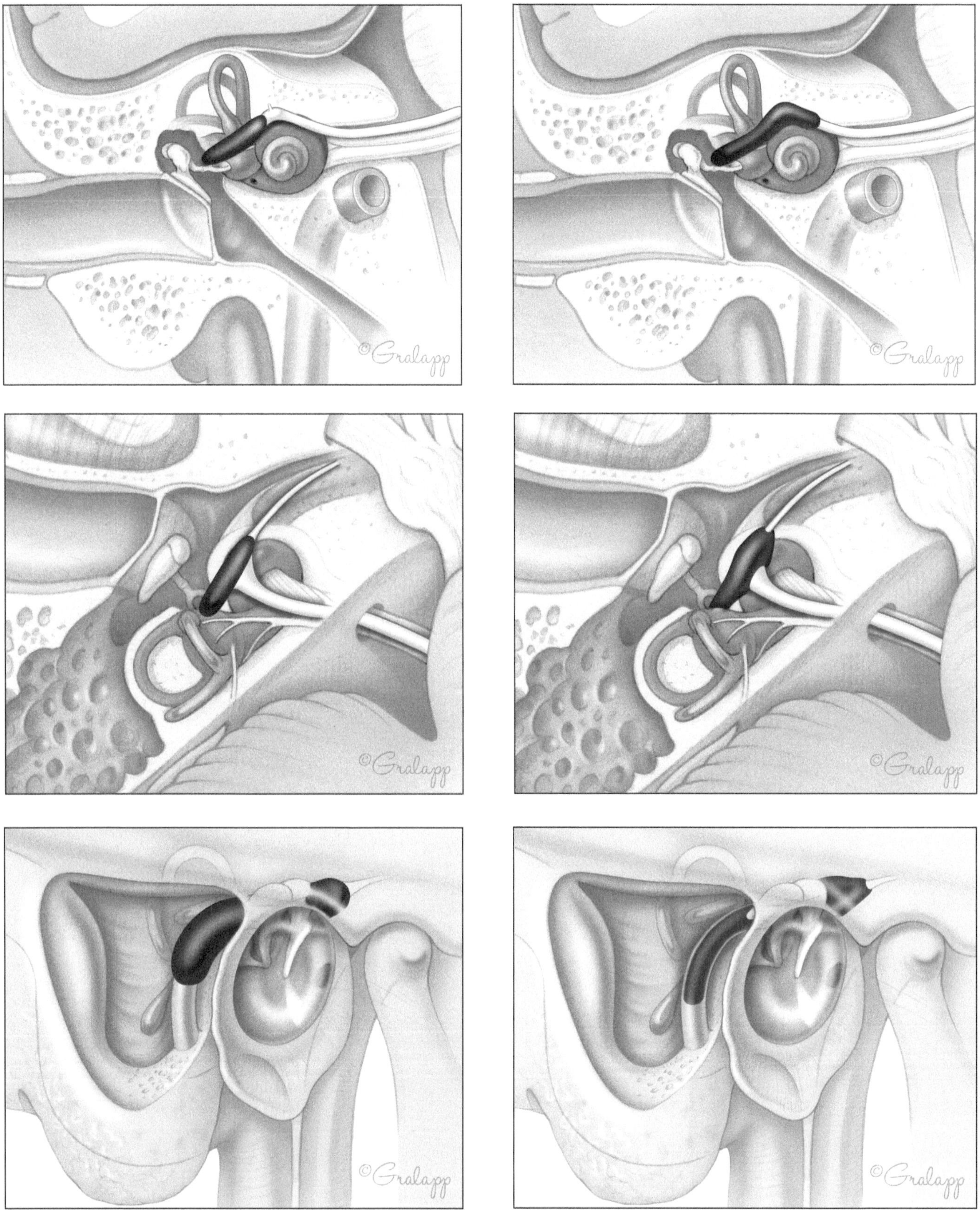

Fig. 1.58 Schwannoma of the facial nerve involving the labyrinthine, geniculate, tympanic, second genu, and upper mastoid segments of the nerve (*left*). The tumor lies entirely confined within the fallopian canal. Schwannoma of the tympanic segment of the facial nerve spanning from the second genu to the lateral aspect of the geniculate ganglion (*center*). The tumor is fusiform and largely conforms to the fallopian canal.

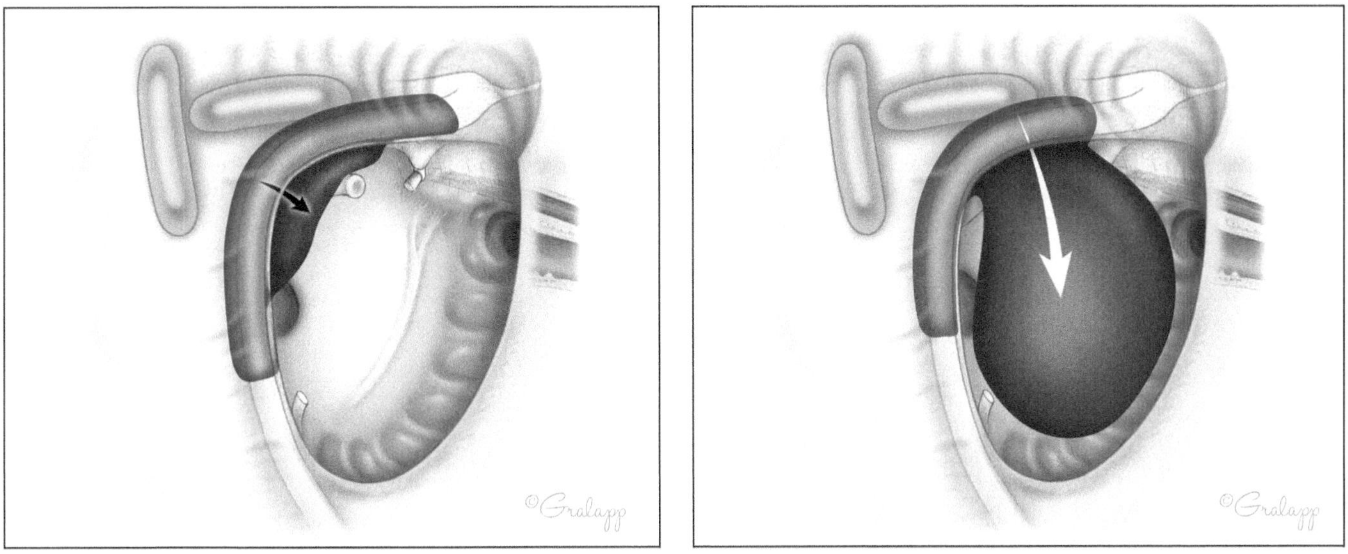

Fig. 1.59 Schwannoma of the tympanic segment of the facial nerve spanning from the second genu to the lateral aspect of the geniculate ganglion. An exophytic mass in the middle ear is present. Such tumors often present with conductive hearing loss accompanied by normal facial function. The tumor may be encountered unexpectedly during a tympanotomy for presumptive otosclerosis.

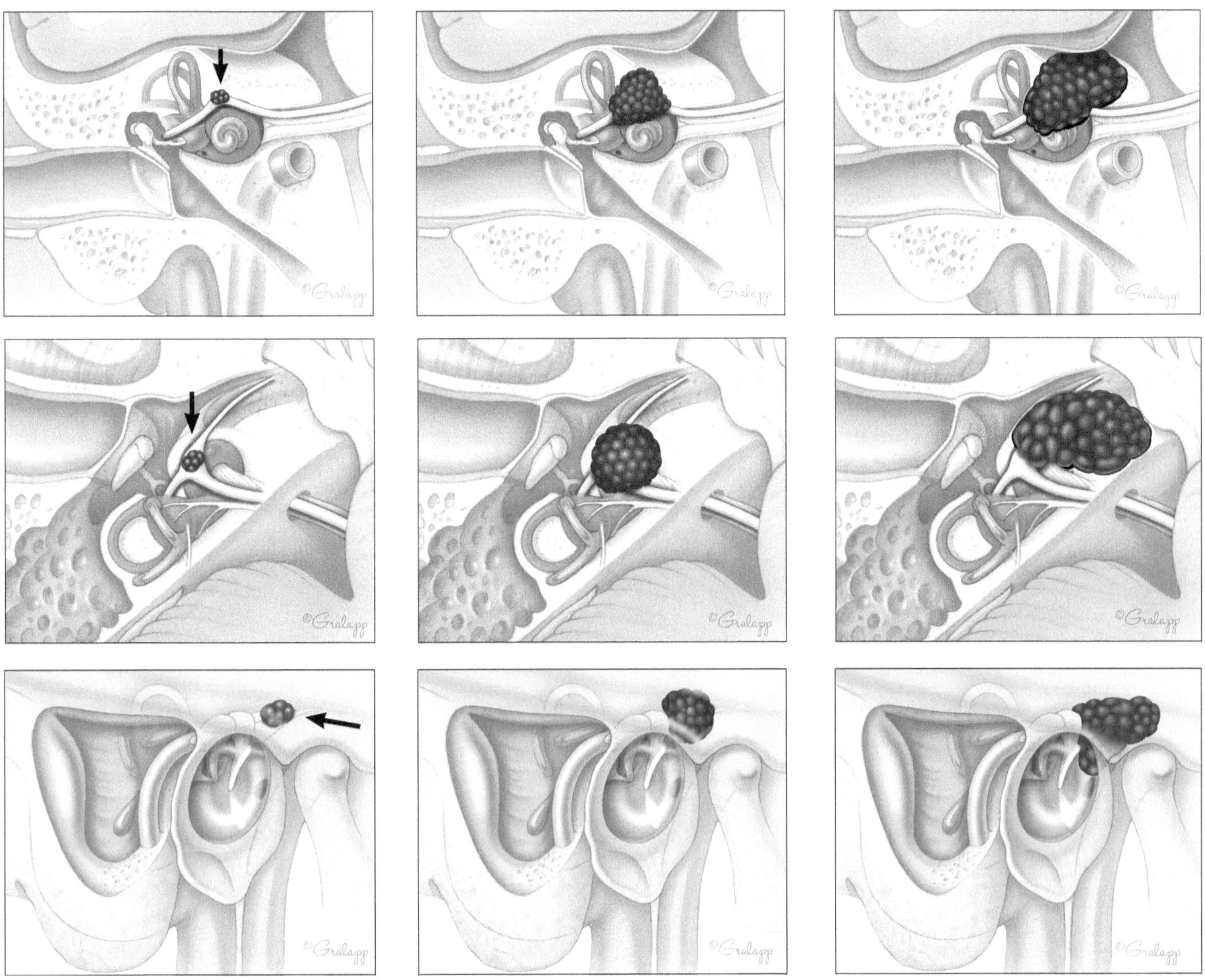

Fig. 1.60 Hemangioma of the geniculate ganglion. Small intraosseous hemangioma situated at the apex of the geniculate ganglion (*left*). Hemangioma involving the entire geniculate ganglion and proximal segment of the greater superficial petrosal nerve. (*Center*) The superior aspect of the cochlea is partially eroded. (*Right*) Geniculate region hemangioma with medially directed growth into the petrous apex. The cochlea is eroded from above.

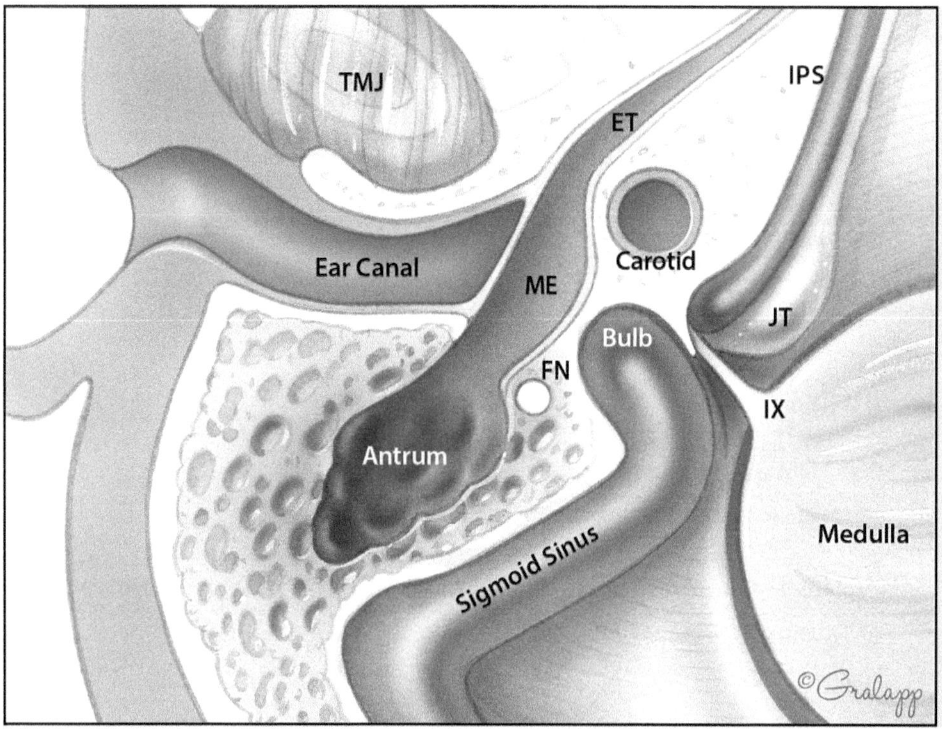

Fig. 1.61 Anatomy of the jugular foramen: axial perspective.

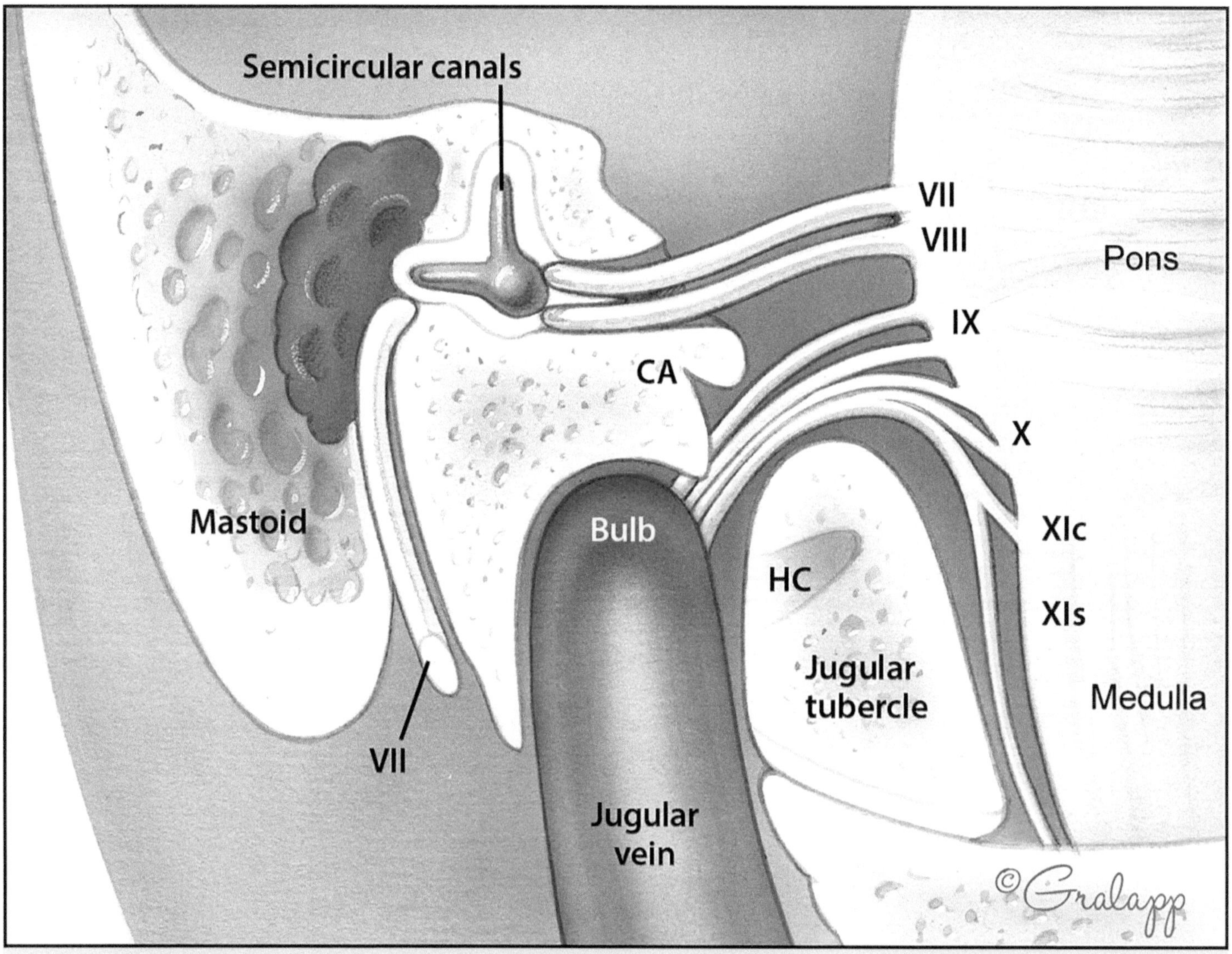

Fig. 1.62 Anatomy of the jugular foramen: coronal perspective.

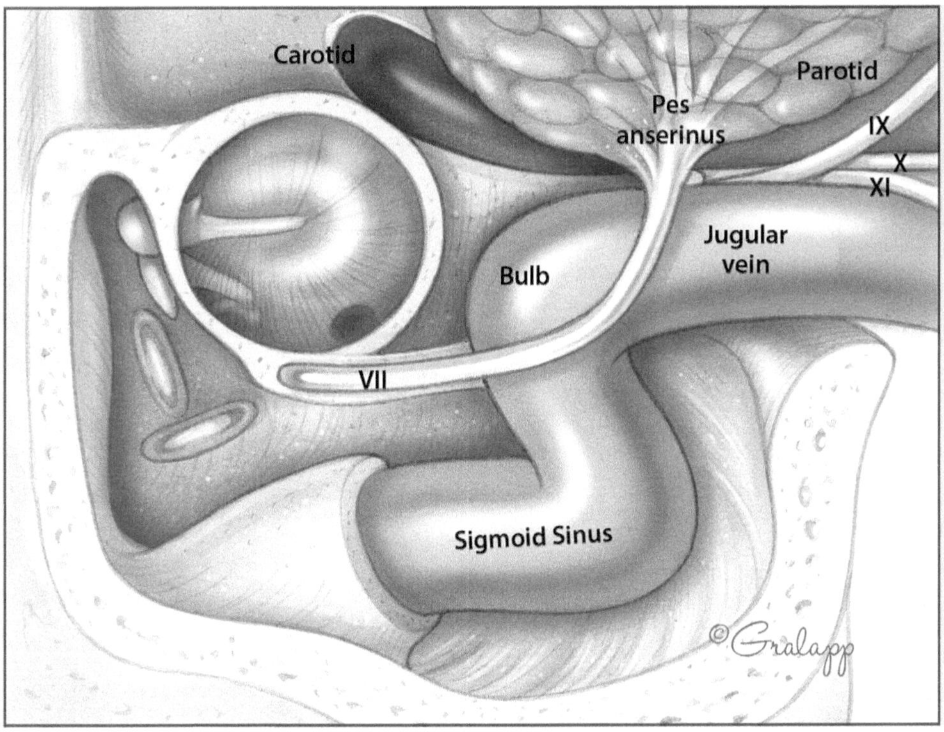

Fig. 1.63 Anatomy of the jugular foramen: lateral perspective.

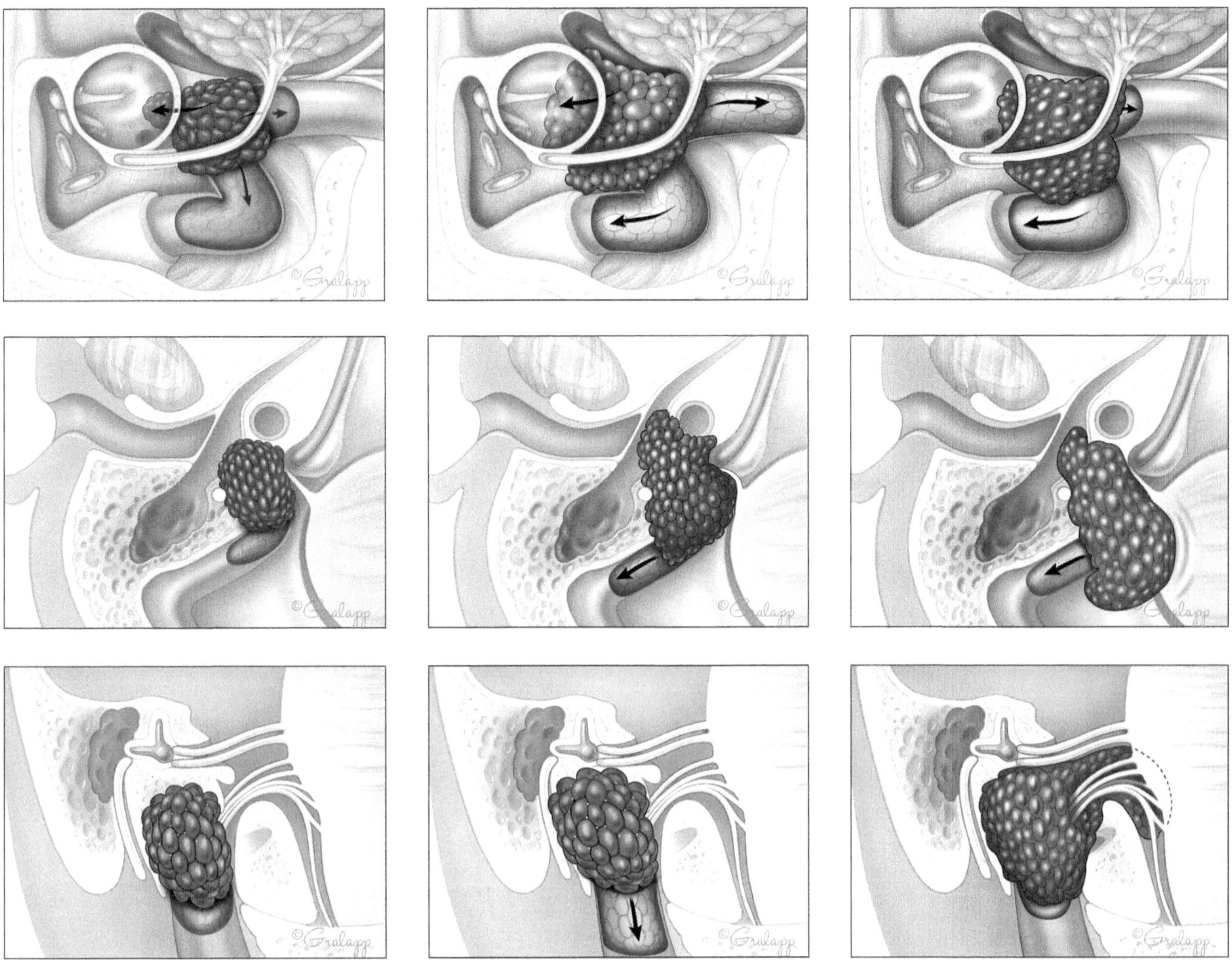

Fig. 1.64 Glomus jugulare tumor. Moderate-size glomus jugulare tumor with a typical extension into the hypotympanum (*left*). The tumor also extends proximally within the lumen of the sigmoid sinus and distally into the upper portion of the jugular vein. (*Center*) More extensive glomus jugulare tumor with erosion of both carotid and fallopian canals. (*Right*) Glomus jugulare tumor with extension into the posterior cranial fossa and upward erosion into the floor of the internal auditory canal.

2 Fundamentals of Ear Surgery

Robert K. Jackler

2.1 Introduction to Ear Surgery

In ear microsurgical training, too little attention is paid to the fundamentals. As a result, even senior-level trainees often struggle with hand stability and suffer bodily contortions due to awkward angles of exposure. The secret of achieving stability and minute control in delicate procedures is less about native talent than it is a learned skill of proper hand, body, and patient positioning. It should be emphasized that many ear microsurgical procedures require deft coordination of both hands working in concert. Surgeons in training tend to rapidly become facile with their dominant hand, but facility with the nondominant hand and coordination between hands requires much practice.

As ear surgeons tend to sit throughout microsurgical procedures, use of proper posture is important as is use of a chair with adequate lumbar support. Far too many otologists pay too little attention to their own ergonomics and suffer chronic back pain as a result. To reduce the incidence of occupational injury, it is recommended that ergonomic training be incorporated in training for the entire surgical team. Otologists should also be cautious about protection from noise exposure emanating from high-powered drill systems.

Further Reading

1. Bolduc-Bégin J, Prince F, Christopoulos A, Ayad T. Work-related musculoskeletal symptoms amongst otolaryngologists and head and neck surgeons in Canada. Eur Arch Otorhinolaryngol 2018;275(1):261–267 PubMed
2. Coskun BU, Cinar U, Seven H, Ugur S, Dadas B. The effects of the incision types in myringoplasty operations on cosmesis. Eur Arch Otorhinolaryngol 2006;263(9):820–822 PubMed
3. Ho TT, Hamill CS, Sykes KJ, Kraft SM. Work-related musculoskeletal symptoms among otolaryngologists by subspecialty: A national survey. Laryngoscope 2018;128(3):632–640 PubMed
4. Inwood JL, Wallace HC, Clarke SE. Endaural or postaural incision for myringoplasty: does it make a difference to the patient? Clin Otolaryngol Allied Sci 2003;28(5):396–398 PubMed
5. Khan I, Mohamad S, Ansari S, Iyer A. Are head bandages really required after middle-ear surgery? A systematic review. J Laryngol Otol 2015;129(8):740–743 PubMed
6. Montague P, Bennett D, Kellermeyer B. How was your otology training? A survey of recent otolaryngology residents. Otol Neurotol 2017;38(10):1535–1539 PubMed
7. Mudry A. The history of the microscope for use in ear surgery. Am J Otol 2000;21(6):877–886 PubMed
8. Vaisbuch Y, Alyono JC, Kandathil C, Wu SH, Fitzgerald MB, Jackler RK. Occupational noise exposure and risk for noise-induced hearing loss due to temporal bone drilling. Otol Neurotol 2018;39(6):693–699 PubMed
9. Vaisbuch Y, Alyono JC, Kandathil C, Wu SH, Fitzgerald MB, Jackler RK. Occupational Noise Exposure and Risk for Noise-Induced Hearing Loss Due to Temporal Bone Drilling. Otol Neurotol 2018;39:693–699
10. Vijendren A, Yung M, Sanchez J, Duffield K. Occupational musculoskeletal pain amongst ENT surgeons - are we looking at the tip of an iceberg? J Laryngol Otol 2016;130(5):490–496 PubMed

2.2 Patient Positioning

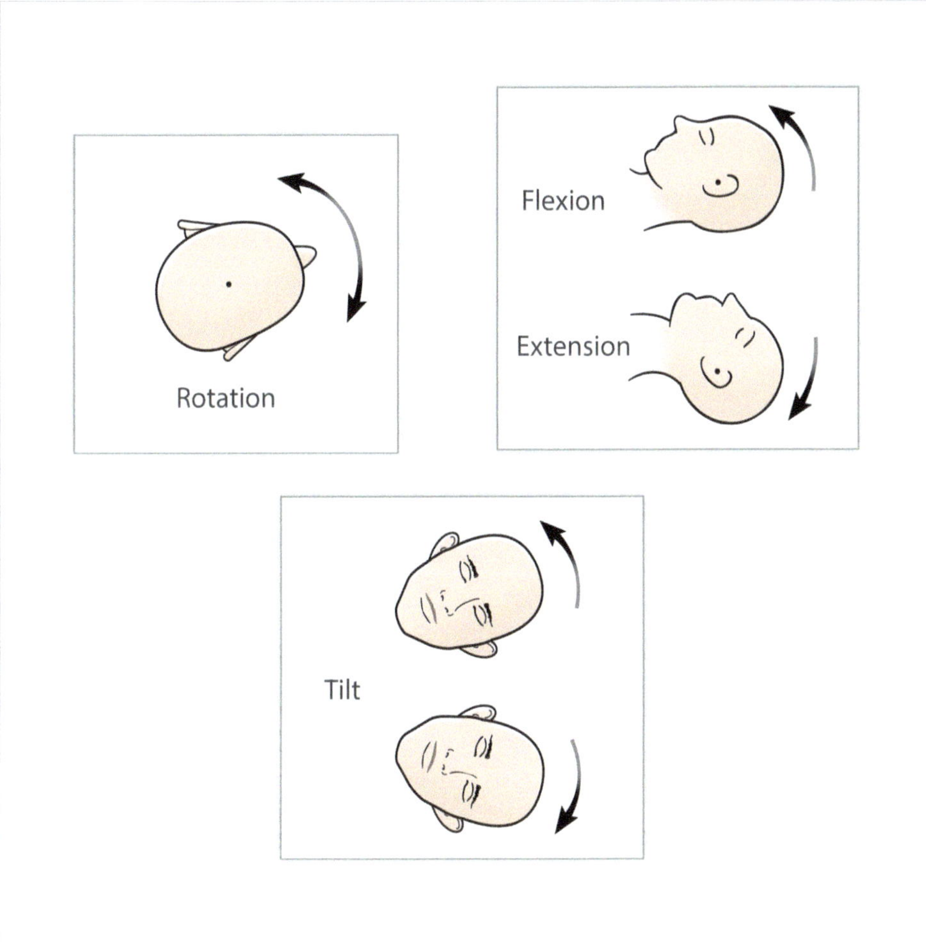

Fig. 2.1 The three variables for positioning of the head in ear microsurgery: rotation, tilt, and flexion–extension.

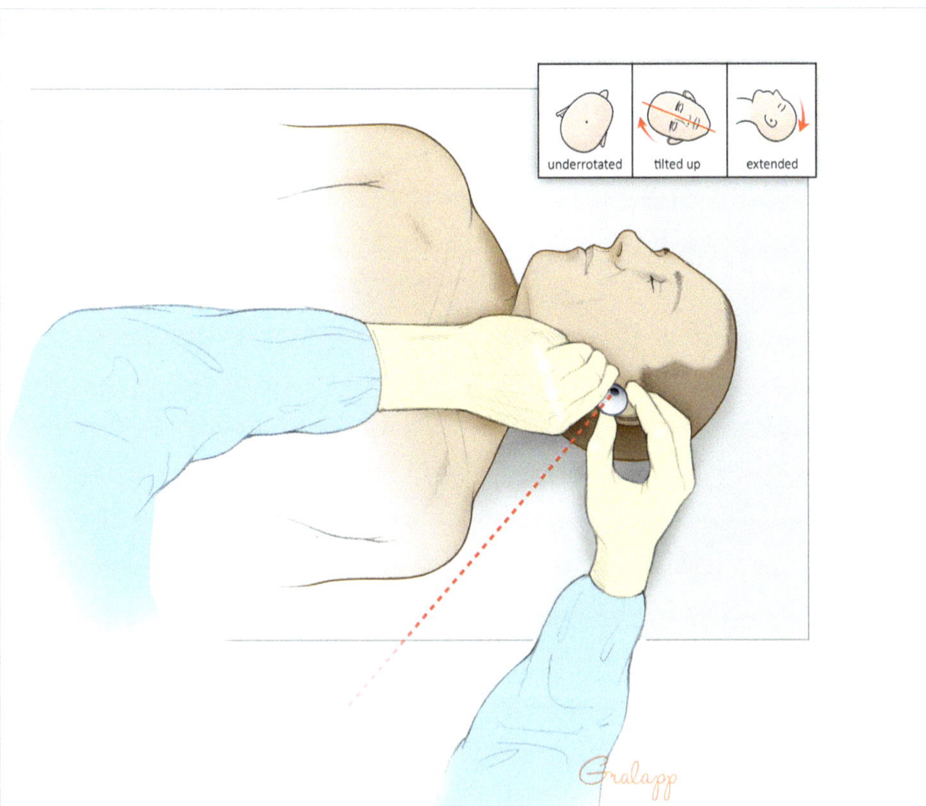

Fig. 2.2 Incorrect positioning with the head under rotated, extended, and tilted. This forces the surgeon to operate at an awkward angle, in the case depicted with the arm on the patient's thorax.

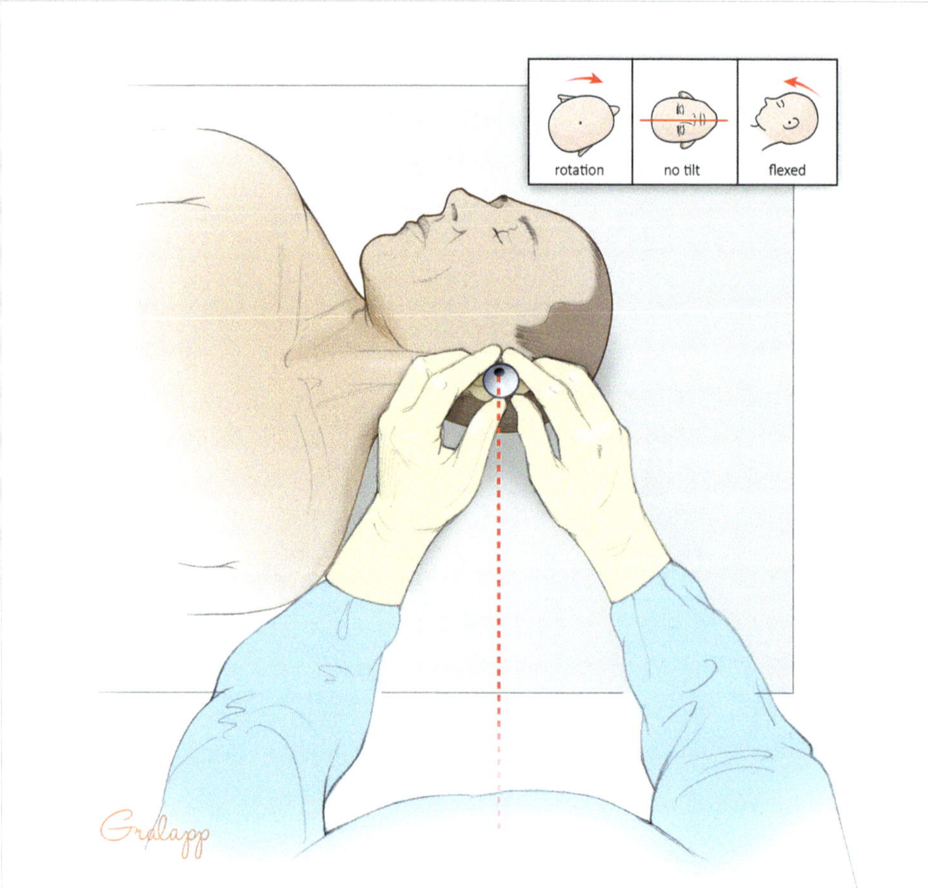

Fig. 2.3 Optimal positioning with the head rotated, flexed, and not tilted.

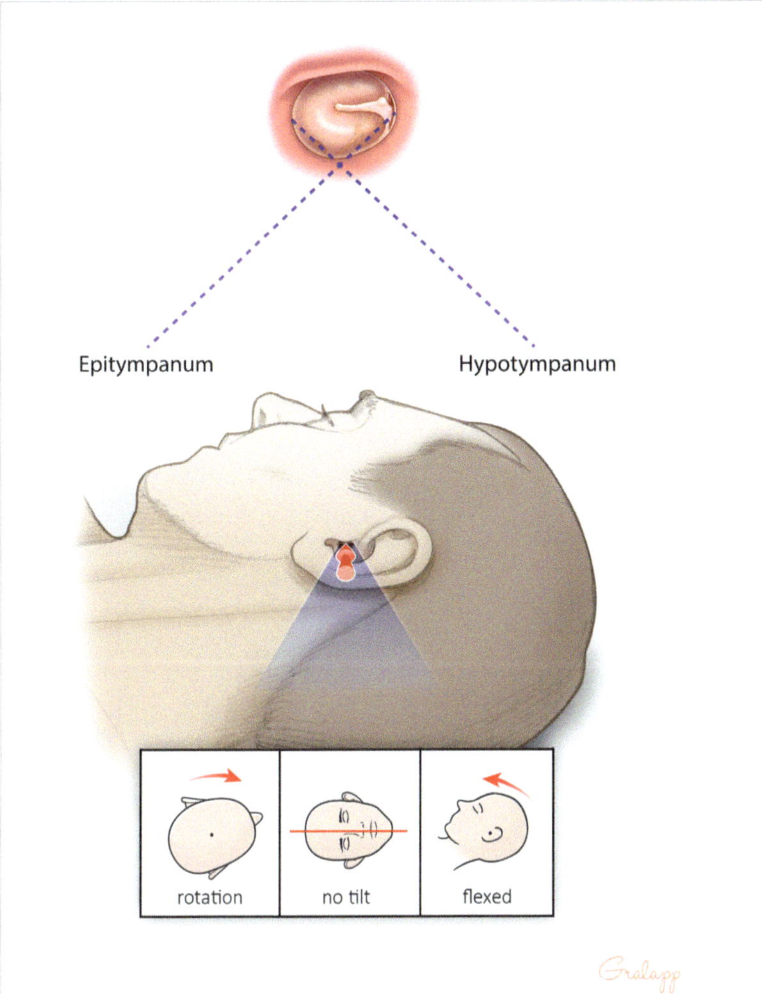

Fig. 2.4 When the patient is positioned well, the surgeon should be able to gaze from the epitympanum to hypotympanum. Suboptimal patient positioning contributes to neck and lower back problems endemic among otologic surgeons.

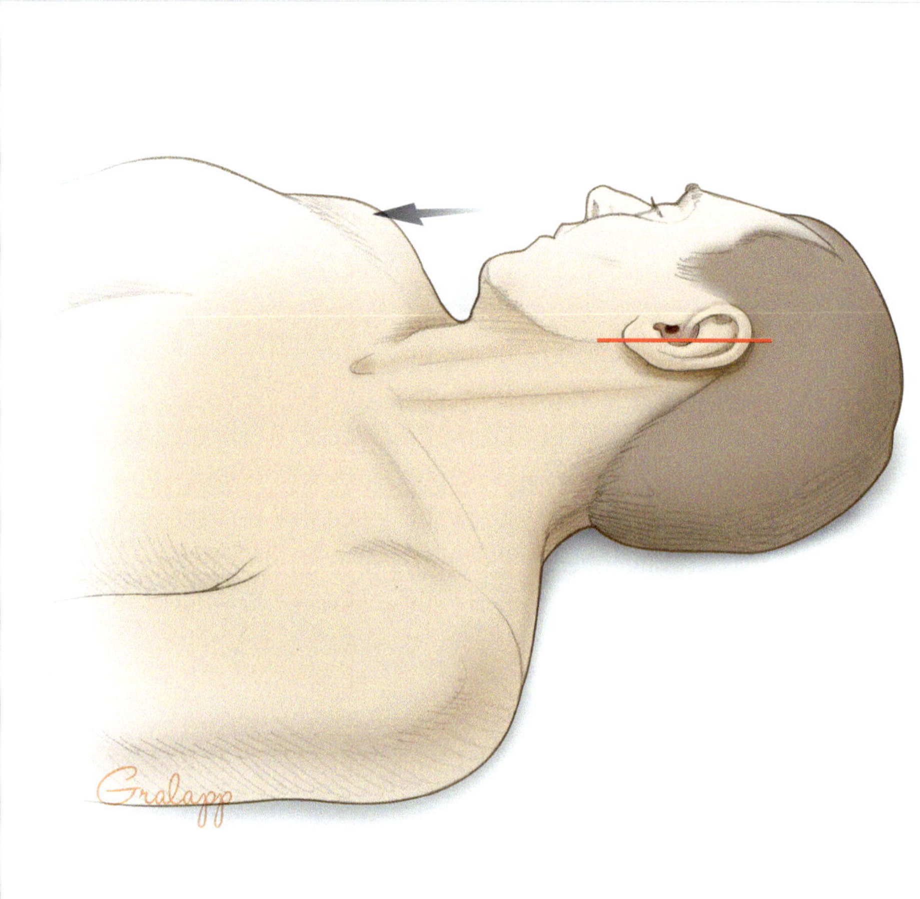

Fig. 2.5 Downwardly deflecting the opposite shoulder helps achieve rotation and flexion needed for optimal positioning.

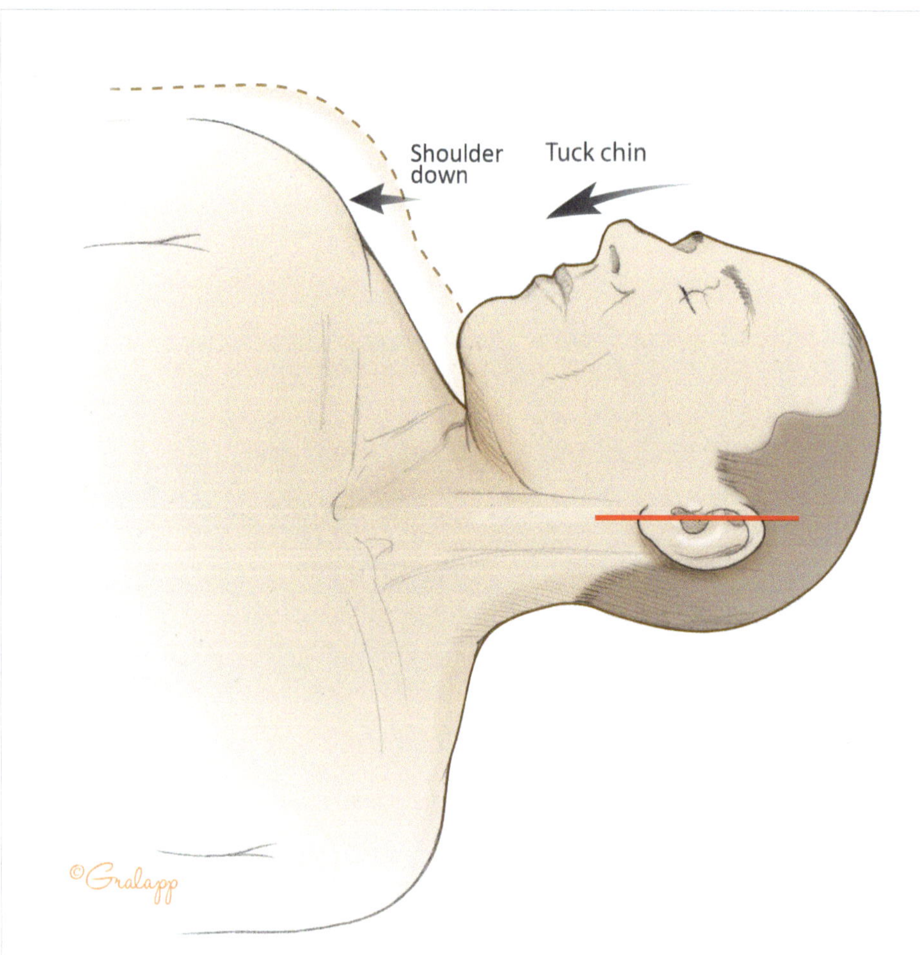

Fig. 2.6 Correct position has head rotated and head flexed with opposite shoulder deflected downward.

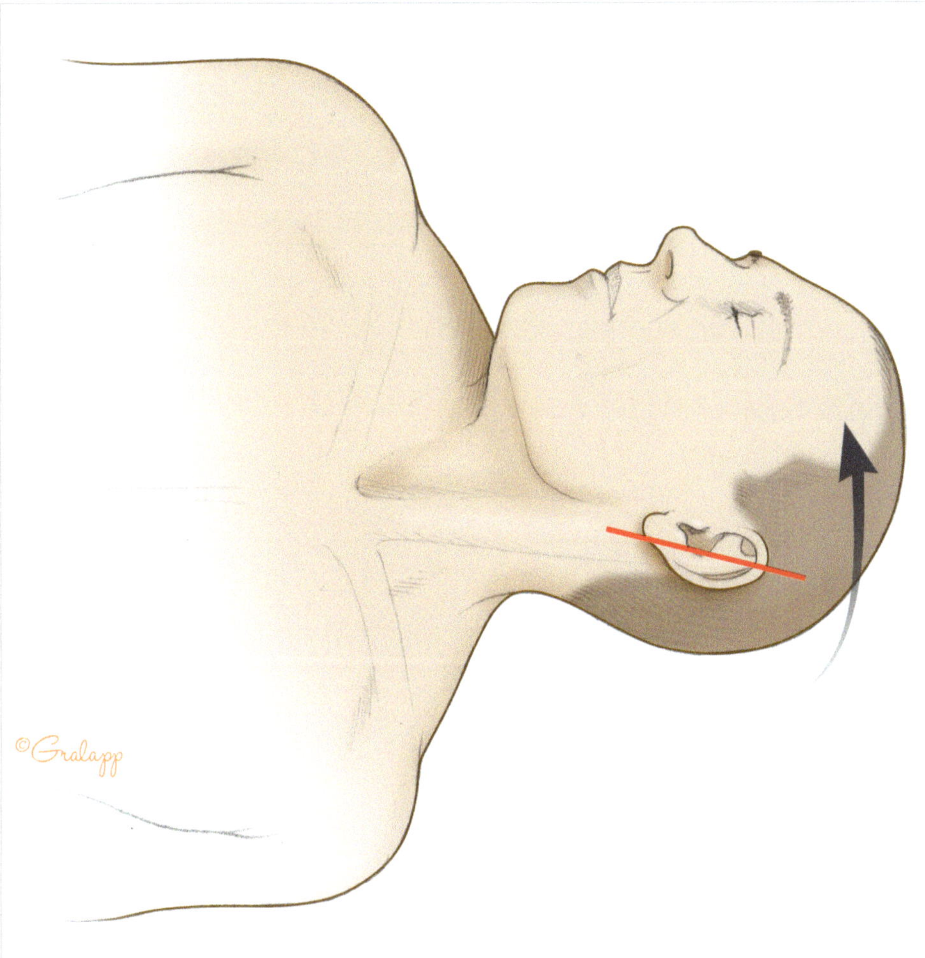

Fig. 2.7 When the opposite shoulder is not pushed down, the head tends to be under-rotated and the neck extended.

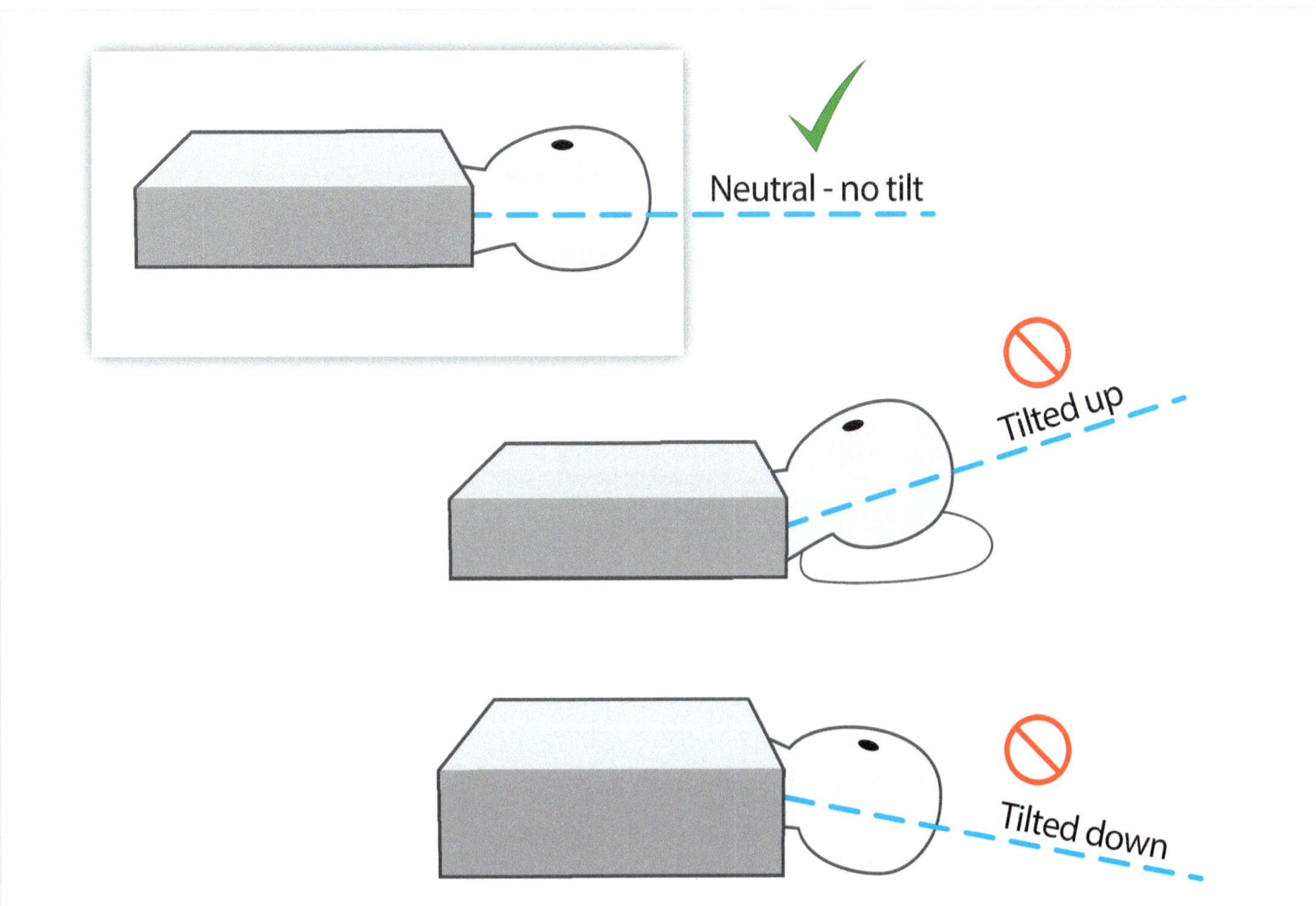

Fig. 2.8 In most ear microsurgery, the head is rotated and flexed, but with the head neutral neither tilted up nor down.

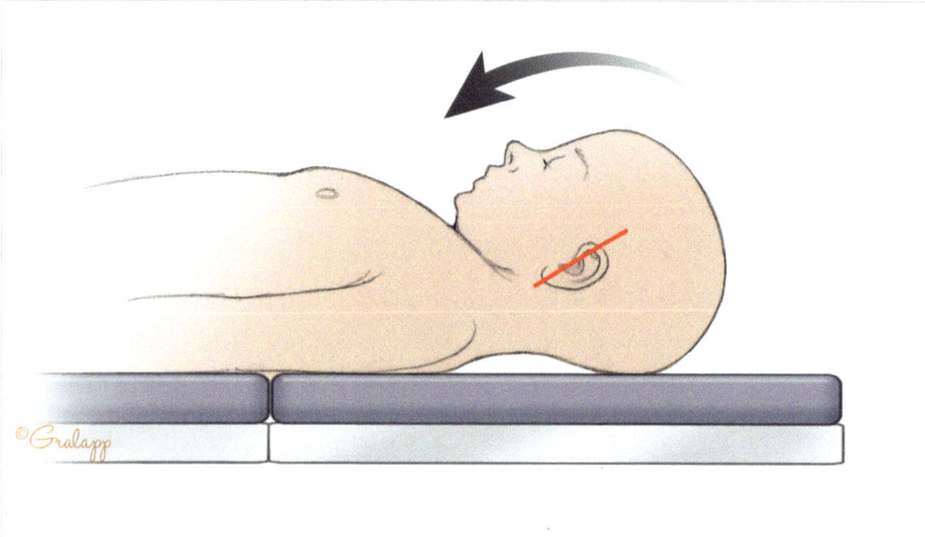

Fig. 2.9 In a child, the head is proportionally larger than the body. This leads to a flexed position.

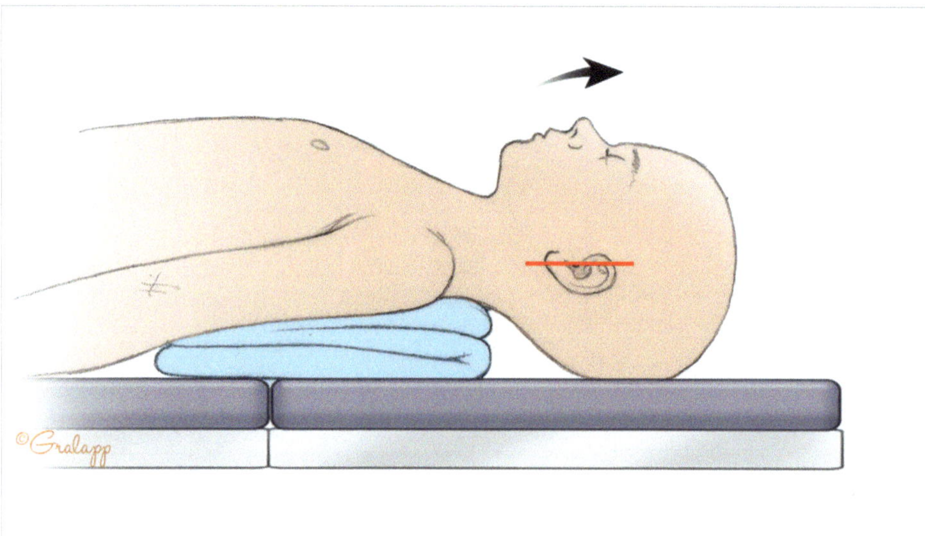

Fig. 2.10 Towels placed under the back can achieve a neutral position.

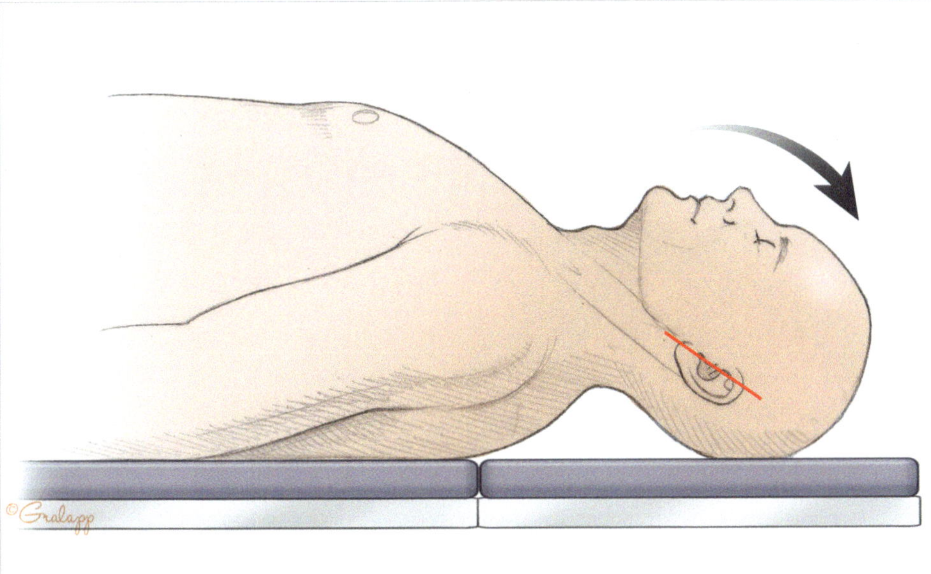

Fig. 2.11 In a barrel-chested adult, the body is proportionally larger than the head.

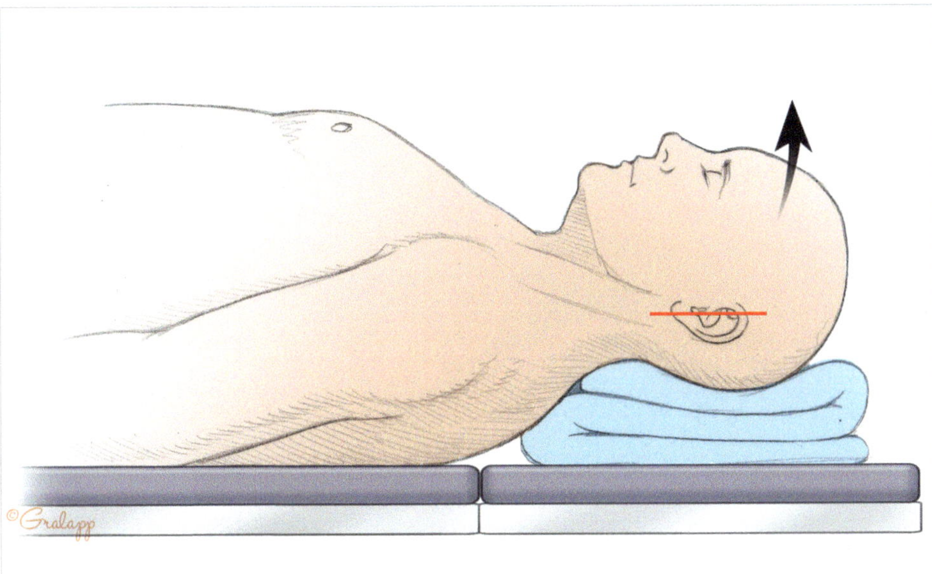

Fig. 2.12 Towels placed under the head can achieve a neutral position.

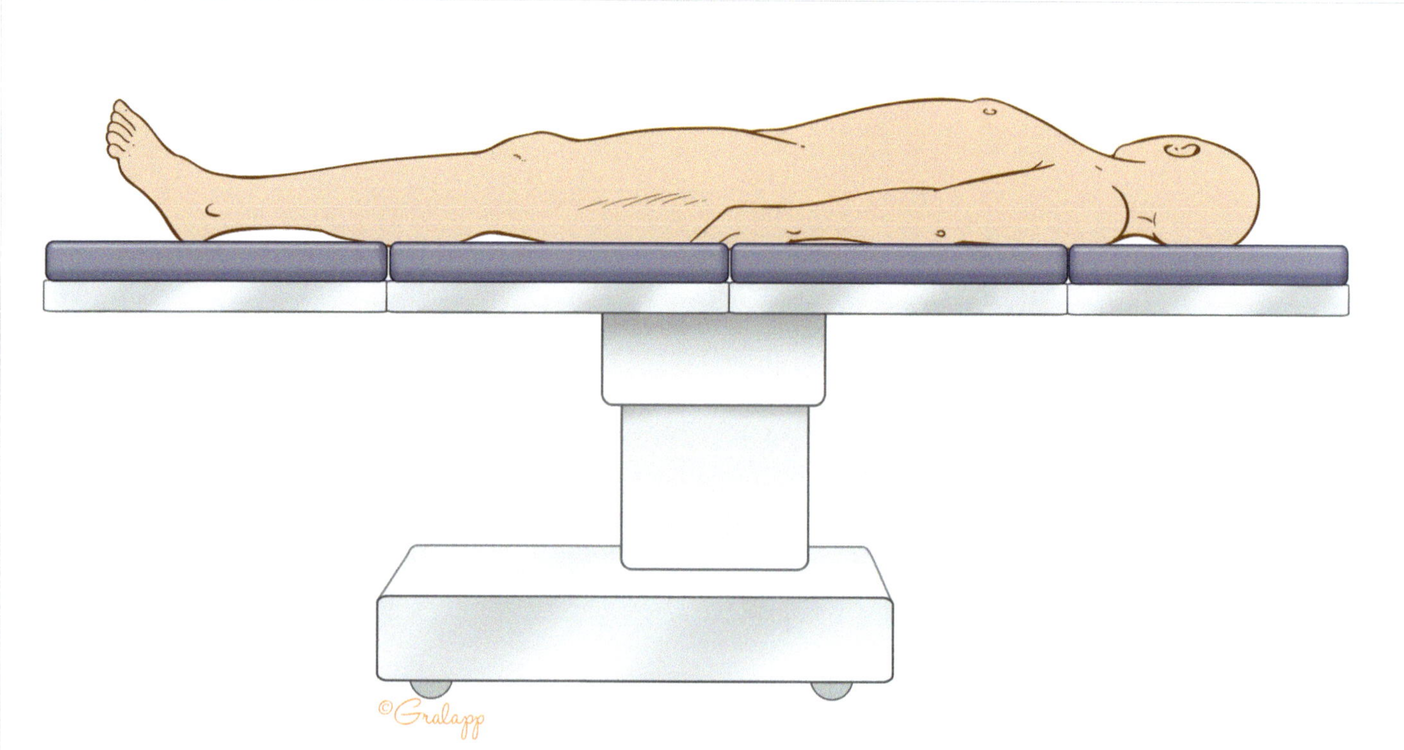

Fig. 2.13 Table positioning for stapes surgery to optimally view the posterior superior quadrant of the middle ear. This is the starting point.

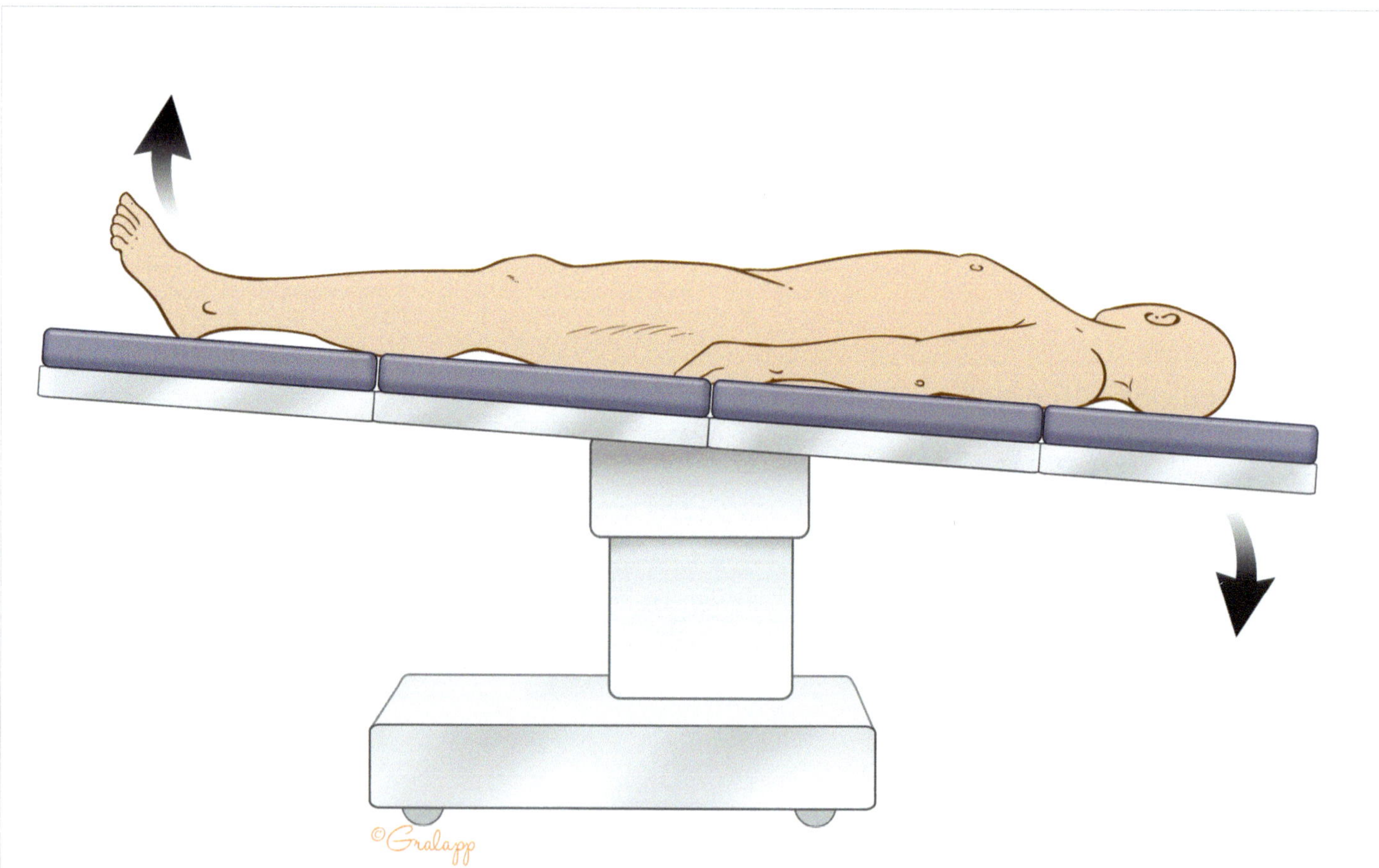

Fig. 2.14 Table positioning for stapes surgery: slight Trendelenburg (head down).

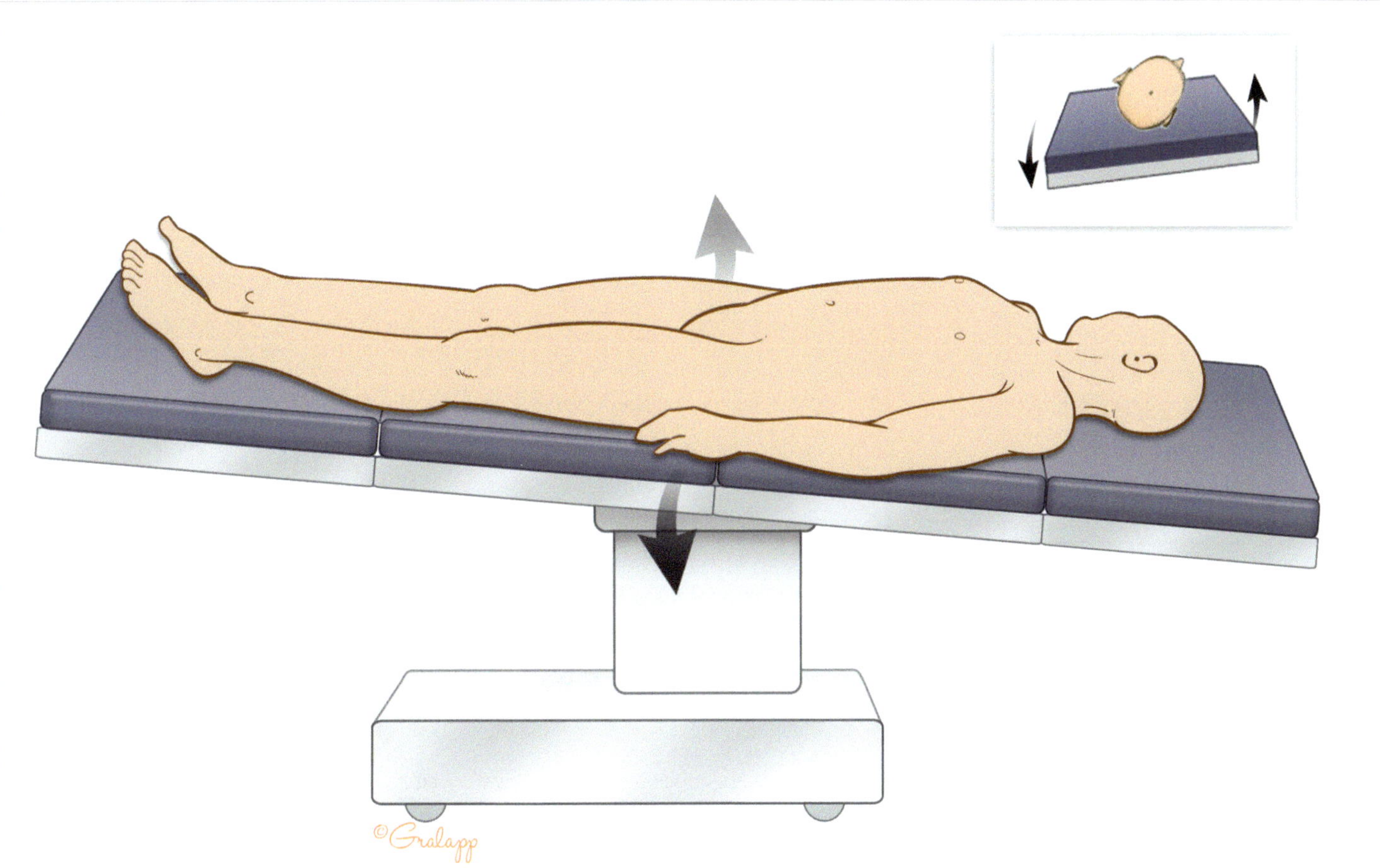

Fig. 2.15 Table positioning for stapes surgery: slight rotation toward the surgeon to optimize angle to the posterior–superior quadrant.

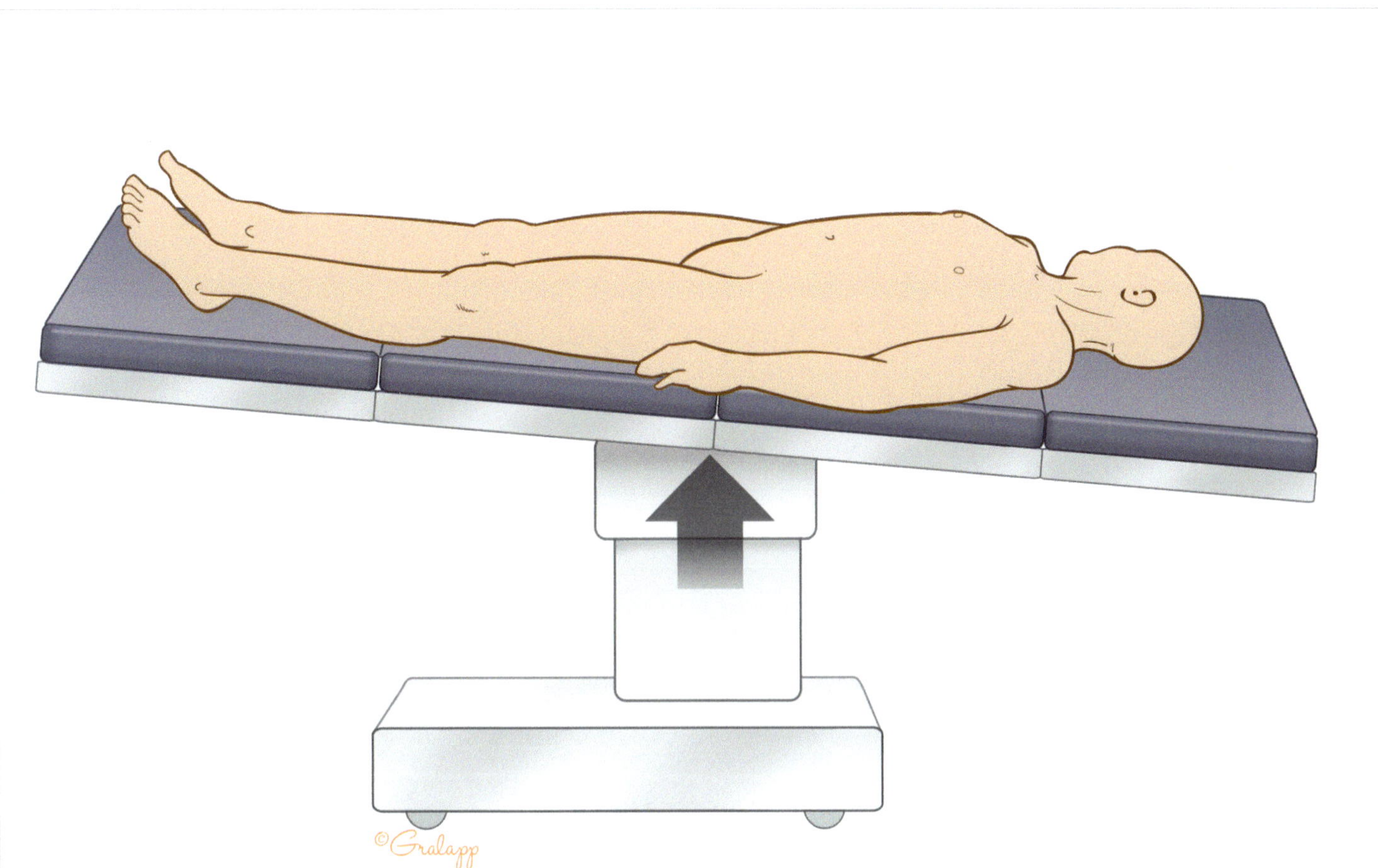

Fig. 2.16 Last step in table positioning for stapes surgery is raising the bed to allow microsurgery at a comfortable height for the surgeon.

2.3 Microinstrument Hand Positioning

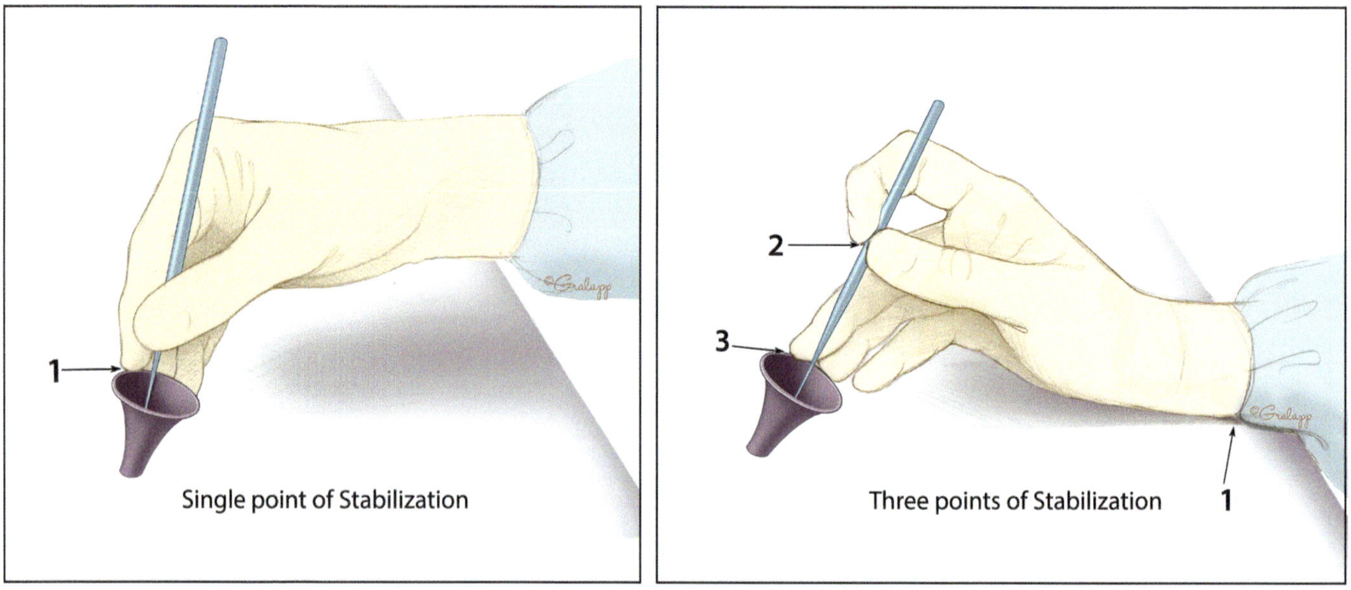

Fig. 2.17 Incorrect hand position for ear microsurgery, which is less stable and limits visibility. The correct hand position has three-point stabilization.

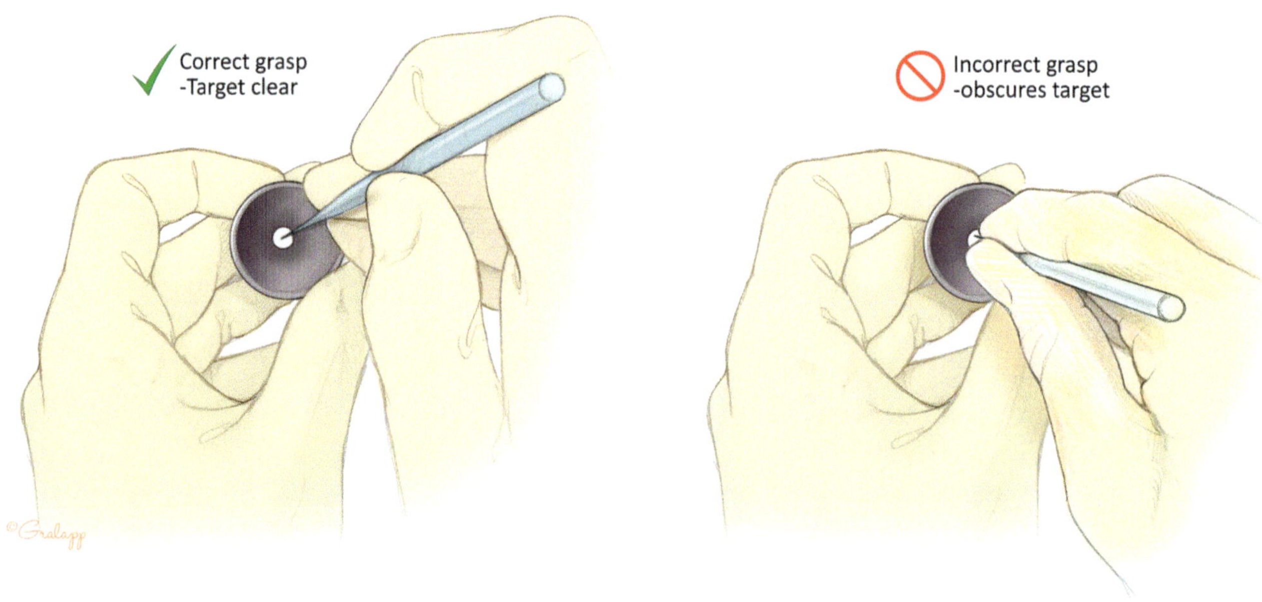

Fig. 2.18 Correct hand position enables both greater stability and two eyed visualization.

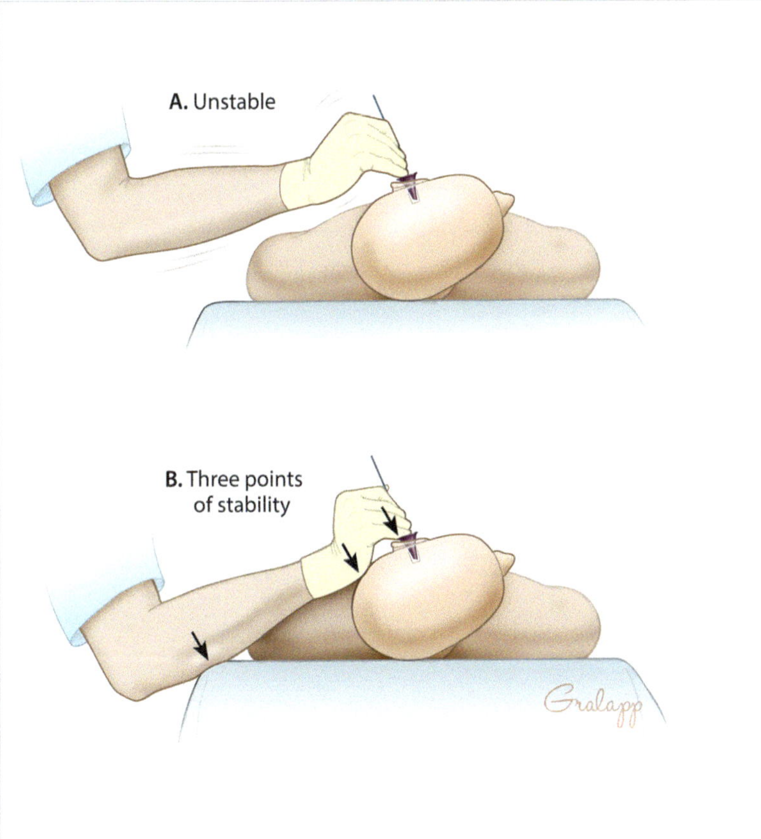

Fig. 2.19 Correct arm and hand position has multiple points of stabilization. Without stabilization of the forearm and wrist ("operating from the elbow"), maintaining steady control of the tip of a microsurgical instrument is very difficult.

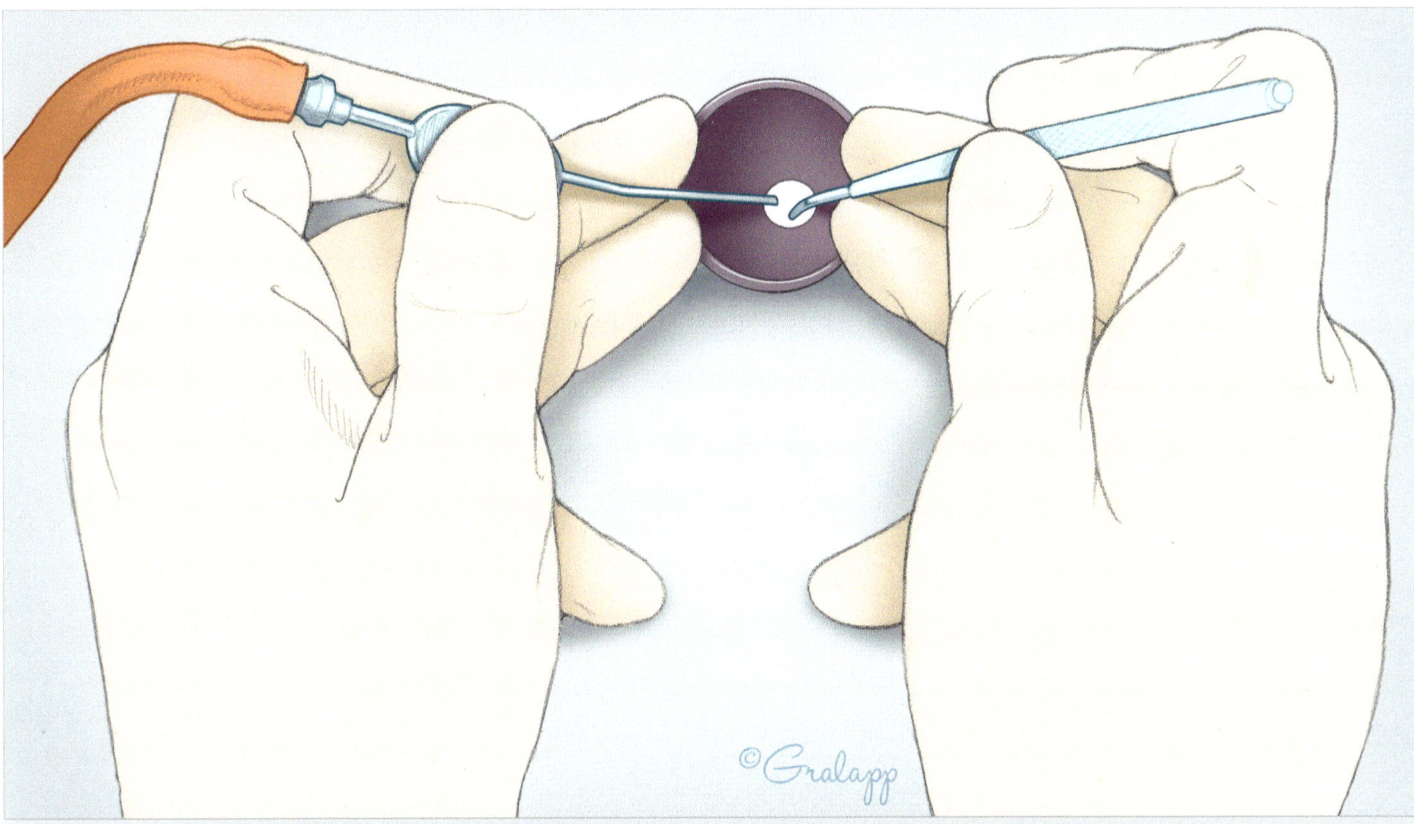

Fig. 2.20 Placement of the surgeon's hands during transcanal microsurgery. The third and fourth fingers of each hand stabilize the speculum. Note that the microinstrument (right hand) and suction (left hand) are held in a manner to both optimize stability and to enable binocular viewing. Some surgeons use a speculum holder to enhance stability, but it is best for all ear surgeons to be trained without use of a holder as such devices may not be available in all settings.

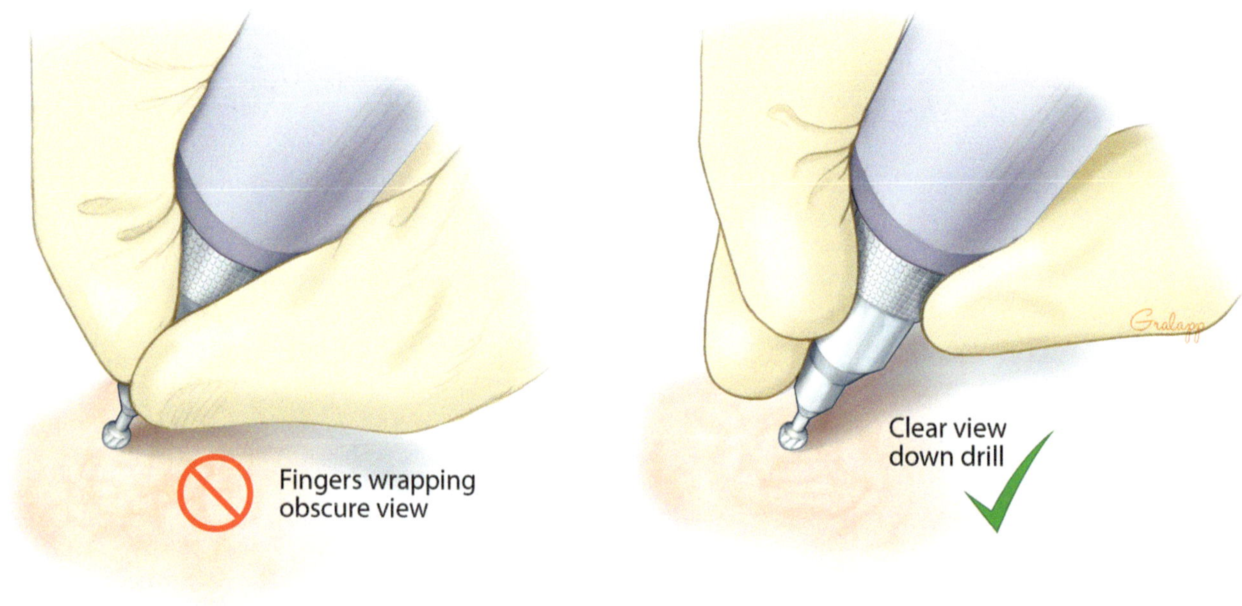

Fig. 2.21 The proper holding of a drill enables binocular visualization.

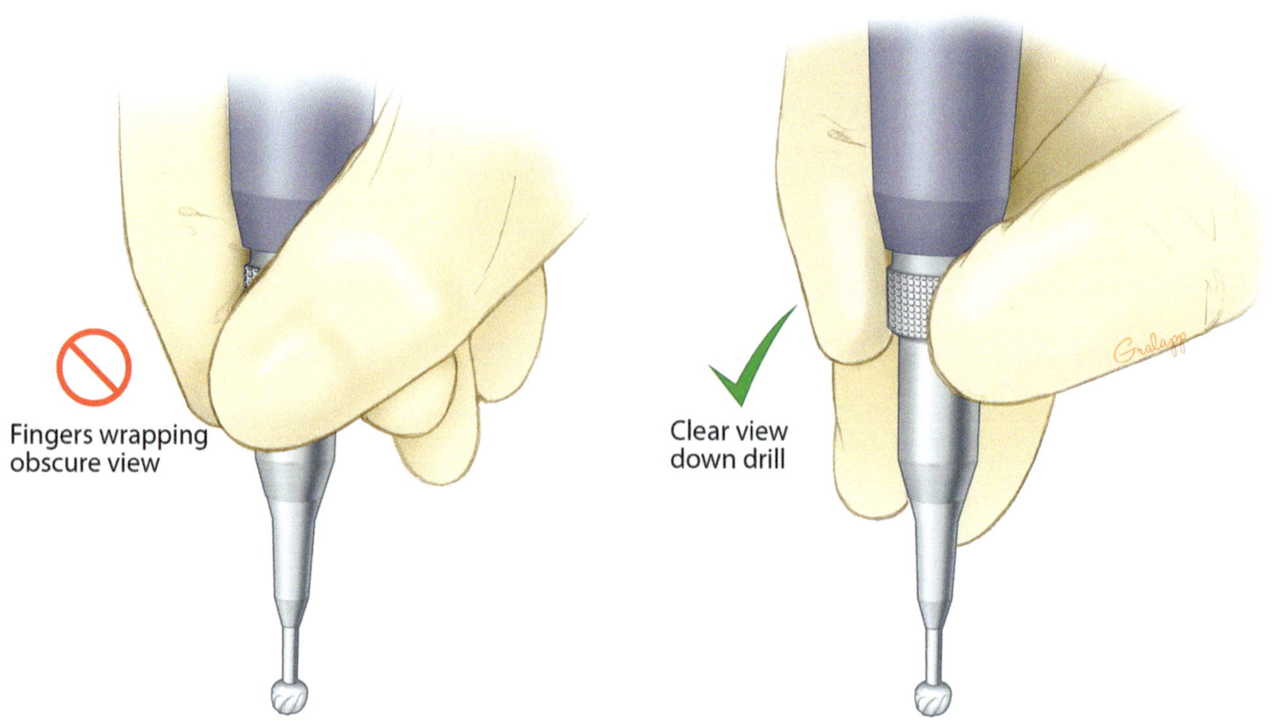

Fig. 2.22 Note that gripping the drill at two points is more stable and also improves visibility down the shaft.

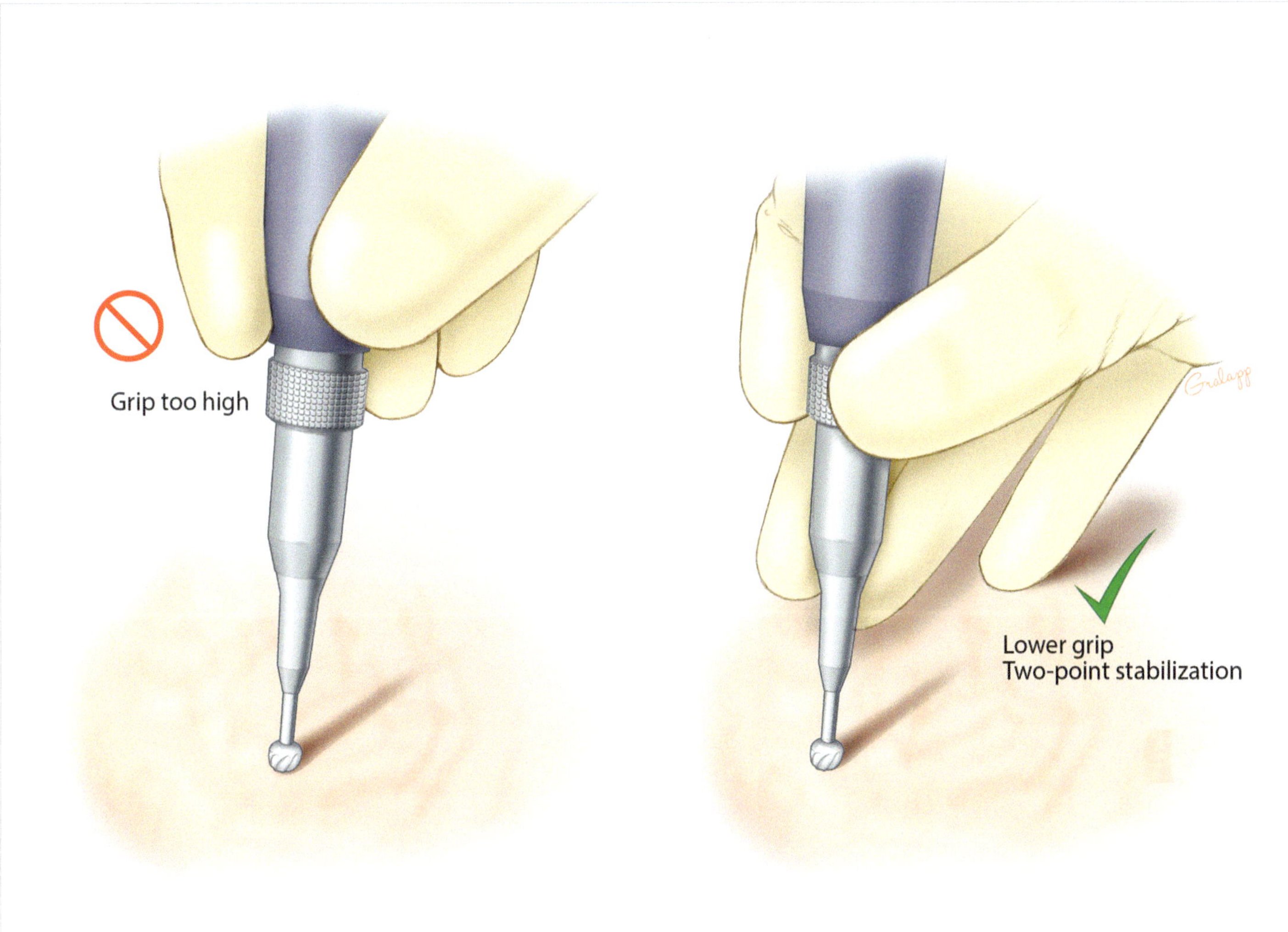

Fig. 2.23 Gripping the drill too far up the shaft reduces control of the burr.

2.4 Ergonomics

Yona Vaisbuch

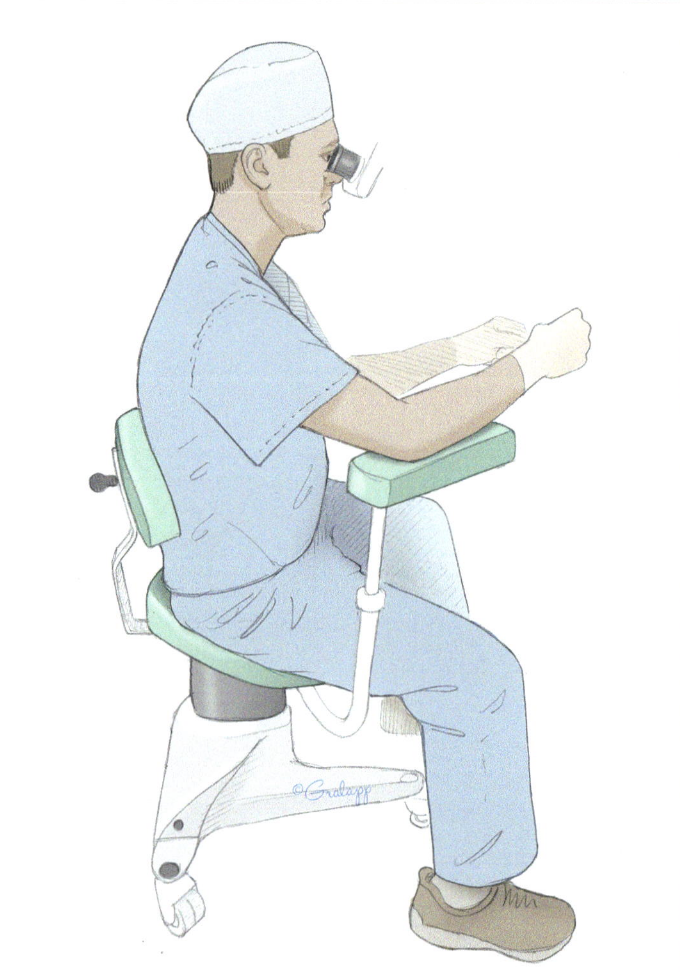

Fig. 2.24 A sizable fraction of ear microsurgeons develop back problems over time. This can be mitigated by using proper posture during microsurgery. This involves upright posture and good lumbar support as shown here. Many surgeons use rests to enhance stability and alleviate arm fatigue.

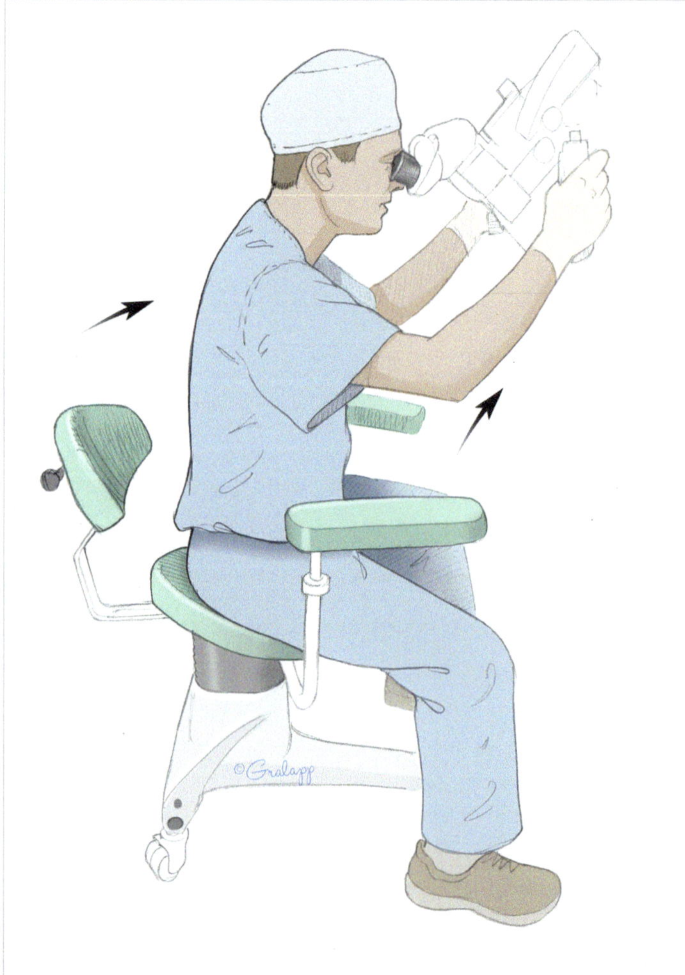

Fig. 2.25 Forward leaning posture lacking in lumbar support puts stress on the lower back.

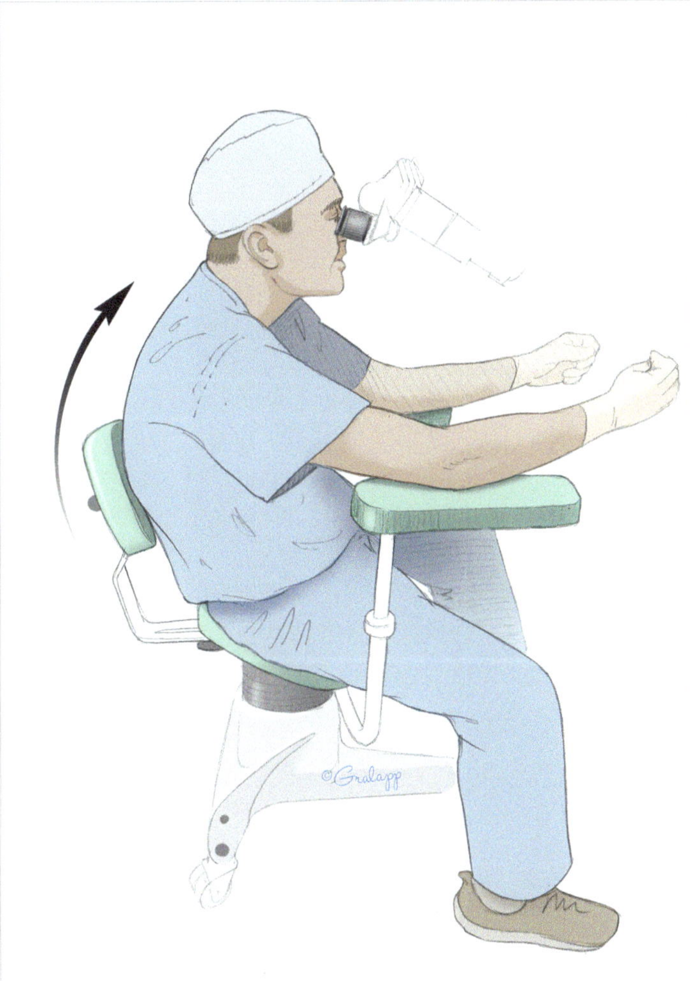

Fig. 2.26 Some otologists were taught to practice the "otological slouch" because theoretically it was a relaxed posture. However, a curved back, rounded shoulders, and a flexed neck is ergonomically unsound and contributes to low back problems.

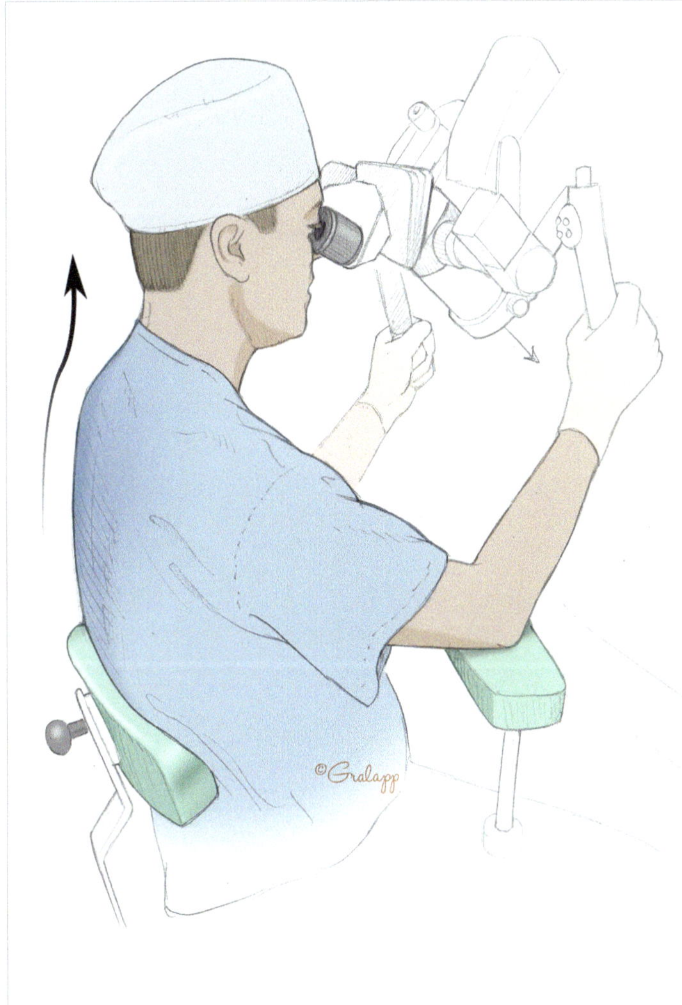

Fig. 2.27 Microsurgeons are also prone to cervical spine problems. Maintaining a neutral neck position when using a microscope reduces strain on the surgeon's neck.

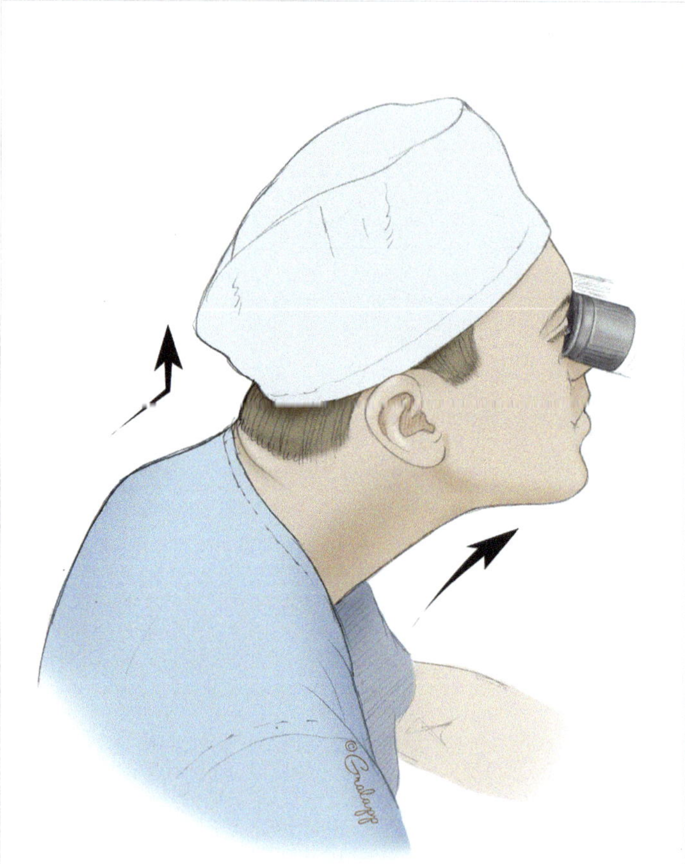

Fig. 2.28 It is often tempting to lean into the microscope optics which results in uncomfortable neck extension and forward thrust.

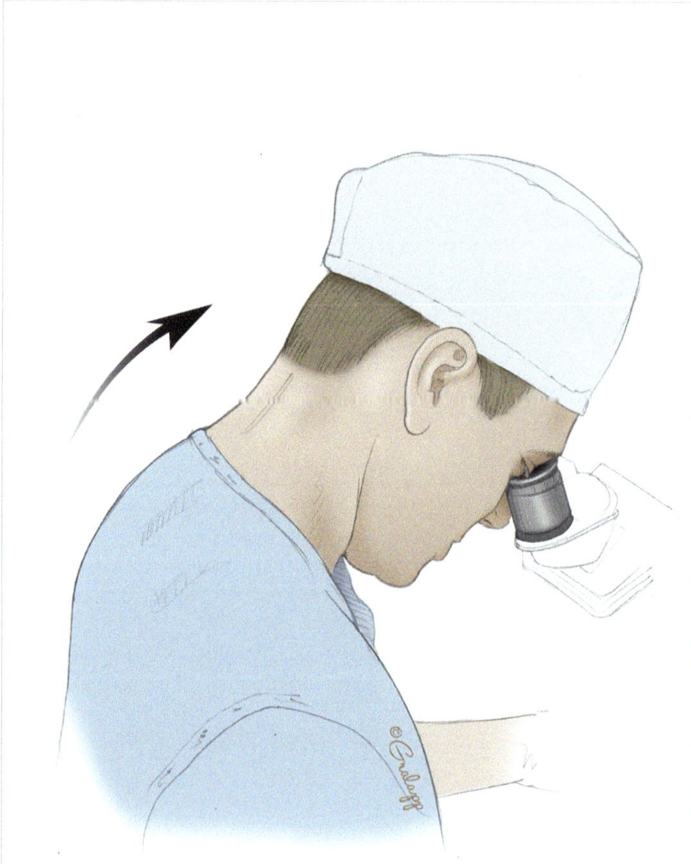

Fig. 2.29 Prolonged flexion of the neck can contribute to chronic neck problems.

2.5 Postauricular Incisions

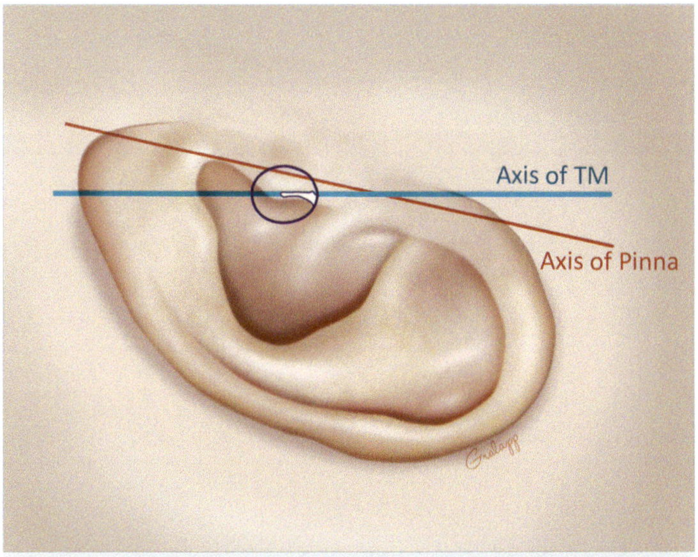

Fig. 2.30 The pinna tilts posterior about 15 degrees with respect to the axis of the malleus.

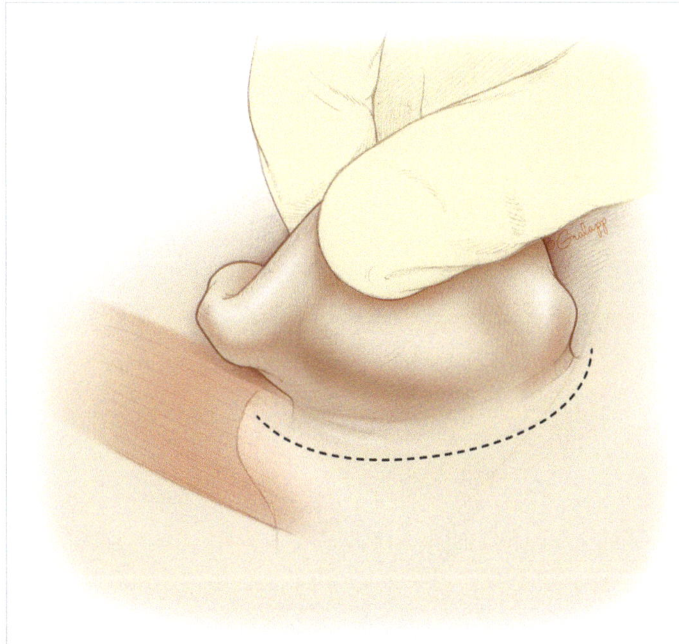

Fig. 2.31 Postauricular incision may be done in the sulcus, but incisions 5 to 10 mm behind the sulcus heal well and are less likely to retract. Note that the incision is carried forward in its superior limb to enable the ear to be turned forward for unhindered access to the structures of the middle ear. Inferiorly, the incision carries over the mastoid tip. In infants and very young children, who have not yet developed a mastoid tip, the incision should not be carried inferiorly to the same degree as it risks facial nerve injury.

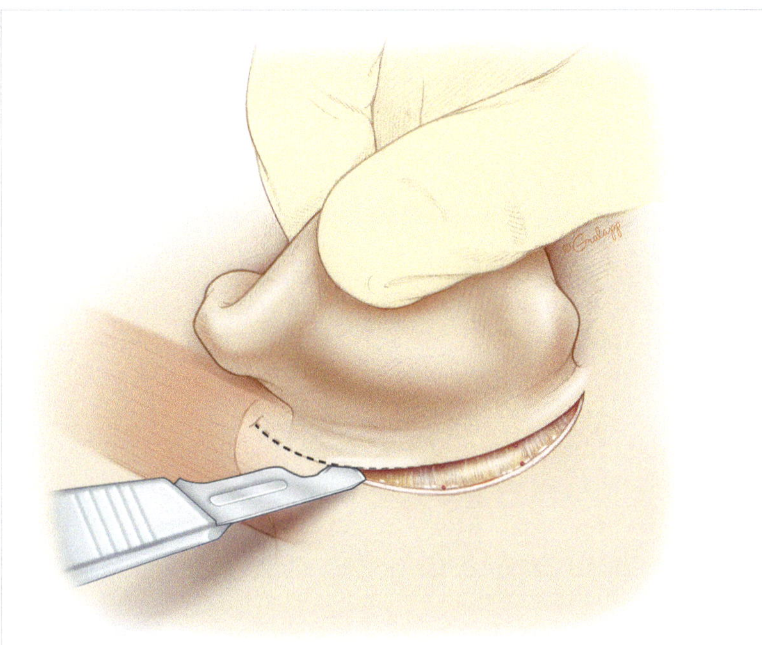

Fig. 2.32 Incision is carried through the dermis with a scalpel. Some surgeons open the skin with electrocautery.

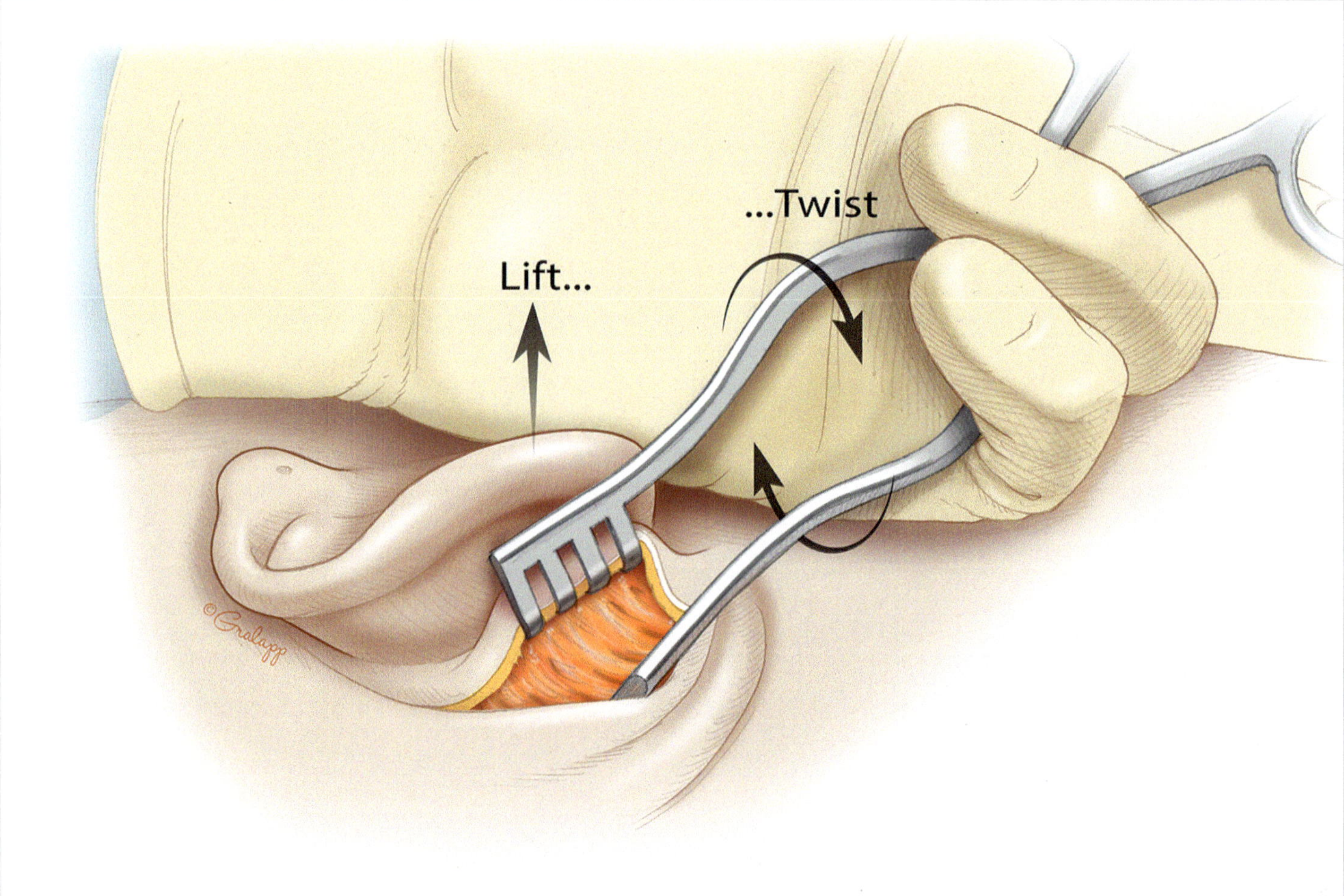

Fig. 2.33 The next goal is to identify the temporalis fascia and linea temporalis. Use of a mastoid retractor to place the tissue under tension aids in this process. The superficial layers can be opened expeditiously with electrocautery.

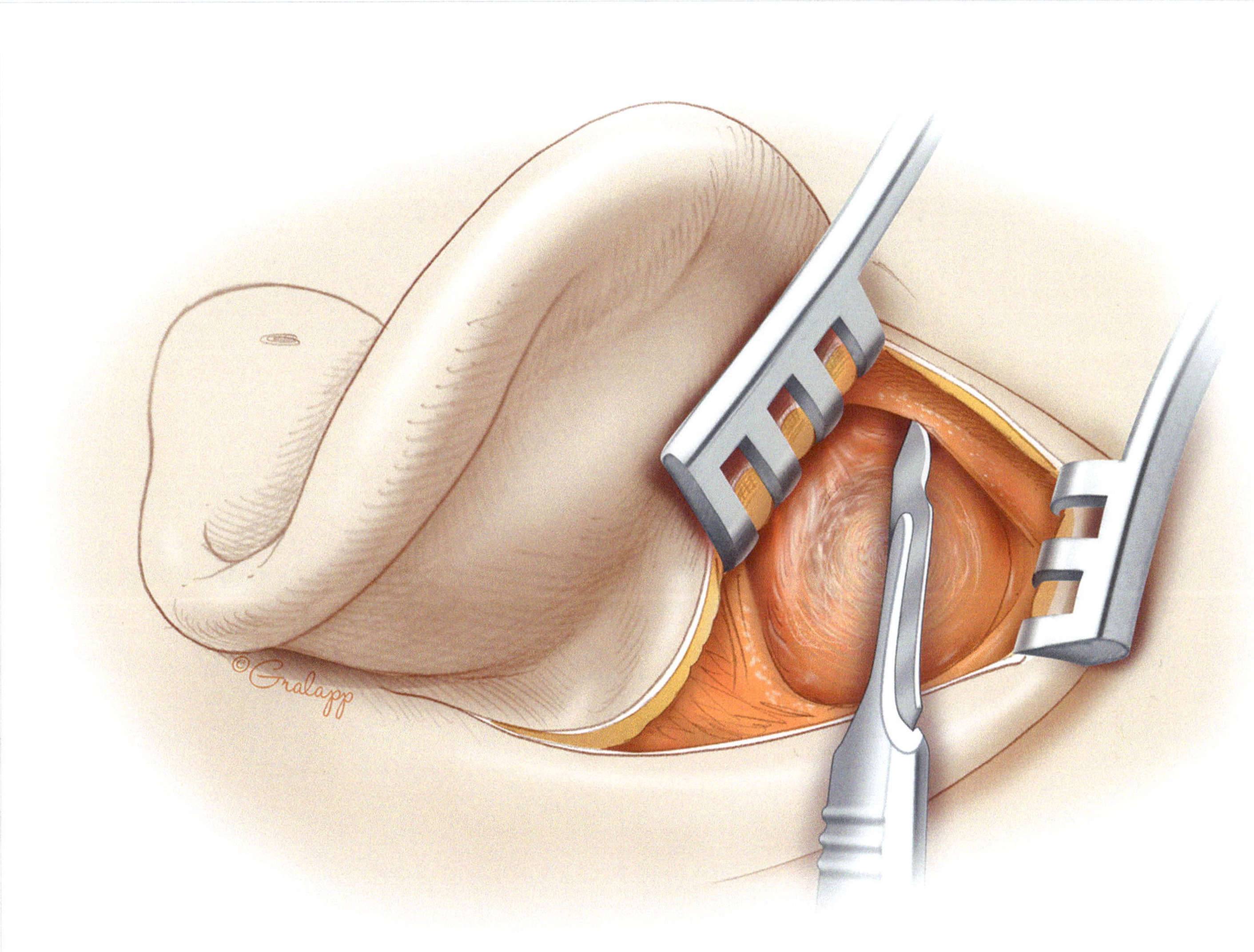

Fig. 2.34 During dissection above the ear, a hood commonly develops, which should be sharply parted.

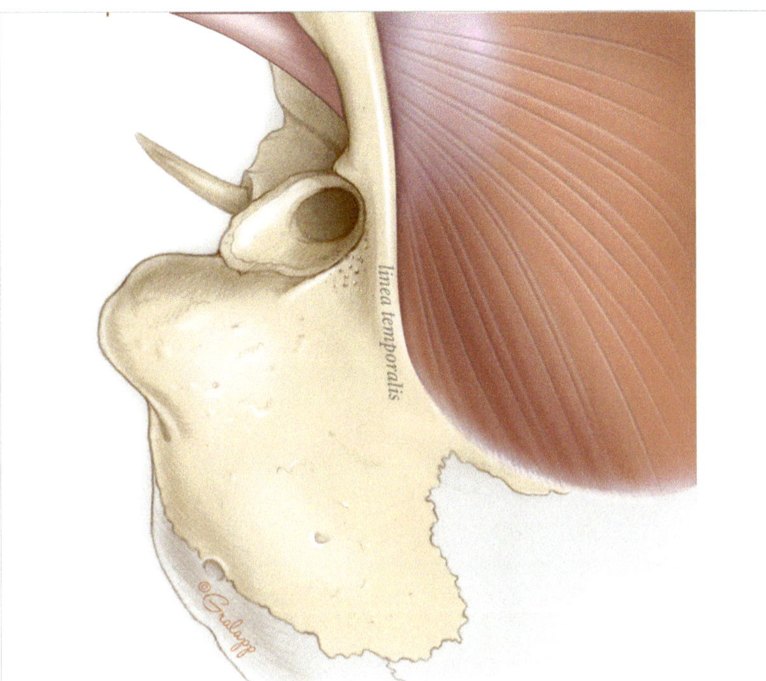

Fig. 2.35 The temporalis muscle lives in a fossa whose lower edge is the linea temporalis: an important landmark in opening the ear from behind.

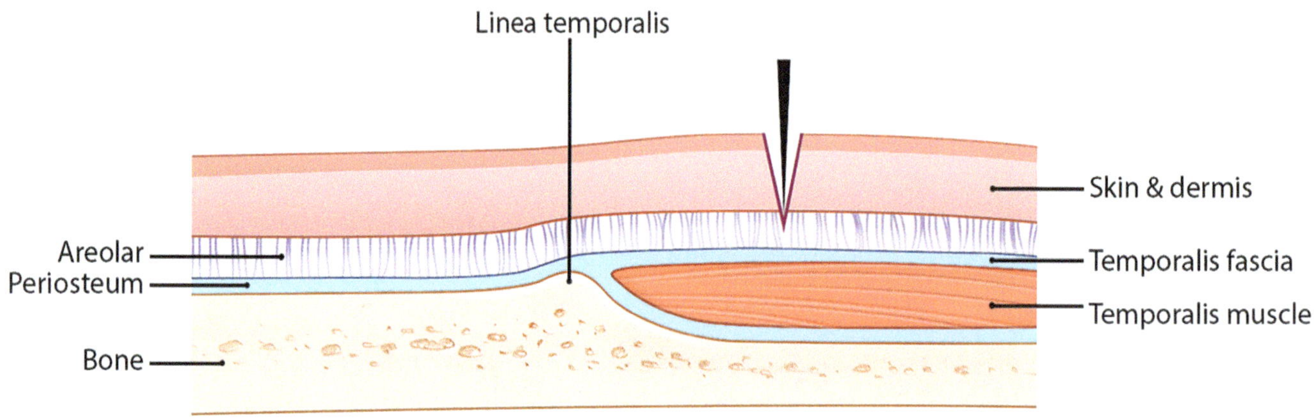

Fig. 2.36 Soft-tissue layers illustrated in relation to the linea temporalis.

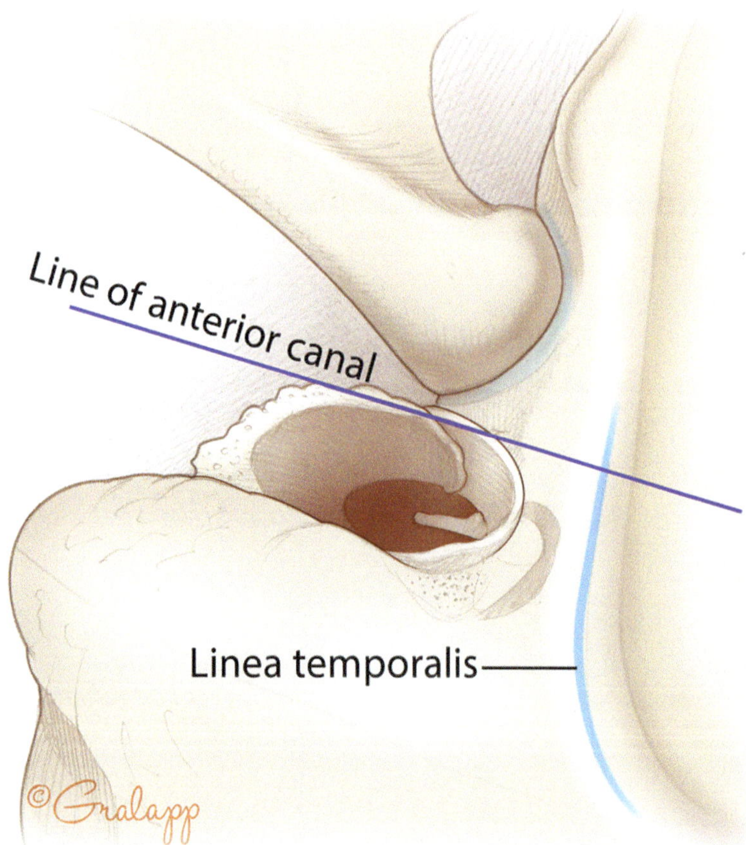

Fig. 2.37 The incision of periosteum along the linea temporalis should be carried forward to the level of the anterior aspect of the ear canal so that the soft tissues rotate forward to enable a full view down the ear canal to the middle ear structures.

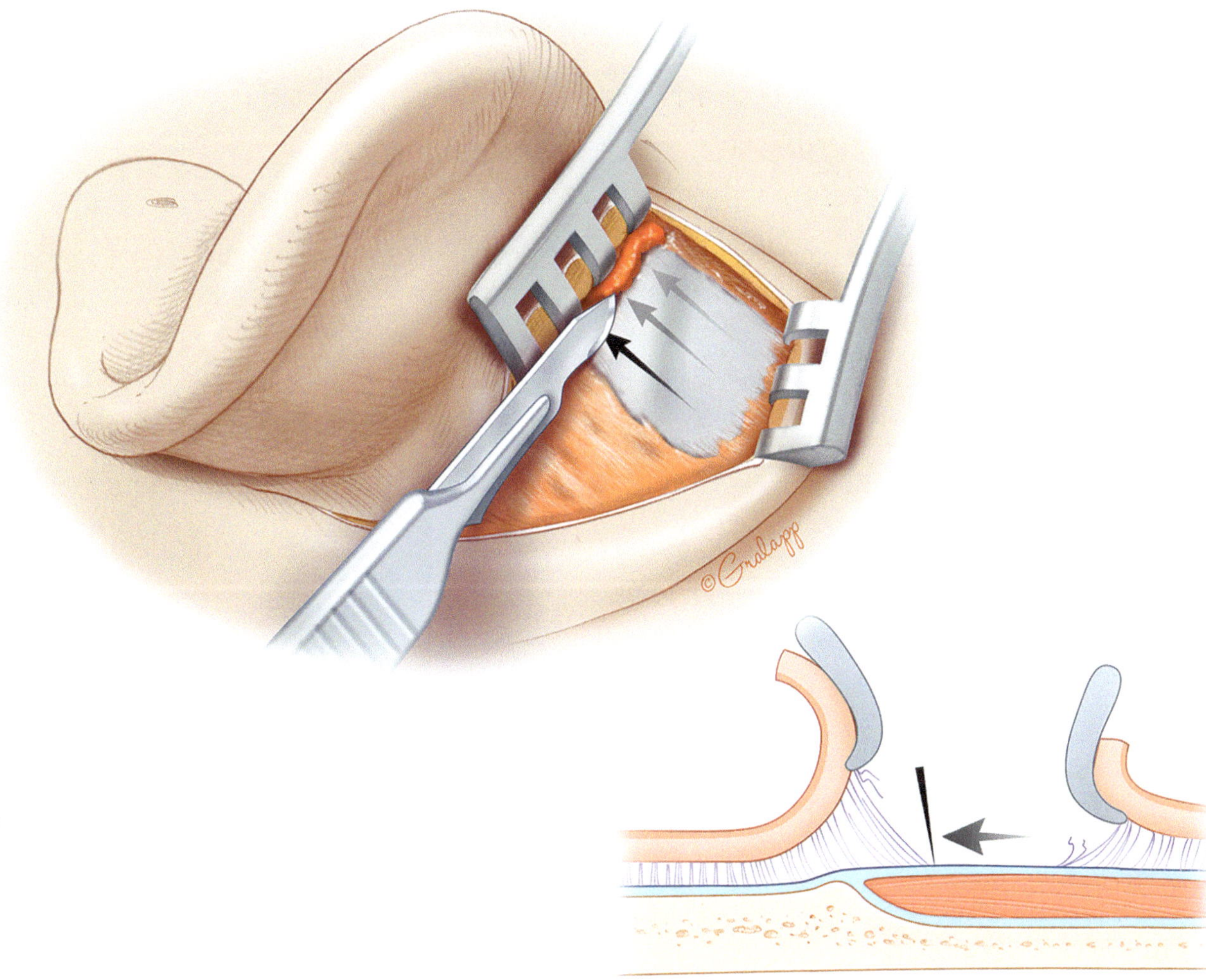

Fig. 2.38 Sweeping with a scalpel while clicking open the mastoid retractor to maintain tension in the soft tissues expedites identification of the temporalis fascia. Note that the scalpel blade is tilted superiorly. If directed inferiorly, it tends to cut into the fascia and can even open the roof of the external auditory canal.

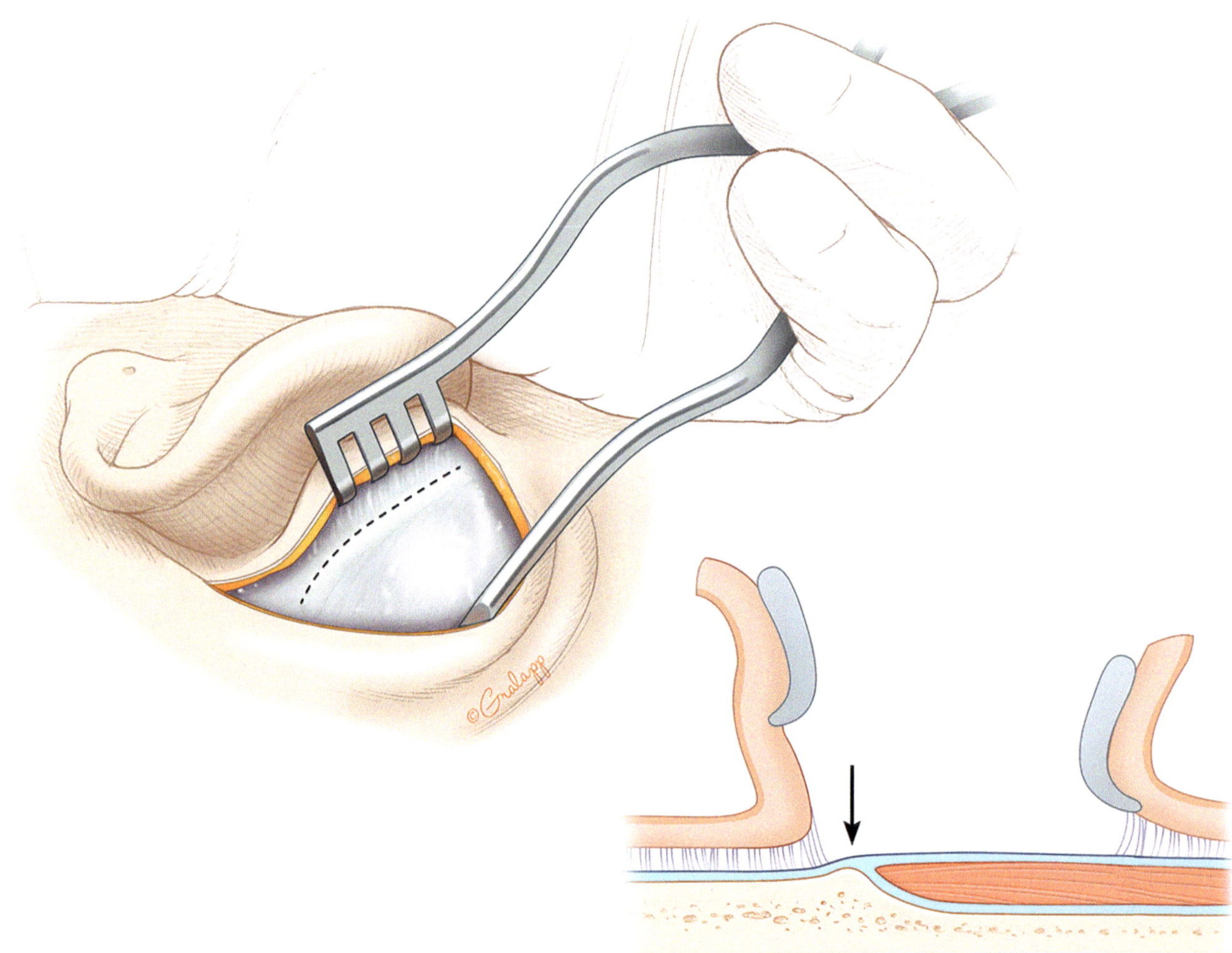

Fig. 2.39 Identification of the linea temporalis, a bony ridge at the lower margin of the temporalis muscle (*dotted line, arrow*).

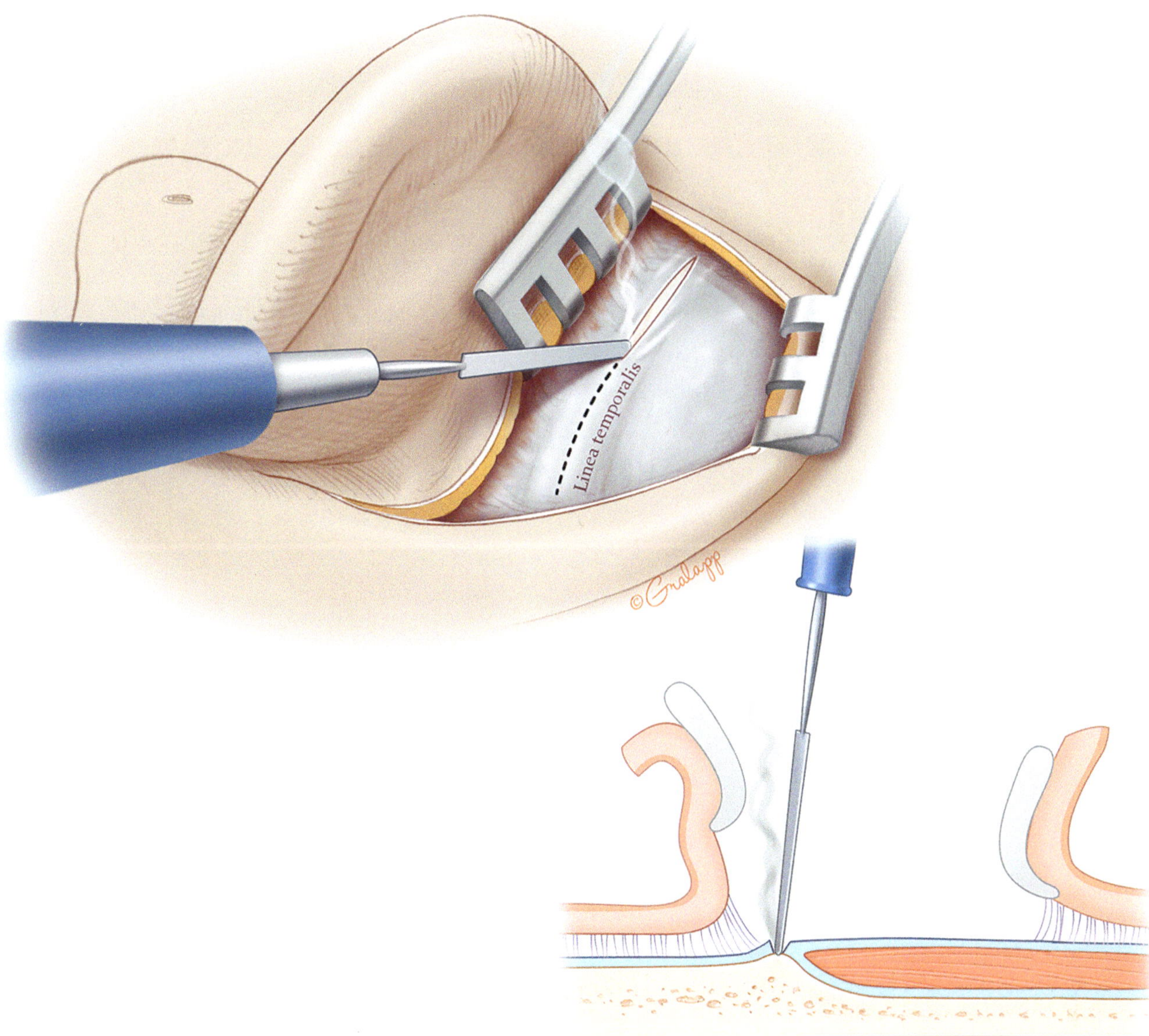

Fig. 2.40 Electrocautery is used to make an incision along the linea temporalis. A posterior branch of the superficial temporal artery often needs to be controlled at the anterior aspect of the incision.

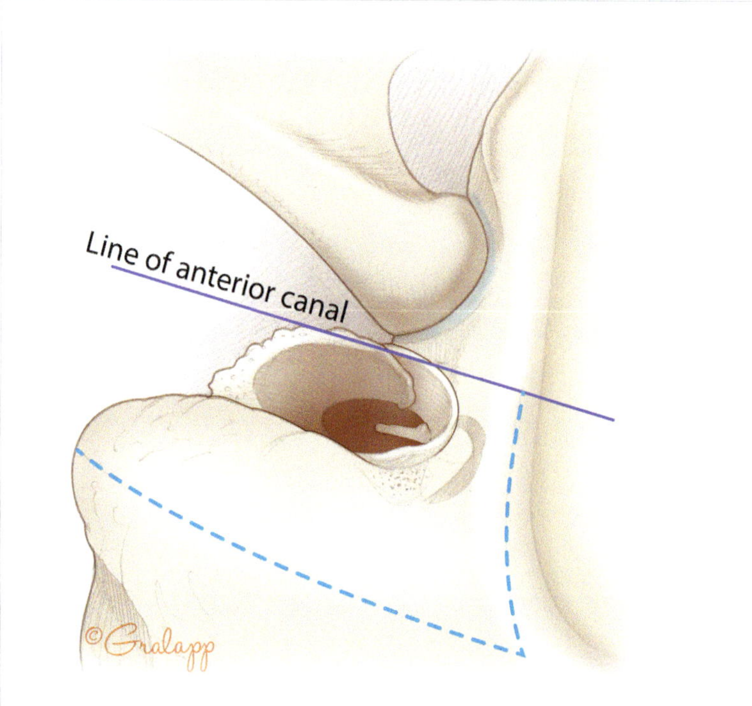

Fig. 2.41 After the superior incision has been completed, if mastoidectomy is planned the periosteum is then opened over the cortex to the mastoid tip. If only postauricular tympanoplasty is planned, then the periosteal incision can be made closely behind the ear canal.

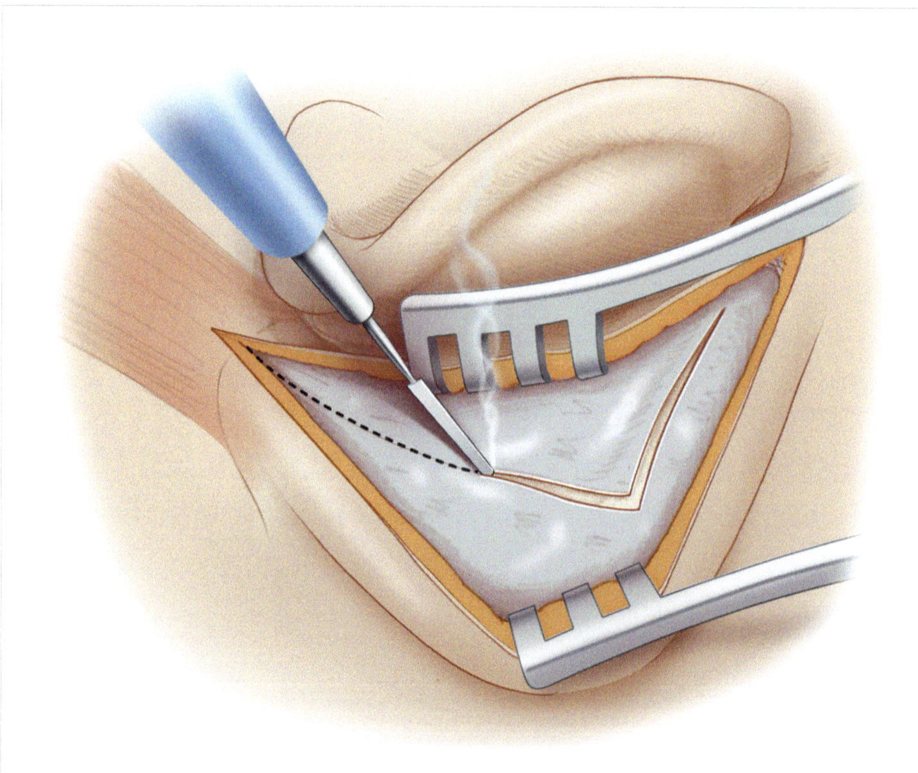

Fig. 2.42 Periosteum is then opened over the cortex to the mastoid tip.

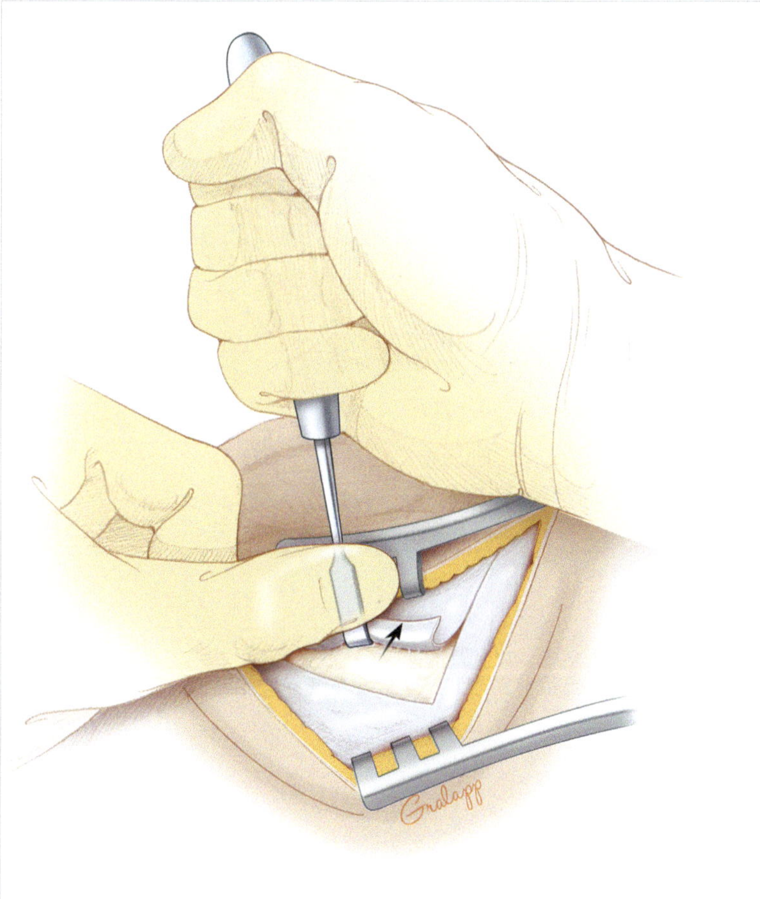

Fig. 2.43 Using a periosteal elevator, the mastoid cortex is exposed first by elevating toward the ear canal. Technique shown employing a Lempert periosteal elevator.

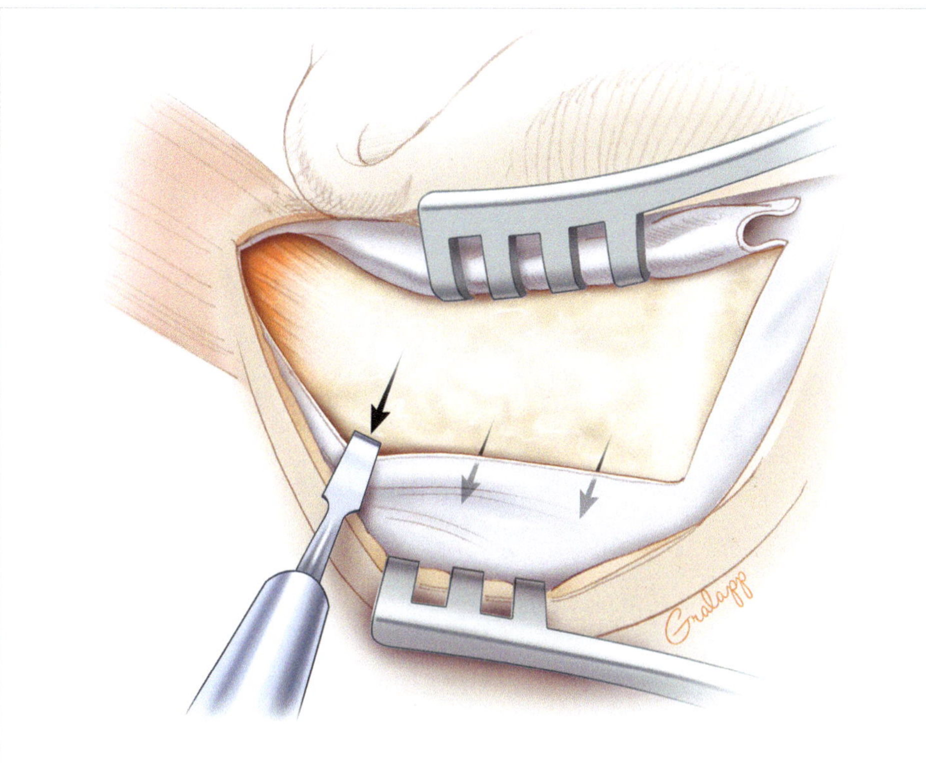

Fig. 2.44 Using a periosteal elevator, the mastoid cortex is exposed posteriorly.

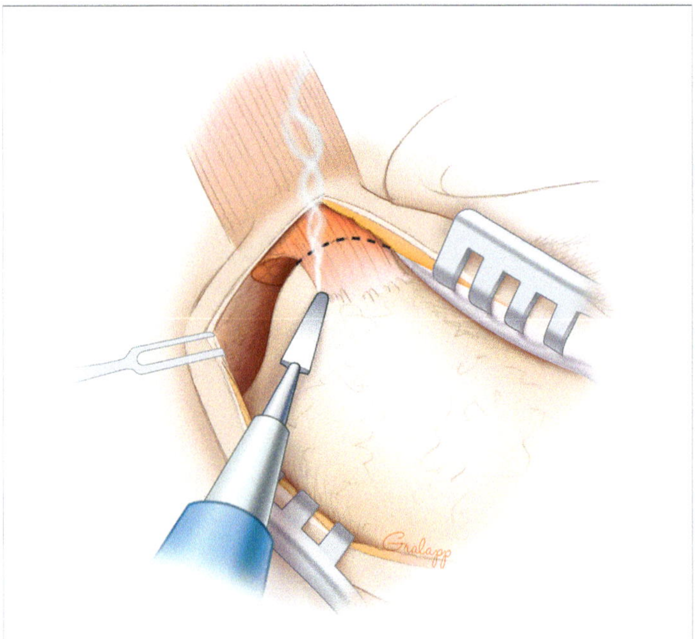

Fig. 2.45 The insertion of the sternocleidomastoid muscle is dissected off the mastoid tip with electrocautery.

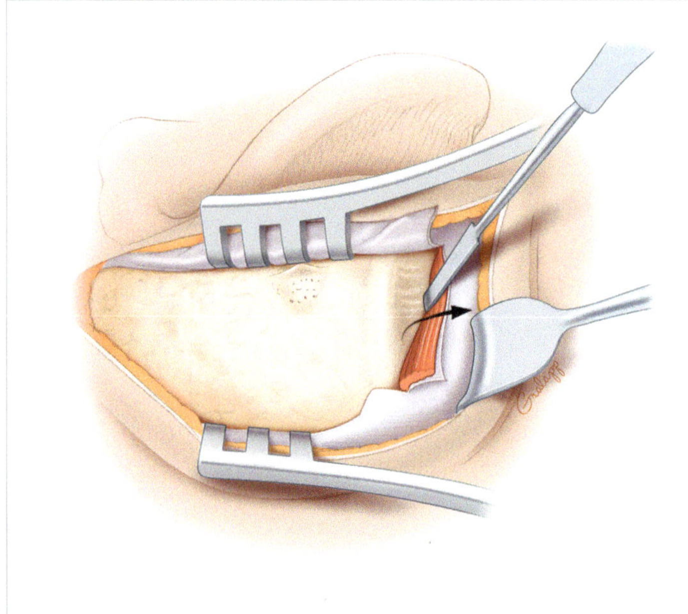

Fig. 2.46 The temporalis muscle is elevated from the linea temporalis. Note that a small relaxing incision is often made posteriorly.

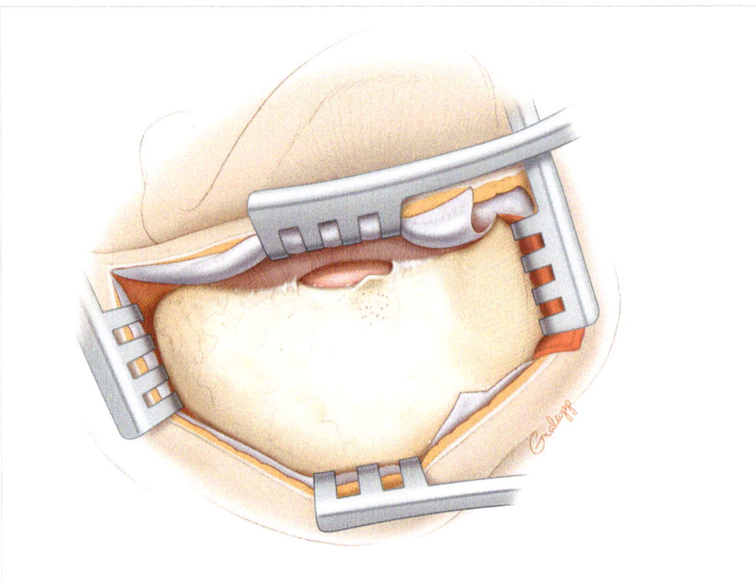

Fig. 2.47 Completed exposure for mastoidectomy. Two retractors are set, one spanning from the ear canal to the sinodural angle. Care must be taken when opening this retractor lest the meatal skin be torn. Liberating the meatal skin from the osseous meatus reduces this likelihood. The second retractor elevates the temporalis muscle and depresses the sternocleidomastoid muscle.

2.6 Postauricular Canal Flap Design

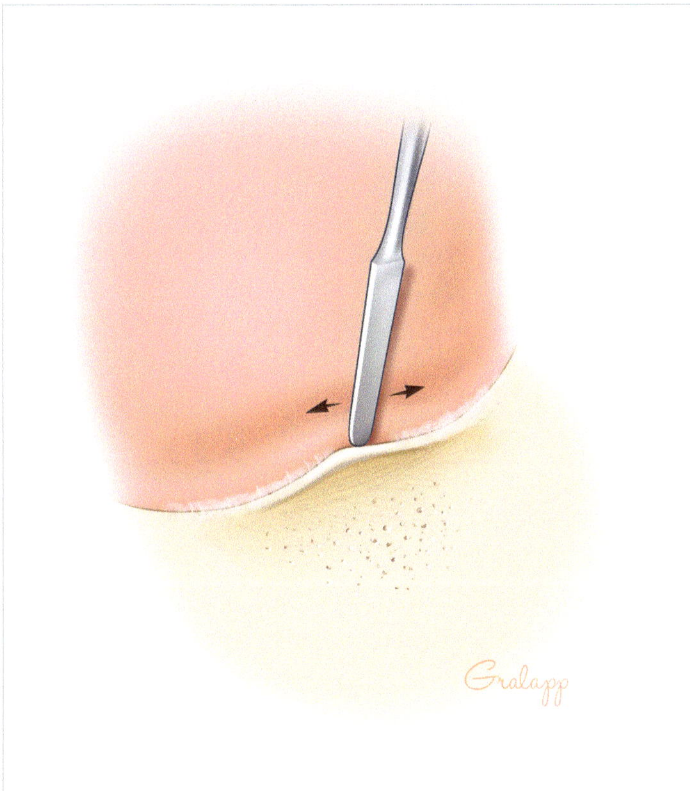

Fig. 2.48 Commencing elevation of the ear canal flap (skin and periosteum) from Henle's spine. Note the cribriform region just posterior to the spine.

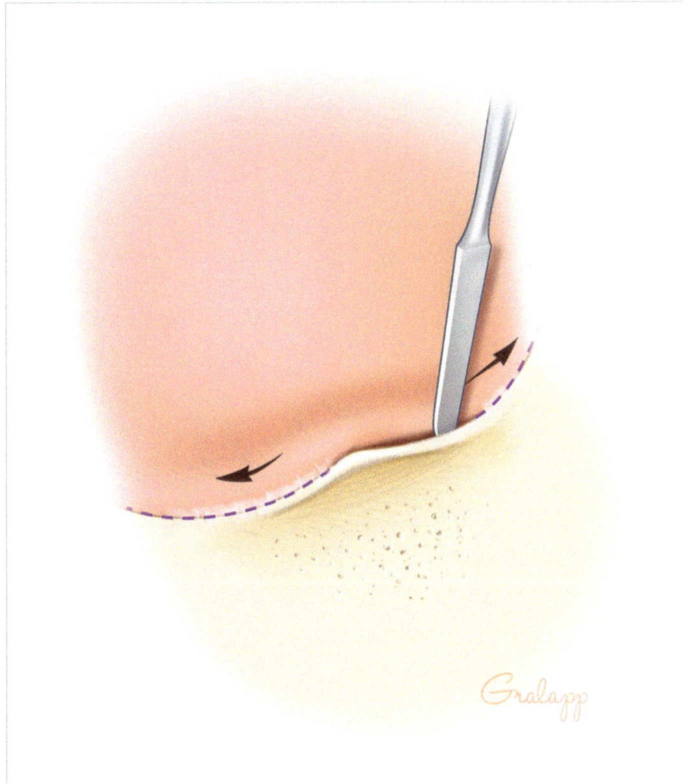

Fig. 2.49 Developing the periosteal plane of the ear canal.

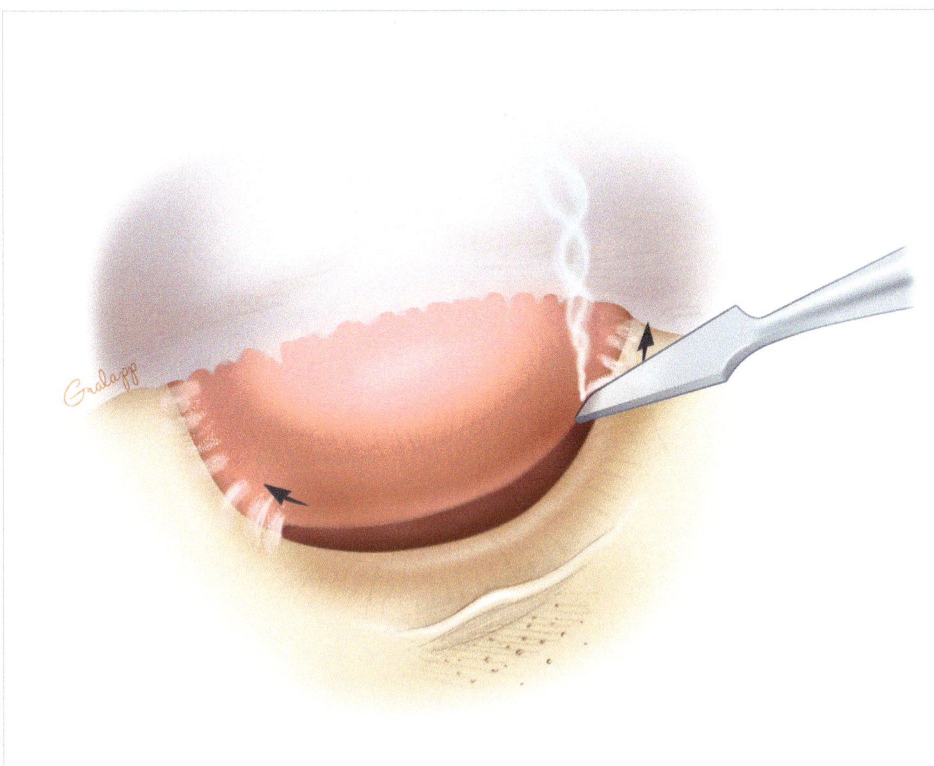

Fig. 2.50 When the flap adheres to the tympanomastoid (inferior) and tympanosquamous (superior) suture lines, a needle point electrocautery may be used to effect sharp elevation.

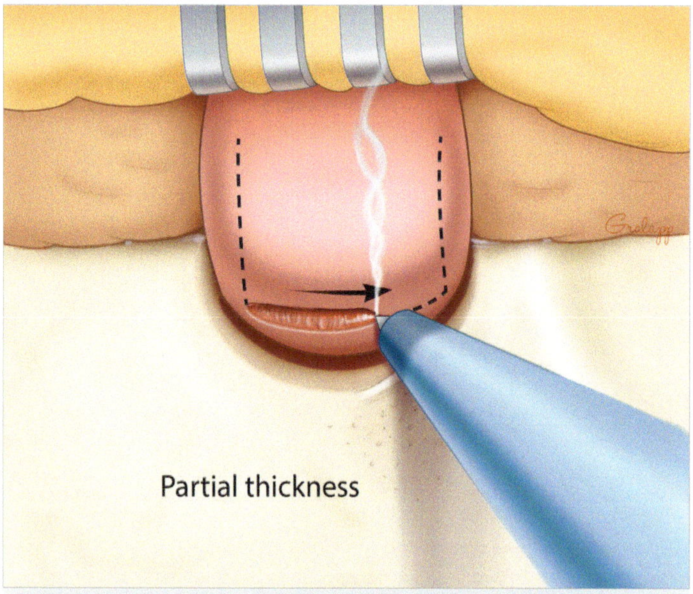

Fig. 2.51 One option for incising the ear canal skin is a posterior ear canal flap (also known as a Koerner's flap). Because ear canal incisions can bleed significantly, the periosteum and dermis is parted with needle point electrocautery.

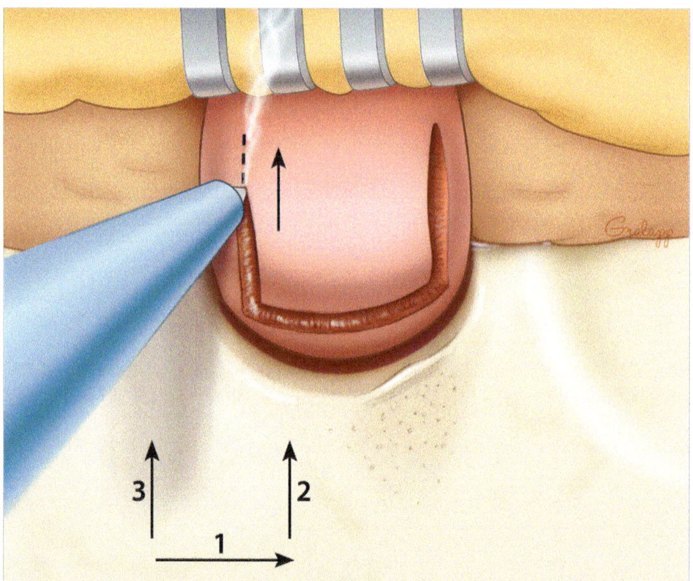

Fig. 2.53 Cutting the vertical limbs of the flap. These are done from medial to lateral so that any bleeding will not obscure continuation of the incision.

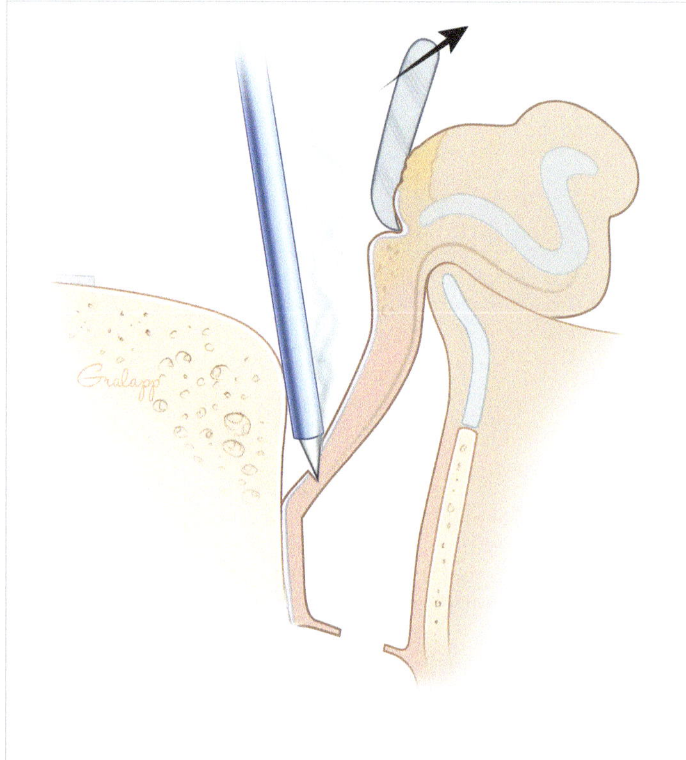

Fig. 2.52 The incision is initiated part way down the osseous canal.

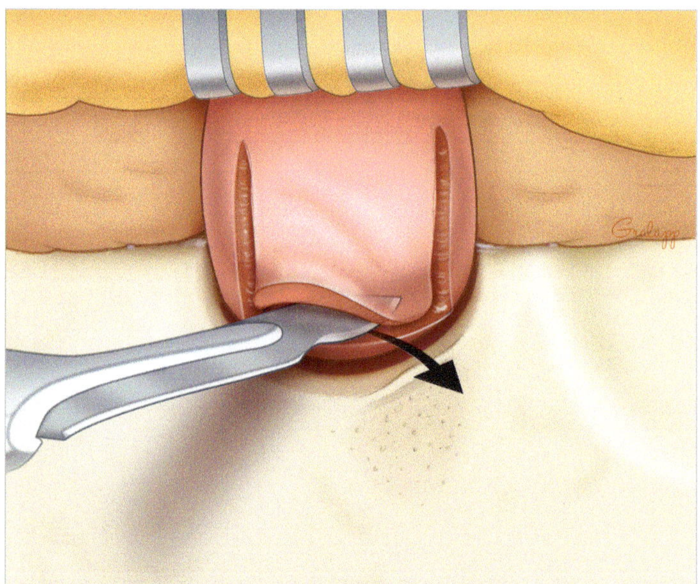

Fig. 2.54 The epidermis is cut sharply with a scalpel.

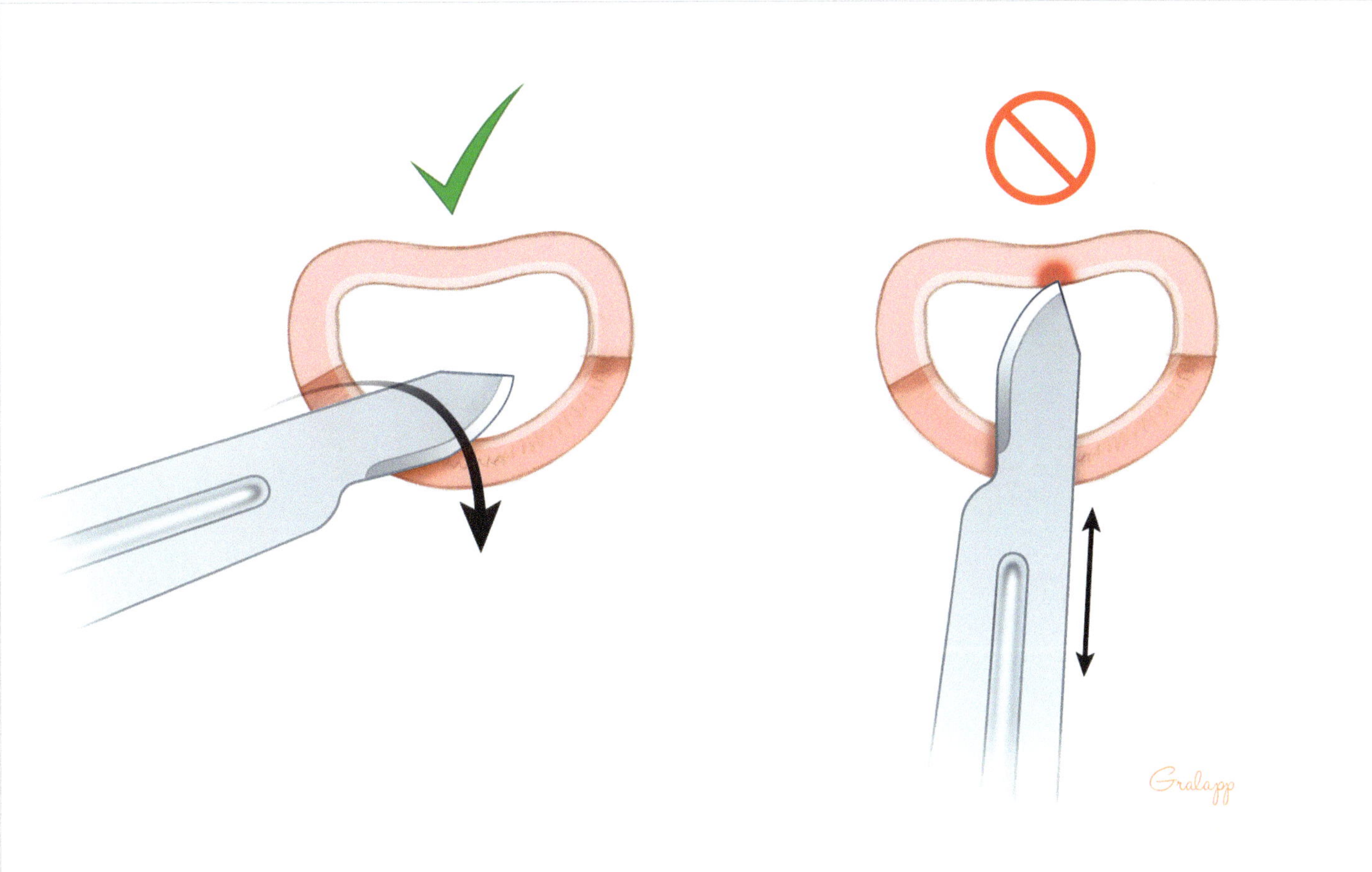

Fig. 2.55 When cutting the skin, it is best to cut toward the surgeon to avoid possibly incising the anterior canal skin.

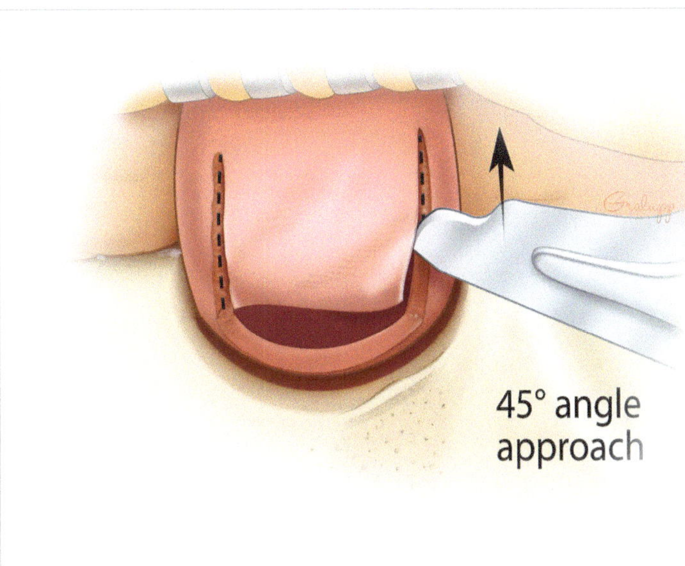

Fig. 2.56 Incising the vertical limbs of the posterior ear canal flap.

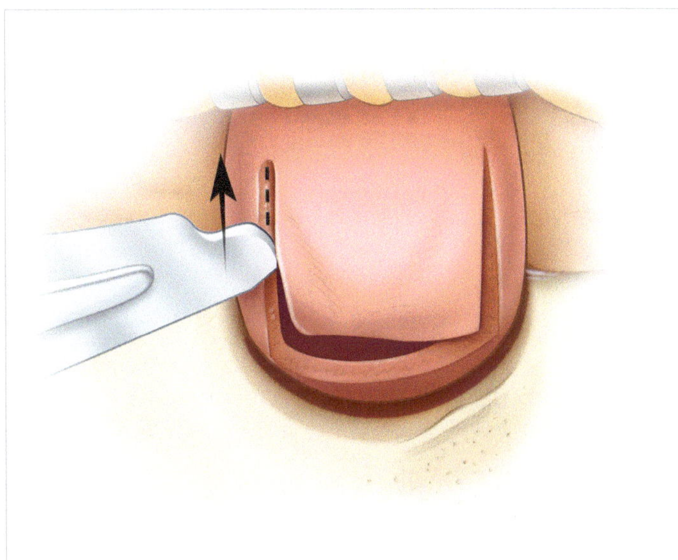

Fig. 2.57 Incising the vertical limbs of the posterior ear canal flap.

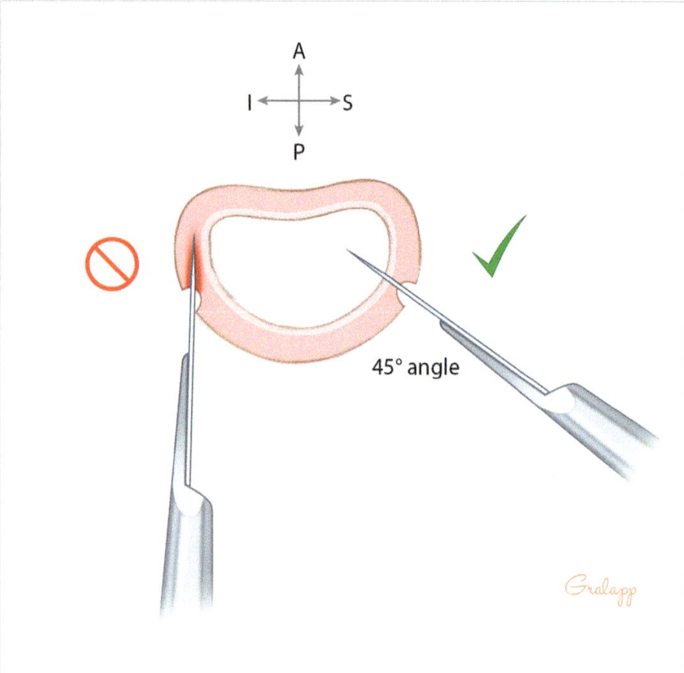

Fig. 2.58 In making the vertical limbs, it is important to angle the cut by 45 degrees lest the incision simply penetrates the soft tissue of the canal and not properly enter the lumen.

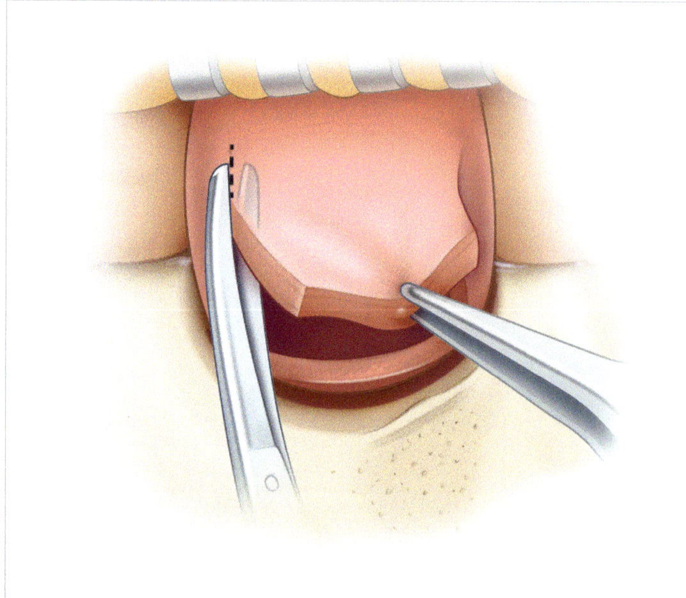

Fig. 2.59 The incisions can be carried laterally using either scalpel or scissors.

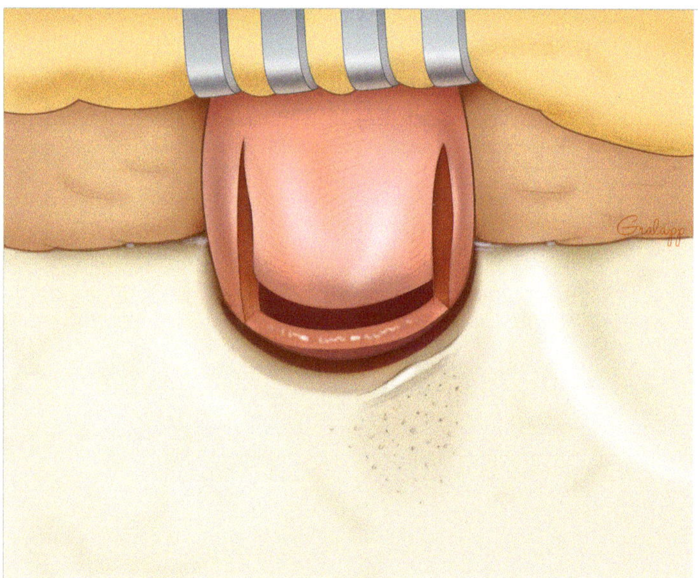

Fig. 2.60 Completed incision of posterior ear canal flap.

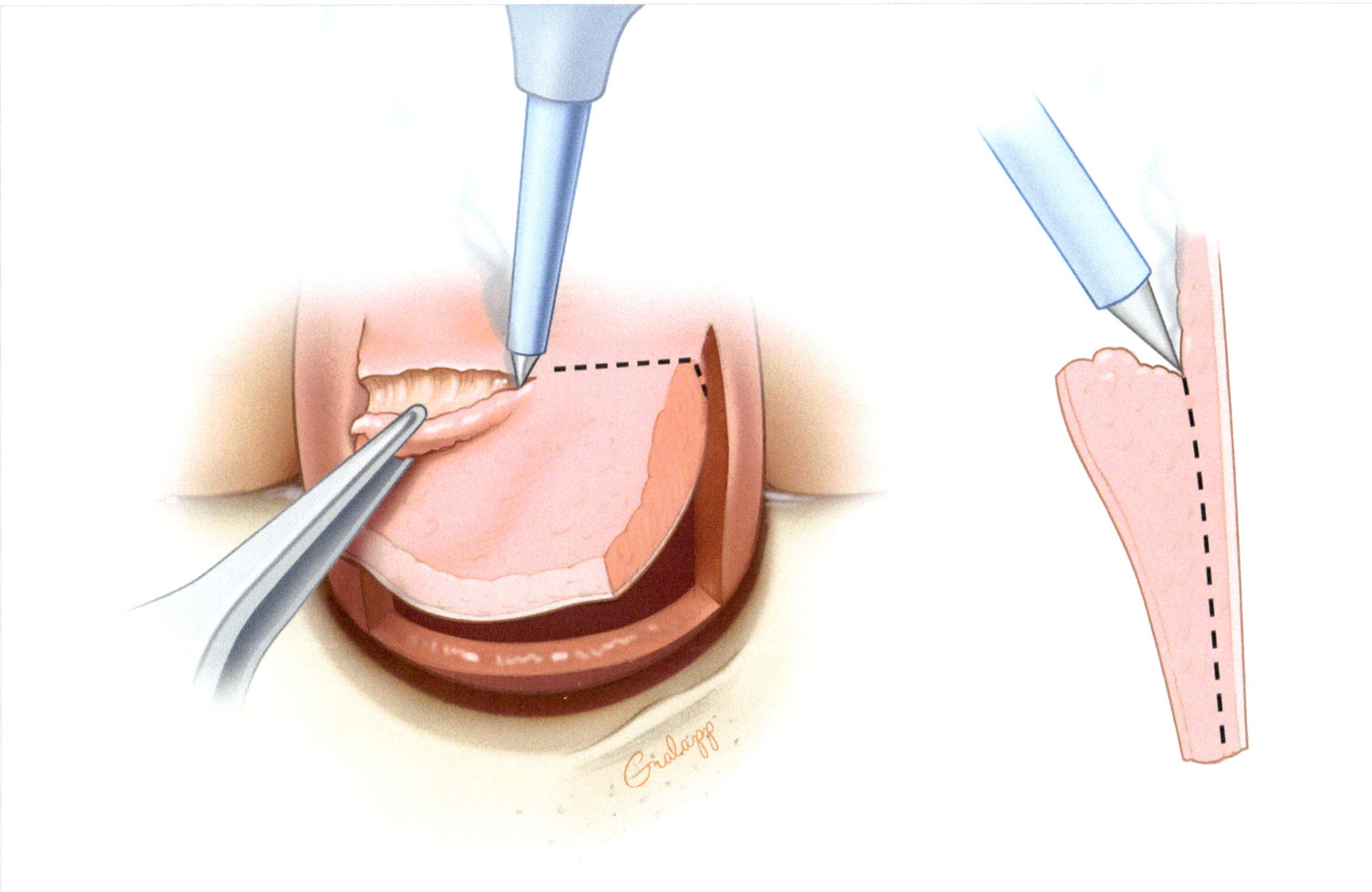

Fig. 2.61 Thinning the flap is an important part of soft tissue canaloplasty.

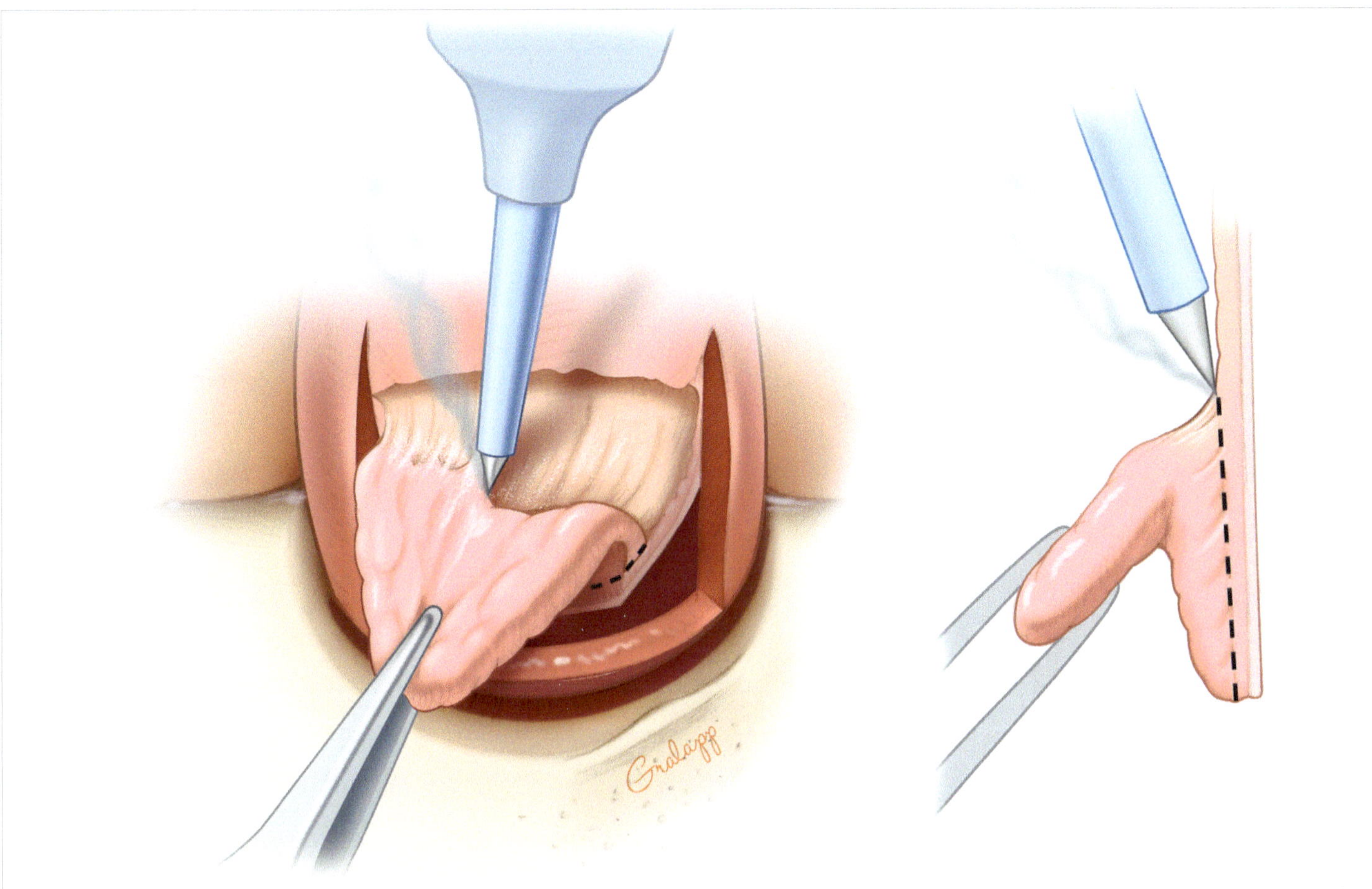

Fig. 2.62 To minimize bleeding, electrocautery may be helpful in thinning the flap.

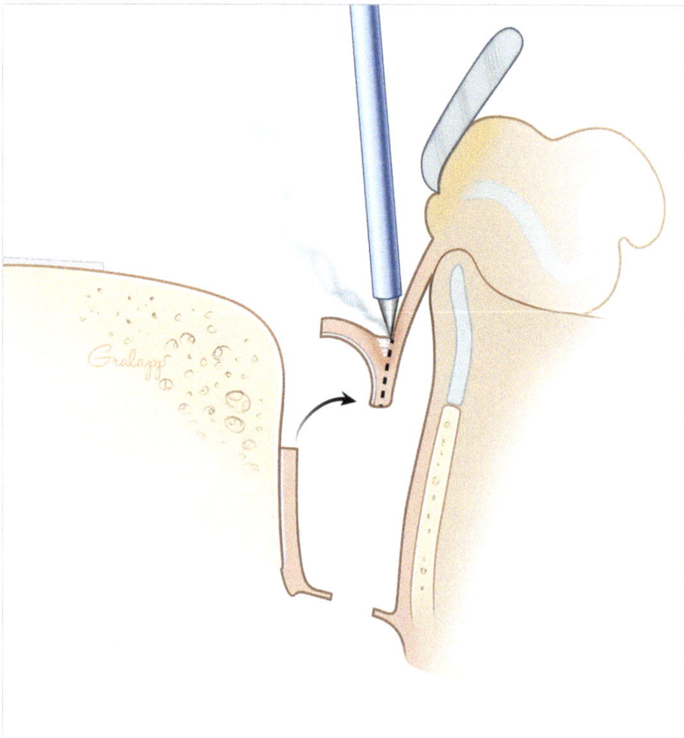

Fig. 2.63 Flap thinning.

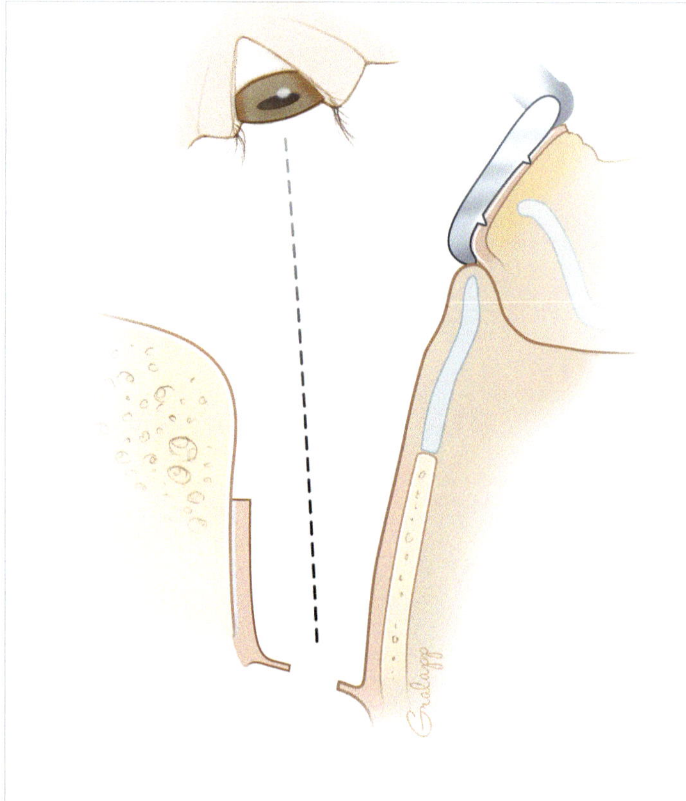

Fig. 2.64 The Koerner's flap is flipped outward and helped under a spiked, flat blade retractor (e.g., Perkin's). This procedure enables a direct view down the ear canal with no overhanging soft tissue to obscure the surgeon's view.

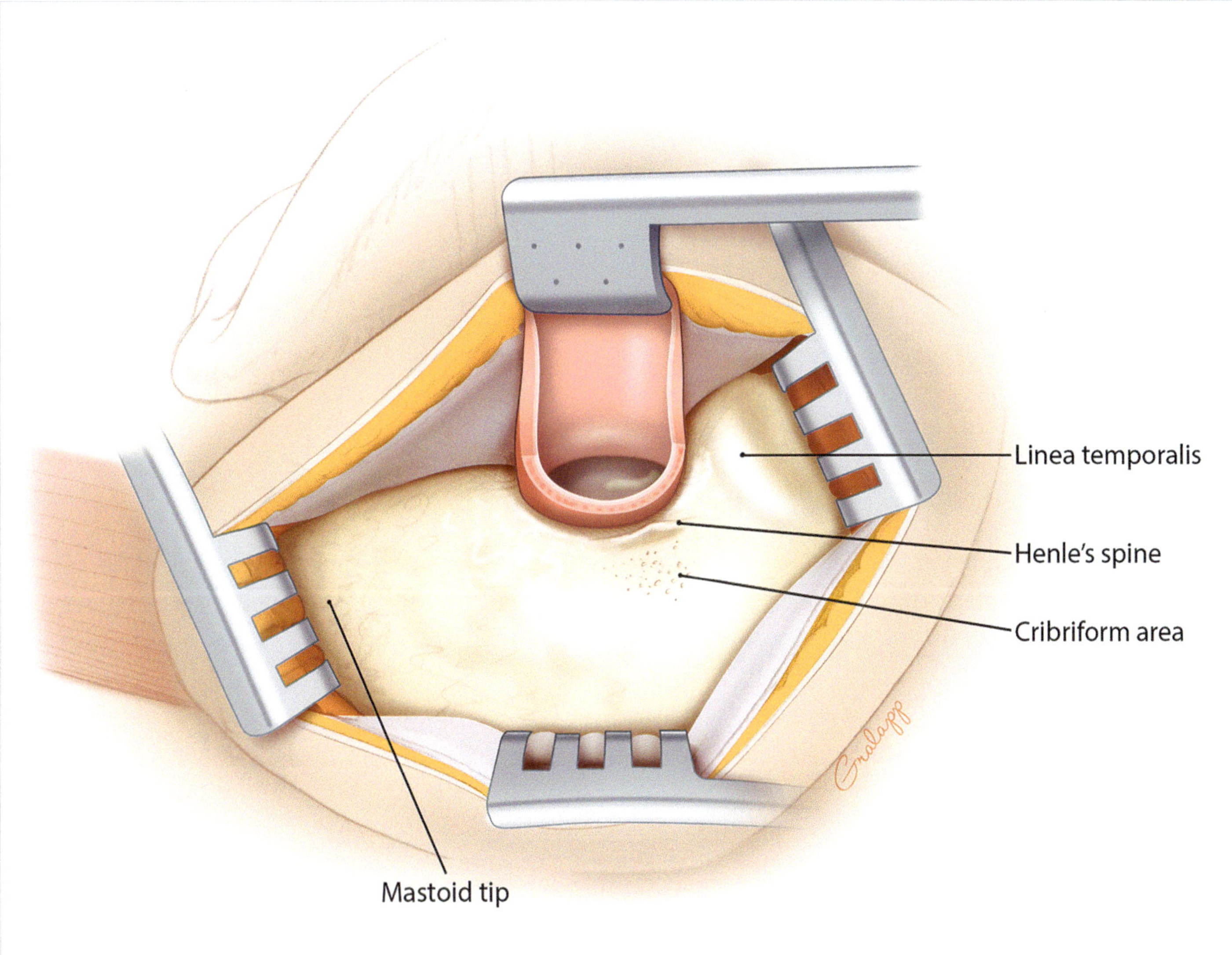

Fig. 2.65 View of the mastoid and ear canal after completion of the posterior ear canal flap.

2.7 Endaural Incision

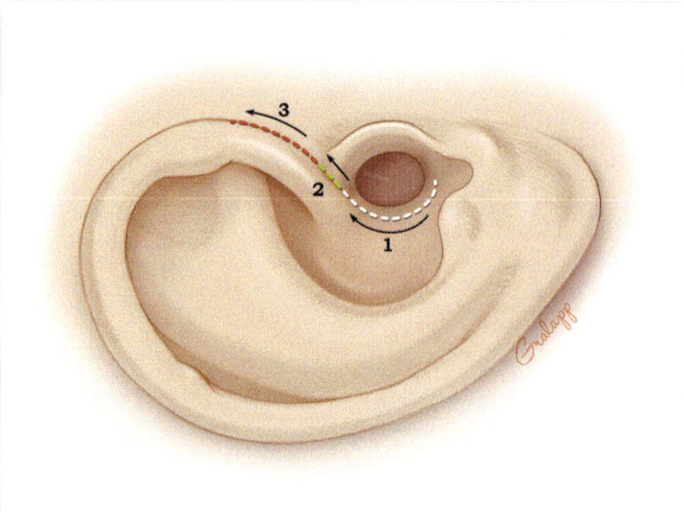

Fig. 2.66 There are three segments to an endaural incision: circumferential, intercartilaginous (between the helical crus and the tragus), and the vertical limb. It is less commonly used today compared to the postauricular incision due to the visibility of the scar and limitation of exposure posteriorly.

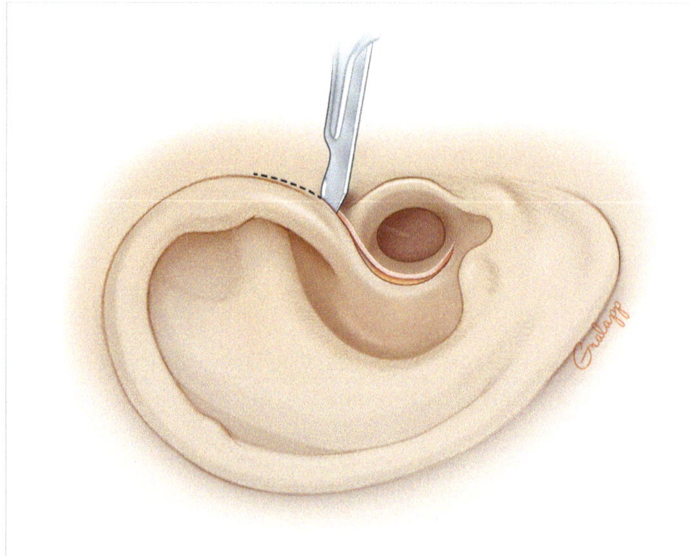

Fig. 2.67 Commencing the endaural incision.

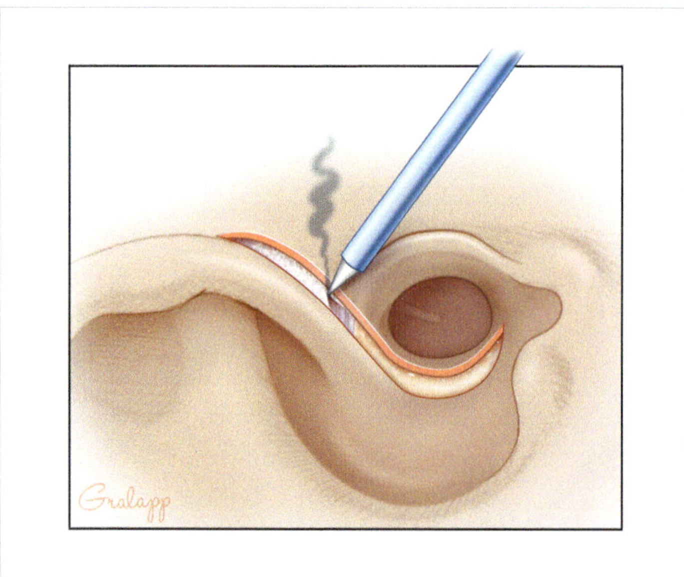

Fig. 2.68 Needle point electrocautery through the dermis to the temporalis fascia superiorly.

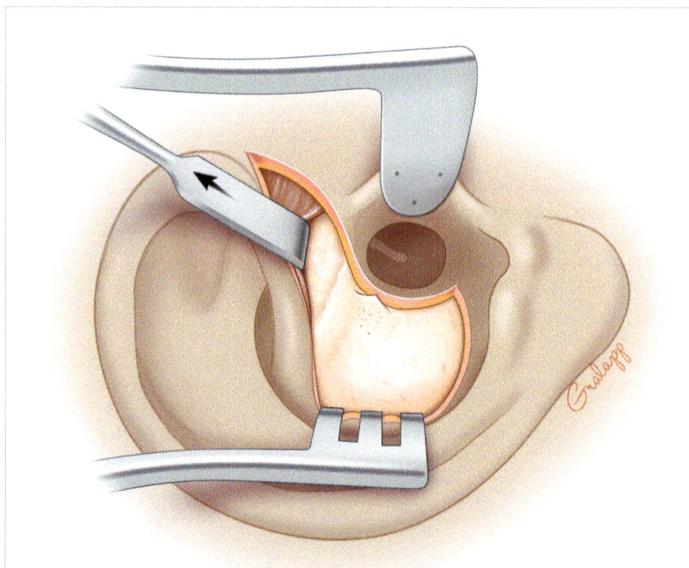

Fig. 2.69 Elevation of the temporalis muscle off the linea temporalis superiorly.

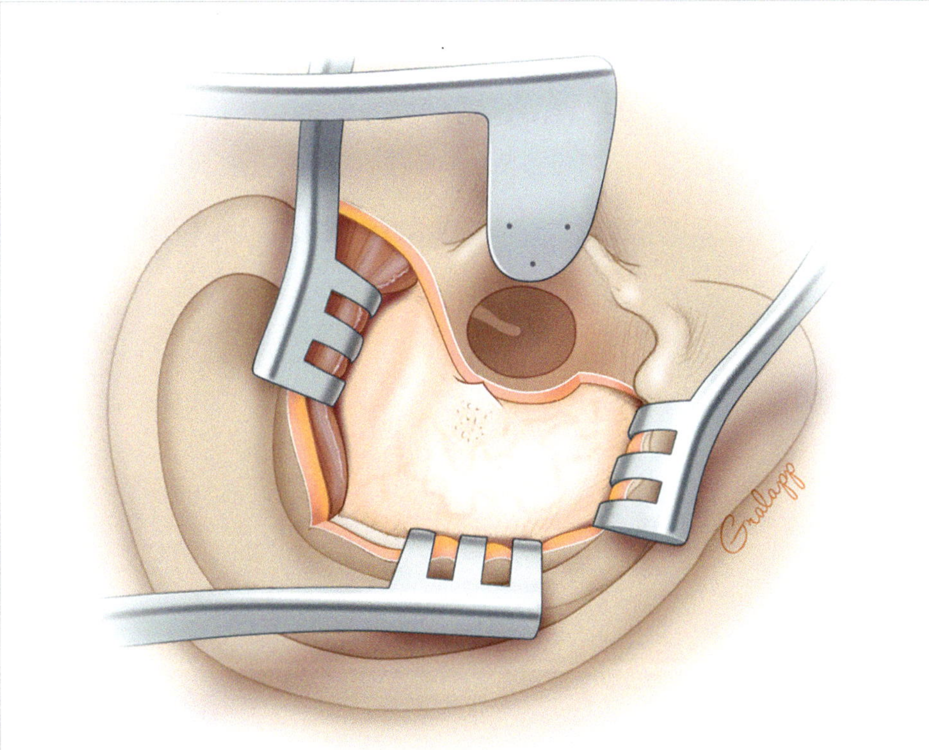

Fig. 2.70 Completed endaural exposure enables tympanomastoid surgery.

2.8 Incision Closure

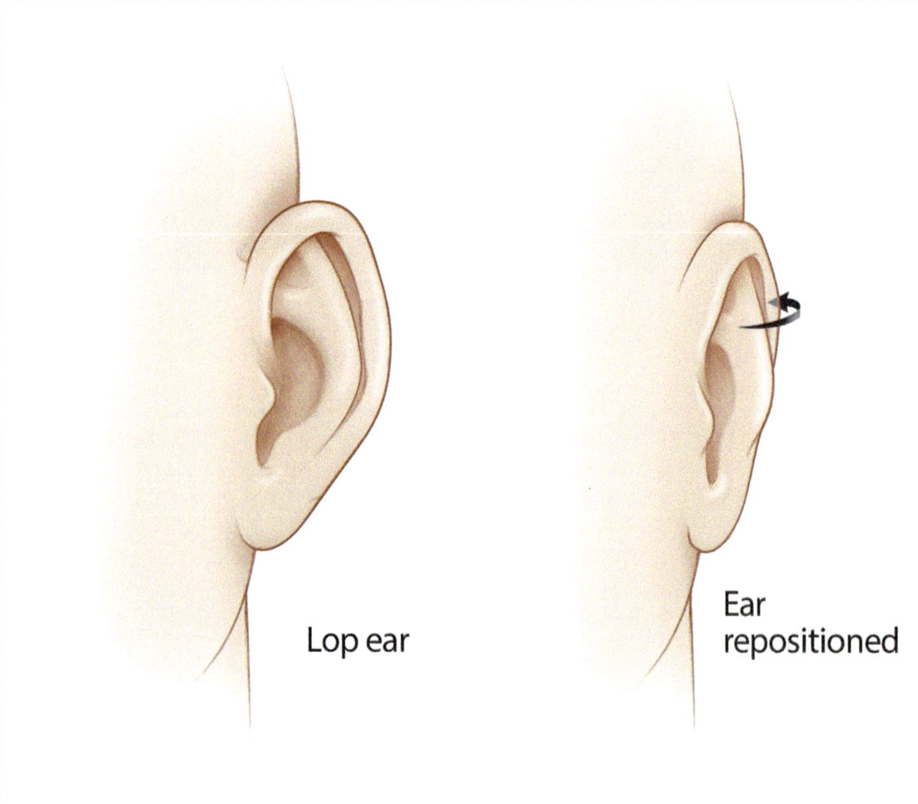

Fig. 2.71 In closing a postauricular incision following tympanomastoid procedures, the pinna may rotate outward and develop a cosmetically undesirable prominence (i.e., lop ear). This is especially the case in children due to the flexibility of their cartilage.

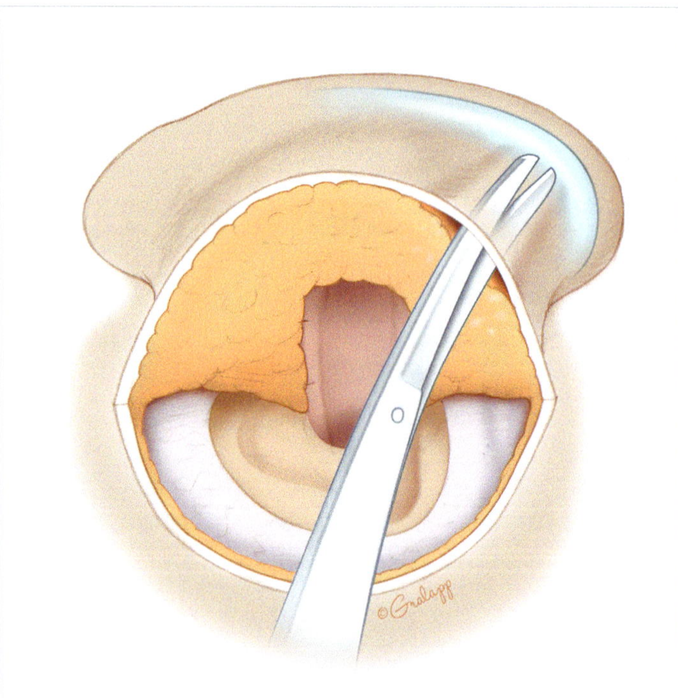

Fig. 2.72 Placement of an anti-lopping suture begins with tunneling to expose antihelical fold.

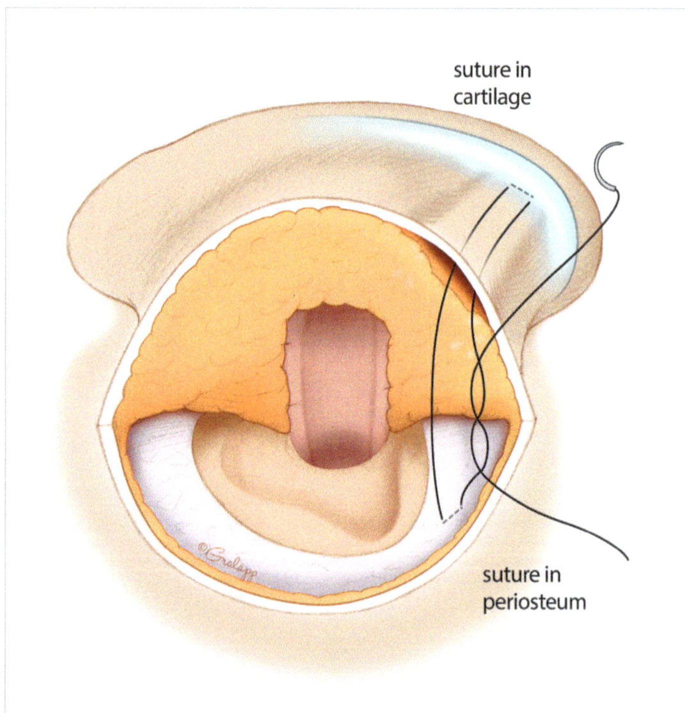

Fig. 2.73 Placement of an anti-lopping suture. To avoid the suture pulling through the perichondrium while tying, the ear is pushed from its ventral side against the head.

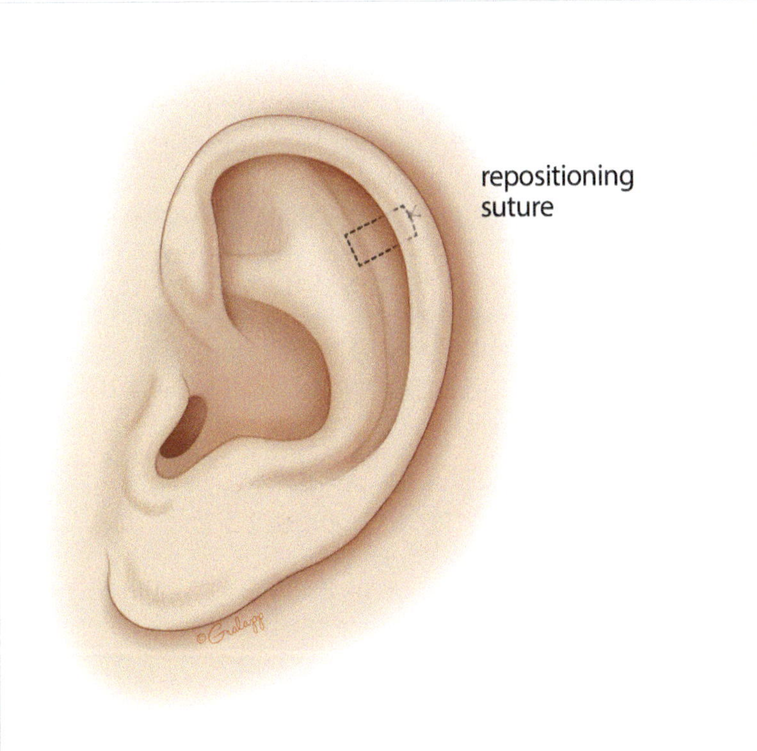

Fig. 2.74 An anti-lopping suture in place.

3 External Ear

Robert K. Jackler

3.1 Introduction to the External Ear

It is more than a little ironic that most patients think of the ear in terms of the pinna, whereas many ear surgeons relegate pinna surgery to their facial plastic surgical colleagues. Nevertheless, the repair of the lop ear, microtia, atresia, auricular injuries, and neoplasia of the auricle rightly lies in the armamentarium of the otologist.

Microtia repair is a technically challenging, multistage procedure best done only by surgeons with specialized training. In microtia repair, with either autologous rib cartilage or high-density polyethylene implants, it is essential that canal atresia or stenosis repair be done in the correct sequence. In autologous rib microtia repair, the canal atresia or stenosis repair is done only after the auricular reconstruction is complete. This is essential to keep the skin flaps pliable and well vascularized. The challenge of microtia repair is maintaining the vascularity of the skin flaps that must drape over the cartilage construct. Two-staged repairs of Firmin and Nagata techniques are very demanding on the skin, and any compromise from previous incisions can be devastating to the outcome. In contrast, for high-density polyethylene implants, the canal must be done before or concurrently with the Microtia repair. The stability of polyethylene implants relies on the vascular supply of the superficial temporal artery supplying the temporal–parietal–facial flap. This flap is elevated after the canal is created. While performing atresia repair, the surgeon must exercise care in avoiding injury to this artery.

Becoming proficient with meatoplasty technique is crucial for ear surgeons who manage chronic ear disease. With proper technique, results should be predictable and reliable and the incidence of restenosis should be low. It is a common misconception that the ear canal is one-third cartilaginous and two-thirds bony. Anteriorly, the cartilage section is elongated, as it merges with the tragus, but posteriorly the conchal bowl sits directly on the mastoid meaning that the cartilaginous canal is composed only of the thickness of the conchal edge: a mere few millimeters.

Most bony ear canal surgery is done as an adjunct to chronic ear surgery. A narrow ear canal exacerbating chronic otitis media left uncorrected will hinder both surgical exposure and access for ongoing care. The most common surgery for primary ear canal disease is removal of exostoses, which tend to happen with repeated exposure to intermittent water immersion such as in surfing and kayaking. While most surgeons remove the exophytic bone with a drill, some experts use small chisels. Restoring patency to an obstructed ear canal can be dangerous as the facial nerve can be injured should the surgeon become disoriented to the alignment of the canal. The rule of thumb in both obstructing exostoses and cases of atresia is to always keep the deepest excavation superior (toward dura) and anterior (toward temporomandibular joint). Minor exposures of the temporomandibular joint capsule are of no consequence, but wide removal of this bony plate is best avoided.

When a very narrow ear canal is restored to normal size, it will not remain so unless there is adequate skin covering. This is especially important in congenital and acquired stenosis as well as in atresia. While small areas of exposed canal bone are common following chronic ear procedures, in cases of extensive osseous exposure, use of a thin split thickness skin graft is necessary. A caution is that full thickness or split thickness of excessive dermal thickness tends to undergo stenosis in ear canal repair. Also, a segment of ear canal which has been circumferentially denuded of its skin coverage is at a high risk of stenosis and should be grafted.

Further Reading

1. Barrett G, Ronan N, Cowan E, Flanagan P. To drill or to chisel? A long-term follow-up study of 92 exostectomy procedures in the UK. Laryngoscope 2015;125(2):453–456 PubMed
2. Brent B. Microtia repair with rib cartilage grafts: a review of personal experience with 1000 cases. Clin Plast Surg 2002;29 (2):257–271, vii PubMed
3. Chen Y, Zhang T. Modified meatoplasty for external auditory canal stenosis with endoaural-conchal incision. Otol Neurotol 2015;36(1):1–3 PubMed
4. Constantine KK, Gilmore J, Lee K, Leach J Jr. Comparison of microtia reconstruction outcomes using rib cartilage vs porous polyethylene implant. JAMA Facial Plast Surg 2014;16 (4):240–244 PubMed
5. Dedhia K, Yellon RF, Branstetter BF IV, Best M. External auditory canal: inferior, posterior-inferior, and anterior canal wall overhangs. Int J Pediatr Otorhinolaryngol 2018;109:138–143 PubMed
6. Firmin F, Dusseldorp J, Marchac A. Auricular Reconstruction. New York, NY: Thieme; 2017
7. Firmin F. State-of-the-art autogenous ear reconstruction in cases of microtia. Adv Otorhinolaryngol 2010;68:25–52 PubMed
8. Gandy JR, Lemieux B, Foulad A, Wong BJ. Modular component assembly approach to microtia reconstruction. JAMA Facial Plast Surg 2016;18(2):120–127 PubMed
9. Goldsztein H, Roberson JB Jr. Anatomical facial nerve findings in 209 consecutive atresia cases. Otolaryngol Head Neck Surg 2013;148(4):648–652 PubMed
10. Hetzler DG. Osteotome technique for removal of symptomatic ear canal exostoses. Laryngoscope 2007;117(1, Pt 2; Suppl 113):1–14 PubMed
11. Huang WJ, Chu CH, Wang MC, Kuo CL, Shiao AS. Decision making in the choice of surgical management for preauricular sinuses with different severities. Otolaryngol Head Neck Surg 2013;148(6):959–964 PubMed
12. Jahrsdoerfer RA, Lambert PR. Facial nerve injury in congenital aural atresia surgery. Am J Otol 1998;19(3):283–287 PubMed
13. Jahrsdoerfer RA, Yeakley JW, Aguilar EA, Cole RR, Gray LC. Grading system for the selection of patients with congenital aural atresia. Am J Otol 1992;13(1):6–12 PubMed
14. Lam HC, Soo G, Wormald PJ, Van Hasselt CA. Excision of the preauricular sinus: a comparison of two surgical techniques. Laryngoscope 2001;111(2):317–319 PubMed
15. Litton WB, Krause CJ, Anson BA, Cohen WN. The relationship of the facial canal to the annular sulcus. Laryngoscope 1969;79(9):1584–1604 PubMed
16. Moss WJ, Lin HW, Cueva RA. Surgical and audiometric outcomes for repair of congenital aural atresia and hypoplasia. JAMA Otolaryngol Head Neck Surg 2016;142(1):52–57 PubMed
17. Nagata S. A new method of total reconstruction of the auricle for microtia. Plast Reconstr Surg 1993;92(2):187–201 PubMed
18. Nguyen TB, Chin RY, Da Cruz M. The semi-lunar meatoplasty. Otol Neurotol 2014;35(7):e208–e210 PubMed
19. Patil S, Ahmed J, Patel N. Endaural meatoplasty: the Whipps Cross technique. J Laryngol Otol 2011;125(1):78–81 PubMed
20. Stephan S, Reinisch J. Auricular reconstruction using porous polyethylene implant technique. Facial Plast Surg Clin North Am 2018;26(1):69–85 PubMed
21. Yeo SW, Jun BC, Park SN, et al. The preauricular sinus: factors contributing to recurrence after surgery. Am J Otolaryngol 2006;27(6):396–400 PubMed

3.2 Otoplasty

Sam P. Most

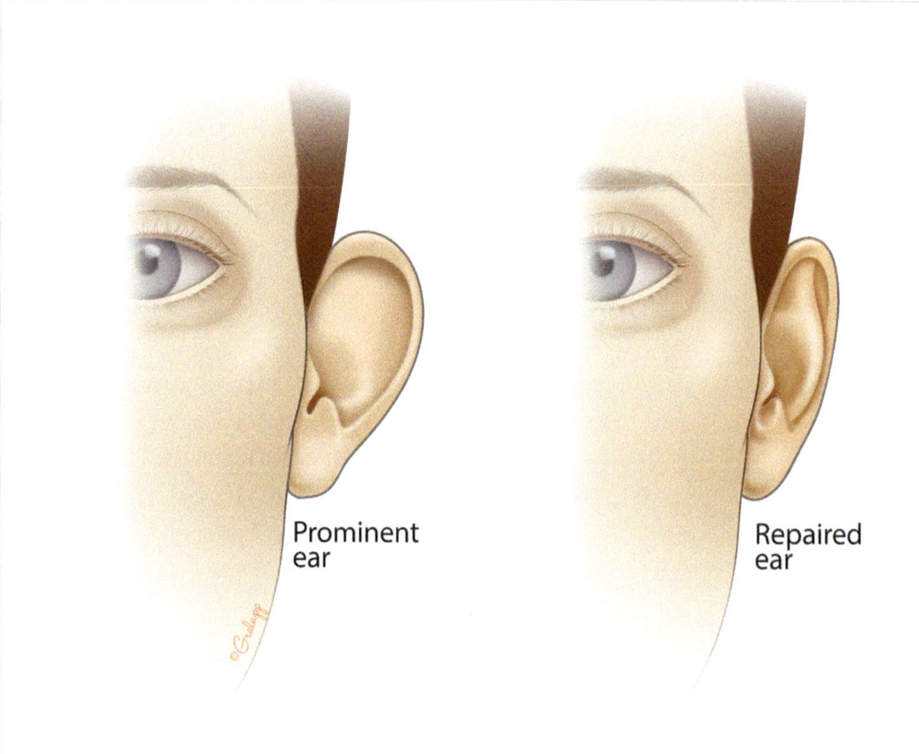

Fig. 3.1 A prominent ear can be caused by lack of an antihelical fold or prominence of the conchal cartilage, or both. Otoplasty can be used to correct both of these, resulting in a less prominent pinna on frontal view.

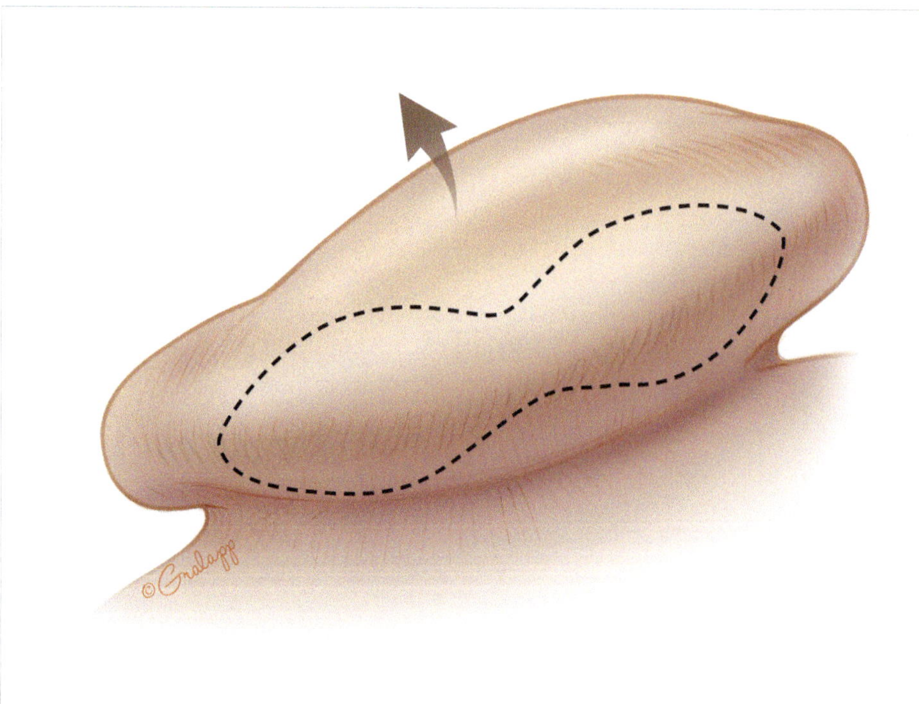

Fig. 3.2 The posterior skin excision is done in elliptical fashion. This helps reduce posterior tethering in the midportion of the pinna, which can contribute to a "telephone ear" deformity.

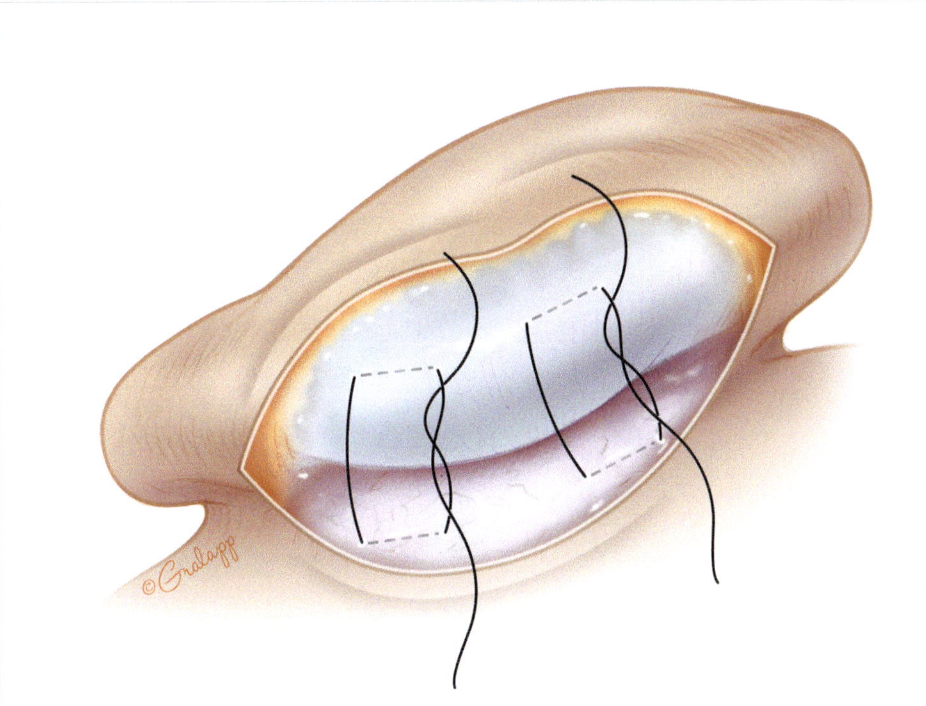

Fig. 3.3 Transcutaneous black nylon sutures are placed to create the superior antihelical fold. These are typically 5-mm wide and separated by 1 cm. The width and tension of the mattress sutures will cause variation in acuity of the antihelical fold.

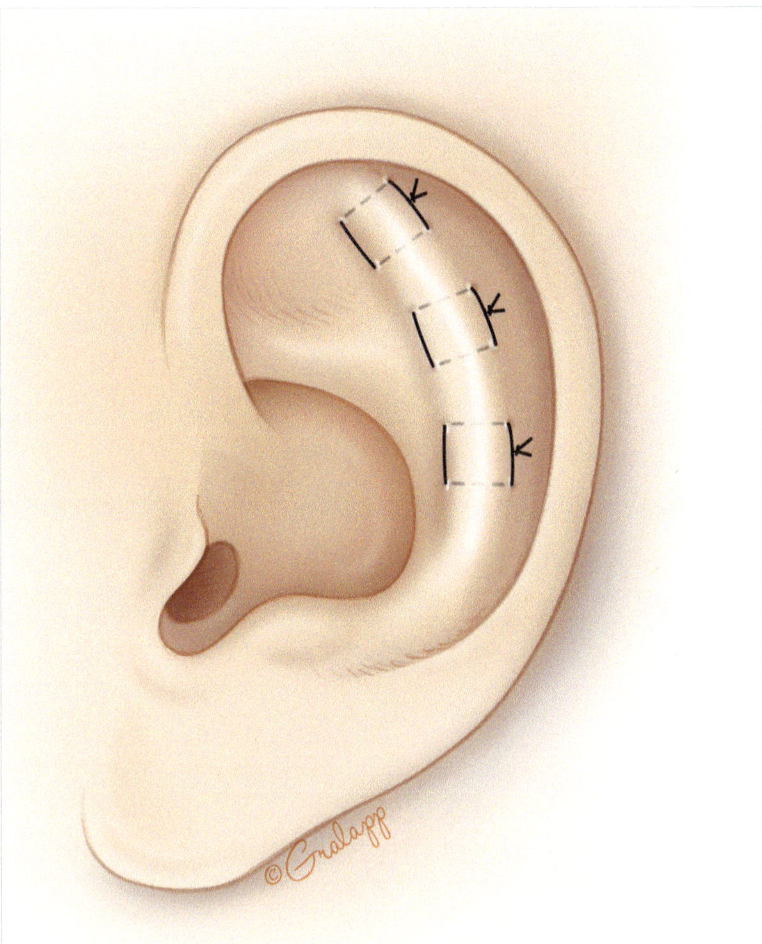

Fig. 3.4 The ear is reflected anteriorly, and the black sutures visualized. Clear nylon mattress sutures are then placed according to the method of Mustardé. Care is taken to avoid violation of the anterior auricular skin.

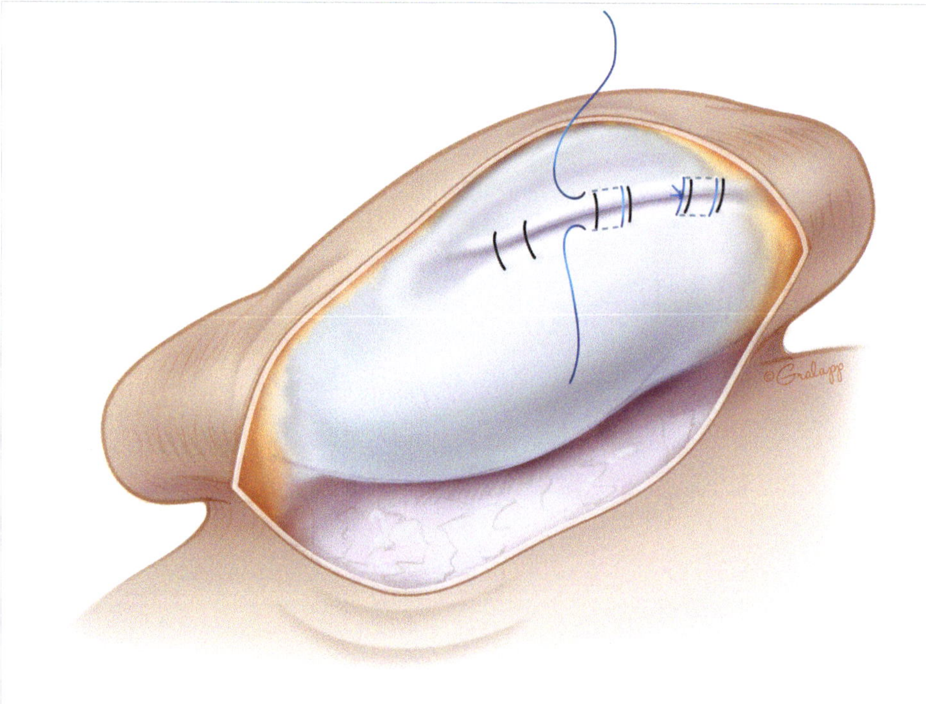

Fig. 3.5 An axial view of pinna demonstrating temporary and permanent suture placement to create the antihelical fold. Note that the permanent suture (shown here in blue) does not violate the skin anteriorly, but does penetrate the perichondrium.

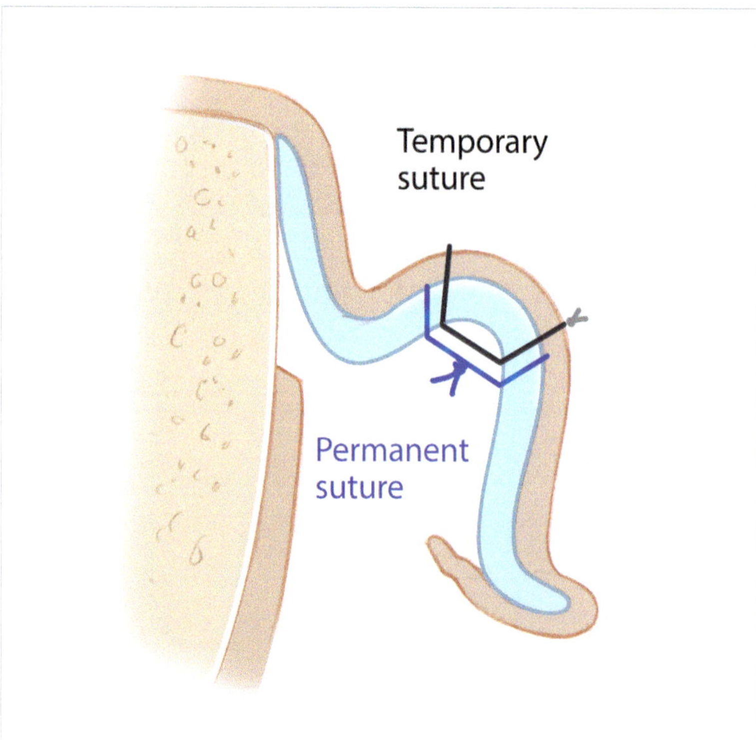

Fig. 3.6 Two permanent mattress sutures are placed through the auricular cartilage and anterior perichondrium, with care taken to avoid violation of the skin, using the method of Furnas. These are then secured to the mastoid periosteum. Anterior displacement of the conchal cartilage is avoided by placing these sutures posteriorly on the mastoid.

3.3 Microtia Repair

Mai Thy Truong and Kay W. Chang

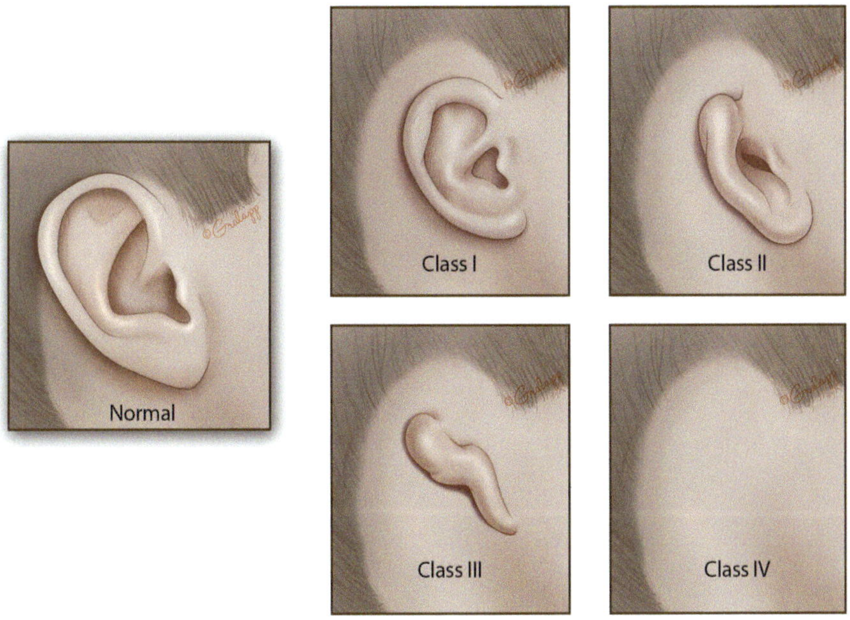

Fig. 3.7 The classes of microtia according to pinna size and subunits affected. For the purpose of this classification, the subunits of the pinna are helix, antihelix, scapha, tragus, antitragus, concha, and lobule. Class 1: a small ear with all of the subunits present, although some may be abnormally shaped; Class 2: a small ear with missing subunits; Class 3: a classic peanut ear with no recognizable subunits except for the lobule; Class 4: anotia (the complete absence of a pinna). Microtia surgery involves multiple stages. Some surgeons employ two stages, others employ three or more. Stages are usually spaced by 3 to 4 months at a minimum. In this chapter, we illustrate a two-staged technique as described by Dr. Francoise Firmin. Foundations from Dr. Burt Brent's four-staged technique and Dr. Satoru Nagata's two-staged technique can be appreciated.

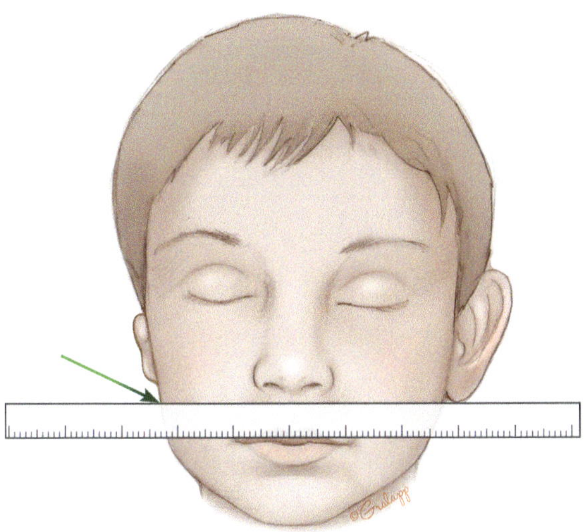

Fig. 3.8 Stage 1 initiates with planning the placement of the reconstructed ear. Standing at the head of the bed, a ruler is used to mark the inferior point of the lobule in symmetry with the nonmicrotia ear. In bilateral microtia, the commissures of the eye and mouth are used as reference points, with the new pinna placed as high as permitted by the demarcation of non–hair-bearing retroauricular skin.

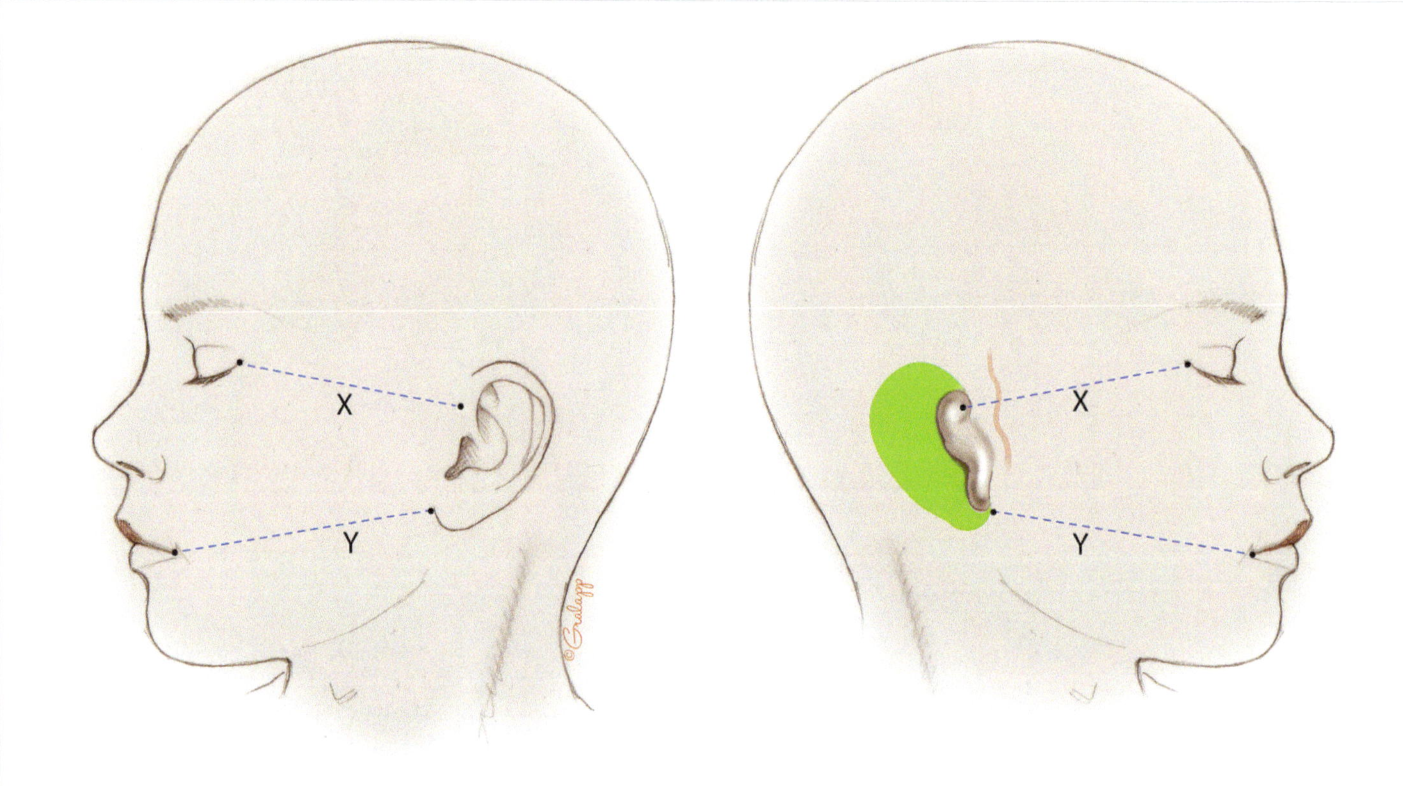

Fig. 3.9 The distances from the lateral canthus of the eye to the root of the helix (X), and the lateral commissure of the mouth and the anterior point of the lobule (Y), are measured on the unaffected side. These measurements are used for placement of the reconstructed ear. The superficial temporal artery is identified with Doppler and marked.

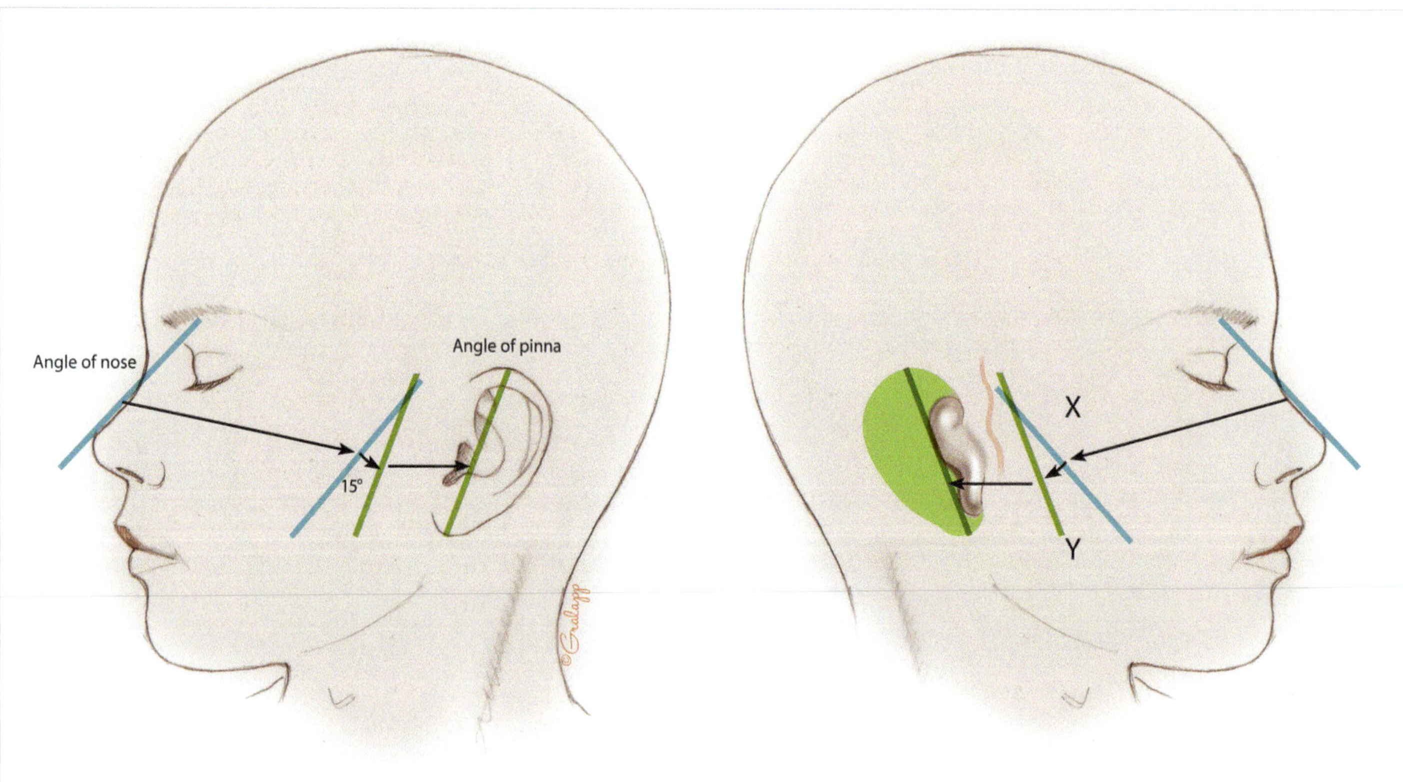

Fig. 3.10 The rotation of the ear. The pinna has a polarity, or an axis of rotation. First, on the nonmicrotia side, the slope of the nose is drawn on the face, and the angle of the pinna is drawn, as determined by the longest measurement of the pinna. The angle between these is measured. On the microtia side, the slope of the nose is repeated, the angle is measured, and the axis of the reconstructed ear is drawn on the face. This becomes a guide for the planned rotation of the reconstructed ear.

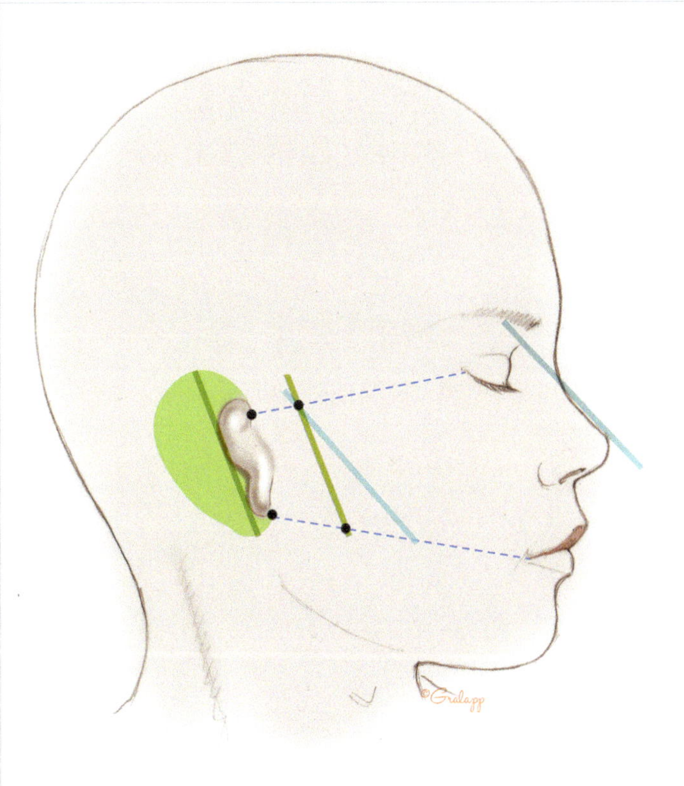

Fig. 3.11 Markings for the planned placement of the reconstructed ear are kept in view throughout the procedure.

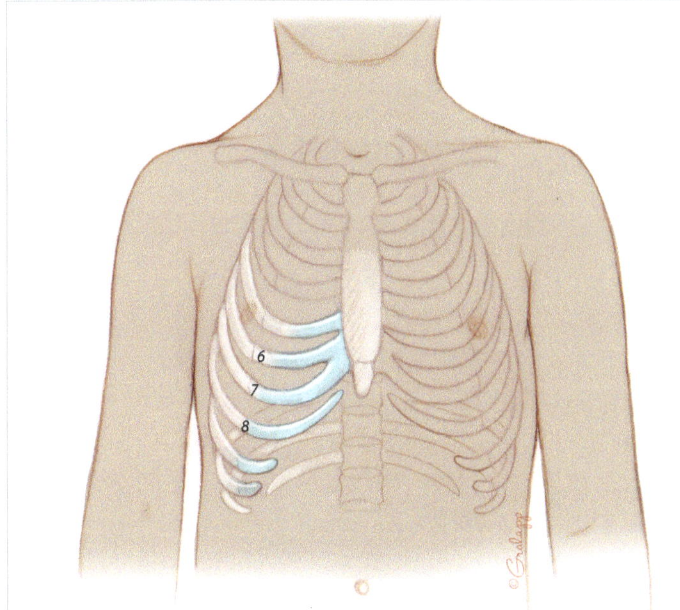

Fig. 3.12 Harvest of rib cartilage is planned from the sixth to ninth cartilage. The ninth cartilage is obtained when prominent. In this technique, cartilage is harvested from the ipsilateral side of the microtia ear.

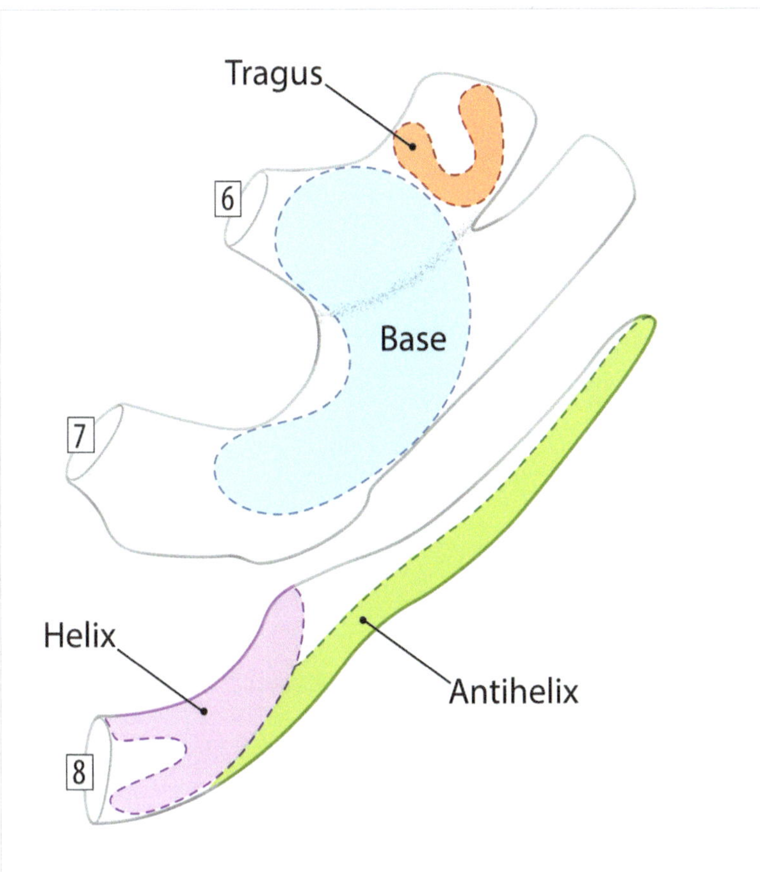

Fig. 3.13 The typical plan for the harvested cartilage for microtia reconstruction of the left ear: The floating eighth rib often serves as the helical rim and, when robust, can also be used for the antihelix. The synchondrosis of the sixth and seventh ribs often provides the base plate. Extra pieces of cartilage serve to become the P1 (Projection 1) piece as described by Dr. Firmin, and banked pieces for the elevation of the ear in the second stage. Banked cartilage pieces are placed in a pocket of the subcutaneous skin of the chest closure secured to the dermis.

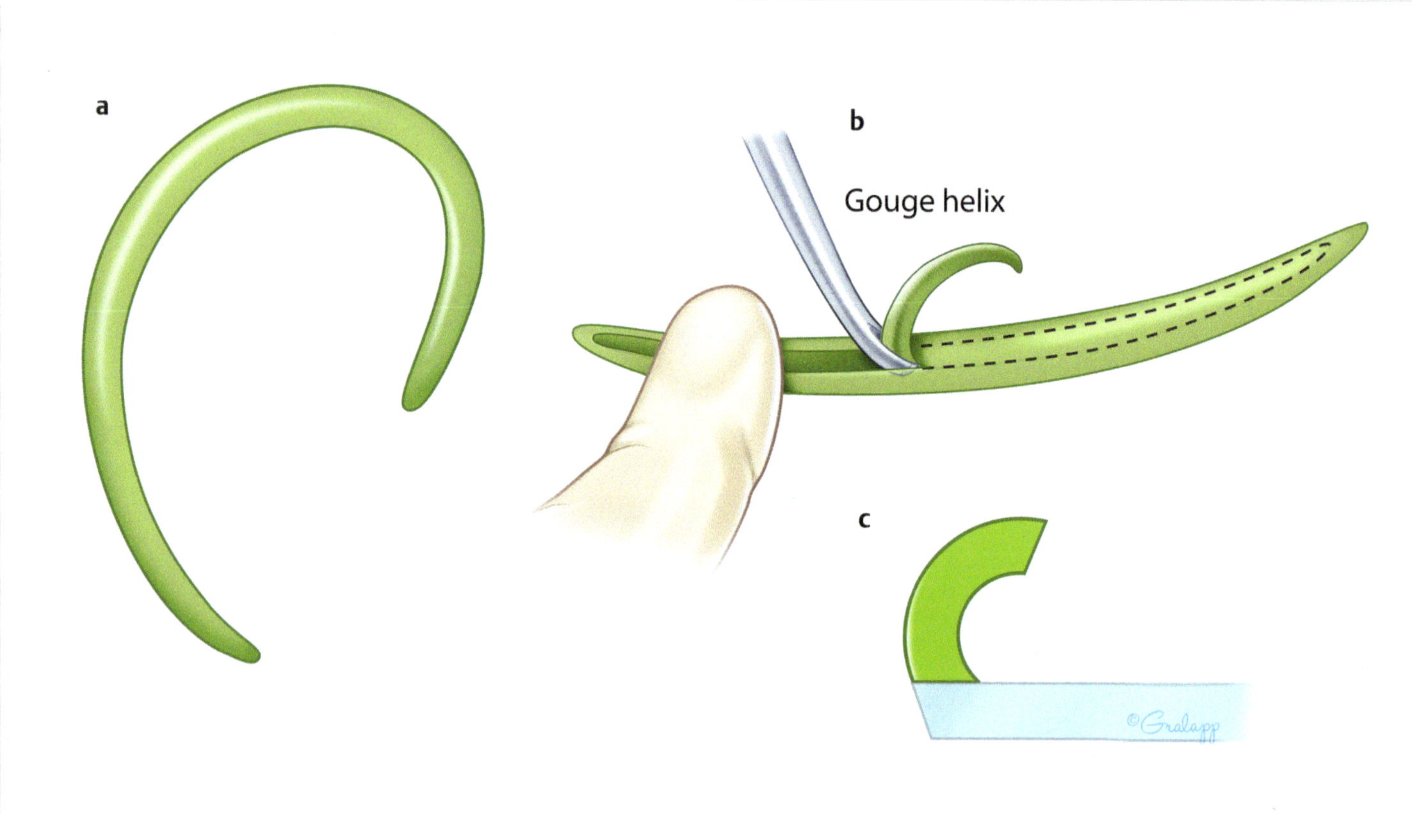

Fig. 3.14 The helix is often carved from the eighth rib cartilage, and is shaped to sit flat on the base plate. The center is gouged to create a curved surface and allow for ease of curvature.

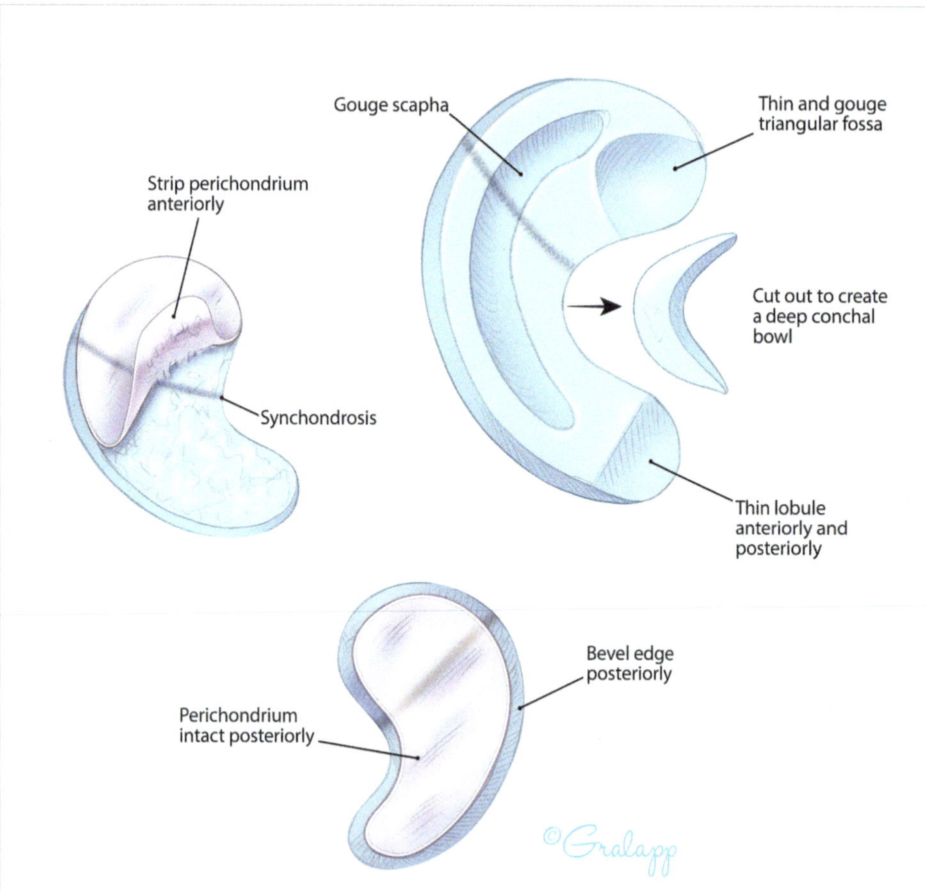

Fig. 3.15 The base plate is prepared by removing the perichondrium on the anterior surface. It is kept intact on the posterior surface. Often, marks are made on the cartilage to delineate the placement of the antihelix and the scapha in the correct orientation. This can be done by inking the cartilage based on a drawing of the opposite ear drawn on X-ray film. The X-ray film is then flipped to show the mirror image, and drawn on paper. The paper is then dipped in water-soluble ink, and stamped on the cartilage. Carving begins with reducing the lobule and gouging the scapha. Then, the triangular fossa can be deepened. Posteriorly, the edge of the cartilage is beveled so that the back surface of the ear is sloped.

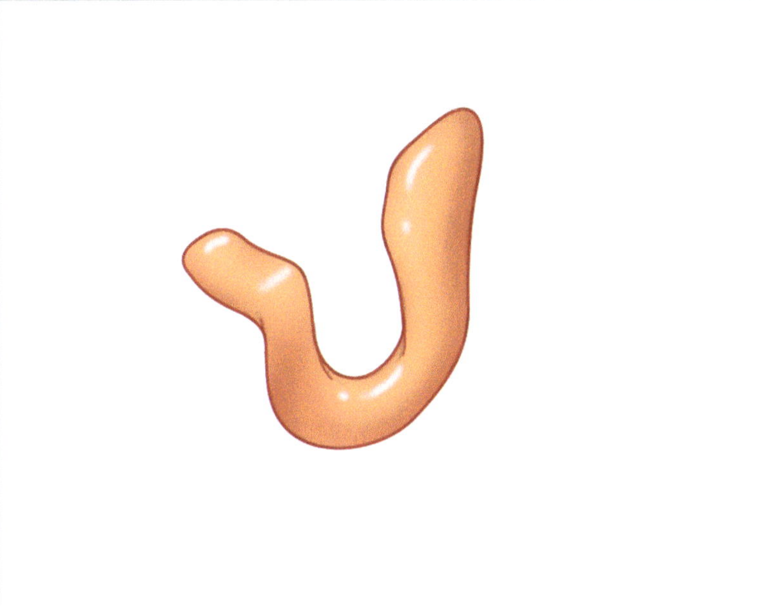

Fig. 3.16 The tragus–antitragus complex is a challenging three-dimensional entity that has convexities and concavities. The intertragal notch is the thinnest portion.

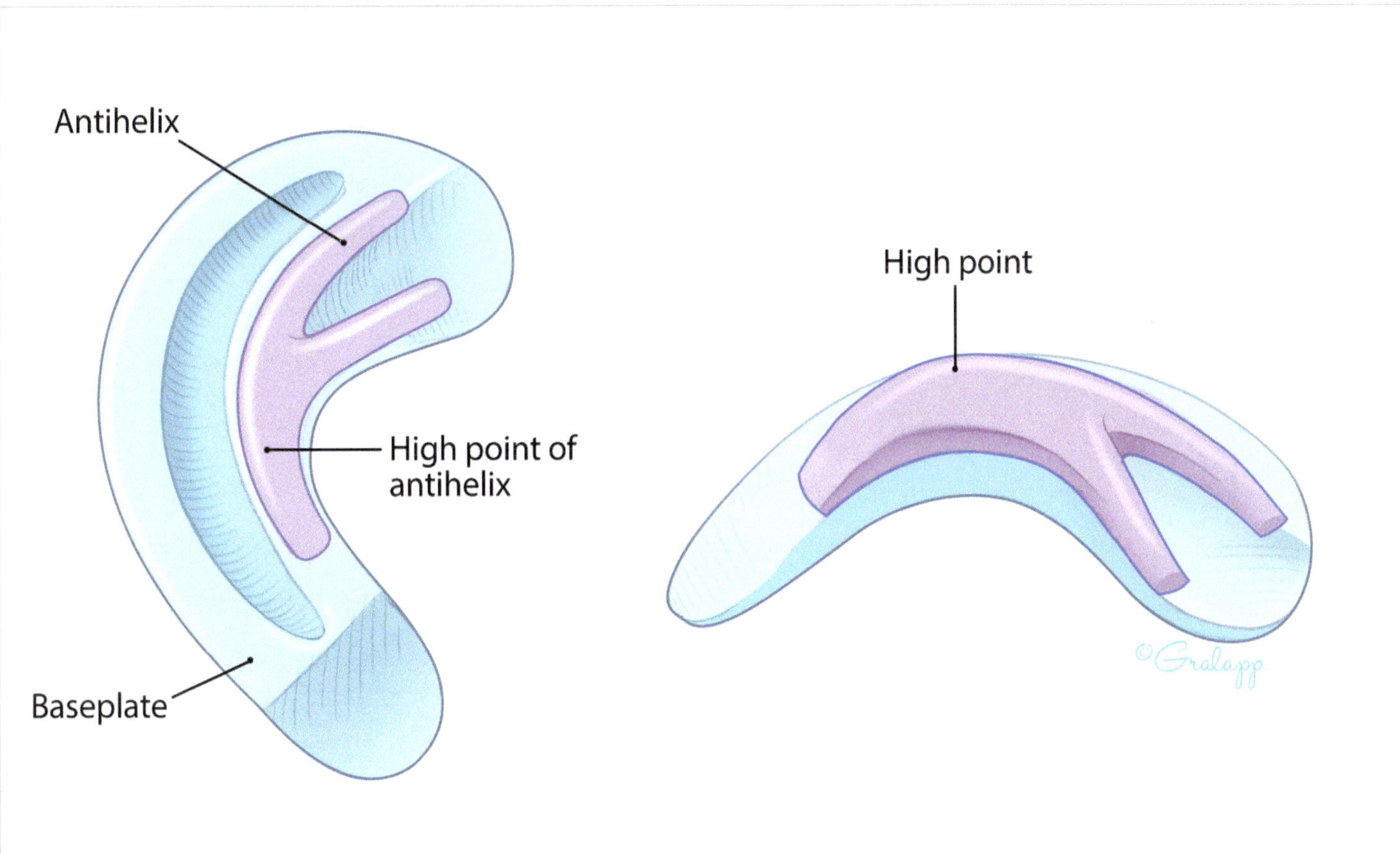

Fig. 3.17 The antihelix is first to be placed on the baseplate.

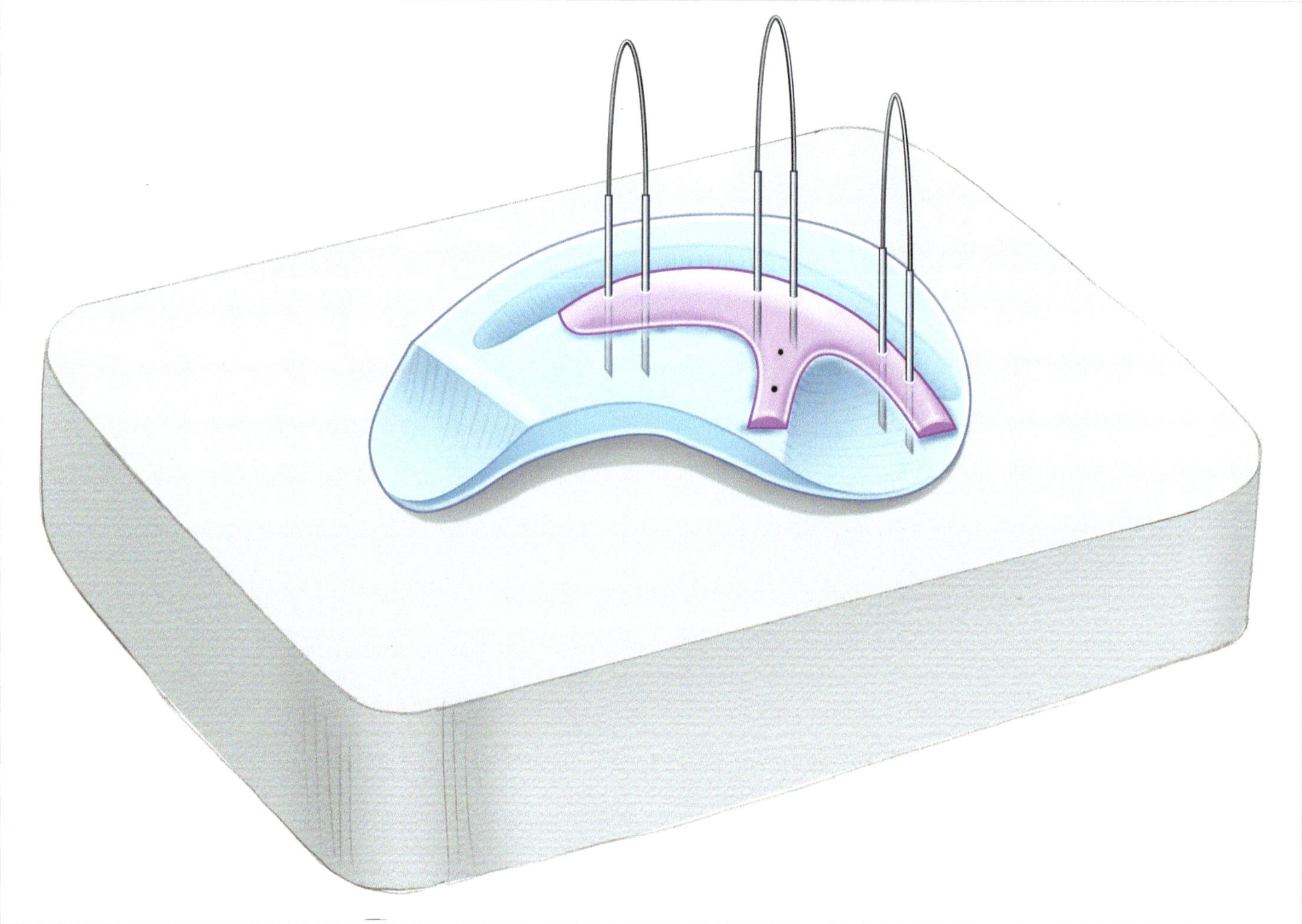

Fig. 3.18 A silicone block is used to secure the cartilage as the individual pieces are constructed together. Double-ended 5.0-steel sutures are used to suture the cartilage. Steel suture is preferred to prevent future migration of cartilage pieces when exposed the tensile strength of the skin. Double-ended steel sutures can be made by hand threading 5.0-steel wire through the eyelet of small, straight cutting needles.

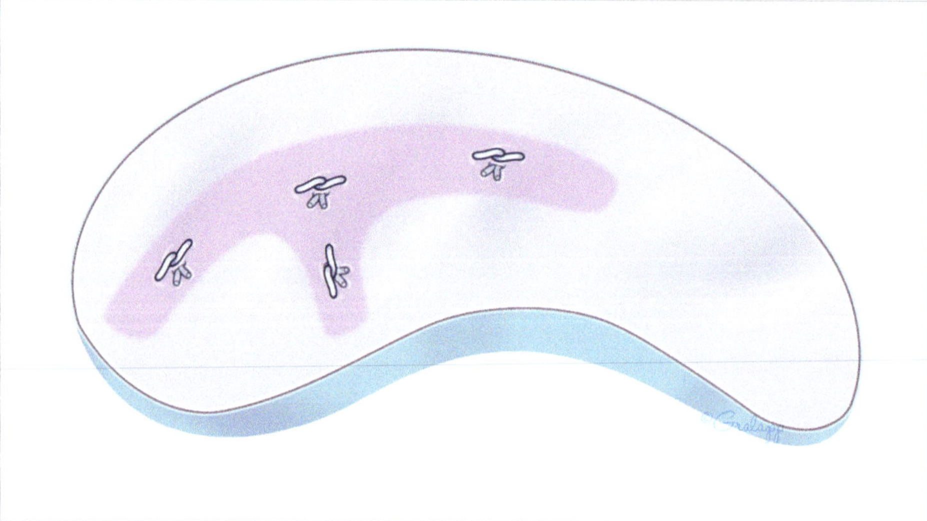

Fig. 3.19 View of the undersurface: the cartilage construct is lifted away from the silicone block, the needles cut, and the wire sutures are twisted together, trimmed, and ends turned down onto the undersurface of the cartilage. As each cartilage piece is added to the construct, the silicone block provides the stability needed for suturing.

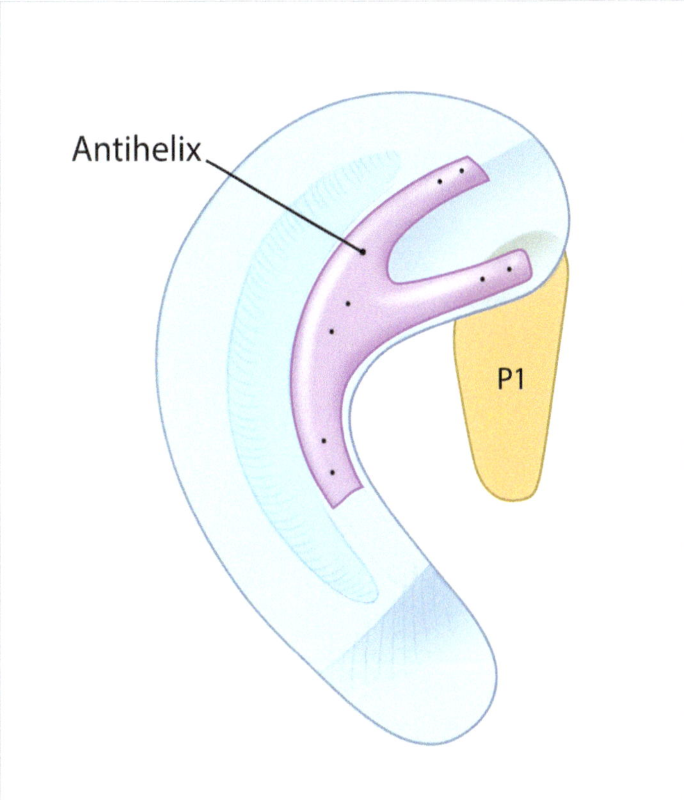

Fig. 3.20 Once the antihelix is placed, the P1 piece is secured to the baseplate in preparation for the helix. The P1 piece allows for the crus of the helix to drop to a lower plane while providing stabilization to the curve of the helix.

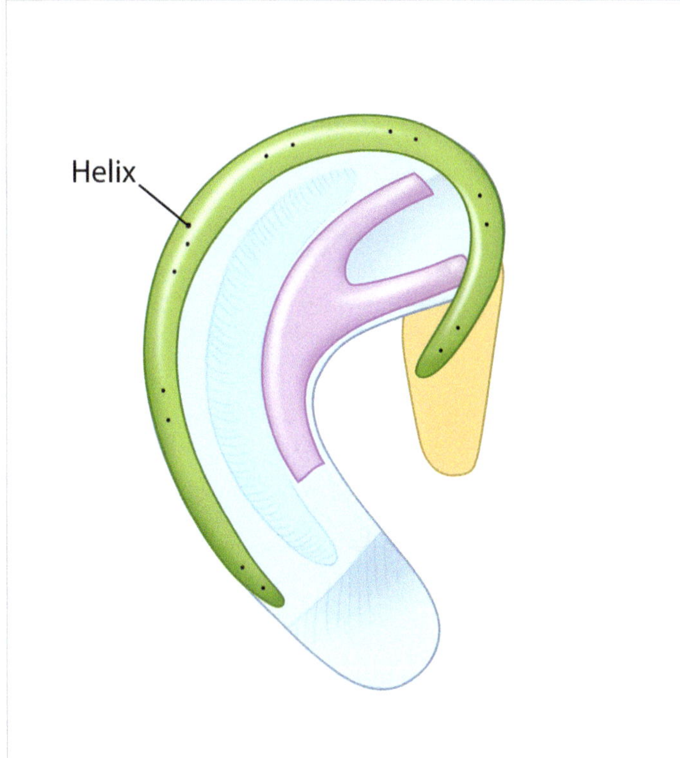

Fig. 3.21 The helix is then secured with steel sutures.

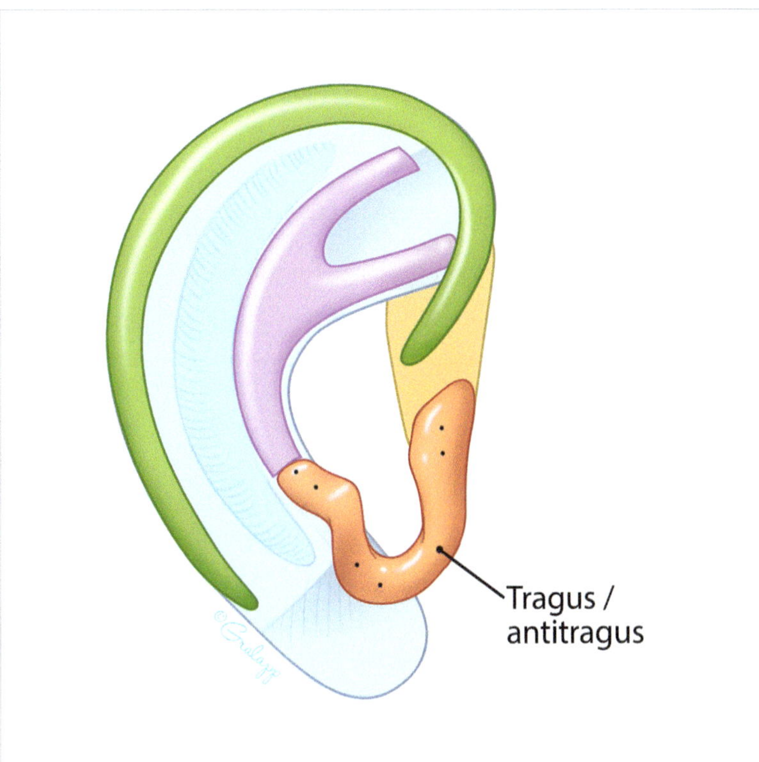

Fig. 3.22 The tragus–antitragus complex is placed and secured to the baseplate and the P1 elevation piece.

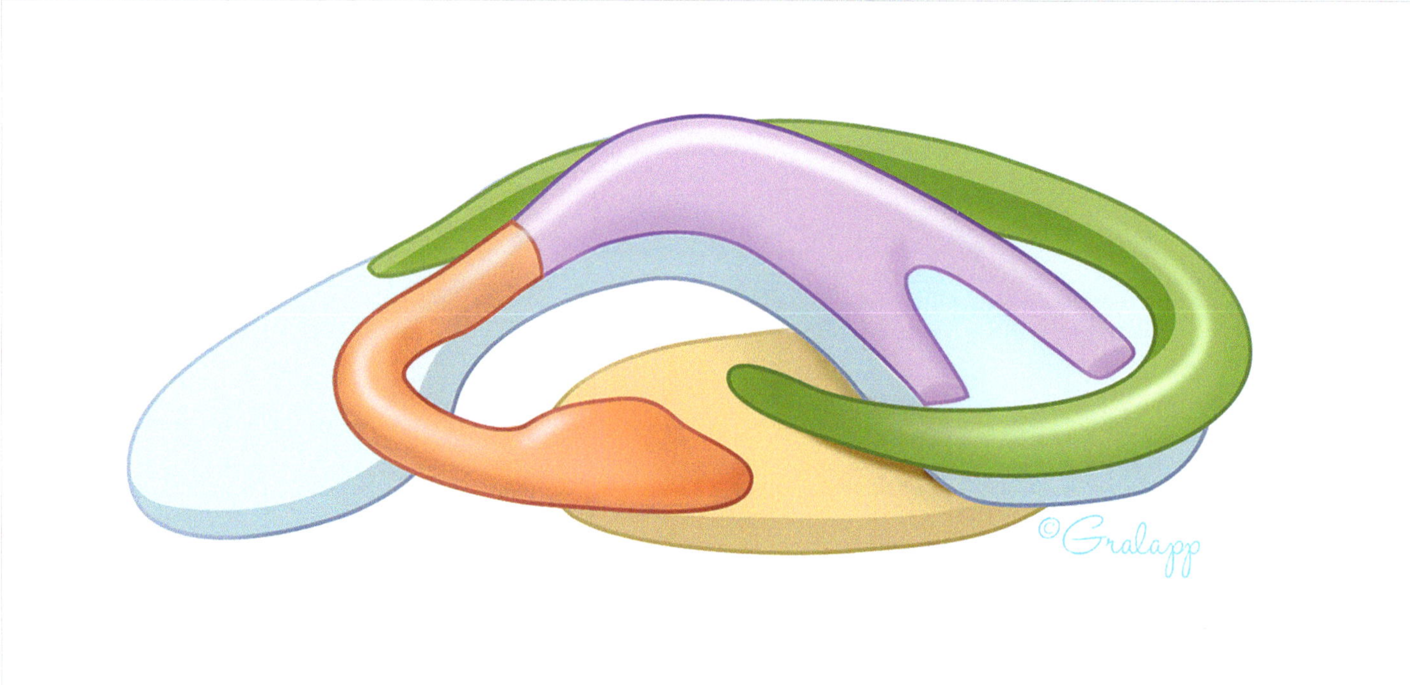

Fig. 3.23 An anterior view allows appreciation of the appropriate contours of the ear construct.

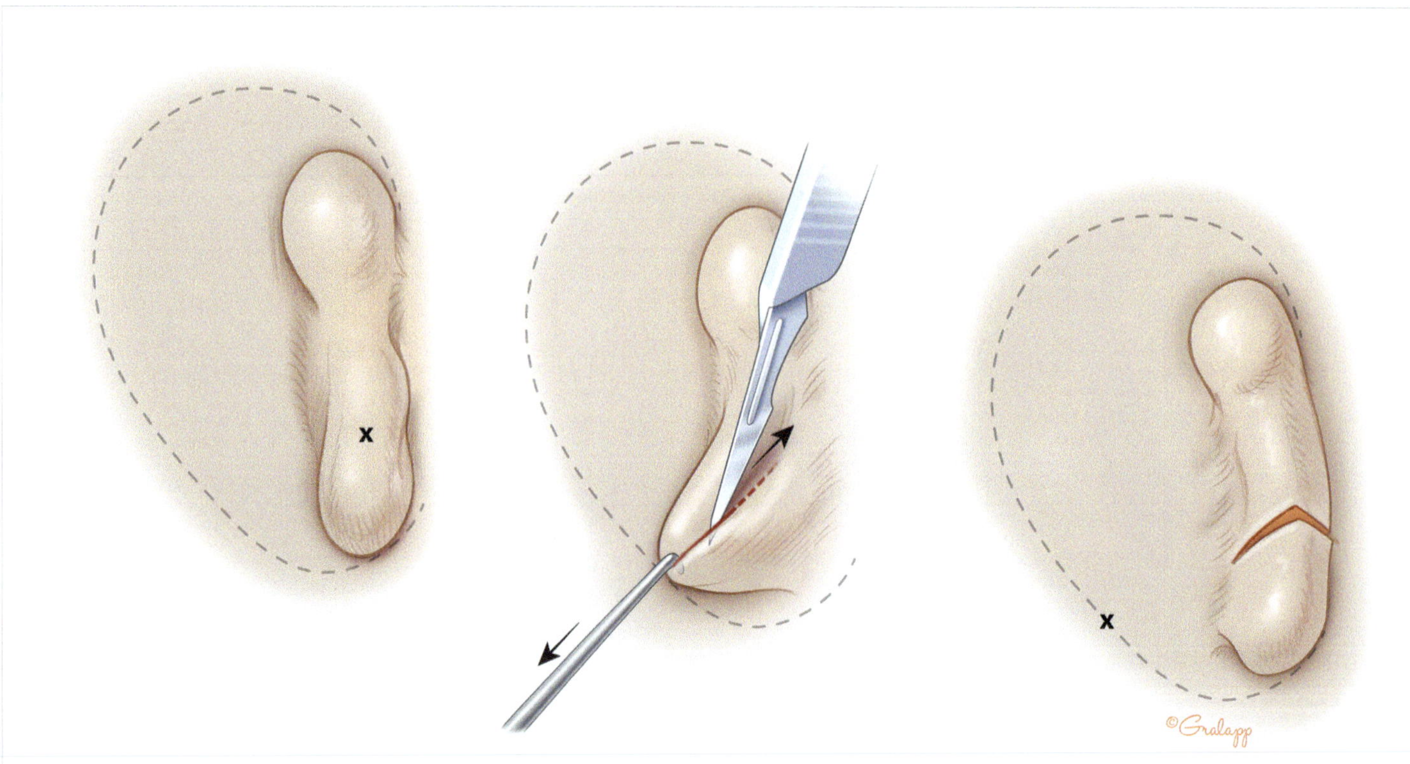

Fig. 3.24 Preparation of the skin for a type 2 skin approach as described by Dr. Firmin. This approach is often chosen for class 3 microtia when the inferior portion of the microtia remnant will be used to make the lobule of the new pinna. With the planned outline for the ear reconstruction drawn relative to the microtia ear, the ear is pulled until a natural point is found where the lobule meets the planned incision with the least amount of tension on the remnant. This is where the lobule will be transposed. The X marks the point where the lobular skin meets the planned point of transposition.

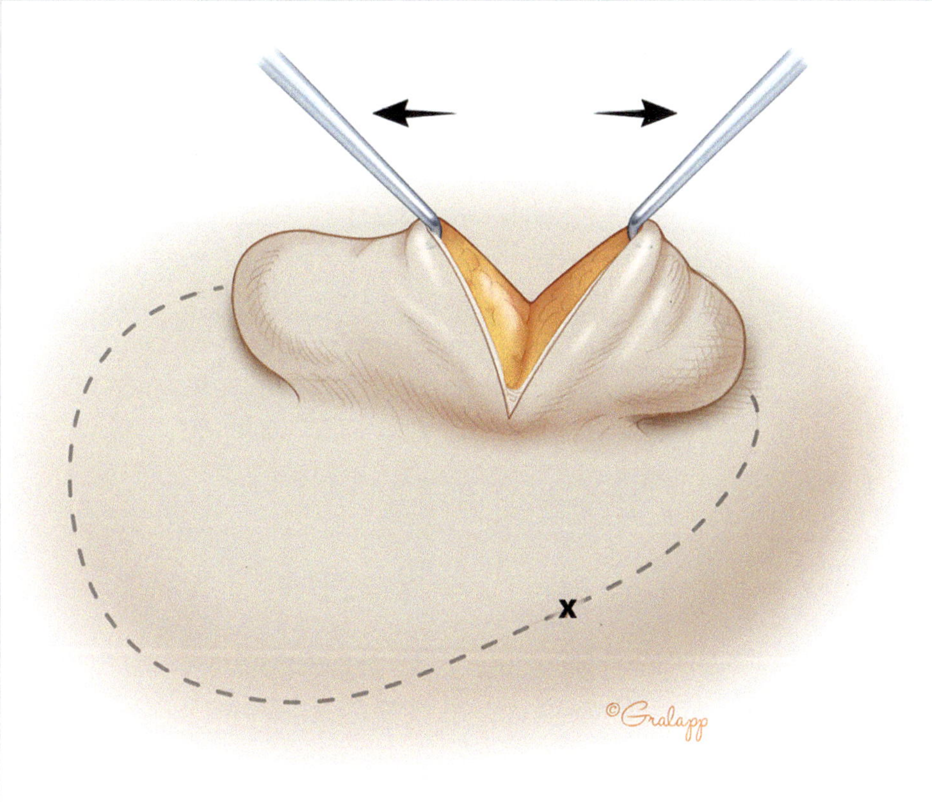

Fig. 3.25 The skin is then divided and a pocket is dissected in the lobule to allow insertion of the cartilage framework. Best results are obtained when the cartilage inserts well into the lobule, near the tip.

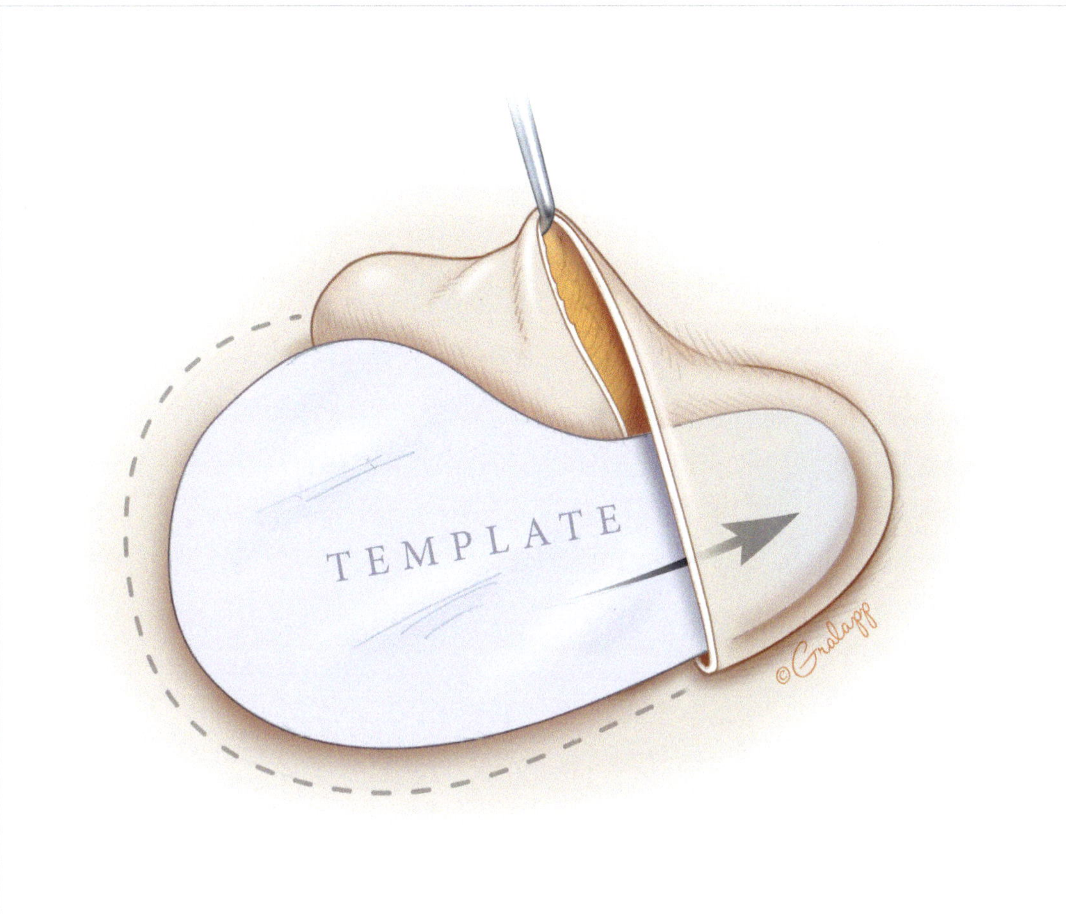

Fig. 3.26 As the lobule is turned to its new location, an X-ray template of the base plate can be used to check the insertion of the lobule.

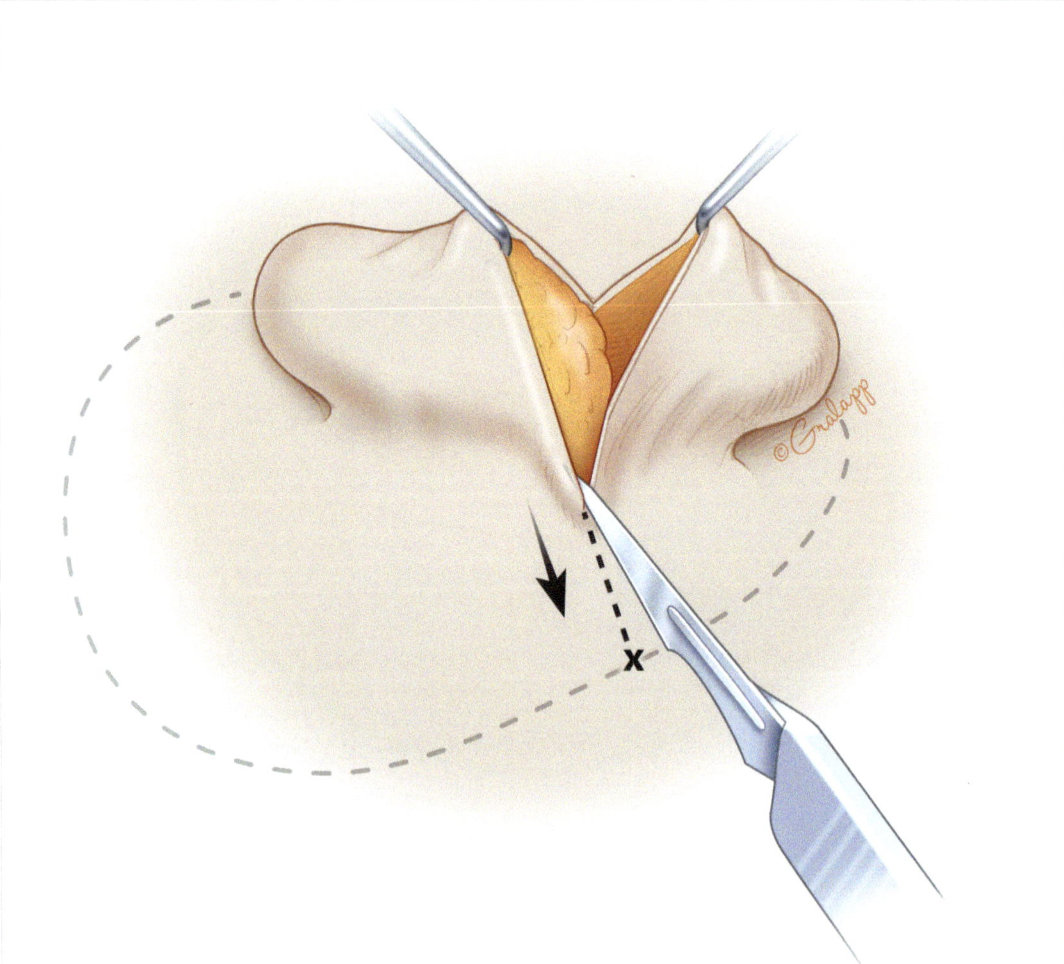

Fig. 3.27 The posterior skin is incised to allow the transposition of the lobule to the new location.

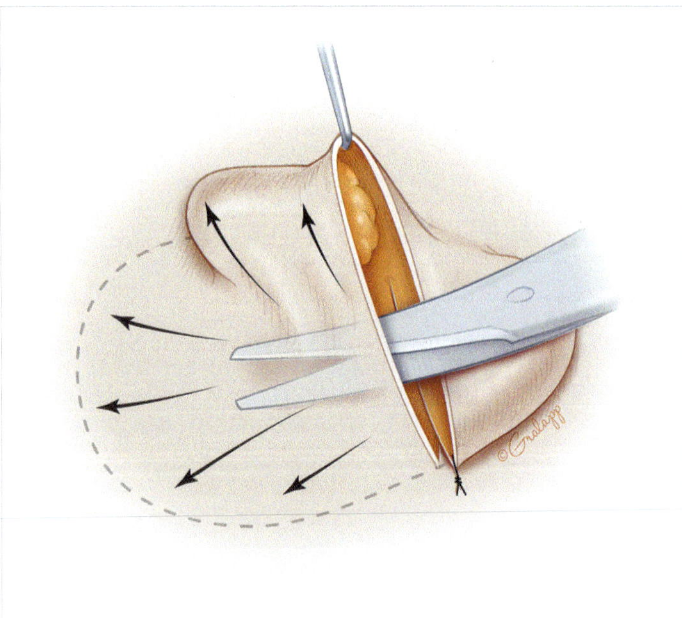

Fig. 3.28 The retroauricular skin is then dissected, and the cartilage remnant is removed from the microtia ear. This skin will drape over the cartilage construct, so care must be used to maintain the skin vascularity and the same thickness throughout.

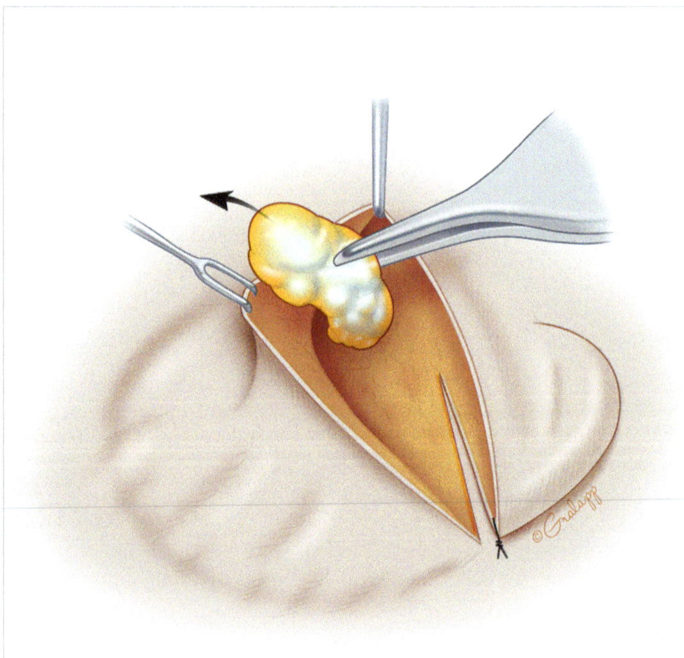

Fig. 3.29 The cartilage remnant is removed. In many cases, dissection of the cartilage remnant is not a trivial dissection and requires a meticulous degloving of the cartilage while maintaining skin flap integrity and vascularity.

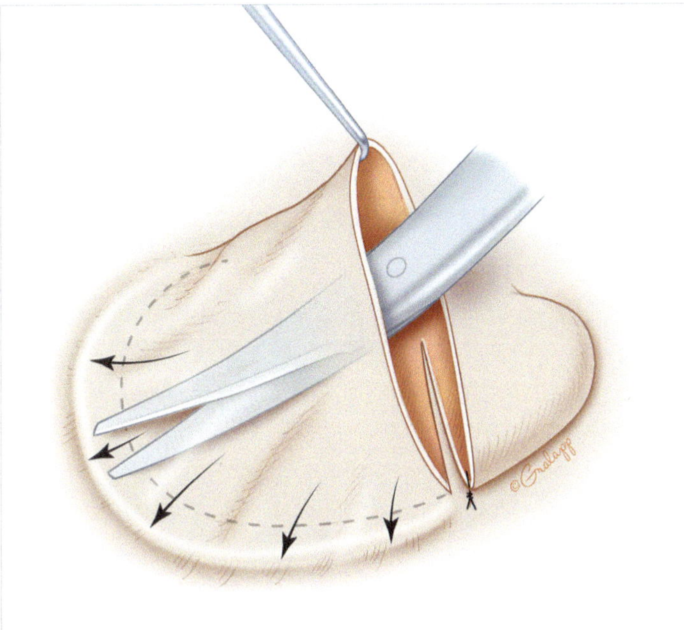

Fig. 3.30 Skin dissection must go beyond the planed placement of the ear to allow for the skin to drape over the contours of the construct, and allow for placement of a posterior drain.

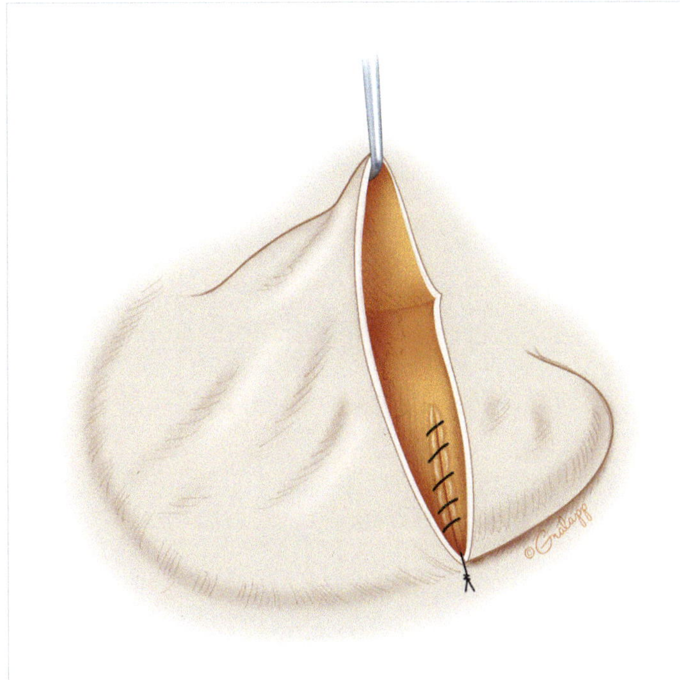

Fig. 3.31 The transposed lobule is then sutured in place posteriorly, known as the "adhesion of the lobule," with a 4-0 absorbable suture.

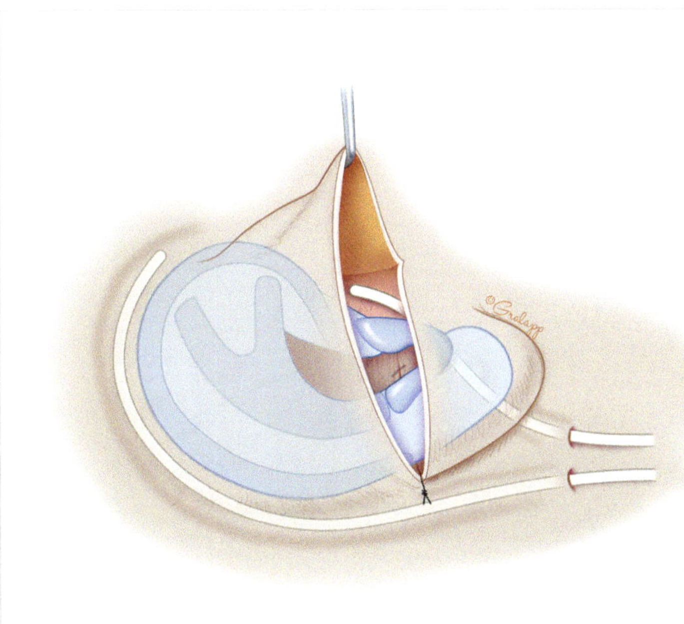

Fig. 3.32 The cartilage construct is inserted into the lobule and placed under the skin. Drains are placed anteriorly and posteriorly to allow suction of the skin to aid resection of excess skin. Typically, 10F Blake drains are used, under low suction, classically maintaining suction with test tubes.

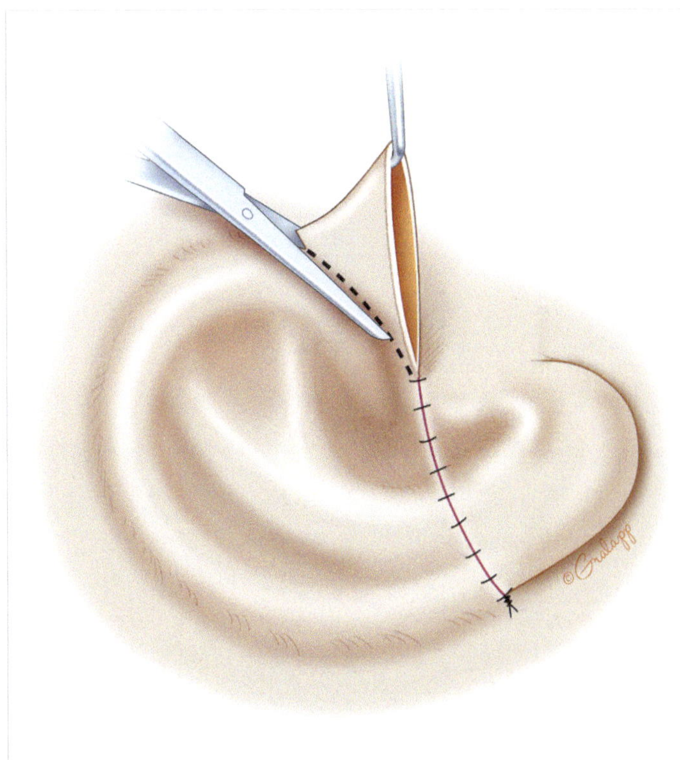

Fig. 3.33 Excess skin is excised. Incisions are hidden in the natural junction of subunits, and trifurcations of the closure are avoided if possible.

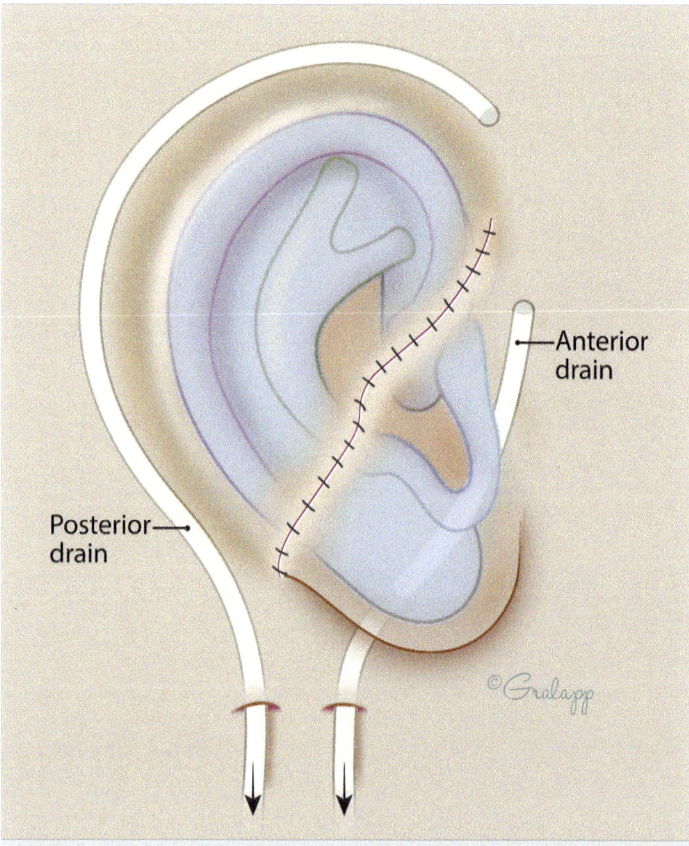

Fig. 3.34 The skin is closed with 6.0 nylon sutures, and the drains are kept to suction for 3 to 5 days. Postoperatively, test tubes are changed every 3 to 4 hours to maintain suction while the construct heals.

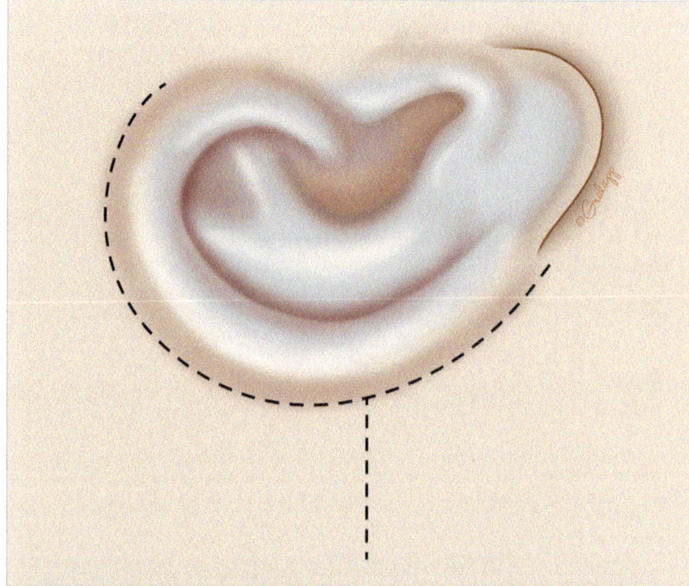

Fig. 3.35 Stage 2: elevation of the ear. The initial step of stage 2 involves planning the retroauricular incision. Care must be taken to be off the edge of the cartilage framework. A releasing incision is designed to allow advancement of the retroauricular skin.

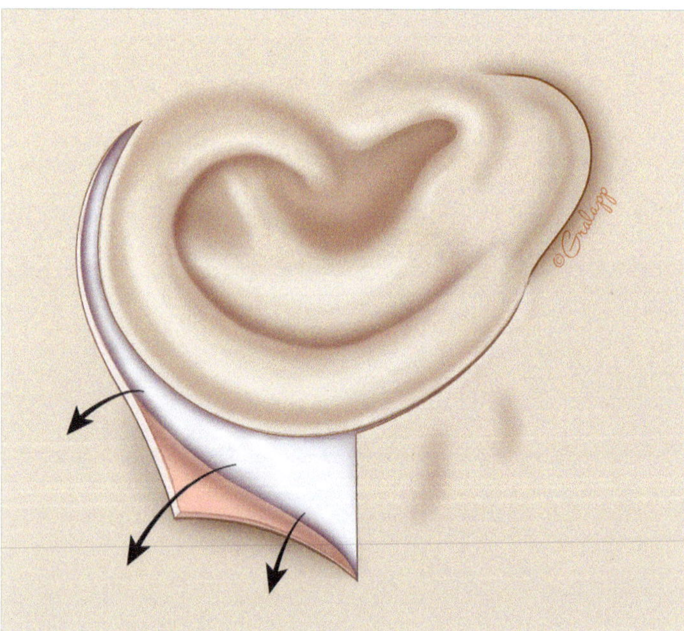

Fig. 3.36 Elevation of the superior flap. It is essential to elevate only skin and leave the fascia and periosteum overlying the cortex intact.

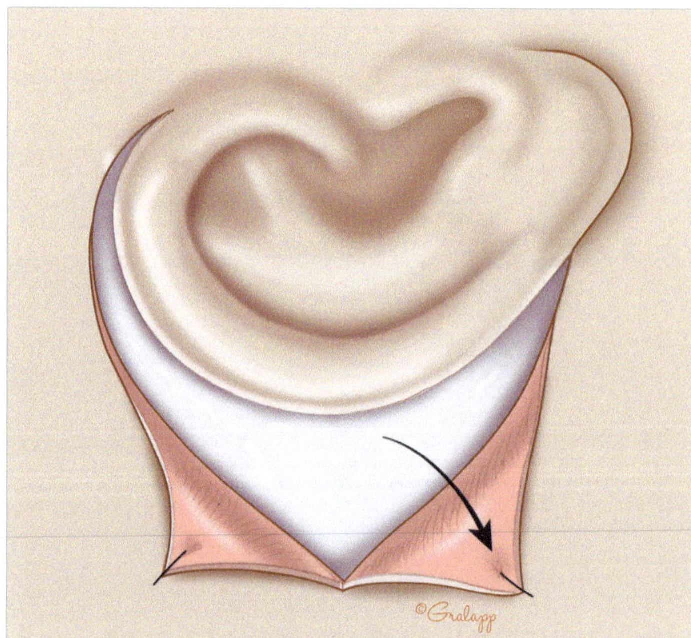

Fig. 3.37 Elevation of the inferior flap. At this step, the areolar tissue overlying the mastoid can be thinned to deepen the sulcus.

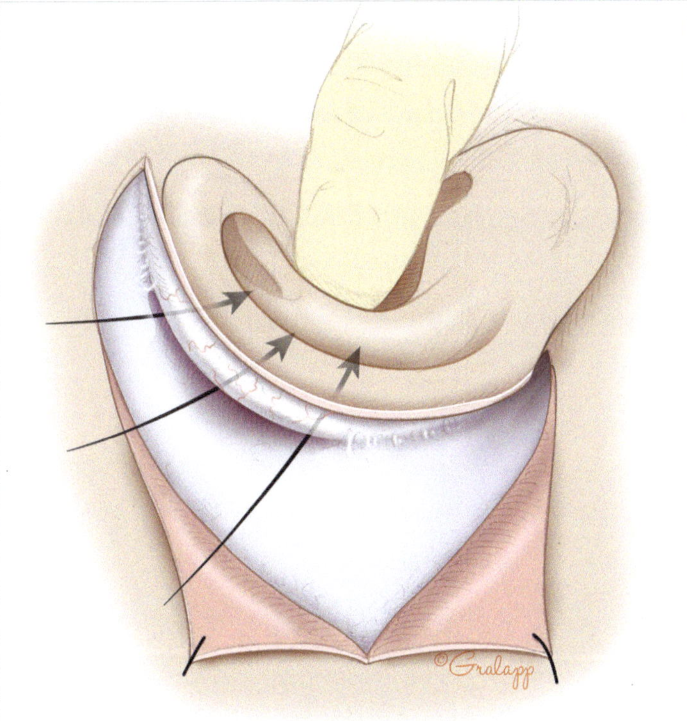

Fig. 3.38 In preparation for creation of a postauricular sulcus, the auricular construct is elevated. It is essential not to interrupt the enveloping tissue surrounding the cartilage. Any exposure of cartilage will likely lead to wound dehiscence, as the skin graft will not integrate with the cartilage.

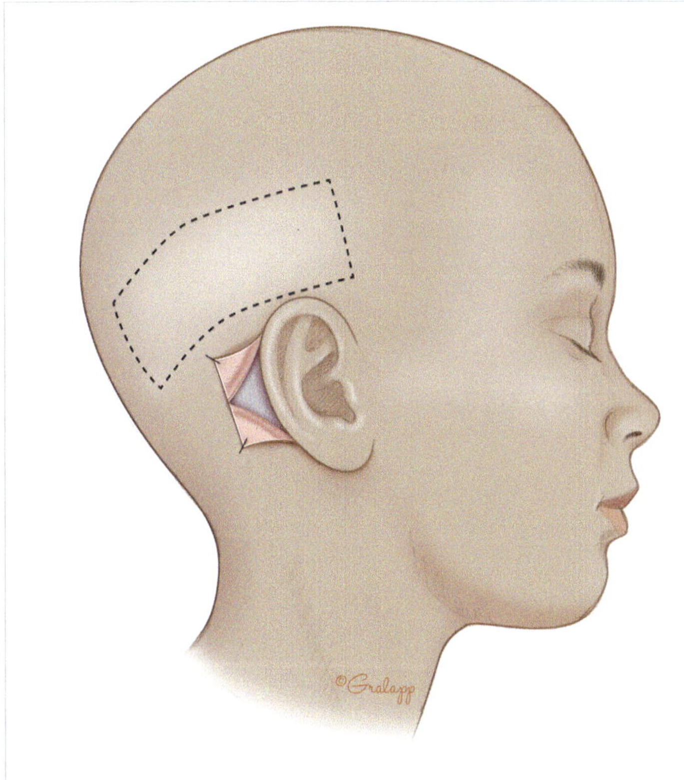

Fig. 3.39 A thin split-thickness skin graft (STSG) is harvested from the hair-bearing scalp as this yields the best texture and color match for the ear. In addition, the donor site will be hidden by hair growth. The typical graft measurement is 5 × 10 cm. Some surgeons harvest skin grafts from the abdomen, groin, arm, or thigh. The graft must be cleaned of hair with gentle wipes from a wet gauze.

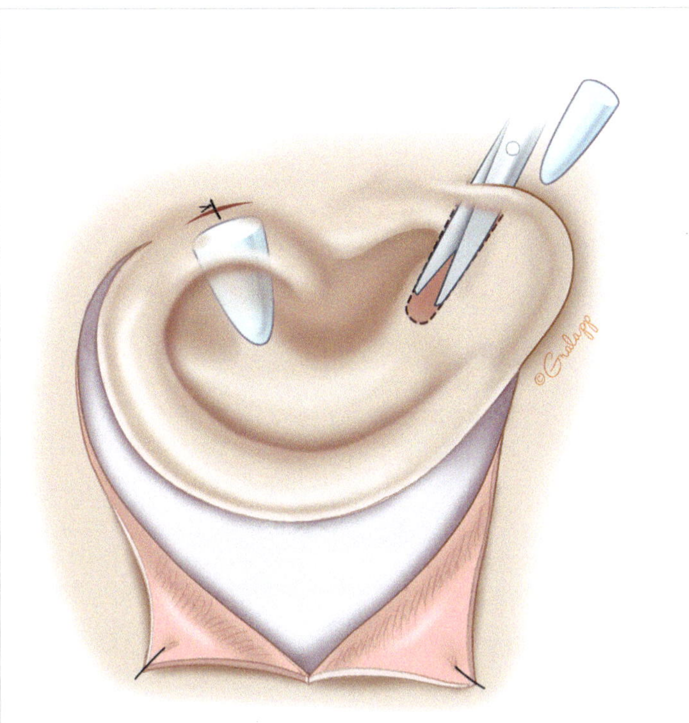

Fig. 3.40 Projection of the ear is achieved through cartilage placed in tunnels, a Type D elevation technique as described by Dr. Firmin. Additionally, cartilage can be tunneled under the antihelix to deepen the conchal bowl (not shown here). This cartilage was banked in a subcutaneous pocket of the chest site during stage 1 and reopened in stage 2.

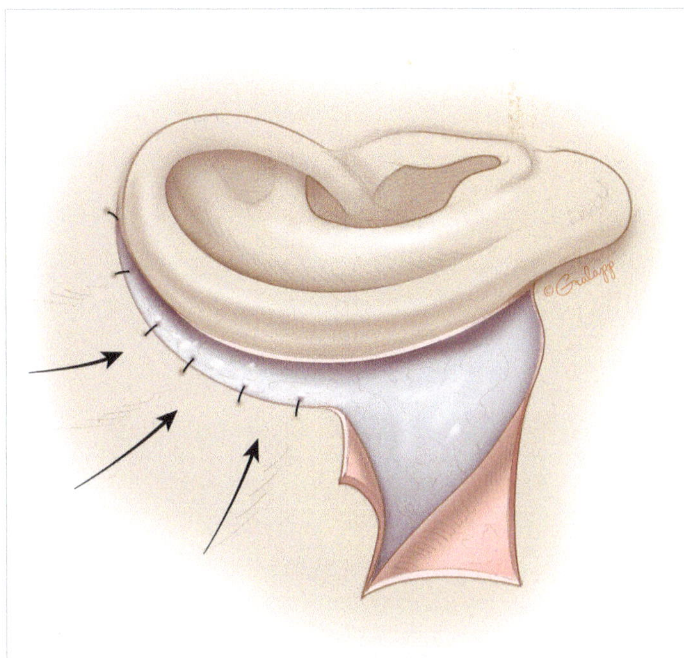

Fig. 3.41 To position the incision behind the pinna and to reduce the size of the skin graft needed, the retroauricular skin flap is advanced and tacked down to the mastoid fascia using 4-0 absorbable suture.

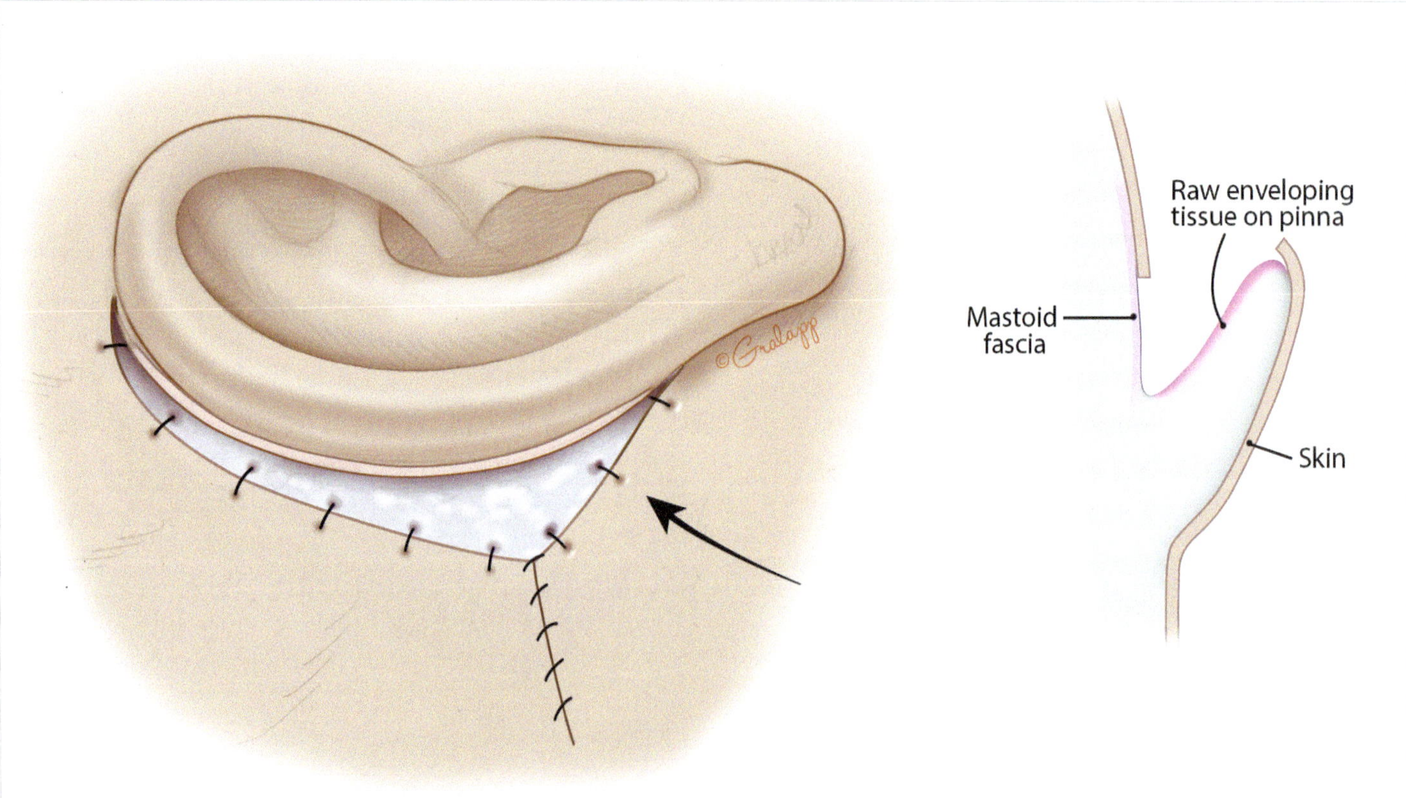

Fig. 3.42 The inferior flap is similarly advanced and the resulting overlap of the skin flaps is resected and sutured closed. An axial view shows the newly created posterior auricular sulcus which must be covered with the skin graft.

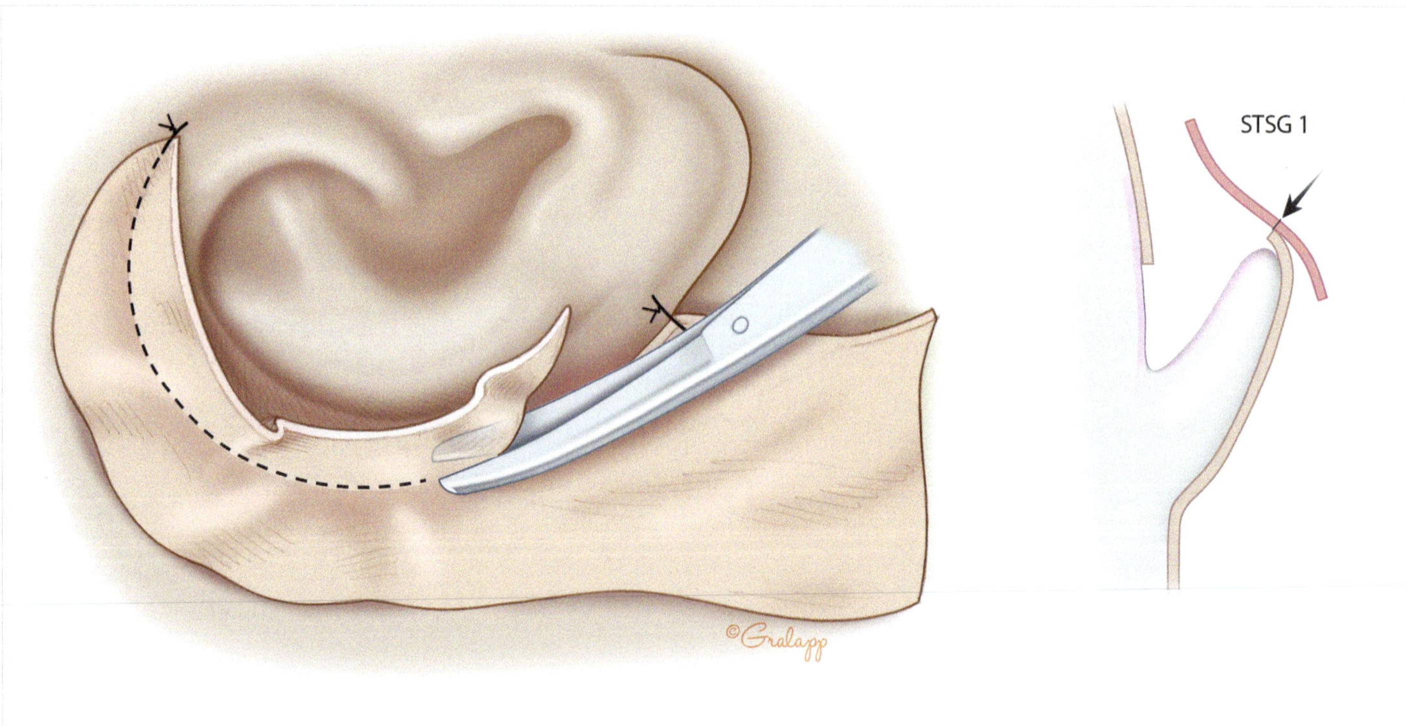

Fig. 3.43 The skin graft is tacked at the superior and inferior aspects of the ear and the anterior rim of the graft is trimmed to give a fresh margin conforming to the shape of the incision. An axial view illustrates how this first skin graft is used to drape the posterior surface of the ear to the sulcus.

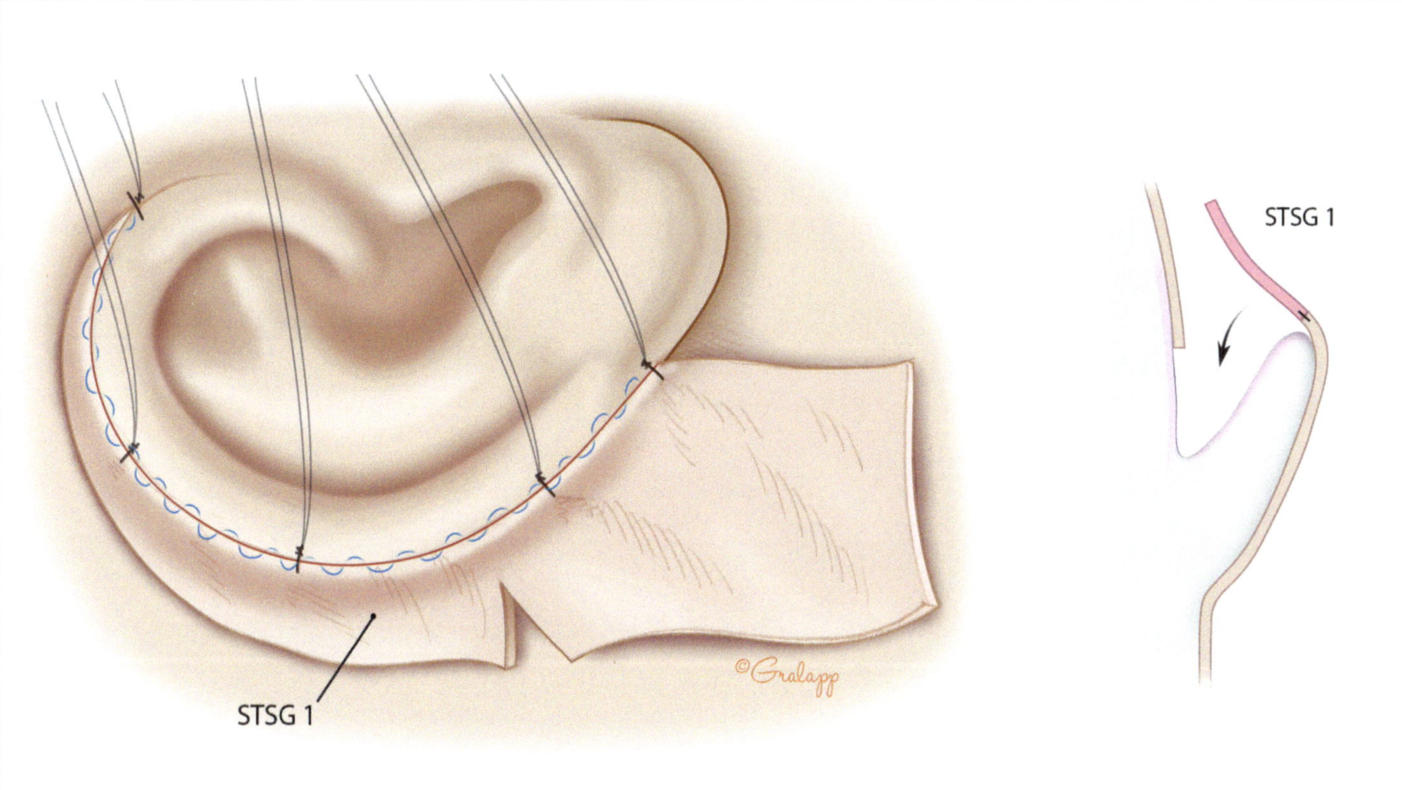

Fig. 3.44 The skin graft is sewn to the anterior margin leaving some of the suture tails long to anchor a bolster once the skin graft is in place. When draping the skin graft toward the postauricular sulcus, it is sometimes necessary to trim a wedge to achieve optimal contour as the skin drapes behind the ear.

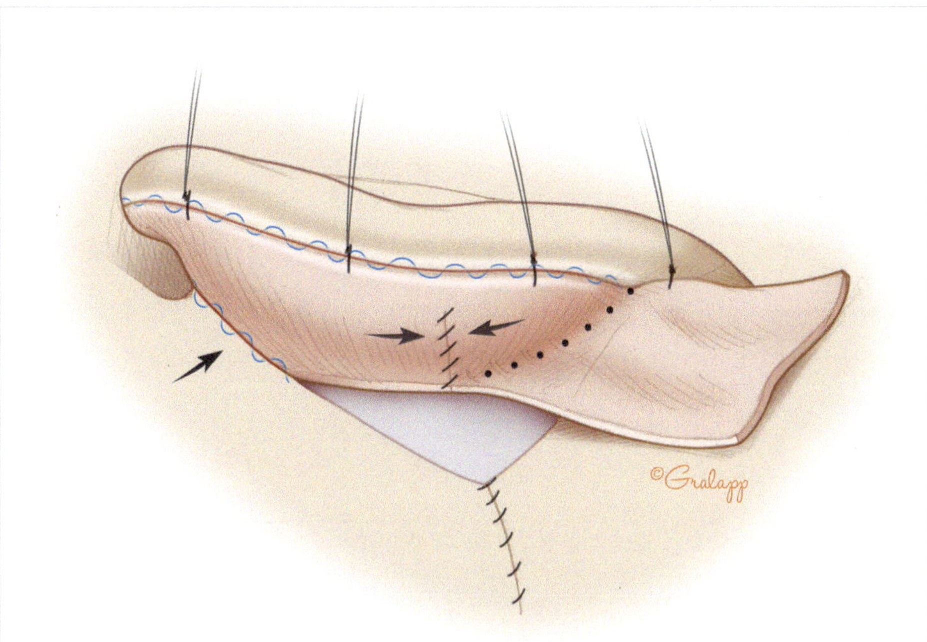

Fig. 3.45 Excess skin graft not needed for the posterior surface of the pinna is trimmed and saved to cover the mastoid defect. This creates a suture line in the sulcus so that the graft does not cross the sulcus. Grafts which cross the sulcus tend to blunt, whereas the suture line tends to create a deeper and more natural sulcus.

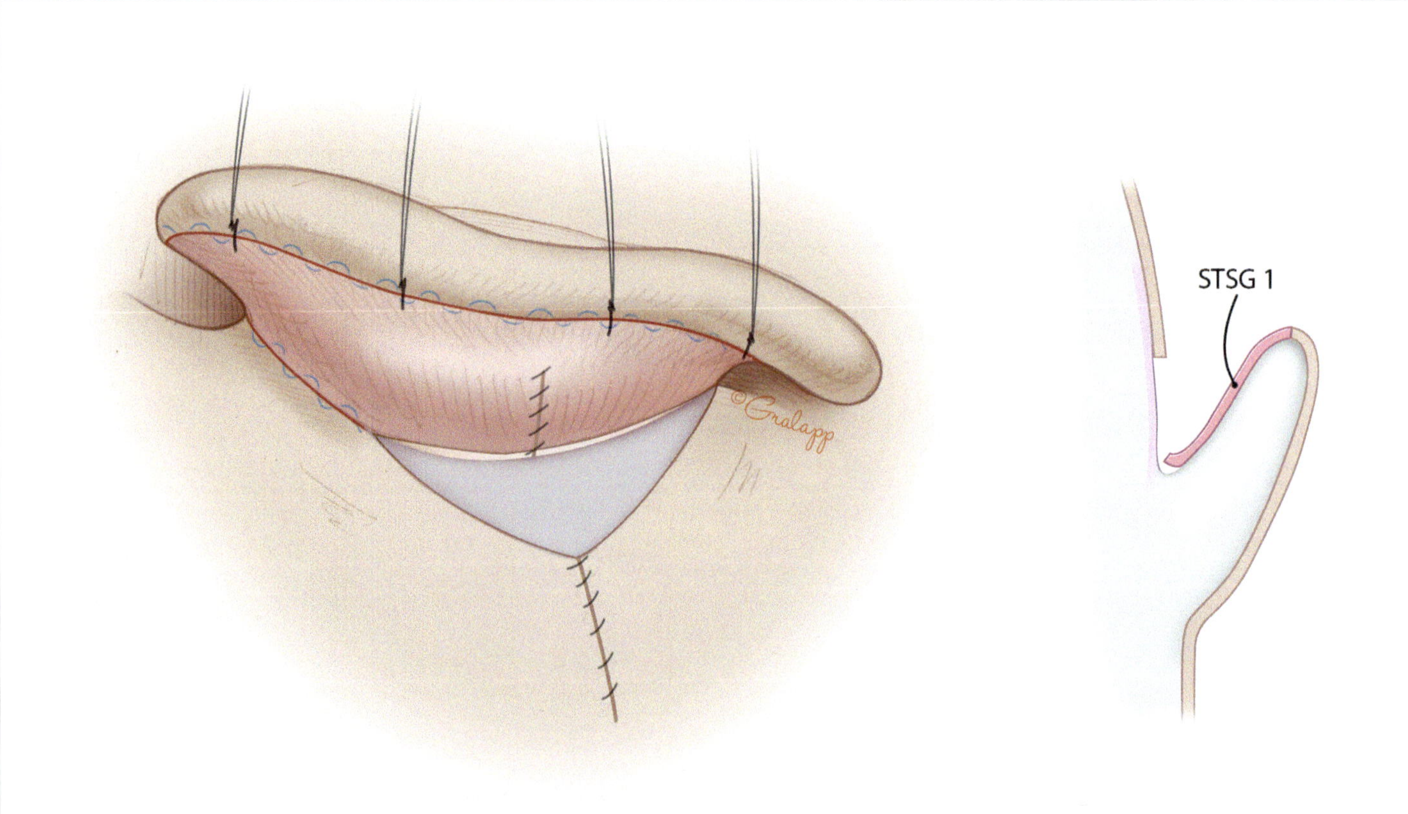

Fig. 3.46 The posterior surface of the construct is covered with skin graft and sutured to the sulcus, leaving a triangular defect on the mastoid that needs skin coverage.

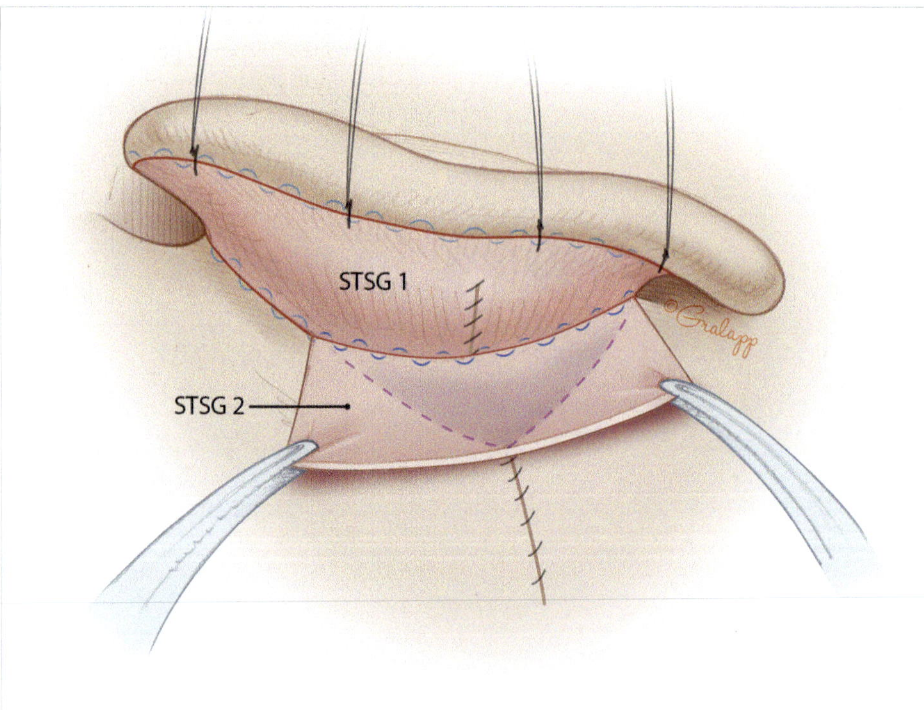

Fig. 3.47 The excess skin is placed over the mastoid defect and secured with clamps before it is cut to shape and sutured in place (STSG 2).

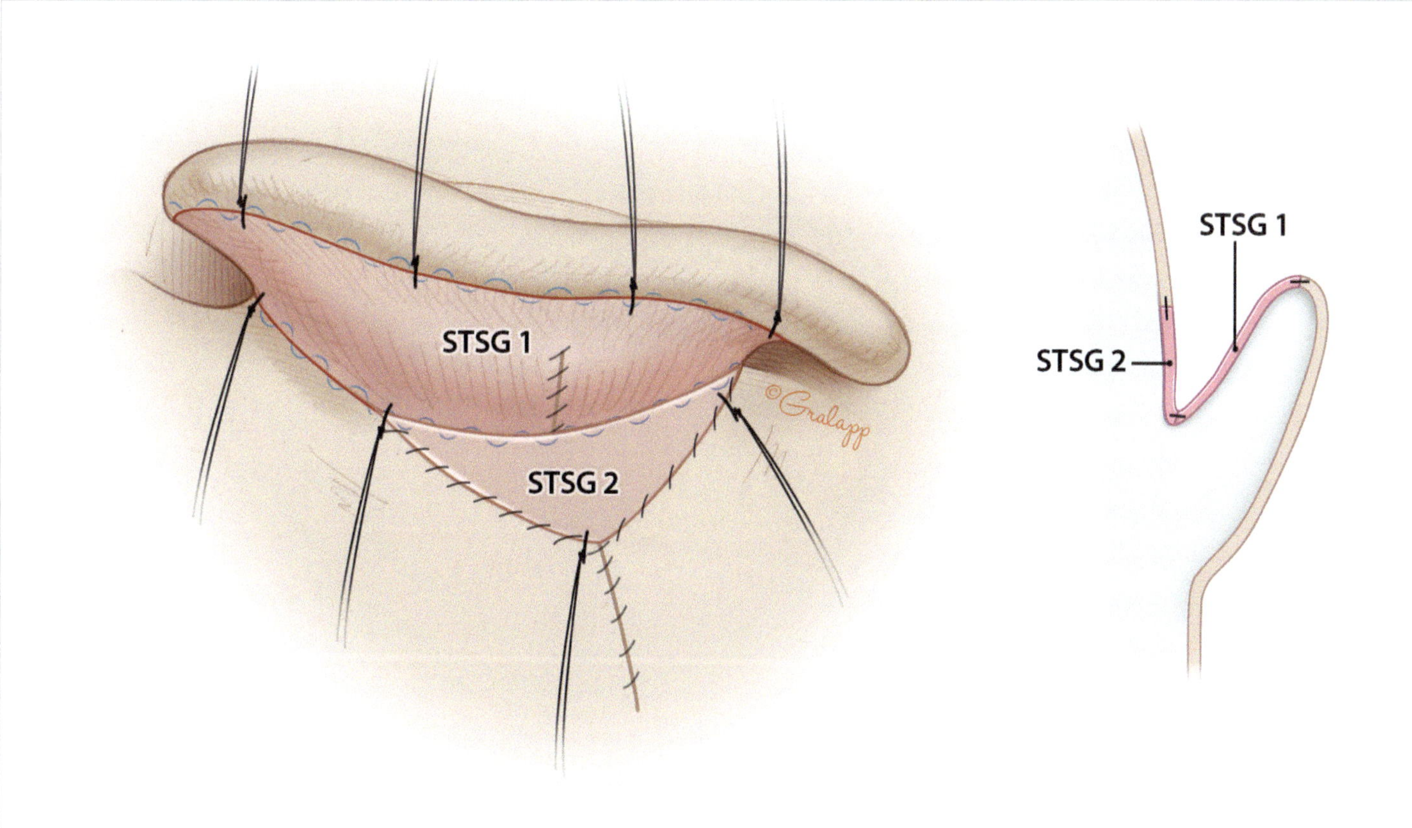

Fig. 3.48 At the completion of stage 2, the ear is elevated, and the postauricular sulcus is created from two pieces of STSG. Bolster sutures are in place.

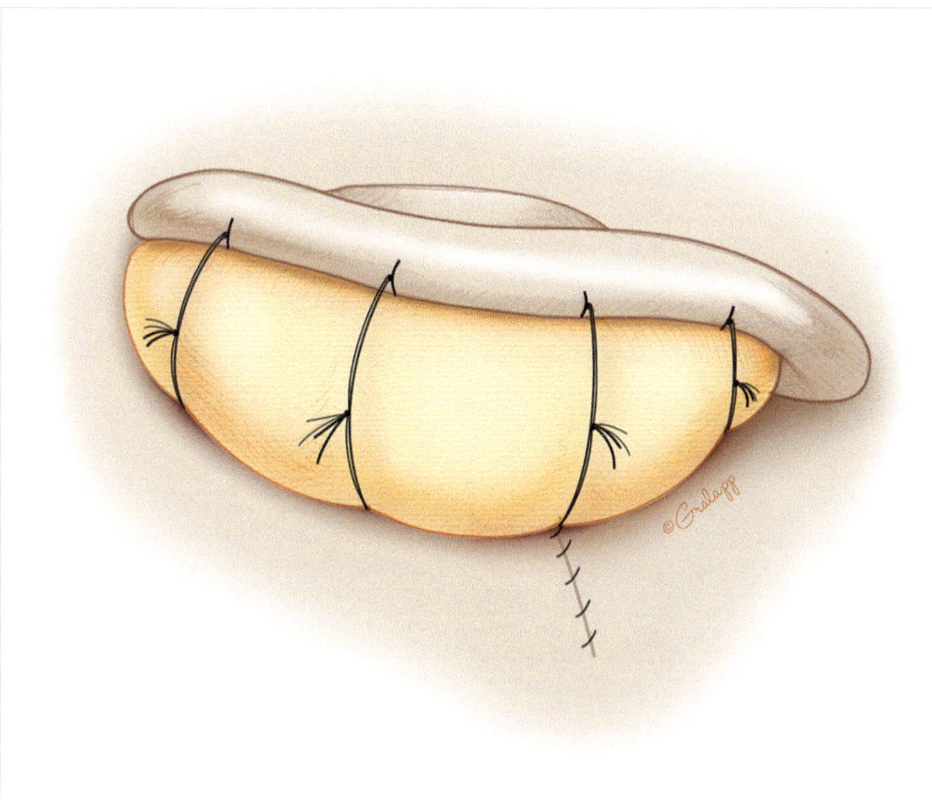

Fig. 3.49 To adhere the skin grafts to the opposing surfaces, some surgeons use either a bolster or a mini-flap drain (e.g., 7 or 10 Fr). Bolsters or drains are left in for 4 days. The skin graft donor site along the scalp is often covered with a topical hemostatic dressing and non-occlusive gauze dressing.

3.4 Repair of Congenital Aural Atresia

Kay W. Chang and Mai Thy Truong

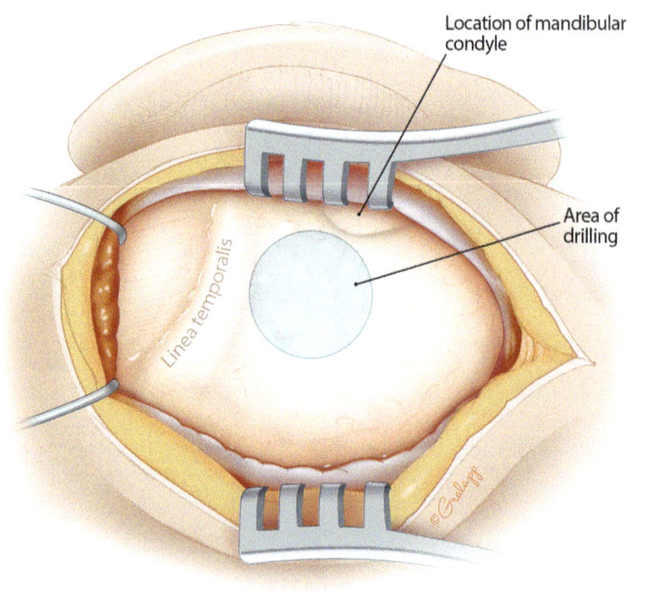

Fig. 3.50 To locate the initial drilling location for the new ear canal in congenital aural atresia, first orient to the glenoid fossa and the linea temporalis.

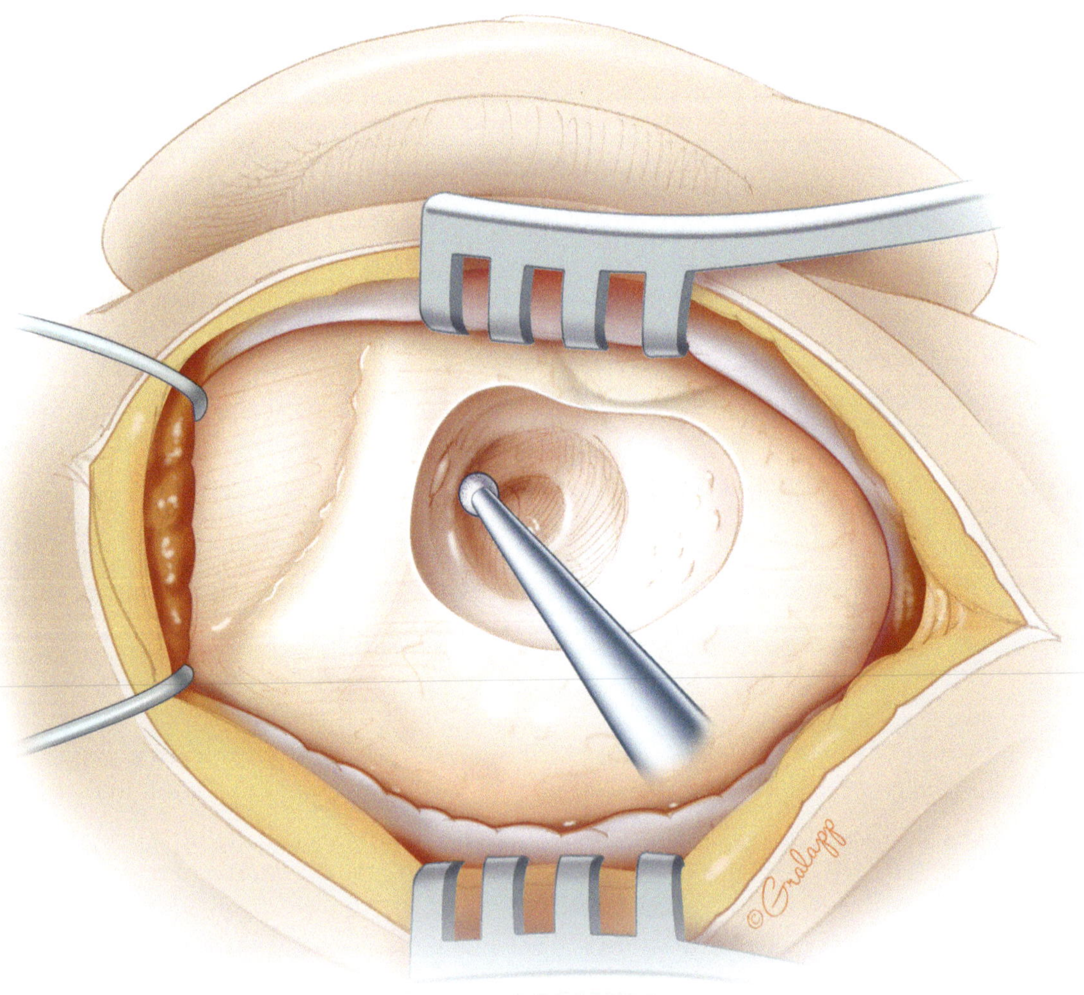

Fig. 3.51 For the safest approach to the tympanum, the deepest point of drill excavation should be kept superior and anterior.

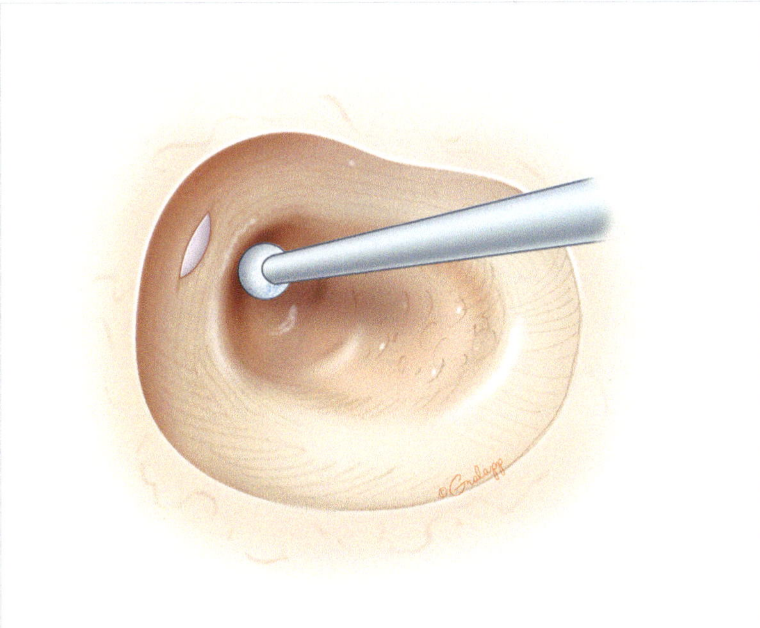

Fig. 3.52 Note the identification of the tegmen dura (usually through a thin sheet of bone) to assure that the neocanal is positioned properly. If the drilling becomes offline, oriented too inferiorly, then the facial nerve may be placed in jeopardy.

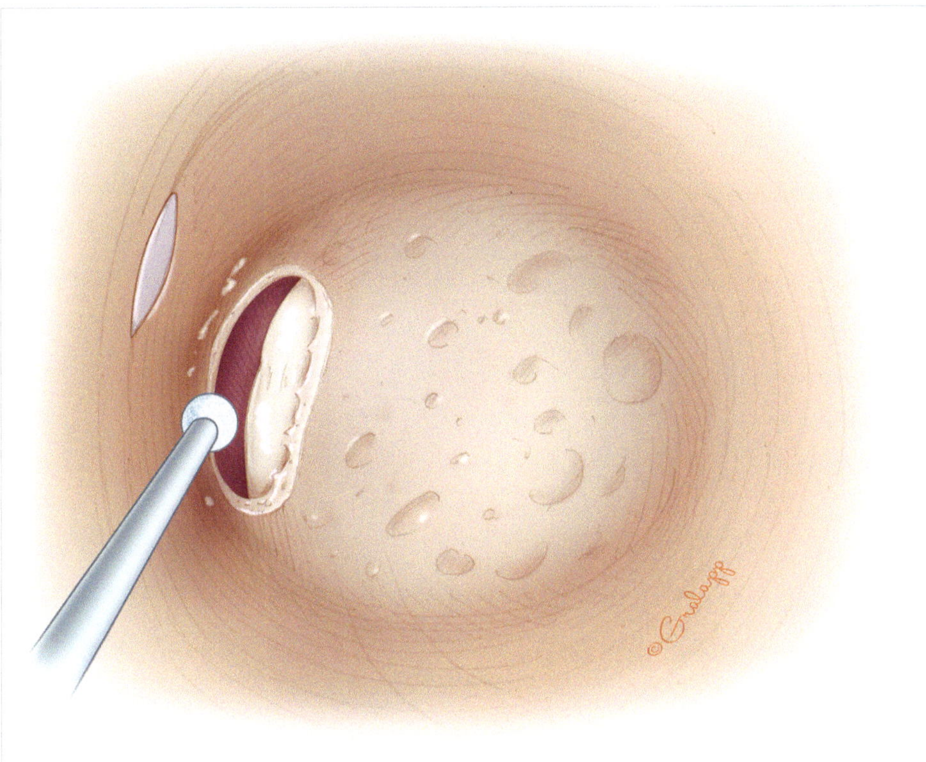

Fig. 3.53 The atresia plate is breached superiorly along the tegmen with identification of the malleus head and incus body, which are fused in patients with atresia.

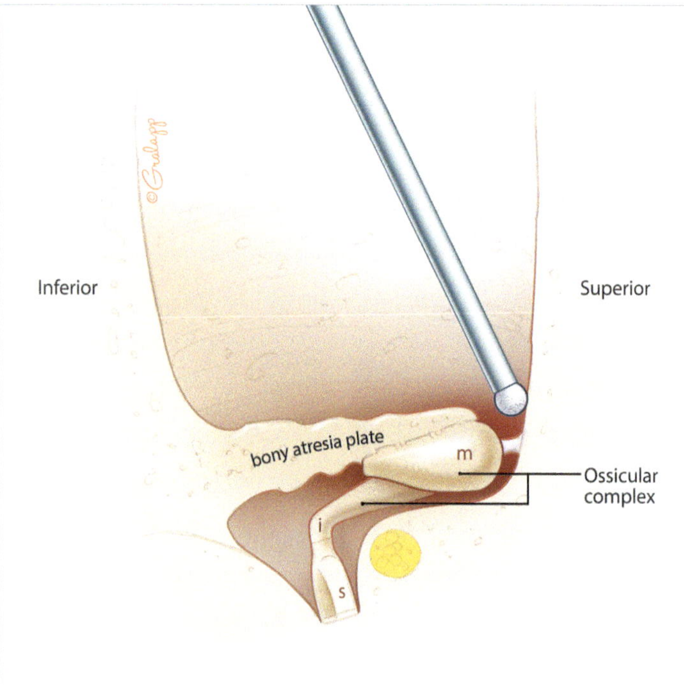

Fig. 3.54 While removing the atretic plate, care must be exerted not to drill on the ossicles, as the transmitted vibration may cause cochlear damage.

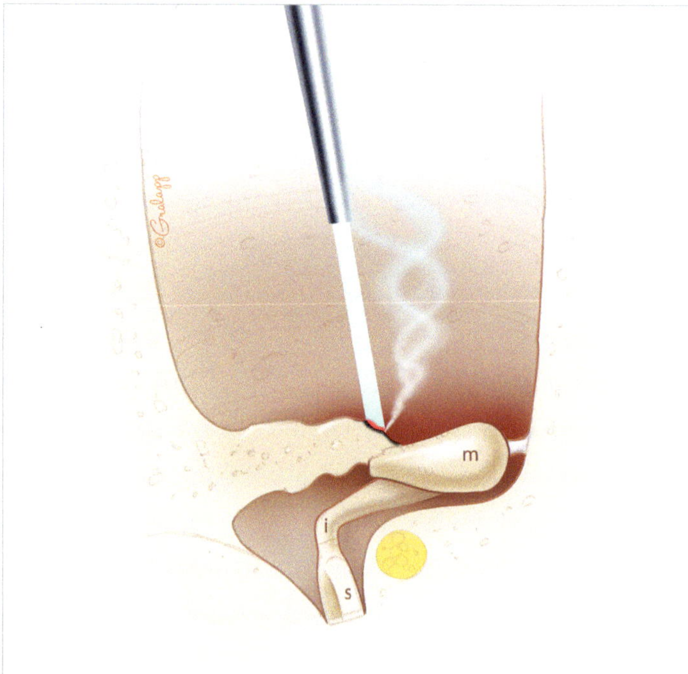

Fig. 3.55 The thinned sheet of atretic bone overlying the ossicles may be removed more safely using a stapes curette rather than a drill. Soft tissue adherent to the ossicles may be vaporized with a laser.

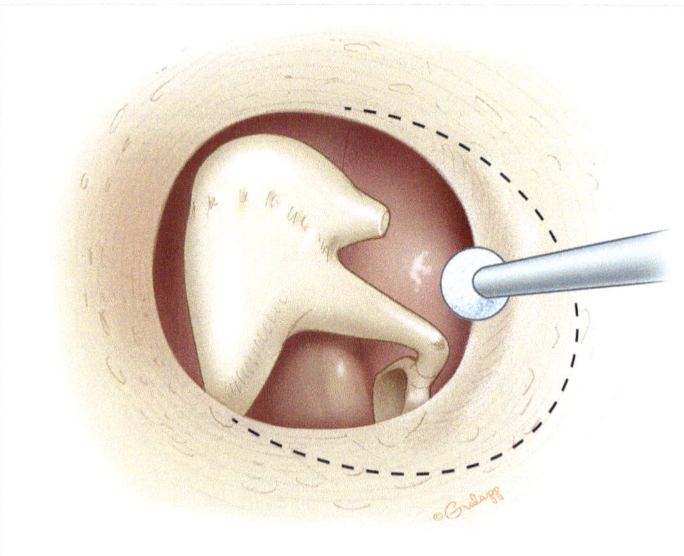

Fig. 3.56 Completing removal of the inferior aspect of the neocanal.

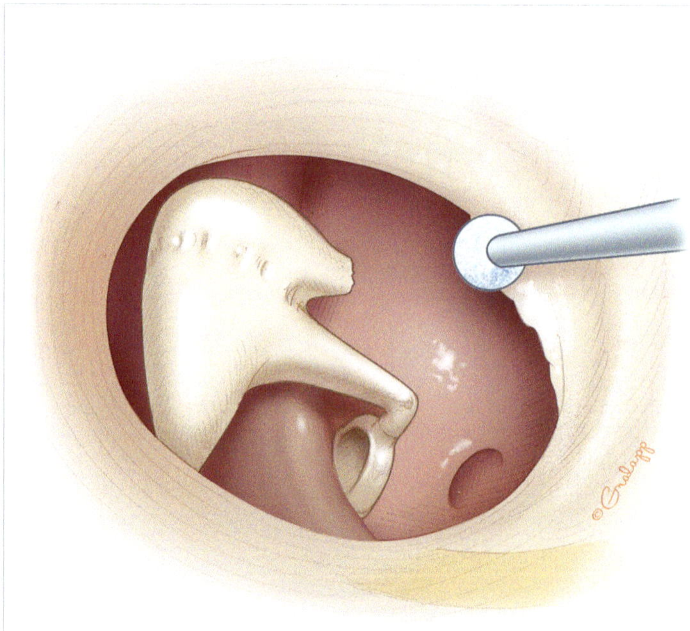

Fig. 3.57 In completing the canal excavation, care must be taken posterior-inferiorly because in atresia, the facial nerve may lie lateral to the tympanic annulus.

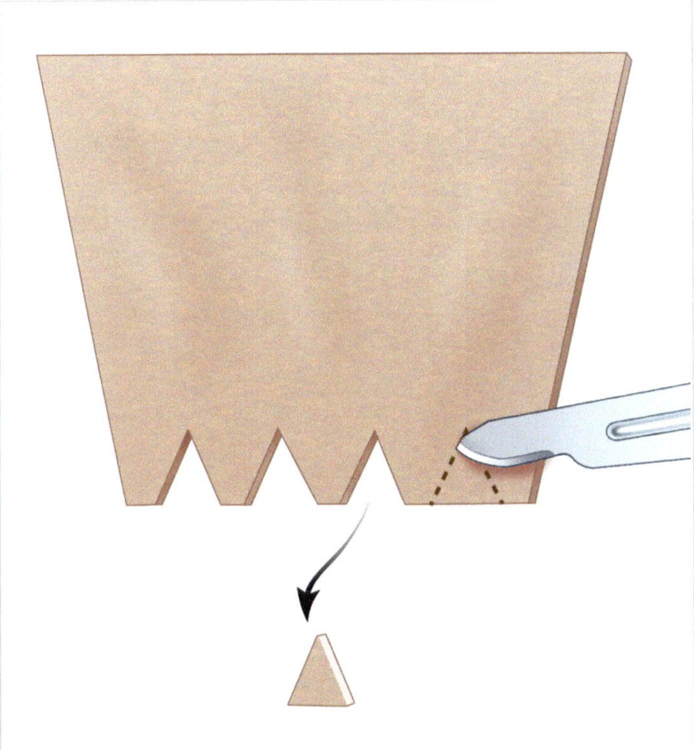

Fig. 3.58 Split-thickness skin graft must be thin to engraft well on the bare bone. If too much dermis remains, it will swell and narrow the canal. Small triangles are removed to enable the graft to contour to the tympanic membrane graft without overlap. Trimming the skin graft is guided by measuring the depth of the newly formed canal and its circumference at both the level of the tympanic annulus and laterally at the bony opening. This can be done by placing a pliable ligature (e.g., silk) as a loop medially and laterally and then using a measuring stick to determine the desired size.

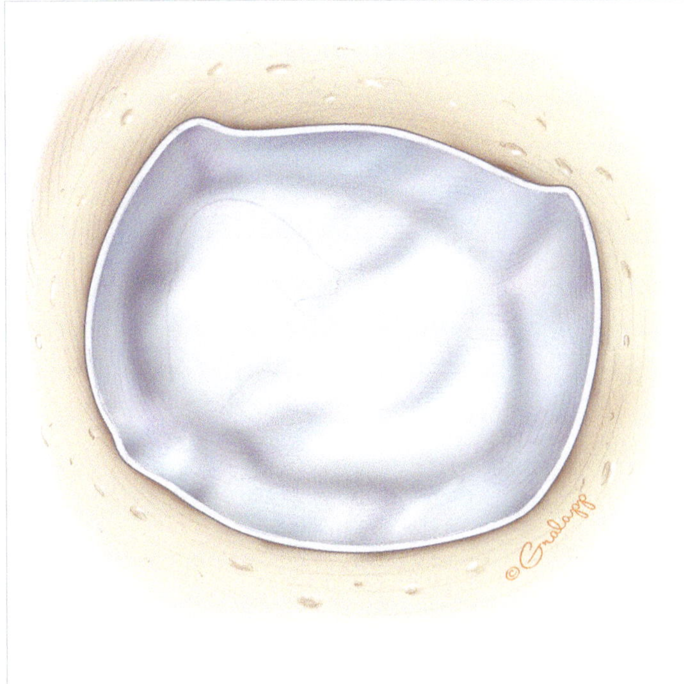

Fig. 3.59 Placement of the temporalis fascia graft which is seated in broad contact with the malleus–incus complex to help prevent lateralization of the graft. The graft should extend on 1 to 2 mm up to the neocanal from the annulus, which encourages graft separation from the ossicles during healing due to lateralization of the newly formed tympanic membrane.

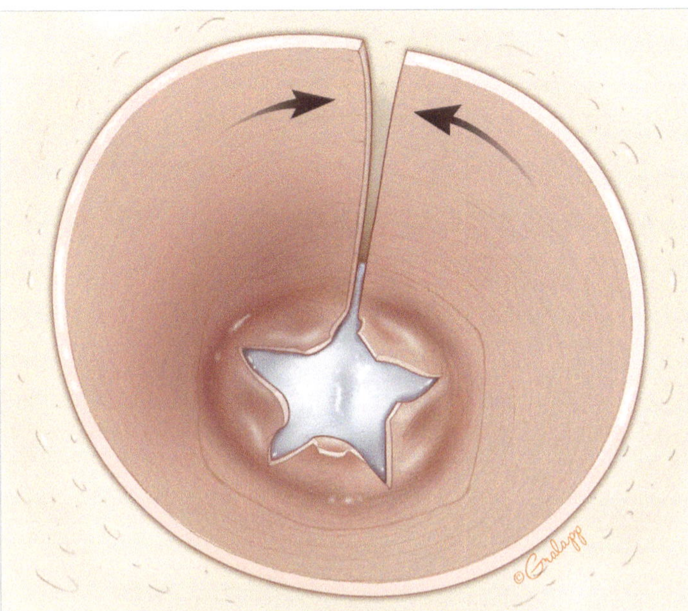

Fig. 3.60 The skin graft is placed with the seam anterior so that any exposed mastoid air cells are fully covered.

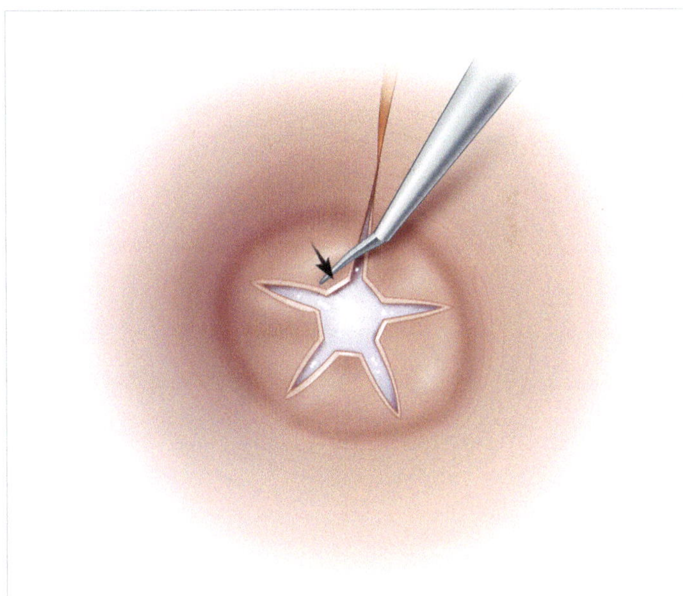

Fig. 3.61 The triangles are smoothed on the fascial graft. Note that the graft is tucked firmly into the margins of the tympanic ring.

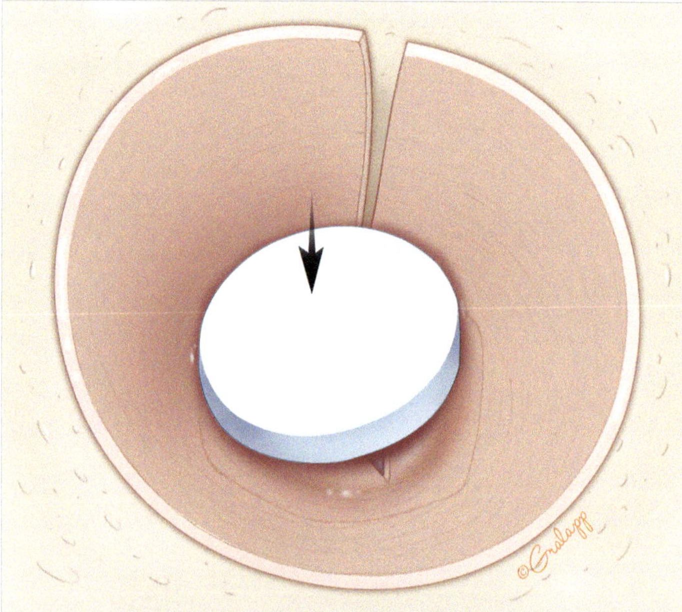

Fig. 3.62 A 0.04-inch thick Silastic disk is trimmed to fit over the graft. This has several advantages: it avoids adherence of the fascia and skin graft to the packing material, encourages the adherence of the graft to the ossicles, and encourages formation of a right angle at the annulus level.

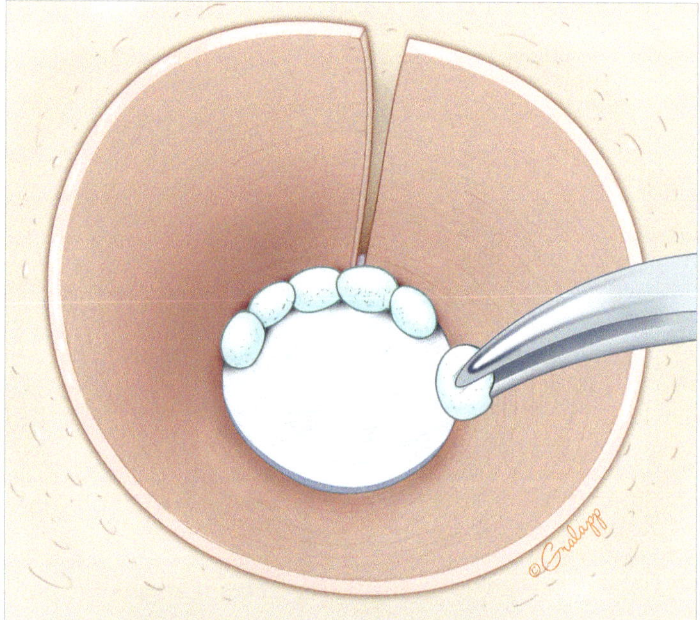

Fig. 3.63 Absorbable gelatin sponge packing may be placed lateral to the Silastic sheet. For ease of removal in a young child, pieces may be larger than depicted here.

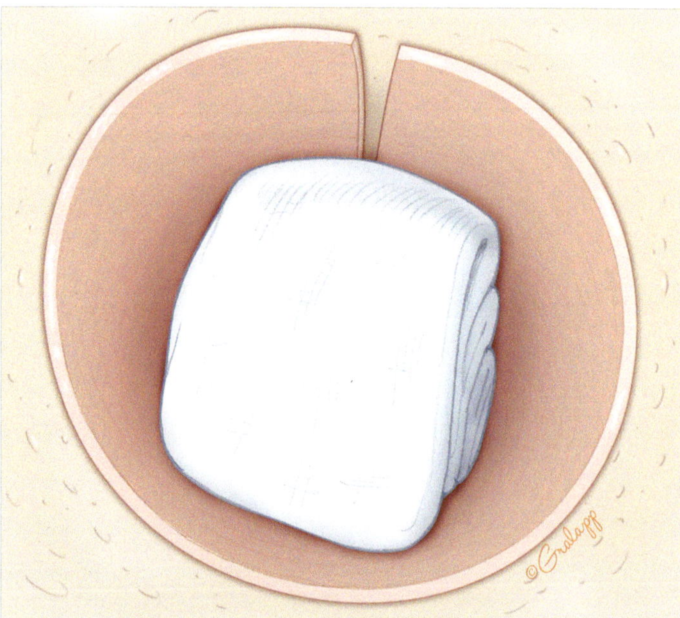

Fig. 3.64 Strip gauze impregnated with antibiotic ointment in place.

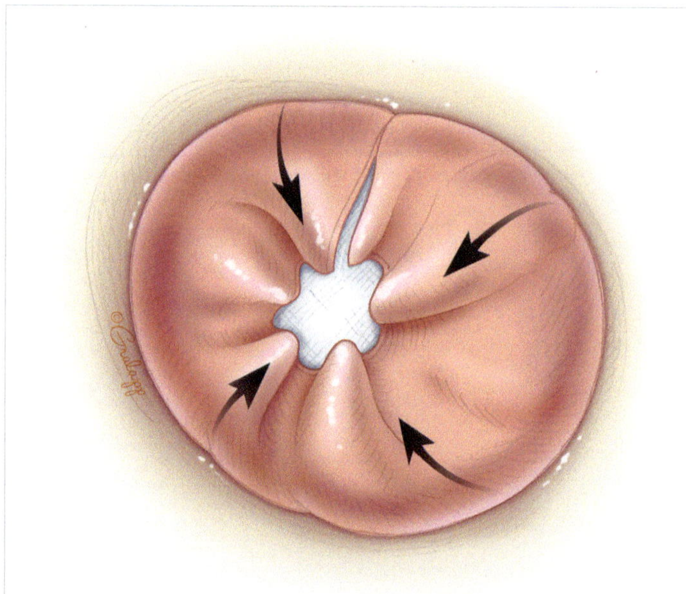

Fig. 3.65 The excess skin graft is folded over in anticipation of meatoplasty.

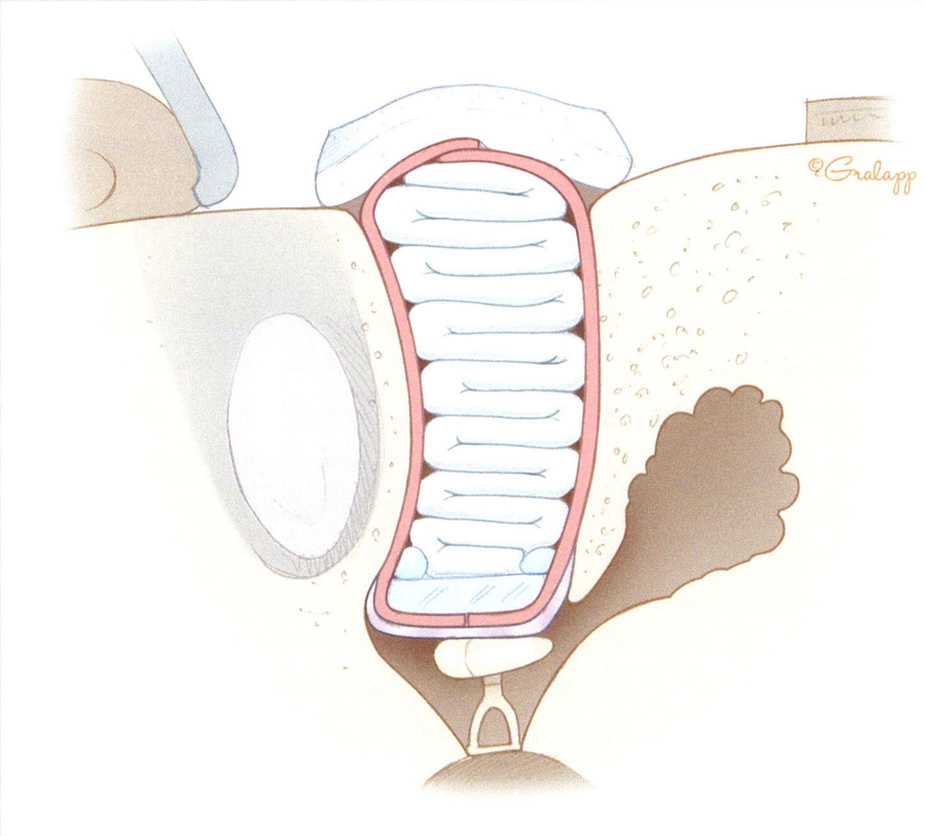

Fig. 3.66 Completed packing.

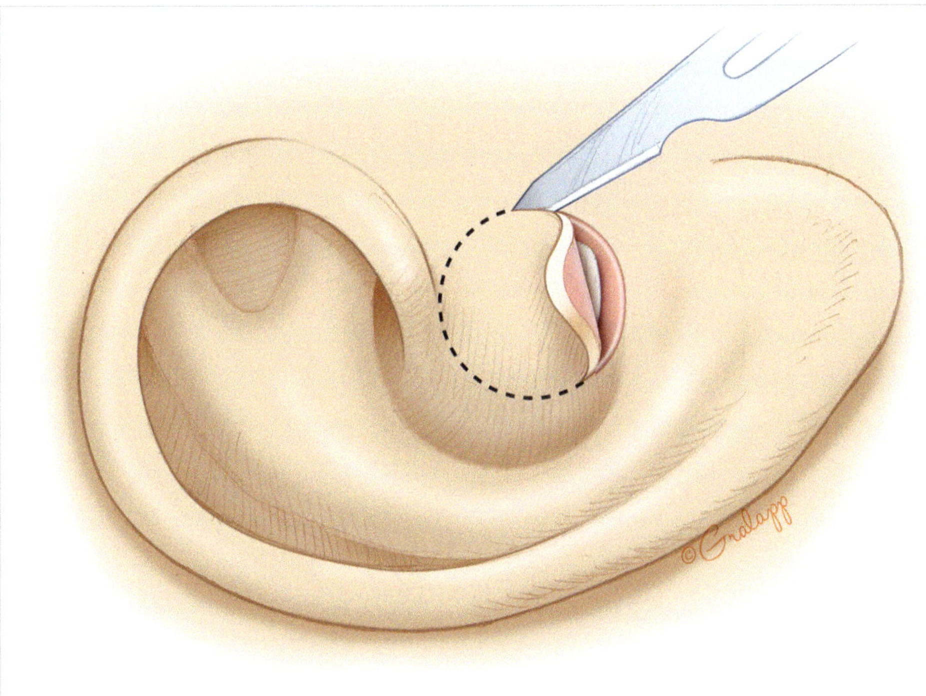

Fig. 3.67 Creation of the meatus.

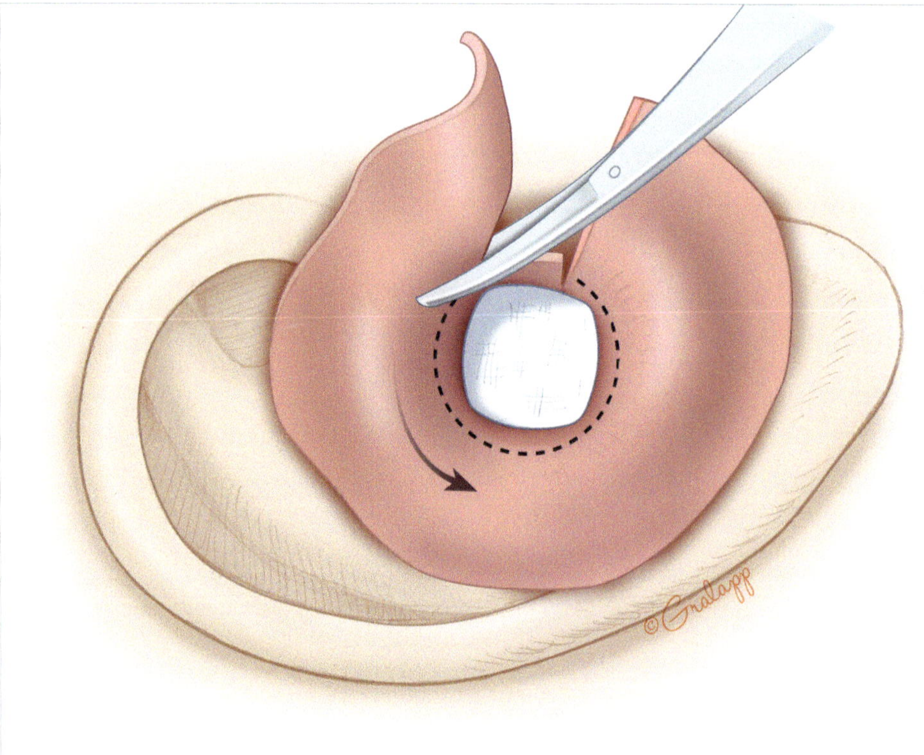

Fig. 3.68 Unfurling of the skin graft, which is trimmed to match the meatal edge.

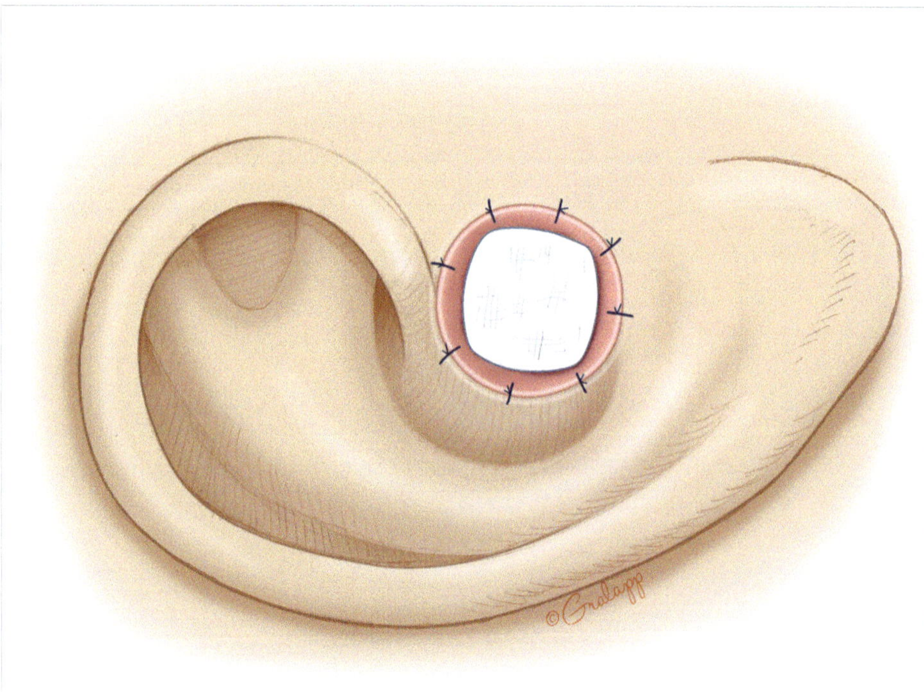

Fig. 3.69 The skin graft is sutured to the meatal skin.

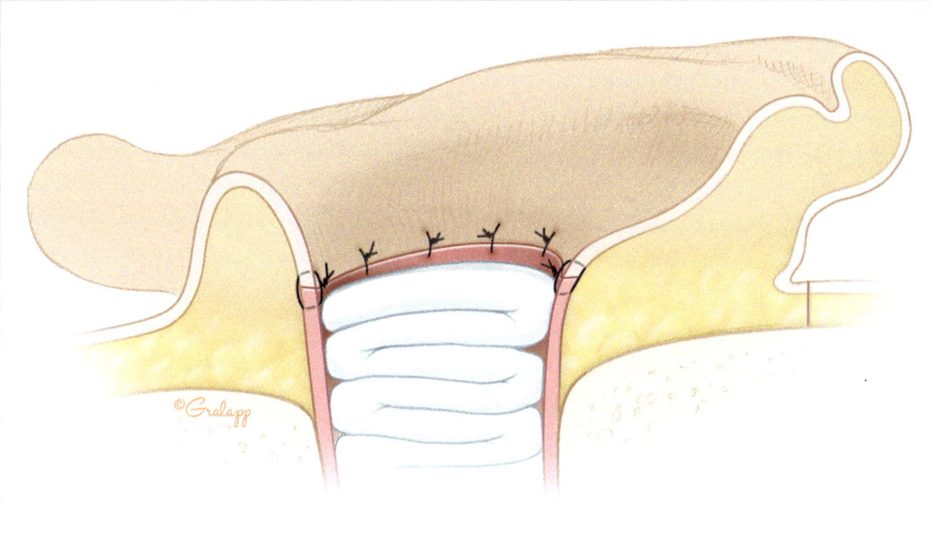

Fig. 3.70 Completed meatal construction.

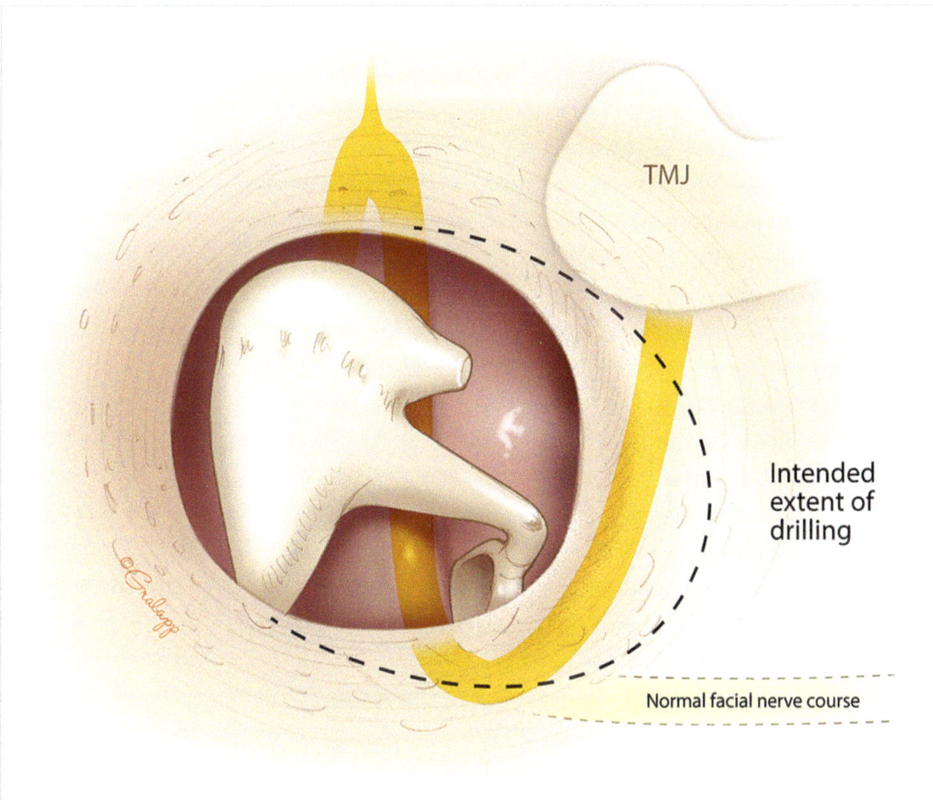

Fig. 3.71 In atresia, the facial nerve may take an anomalous course. In one example, the second genu, which is usually a 90-degree bend, turns 180 degrees and exits the temporal bone via the glenoid fossa. When beginning atresia surgery, it is important not to mistake the glenoid for the ear canal, as deep dissection into the posterior aspect of the glenoid may injure the anomalous facial nerve.

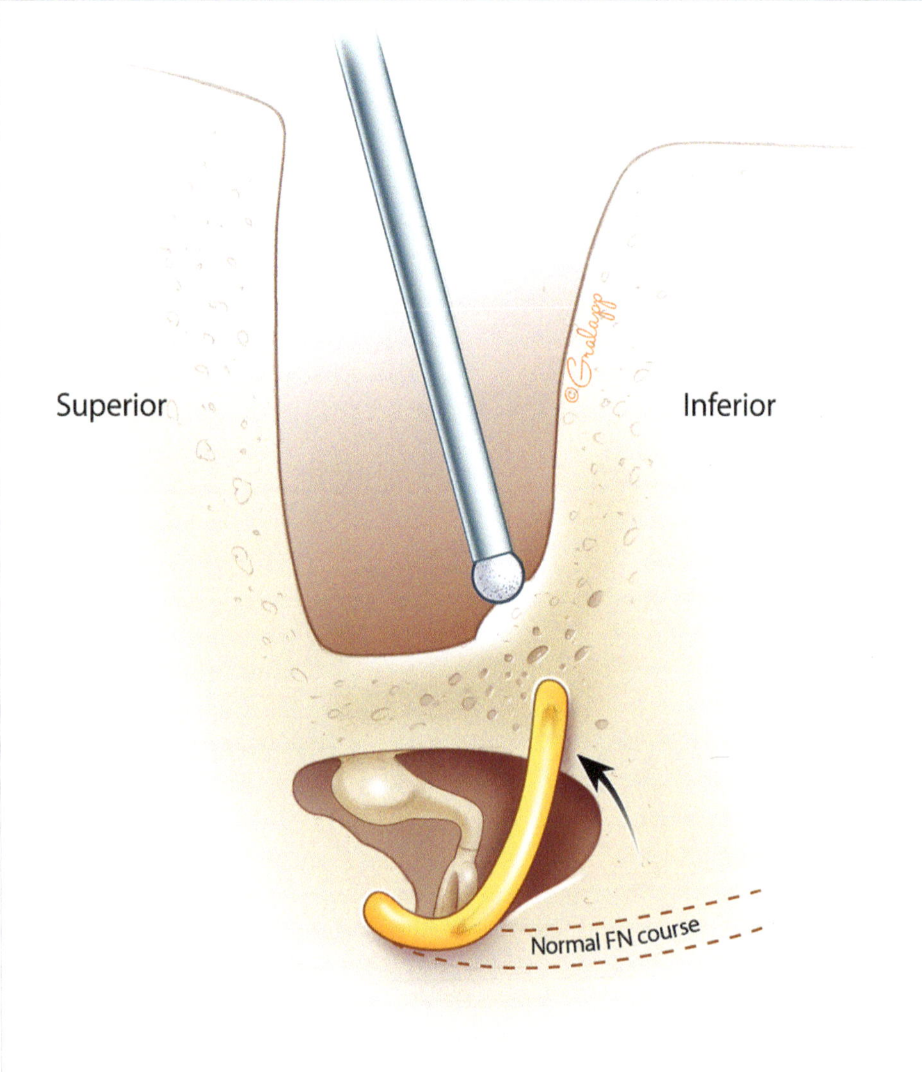

Fig. 3.72 In some cases of atresia, the facial nerve may turn precipitously laterally and present in the ear canal superficial to the medial aspect of the tympanic plate. It is prudent to use facial nerve monitoring and to use diamond burrs and copious irrigation while completing the deep portion of the canal excavation. (Modified after Jahrsdoerfer RA, Lambert PR. Facial nerve injury in congenital aural atresia surgery. *Am J Otol* 1998: 283–287.)

3.5 Postauricular Meatoplasty

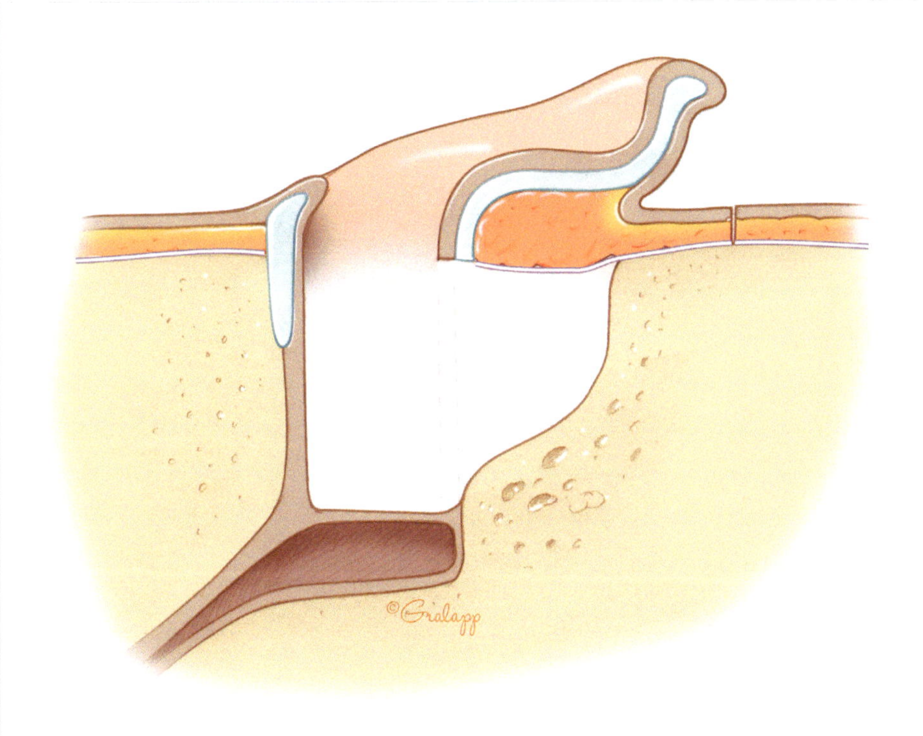

Fig. 3.73 In canal wall down surgery, which exteriorizes the mastoid cavity, creation of an adequate meatus is an essential component of the procedure. The illustration depicts an unmodified meatus in relation to a canal wall down cavity. The natural meatus will not afford sufficient exposure for cleaning and will tend to foster moisture accumulation. The art of reliable meatoplasty is technically quite straightforward, but is often insufficiently taught during training. Using proper techniques, the surgeon should be able to create the desired size of meatus in a high percentage of cases.

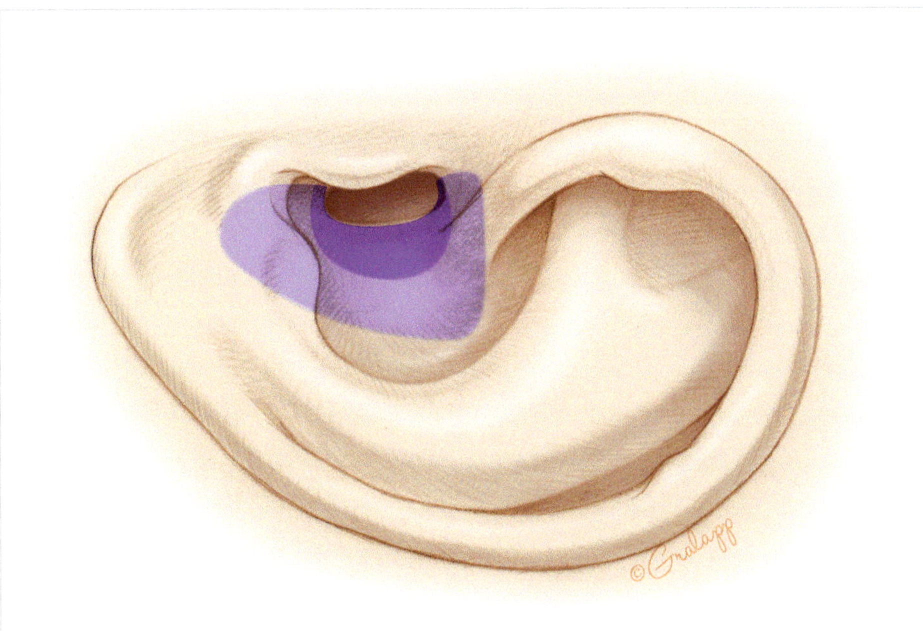

Fig. 3.74 Creation of an adequately sized meatus is an essential component of chronic ear surgery. In canal wall down surgery, the size of the meatus needed depends on the size of the cavity. The meatus (*dark blue*) is matched to allow access to a small cavity (*light blue*).

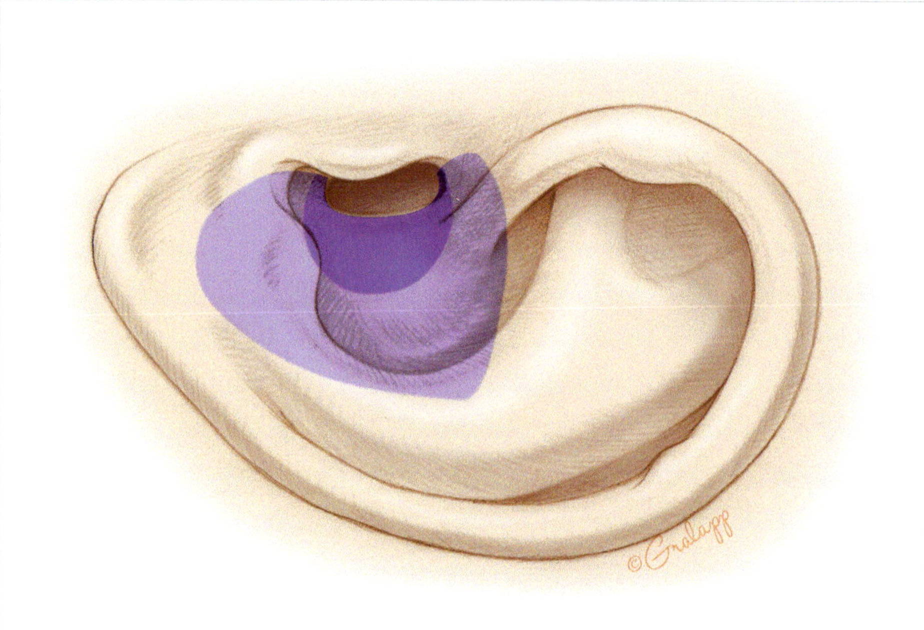

Fig. 3.75 In canal wall down surgery, the size of the meatus needed depends on the size of the cavity. The meatus (*dark blue*) is matched to allow access to a large cavity (*light blue*).

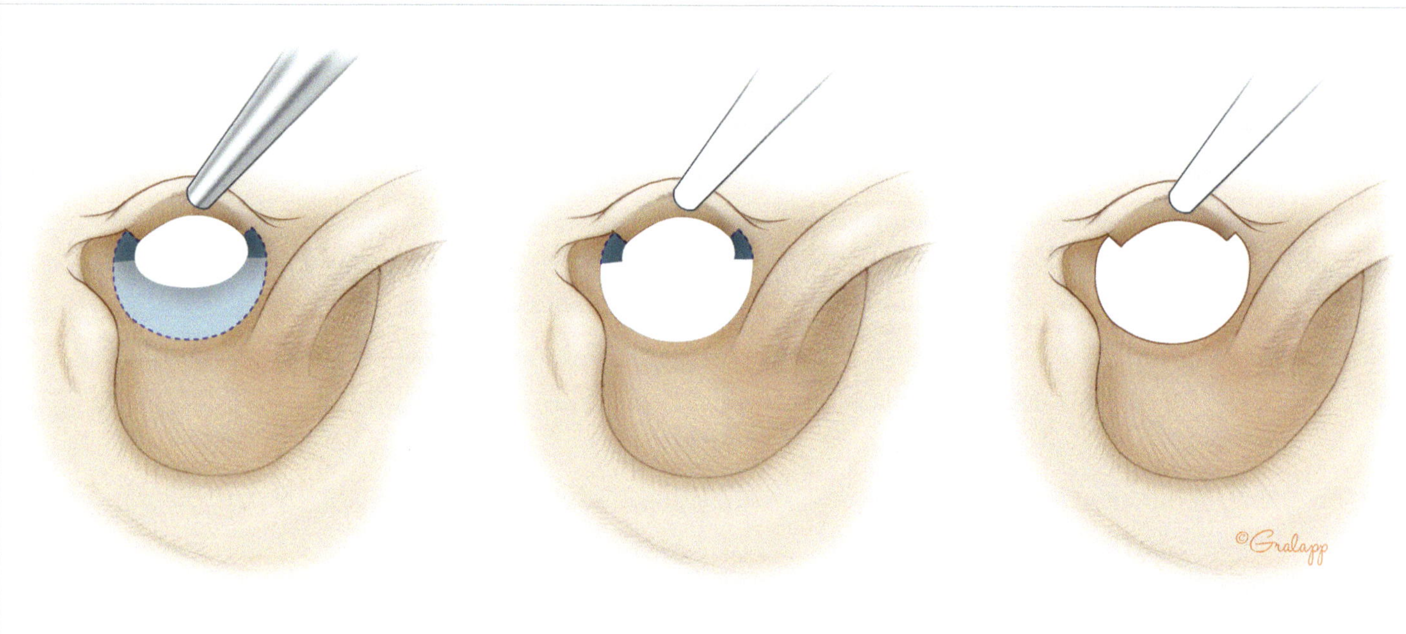

Fig. 3.76 The meatoplasty procedure has two components: the posterior meatus (*light blue*) and the anterior meatus (*dark blue*).

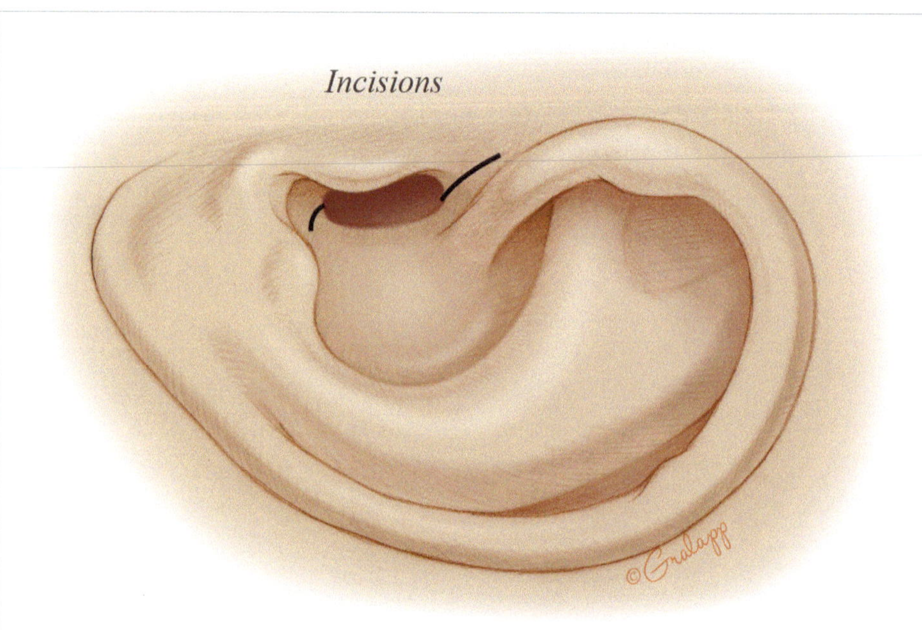

Fig. 3.77 The incisions used in meatoplasty.

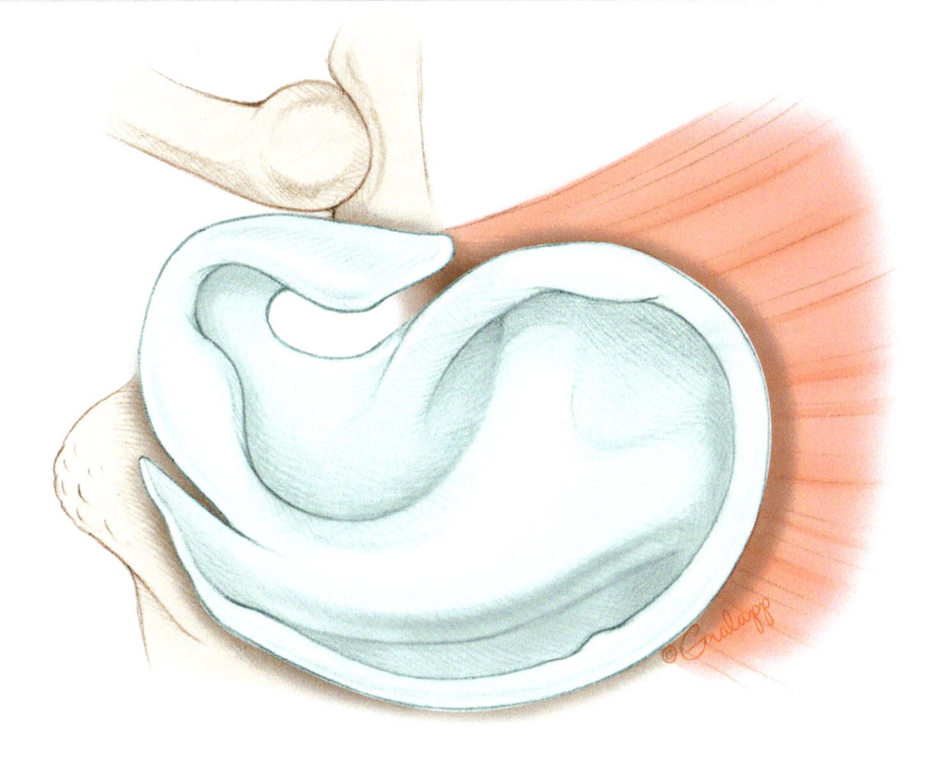

Fig. 3.78 The superior incision is made in the incisura: the interval between the anterior crus of the helix and the superior aspect of the tragus. The inferior incision tracks toward the conchal edge.

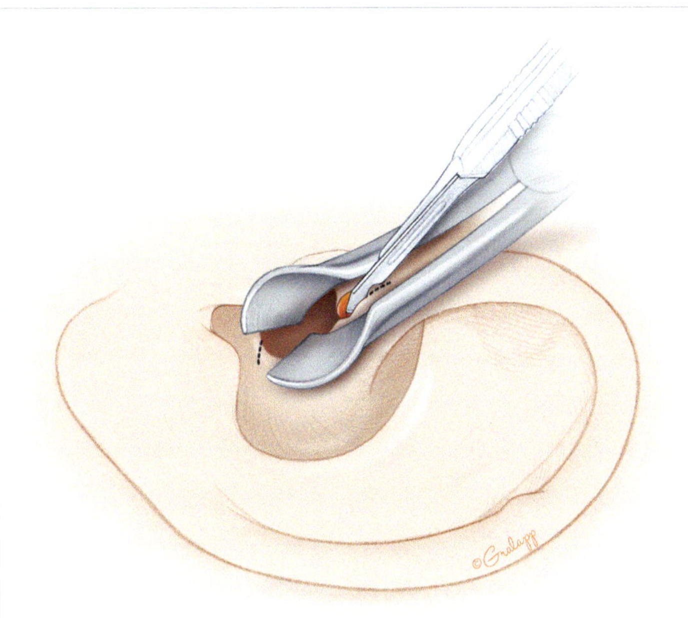

Fig. 3.79 The skin incisions are made with a scalpel.

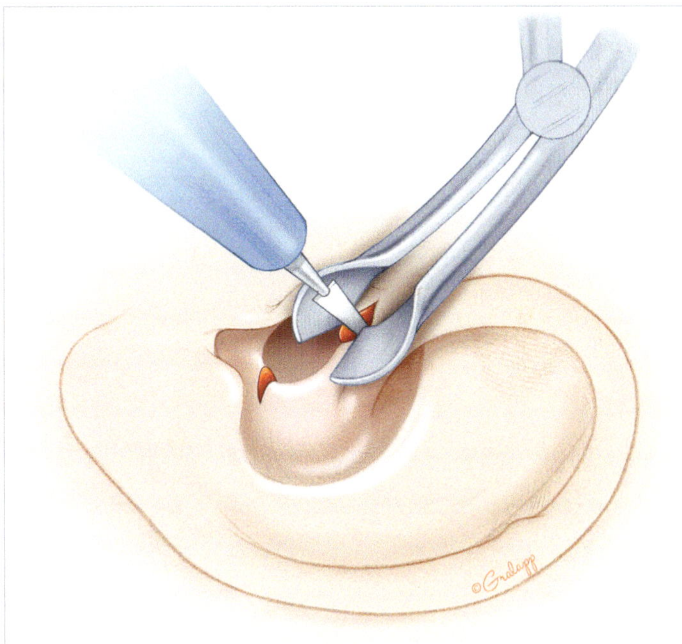

Fig. 3.80 To reduce bleeding, electrocautery is used to deepen the incision. A nasal speculum can be used to spread apart the exposure.

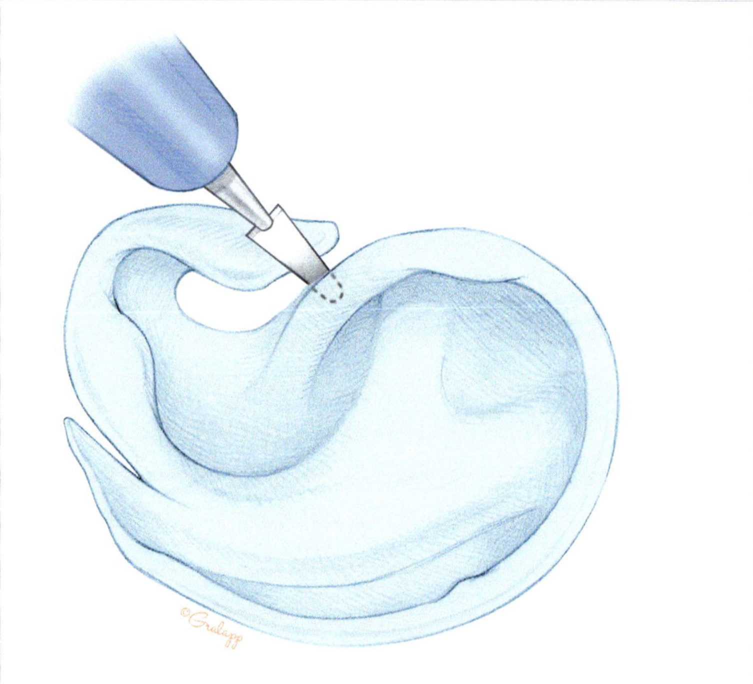

Fig. 3.81 Note that the dissection is directed posteriorly toward the cavity.

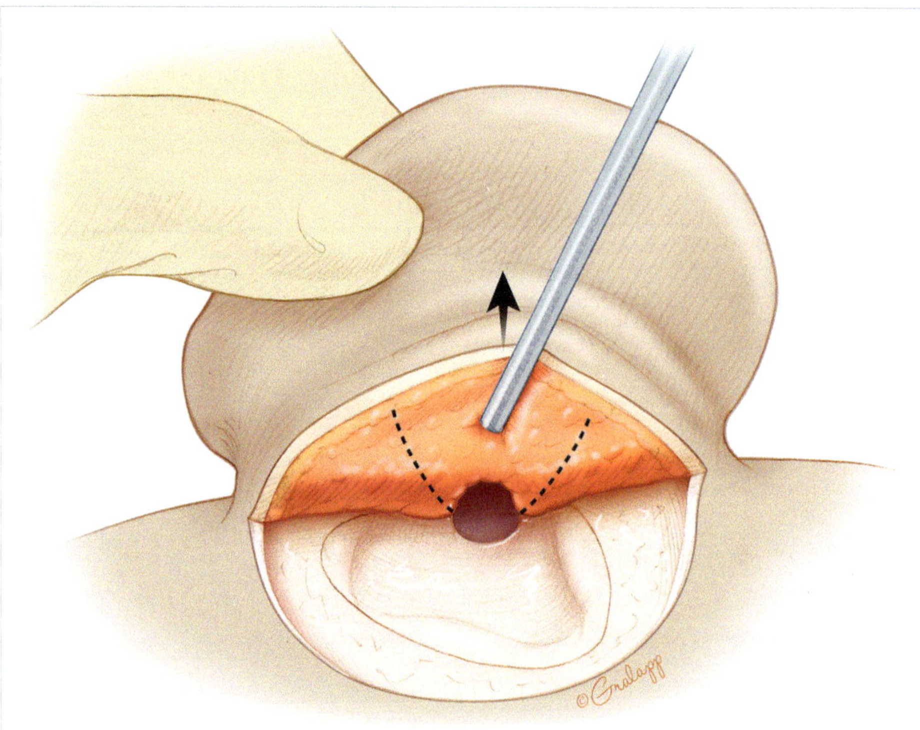

Fig. 3.82 Incisions to commence debulking postauricular soft tissues as part of the soft-tissue meatoplasty.

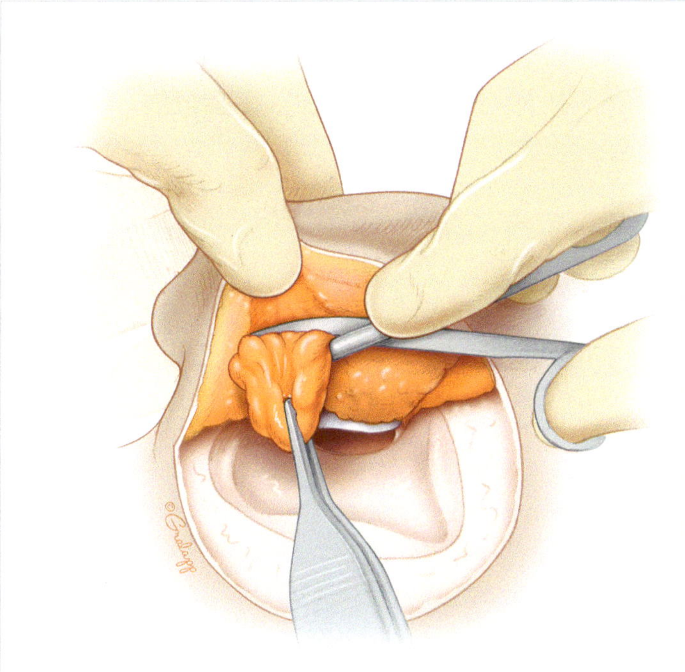

Fig. 3.83 The postauricular soft tissue is debulked.

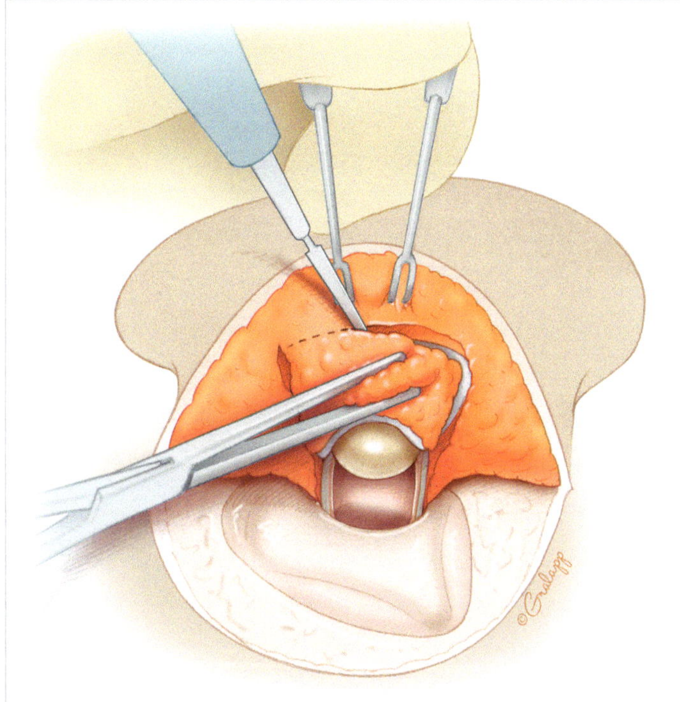

Fig. 3.84 To give tension to its posterior aspect of the now enlarged meatus, the surgeon's middle finger is placed through the meatus. Two double-pronged skin hooks elevate and stabilize the postauricular tissues. With electrocautery or scissors, the tissue is further thinned.

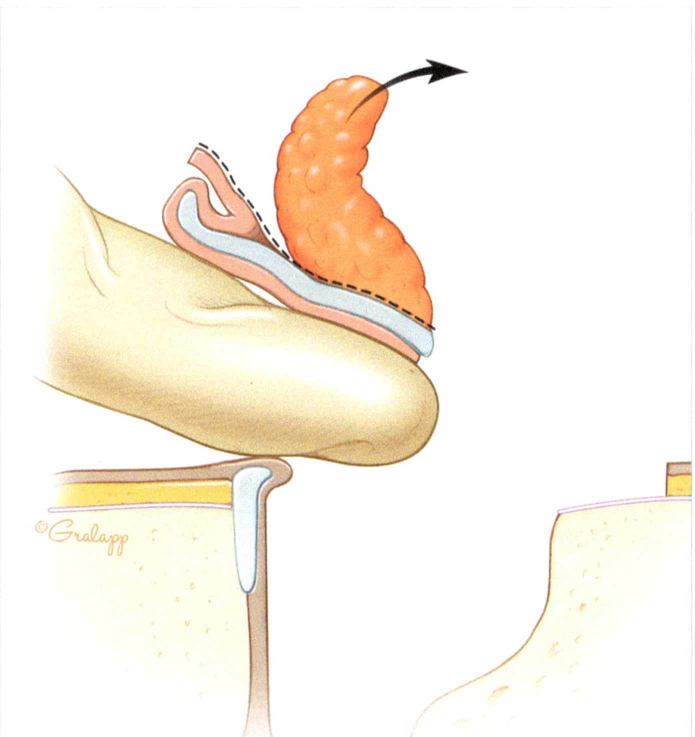

Fig. 3.85 Schematic view of thinning the postauricular soft tissue toward the conchal cartilage.

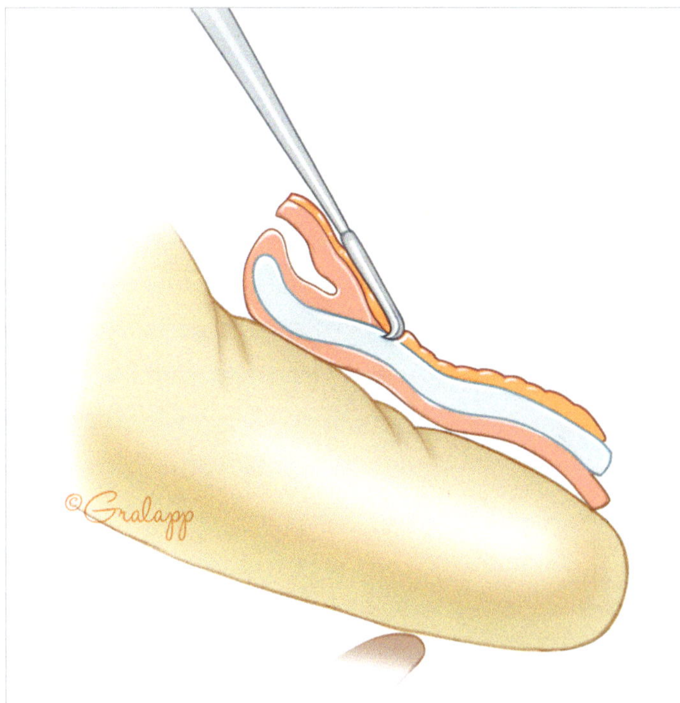

Fig. 3.86 Schematic view of completed postauricular soft-tissue thinning.

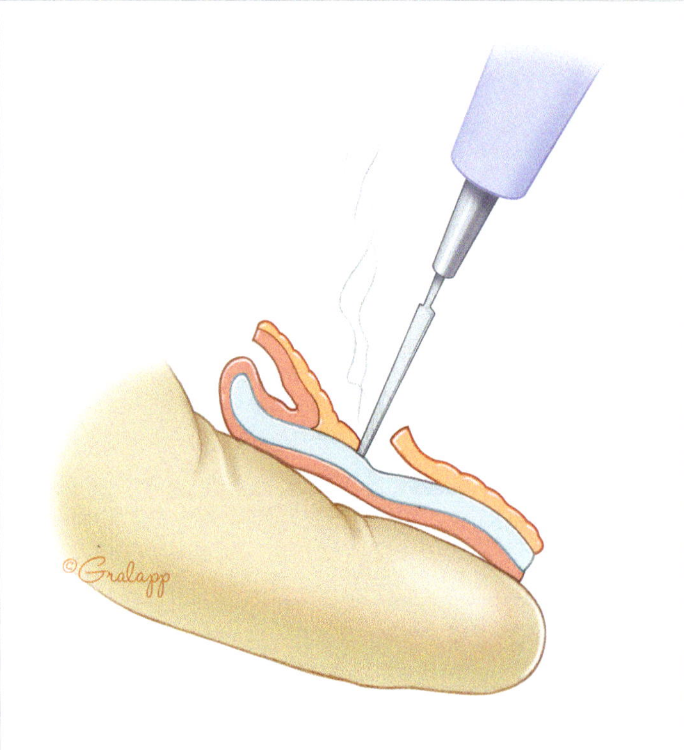

Fig. 3.87 Incision is made through the perichondrium to exposure the conchal cartilage.

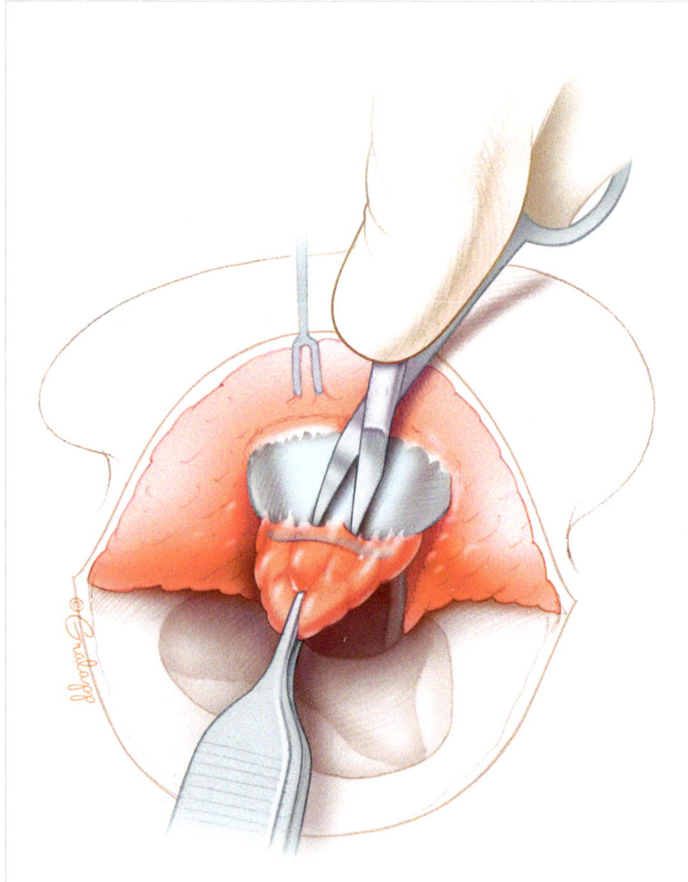

Fig. 3.88 The perichondrium is dissected off the undersurface of the conchal bowl until its free edge is reached.

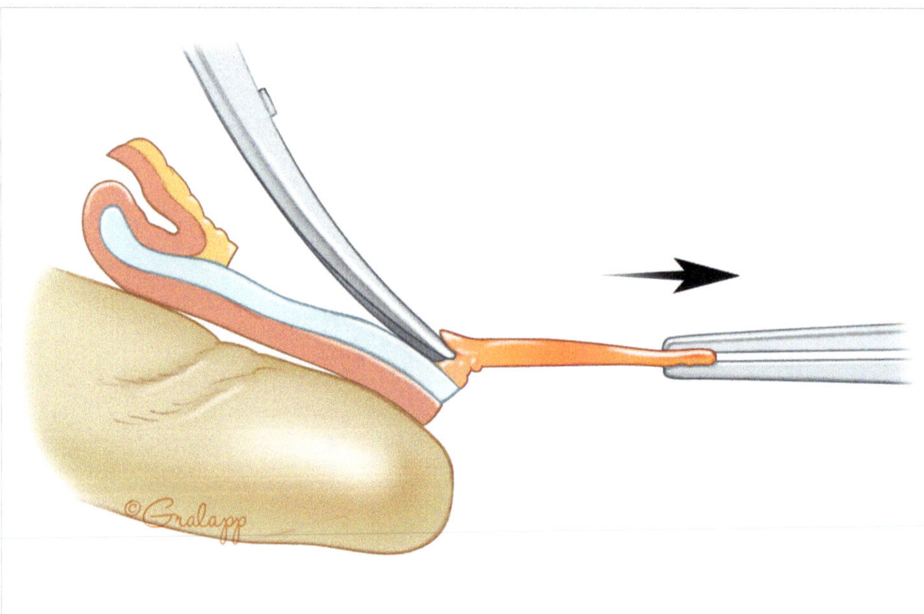

Fig. 3.89 Schematic view of the perichondrial dissection from the undersurface of the concha.

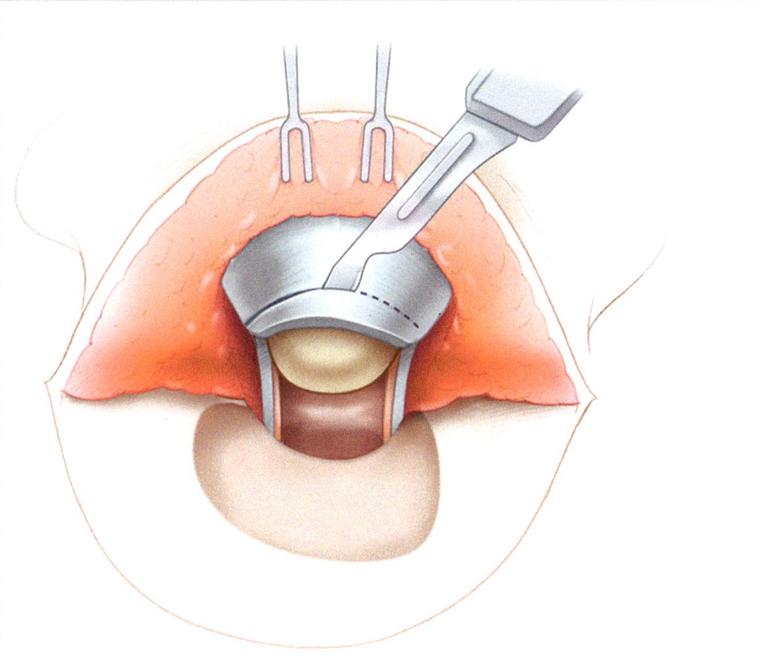

Fig. 3.90 Pushing outward with the finger, the cartilage is incised part way through its thickness. The amount of cartilage to be removed depends on the size of the meatus desired.

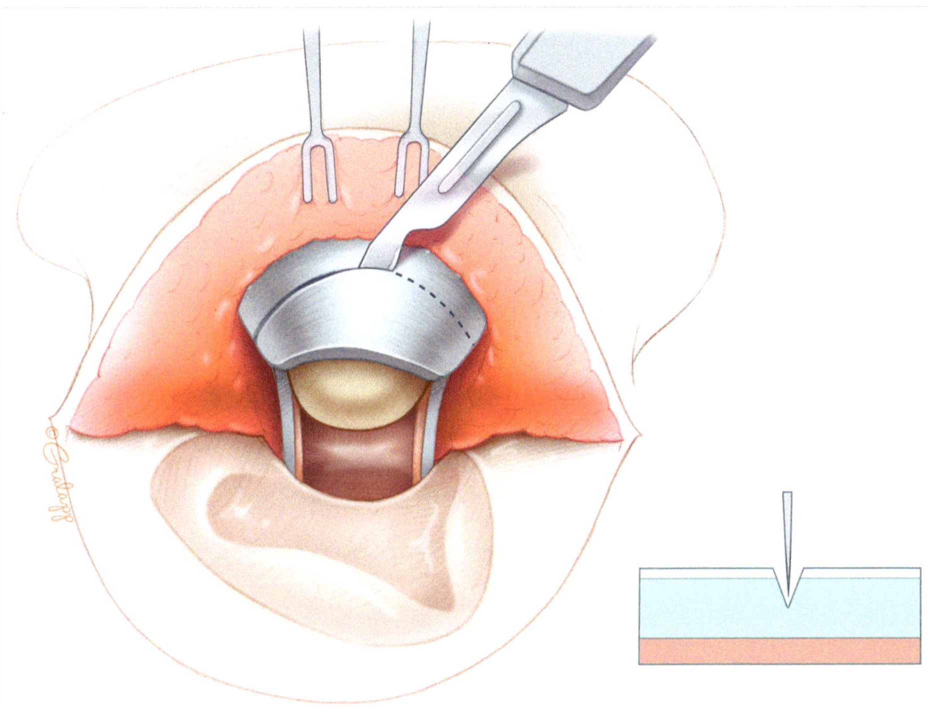

Fig. 3.91 In a larger cavity, a greater extent of cartilage is excised. Note the scalpel incision is partial thickness. Scissors easily complete the rest of the cartilage transection and are less likely than a knife to perforate the underlying perichondrial leaf.

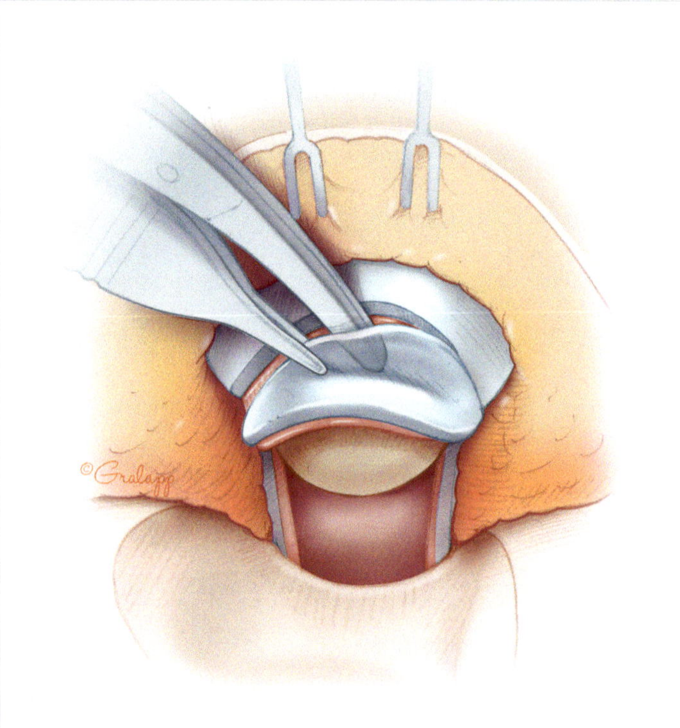

Fig. 3.92 Dissection of the conchal cartilage off the underlying perichondrium.

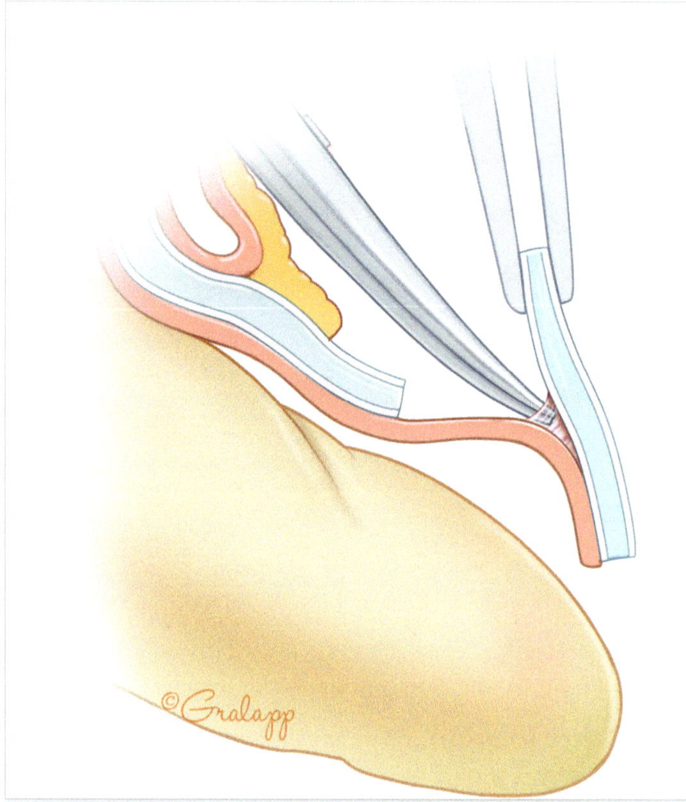

Fig. 3.93 Schematic of the dissection of the cartilage off the underlying perichondrium.

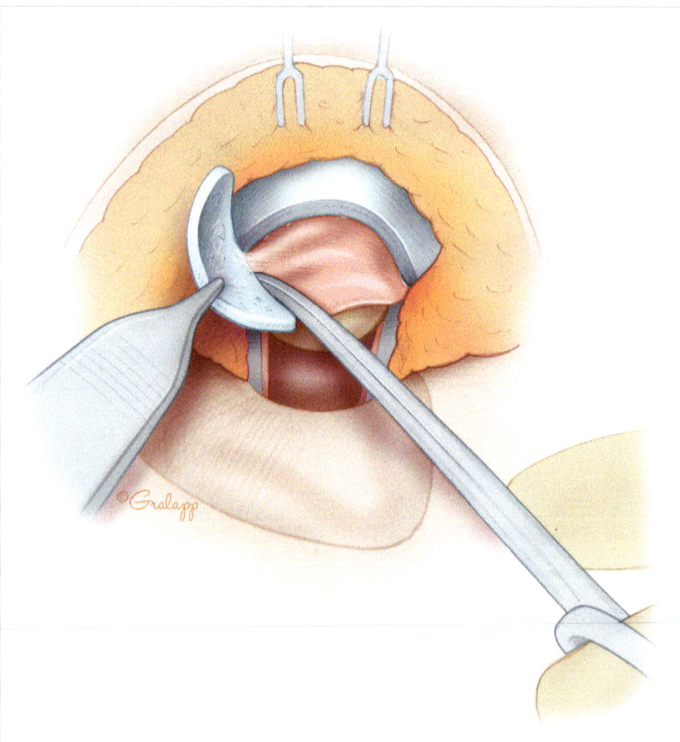

Fig. 3.94 Removal of the conchal cartilage from the meatal skin.

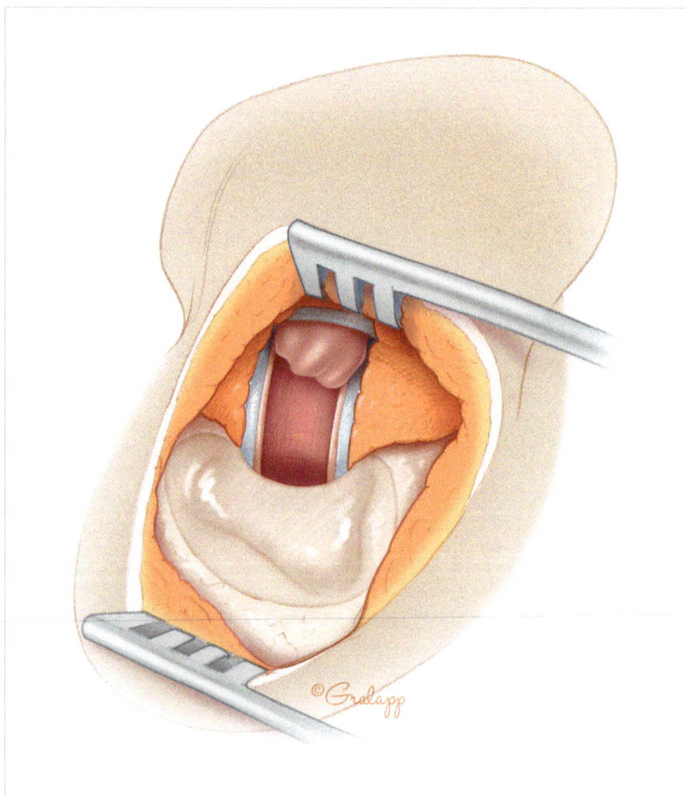

Fig. 3.95 Anterior meatoplasty is needed to balance the size of the anterior meatus with the now larger posterior meatus.

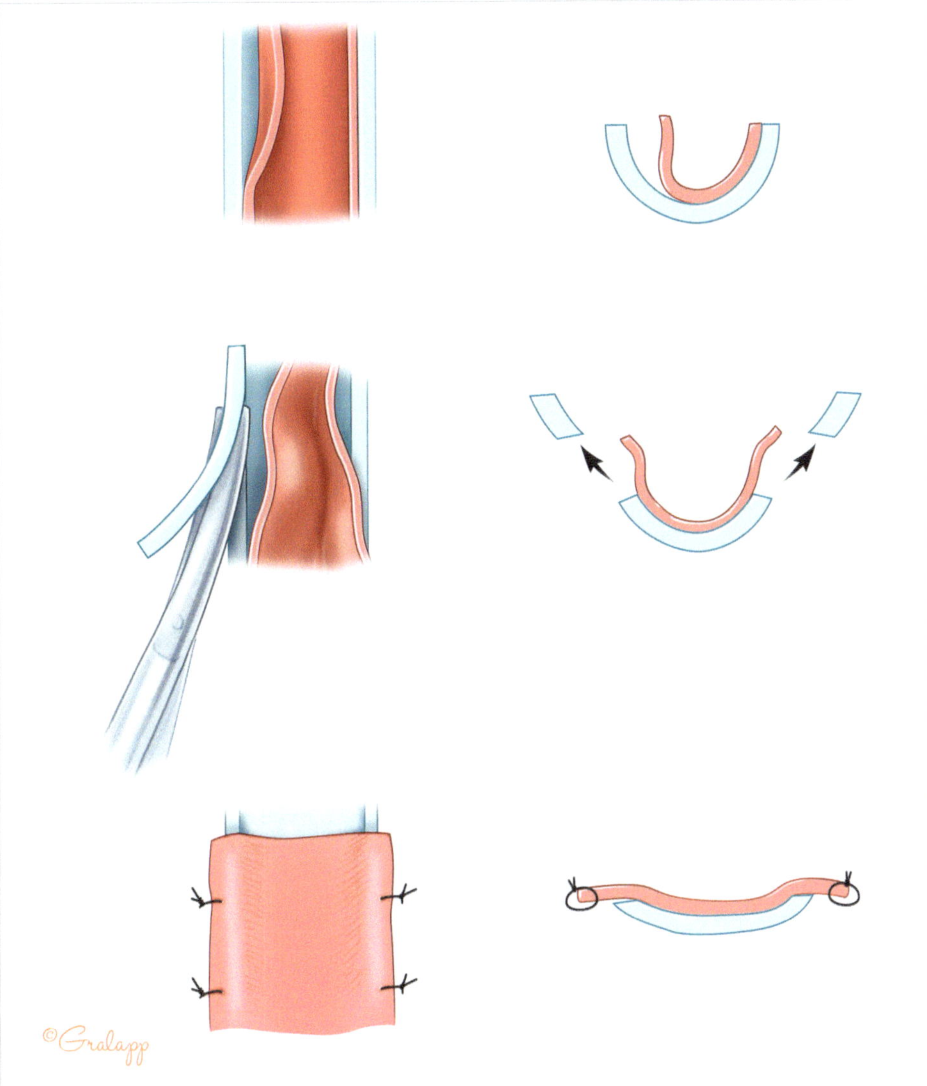

Fig. 3.96 The goal of anterior meatoplasty is to flatten the curvature of the **C**-shaped anterior meatus. The skin is dissected off the cartilage, which is then trimmed flush with the anterior face of the meatus. A couple of tacking stitches are often helpful in securing the anterior skin flap in the desired location.

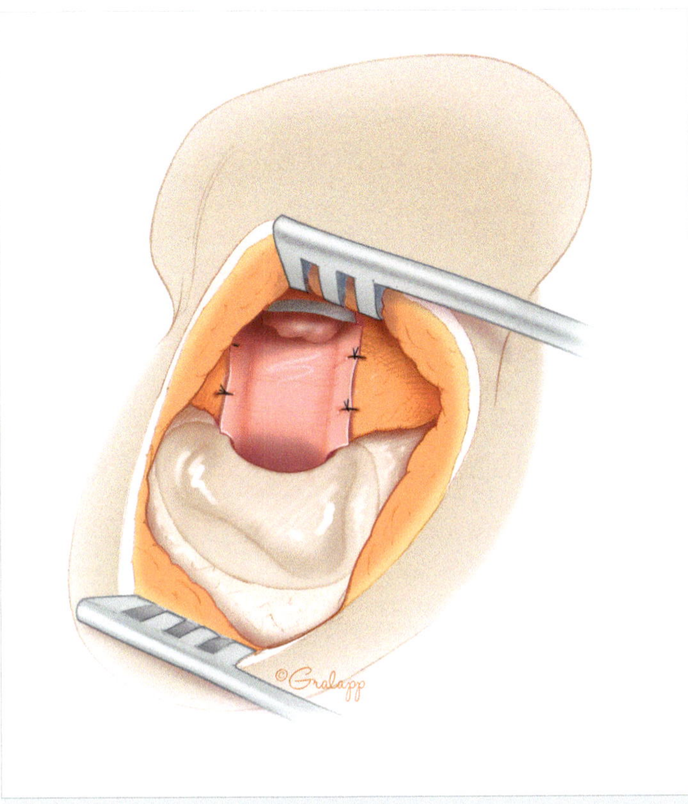

Fig. 3.97 Completed anterior meatoplasty.

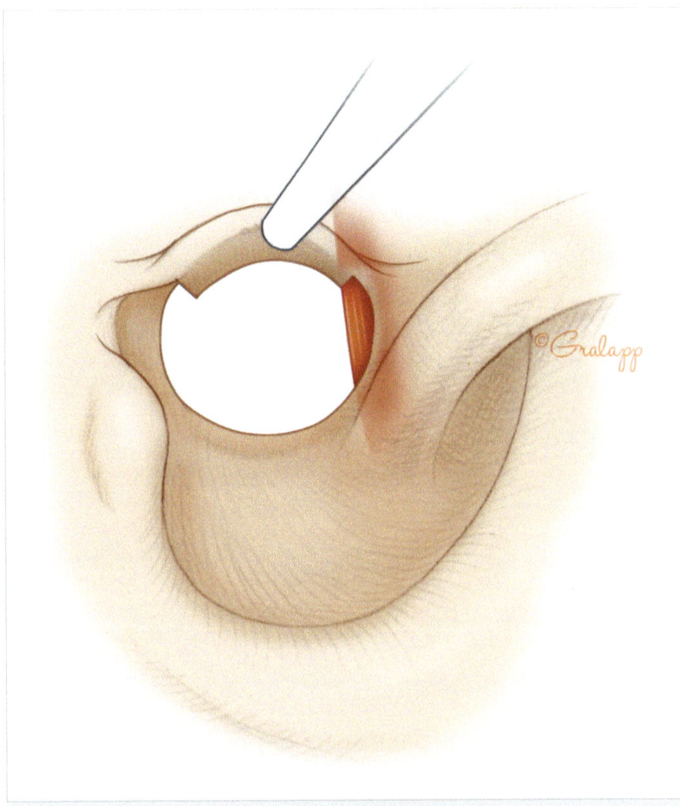

Fig. 3.98 The lower aspect of the temporalis muscle often impinges on the superior aspect of the enlarged meatus.

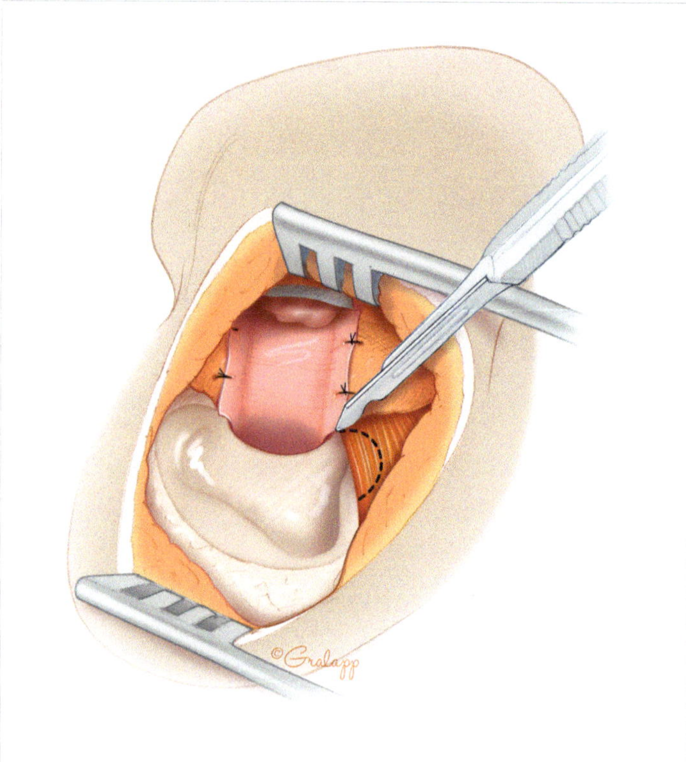

Fig. 3.99 The lower aspect of the temporalis muscle is resected so that it will not impinge on the surgically enlarged meatus.

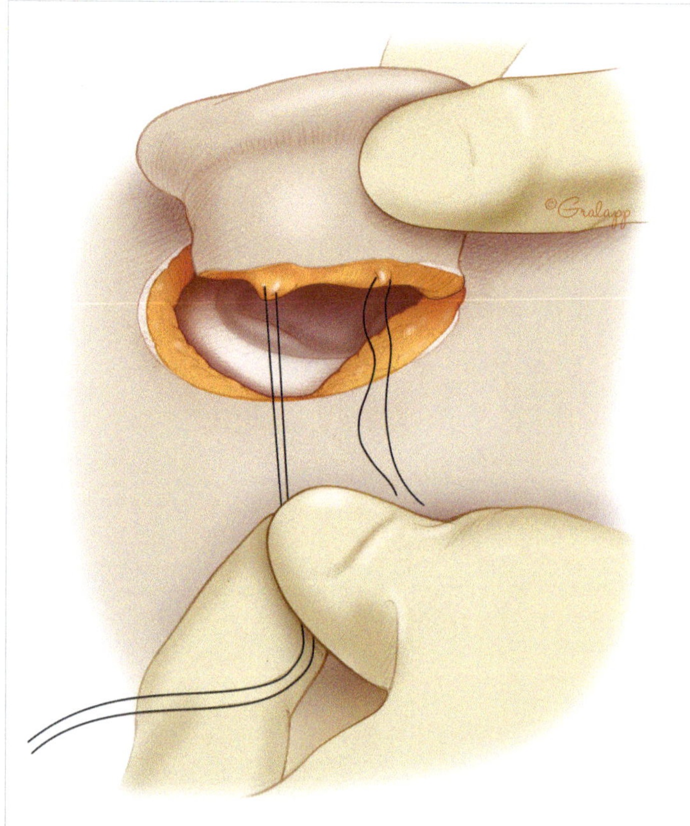

Fig. 3.100 Placement of the initial closure sutures is key to obtaining a proper shaped meatus. Placed through the deep tissue just lateral to the conchal cartilage excision, 2–0 sutures are placed at the upper and lower aspects of the meatus.

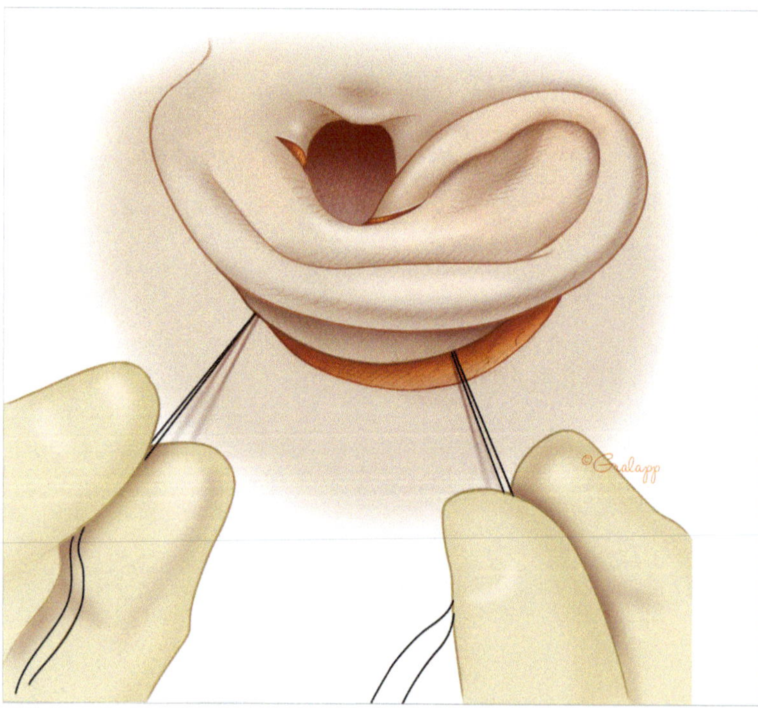

Fig. 3.101 The sutures are anchored in the deep tissue at the back of the incision. Before tying, these are pulled taught to see how they affect the shape of the meatus. The goal is to drape the meatal skin over the trimmed edge of the conchal bowl. If draping is suboptimal, sometimes the skin incision needs to be extended.

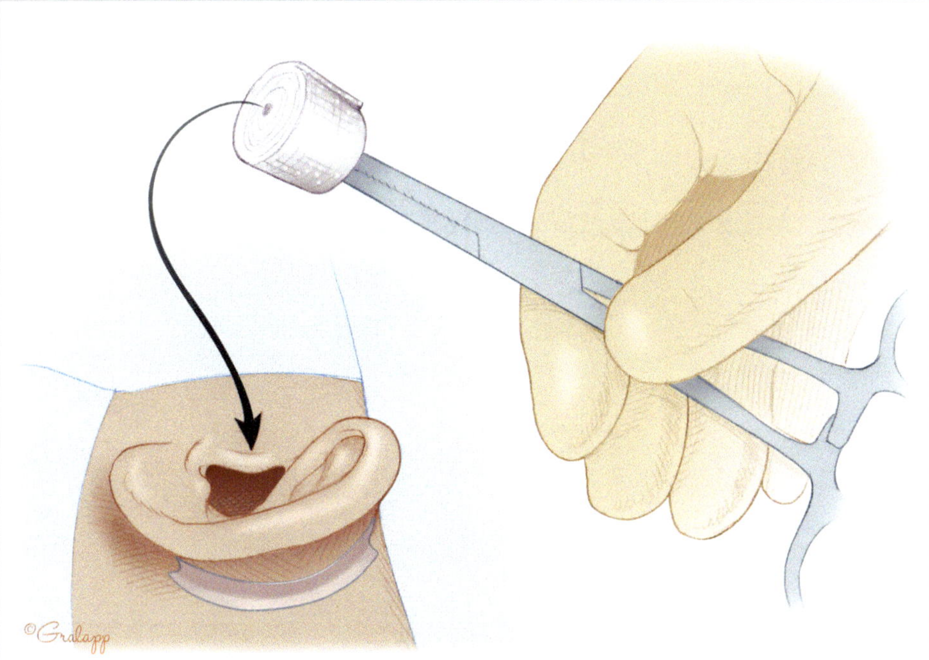

Fig. 3.102 Packing is used to co-apt the meatal skin flap with the newly reshaped conchal margin. Depicted is a 0.5-inch antibiotic-impregnated strip of packing gauze wound around a clamp. While this so-called meatal roll works well, other methods such as a large Merocel sponge are also effective.

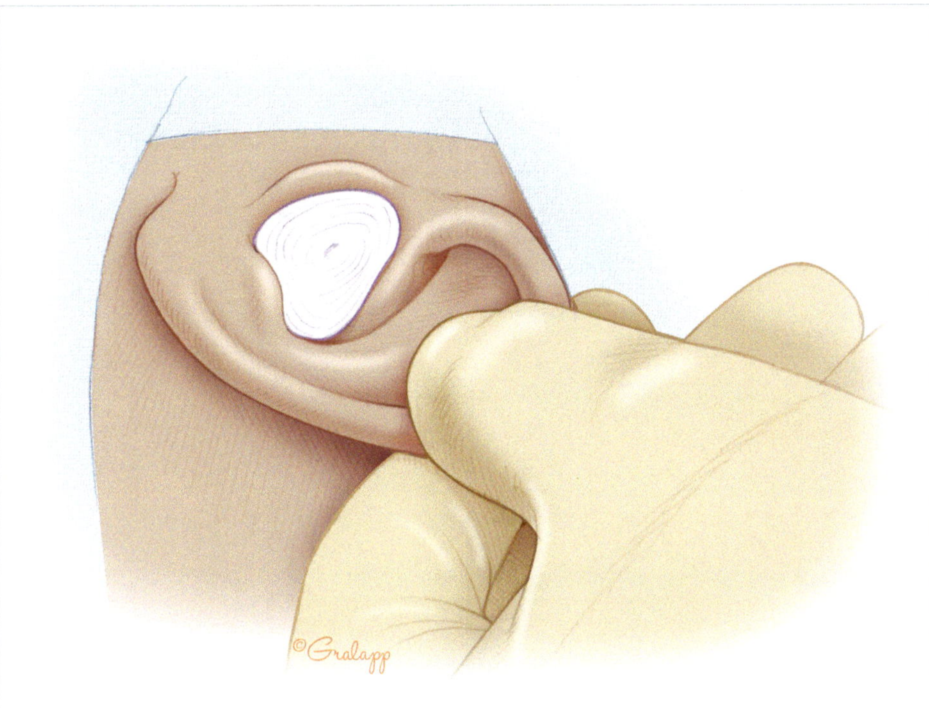

Fig. 3.103 Meatal packing in place. This can be removed as early as a few days later.

3.6 Endaural Meatoplasty

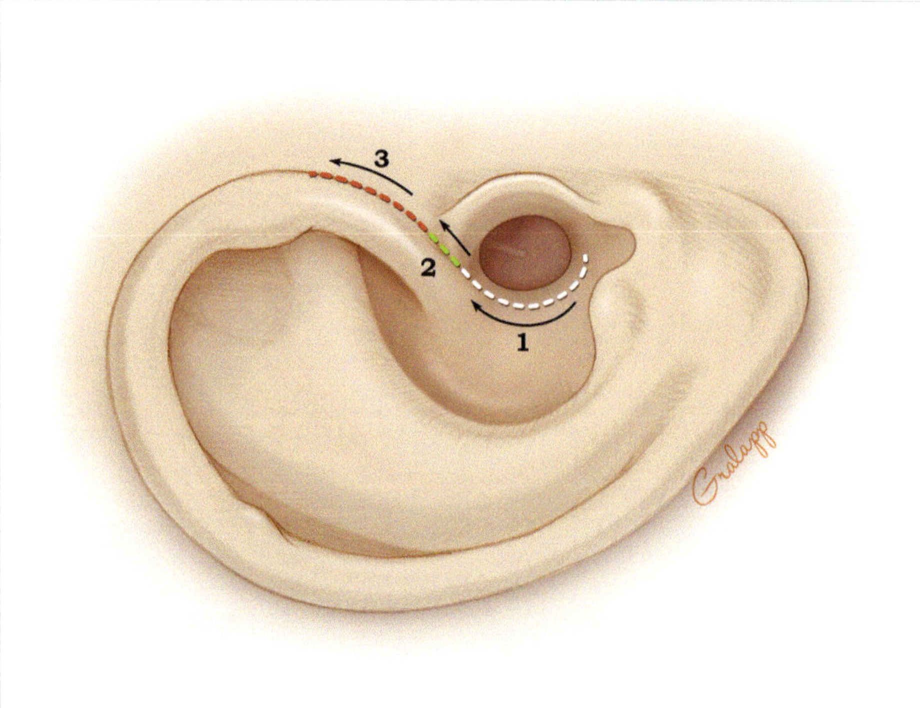

Fig. 3.104 Incision for endaural meatoplasty.

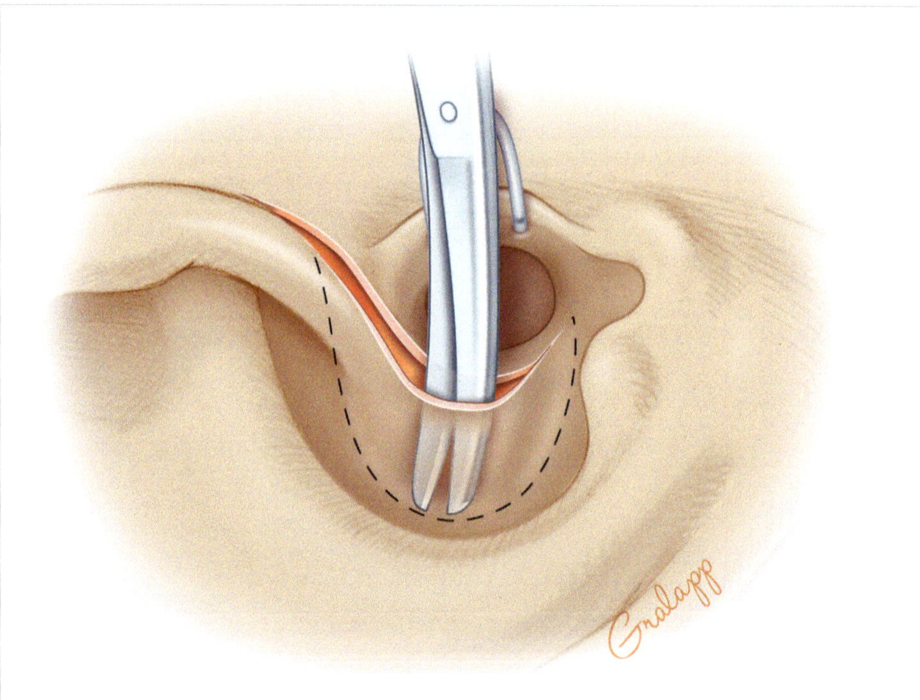

Fig. 3.105 Elevation of conchal skin off conchal cartilage.

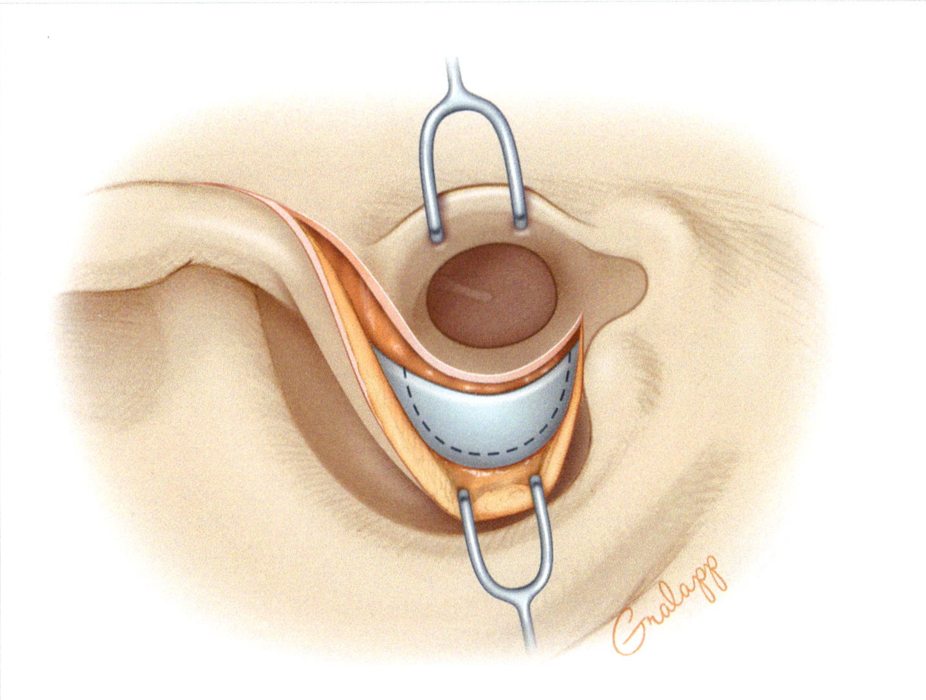

Fig. 3.106 Completed exposure of conchal cartilage. Dotted line is cartilage incision which is placed according to desired meatal size.

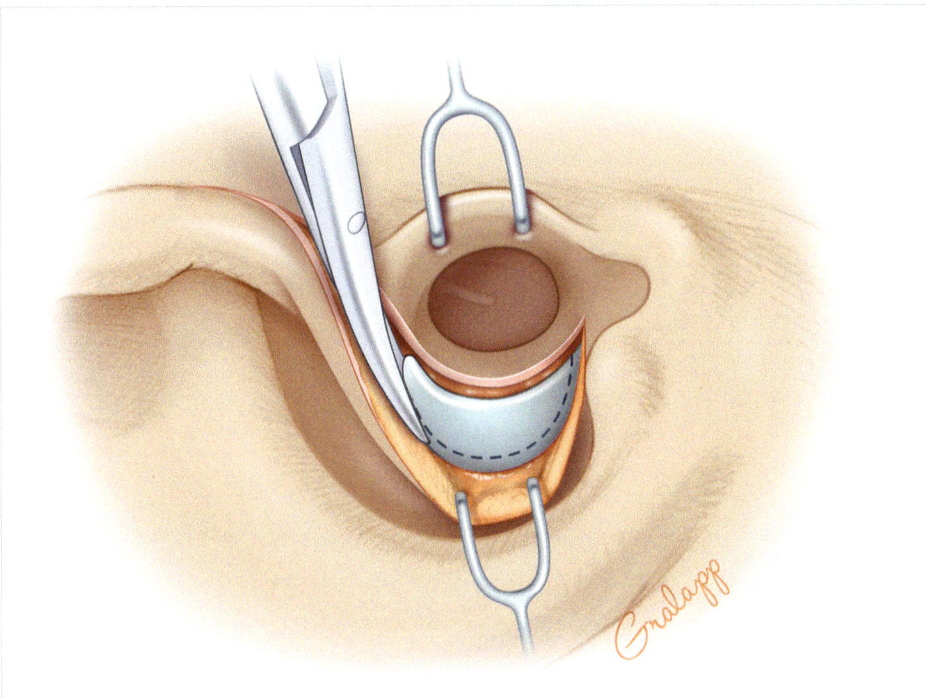

Fig. 3.107 Excision of a rim of conchal cartilage.

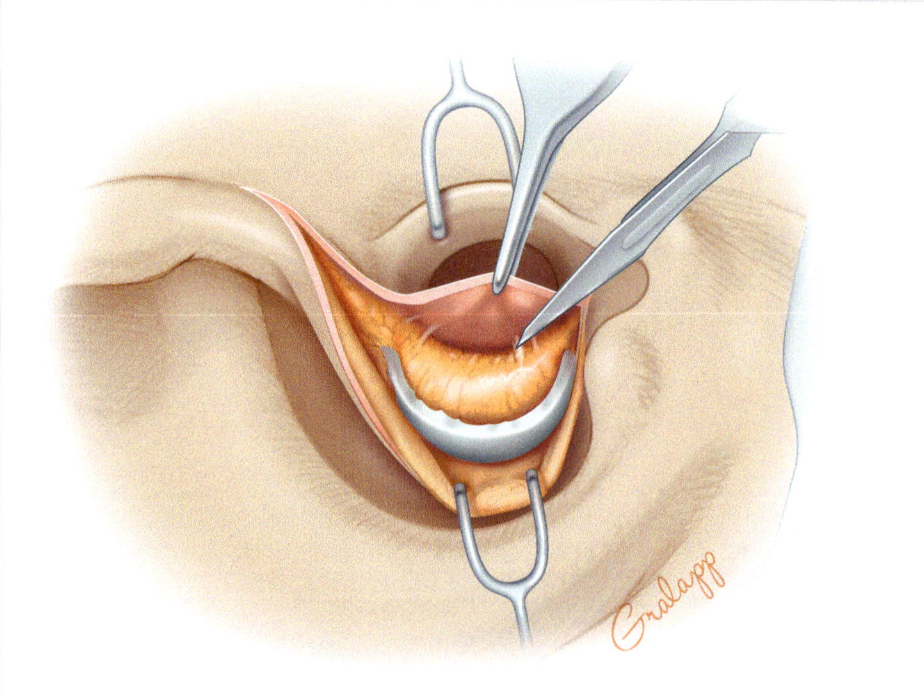

Fig. 3.108 Elevation of soft tissue deep to the excised conchal cartilage from the ear canal skin.

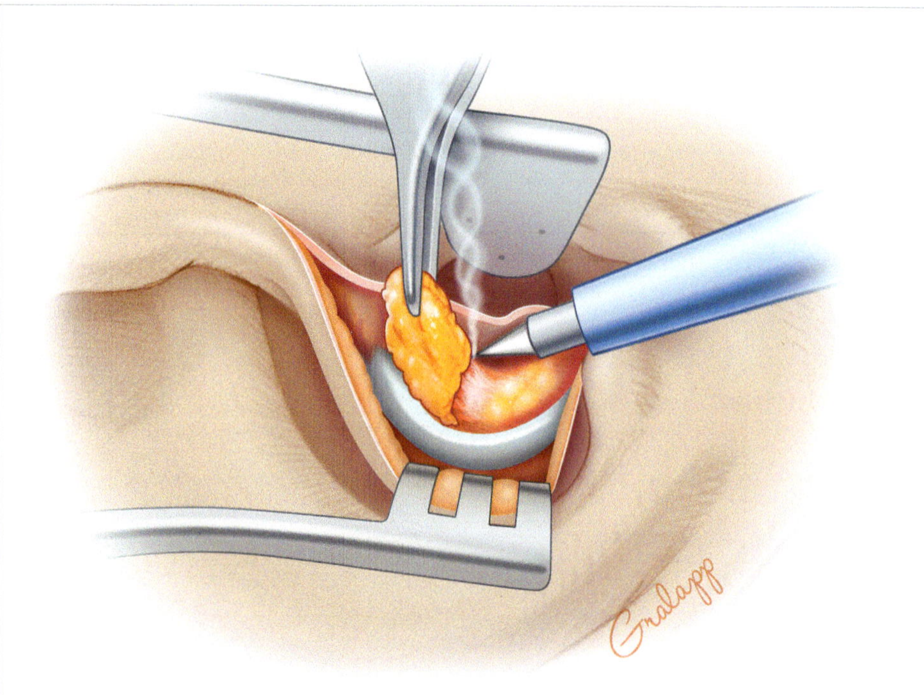

Fig. 3.109 Debulking of soft tissue.

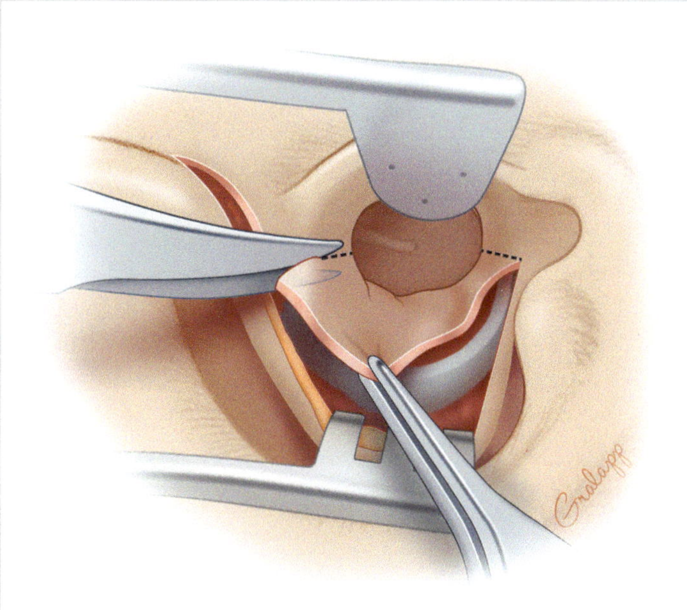

Fig. 3.110 Superior and inferior incisions to enable flap advancement for skin closure.

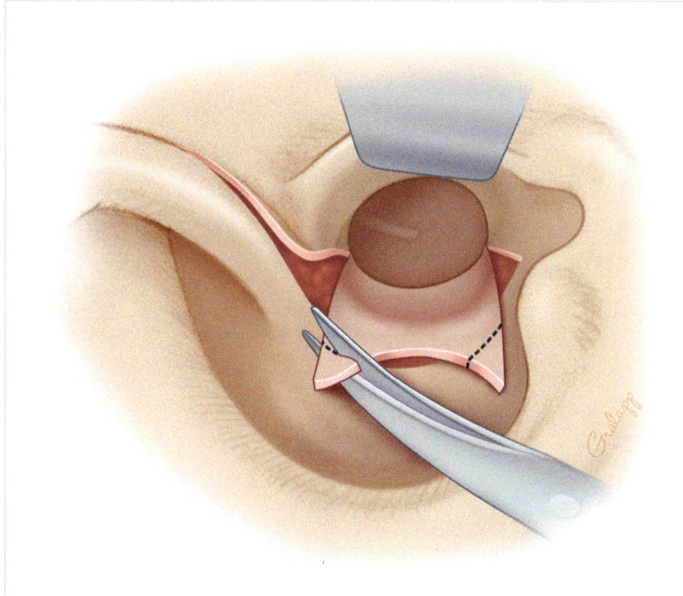

Fig. 3.111 Trimming the extra skin to conform the canal skin to the curved conchal skin.

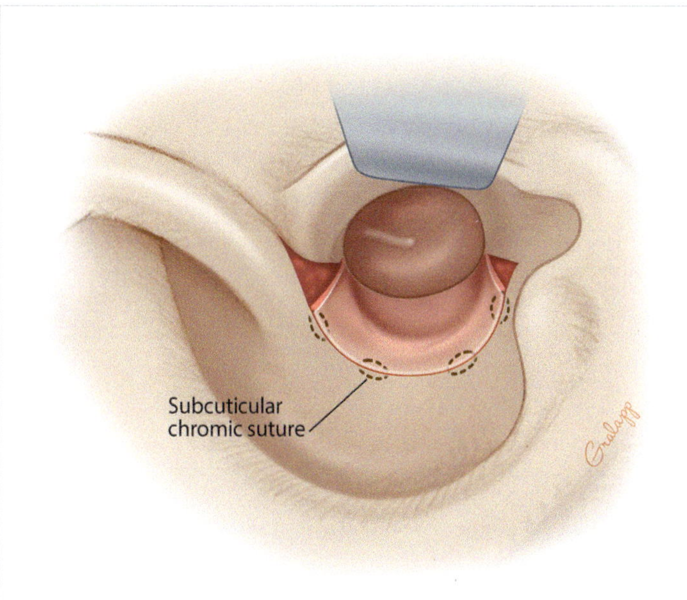

Fig. 3.112 Skin closure.

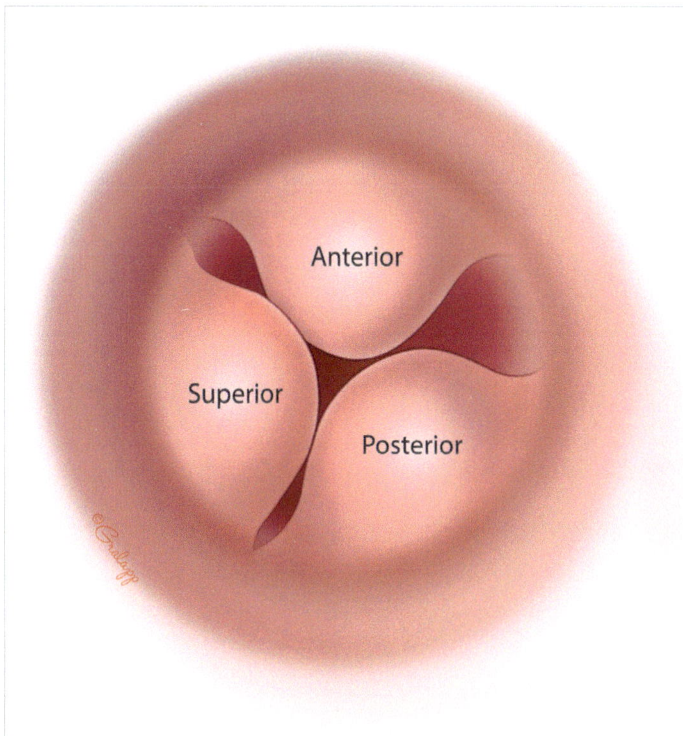

Fig. 3.113 Exostoses of the ear canal are characteristically multiple. Surgery is indicated only when they are advanced and become obstructive or become stubbornly infected. Most surgeons prefer a postauricular approach, although a transcanal approach may be feasible with a large diameter canal.

3.7 Exostoses of the Ear Canal

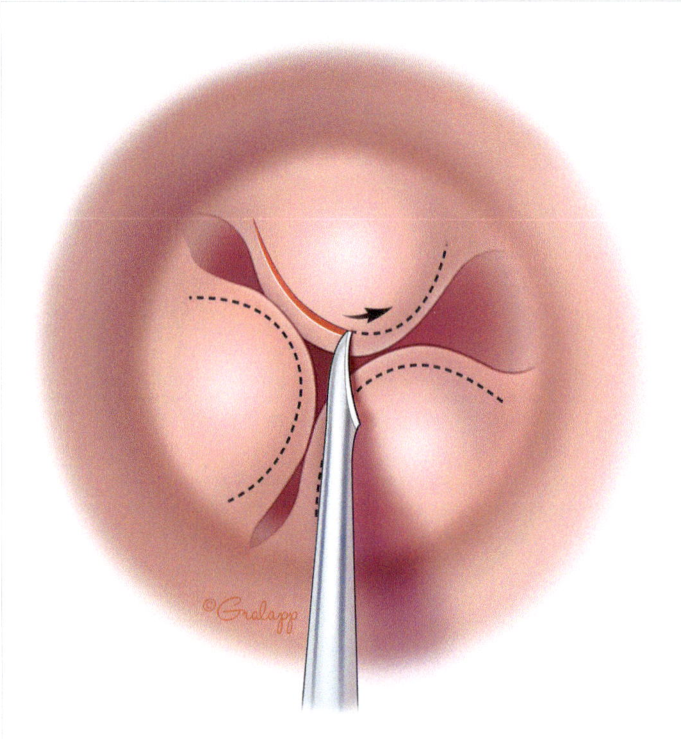

Fig. 3.114 Incisions are designed to preserve as much skin as possible.

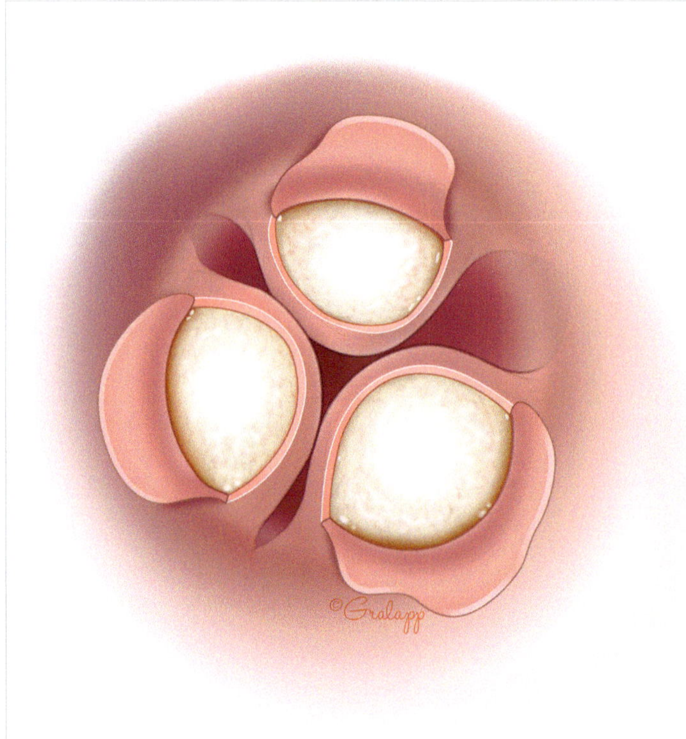

Fig. 3.115 Flaps are developed by elevating the skin off the exostoses in retrograde fashion.

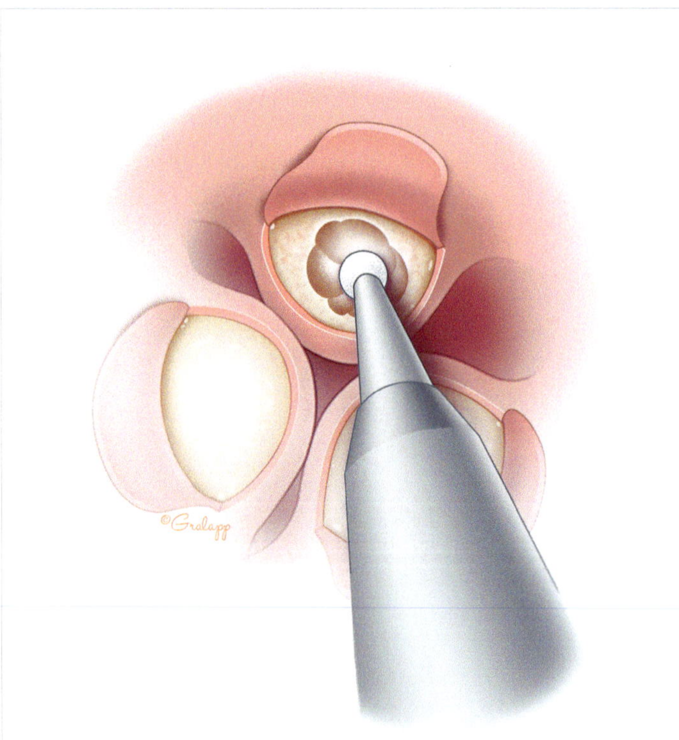

Fig. 3.116 A diamond burr is used to hollow out the exostosis. Some surgeons prefer using a microchisel. It is important to remove the anterior and superior exostoses first to allow orientation to the tympanic membrane.

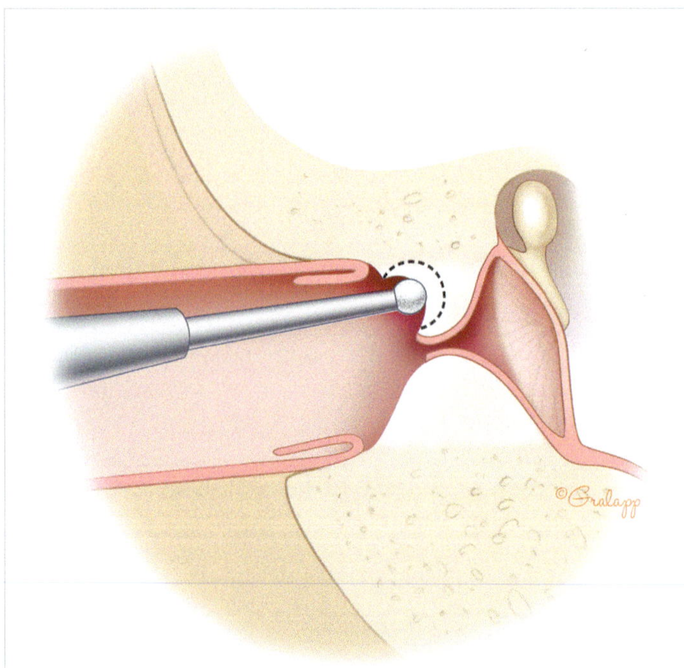

Fig. 3.117 Hollowing out the exostosis.

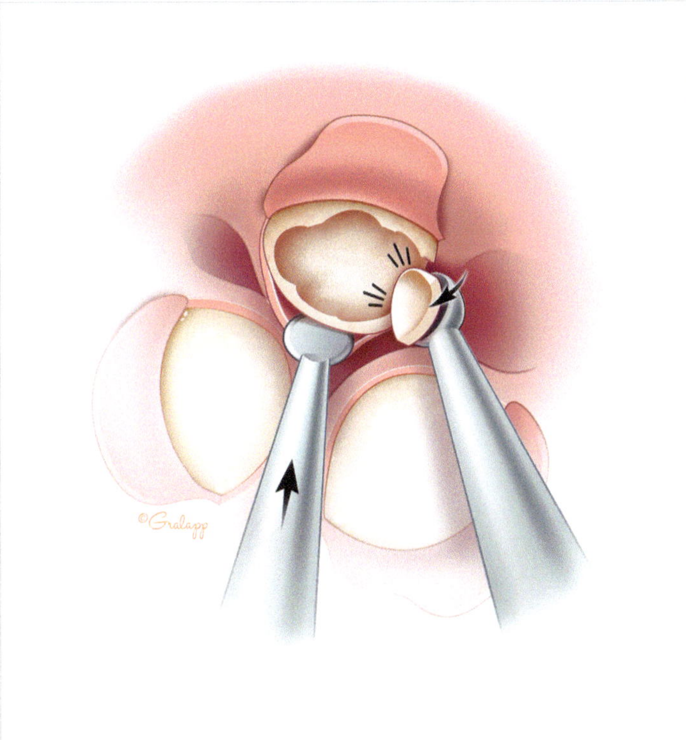

Fig. 3.118 Curetting the thin rim of remaining bone. This maneuver helps conserve the canal skin.

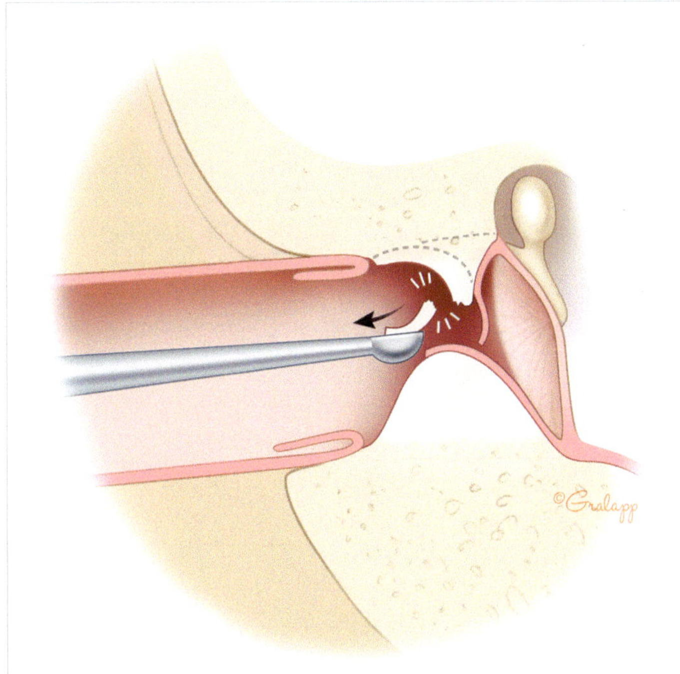

Fig. 3.119 Curetting the rim of the exostosis off the underlying meatal skin.

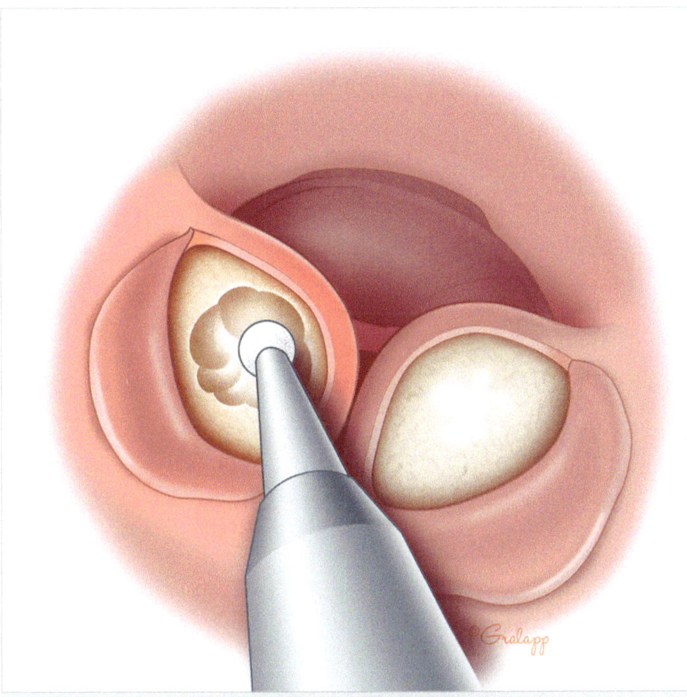

Fig. 3.120 The superior exostosis is removed next.

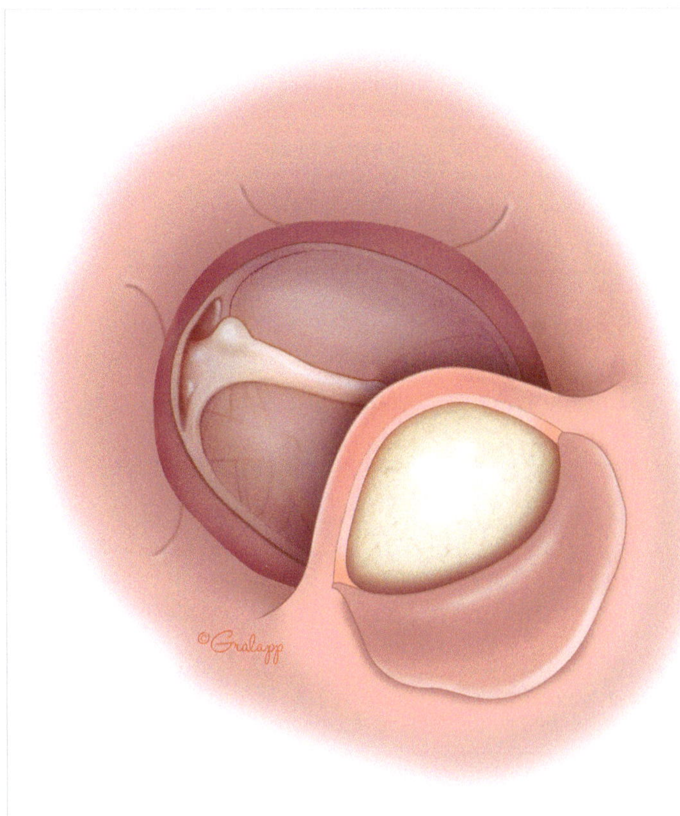

Fig. 3.121 The inferior exostosis is removed last, only after a clear visualization of the posterior tympanic annulus is obtained for orientation.

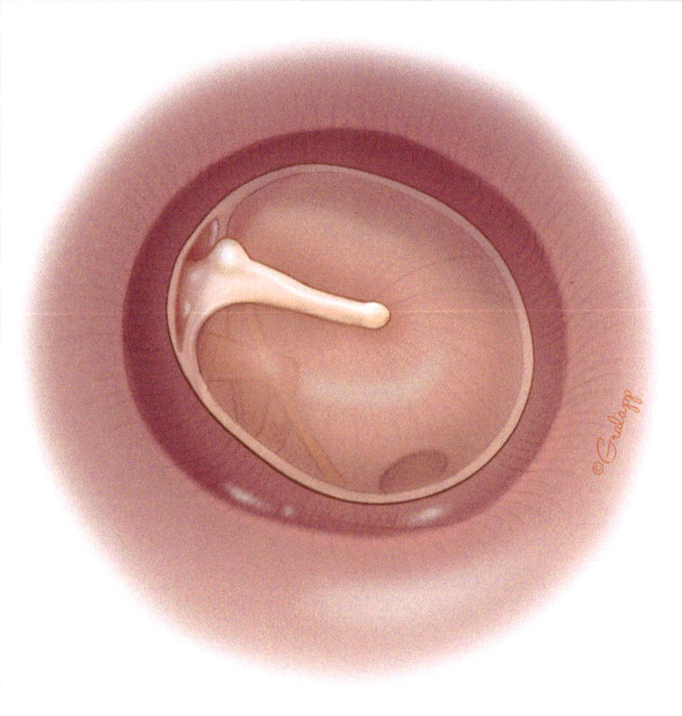

Fig. 3.122 The extent of canaloplasty should be slightly greater than the annulus margin.

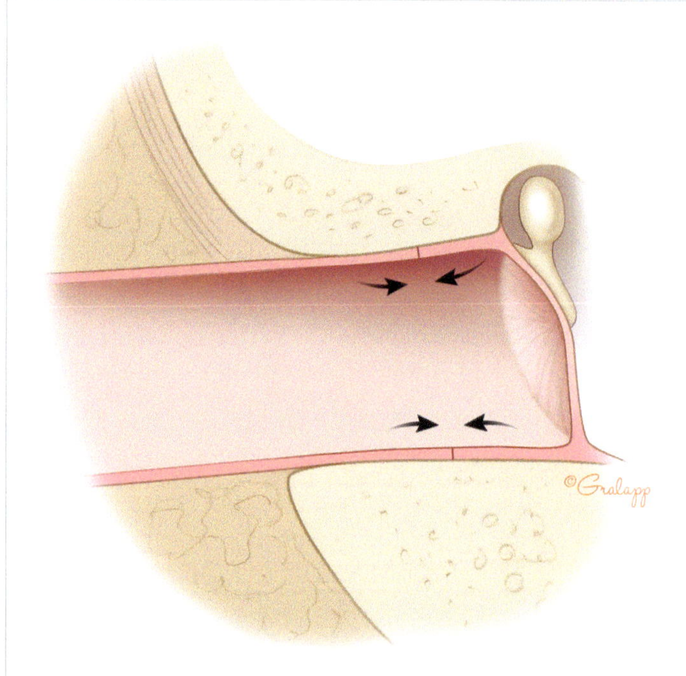

Fig. 3.123 The skin flaps are laid together. It is almost never as neat as illustrated here. Minor areas of exposed bone are common, but heal well if patchy and not circumferential. It is uncommon to need a split-thickness skin grafting.

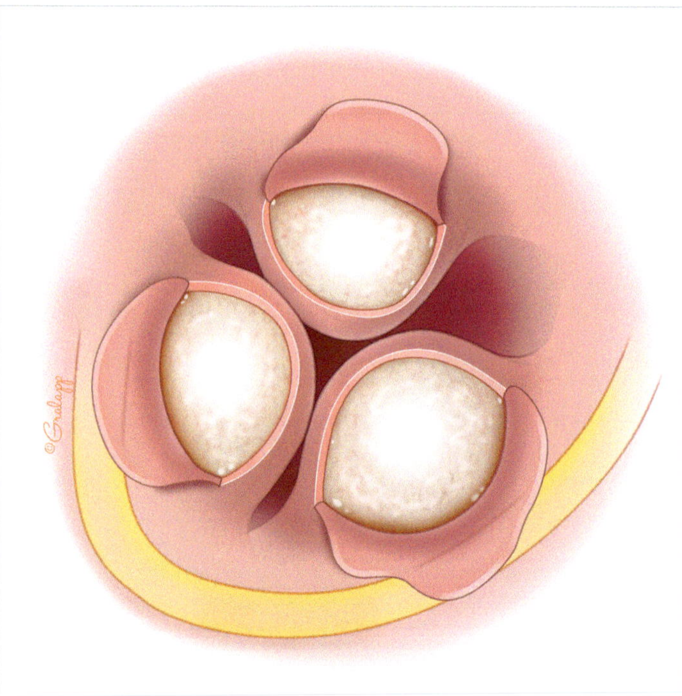

Fig. 3.124 Note the relationship of the facial nerve to the posterior-inferior exostosis. While the nerve lies well deep to the superior exostosis, inferiorly the nerve may occasionally lie lateral to the tympanic annulus. A risk of iatrogenic facial nerve injury in exostosis removal exists if the surgeon does not work first anteriorly to become oriented to the tympanic membrane and becomes disoriented and drills off axis.

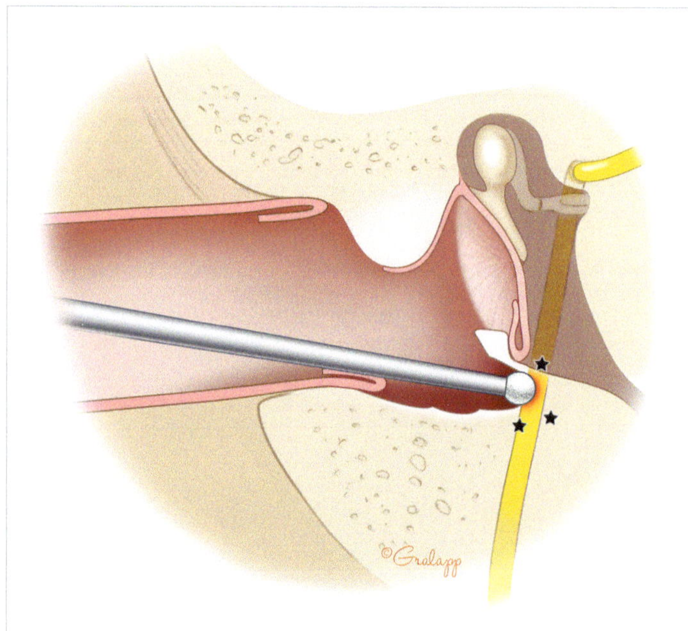

Fig. 3.125 Mechanism of facial nerve injury in exostoses removal. This is avoidable by first orienting to the tympanic membrane by first removing the anterior and superior exostoses.

3.8 Anterior Canaloplasty

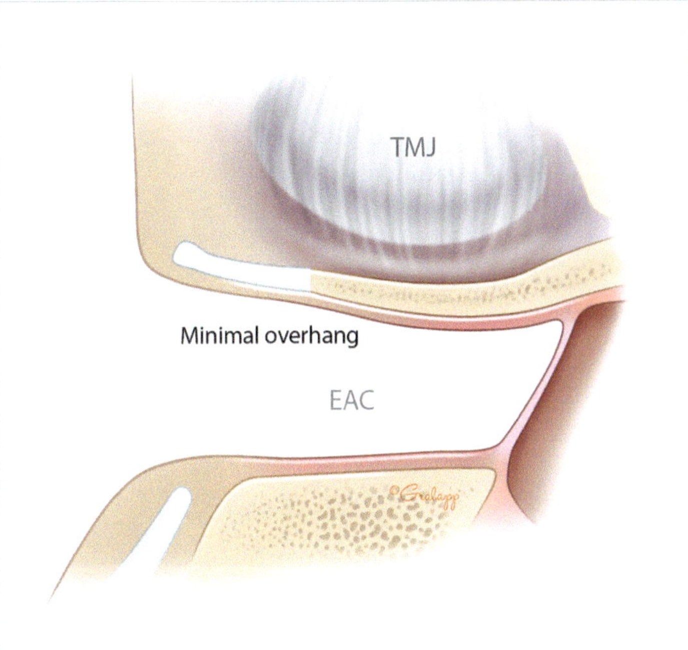

Fig. 3.126 Anterior ear canal with minimal overhang.

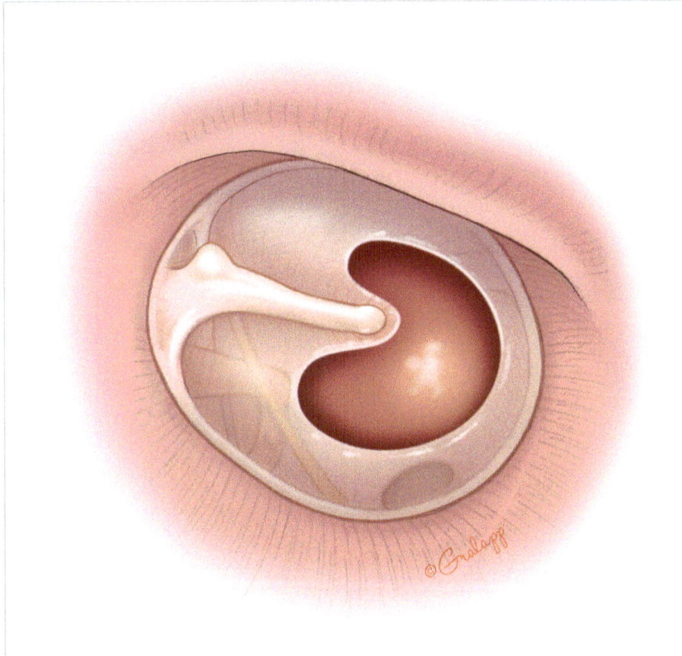

Fig. 3.127 Anterior ear canal with minimal overhang.

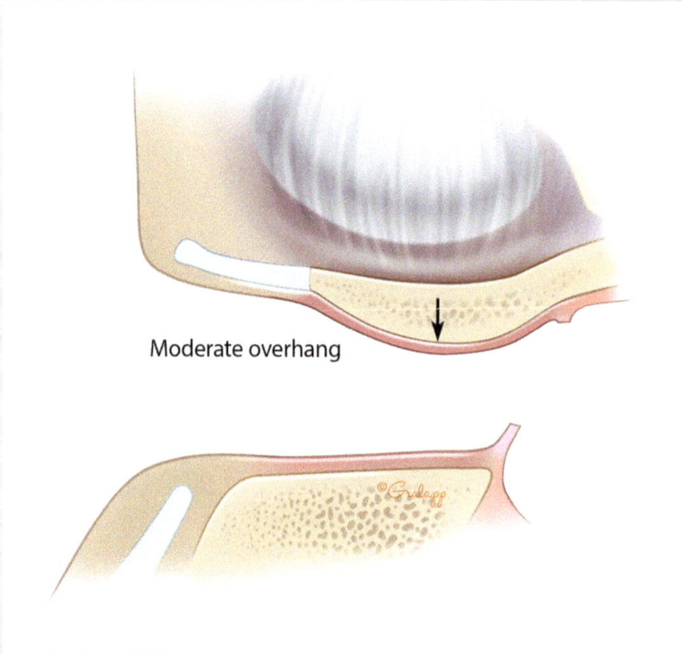

Fig. 3.128 Anterior ear canal with moderate overhang. EAC, external auditory canal; TMJ, temporomandibular joint.

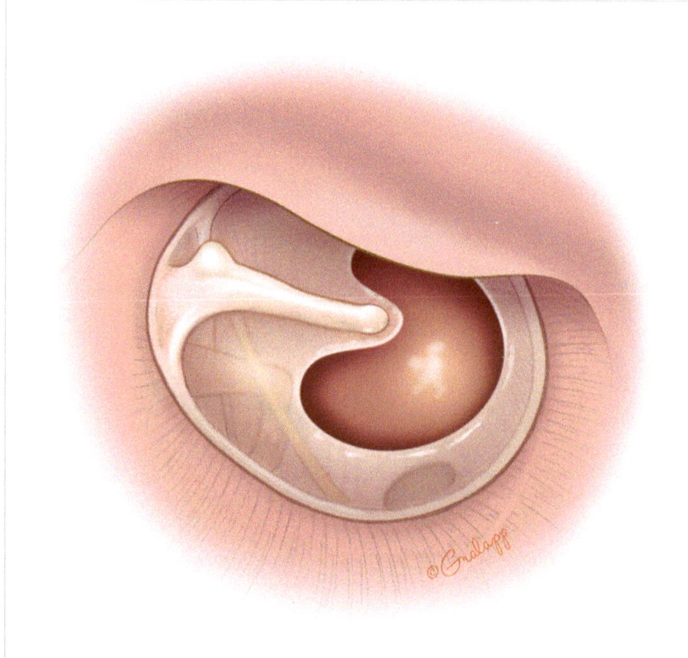

Fig. 3.129 Anterior ear canal with moderate overhang.

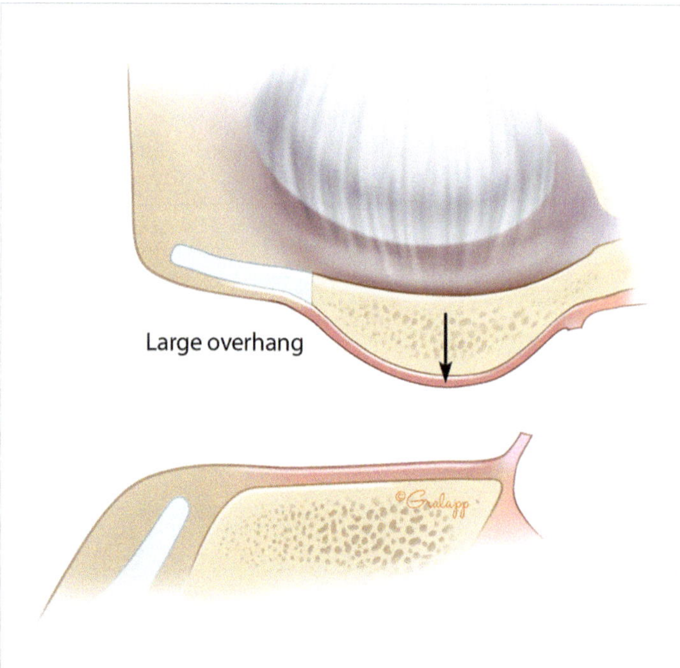

Fig. 3.130 Anterior ear canal with major overhang obscuring the anterior portion of the tympanic membrane.

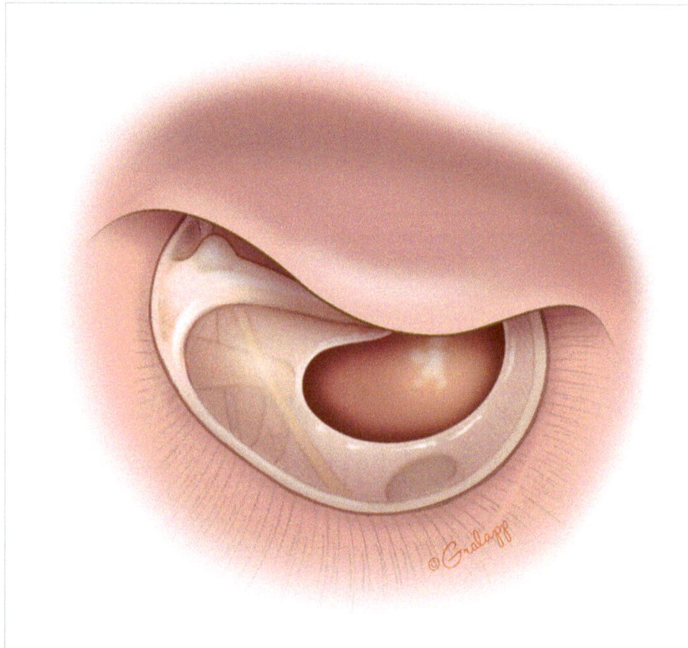

Fig. 3.131 Anterior ear canal with major overhang obscuring the anterior portion of the tympanic membrane.

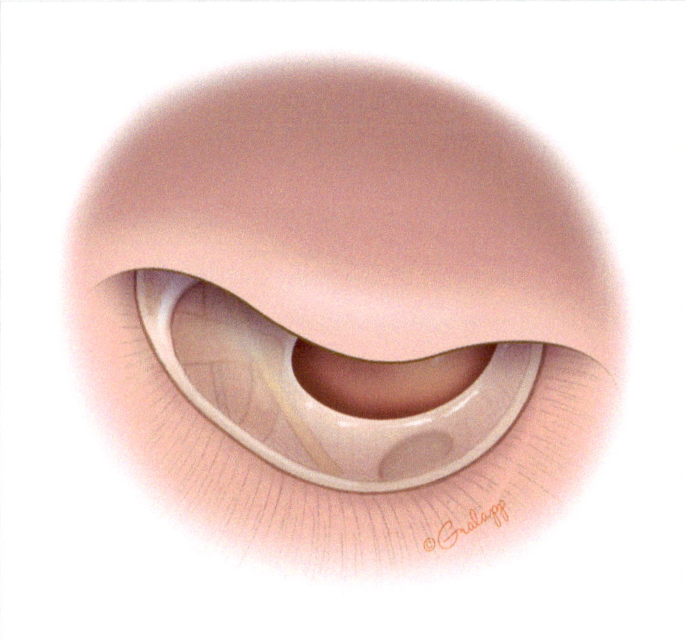

Fig. 3.132 Anterior ear canal with major overhang obscuring the anterior portion of the tympanic membrane.

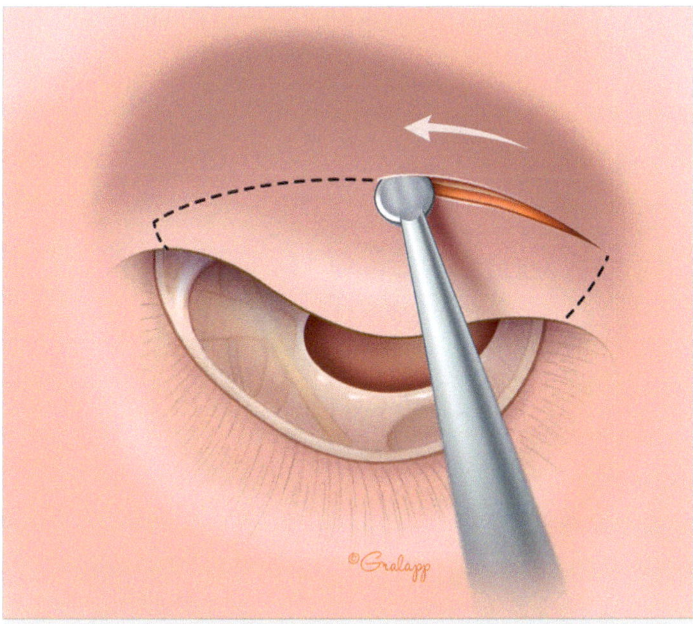

Fig. 3.133 Anterior canal incision.

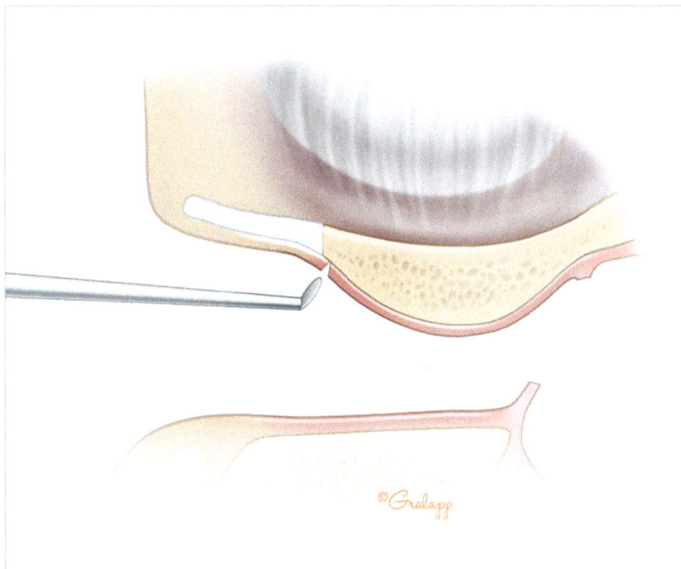

Fig. 3.134 Anterior canal incision.

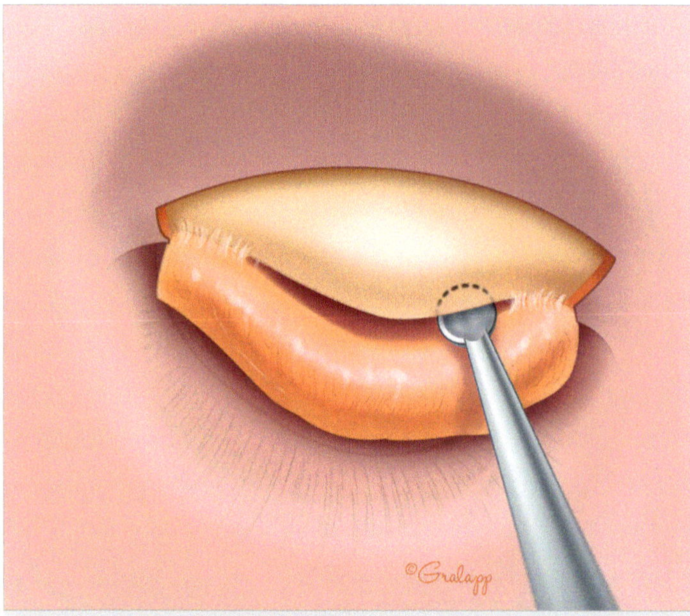

Fig. 3.135 Elevation of canal skin flap.

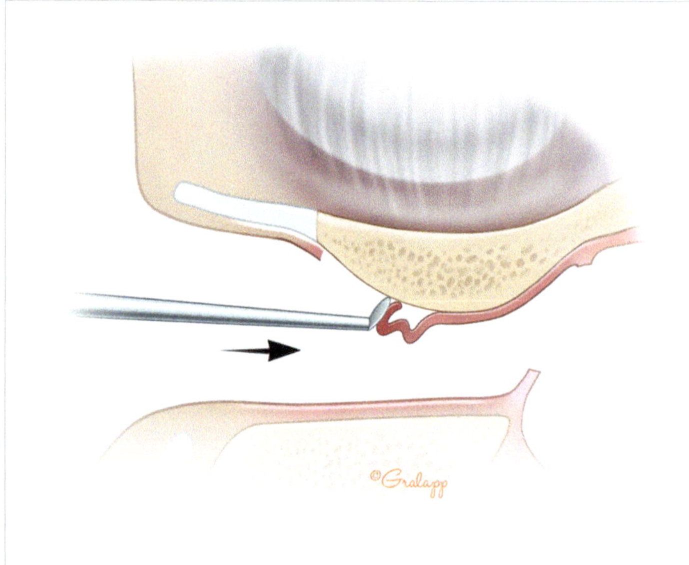

Fig. 3.136 Elevation of canal skin flap.

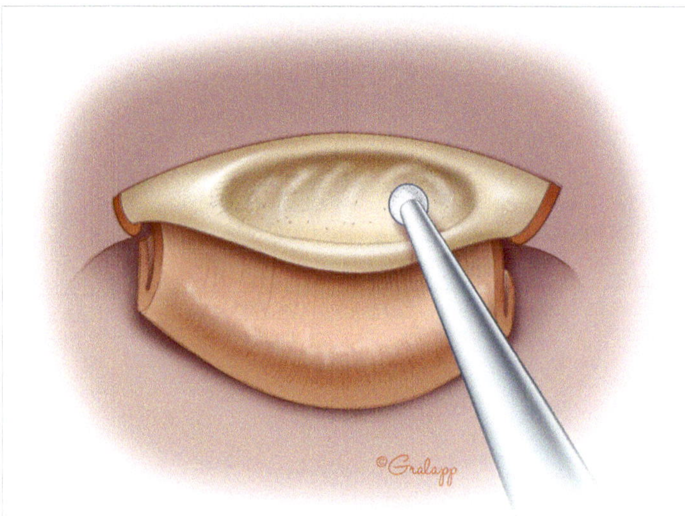

Fig. 3.137 Excavation of canal overhang.

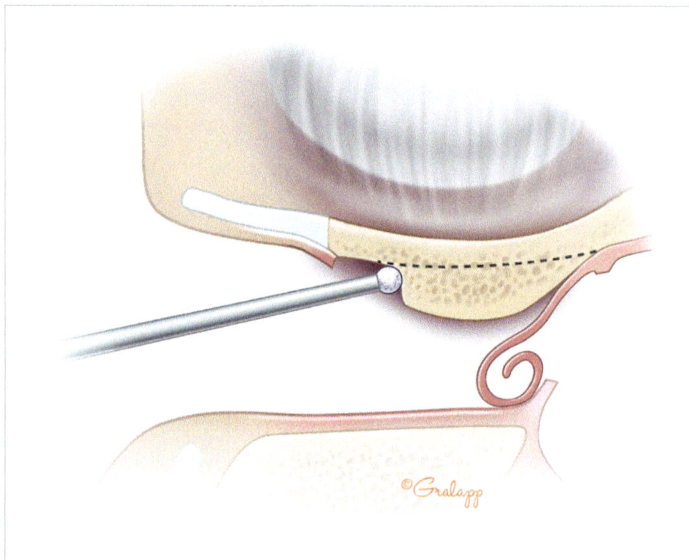

Fig. 3.138 Excavation of canal overhang.

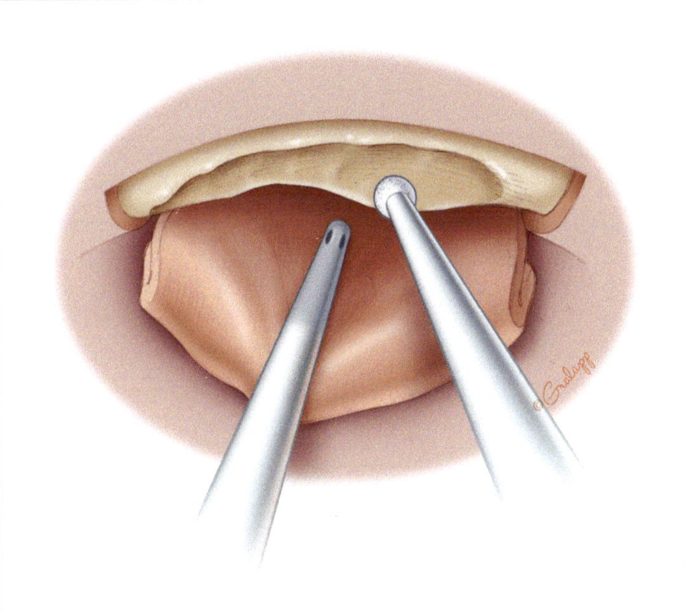

Fig. 3.139 Continued excavation of canal overhang. Note use of fenestrated suction to retract skin flap.

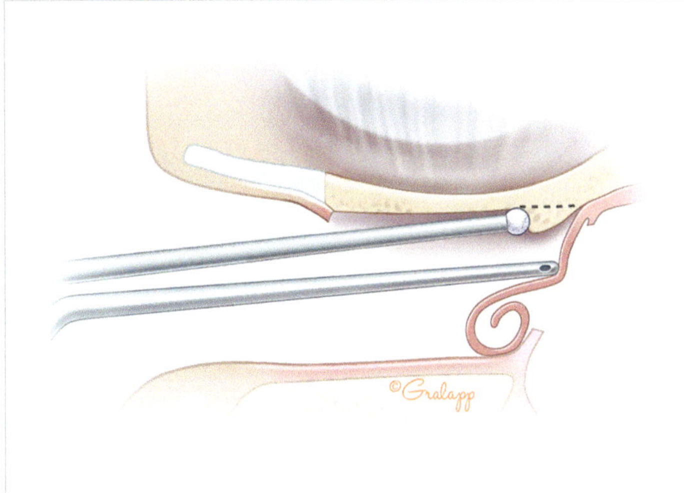

Fig. 3.140 Continued excavation of canal overhang. Note use of fenestrated suction to retract skin flap.

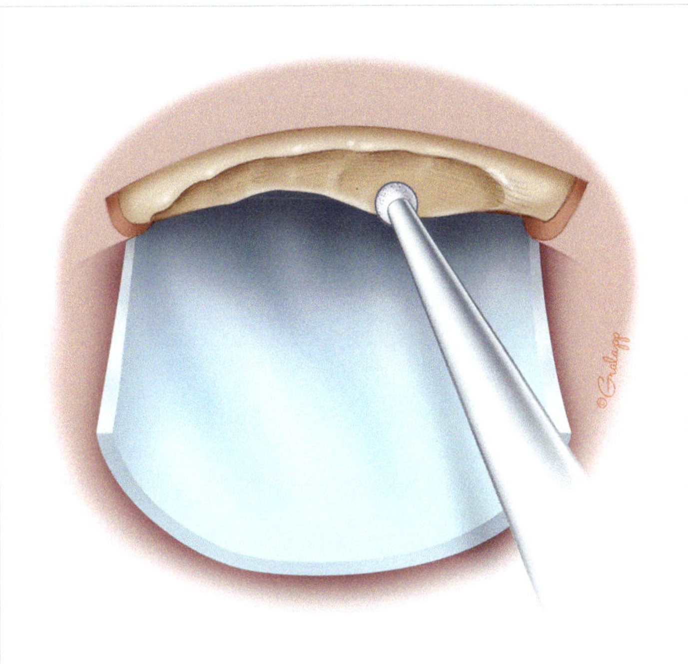

Fig. 3.141 Some surgeons use a thin silicon rubber sheet to protect the skin flap while drilling.

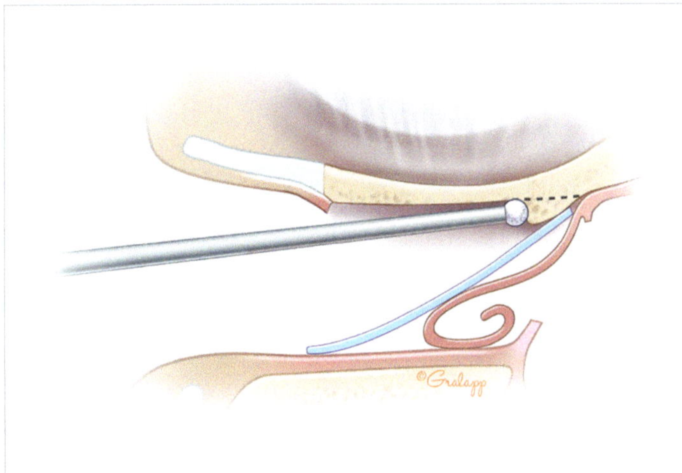

Fig. 3.142 Some surgeons use a thin silicon rubber sheet to protect the skin flap while drilling.

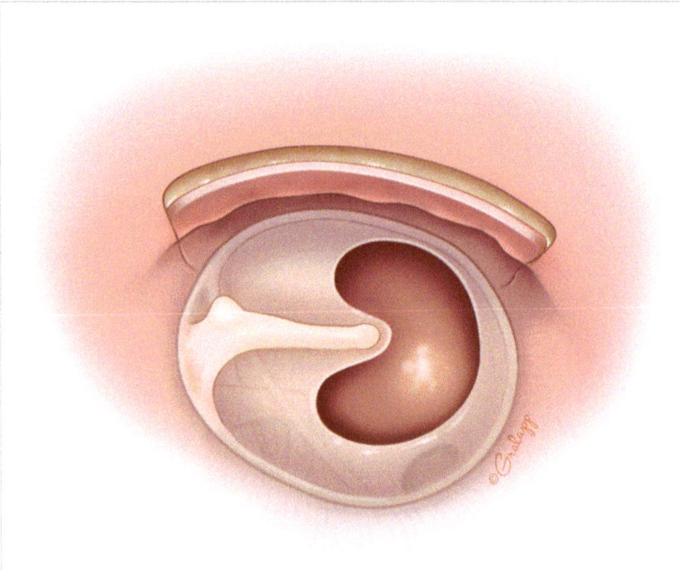

Fig. 3.143 Replacement of the skin flap shows full visualization of the tympanic membrane.

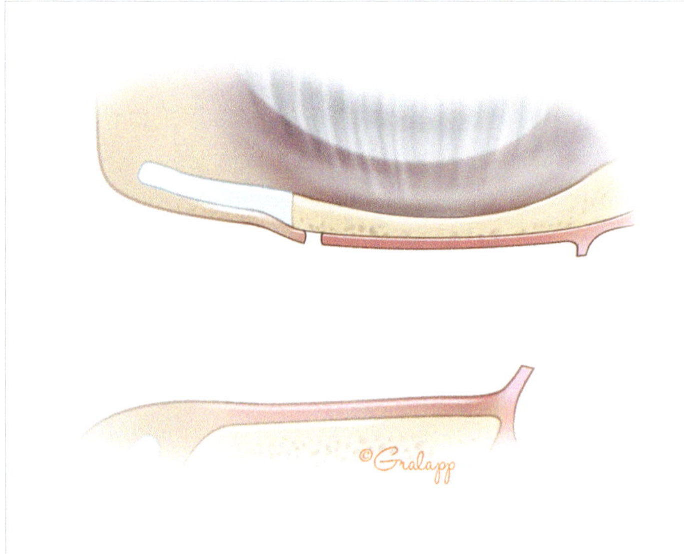

Fig. 3.144 Replacement of the skin flap shows full visualization of the tympanic membrane.

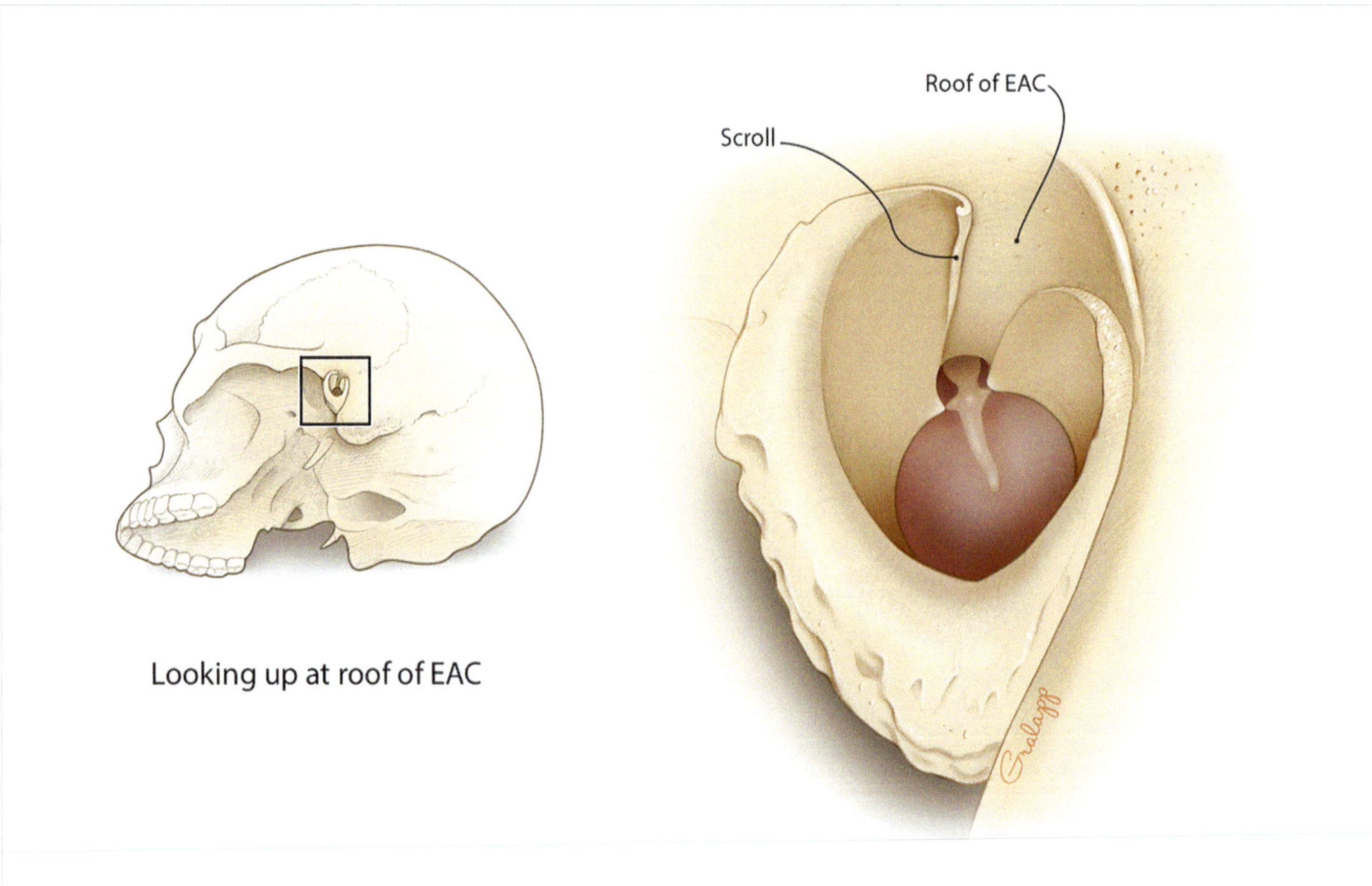

Fig. 3.145 The tympanic bone is an incomplete ring which is open superiorly. At the level of the epitympanum, this aperture is called "the notch of Rivinus." The scroll is a curled edge of the tympanic bone anterosuperiorly which is most prominent just inside the bony canal. The scroll must be removed to provide optimal view of the epitympanum.

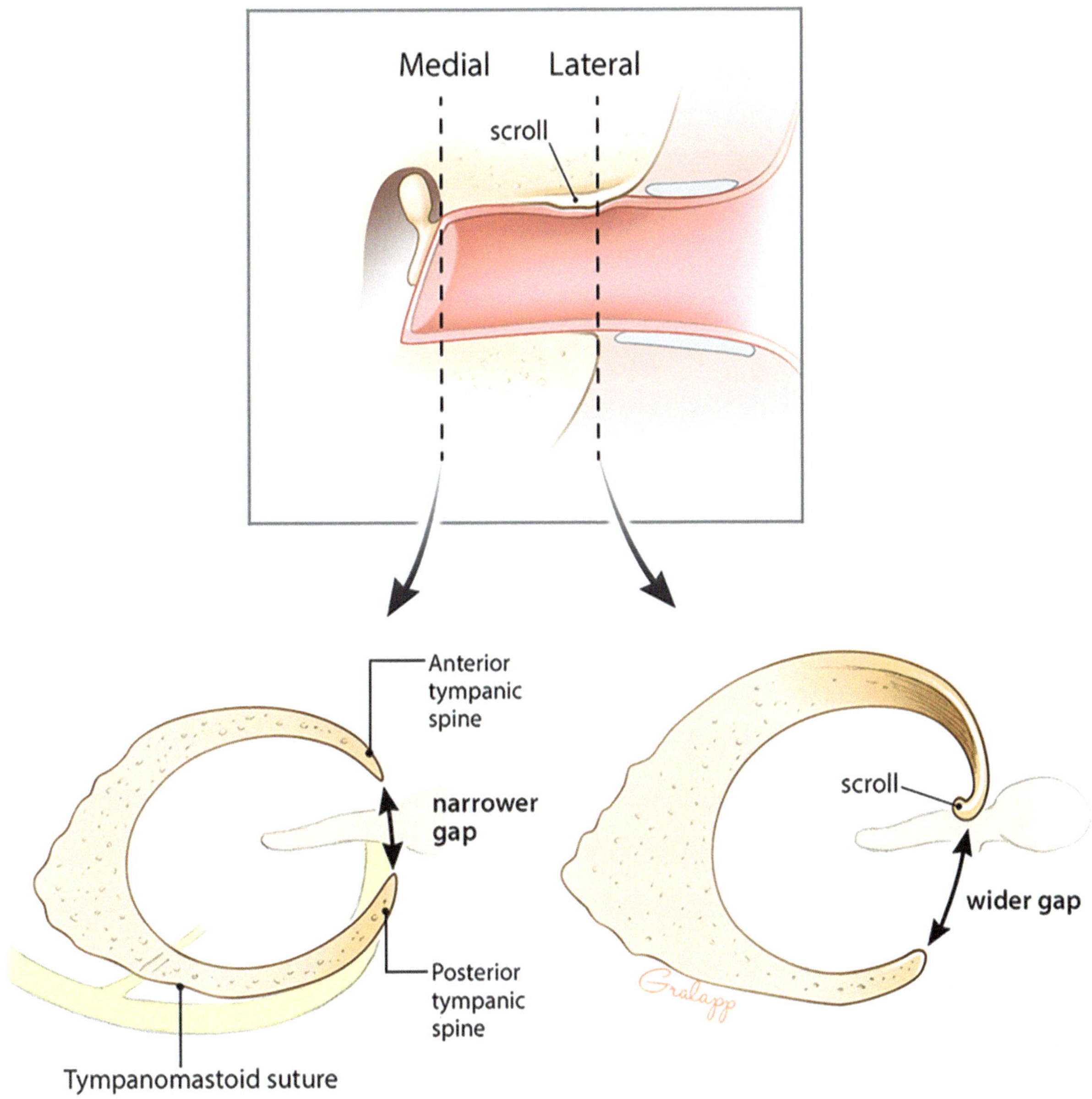

Fig. 3.146 The tympanic bone has a different shape at the annular level and at the bony cartilage junction. The scroll only exists laterally.

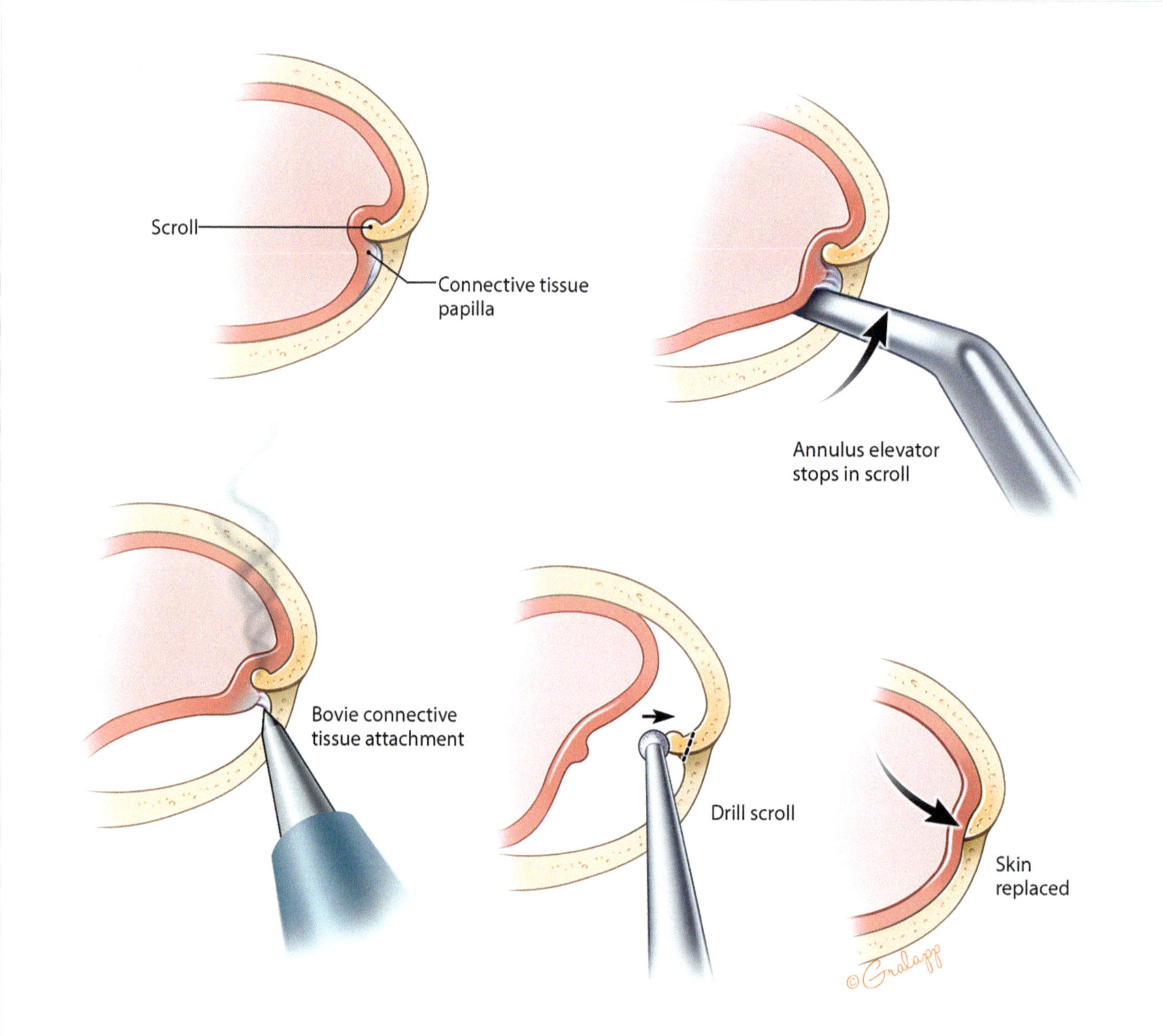

Fig. 3.147 Mechanical elevation of the canal skin from the scroll can be tedious due to dense attachment. It can be achieved rapidly with needle point electrocautery. Once exposed, a diamond burr is used to remove it.

3.9 Preauricular Cyst Excision

Mai Thy Truong

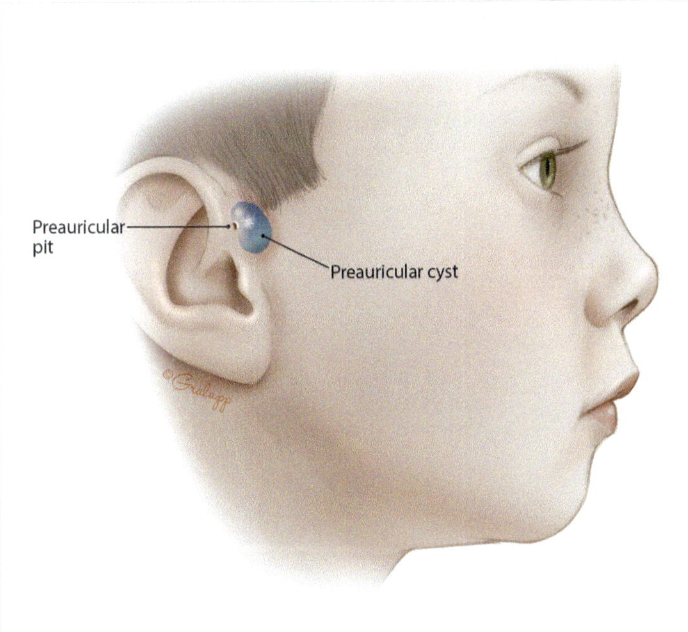

Fig. 3.148 During embryogenesis, the pinna forms from six hillocks: three anterior and three posterior to the external auditory meatus. Preauricular pits result from errors in embryology. As the crus of the helix separates from the tragus, and the incisura deepens between the 1st and 2nd Hillocks of His, a pit can remain. The depth of the sinus varies from person to person. Some are shallow and cause neither drainage nor infection. If the sinus tract becomes obstructed, it may enlarge to form a cyst. These cysts typically adhere to the helical cartilage and sometimes penetrate it. Although commonly limited to the preauricular region, in rare cases tracts can dive either through or beneath the auricular cartilage and may present as a postauricular abscess. They may also be associated with a first branchial cleft fistula that continues parallel to the ear canal or descends deeply into the parotid and even into the upper neck.

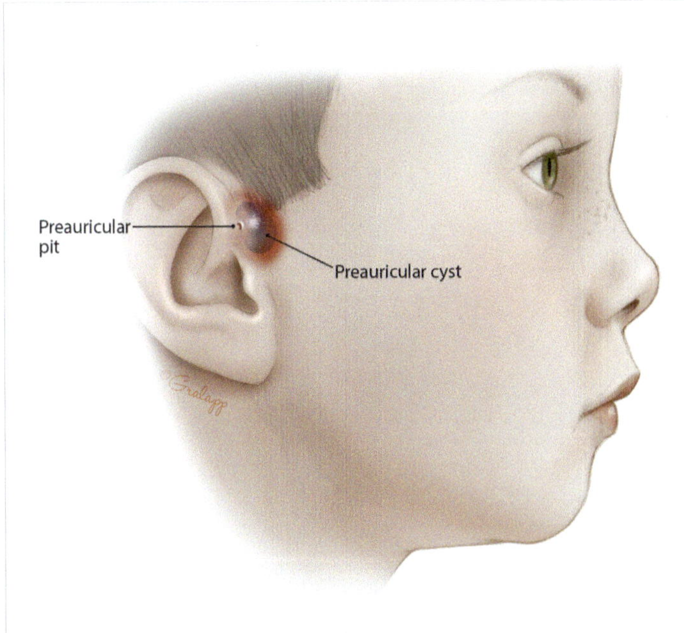

Fig. 3.149 Preauricular cysts are prone to recurrent infections. When they have been repeatedly infected, especially when they have been incised and drained, considerable scarring to adjacent tissues as well as the overlying skin may be present.

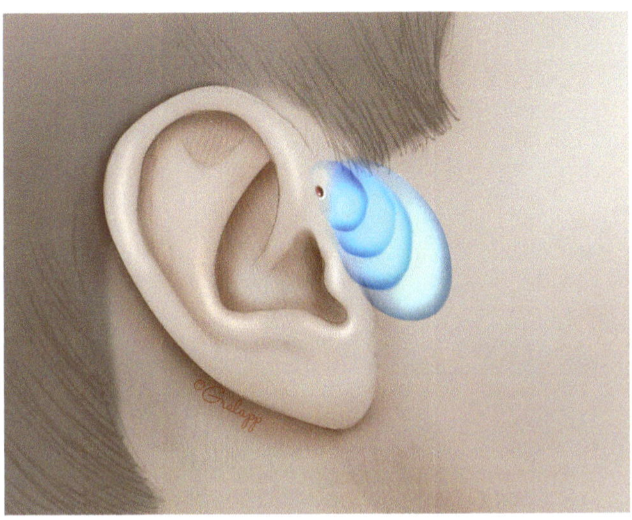

Fig. 3.150 Growth pattern of preauricular cysts. Skin changes sometimes appear discontinuous to the pit.

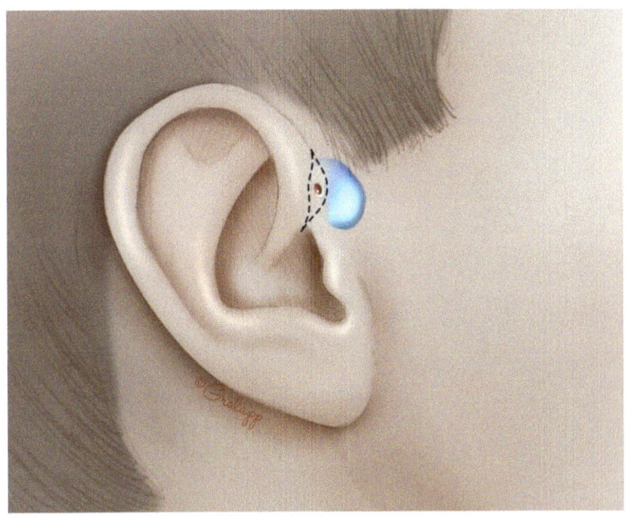

Fig. 3.151 Incision for excision of a small preauricular cyst. The scar aligns with the front edge of the helical crus. The extent of the cyst can sometimes be palpable, although if deflated after recent infection the extent may be difficult to discern. The size of the affected area in previous infections can also clue the surgeon to the approximate size of the cyst.

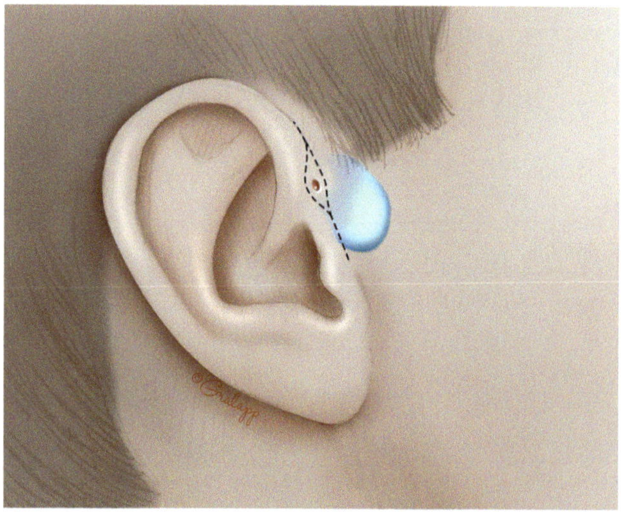

Fig. 3.152 Incision for excision of a moderate sized preauricular cyst.

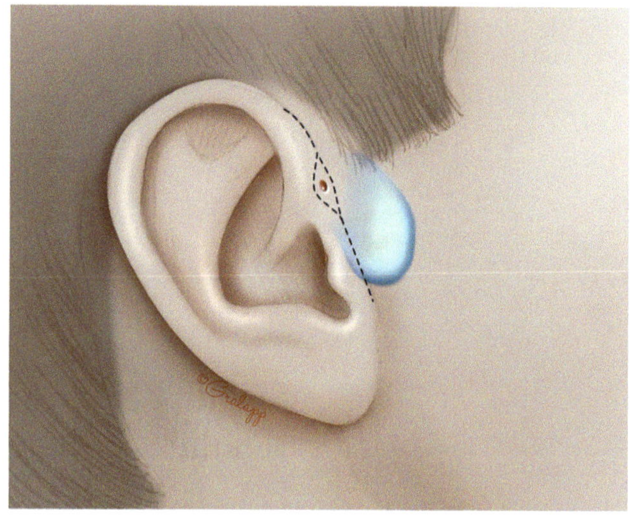

Fig. 3.153 Incision for excision of a large preauricular cyst may align with the pretragal crease or be carried up onto to the tragal crest.

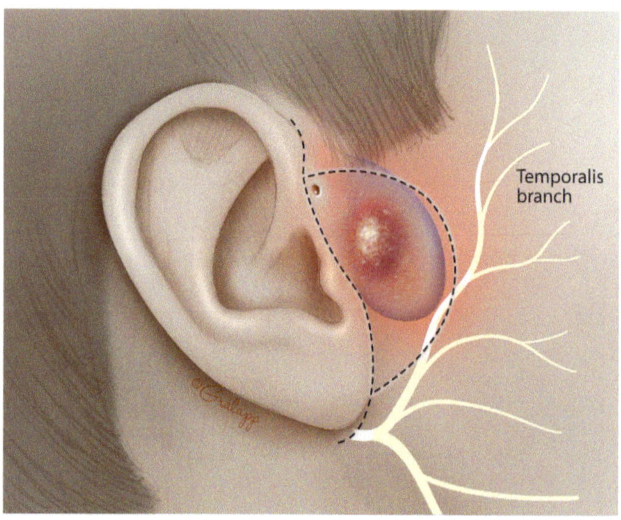

Fig. 3.154 Excision of multiply infected, large preauricular cysts can present technical challenges. When the preauricular skin is abnormal due to recurrent infection and/or repeated drainage, the overlying skin should be removed together with the pit. In this situation, rather than try to follow the contours of the cyst, it is best to establish the plane on the temporalis fascia superiorly and dissect the infected cyst off the fascia en bloc with a cuff of surrounding scar tissue. The temporalis fascia, more specifically the superficial layer of the deep temporal fascia, continues inferior to the zygoma as parotid-masseteric fascia. So long as this fascial layer is not violated, the facial nerve is safe. Because the anterior margin of larger preauricular cysts may approach the temporal branch of the facial nerve, it is prudent to use electrophysiological monitoring. Closure of this wound is done with a face-lift technique. As the closure is often tight, undermining the facial skin may be needed to create the mobility to enable primary closure. Absolute hemostasis is required, especially as many branches from the superficial temporal artery are in this path.

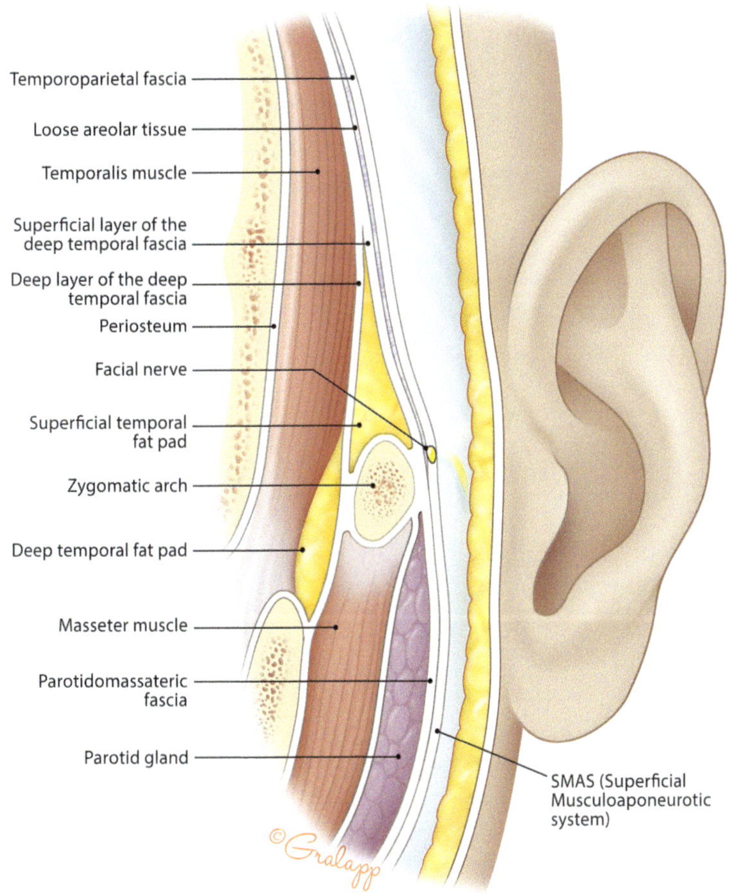

Fig. 3.155 The temporalis fascia, more specifically the superficial layer of the deep temporal fascia, continues inferior to the zygoma as parotid-masseteric fascia. So long as this fascial layer is not violated, the facial nerve is safe.

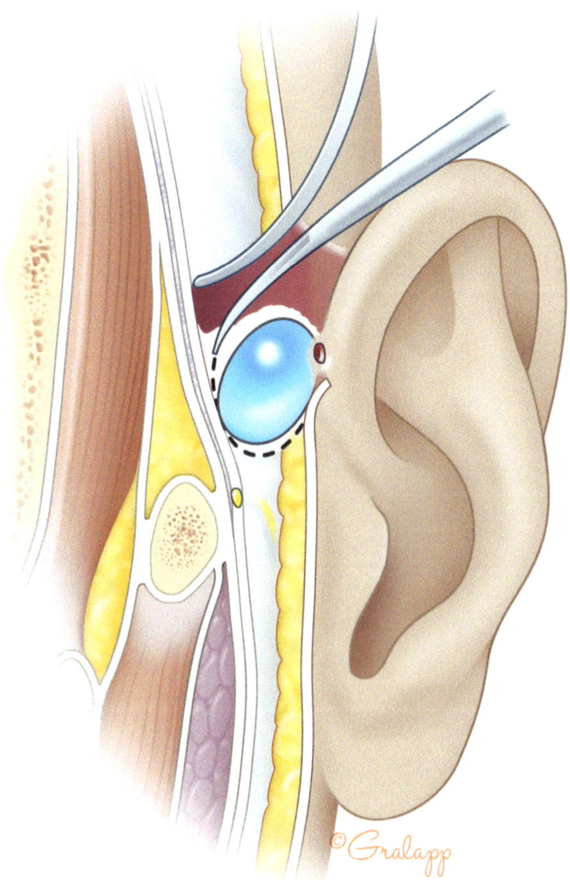

Fig. 3.156 In large preauricular cysts, especially those that have been infected numerous times, dissection of the cyst with a surrounding cuff of tissue off the temporalis fascia is the best strategy for achieving total removal.

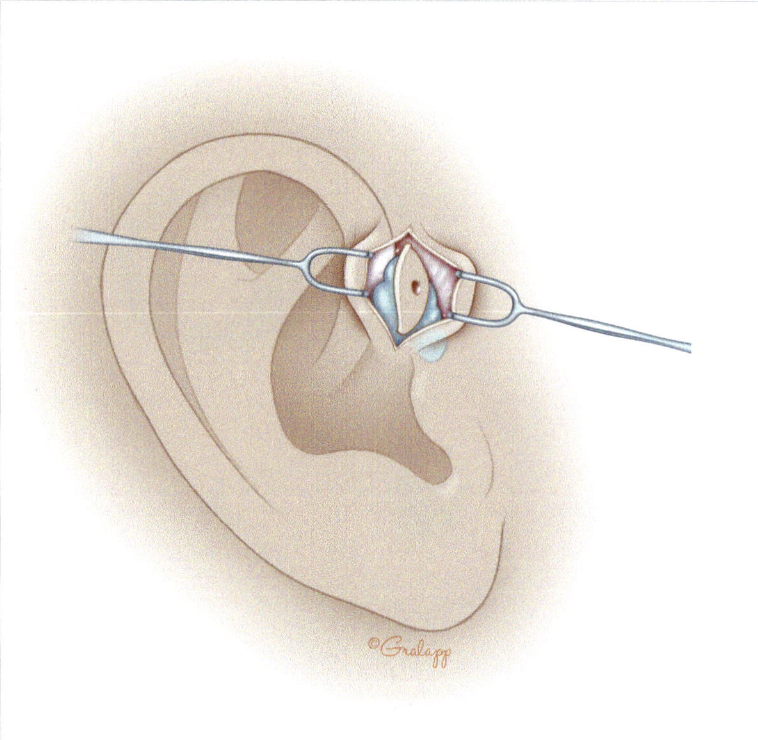

Fig. 3.157 After an elliptical incision through the skin and dermis, dissection is first focused superiorly. The interface of the cyst with the helical cartilage is first identified and followed off the edge toward the temporalis fascia anteriorly. Once these superior borders of the cartilage and fascia are identified, the cyst is then circumferentially dissected.

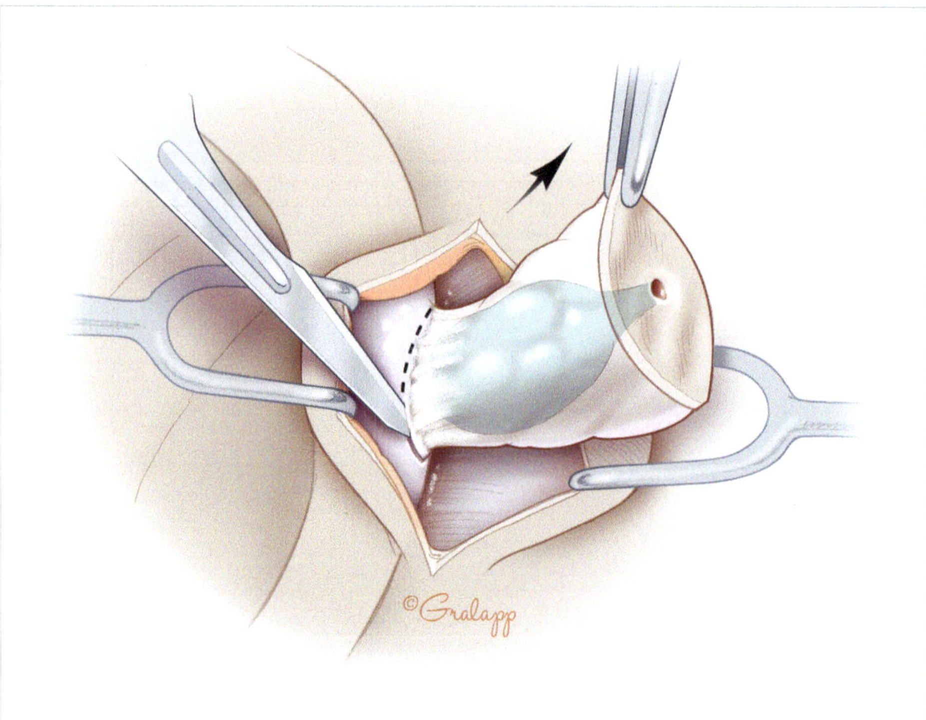

Fig. 3.158 Following the surface of the cyst, its attachment to the helical crus is defined. To decrease the risk of recurrence, the cartilage in contact with the cyst should be excised and removed with the cyst. The surface of the cartilage is exposed peripherally around the cyst, allowing for an elliptical incision on the cartilage. While removing cartilage, it is important not to violate the skin of the cymba concha which underlies it.

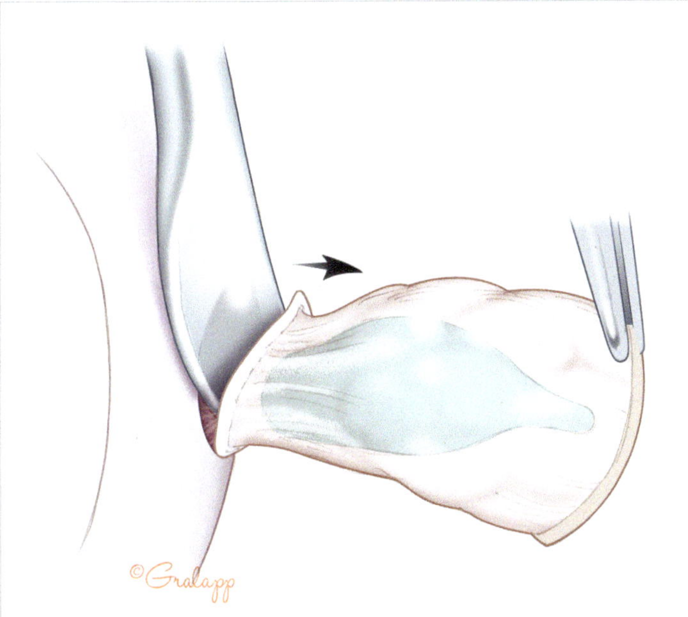

Fig. 3.159 A freer elevator or scalpel can facilitate the removal of the cartilage from the undersurface of the skin of the cymba concha.

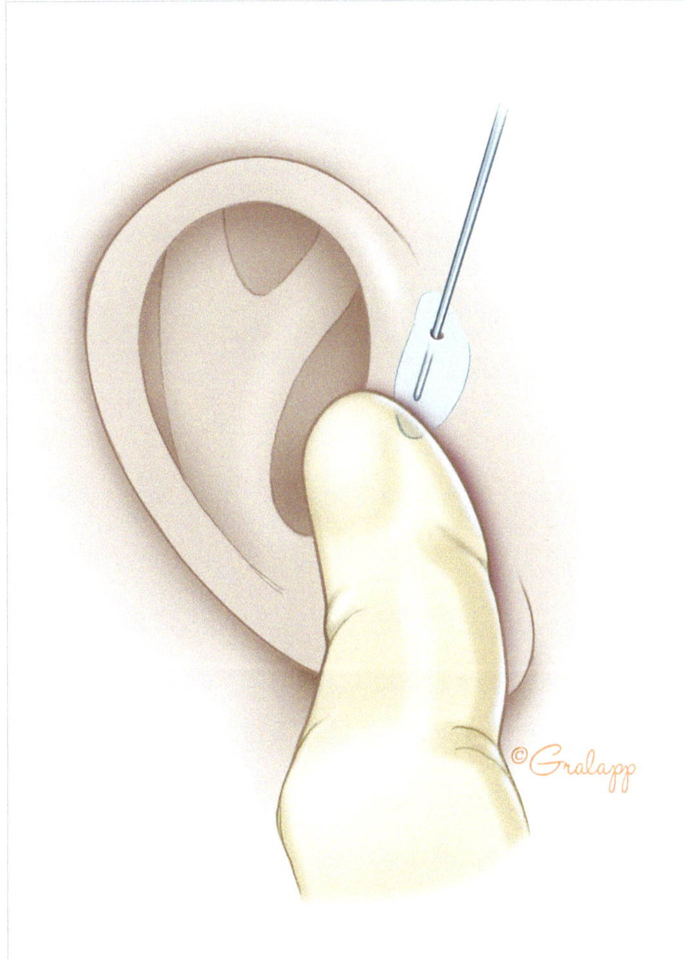

Fig. 3.160 Some surgeons use a lacrimal probe and methylene blue dye to map out the extent of the cyst. The lacrimal probe is used first to gently dilate the opening to allow the introduction of methylene blue. If this is done aggressively, a false passage can be made, allowing the extravasation of methylene blue into normal tissues. Typically, lacrimal probes from size 0 up to no larger than size 1 are used. Methylene blue can often guide the dissection and allow reassurance of complete removal when the cyst is adequately dyed.

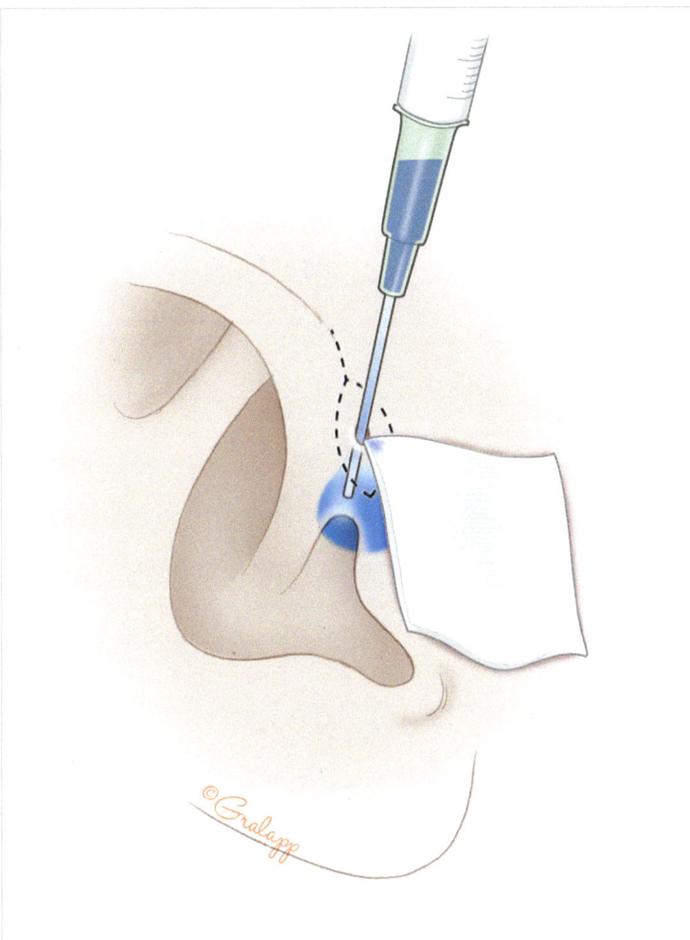

Fig. 3.161 Methylene blue is injected with a 1-mL TB syringe via a 24-gauge Angiocath to allow for controlled introduction. The corner of an alcohol wipe can be kept at the opening to collect any excess methylene blue. Very little dye is often needed to stain the cyst, and a gentle tap of the syringe is recommended over a push.

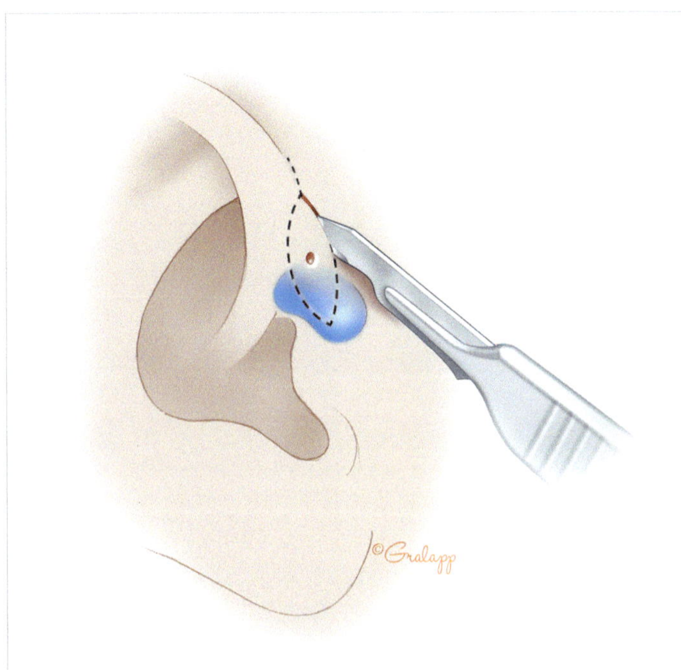

Fig. 3.162 Once the blue has dyed the cyst, the removal continues as in Fig. 3.157. If methylene blue seeps from the pit during the early dissection, it is merely suctioned away from the pit.

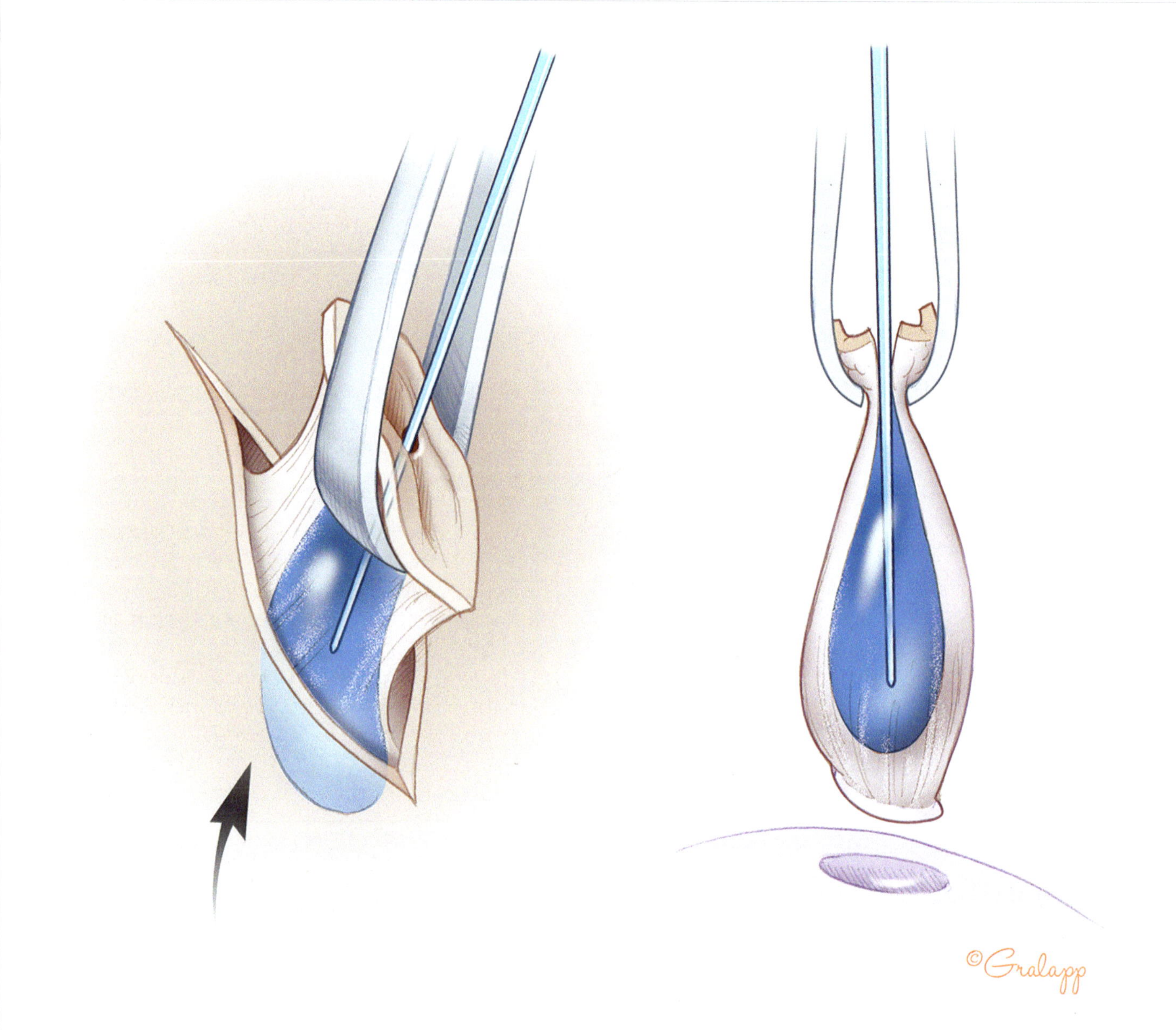

Fig. 3.163 Once the ellipse has been cut and the cyst begins to be freed, the lacrimal probe can be reintroduced. The probe has dual purposes: to plug the pit to reduce extravasation of dye and also to palpate the extent of the cyst. A small Allis clamp secures the lacrimal probe while establishing traction while dissecting the cyst. Care must be taken to not rotate the Allis clamp along its axis as torsion may lead to a rupture of the cyst.

4 Stapes Surgery

Robert K. Jackler

4.1 Introduction to Stapes Surgery

Many otologists would describe stapes surgery as among the most satisfying of all ear operations. The procedure is elegant, technically sophisticated, and most patients are highly appreciative for their improved hearing. It is also among the most perilous. For such a miniscule area, the number of variations and anomalies the otologist might encounter are numerous and can tax even the most experienced ear microsurgeon. When a tympanoplasty fails, it can usually be successfully redone. When stapes surgery goes wrong, it can result in irremediable consequences such as deafness, vertigo, and even facial paralysis. Success in surgery is less about technical virtuosity than it is about mental preparedness, the exercise of sound judgment, and knowing one's limits. The better prepared a surgeon is, the more likely to achieve success and avoid preventable complications.

One important goal in creating these illustrations was to help the novice surgeon gain competence, efficiency, and finesse with the routine aspects of stapes surgery. During training, the learning curve for stapes procedures is steeper than for most ear procedures. Stapes procedures require the surgeon to have a clear plan of the technical maneuvers which, in turn, have to occur in specific sequence. Our illustrations are intended to guide the inexperienced surgeon to learn the principles of obtaining adequate exposure by designing and raising a tympanomeatal flap of the proper size and shape as well as avoiding flap tears or disruption of the tympanic membrane. The fledgling surgeon must master hand positions that afford high levels of stability and also master the skill of two-handed surgery. Beginning surgeons rapidly become facile with their dominant hand, but development of nondominant hand skill takes time and practice. Many of the maneuvers in stapes surgery are completed most effectively when exposure is adequate for binocular viewing. The methods of obtaining adequate exposure of the oval window and incus are central to making the procedure go smoothly. We have made an effort to show a diversity of technical options for opening the footplate (small and large fenestra, microdrill, laser, and pick) as well as illustrating some of the most commonly used stapes prostheses.

The second major goal of these illustrations was to provide stapes surgeons with the intellectual framework to be prepared for the myriad uncommon variants and technical challenges which inevitably arise from time to time. The majority of these (e.g., overhanging facial nerve, narrow niche, deficient incus, thick footplate) are usually not knowable preoperatively by the surgeon. Chances are that when surgeons first encounter a stapes gusher or biscuit footplate, for example, they will be on their own, never having faced these challenges during training. The only way to prepare is through mental preparedness and formulation of a plan, much as an airline pilot does in anticipation of rare emergencies. Illustrations are one means of helping surgeons to recognize and deal with uncommon variants and technical challenges.

Further Reading

1. Bernardeschi D, Canu G, De Seta D, et al. Revision stapes surgery: a review of 102 cases. Clin Otolaryngol 2018;43 (6):1587–1590 PubMed
2. de Sousa C, Gooycoolea MV, Sperling NM. Otosclerosis: Diagnosis, Evaluation, Pathology, Surgical Techniques, and Outcomes. San Diego: Plural Publishing; 2014
3. Eshraghi AA, Telischi FF. Otosclerosis and stapes surgery. Otolaryngol Clin North Am 2018;51(2)
4. Goderie TPM, Alkhateeb WHF, Smit CF, Hensen EF. Surgical management of a persistent stapedial artery: a review. Otol Neurotol 2017;38(6):788–791 PubMed
5. Gros A, Vatovec J, Zargi M, Jenko K. Success rate in revision stapes surgery for otosclerosis. Otol Neurotol 2005;26 (6):1143–1148 PubMed
6. Khorsandi A MT, Jalali MM, Shoshi D V. Predictive factors in 995 stapes surgeries for primary otosclerosis. Laryngoscope 2018;128(10):2403–2407 PubMed
7. McManus LJ, Dawes PJ, Stringer MD. Clinical anatomy of the chorda tympani: a systematic review. J Laryngol Otol 2011;125(11):1101–1108 PubMed
8. Nazarian R, McElveen JT Jr, Eshraghi AA. History of otosclerosis and stapes surgery. Otolaryngol Clin North Am 2018;51 (2):275–290 PubMed
9. Rask-Andersen H, Schart-Morén N, Strömbäck K, Linthicum F, Li H. Special anatomic considerations in otosclerosis surgery. Otolaryngol Clin North Am 2018;51(2):357–374 PubMed
10. Vincent R, Rovers M, Zingade N, et al. Revision stapedotomy: operative findings and hearing results. A prospective study of 652 cases from the Otology-Neurotology Database. Otol Neurotol 2010;31(6):875–882 PubMed
11. Vincent R, Sperling NM, Oates J, Jindal M. Surgical findings and long-term hearing results in 3,050 stapedotomies for primary otosclerosis: a prospective study with the otology-neurotology database. Otol Neurotol 2006;27(8, Suppl 2): S25–S47 PubMed

4.2 Overview of Stapes Surgery

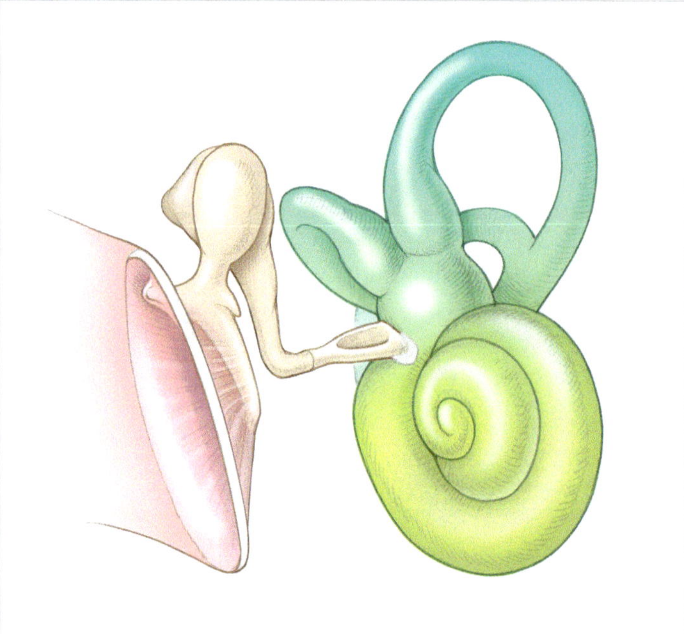

Fig. 4.1 Schematic coronal view of the middle and inner ear showing a fixed stapes due to an otosclerotic plaque at the anterior margin of the oval window.

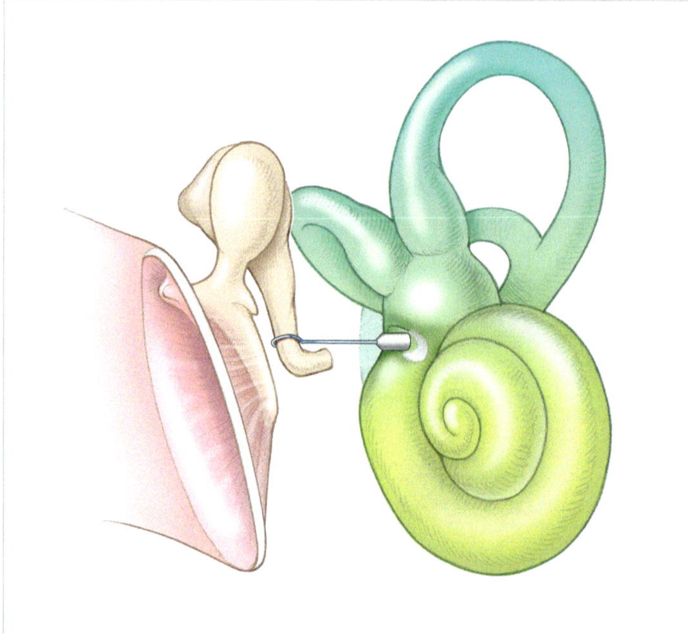

Fig. 4.2 Schematic illustrating small fenestra stapedotomy with a Teflon-wire prosthesis.

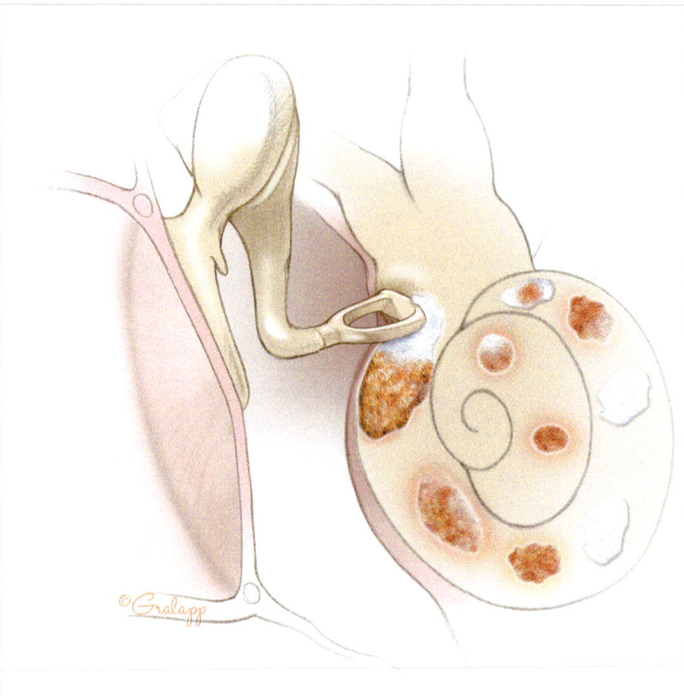

Fig. 4.3 Otosclerosis is a disease of the otic capsule. In its active phase, known as otospongiosis, highly vascular lesions resorb bone surrounding the inner ear, most often in a patchy pattern. The active lesions mature into calcified otosclerotic plaques which are responsible for stapes fixation.

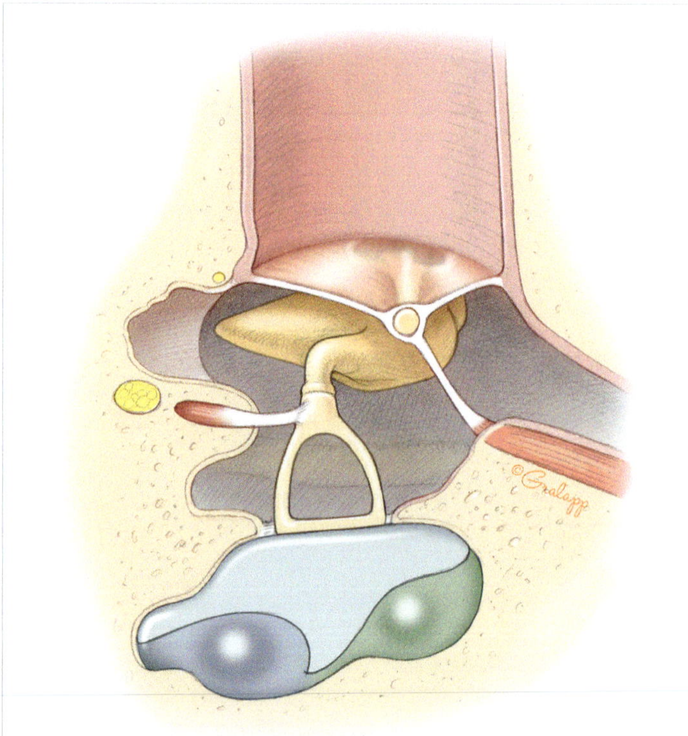

Fig. 4.4 Schematic view of the middle and inner ear displayed via a perspective looking upward from the hypotympanum. This projection was chosen as a means of introducing the concepts of stapes surgery in a perspective which enables simultaneous viewing of the ear canal, middle ear, stapes, vestibule, utricle (*blue*), and saccule (*green*).

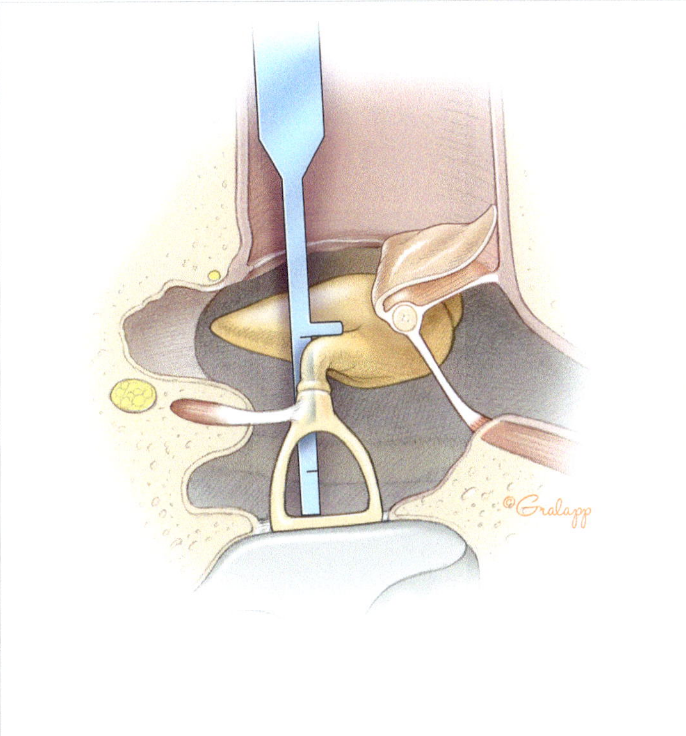

Fig. 4.5 The tympanomeatal flap (canal skin and eardrum) has been raised and reflected anteriorly to expose the posterior half of the middle ear. To aid in selection of the proper length prosthesis, the distance from the lateral surface of the incus to the footplate is being measured.

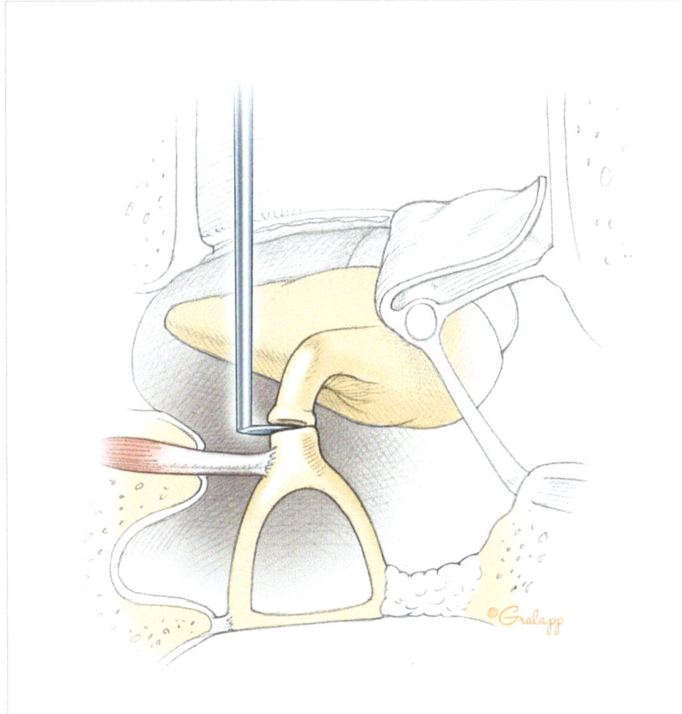

Fig. 4.6 Division of the joint between the incus and stapes using an incudostapedial joint knife.

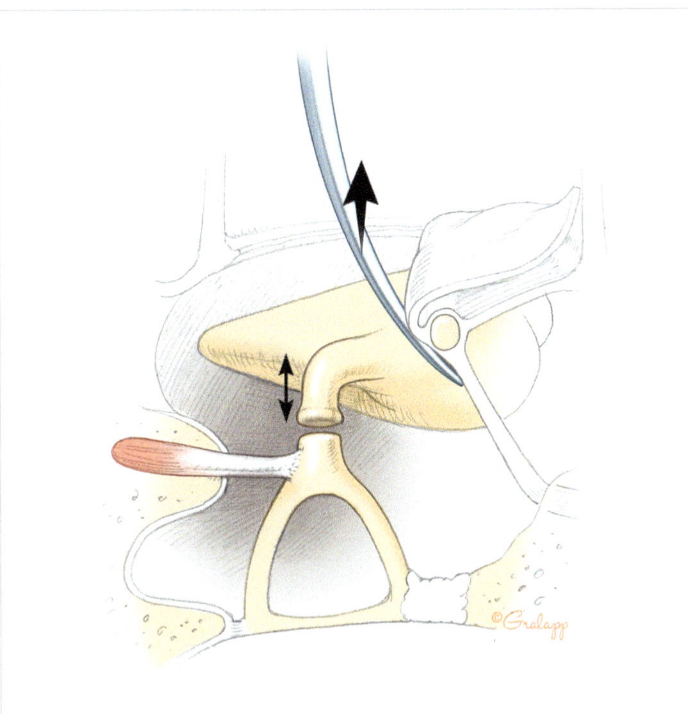

Fig. 4.7 After division of the joint, mobility of the lateral ossicles (malleus and incus) is tested.

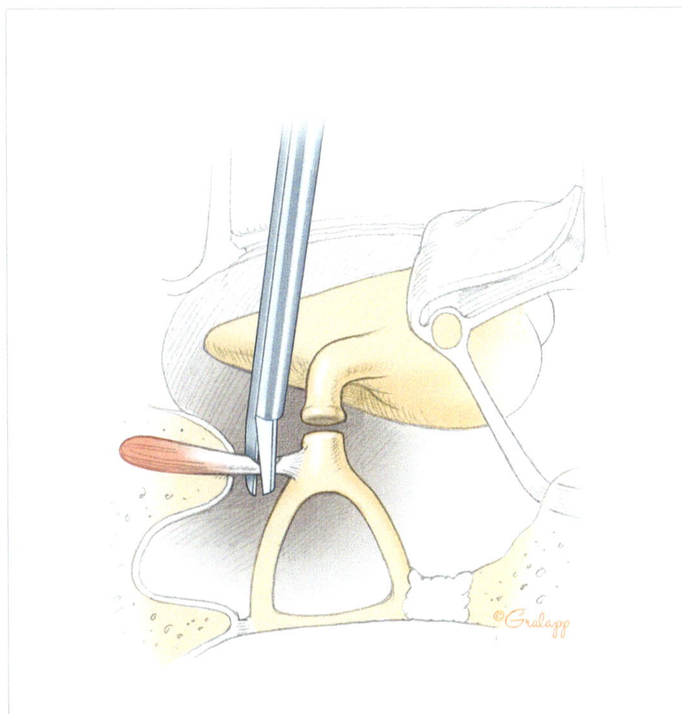

Fig. 4.8 Section of the stapedius muscle with microscissors.

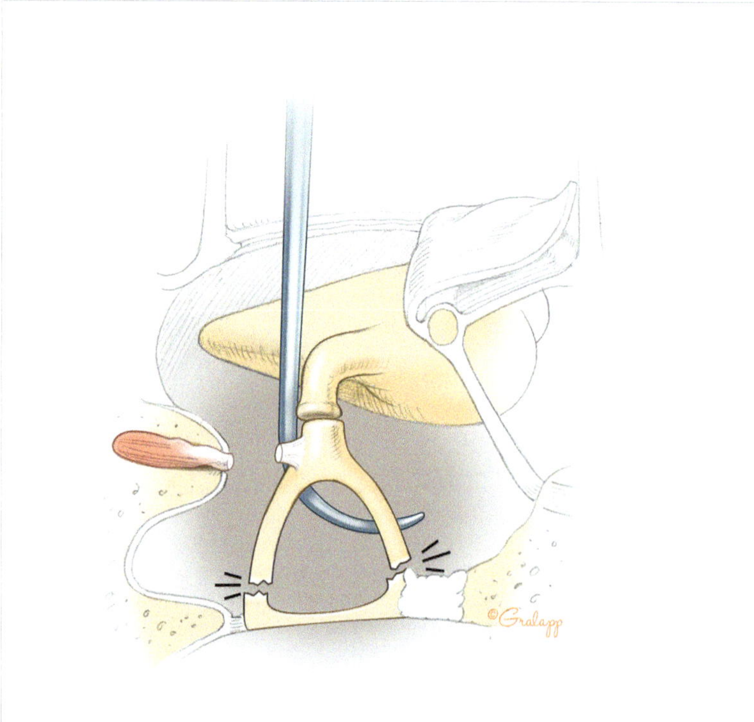

Fig. 4.9 Removal of the stapes superstructure using a curved needle.

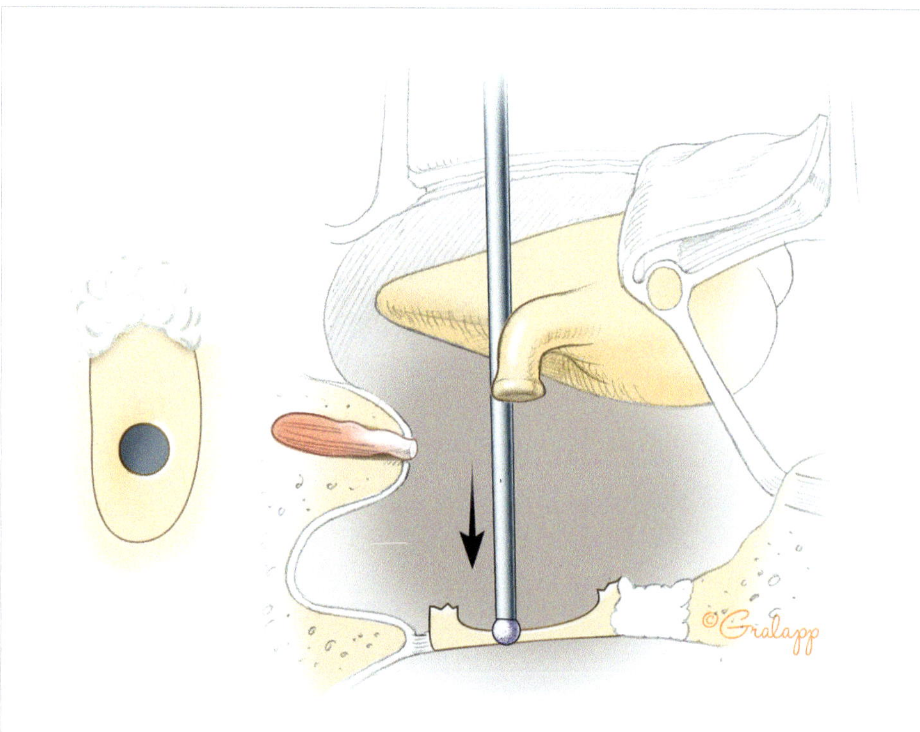

Fig. 4.10 Creation of a small fenestra stapedotomy with a microdrill.

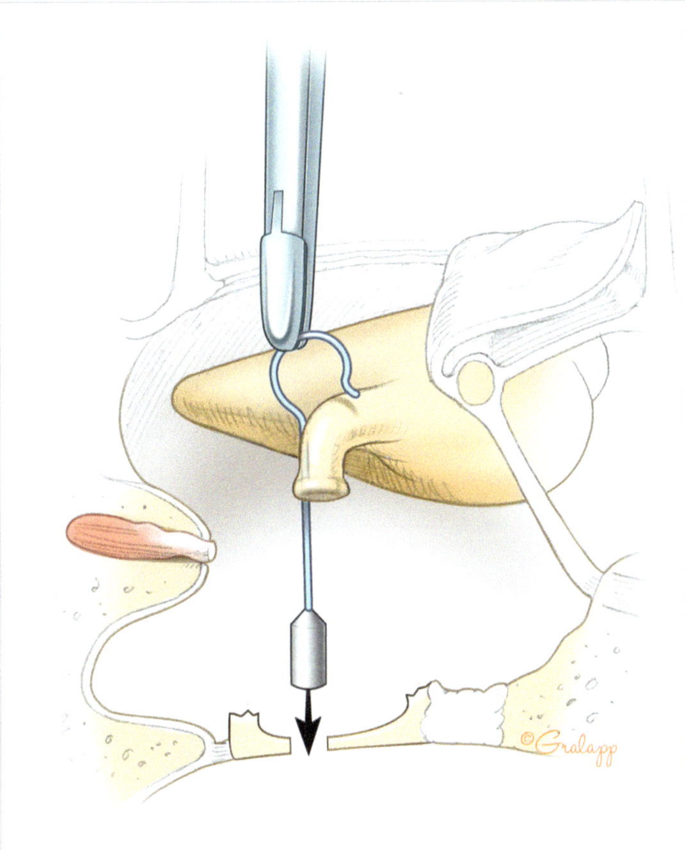

Fig. 4.11 Placement of a stapedotomy piston.

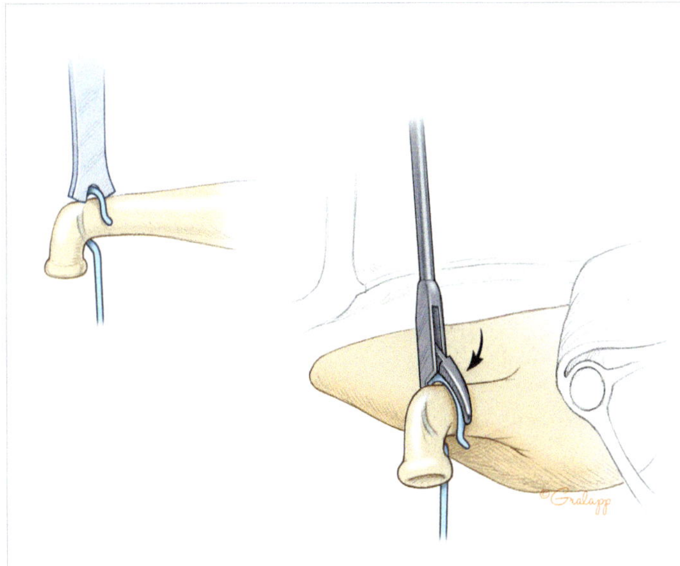

Fig. 4.12 Positioning of the shepherd's crook on the incus with a notched chisel (strut guide) and closing the wire with a crimper.

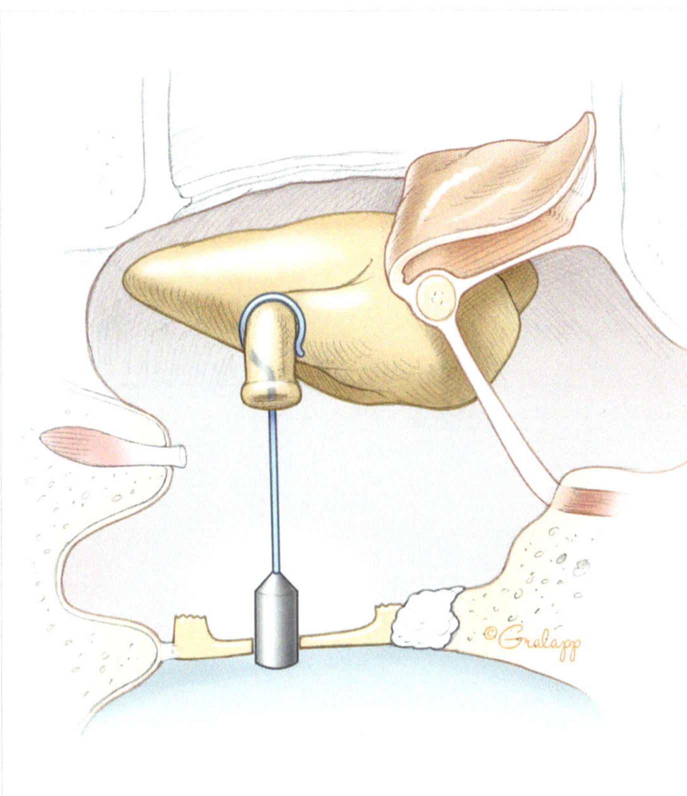

Fig. 4.13 Completed placement of the stapes piston through the stapes fenestra into the vestibule.

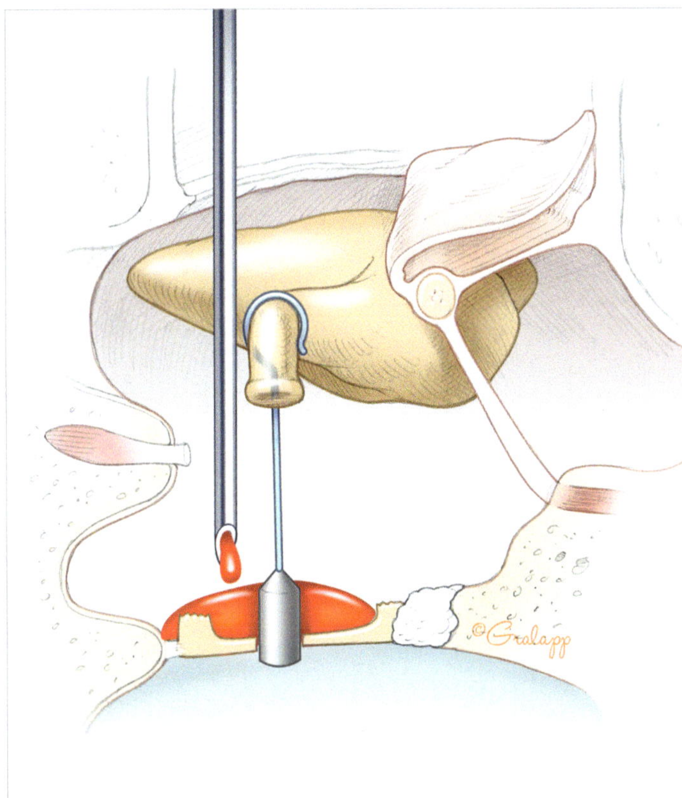

Fig. 4.14 Sealing around the prosthesis with blood.

4.3 Exposure

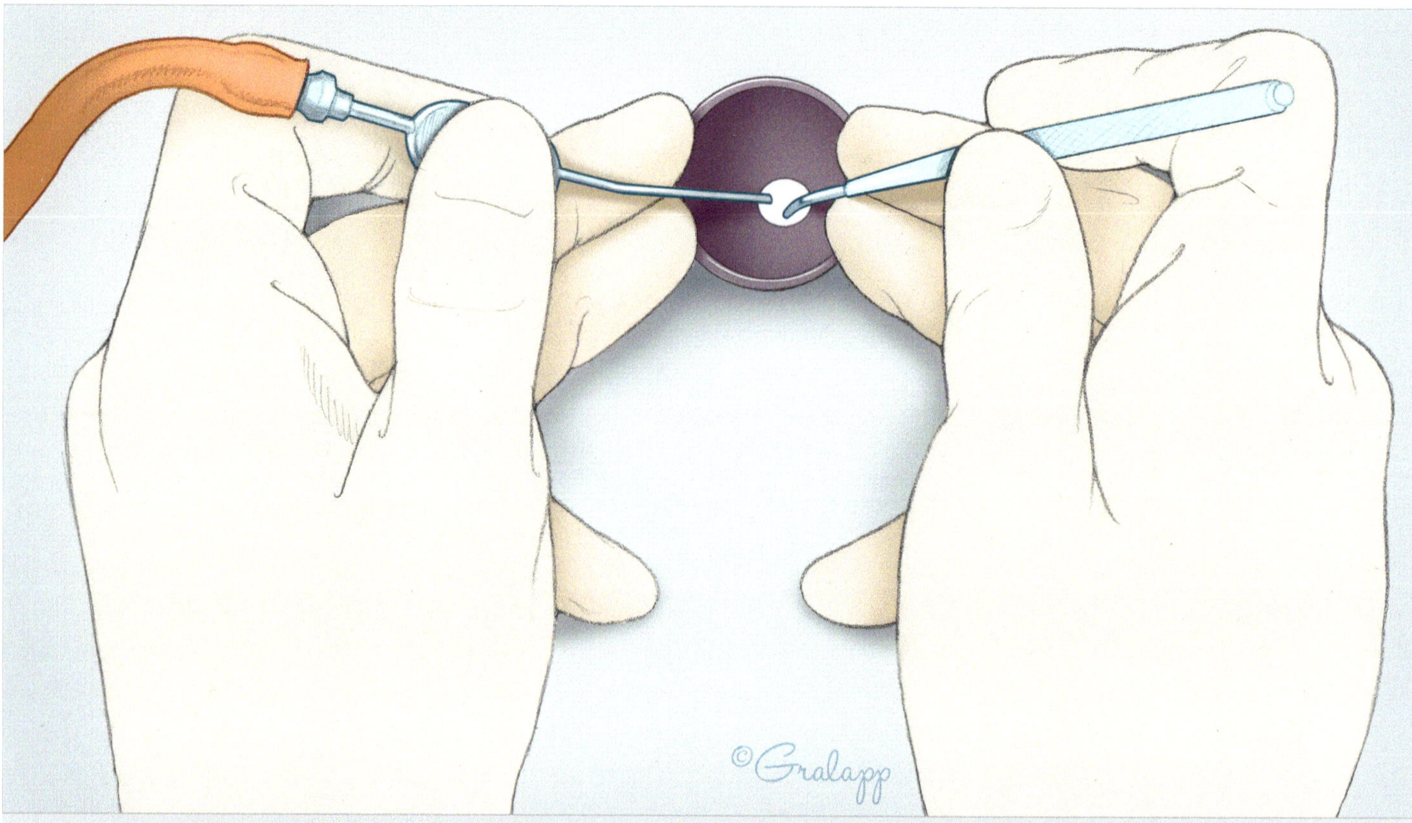

Fig. 4.15 Placement of the surgeon's hands during transcanal stapes microsurgery. The third and fourth fingers of each hand stabilize the speculum. Note that the microinstrument (right hand) and suction (left hand) are held in a manner to both optimize stability and to enable binocular viewing. Some surgeons use a speculum holder to enhance stability.

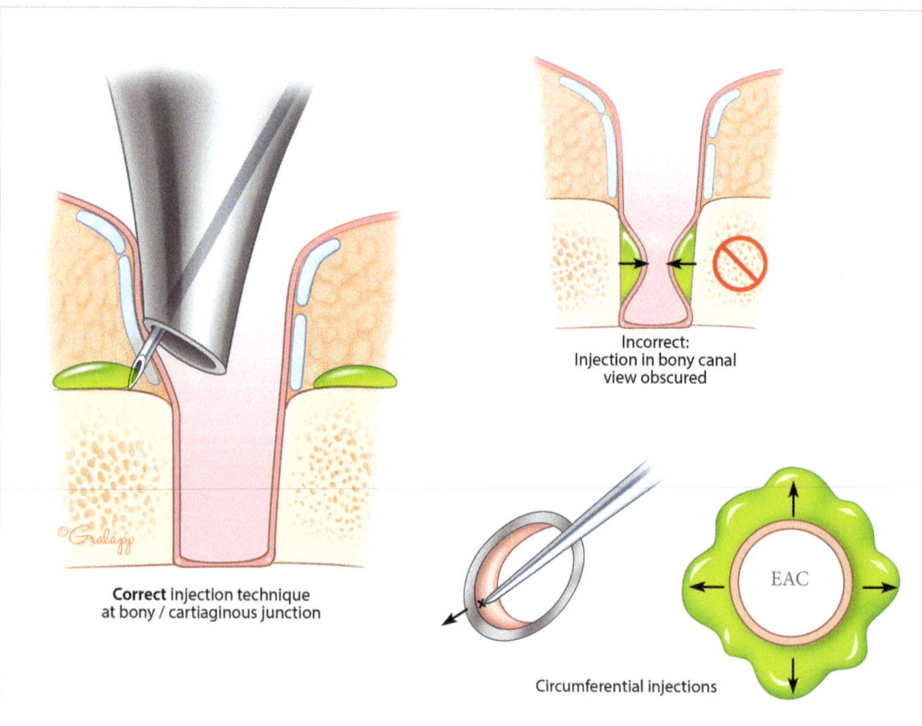

Fig. 4.16 Injection of lidocaine with epinephrine into the ear canal has two purposes: anesthesia and vasoconstriction. Using the speculum to offset the cartilaginous canal, circumferential injections are placed around the bony cartilaginous junction. To avoid transient postoperative facial paralysis, a smaller volume of anesthetic is injected anteriorly. It is usually best to avoid injection in the bony canal, other than raising a bleb under the vascular strip, to avoid narrowing the lumen and hindering exposure.

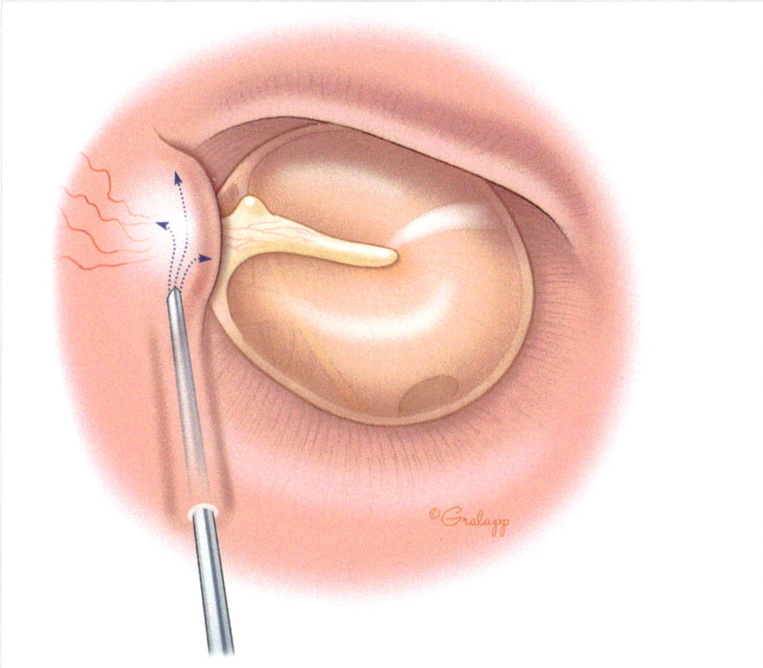

Fig. 4.17 Injection of lidocaine with epinephrine via a 27-gauge needle in the posterior-superior ear canal resulting in vasoconstriction of the "vascular strip."

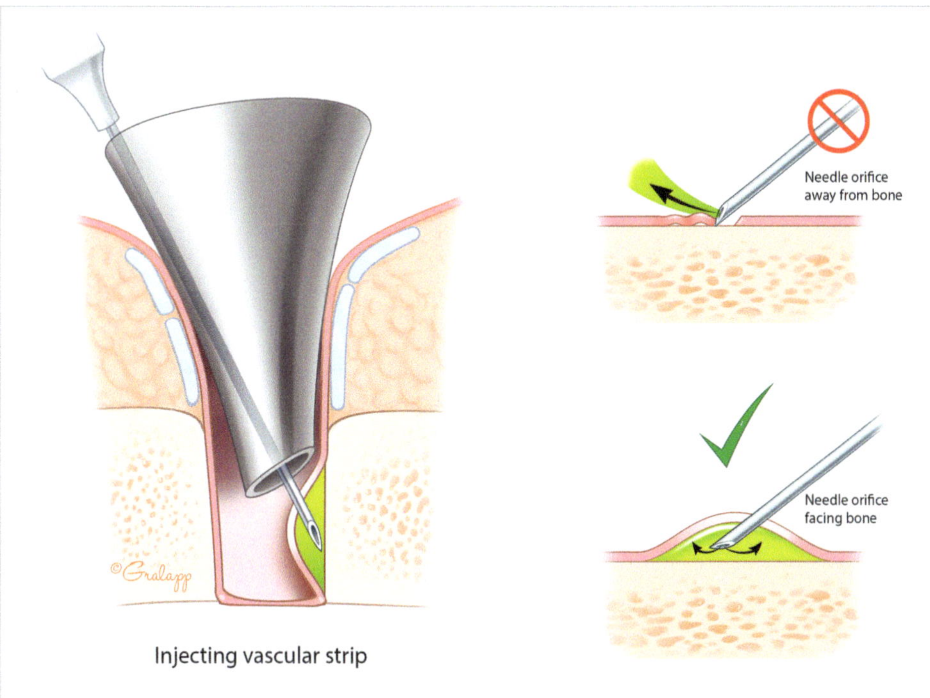

Fig. 4.18 During vascular strip injection, the bevel of the needle must face the bone.

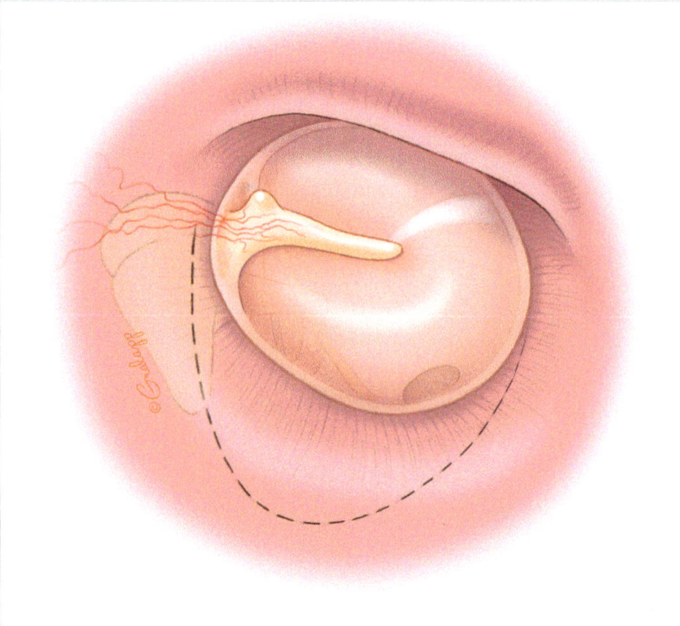

Fig. 4.19 Operative view of the ear canal and ear drum as seen in a transcanal approach. Dotted line represents the canal incision of a tympanomeatal flap. The flap is longer superiorly to cover the scutectomy defect. Note that the optimal incision is not "12 to 6" but rather more like 1 o'clock to 7 o'clock on an imaginary clock face in which the malleus sits at 12 noon. For the flap to properly fold on itself exposing the posterior superior quadrant, it is best to carry the incision slightly beyond the malleus.

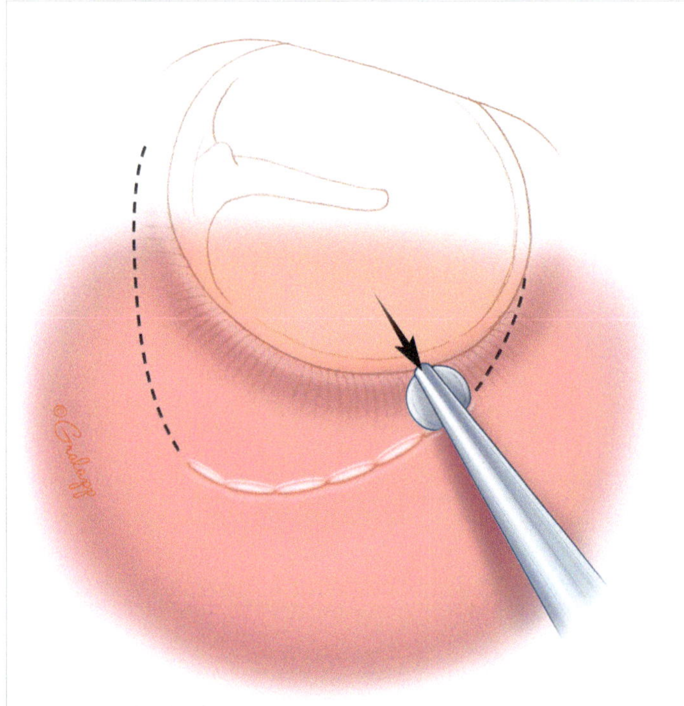

Fig. 4.20 The incision line is first crushed with a round stapes knife. This maneuver squeezes closed blood vessels and thereby reduces bleeding. It also helps minimize flap tearing during incision.

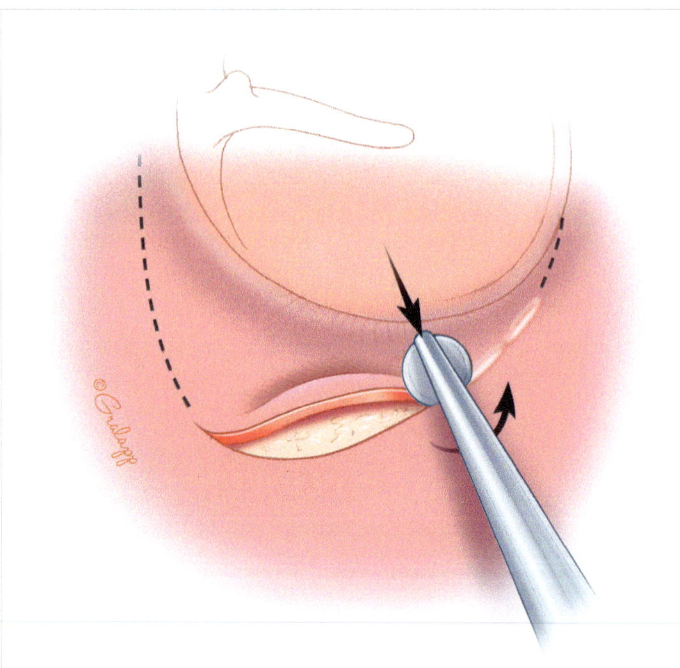

Fig. 4.21 Using a twisting motion, the incision is created with a stapes knife.

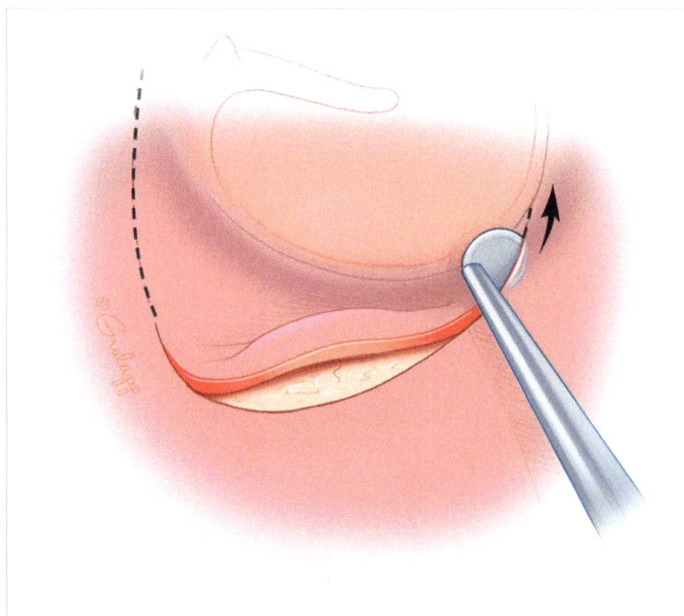

Fig. 4.22 The incision is carried inferiorly. As the stapes exposure is in the superior quadrant, the inferior portion of the flap can be kept quite short.

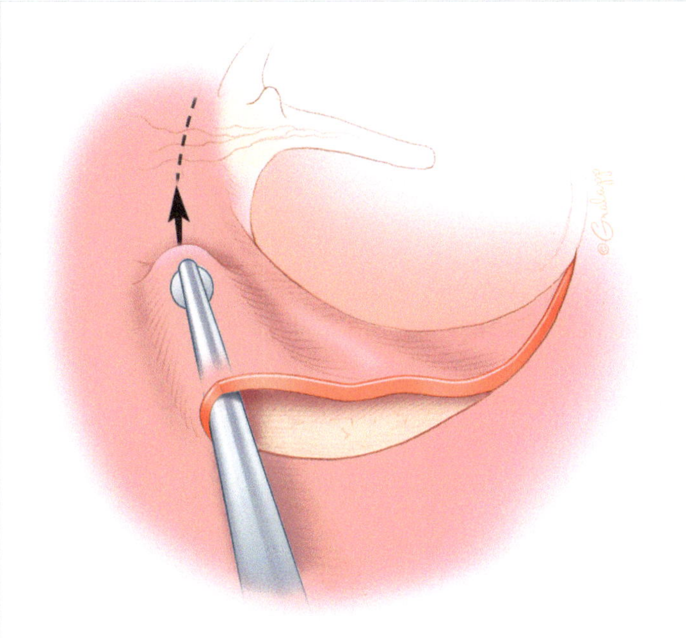

Fig. 4.23 Using either a stapes knife or annulus elevator, a tunnel is created under the so-called vascular strip, the portion of the flap most likely to bleed.

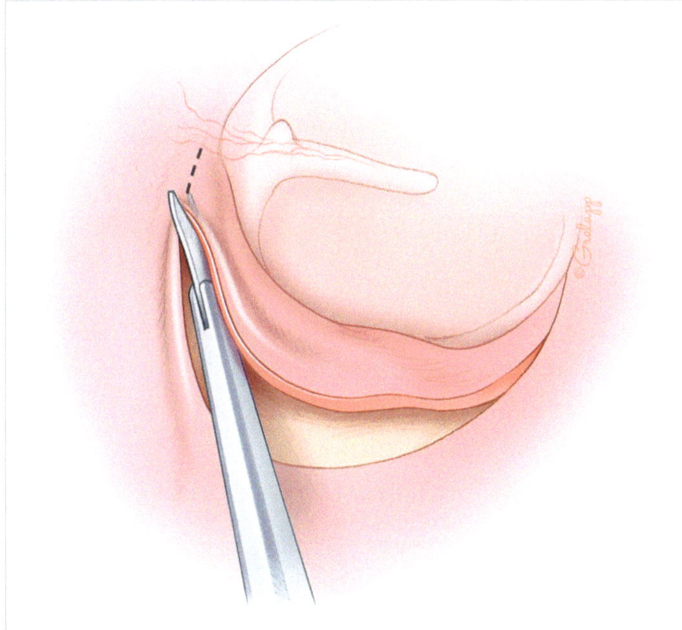

Fig. 4.24 Cutting the vascular strip with scissors squeezes vessels closed and thereby reduces bleeding. It also creates a neatly designed flap without irregular edges. Some surgeons prefer to cut the entire flap with a stapes knife.

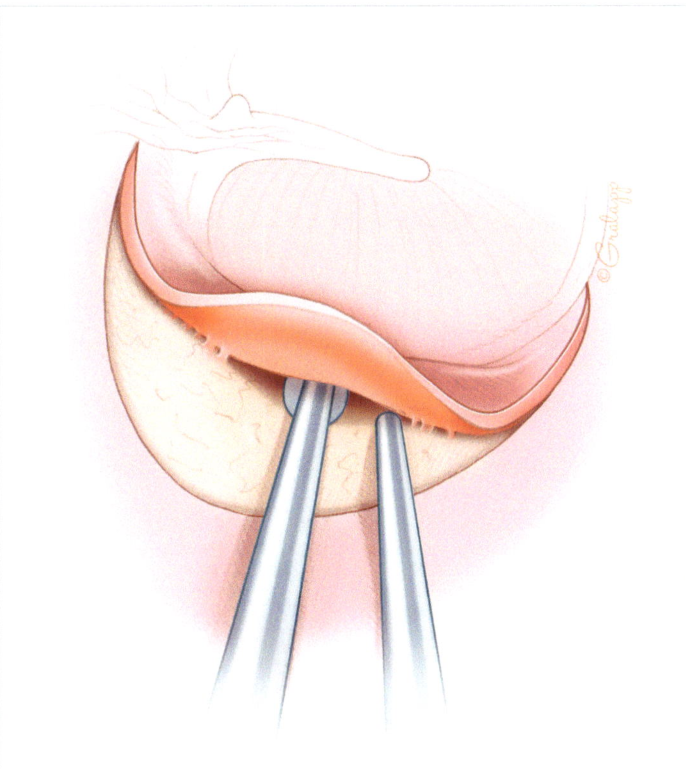

Fig. 4.25 The flap is raised to the level of the tympanic annulus. Care must be taken to avoid traumatizing the flap by aspirating it with the suction. The suction is best kept above the stapes knife blade.

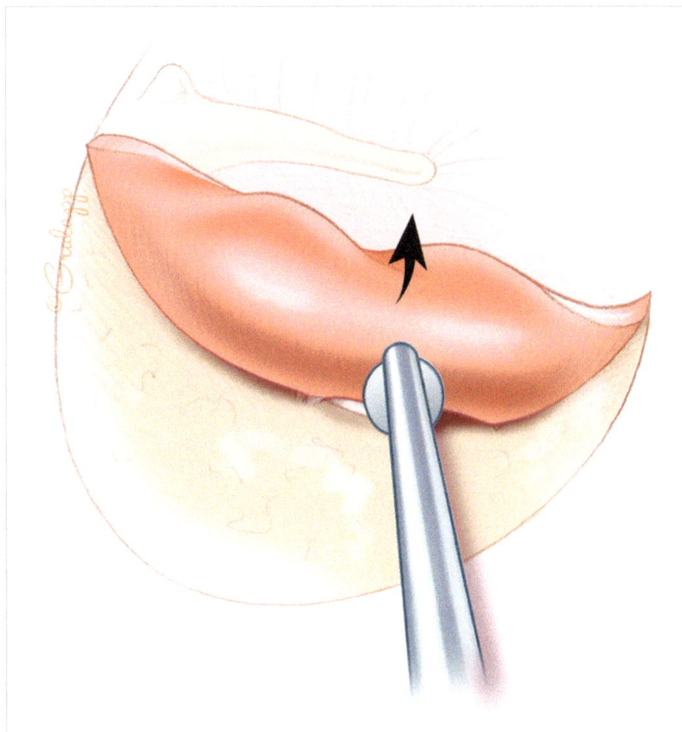

Fig. 4.26 To avoid potential disturbance to the ossicles, the middle ear is first entered inferiorly. The stapes knife lifts the tympanic annulus out of its bony groove. With gentle downward and inward pressure, the knife can then safely fall over the margin into the posterior tympanic space.

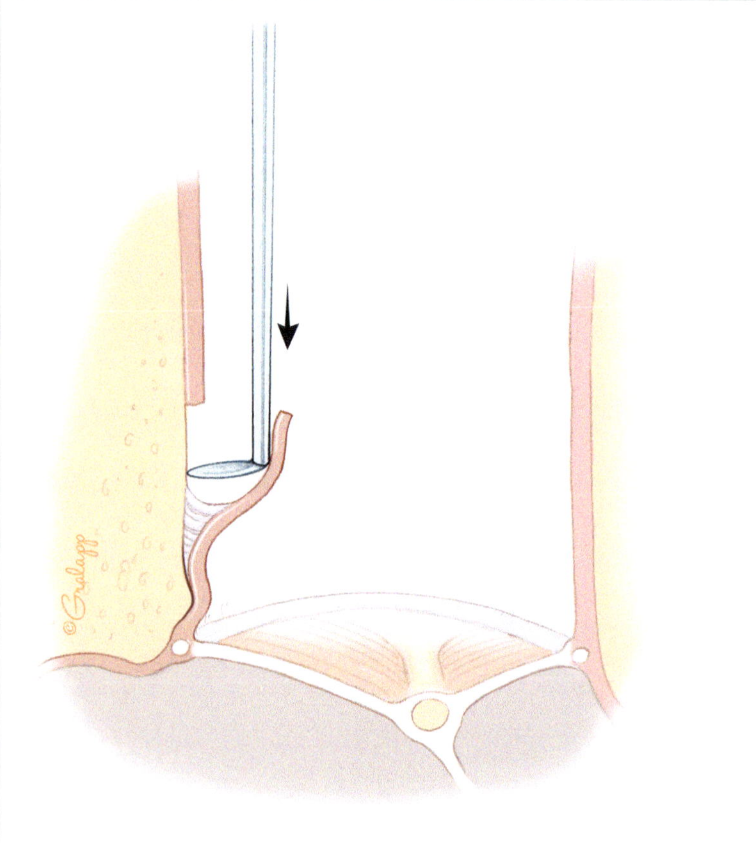

Fig. 4.27 A bony prominence is often encountered slightly lateral to the tympanic membrane level.

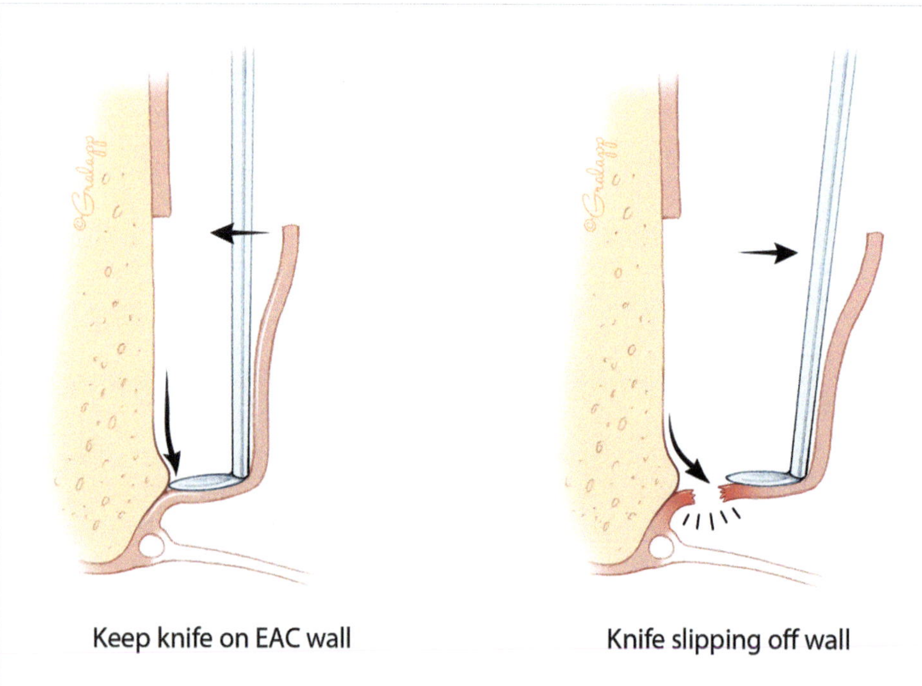

Fig. 4.28 To avoid tearing of the flap or tympanic membrane, it is necessary to maintain continuous pressure with the stapes knife against the bony canal. Allowing the stapes knife to disengage from the canal wall risks tearing the flap. EAC, external auditory canal.

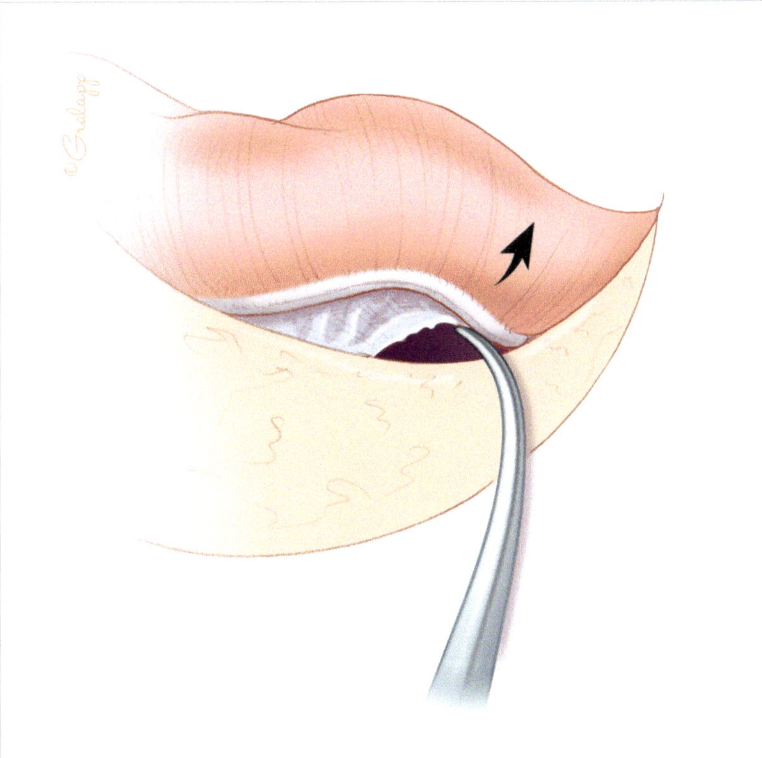

Fig. 4.29 The tympanic mucosa is lysed with a curved needle. When done under local, lidocaine is infused into the middle ear to anesthetize the tympanic mucosa. To avoid anesthetizing the labyrinth with resultant postoperative vertigo, lidocaine should be promptly suctioned from the middle ear, especially from the round window niche where it tends to accumulate.

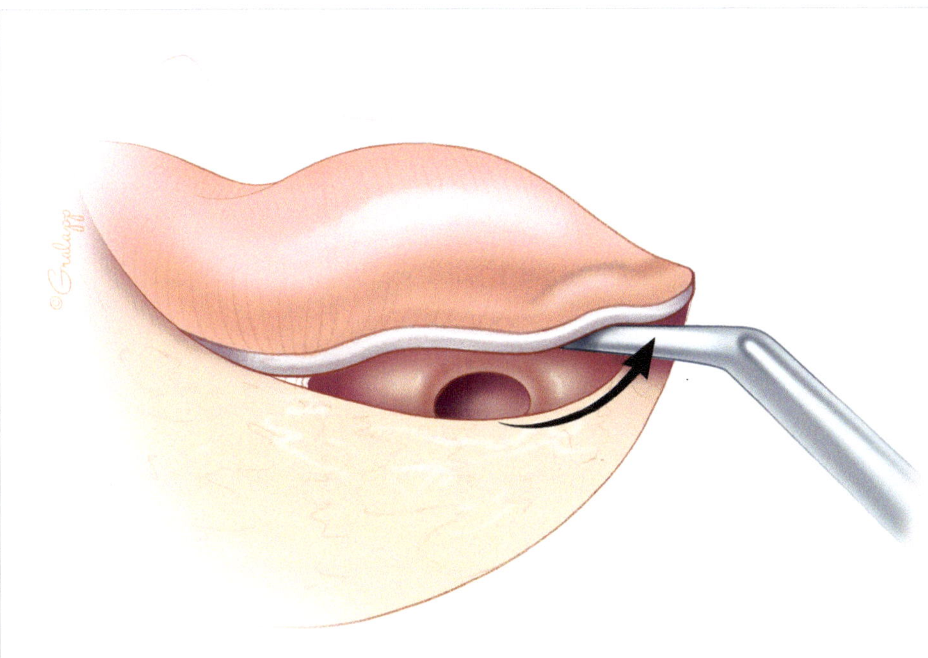

Fig. 4.30 Elevation of the tympanic annulus inferiorly using an annulus elevator. To avoid tearing, it is important to maintain firm pressure against the bone. Elevation is with the side of the shaft, not the tip of the instrument. When under local, this maneuver is often incompletely anesthetized.

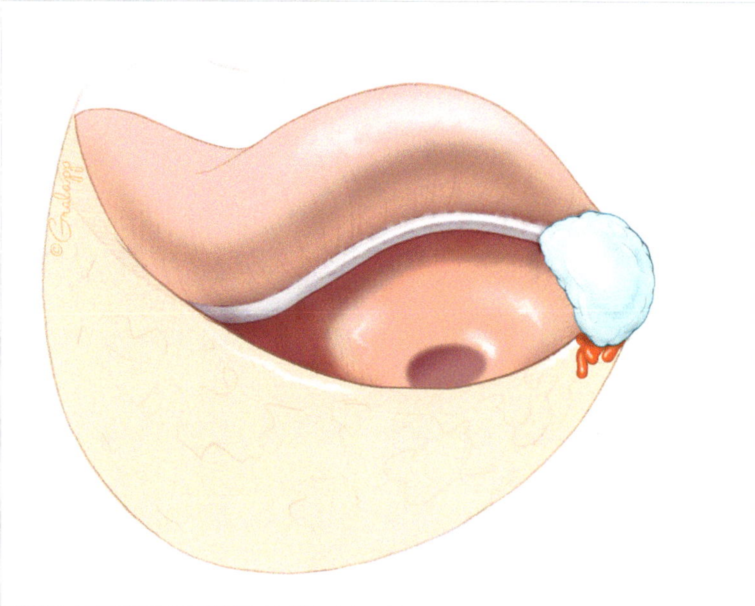

Fig. 4.31 Bleeding from the inferior edge is common after this maneuver. Application of a small cube of epinephrine-soaked absorbable gelatin sponge readily controls.

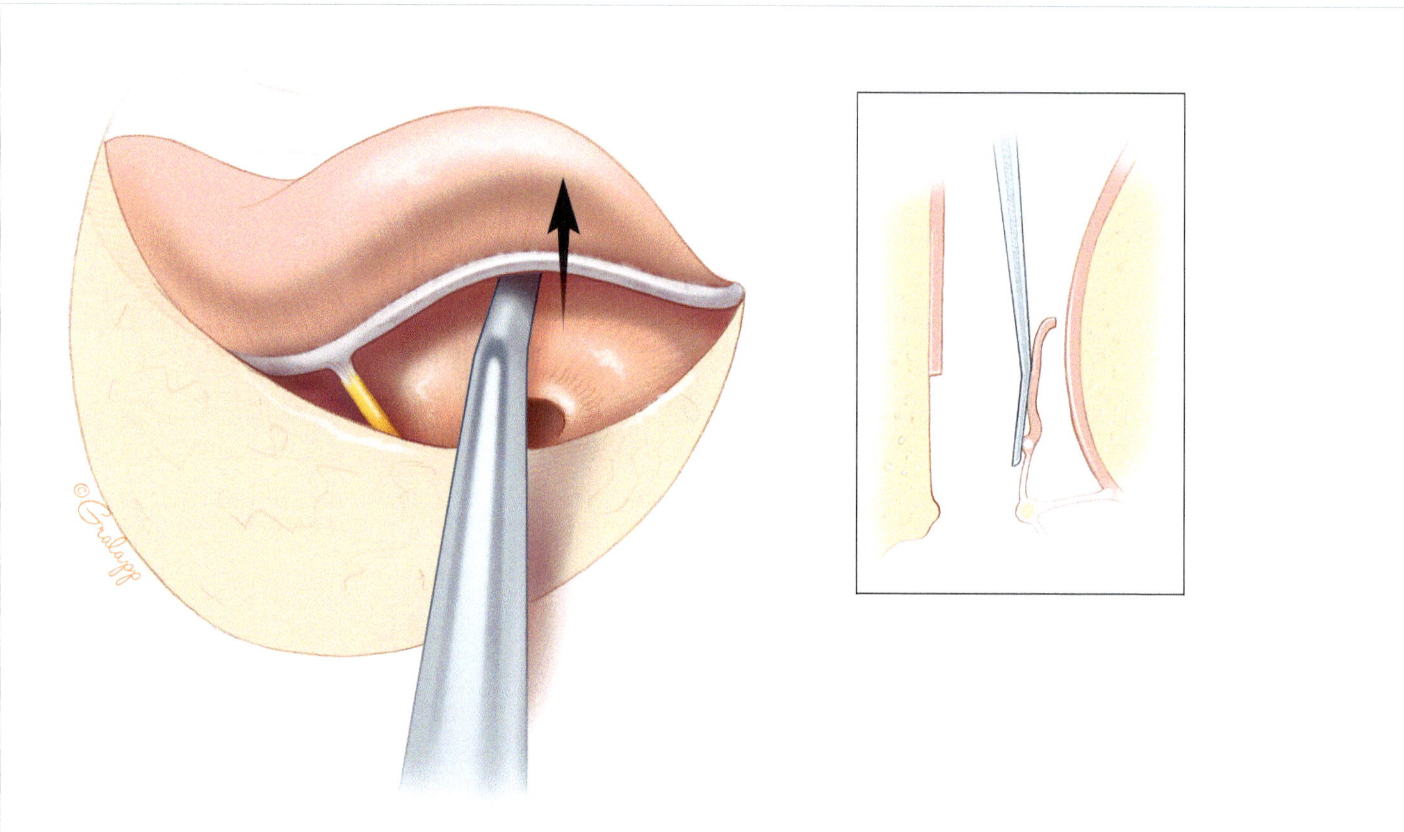

Fig. 4.32 It is important to have the middle ear exposure remain adequately open throughout the surgery. Using the back of the annulus elevator, the flap can be pushed against the anterior canal wall where surface tension will adhere to it.

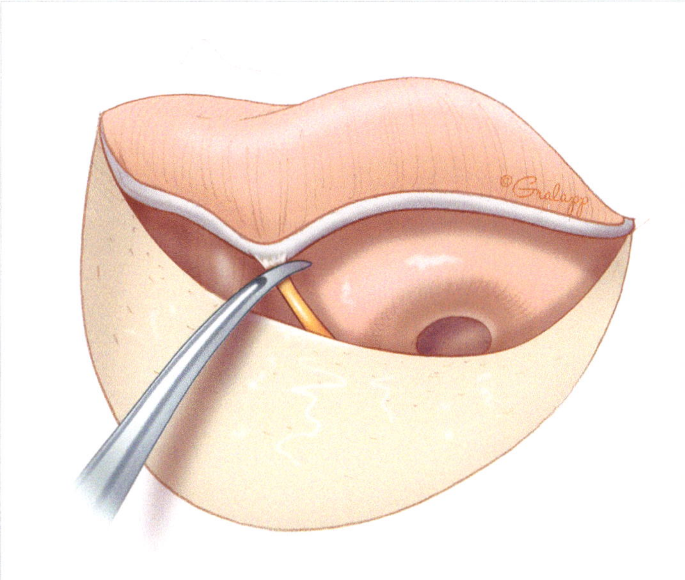

Fig. 4.33 Elevation of the annulus superiorly is done with a curved needle. The chorda tympani nerve is identified and dissected free.

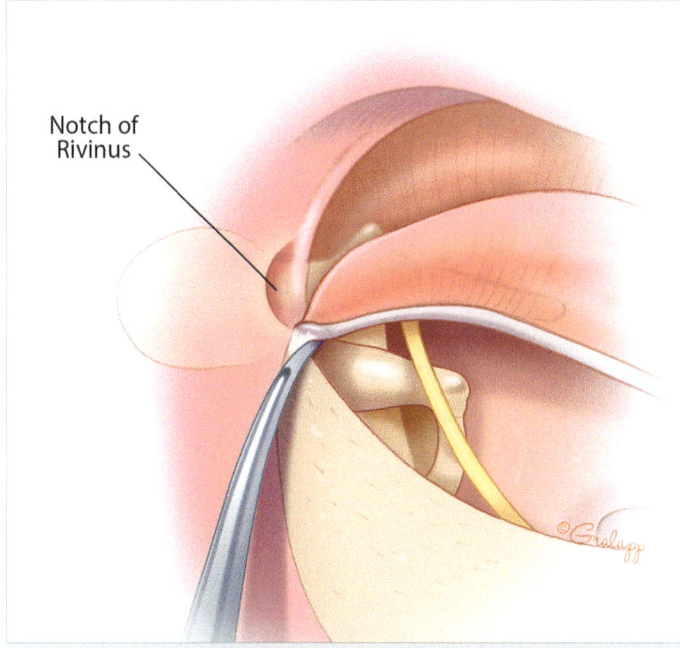

Fig. 4.34 Elevation needs to be carried superiorly until the flap is free from the notch of Rivinus. This ensures that the flap will fold over the malleus handle and thus give sufficient exposure of the incus long process to enable crimping.

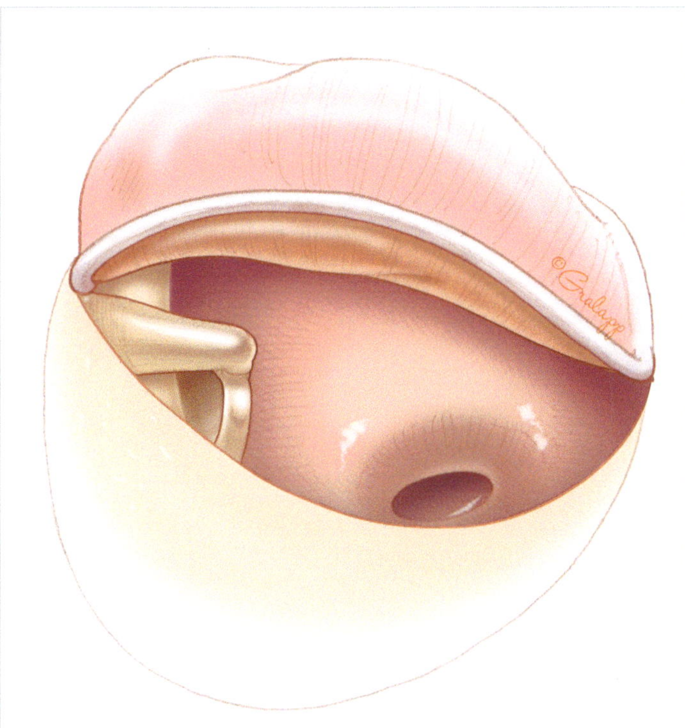

Fig. 4.35 Completed flap elevation. Note that flap is folded on the umbo and that a space is available anterior to the incus. If the flap does readily retain this position, further elevation superiorly or inferiorly is needed.

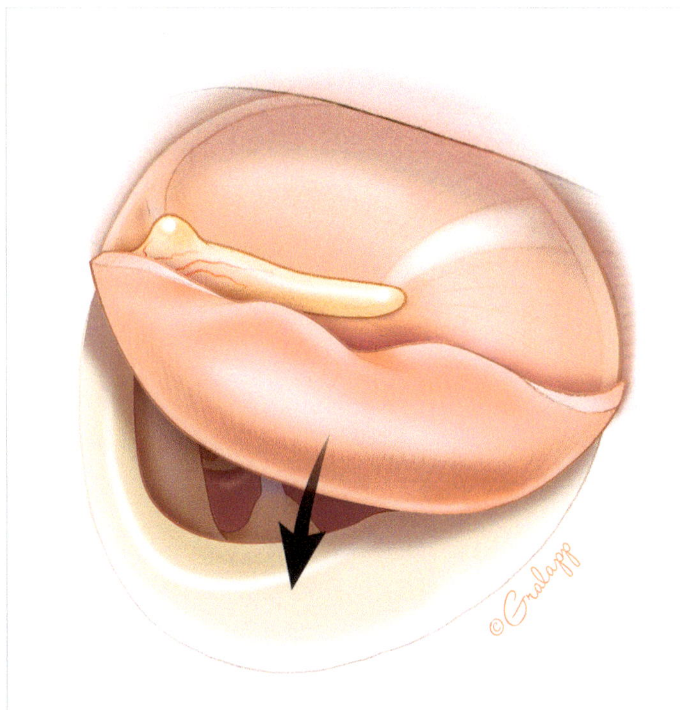

Fig. 4.36 When the flap sags and limits the tympanotomy exposure, sometimes a blood clot may have formed under the flap. Its evacuation restores adequate exposure.

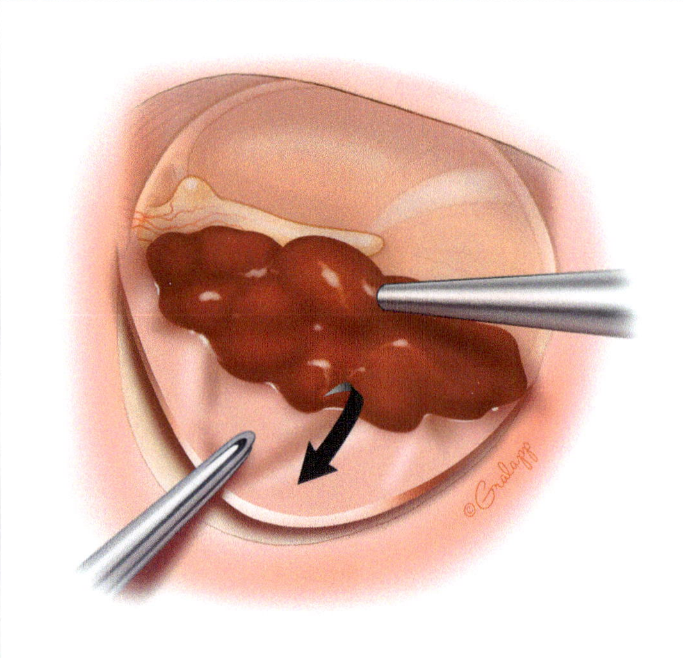

Fig. 4.37 When the flap sags and limits the tympanotomy exposure, sometimes a blood clot may have formed under the flap. Its evacuation restores adequate exposure.

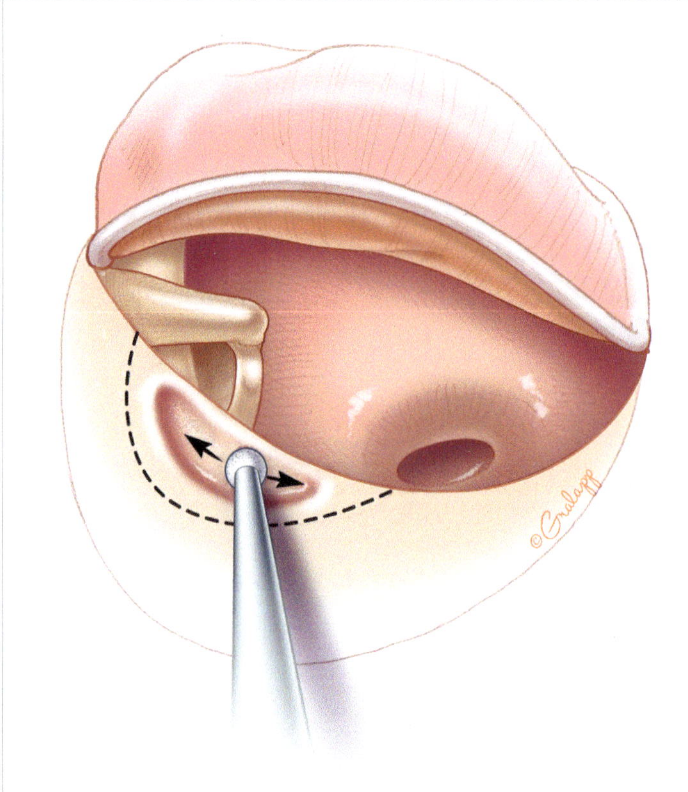

Fig. 4.38 Most commonly the scutum (posterior ear canal overhang) allows at least a partial view of the stapes superstructure. It must be removed to provide full access to the oval window. Scutum removal may be done with either a curette or microdrill or a combination of the two.

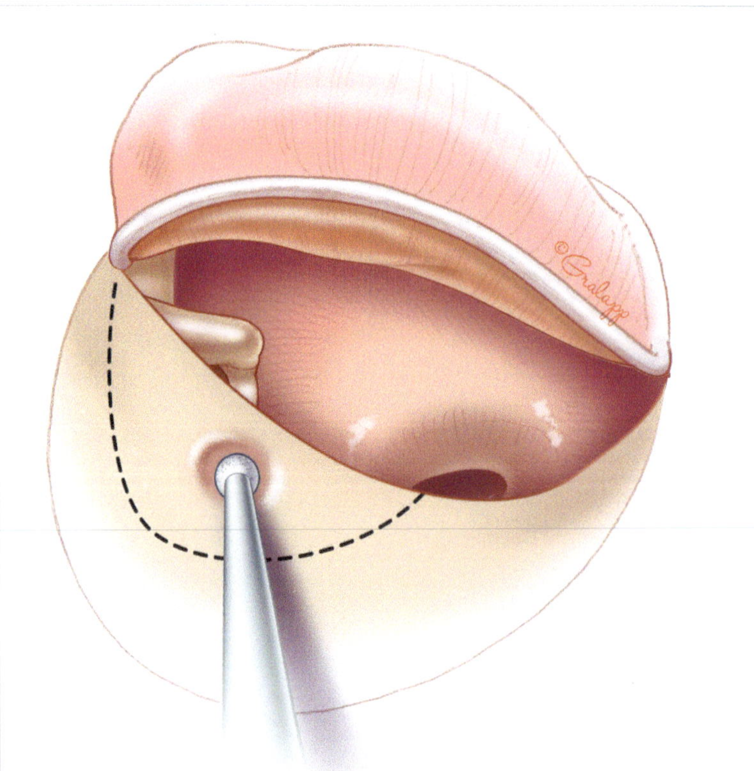

Fig. 4.39 A long scutum may fully obscure the stapes and require a greater degree of bone removal. Curettage of such a thick scutum can require considerable effort.

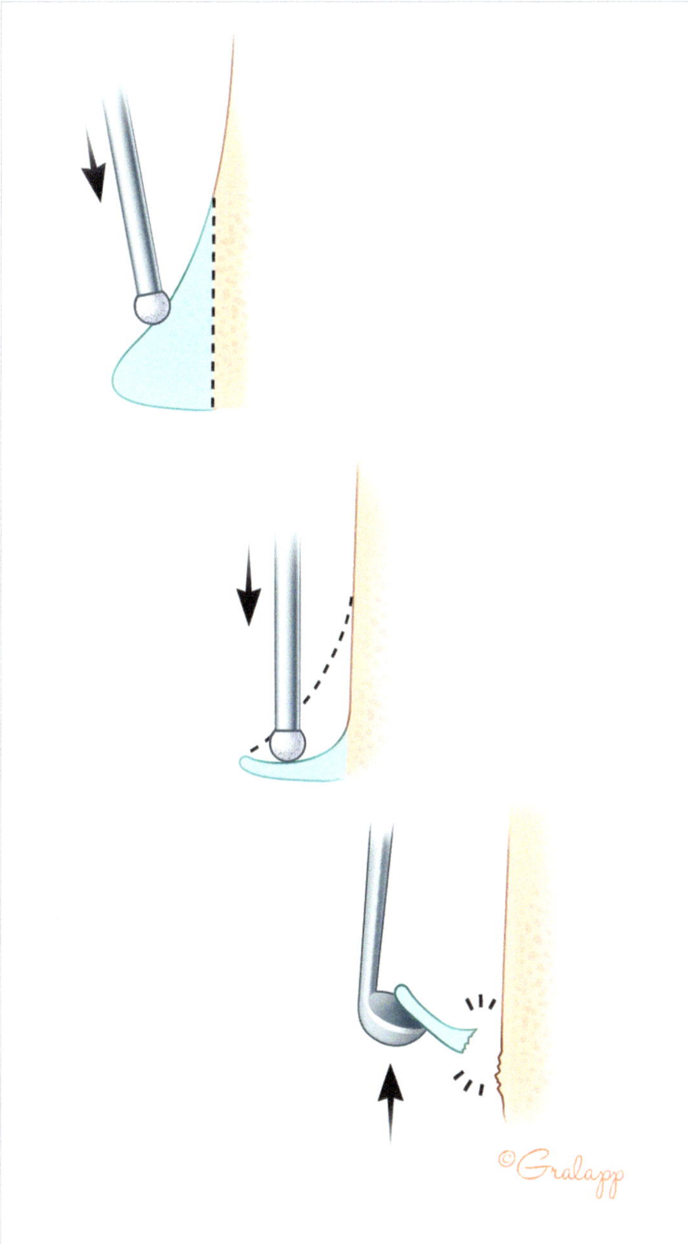

Fig. 4.40 Combined technique in which the scutum is first thinned with a drill (e.g., 2.3-mm diamond) and then a curette removes the last shell. A diamond burr is slightly slower compared to a cutting burr, but is less likely to injure the chorda tympani, flap, or tympanic membrane.

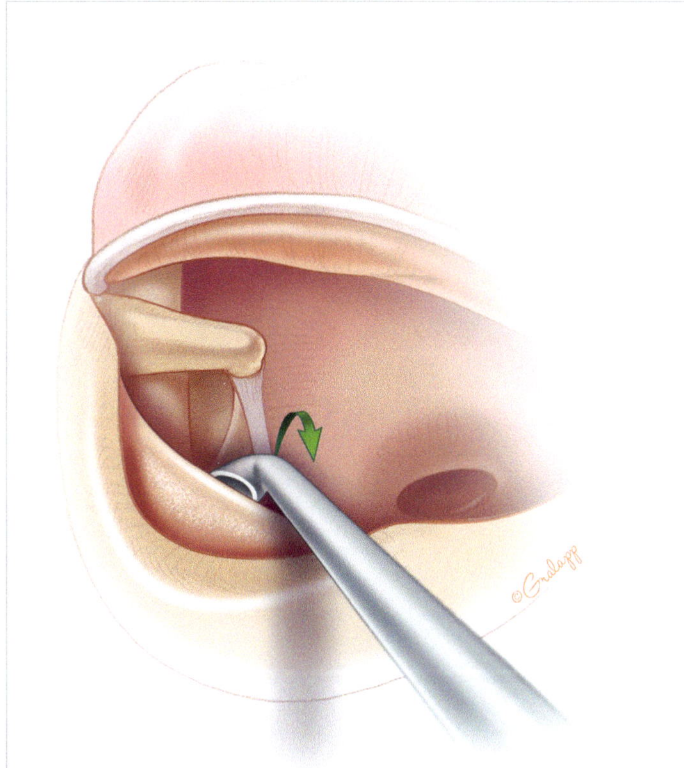

Fig. 4.41 Use of a stapes curette to remove the scutum. The curette is firmly braced against the speculum to create a fulcrum effect. The motion is rotational and outward, never inward. A sudden release of inwardly directed force could lead to incus dislocation. Effective use of the curette takes practice and may be challenging for the novice. Considerable force is needed to fracture pieces of bone. When chipping away bone, it is important to prevent the curette from lurching outward where it can tear the canal skin and trigger bleeding.

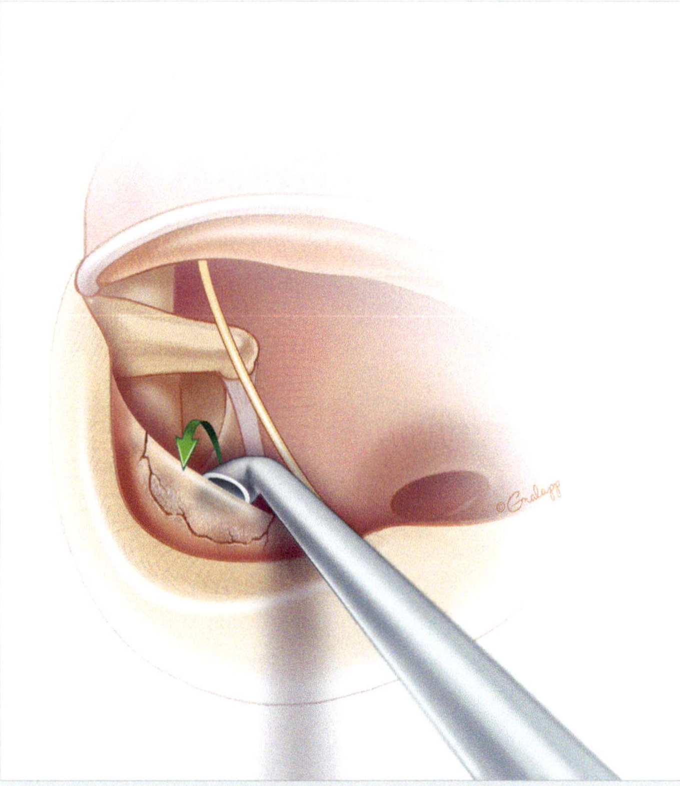

Fig. 4.42 Curetting outward and away from the incus. Sometimes, the scutum breaks away in a single piece. More commonly, it is nibbled away in a series of small bone fragments.

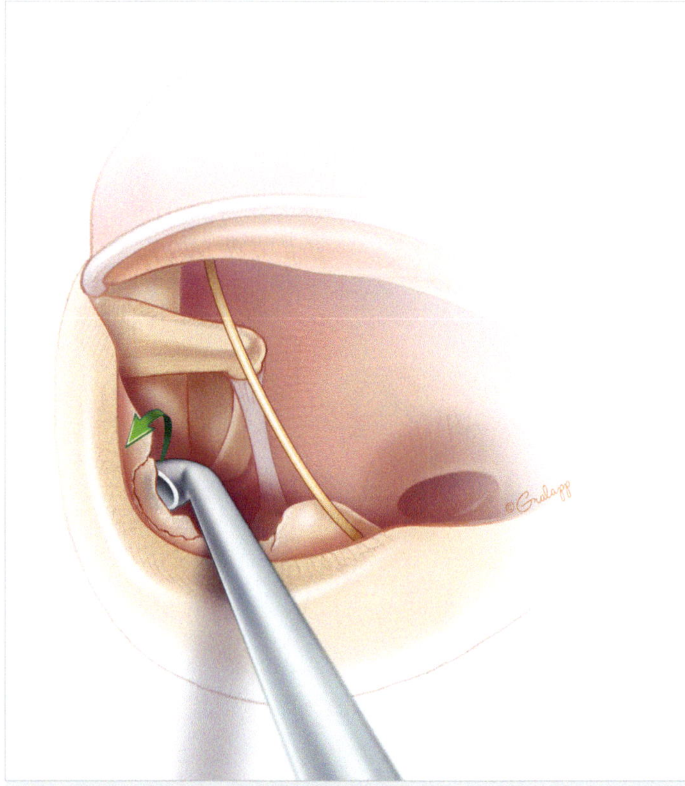

Fig. 4.43 Removal of the last ridge needed for adequate exposure of the stapes. Curetting is complete when the facial nerve is in full view superiorly and the junction of the stapes tendon and pyramid are visible posteriorly.

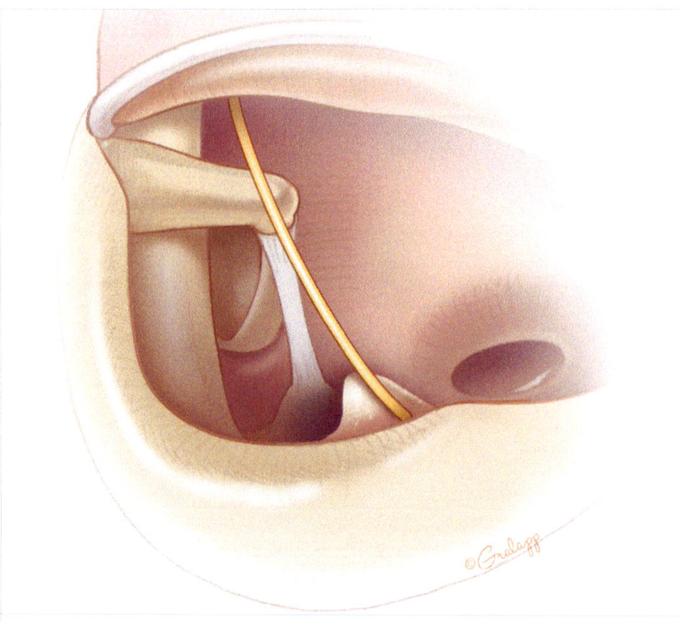

Fig. 4.44 A bony prominence often exists under the entry of the chorda tympani. When the bone hinders exposure of the posterior aspect of the footplate, it must be removed. This must be done carefully to reduce the risk of injury to the chorda tympani.

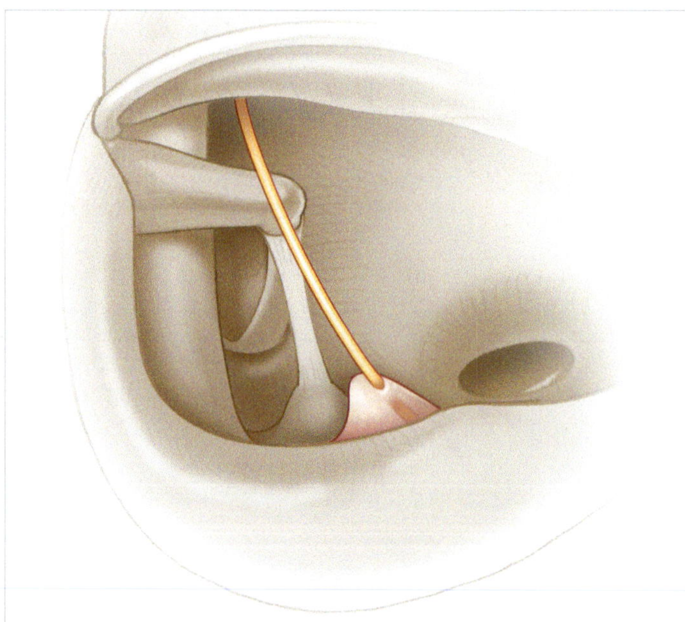

Fig. 4.45 The chorda tympani sometimes traverses a bony prominence.

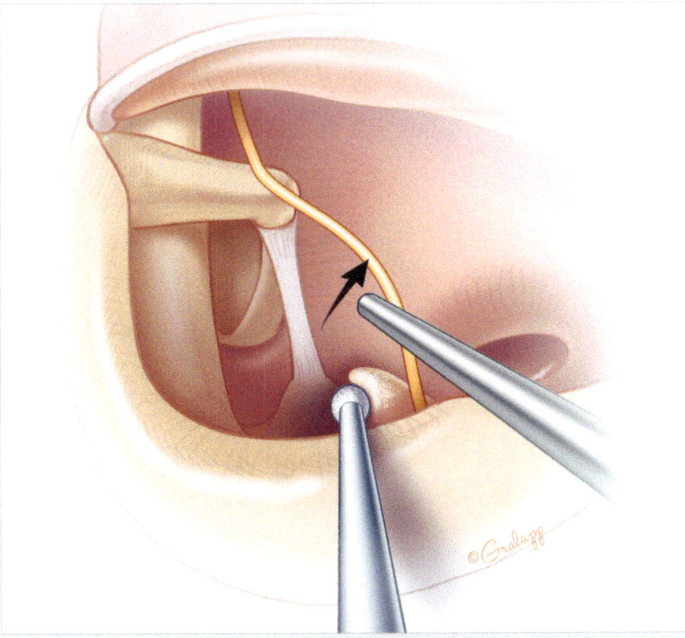

Fig. 4.46 A 1-mm diamond burr is used to partially remove the prominence.

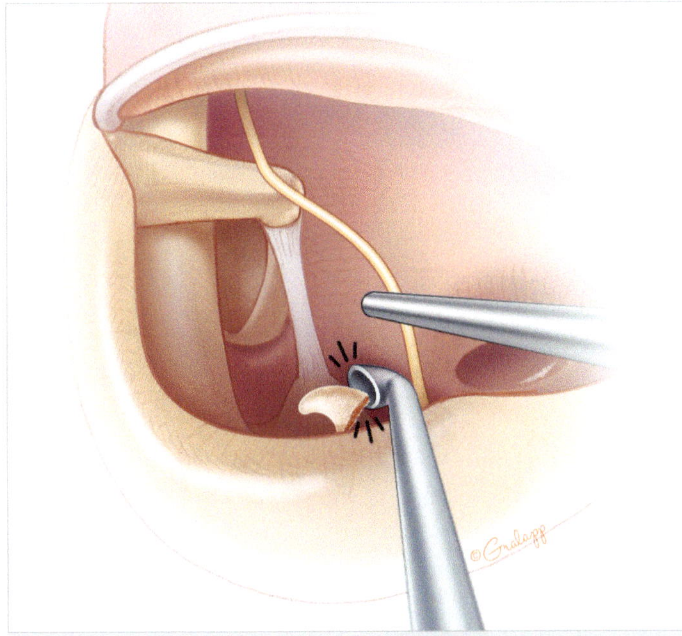

Fig. 4.47 A curette is used to remove the remaining shell.

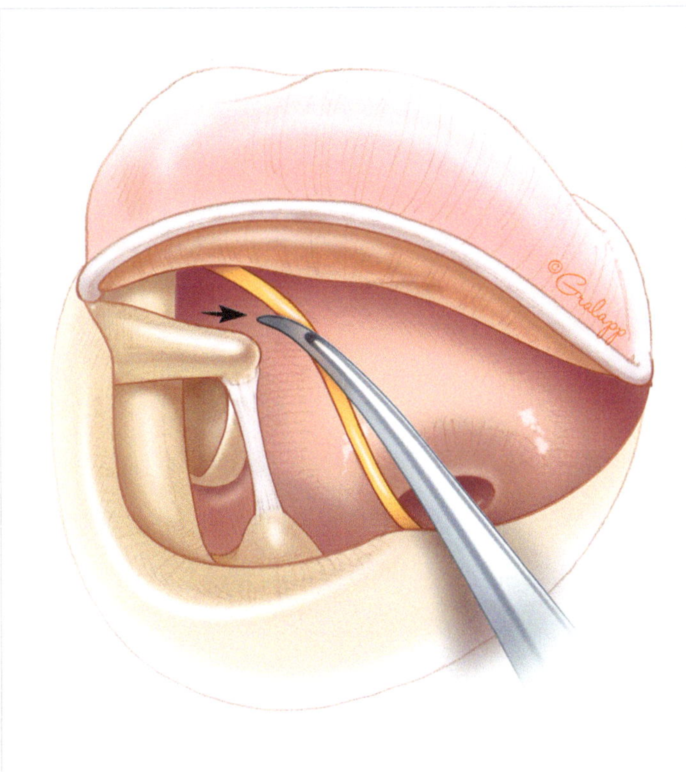

Fig. 4.48 Exposure for stapes surgery is adequate when both the facial nerve and the junction of the stapes tendon with the pyramid are visible. It is important not merely to be able to see the stapes, but to have sufficient room to bring instruments into action from superior, posterior, and inferior directions. Mesenteries (often erroneously called "adhesions" when the mucosal folds are actually embryological remnants) often need to be lysed between the incus long process and the malleus. Establishing exposure anterior to the incus is essential for later placement of the prosthesis.

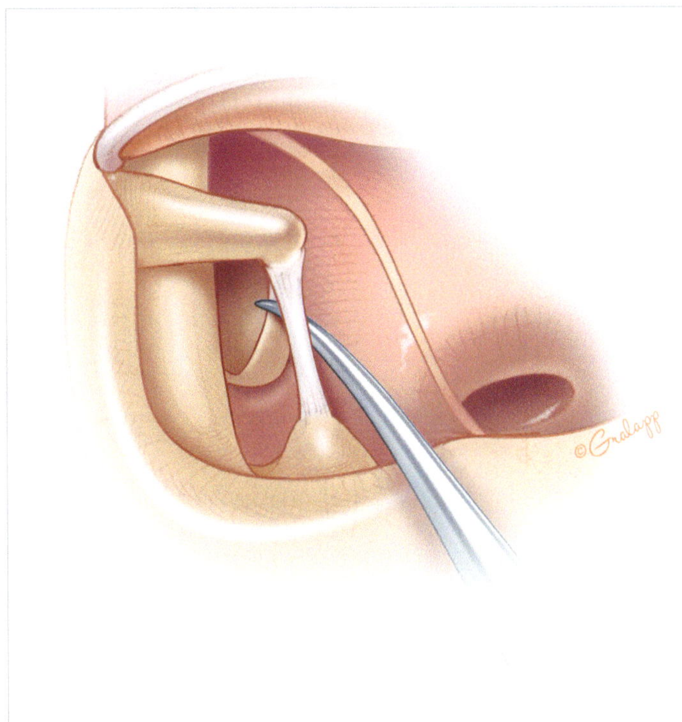

Fig. 4.49 Palpation of the stapes superstructure to confirm fixation. This should be done gently, as excessive force could mobilize a lightly fixed footplate.

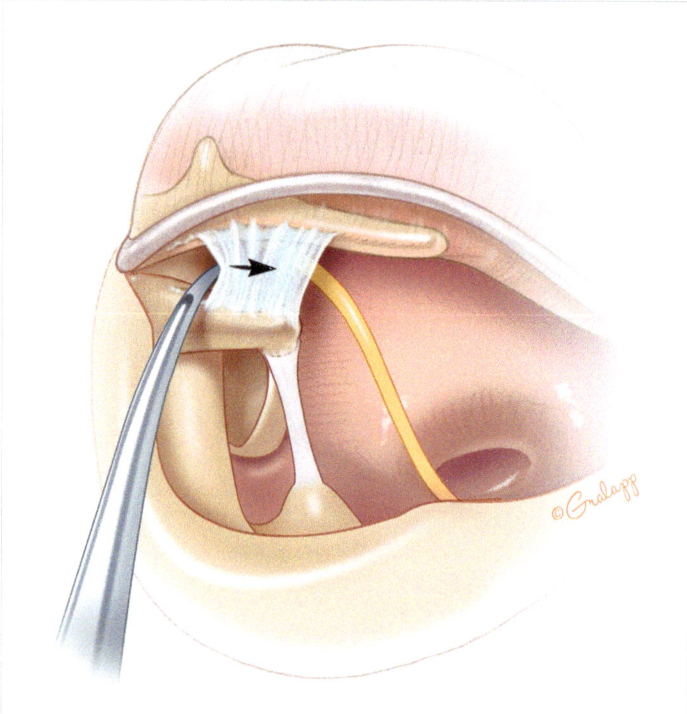

Fig. 4.50 The so-called adhesions are common in the middle ear. During stapes surgery, they are most commonly embryological remnants. To enable later placement of the prosthesis on the incus, the intraosseous ligament needs to be lysed.

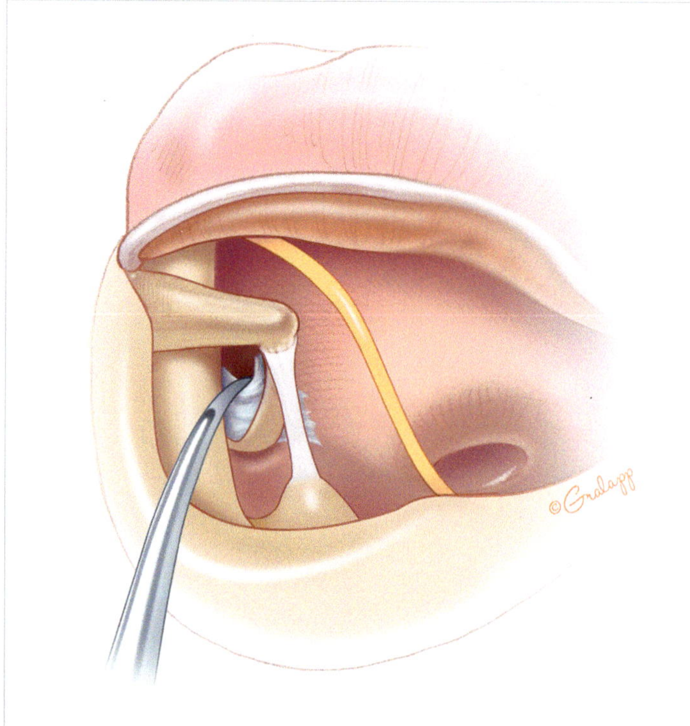

Fig. 4.51 Mucosal folds often overlie the footplate. If visible at this point (sometimes they are obscured by the superstructure), then these should be lysed with a needle or hook.

4.4 Stapedotomy

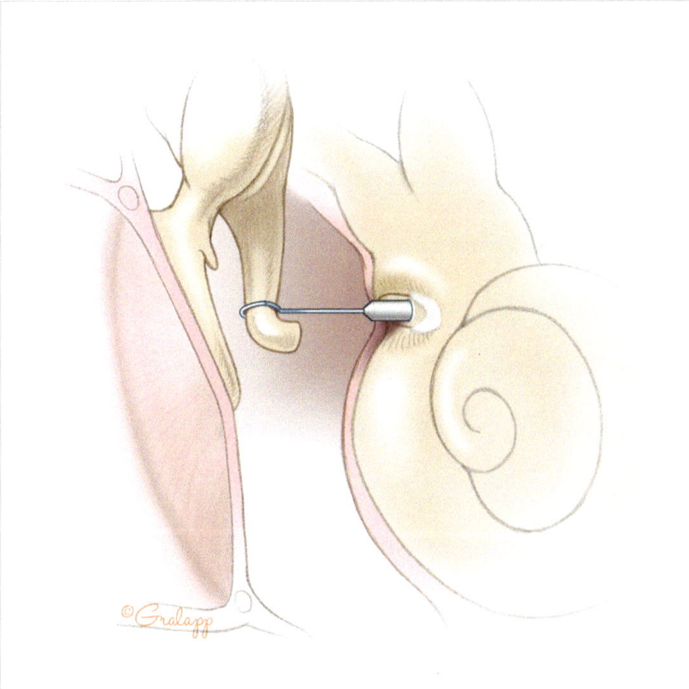

Fig. 4.52 Small fenestra technique.

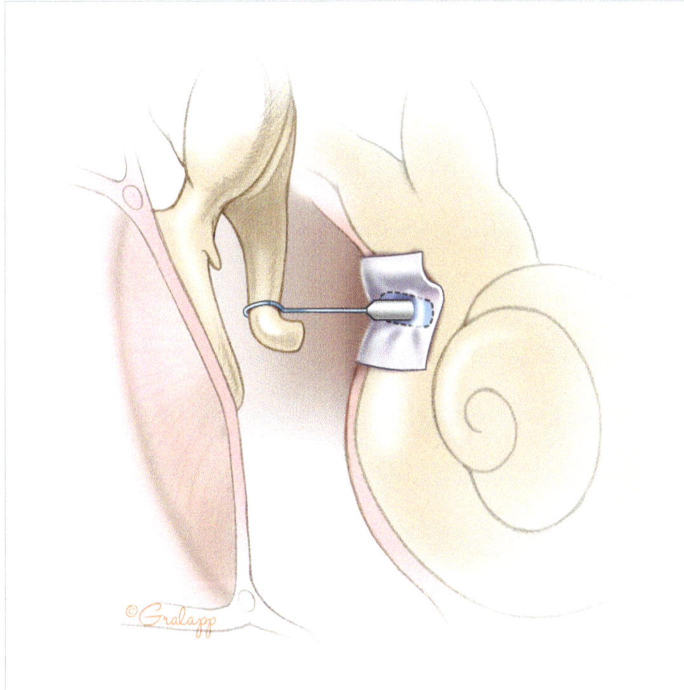

Fig. 4.53 The large fenestra operation requires placement of a membrane across the oval window, most commonly tragal perichondrium, temporalis fascia, or vein harvested from the dorsum of the hand.

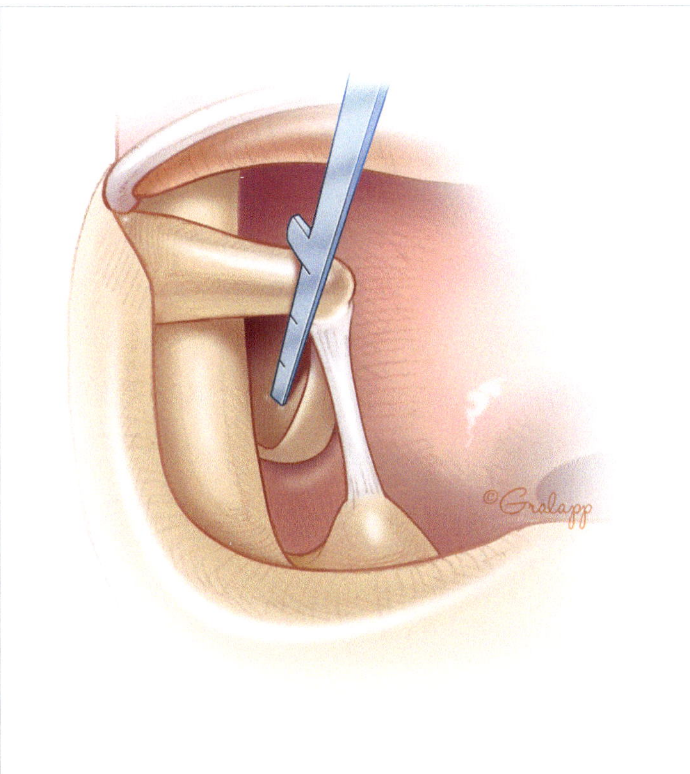

Fig. 4.54 For sizing of the prosthesis, it is necessary to measure from the lateral aspect of the incus to the footplate. Note that the instrument is directly posteriorly, an angle which may require the malleable instrument to be slightly bent. To achieve the proper angle, the instrument shaft has to lean on the anterior wall of the speculum. Correct measurement is between the center and posterior one-third of the footplate. The measurement is 4.5 mm in the majority of cases. The maneuver must be done delicately to avoid perforation of the footplate.

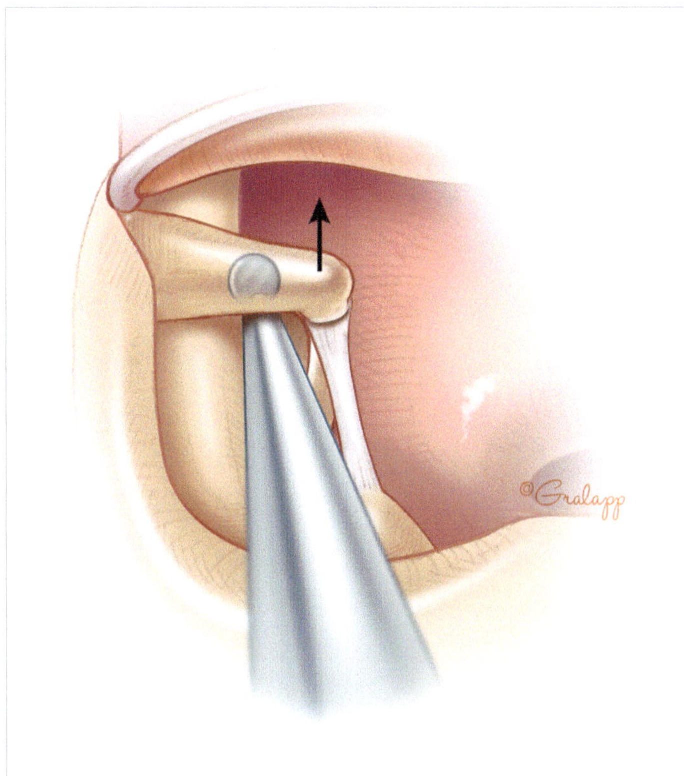

Fig. 4.55 Before cutting the incudostapedial joint, it is helpful to visually identify it. Slight outward pressure on the incus with the incudostapedial joint knife demonstrates the thin gray line of the joint.

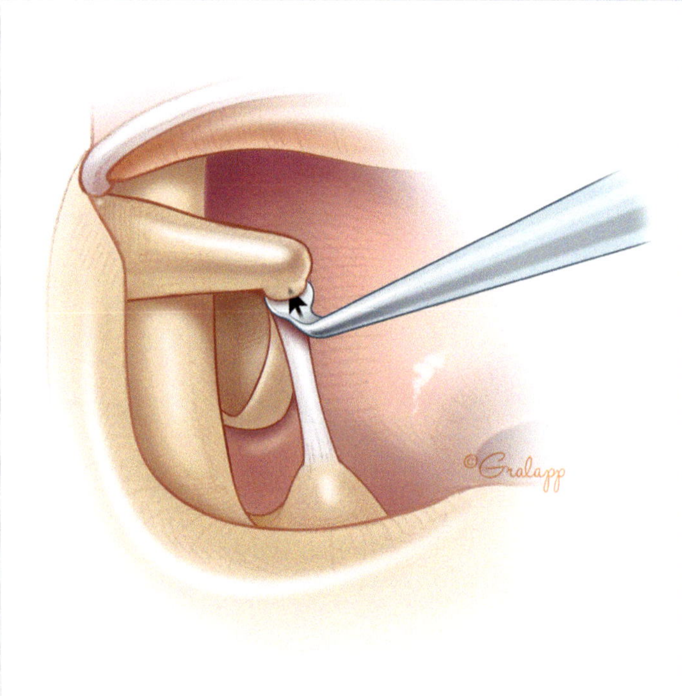

Fig. 4.56 The joint is cut with a gentle "worming" motion in the anterior direction. During this maneuver, gentle outward lifting of the incus is best while strictly avoiding a downward pressure on the stapes capitulum.

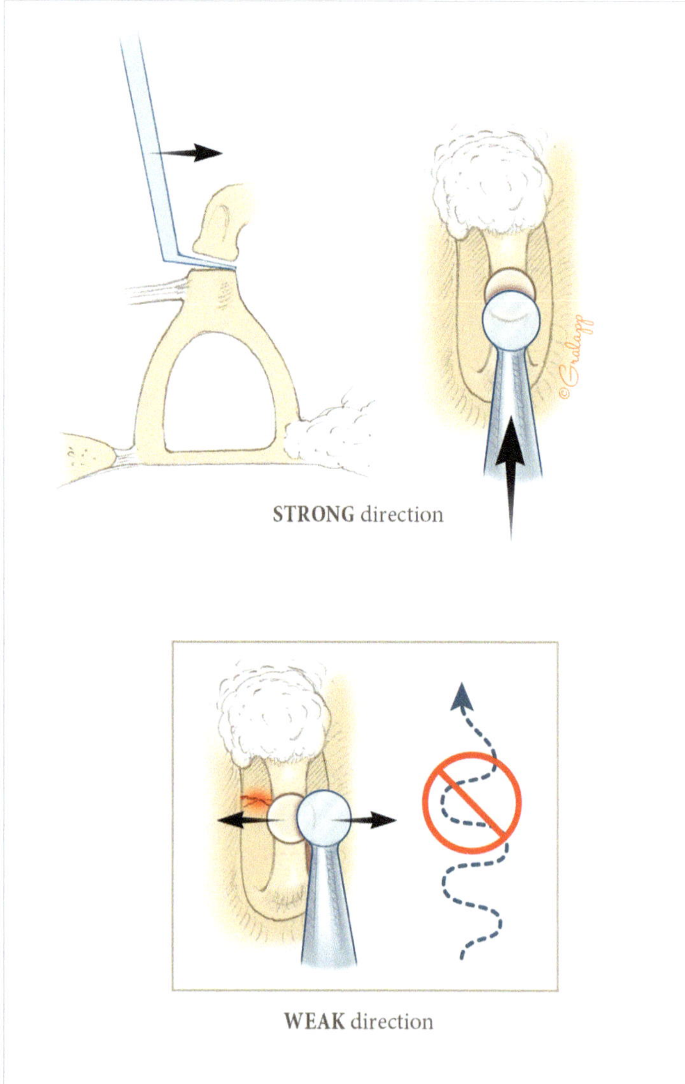

Fig. 4.57 The force vector used while dividing the joint should be primarily anteriorly directed. As the footplate is fixed anteriorly but remains mobile posteriorly, side-to-side motion risks creating a transverse fracture in the footplate.

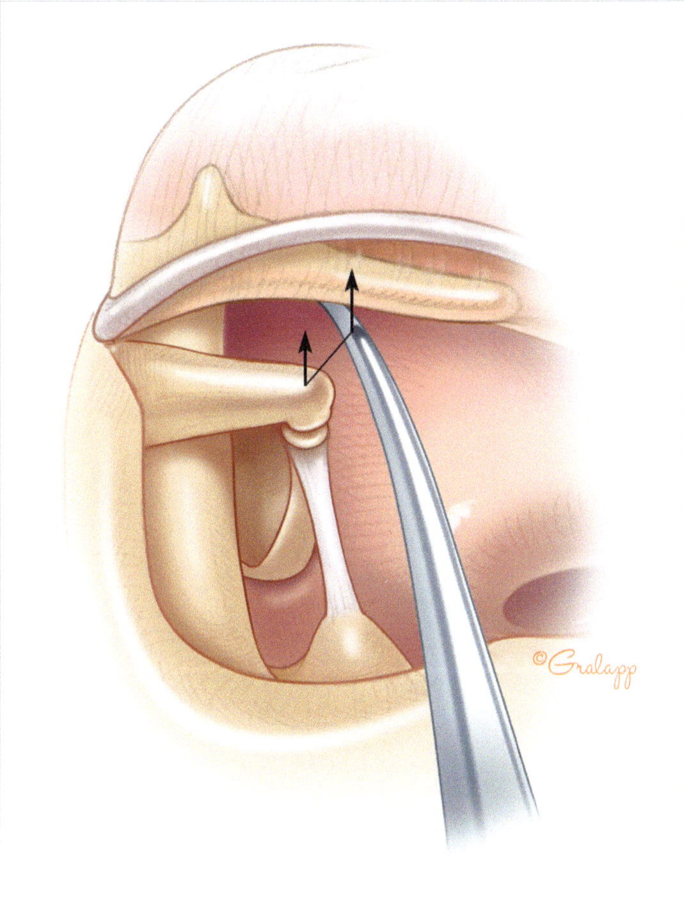

Fig. 4.58 After cutting the incudostapedial joint, mobility of the lateral ossicular chain is tested by pushing gently outward on the malleus. In about 1 of 200 stapes explorations, the lateral ossicular chain will prove to be fixed.

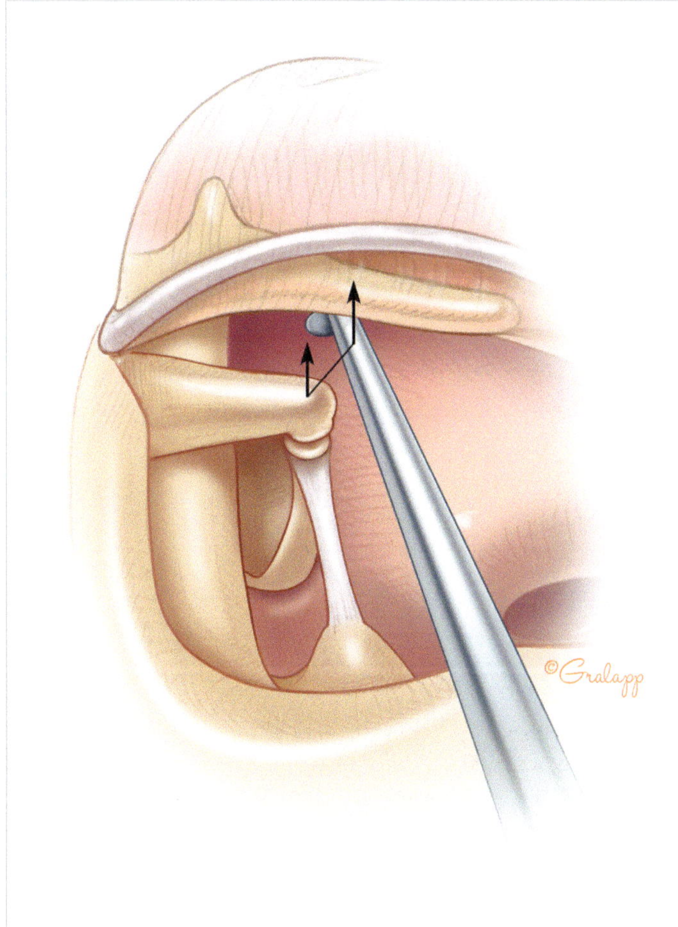

Fig. 4.59 A convenient way of testing lateral chain mobility, which avoids an instrument swap, is using the shaft of the joint knife.

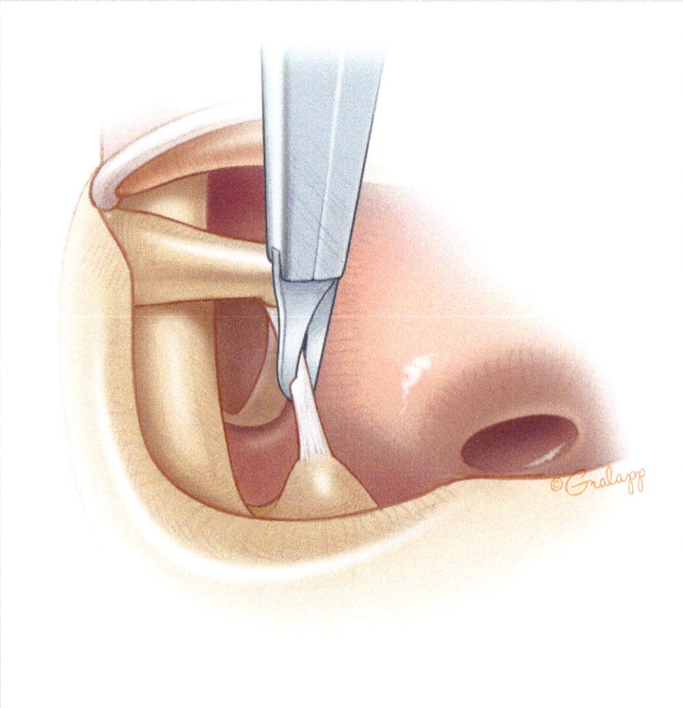

Fig. 4.60 Division of the stapedial muscle tendon using microscissors (e.g., Bellucci). To avoid cutting the posterior stapes crus, the trajectory of the scissors should be posteriorly directed. This is achieved by leaning the shaft of the scissors on the anterior side of the speculum.

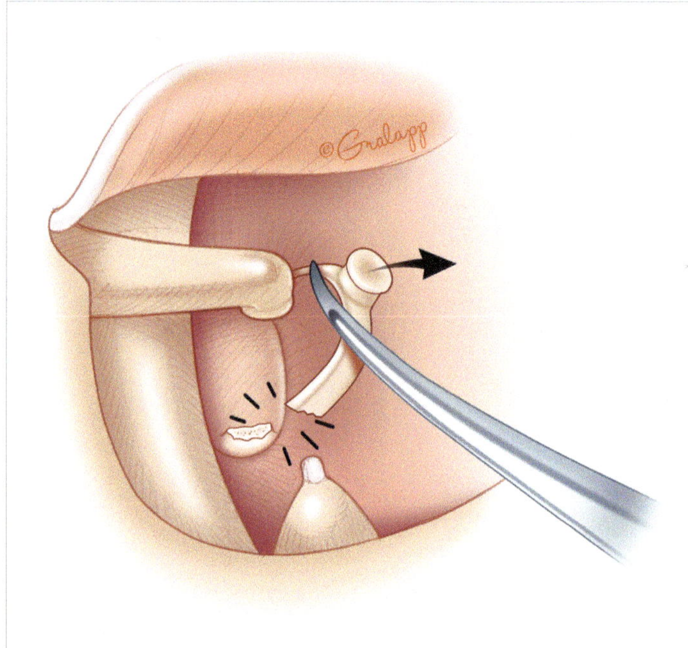

Fig. 4.61 Removal of the stapes superstructure through down fracture toward the promontory. This maneuver should always be conducted away from the facial nerve. The curved needle (e.g., Rosen) should contact both crura, but preferentially apply force to the anterior crus. Excessive pressure on the posterior crus will potentially lead to transverse footplate fracture. Note that this maneuver has to be done briskly. A slowly building motion may mobilize the footplate, while a quick snapping motion will have the desired effect of fracturing the bases for both crural arches as desired. After removing the stapes superstructure, it is important to recheck that the footplate remains intact and fixed. Niche bleeding can be controlled by placing a small pledget of epinephrine-soaked absorbable gelatin sponge in the niche for a minute or two.

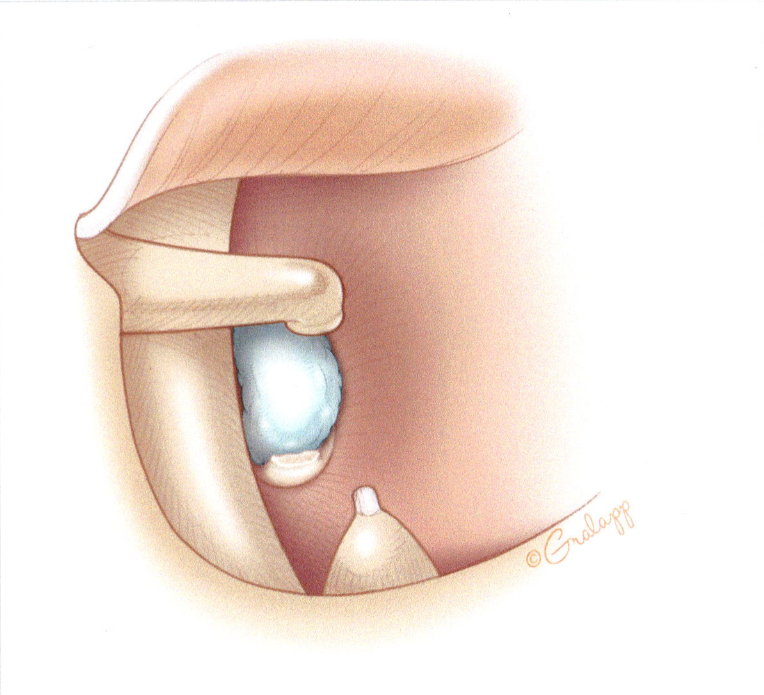

Fig. 4.62 After removing the superstructure, epinephrine-soaked absorbable gelatin sponge is placed in the oval window for a minute or so to constrict vessels before opening the footplate.

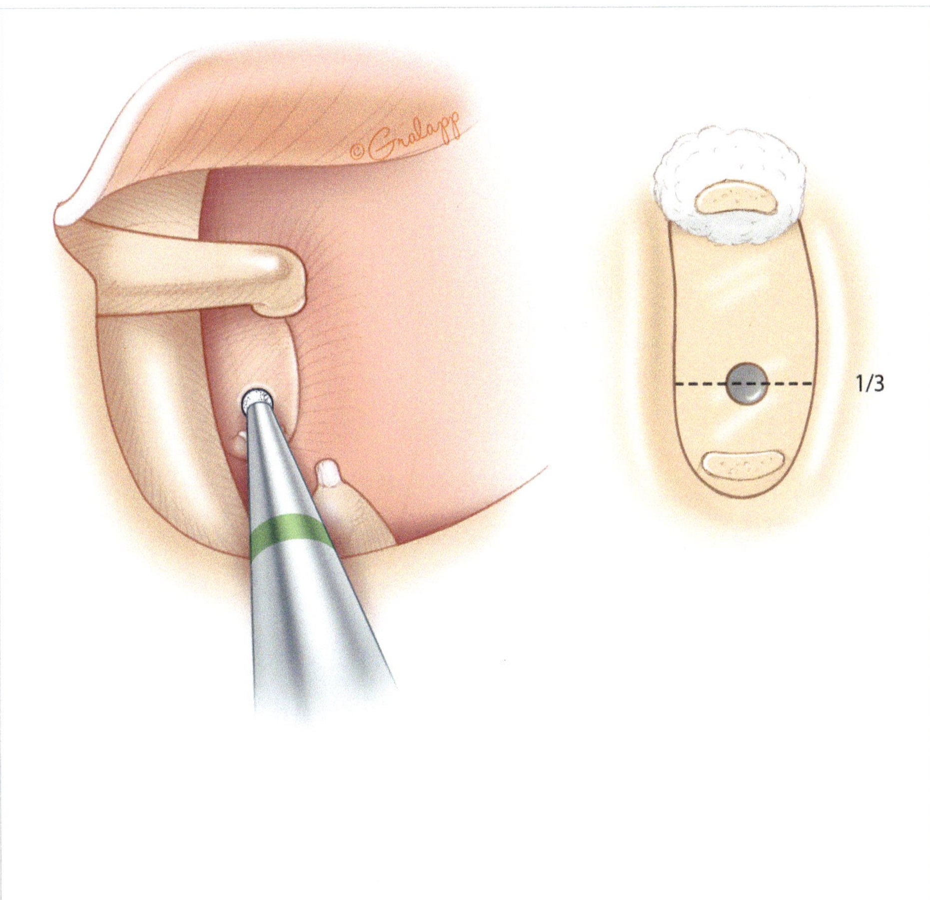

Fig. 4.63 Creation of a small fenestra stapedotomy with a burr slightly larger than the intended prosthesis (e.g., 0.7 mm for a 0.6-mm piston). It is best to use a diamond burr with a thin, blue footplate as a cutting burr is more likely to shatter the footplate. Optimal position of the fenestra is in the posterior central region of the footplate as the vestibule is deepest in this region. Because this procedure is delicate and potentially dangerous, a mere extra 1 mm of penetration can kill the ear, certain precautions are recommended. It is wise to remind everyone in the room to be quiet and strictly be warned to avoid touching the patient or operating table. The surgeon's hand needs to be comfortable, well supported, and absolutely stable. The burr should be running at full speed. To avoid skipping of the drill along the bone, the foot pedal is not engaged and drill rotation not begun while the drill is touching the footplate, but rather while hovering in the air just over the footplate. The drilling motion is a quick, subtle inward motion with the goal of having the burr penetrate to its meridian (i.e., widest point) and not beyond. Contact with the footplate should be brief. A fenestrometer is used to ascertain the adequacy of the fenestra (see illustration in laser stapes surgery). If too small, then an additional edge of the shape of a crescent moon is drilled to enlarge the fenestra.

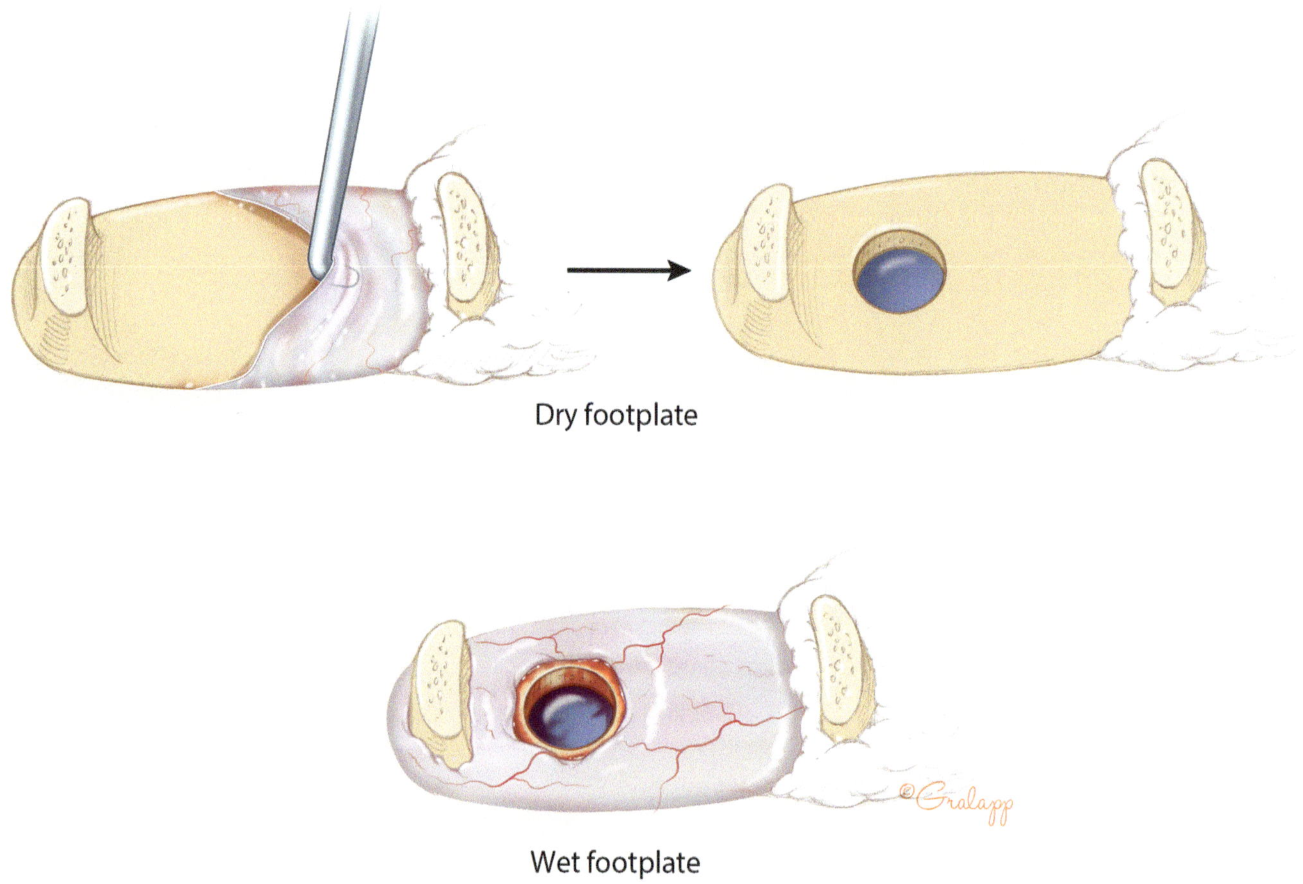

Fig. 4.64 Prior to fenestration, some surgeons remove the footplate mucosa. Once the bleeding has ceased, the fenestra can be created without stirring up bleeding. With the mucosa intact, oozing often occurs which can hinder placement of the prosthesis.

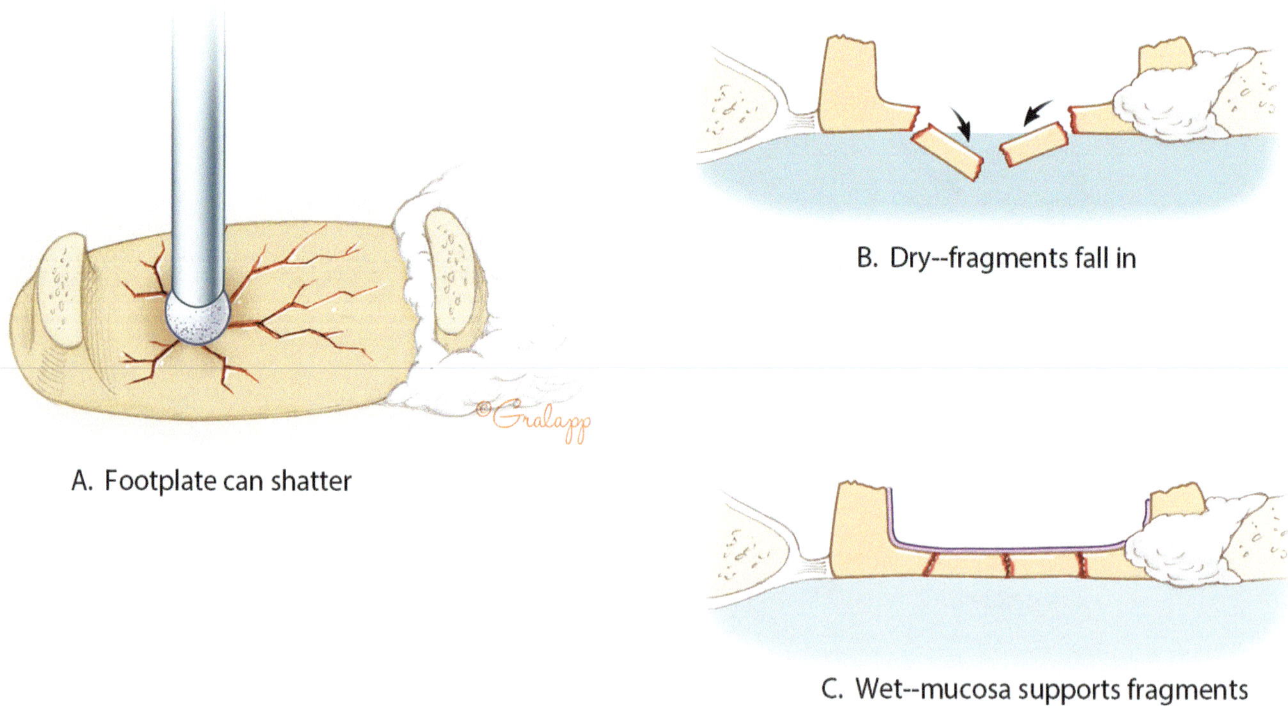

Fig. 4.65 Despite the greater potential for niche bleeding, many surgeons prefer to leave the footplate mucosa intact. Should the footplate shatter during drilling, the mucosa retains the fragments at the oval window level. Without tethering mucosa, these tend to fall into the vestibule.

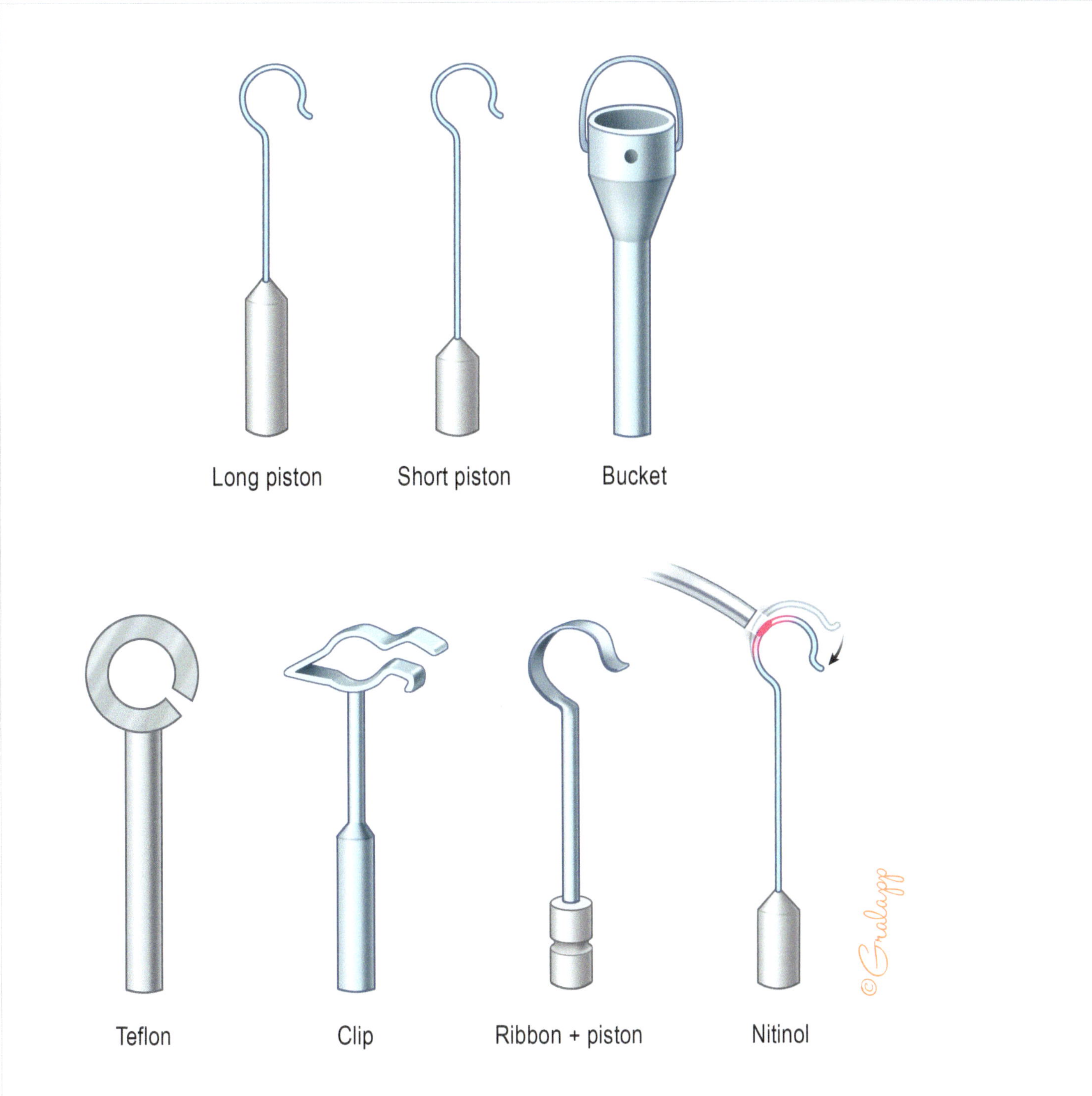

Fig. 4.66 A wide variety of stapes prostheses are available. The major types are depicted here. Most common materials used are titanium, nonmagnetic stainless steel, and Teflon. Many carry the names of their inventors.

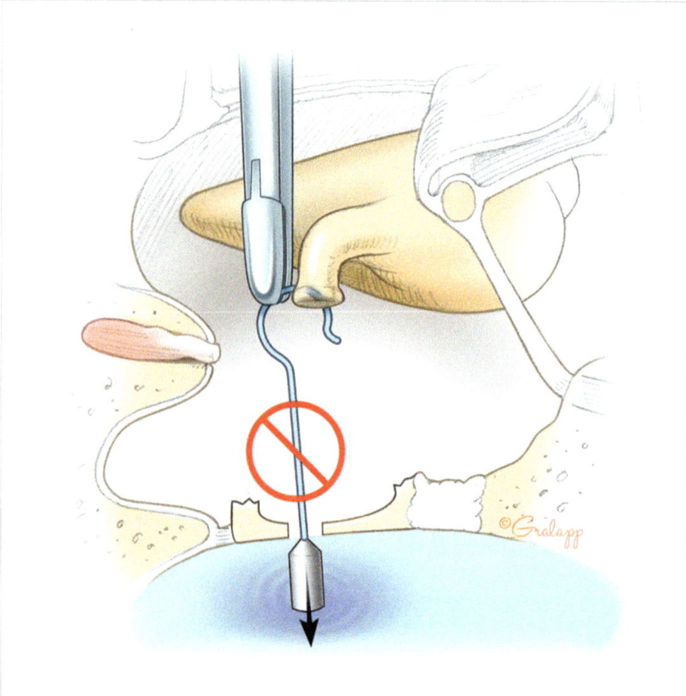

Fig. 4.67 The prosthesis is inserted with a smooth alligator. It is important that the shepherd's crook engage the incus-long process lest the prosthesis overly penetrate the vestibule.

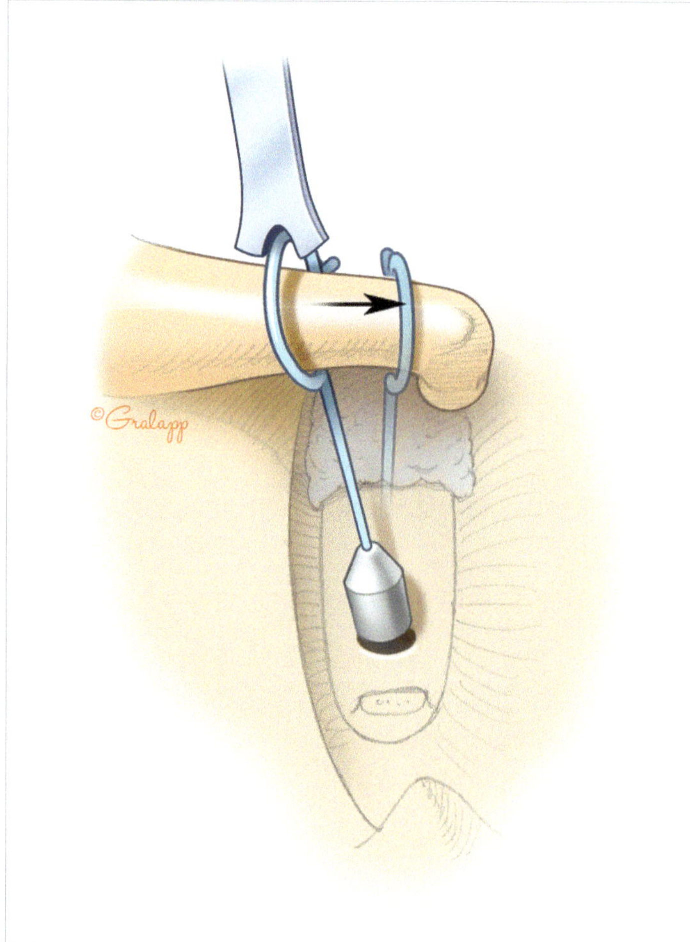

Fig. 4.68 In preparation for crimping, a notched chisel (also known as strut guide) is used to move the prosthesis into position.

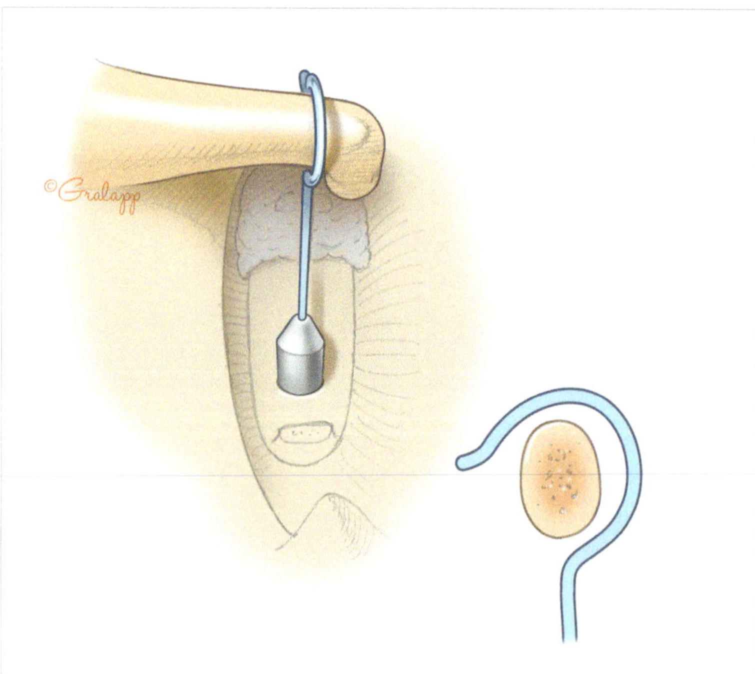

Fig. 4.69 Using a smooth alligator, the prosthesis is seated in position. It is important to have the shepherd's crook engage both the incus and the piston to the fenestra. If the wire misses the incus, the piston can penetrate the vestibule too deeply.

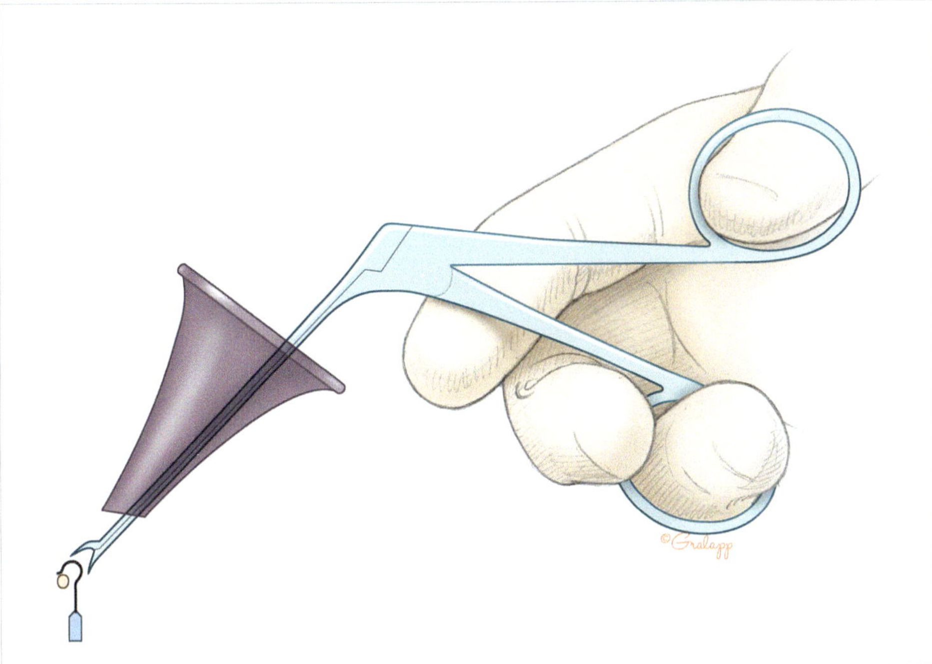

Fig. 4.70 Crimping of the prosthesis on the long process of the incus is a delicate maneuver. The crimper must be stabilized on the wall of the speculum.

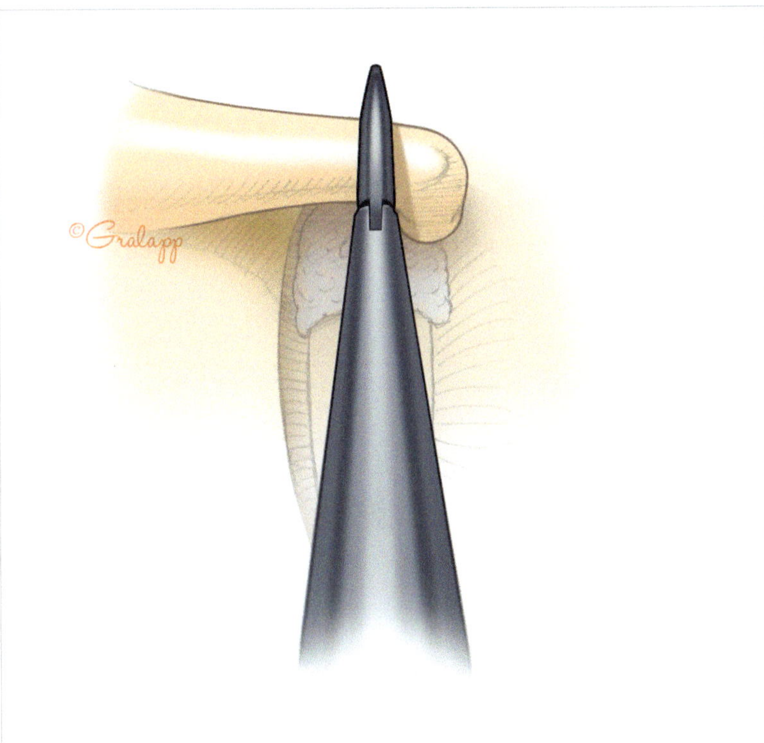

Fig. 4.71 The crimper must be aligned perfectly with the wire. If misaligned, the prosthesis will not crimp but will instead twist off to one side.

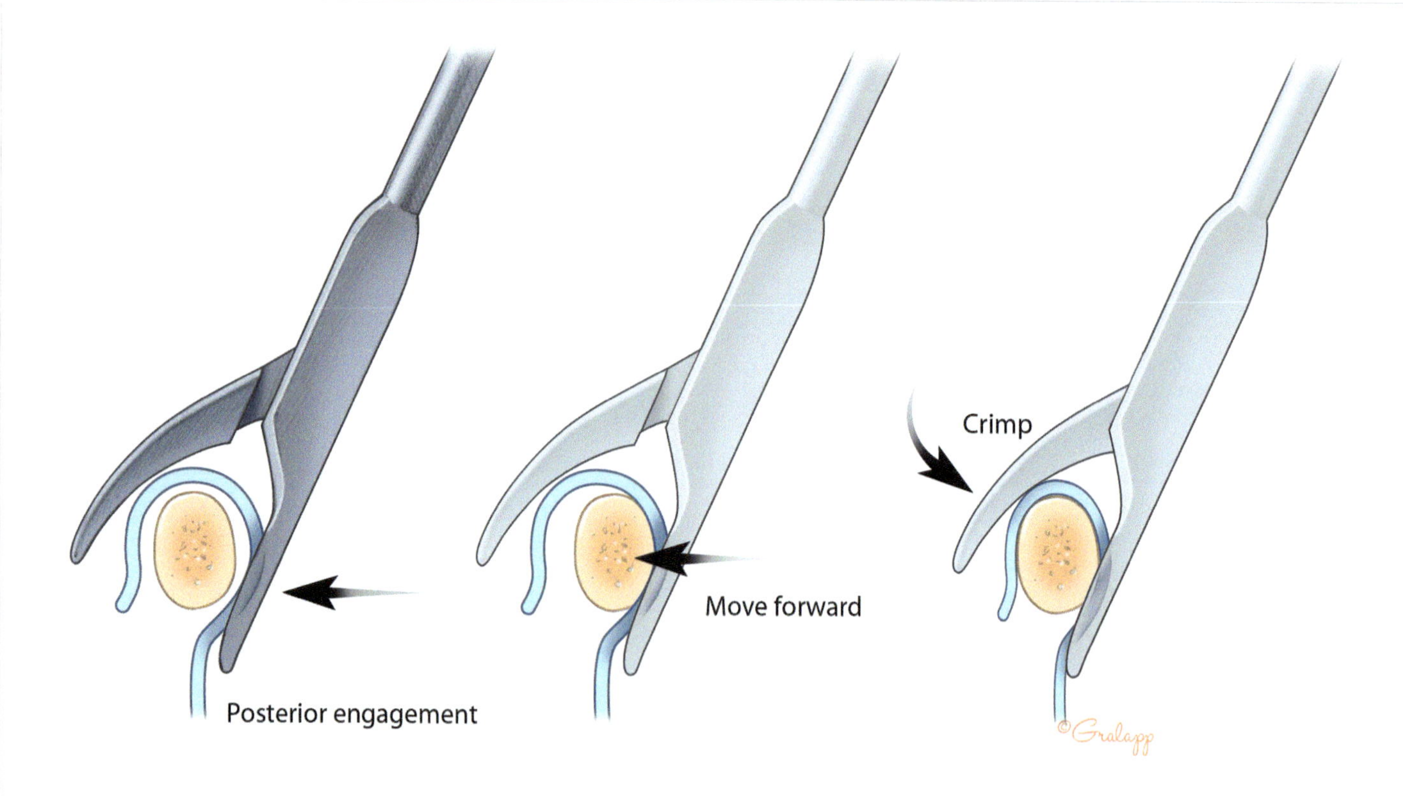

Fig. 4.72 It is important to understand the crimper's action. The back tine should be held stable while the front tine actively closes onto the incus.

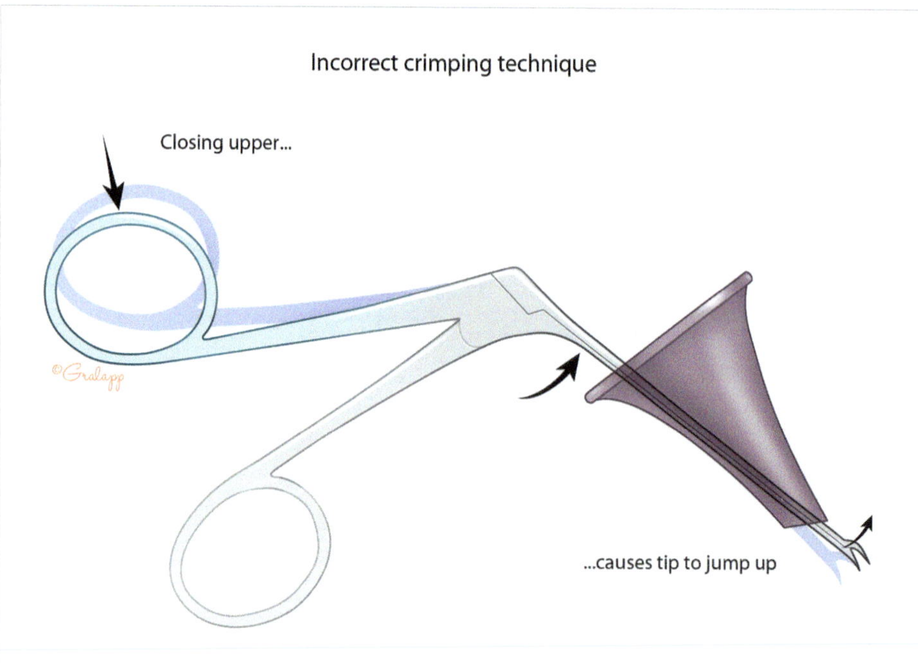

Fig. 4.73 Incorrectly moving the thumb side will cause the tip of the crimper to move forward putting force on the incus.

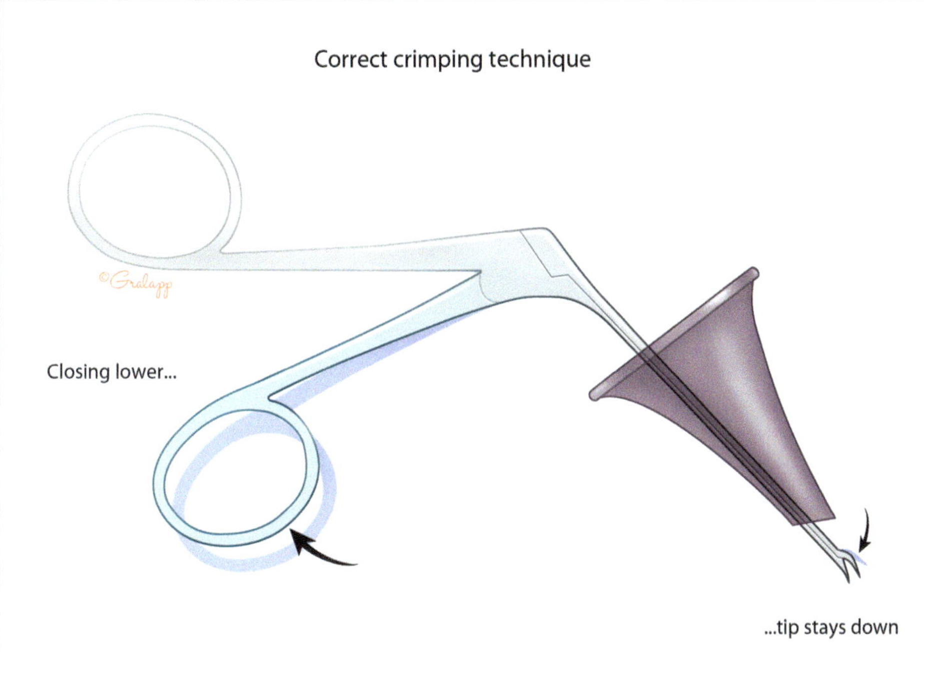

Fig. 4.74 Proper crimping motion stabilizes the incus and allows the anterior tine to close the wire.

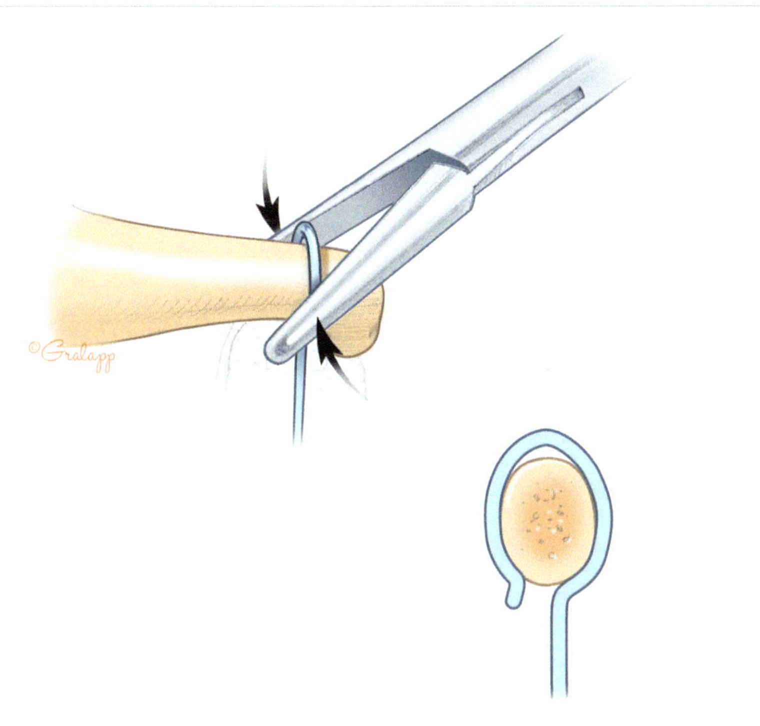

Fig. 4.75 The loop closure after crimping is often too loose. To tighten, the loop is moved to the narrowest point of the incus shaft and then cinched down with a smooth alligator. The closed loop can then be slid down the incus slightly toward the lenticular process to fit snugly.

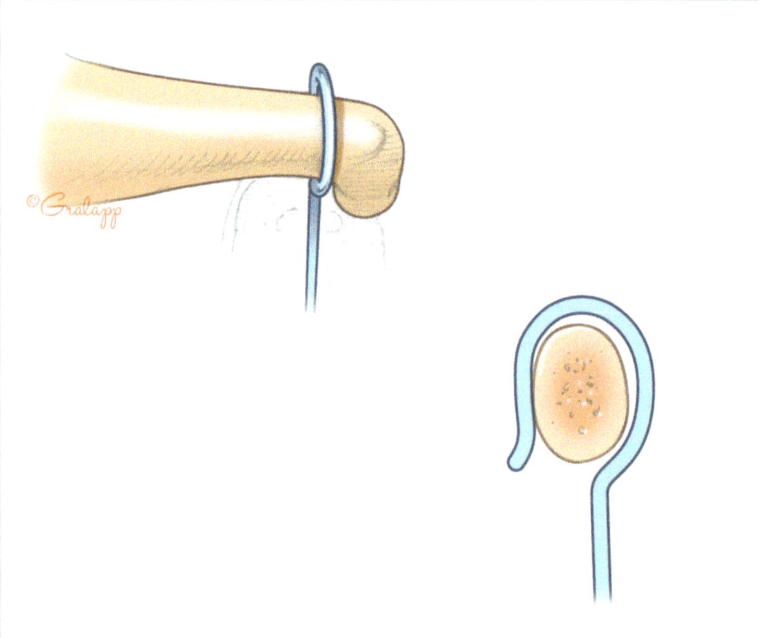

Fig. 4.76 An ideal crimp is not hermetically tight around the incus, as this may lead to later incus necrosis. The usual crimp may have a slight play to it.

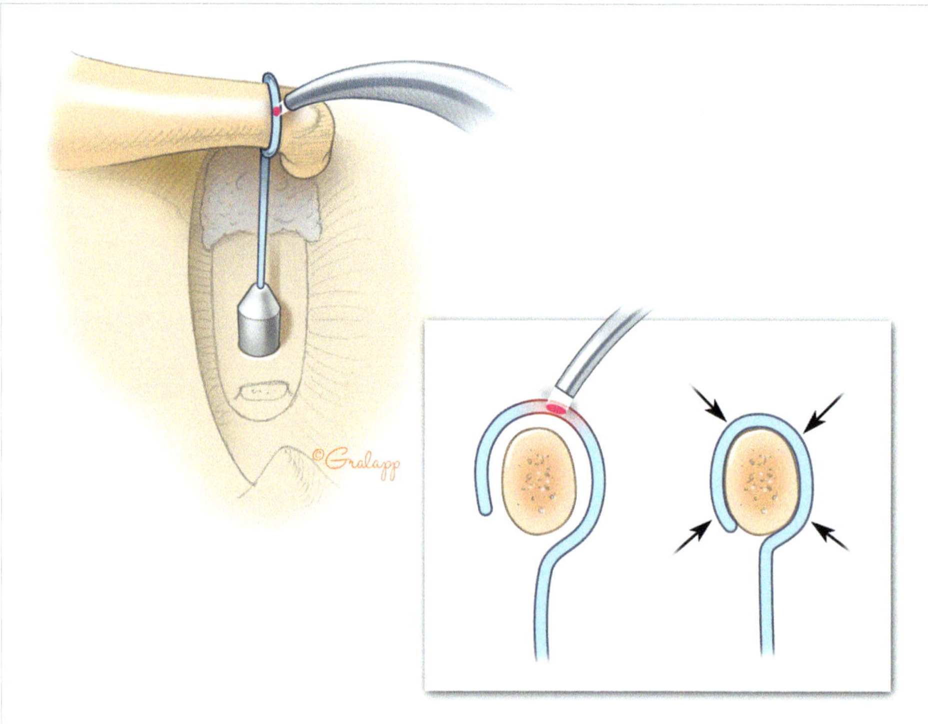

Fig. 4.77 Nitinol prostheses avoid the need for mechanical crimping. The heat-activated metal crimps to the incus with the application of laser energy.

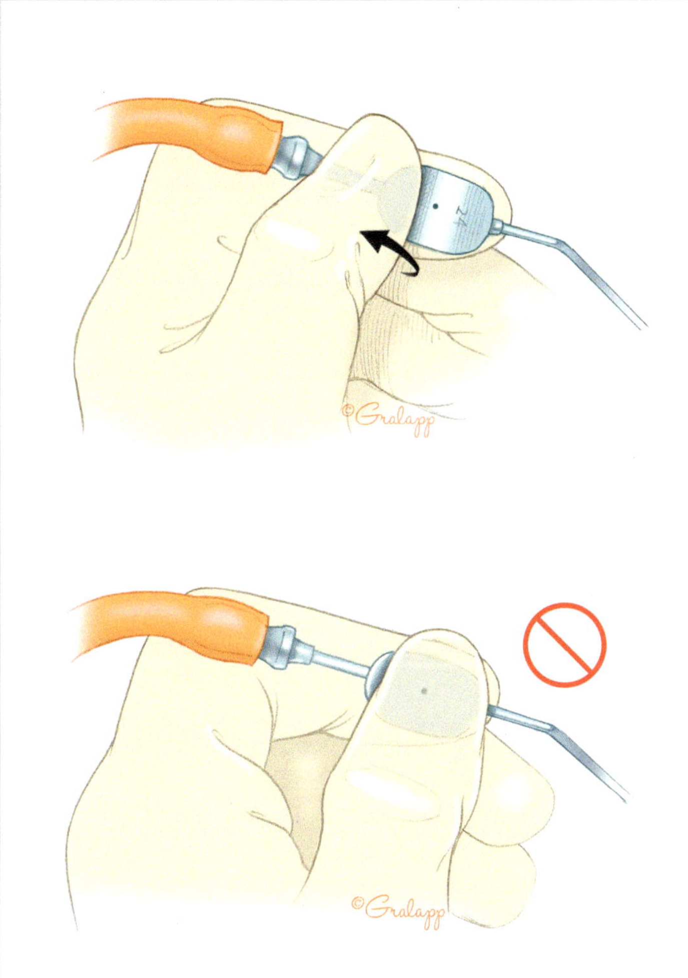

Fig. 4.78 Removing blood from the vicinity of an open oval window must be done with great care. It is best to use a very small suction (e.g., a no. 24 needle), turned down low, with the surgeon's thumb off the hole. When needed to remove tenacious clot, the thumb can briefly roll over the hole to momentarily enhance suction force. As a general rule, it is best whenever possible to remove liquid blood from the footplate before it has the opportunity to clot.

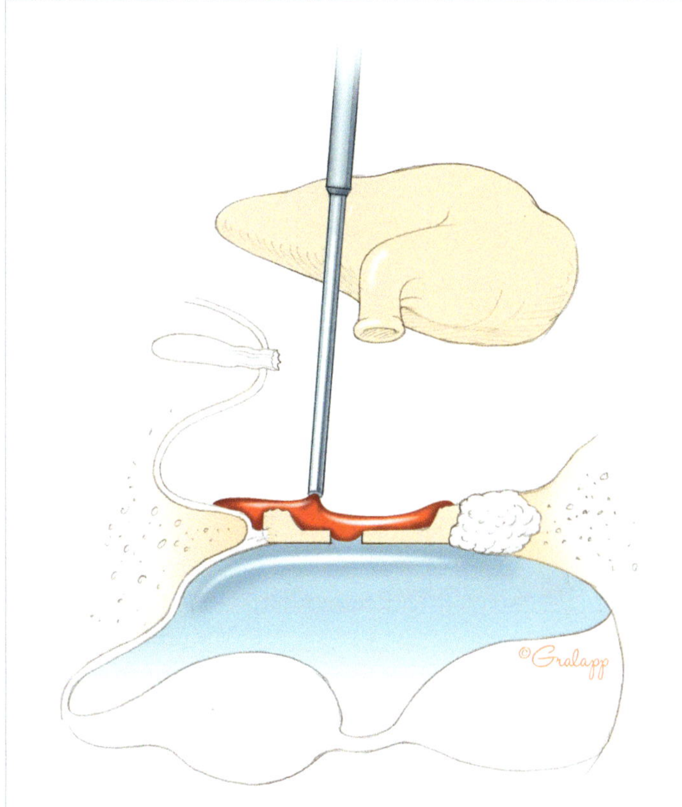

Fig. 4.79 Blood is suctioned from the footplate by vacuuming anterior or posterior to the fenestra.

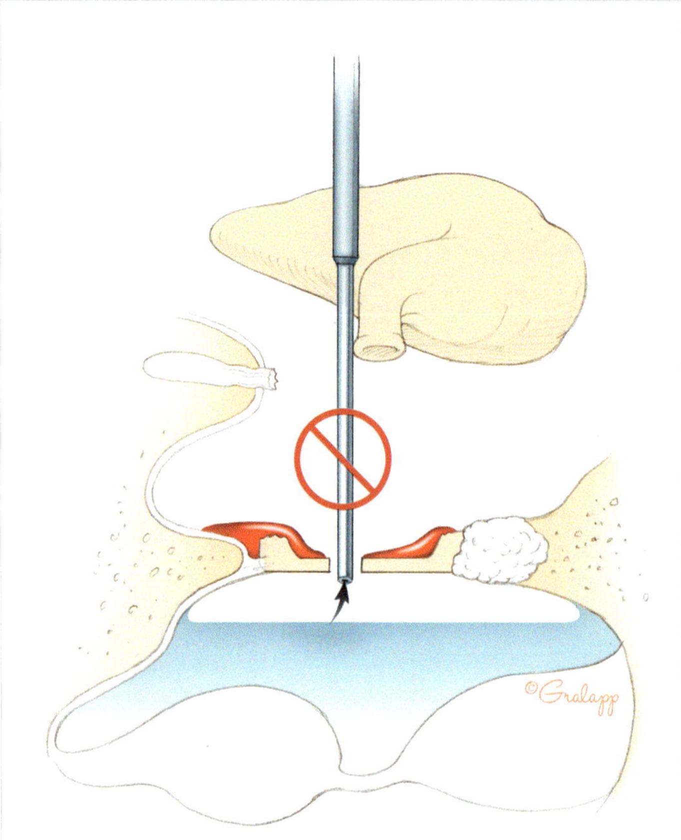

Fig. 4.80 Suctioning directly over the fenestra can remove perilymph leading to a dry vestibule. This may result in sensory loss and postoperative vertigo. When air is in the vestibule, some surgeons refill it with saline, but perilymph typically replenishes spontaneously via the cochlear aqueduct. Injury to the utricle or saccule, admixing endolymph with perilymph, is a much more serious injury.

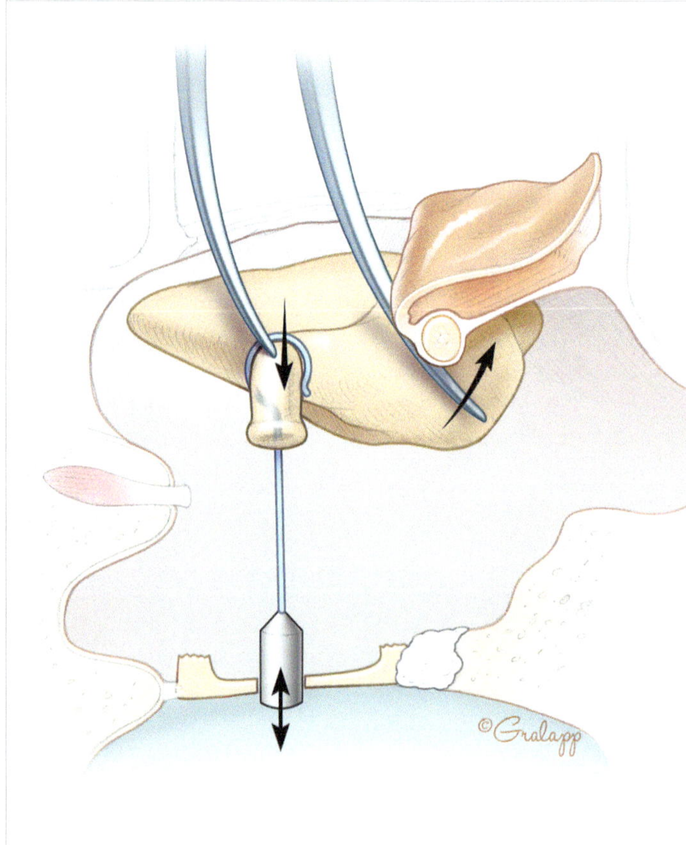

Fig. 4.81 Once the prosthesis is seated and crimped, its mobility is tested by gently moving either the incus or malleus handle. To avoid trauma to the inner ear, this maneuver is done only once or twice. The author does not use the round window reflex, as it is unnecessary and risks traumatizing the inner ear.

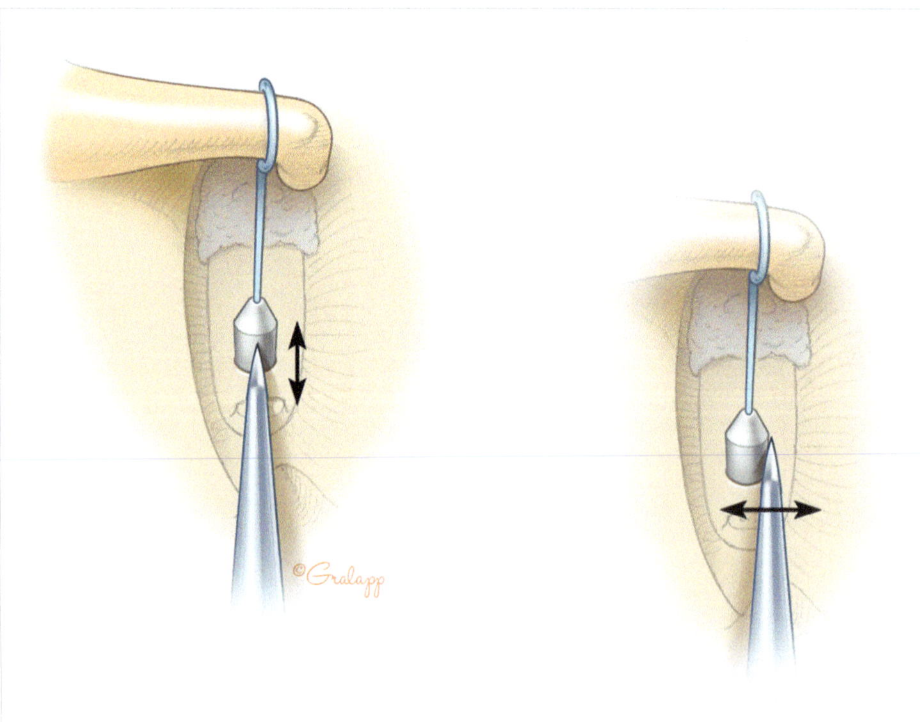

Fig. 4.82 A needle or hook tests the adequacy of the piston's depth of insertion.

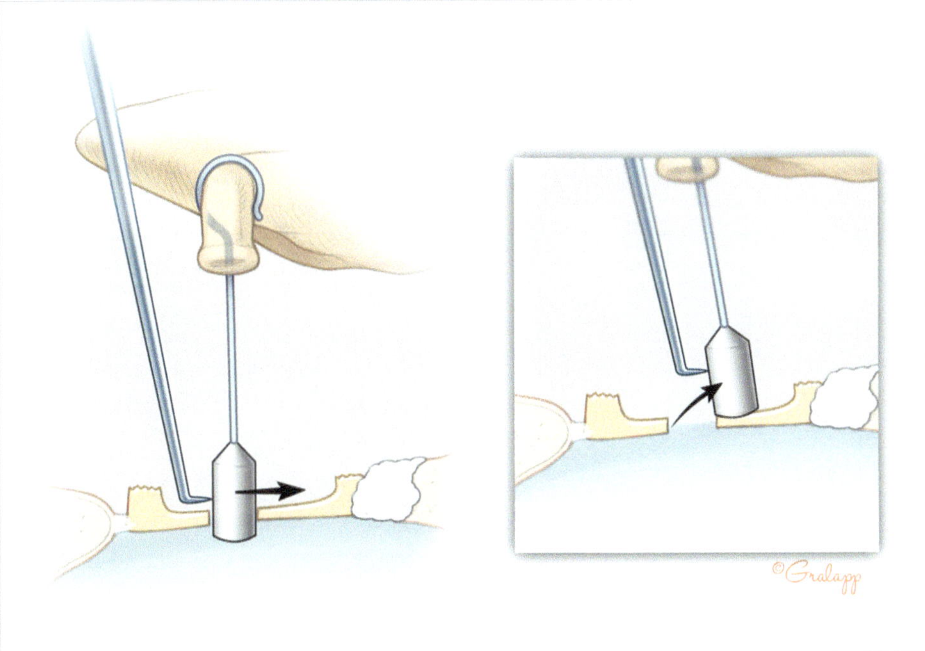

Fig. 4.83 While a well-placed prosthesis will retain under gentle pressure (left), a shallowly placed prosthesis will pop out when subjected to stress (right). If this occurs, the prosthesis is replaced with another 0.25 mm longer.

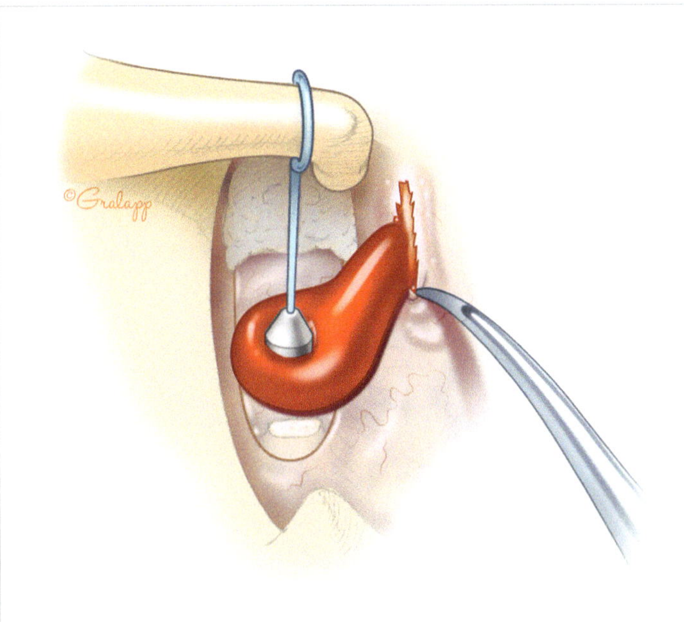

Fig. 4.84 A blood seal can usually be stimulated by scratching the promontory mucosa. If insufficient bleeding occurs with the method, then venous blood from the arm is an alternative source.

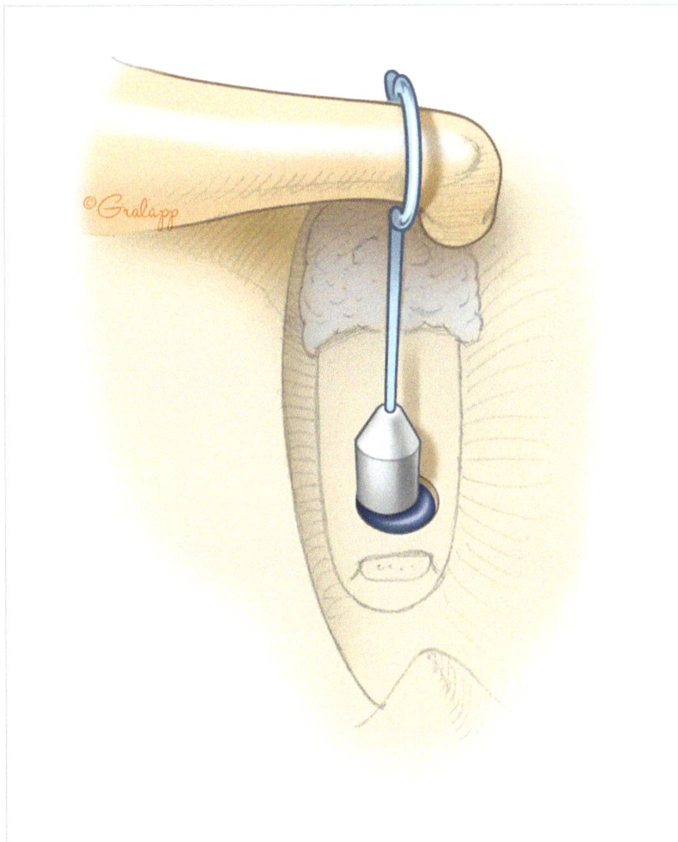

Fig. 4.85 The ideal fenestra size is just slightly larger than the piston (e.g., 0.7 mm for a 0.6-mm piston). When the fenestra appears slightly larger than ideal, the gap should be sealed.

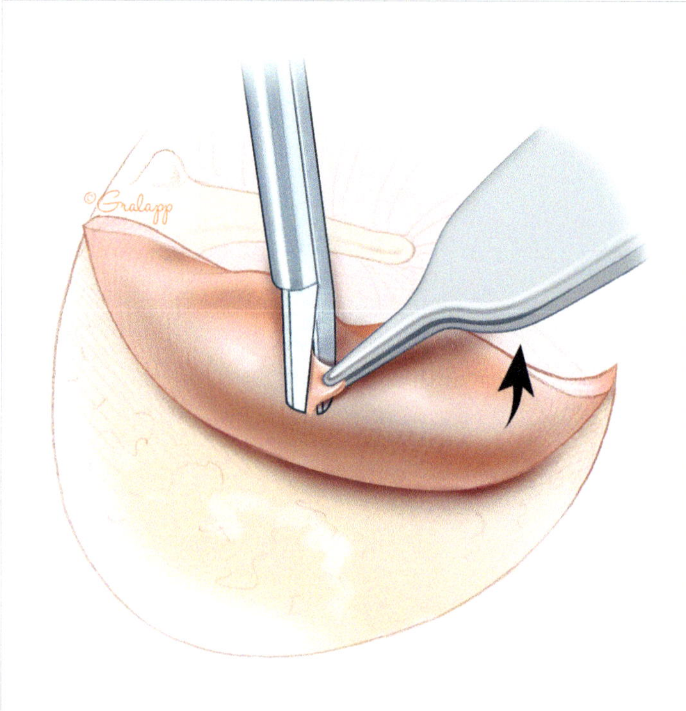

Fig. 4.86 To seal a slightly too large fenestra, a pinch of connective tissue can be harvested from the flap superiorly (vascular strip).

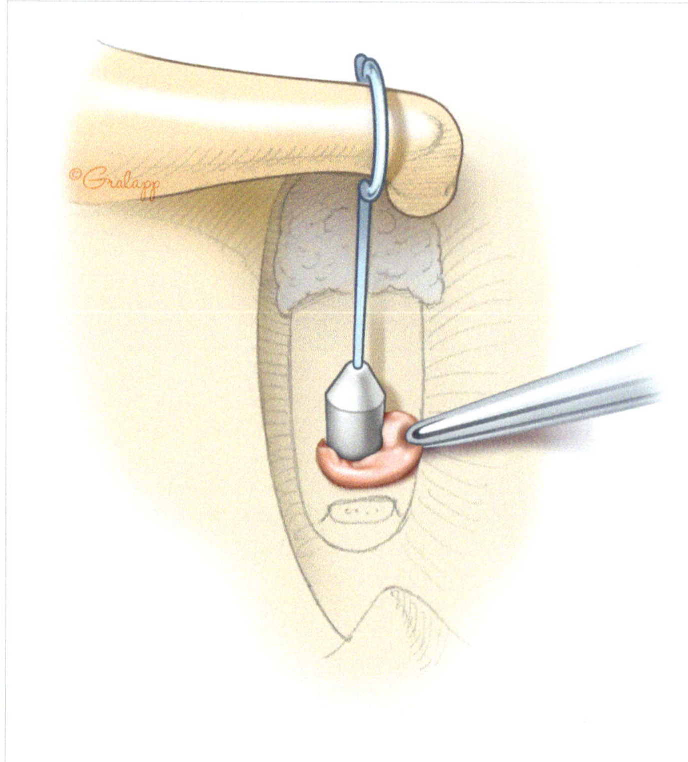

Fig. 4.87 Seating of the connective tissue to seal the oval window. A larger fenestra necessitates a connective tissue sheet beneath the prosthesis.

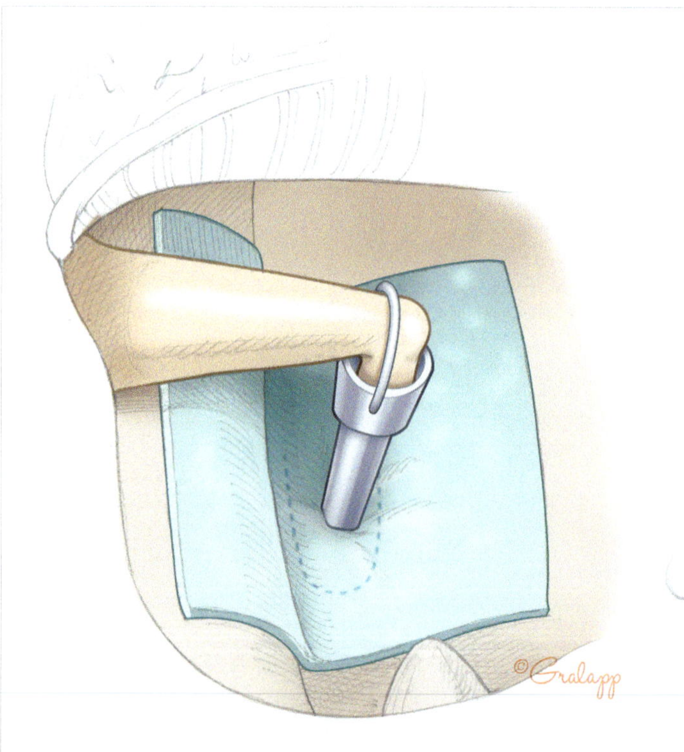

Fig. 4.88 A bucket handle prosthesis requires no crimping, and the loop is simply pulled over the incus. A tissue membrane is shown sealing a large fenestra.

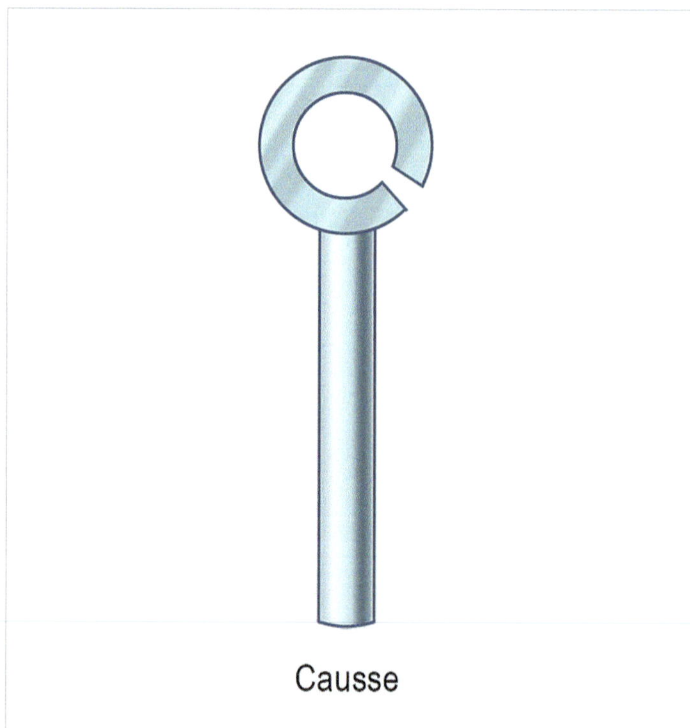

Fig. 4.89 A Teflon prosthesis of the Causse type.

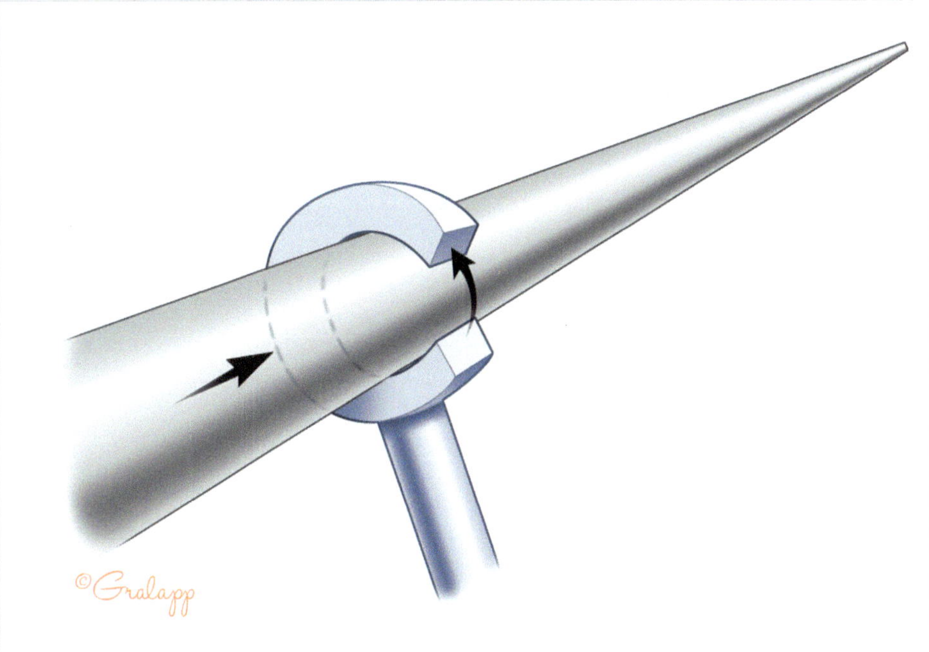

Fig. 4.90 The loop is dilated to accommodate the incus-long process.

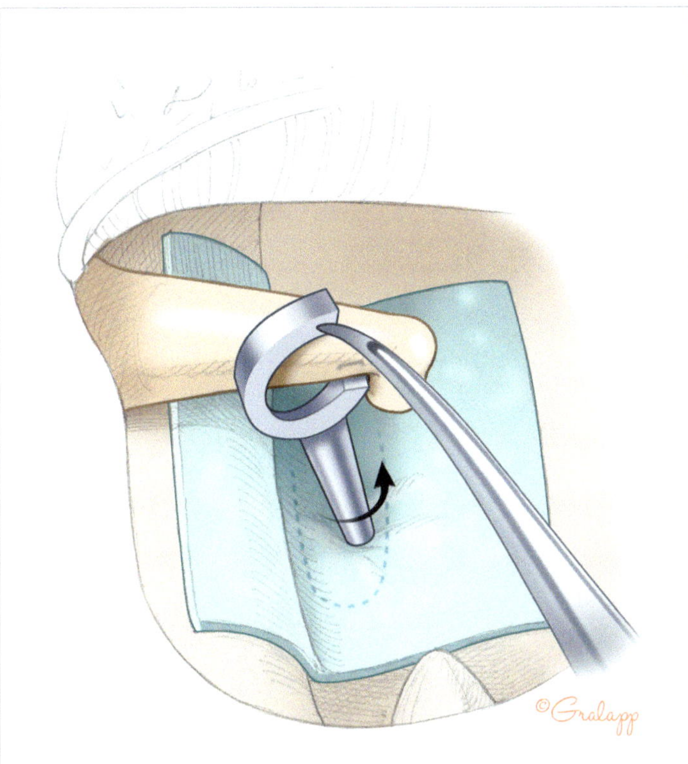

Fig. 4.91 The prosthesis is rotated to engage the incus.

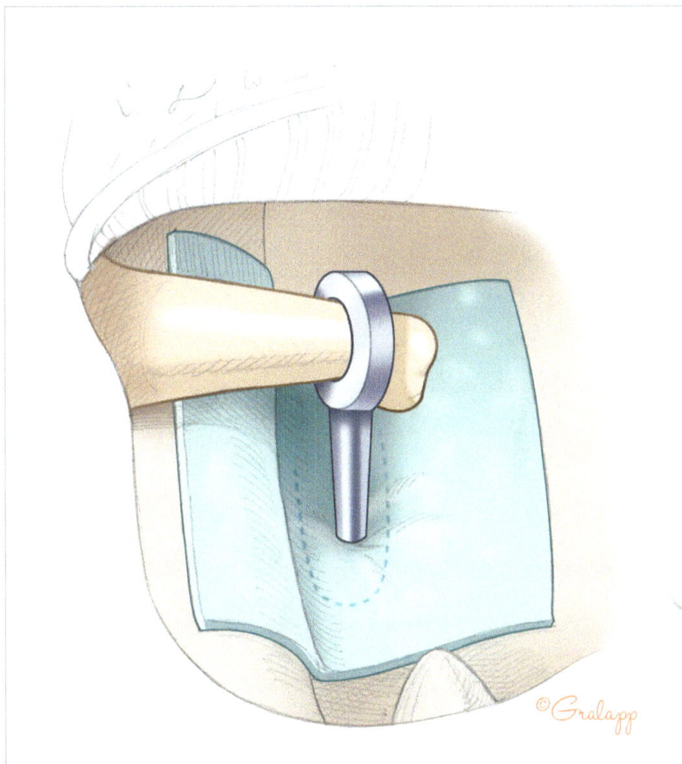

Fig. 4.92 The Teflon loop prosthesis is seated into the fenestra.

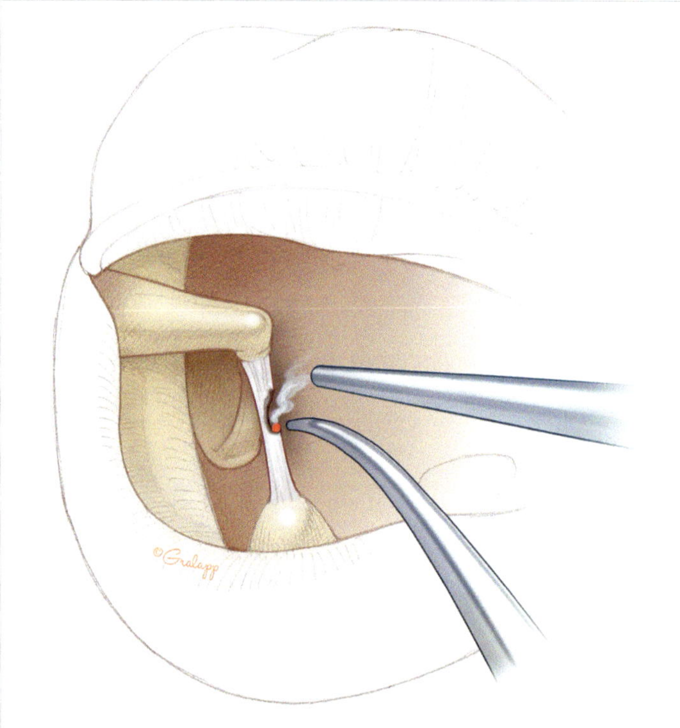

Fig. 4.93 In laser stapes technique, the stapedial tendon is divided with the laser. The illustration depicts a handheld laser fiber delivery system, which is favored in most centers over micromanipulator systems. One advantage of the handheld laser fiber is its divergent beam which dissipates laser energy away from the tip thus reducing the risk of overshoot injury. The fiber can also be brought in from various angles, whereas a micromanipulator beam is restricted to line of sight.

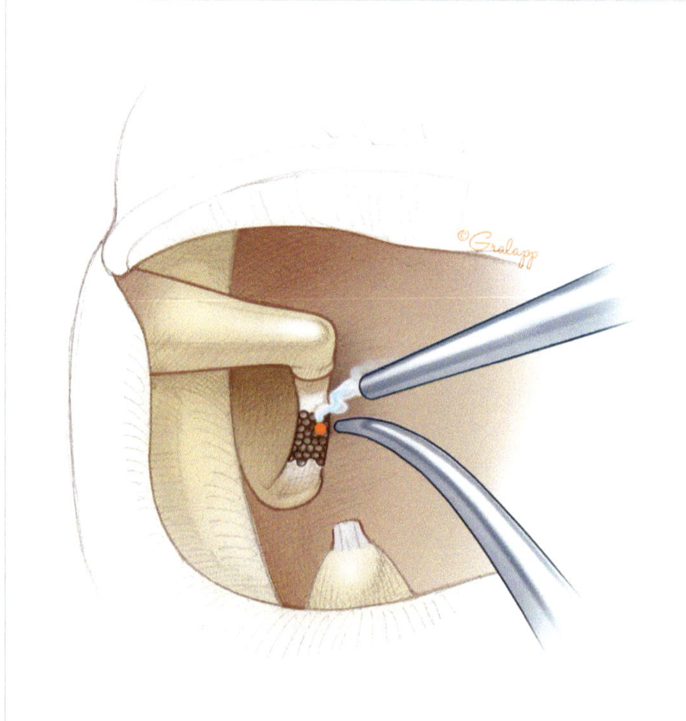

Fig. 4.94 Charring of the posterior crus with multiple, overlapping laser bursts.

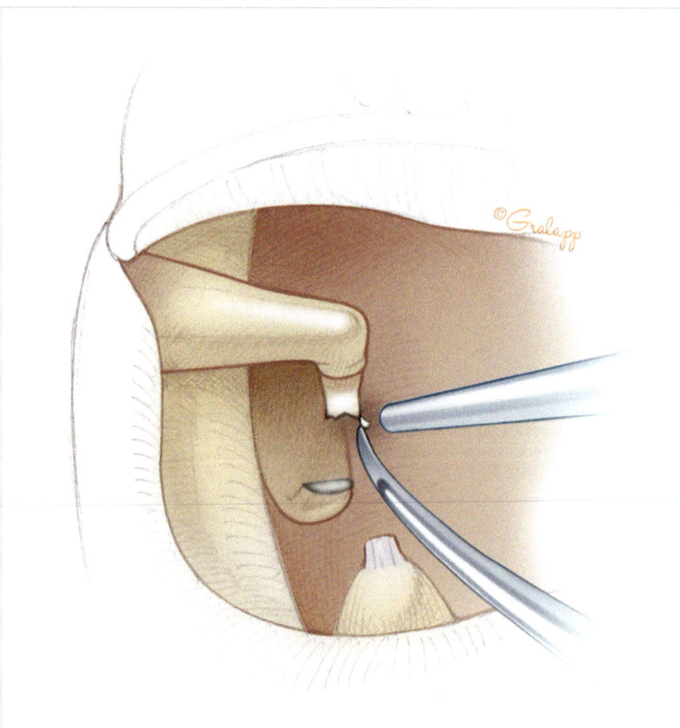

Fig. 4.95 The charred posterior crus is chipped away.

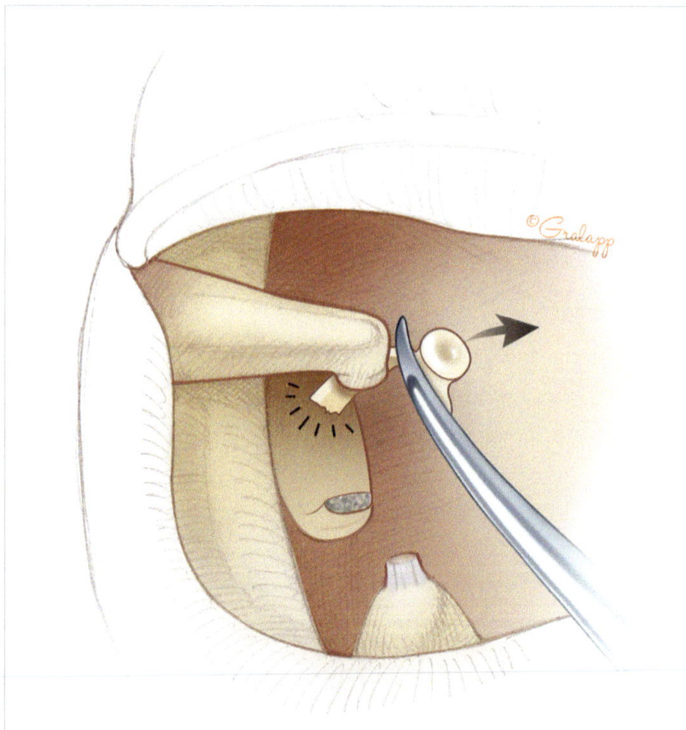

Fig. 4.96 In most cases, it is difficult to target the anterior crus with the laser; so, it is snapped off mechanically.

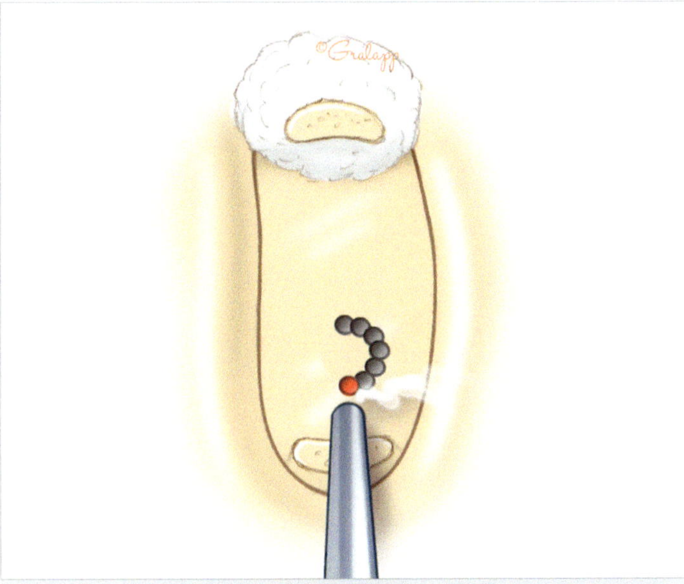

Fig. 4.97 Small fenestra stapedotomy with a laser is usually created with a rosette of overlapping pulses. As the unpigmented footplate may act like a laser mirror, the process may require initiation by allowing a drop of blood to form on the footplate. To catalyze energy absorption, each successive laser shot overlaps the char from the last one slightly.

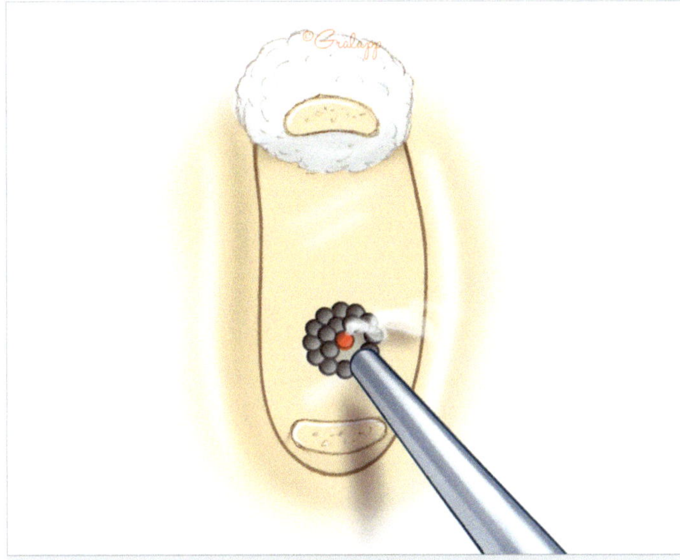

Fig. 4.98 The rosette is completed by charring the entire area to be removed.

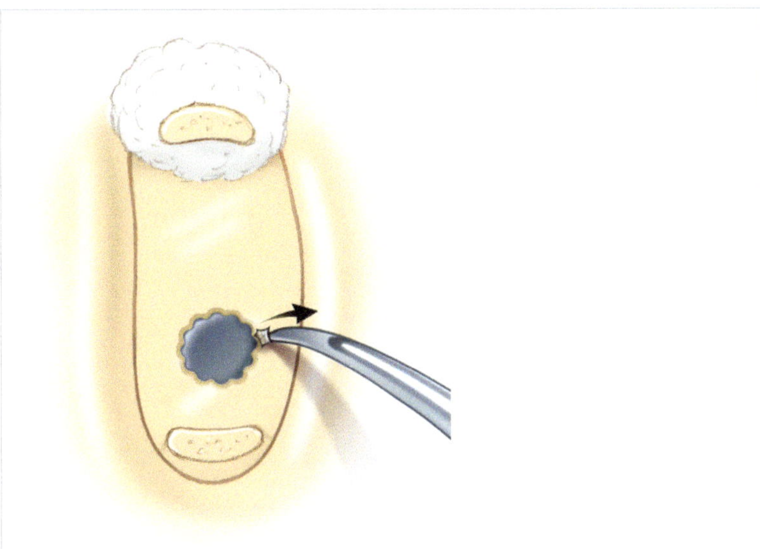

Fig. 4.99 The char overlying the fenestra is then picked away. Other surgeons simply push the piston through the char.

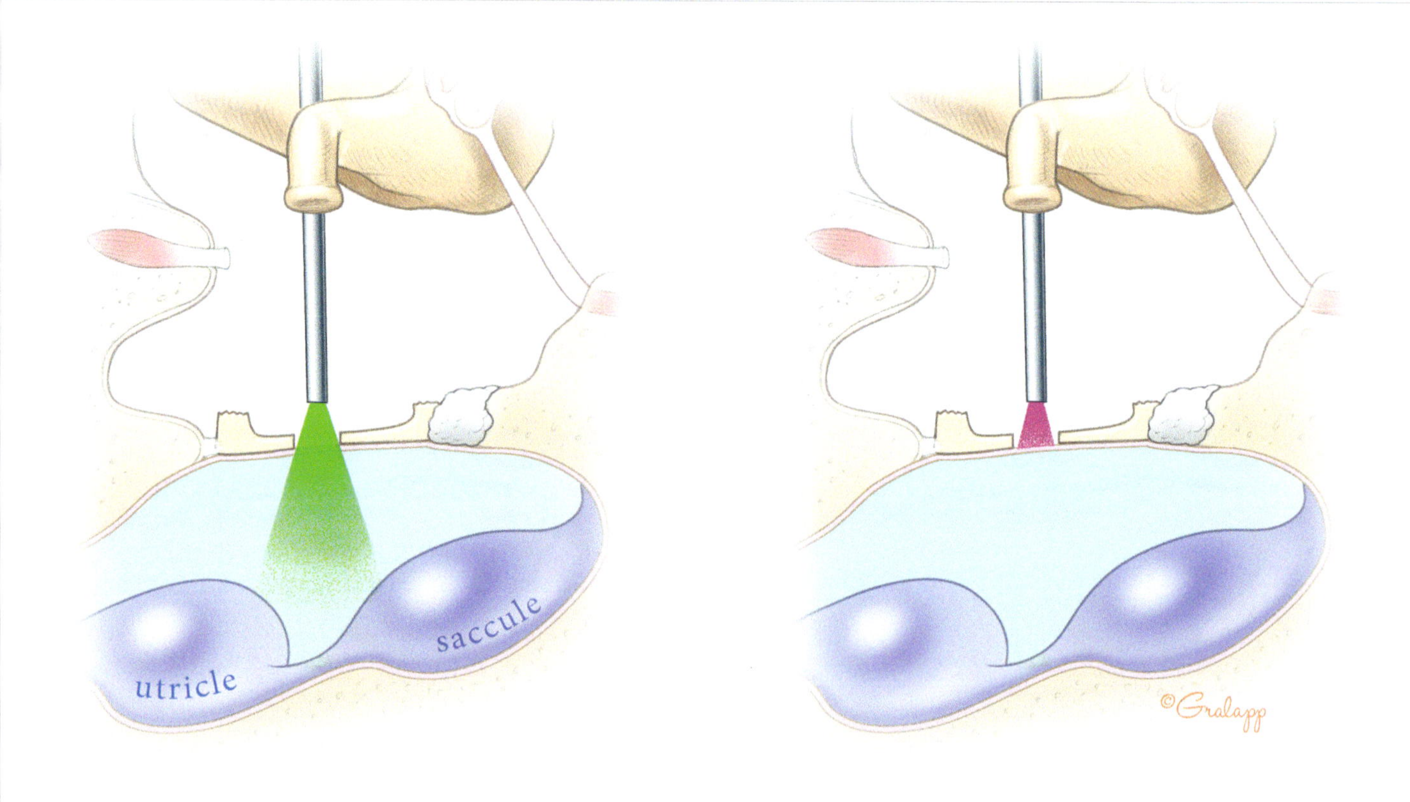

Fig. 4.100 Visual spectrum laser (e.g., argon) shown in green passes through perilymph and may transfer energy to the endolymphatic membrane of the utricle and saccule. The CO_2 laser is not visible to the human eye, but is shown in *magenta* here for clarity. CO_2 laser energy is absorbed by the perilymph thus heating this fluid.

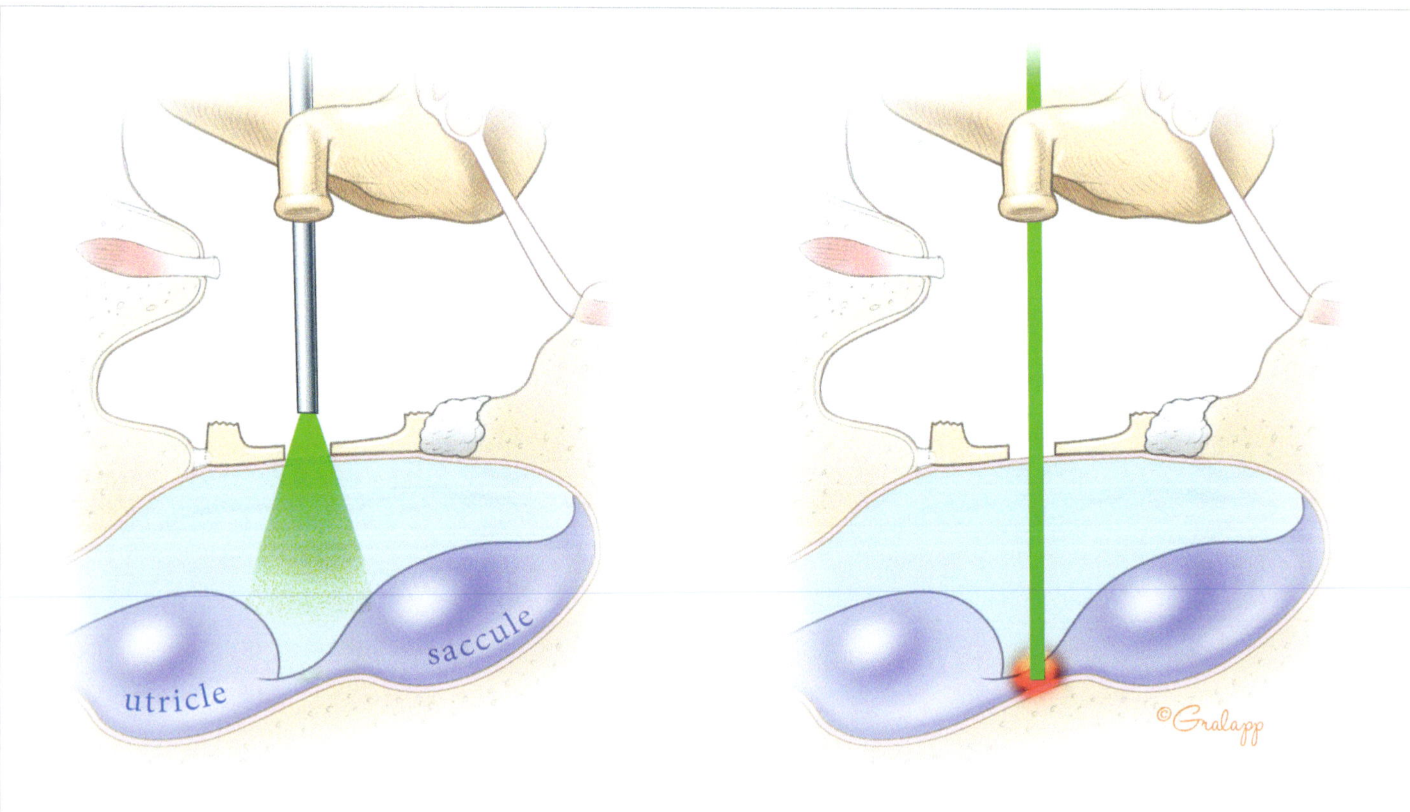

Fig. 4.101 Energy emitted from a handheld laser (*left*) is divergent and disperses so that overshoot injury is less likely. A beam from a microscope-mounted micromanipulator remains collimated and this has greater risk of overshoot injury.

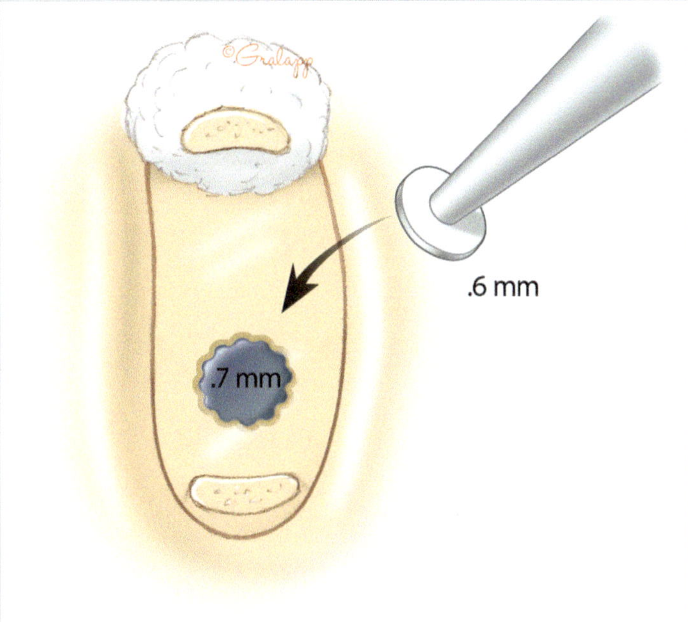

Fig. 4.102 A fenestrometer (e.g., 0.6 mm) can be used to evaluate the adequacy of the fenestra. The ideal fenestra is 0.1 mm in diameter wider than the piston.

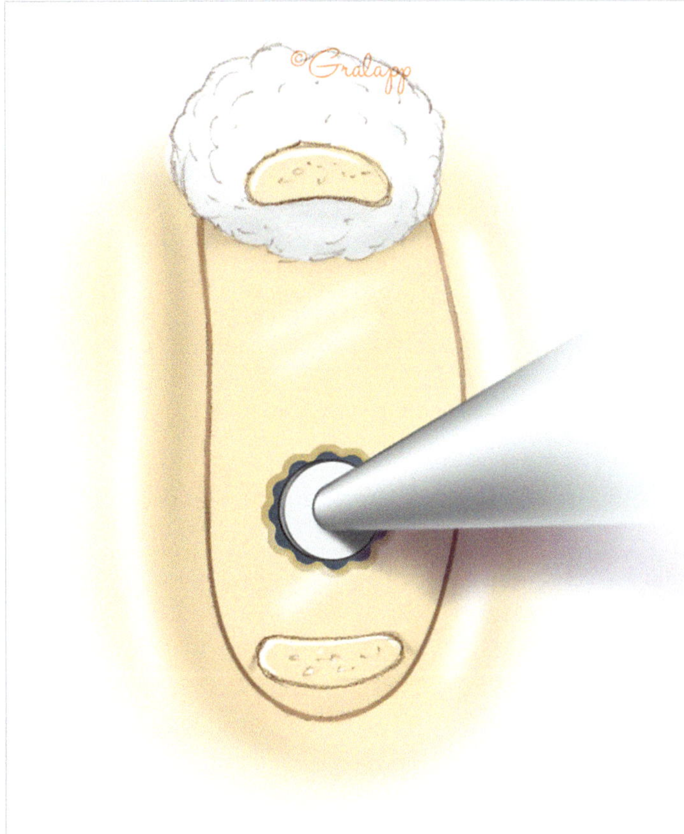

Fig. 4.103 The fenestrometer is for visual reference only; it is best kept superficial to the fenestra.

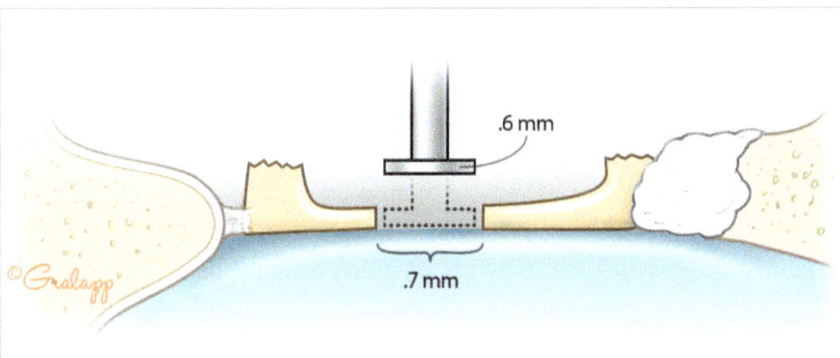

Fig. 4.104 Placing the fenestrometer within the fenestra risks damage to the footplate.

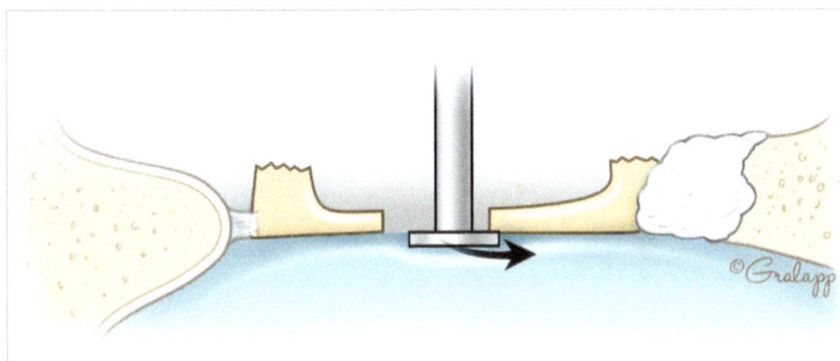

Fig. 4.105 Once beneath the plane of the fenestra, it is difficult to remove without chipping away additional bone from the fenestra margins.

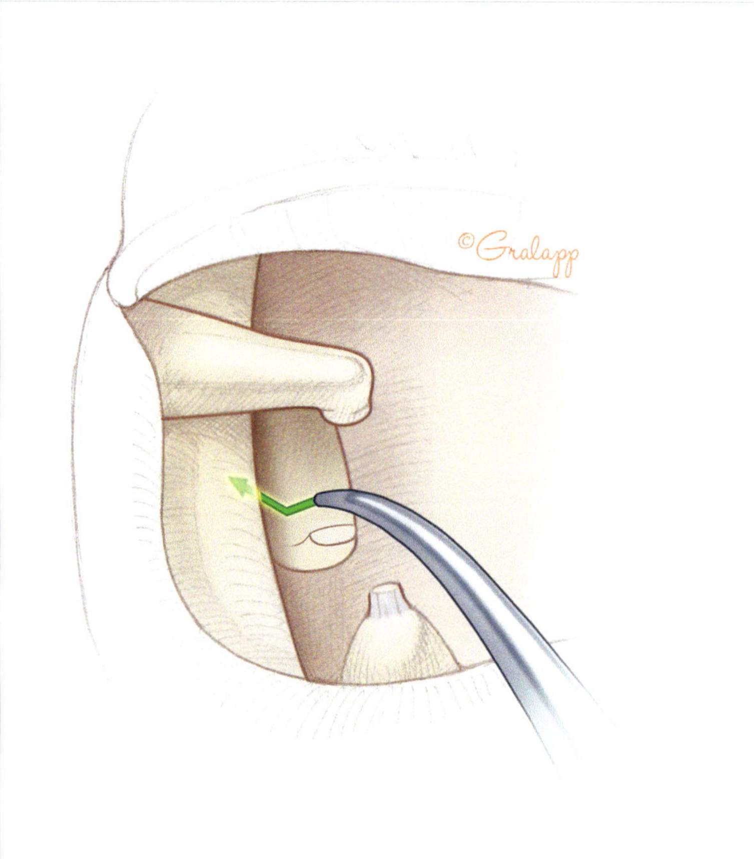

Fig. 4.106 The footplate can act like a mirror reflecting laser energy which becomes deposited elsewhere in the middle ear.

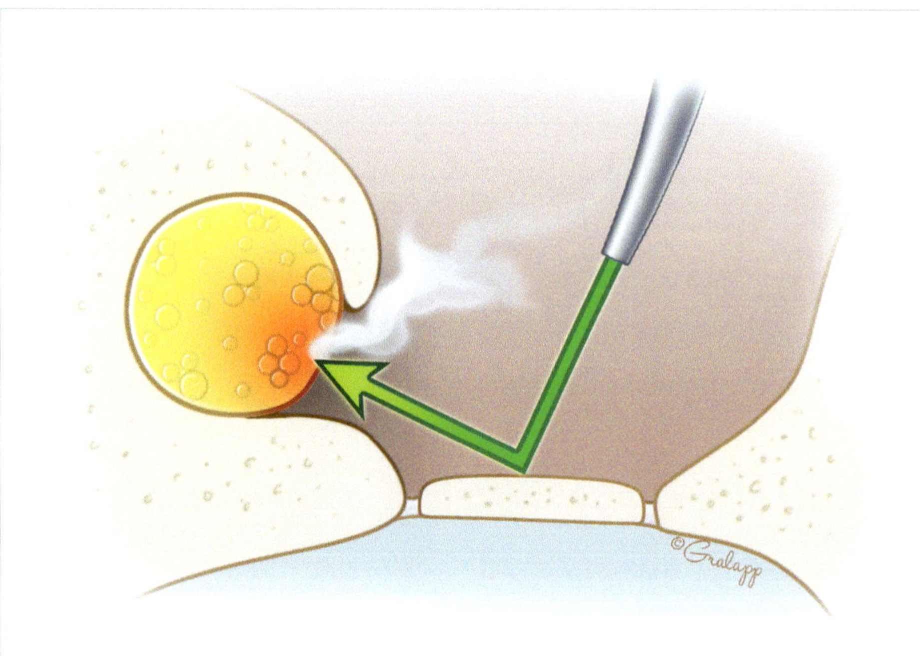

Fig. 4.107 Facial nerve injury has occurred when the surgeon inadvertently heated the adjacent facial nerve which is often dehiscent on its undersurface facing the footplate.

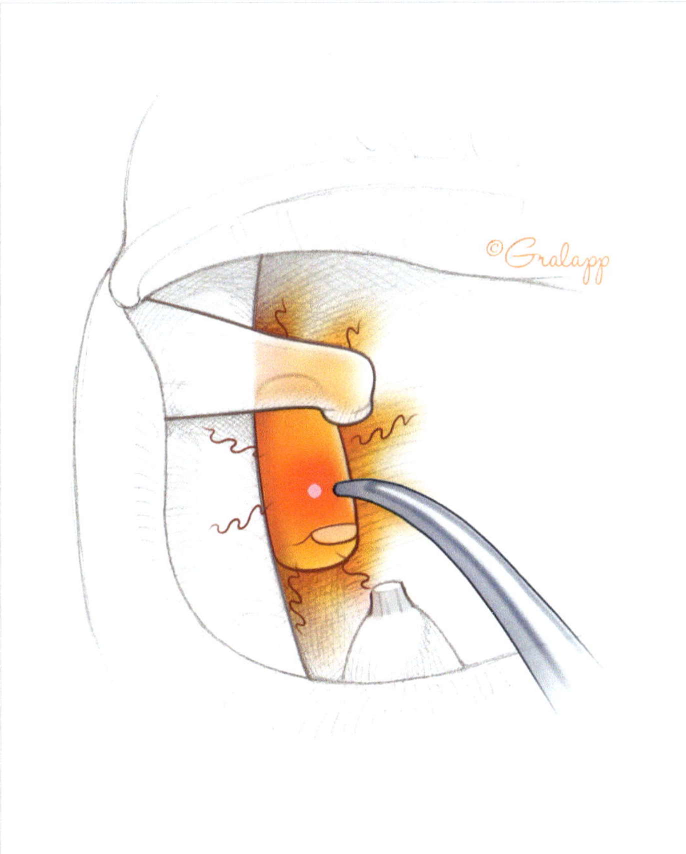

Fig. 4.108 Both repeated laser impulses which fail to char the footplate (i.e., a large fraction of the energy is reflected) and excessive laser power may contribute to the risk of facial nerve or inner ear thermal injury.

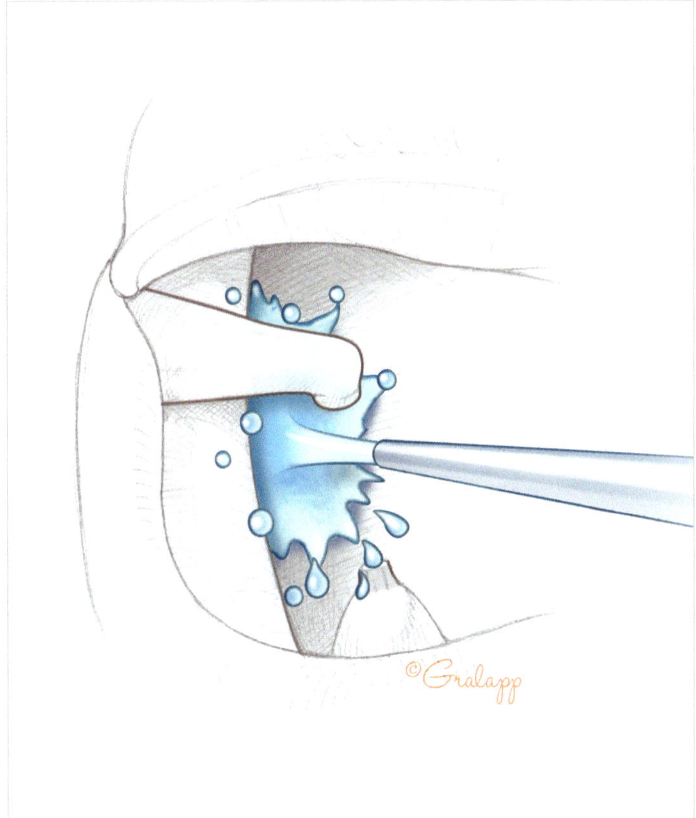

Fig. 4.109 When delivering laser pulses to the footplate, it is wise to periodically flush with cool saline as a means of mitigating unwanted heat buildup.

4.5 Stapedectomy

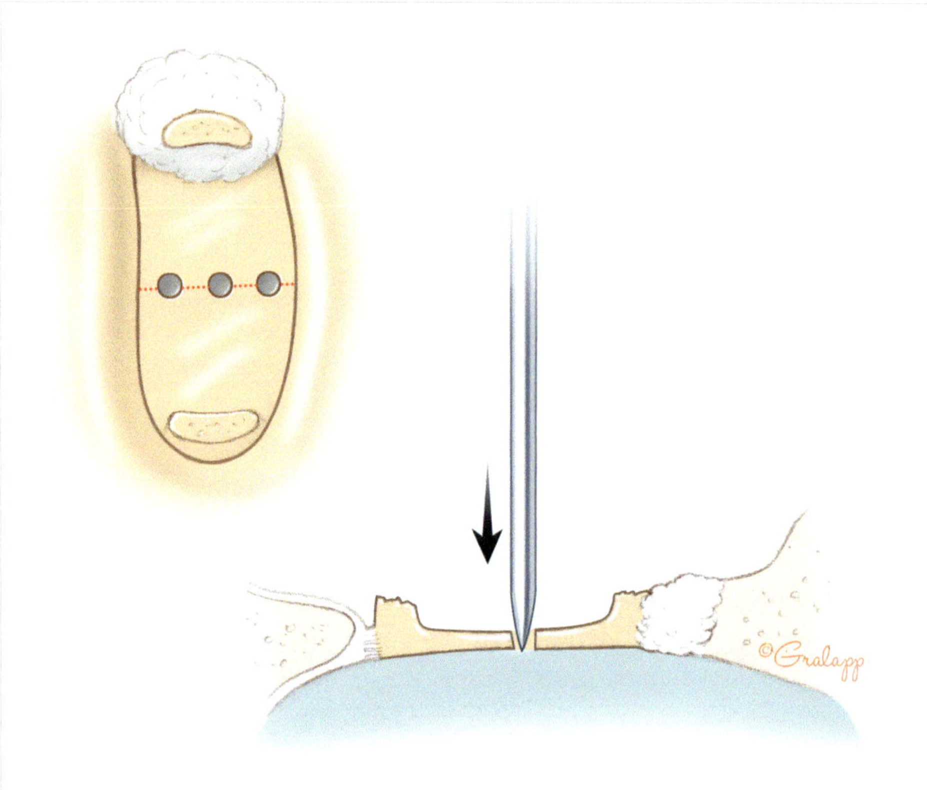

Fig. 4.110 In traditional large fenestra technique, one-half or more of the footplate is removed. A sharp straight needle is used to create a series of footplate perforations across the meridian of the footplate. Some surgeons keep a sharpening stone on their set to remove any barbs from the needle before this maneuver. A dull needle might crack the footplate.

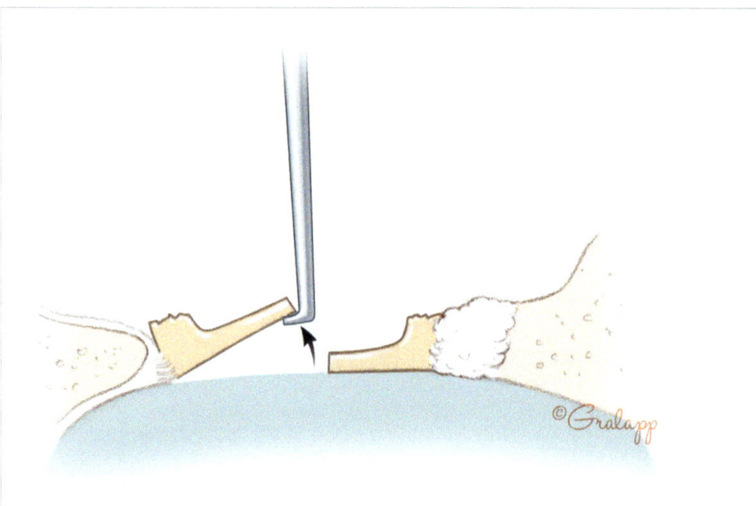

Fig. 4.111 A hook is used to extract the posterior half of the footplate.

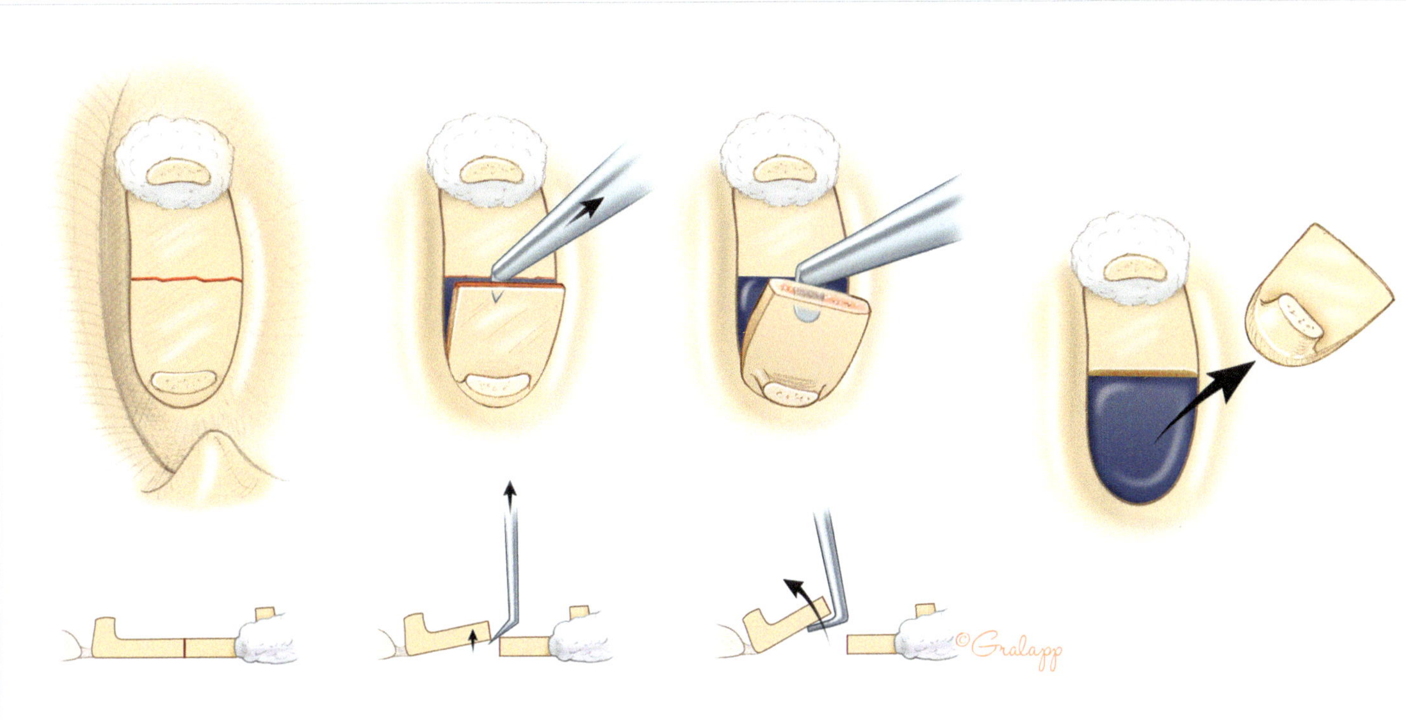

Fig. 4.112 When the footplate crack is thin and nondisplaced, an obtuse (45-degree) hook is needed as a crack opener. This is the most useful tool to have on a stapes set. Once the posterior half has been elevated, a broad 90-degree hook (e.g., Hough hoe) can be used. When access is adequate, it is better to use a broad surfaced hook rather than a pointed one, as the latter can chip fragments of bone rather than lift the segment whole.

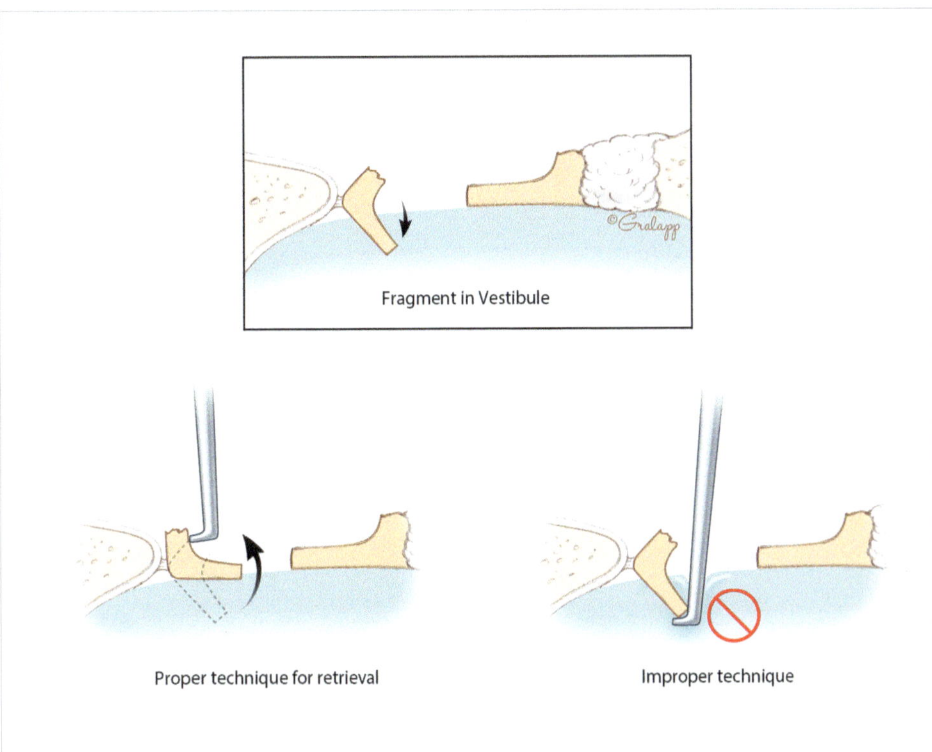

Fig. 4.113 When a footplate fragment begins to fall into the oval window, it is a central axiom of stapes surgery not to reach into the vestibule. Often the fragment can be retrieved by engaging the crural base remnant with a hook.

4.6 Challenges in Stapes Surgery

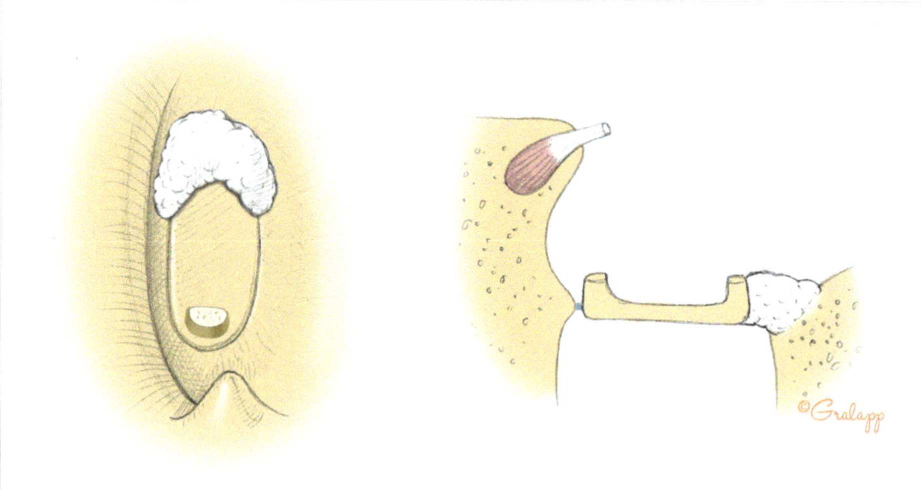

Fig. 4.114 Anterior fixation of the footplate is most commonly encountered.

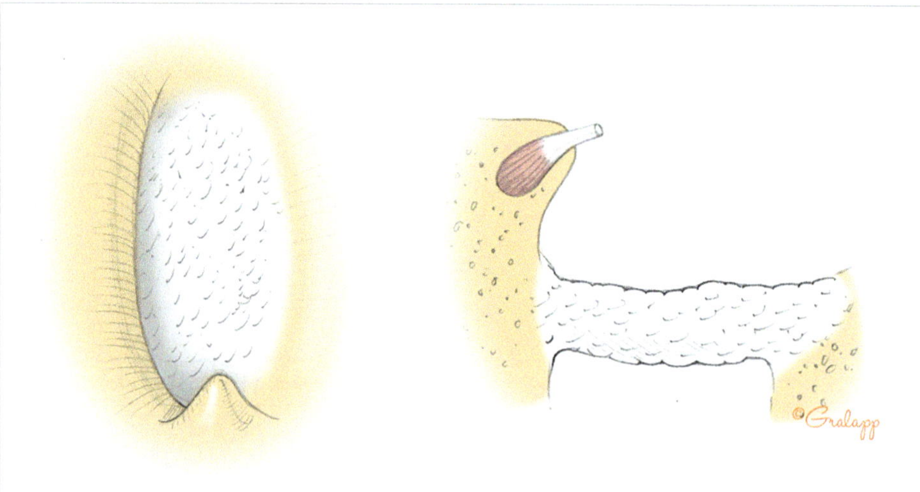

Fig. 4.115 An obliterative footplate is thick and tightly fixed. The footplate appears chalky white and blood tends to accumulate in its center.

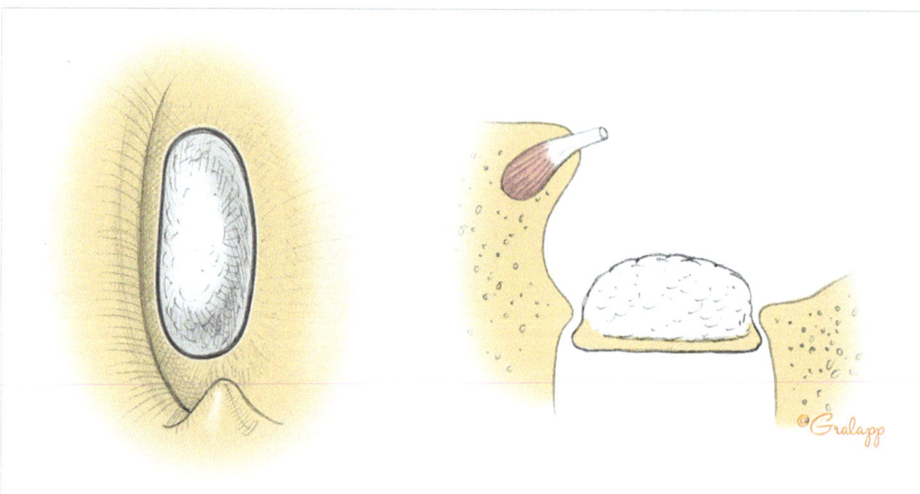

Fig. 4.116 A biscuit footplate is thick and white, but is lightly fixed. Blood pools peripherally around the annular ligament. A flange may be present on the vestibule side which makes its extraction difficult.

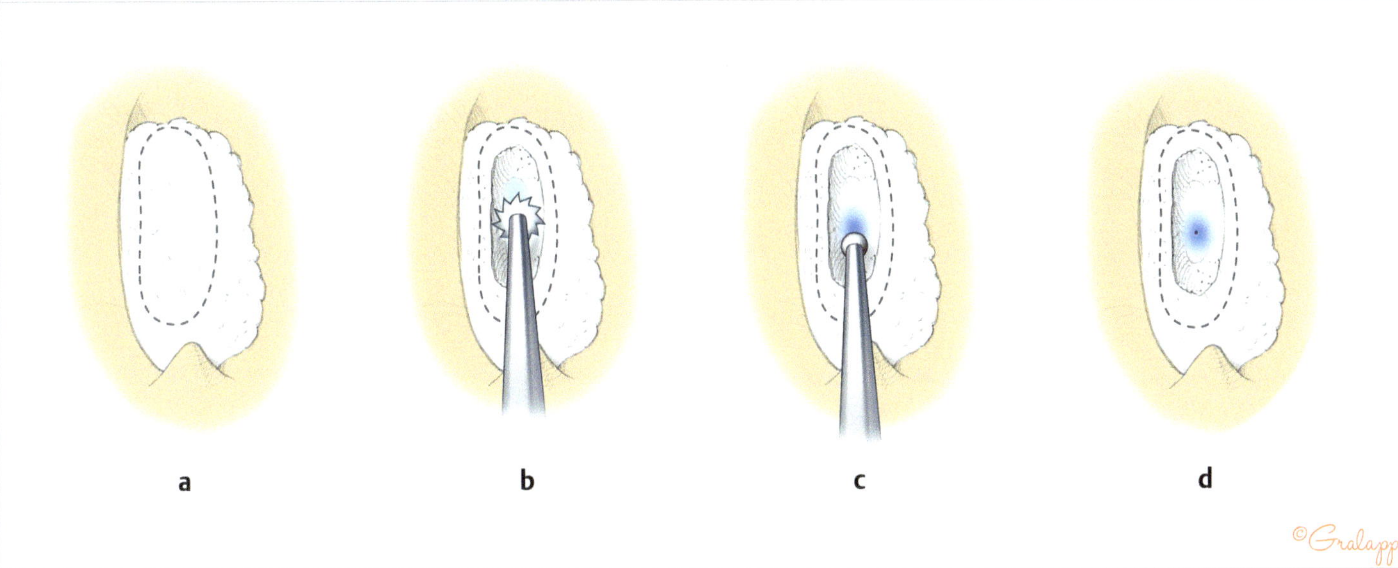

Fig. 4.117 Managing obliterative otosclerosis is quite straightforward. Using a cutting burr (e.g., 0.8 mm), the footplate is thinned until a blue region has been created. A routine small fenestra opening may then be formed with a diamond burr through the thin area.

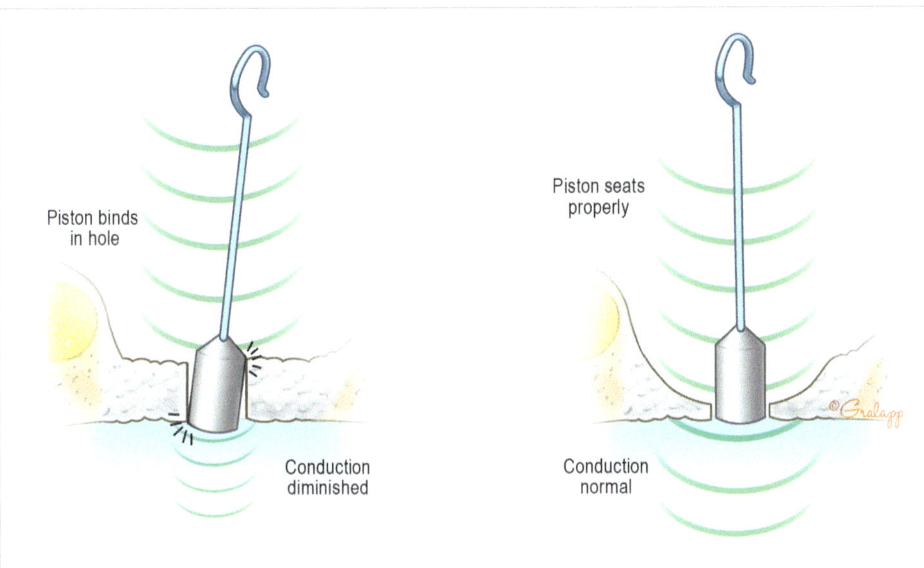

Fig. 4.118 In reducing the thickness of the footplate in obliterative otosclerosis, it is important to create an adequate thin area. If the opening is too narrow (*left*), then the prosthesis will rub if it is even slightly off line with the opening.

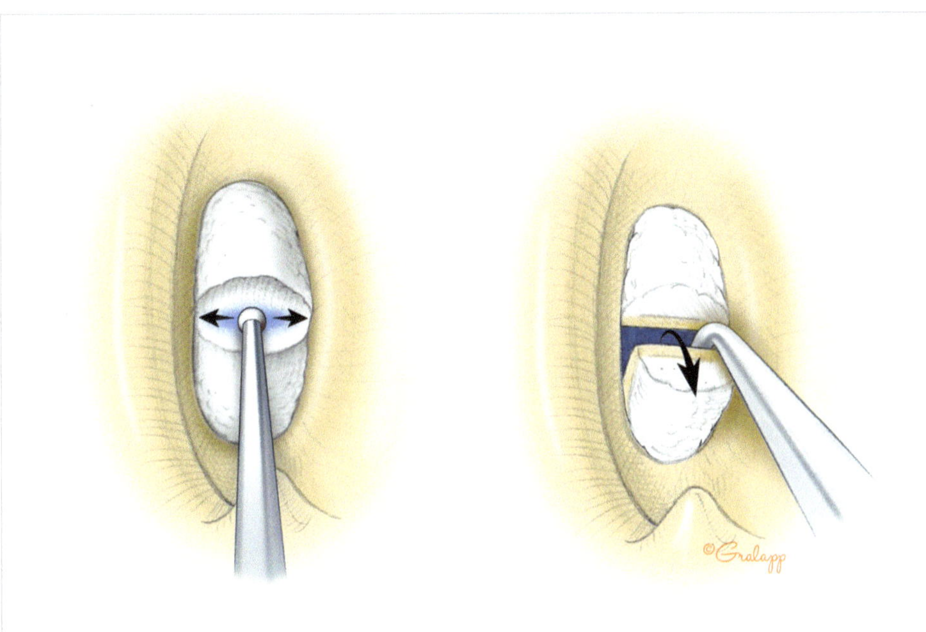

Fig. 4.119 Dealing with a biscuit footplate is one of the great challenges in stapes surgery. The problem is that when drilling starts, it tends to become mobile. Drilling on a mobile footplate is forbidden due to risk of sensory loss. Once mobilized, manipulation tends to depress the biscuit footplate into the vestibule. Under favorable circumstances, the thick footplate can be bisected and the posterior half delivered.

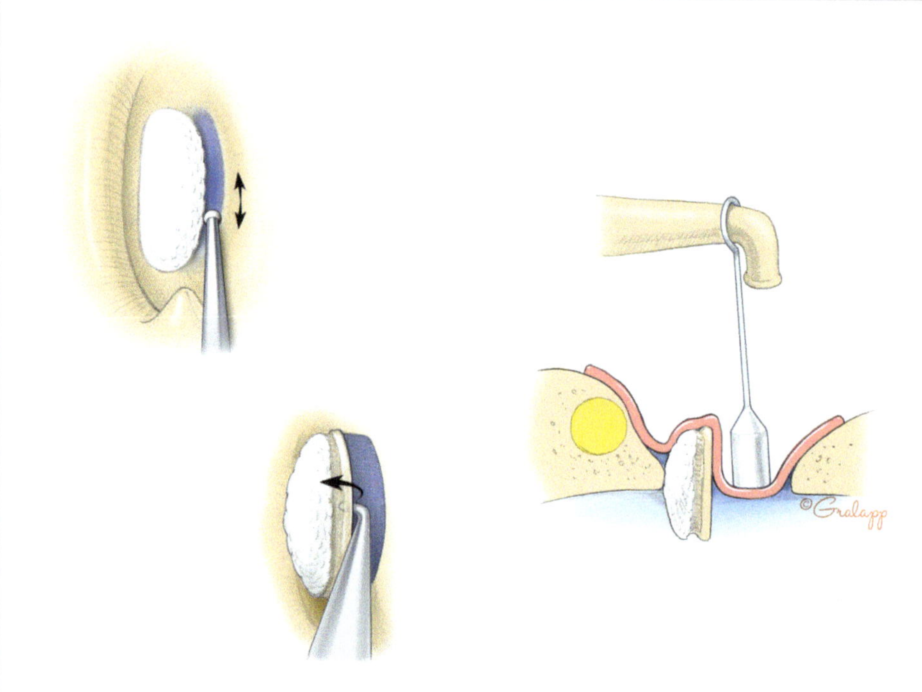

Fig. 4.120 One technique for dealing with a biscuit footplate is the so-called log roll maneuver. A thin trough is drilled on the promontory side (to overcome restriction from the inner flange) and the footplate is rolled up on its side.

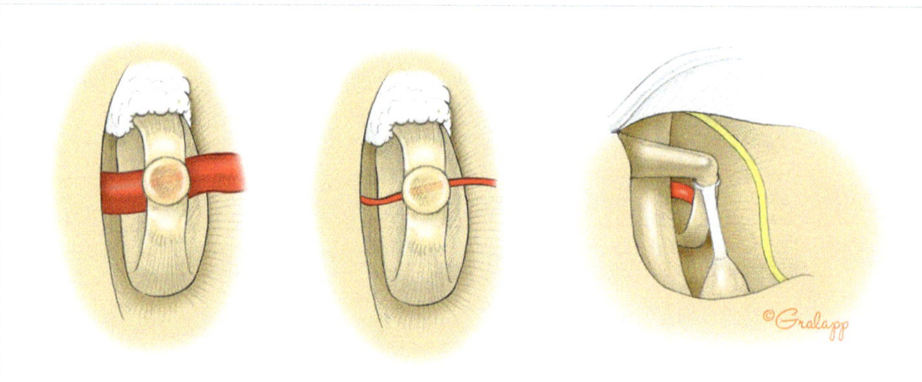

Fig. 4.121 If the surgeon encounters a large persistent stapedial artery, then it is best to stop the procedure and recommend amplification. A vestigial stapedial artery remnant is quite common and should not deter completion of the procedure.

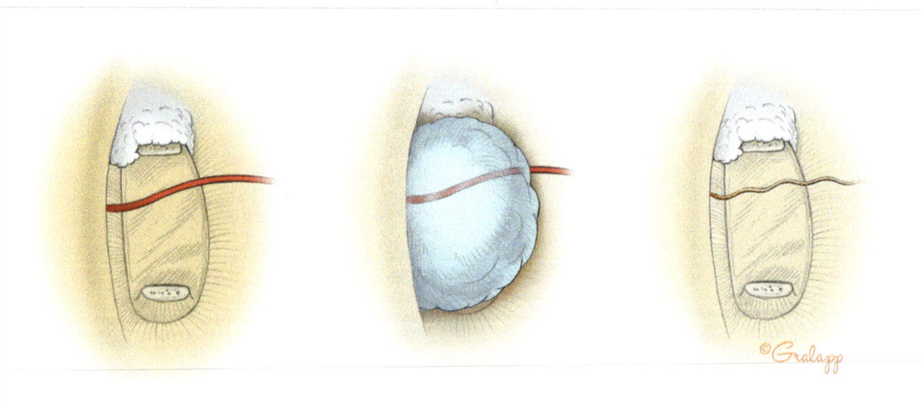

Fig. 4.122 Placing an epinephrine (1:1,000) soaked absorbable gelatin sponge pledget can help shrink the stapes artery remnant. The fenestra can usually be placed posterior to the vestigial artery without disturbing it.

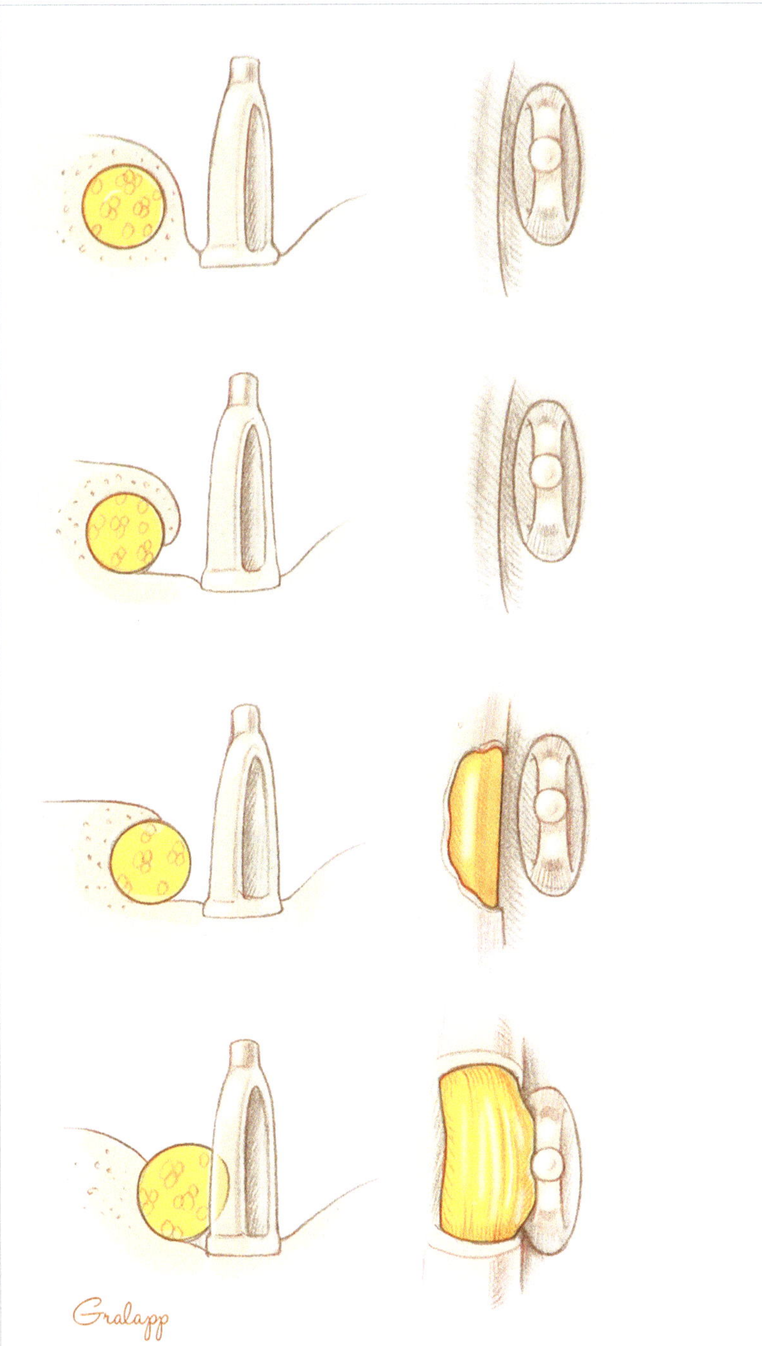

Fig. 4.123 The facial nerve is situated immediately superior to the oval window. It is often dehiscent on its lower medial, out of the surgeon's line of sight. Occasionally, it lies fully dehiscent (i.e., lacking any bony covering). Rarely, the facial nerve may prolapse from its canal and even impinge on the stapes arch. In such cases, the surgeon must determine whether the conductive hearing loss is due to stapes fixation or merely from the facial nerve leaning on the crura.

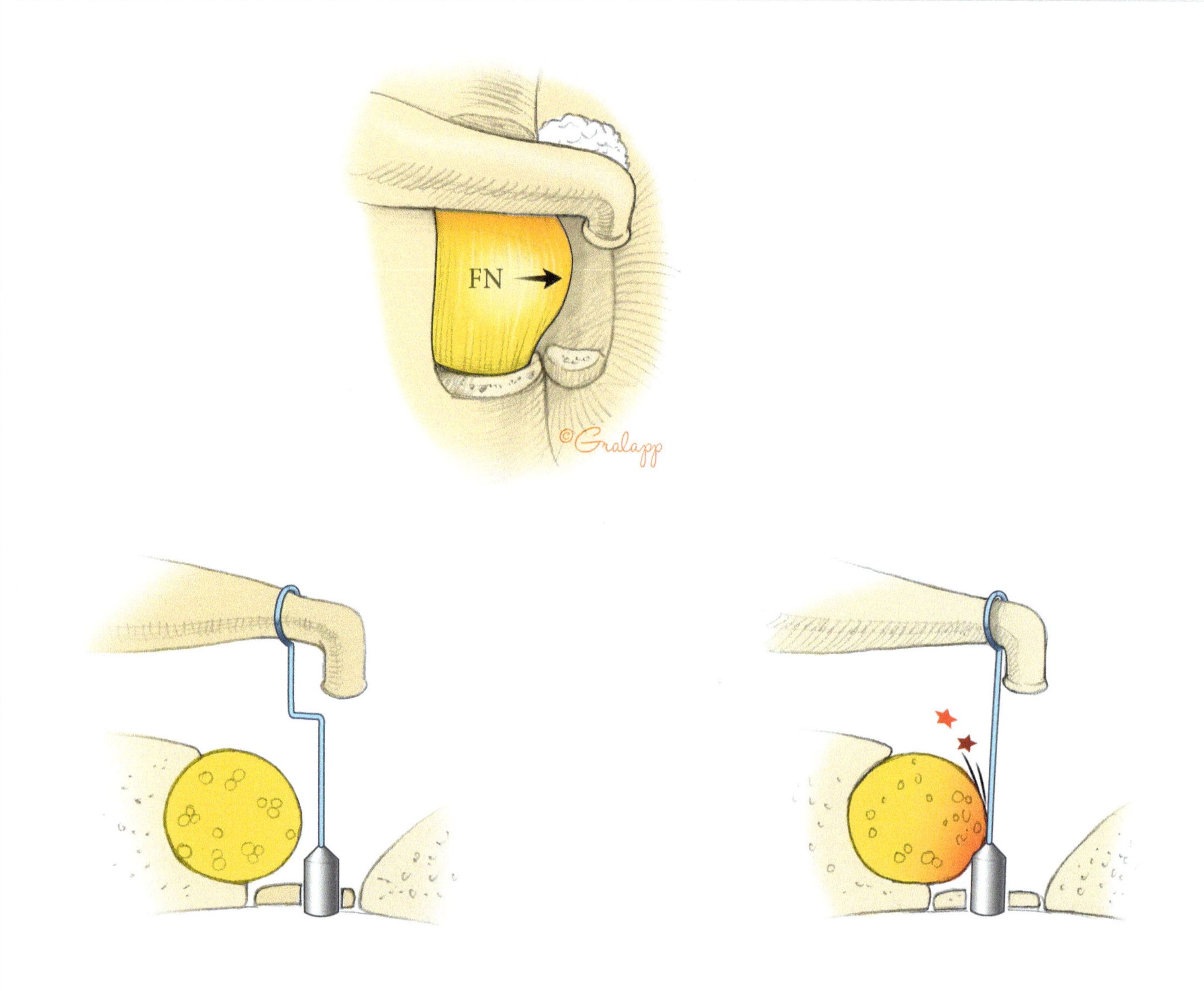

Fig. 4.124 While a severely protruding facial nerve renders stapes surgery impossible, minor degrees of prolapse can be accommodated by routing the wire around the nerve using the double bend technique.

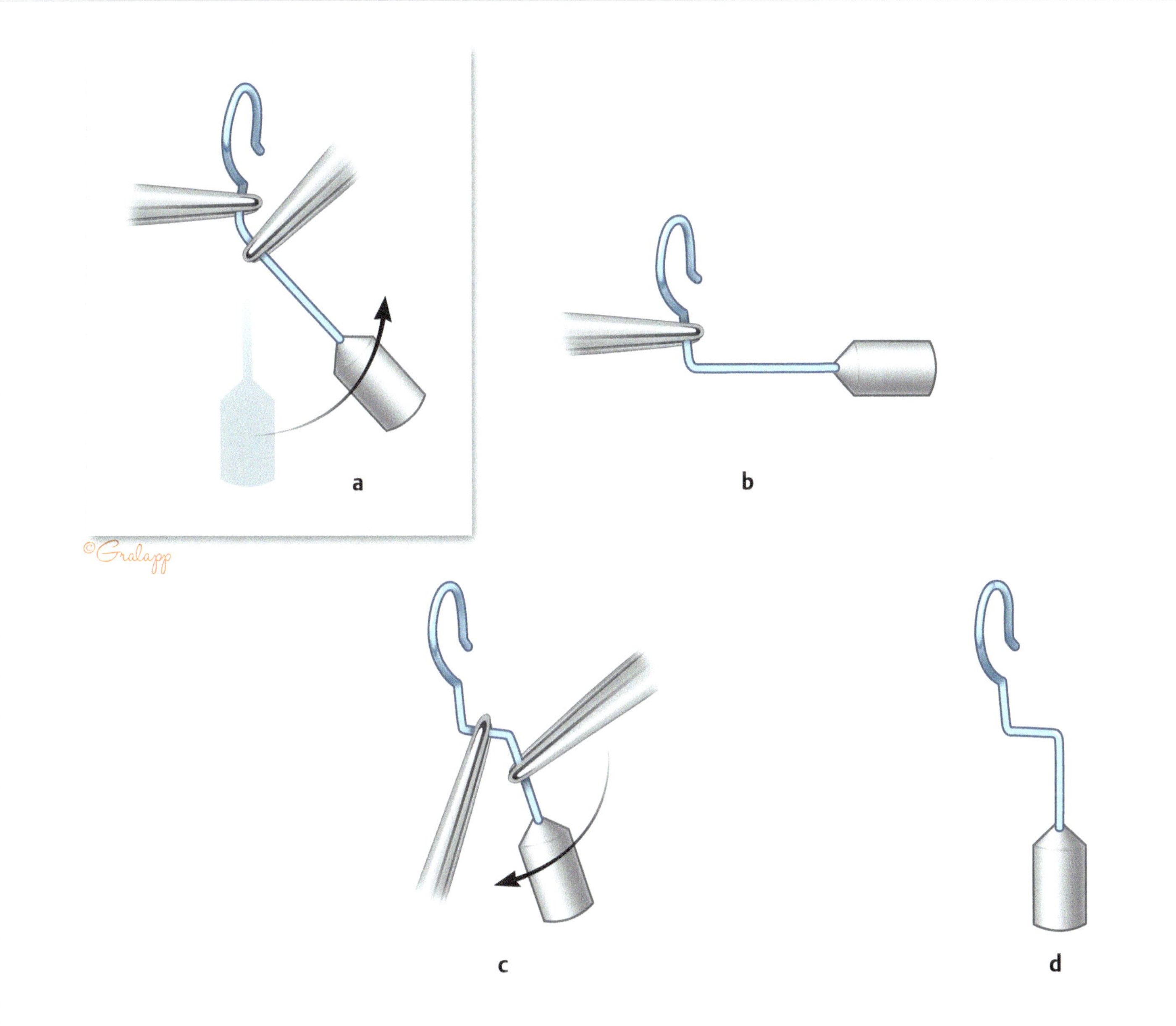

Fig. 4.125 To route the wire around a dehiscent facial nerve, the double-bend technique may be used. This requires adding 1 mm to the length of the wire. Using two smooth alligators, two bends are created as depicted.

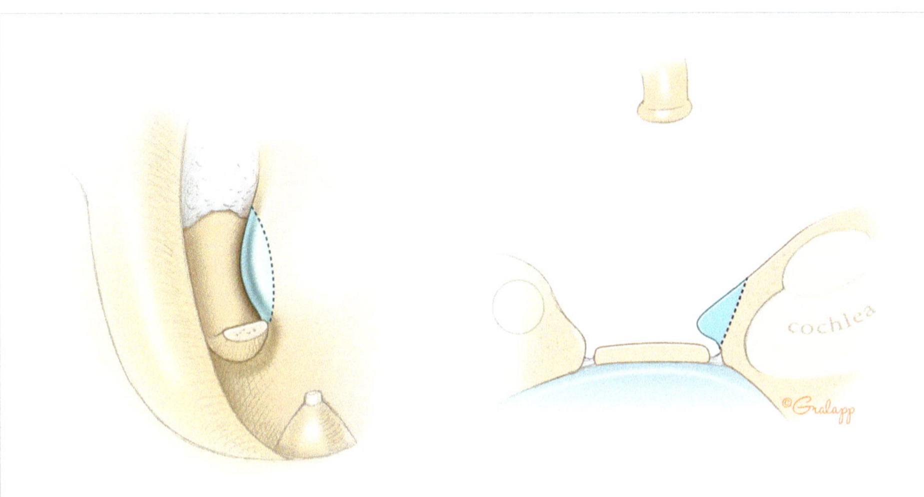

Fig. 4.126 An oval window may be narrowed by a promontory scroll which limits access for footplate fenestration.

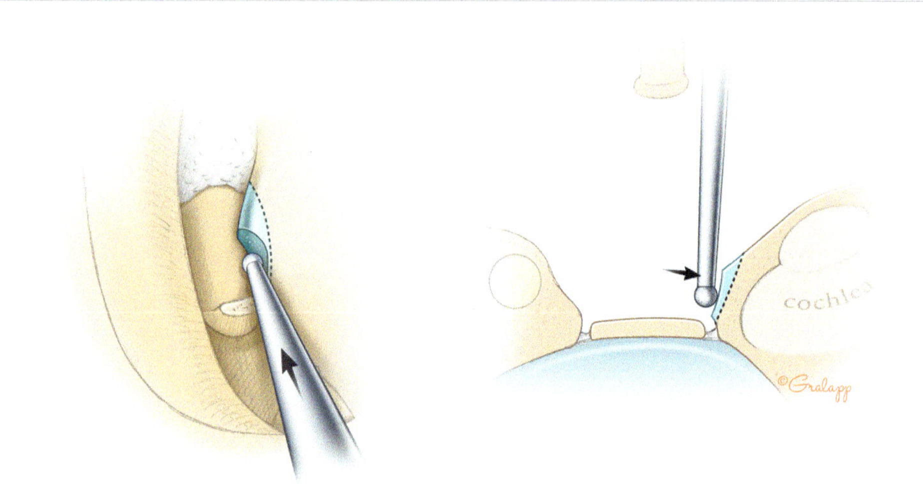

Fig. 4.127 Using a diamond burr, the promontory scroll can be removed slightly inferior to the level of the annular ligament with no fear of entering the cochlea.

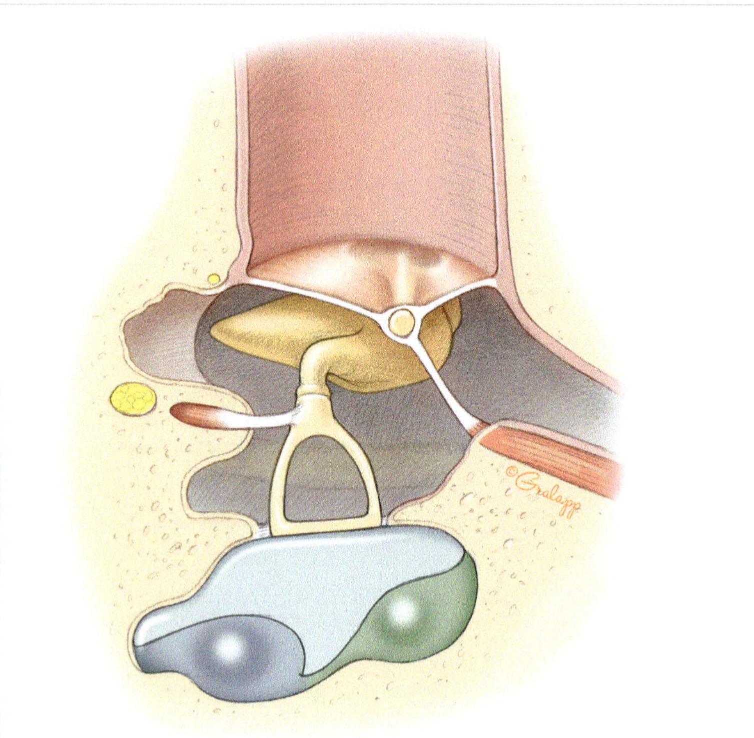

Fig. 4.128 The normal relationship of the utricle (*blue*) and saccule (*green*) to the footplate. The distance from footplate to the utricle is approximately 2 mm, while the space to the saccule is about 1.25 mm.

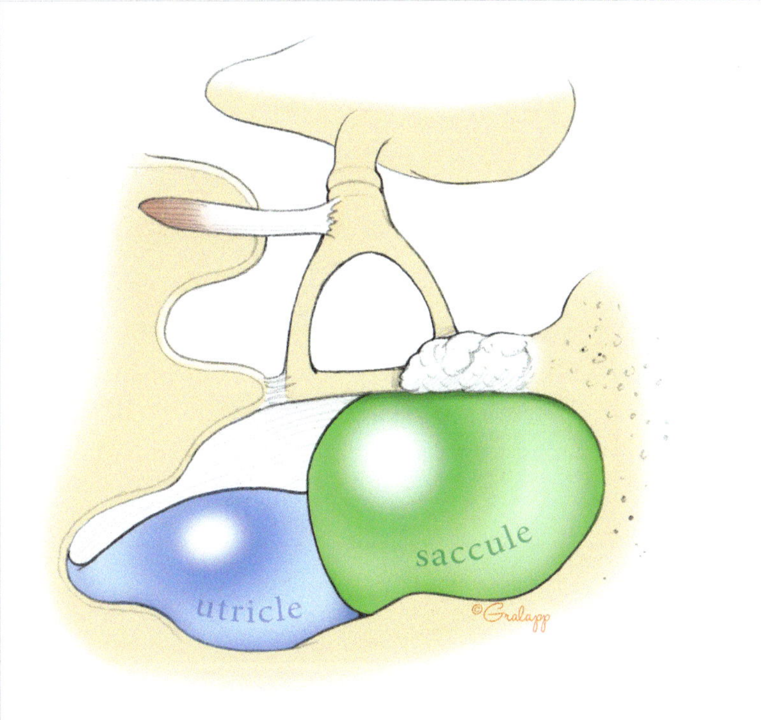

Fig. 4.129 In endolymphatic hydrops (e.g., Meniere's disease), the saccule may swell against the undersurface of the footplate. For this reason, hydropic symptoms contraindicate stapes surgery. Hydrops and otosclerosis may coexist, as depicted here, perhaps due to otosclerotic involvement of the vestibular aqueduct.

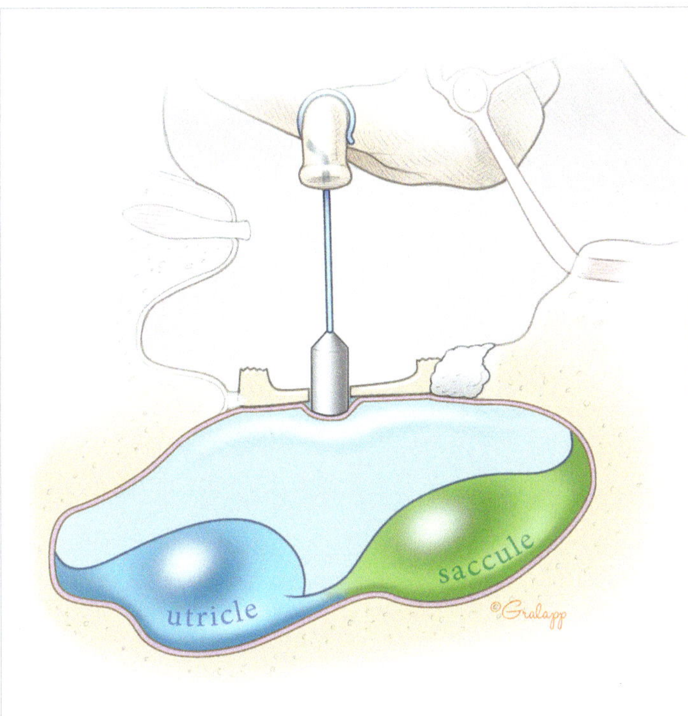

Fig. 4.130 The normal position of a stapes piston in the vestibule. The piston should be only approximately 0.5 mm into the vestibule. Over time, the endosteal membrane reforms underneath the piston. Once this membrane has reformed, the piston does not directly contact perilymph. It can be thought of as residing in a diverticulum of the middle ear.

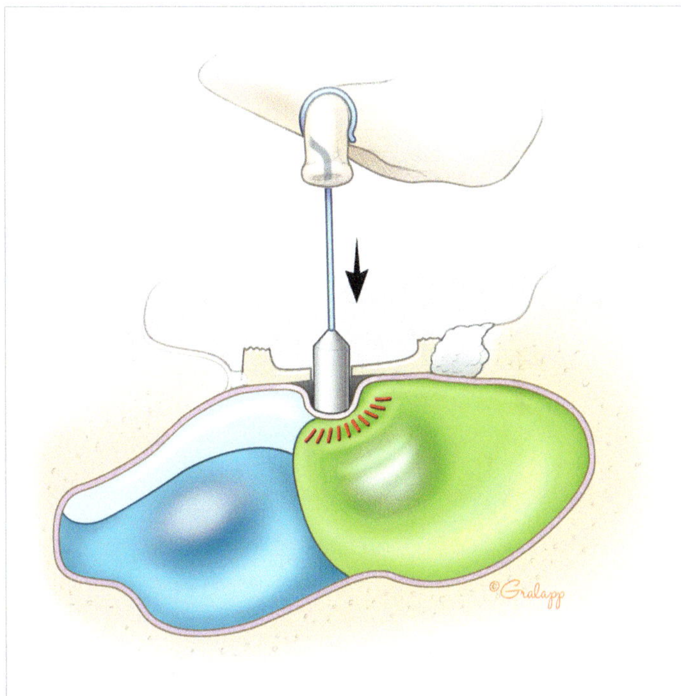

Fig. 4.131 Stapes surgery is contraindicated in hydrops due to risk of the piston traumatizing the otolithic organs. Among other complications, this can lead to Tullio's phenomenon (vertigo with loud noise).

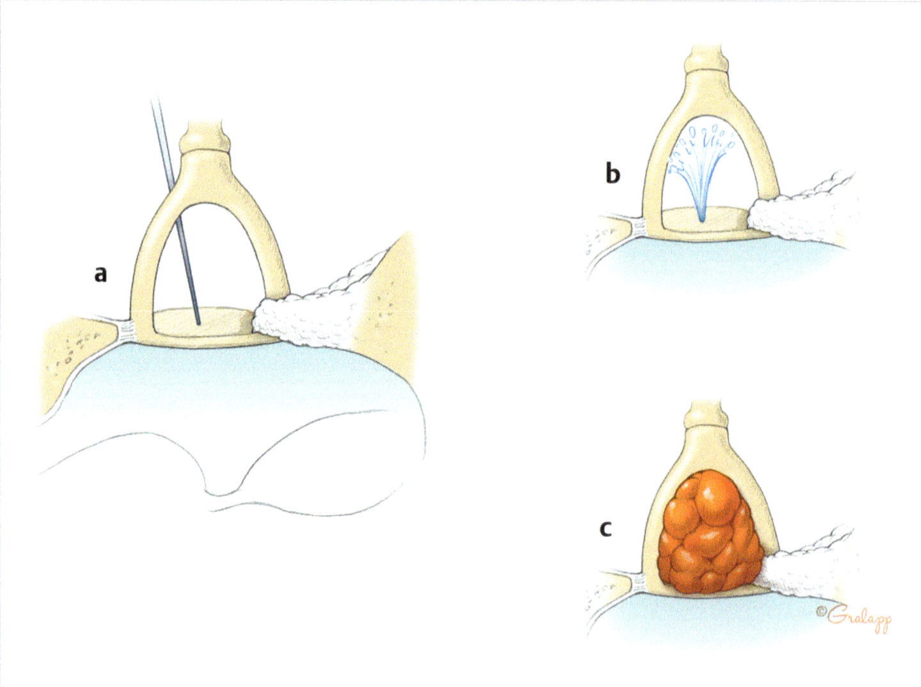

Fig. 4.132 In rare instances, the inner ear may have CSF pressure within it. This may occur in certain inner ear malformations (e.g., large vestibular aqueduct) as well as the X-lined gusher syndrome. In congenital conductive hearing loss, a CT scan should be obtained to rule out inner ear malformation. Stapes surgery is contraindicated in inner ear malformation as the audiogram may reflect a pseudoconductive hearing loss and the risk of hearing loss is high. In conductive loss existing since early in life (whether in a child or adult), creation of a control hole (**a**) may help detect a gusher. Should a gusher occur (**b**), a soft-tissue plug can be placed beneath the stapes arch (**c**).

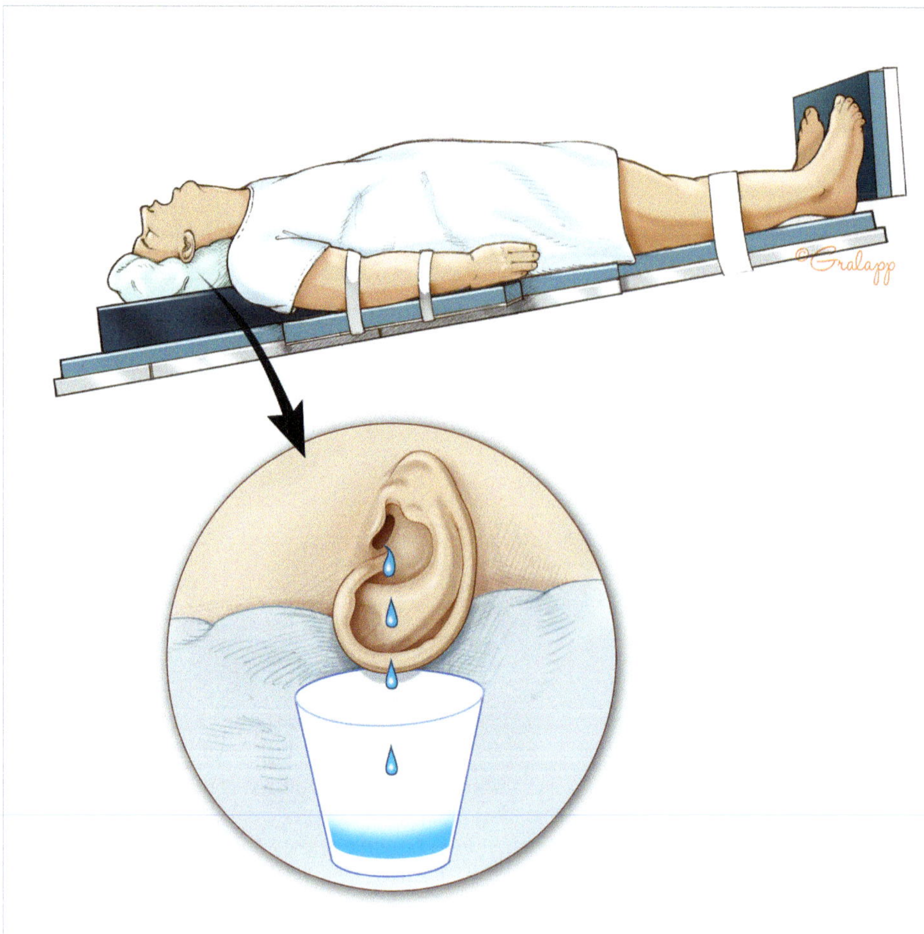

Fig. 4.133 In true stapes gusher, brisk CSF flow prohibits orderly microdissection. Rather than packing the oval window in panicked fashion with poor visualization, it is better to drop the head into Trendelenburg and allow the CSF to escape.

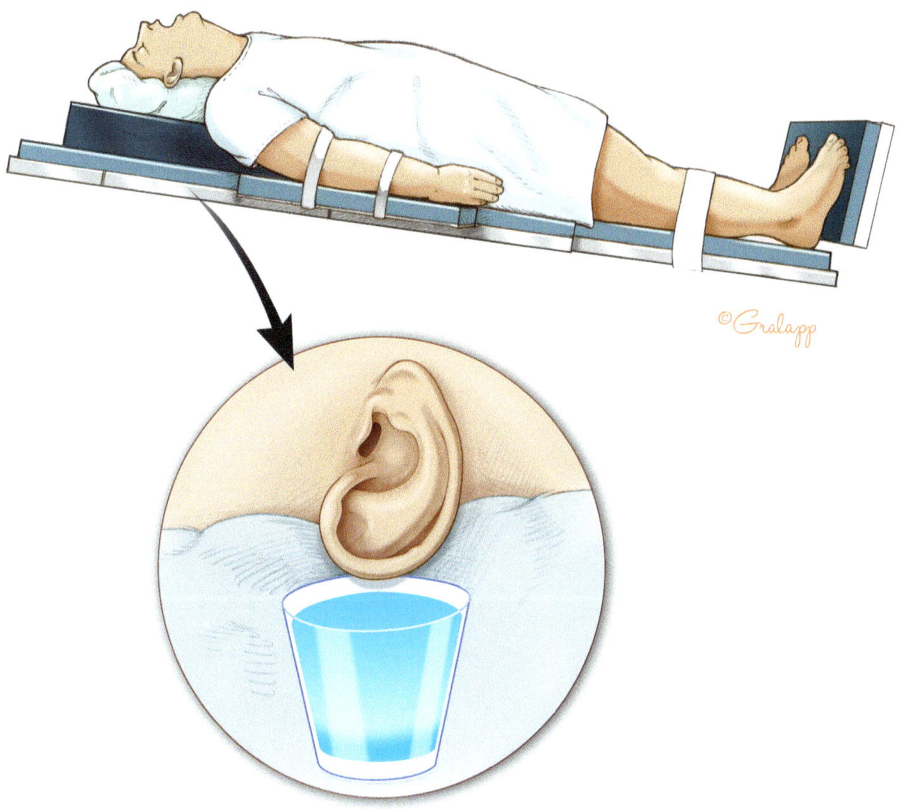

Fig. 4.134 When the drainage has ceased, the head is elevated into reverse Trendelenburg. The surgeon can then complete the soft-tissue closure of the oval window in a dry field. A lumbar subarachnoid drain may be placed.

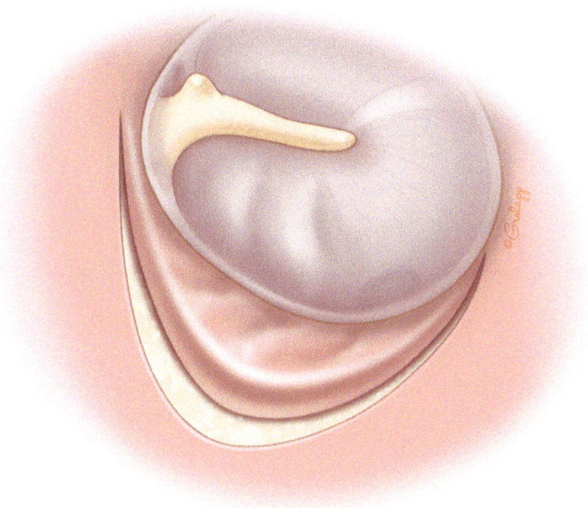

Fig. 4.135 The edge of the tympanomeatal flap is curled under.

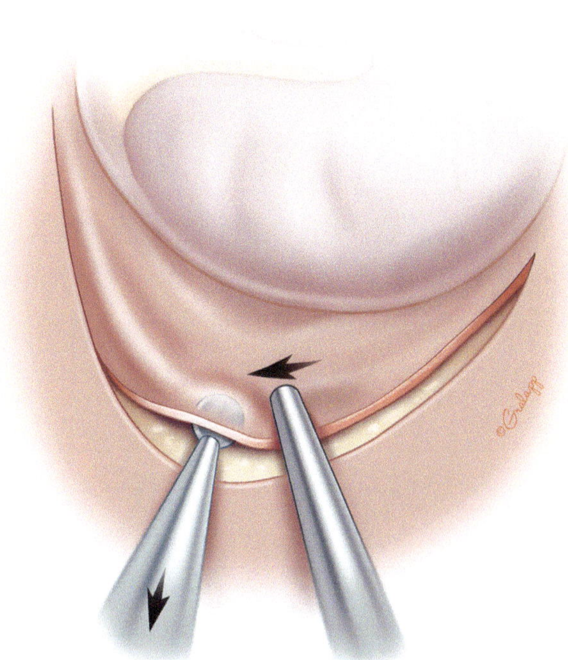

Fig. 4.136 A joint knife may be used to unfurl the edge to ensure the flap lies flat against the bony canal.

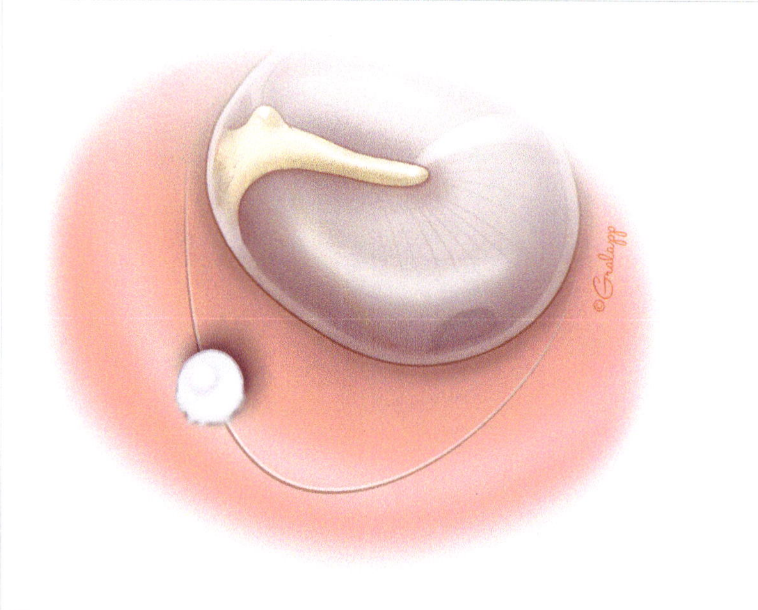

Fig. 4.137 Infolding of the tympanomeatal flap edge can lead to formation of a keratin pearl.

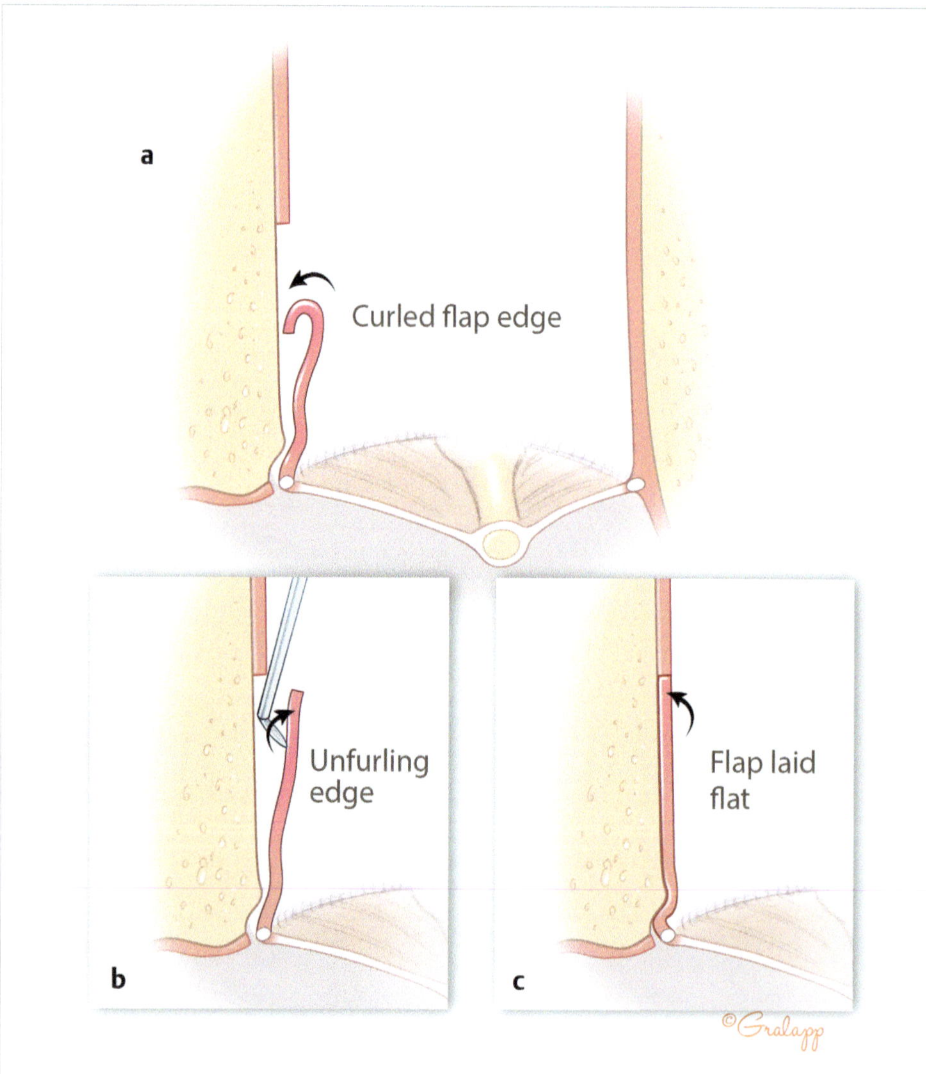

Fig. 4.138 After repositioning the flap, a joint knife may be used to unfurl the curled edge to ensure the flap lies flat against the bony canal.

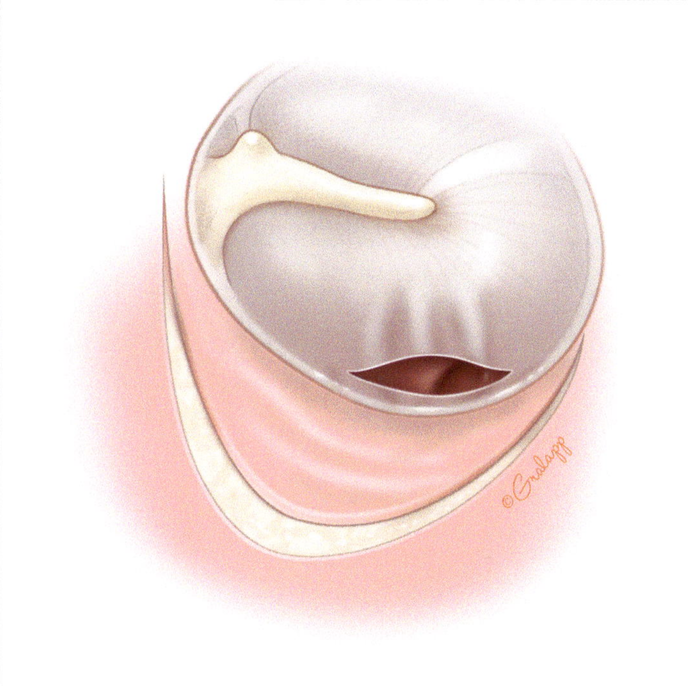

Fig. 4.139 Tympanic membrane tear sustained during flap elevation.

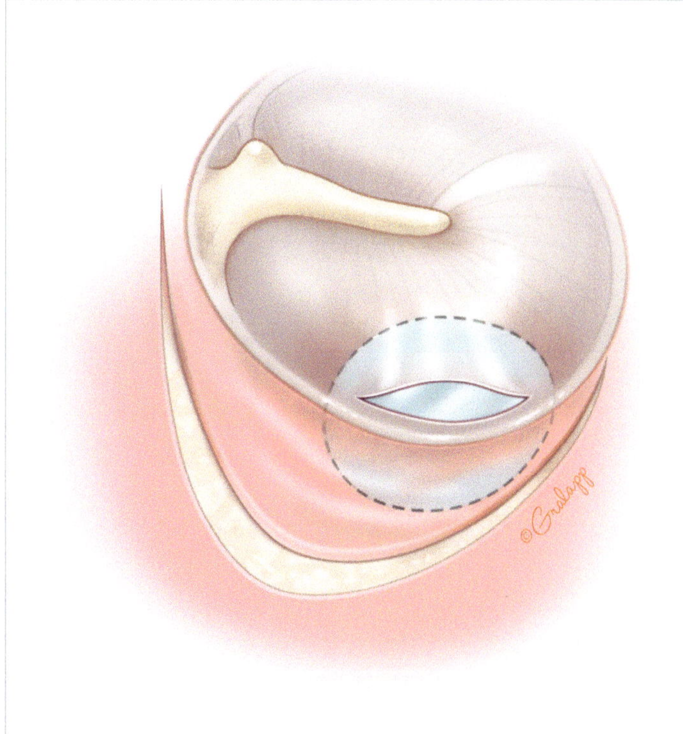

Fig. 4.140 As the incision has devascularized the posterior aspect of the tympanic membrane, spontaneous healing is not assured. The tympanic membrane is best repaired with a perichondrial or fascial graft placed medial to the tear.

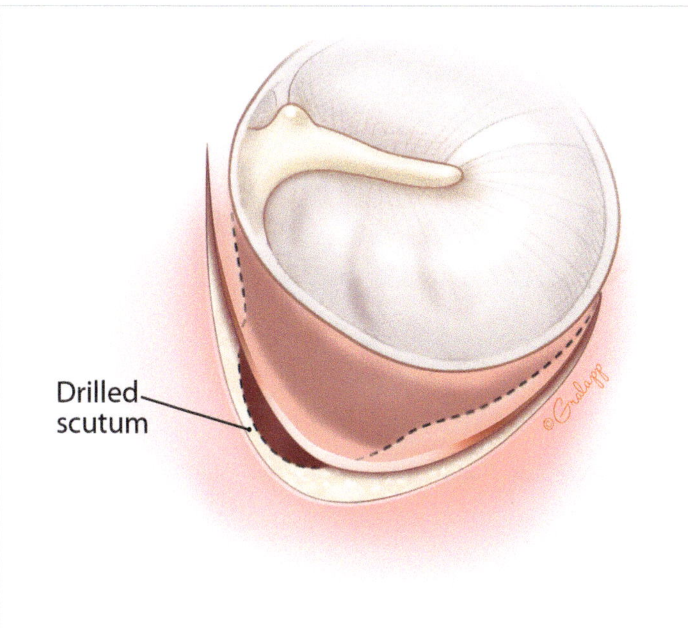

Fig. 4.141 Marginal dehiscence of the flap due to either too short of a flap design or a long scutum necessitating more extensive bone removal than the flap can cover.

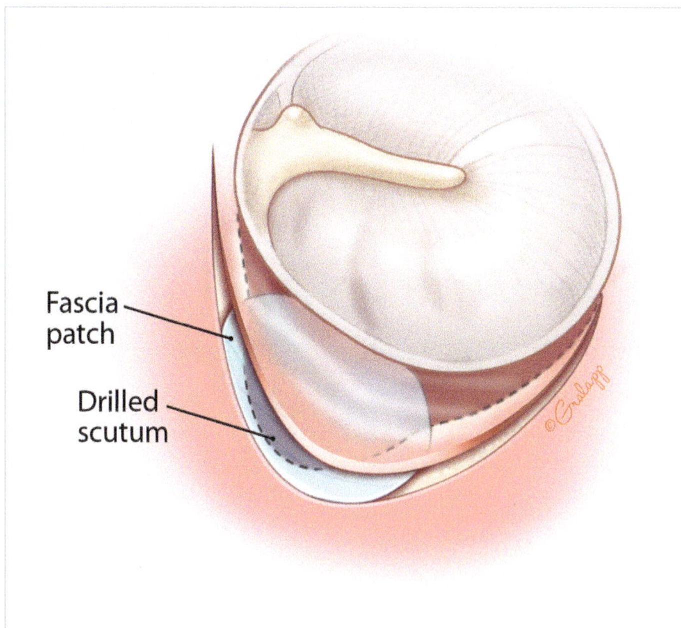

Fig. 4.142 Marginal dehiscence should be repaired with a perichondrial or fascial graft.

4.7 Deficient Incus

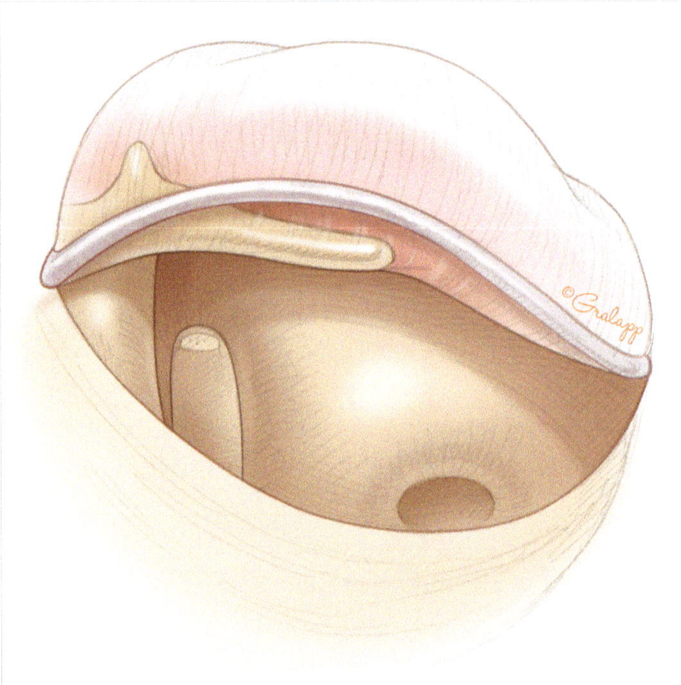

Fig. 4.143 An absent or insufficient incus represents a technical challenge in stapes surgery.

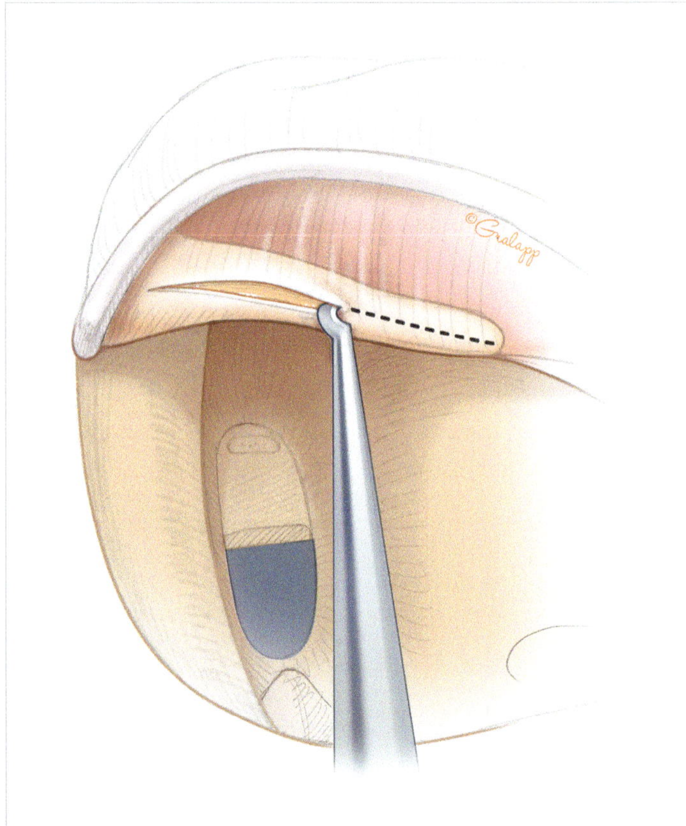

Fig. 4.144 Incision is made in the posterior aspect of the umbo with either a myringotomy knife or laser.

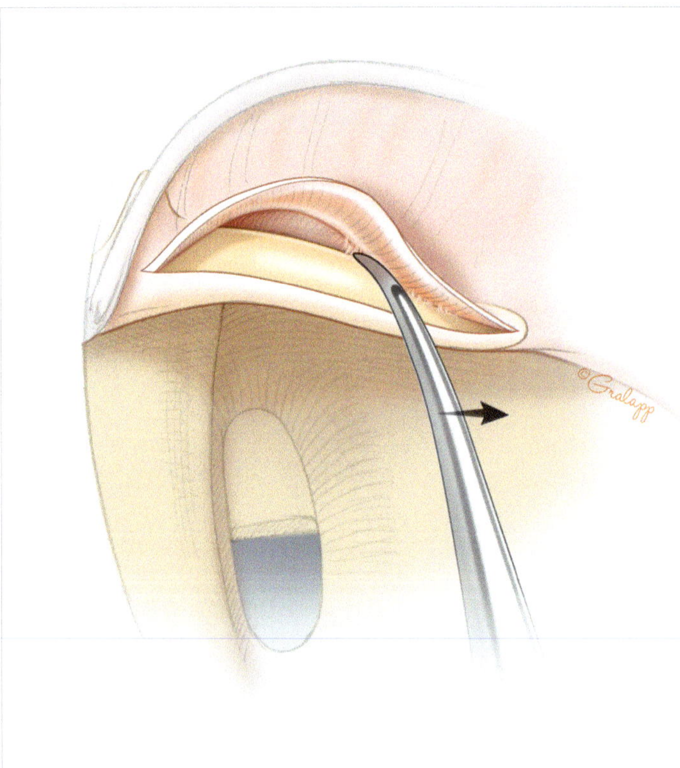

Fig. 4.145 A pocket is raised from the malleus short process to the umbo to accommodate the prosthesis, exercising care to avoid tympanic membrane disruption.

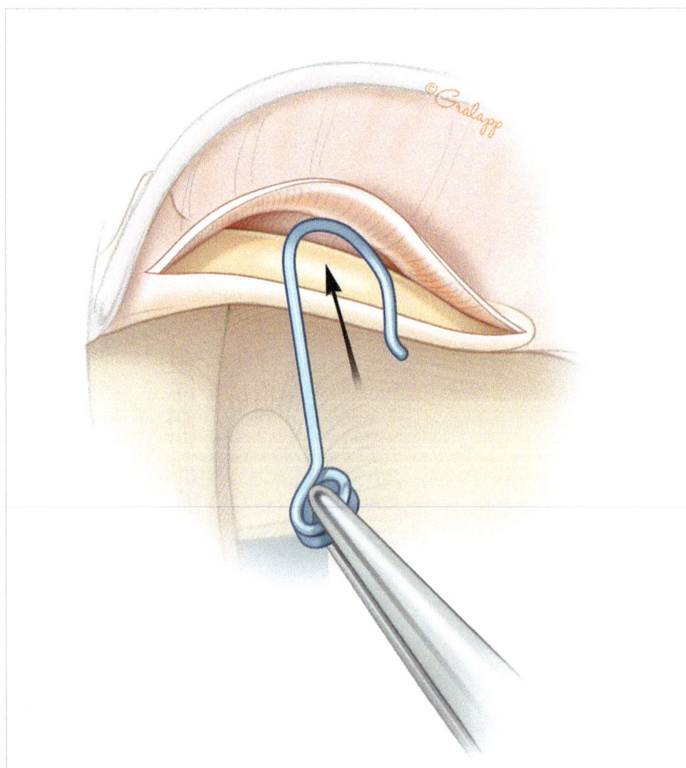

Fig. 4.146 Technique of inserting an incus replacement wire (Sheehy IRP).

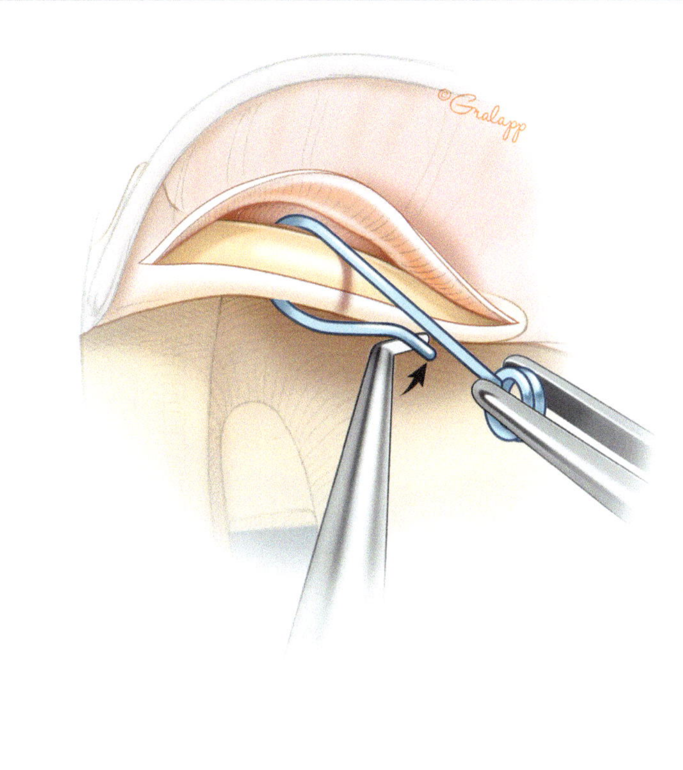

Fig. 4.147 The IRP is tied around the malleus with a hook while the prosthesis is stabilized with an alligator.

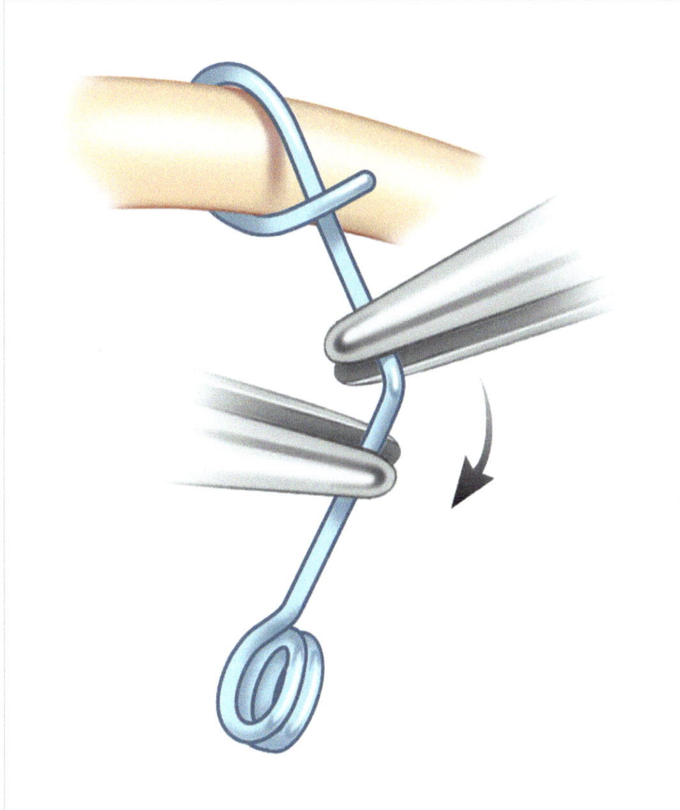

Fig. 4.148 To avoid the need for various lengths, a long prosthesis is used which is bent before positioning above the oval window.

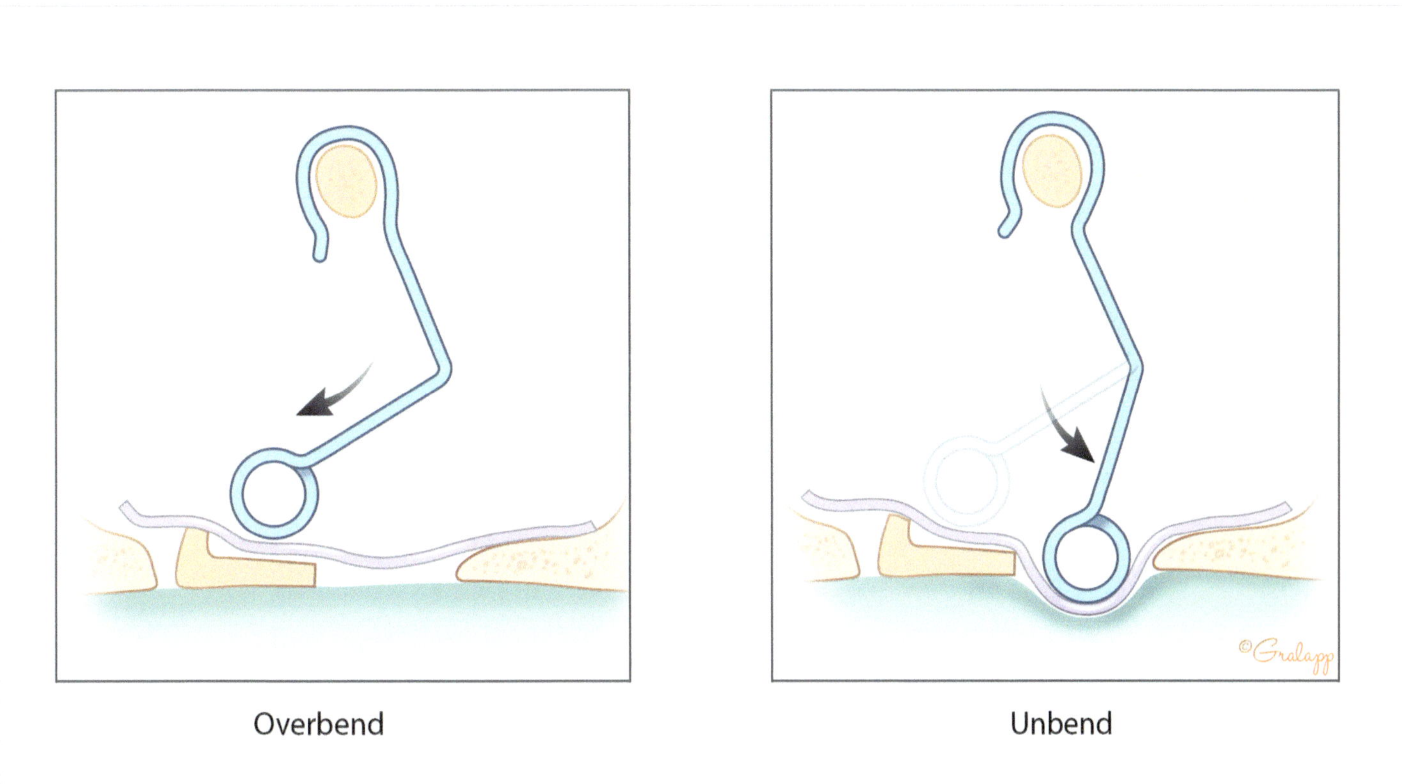

Fig. 4.149 The bend is progressively straightened until the desired tension is achieved.

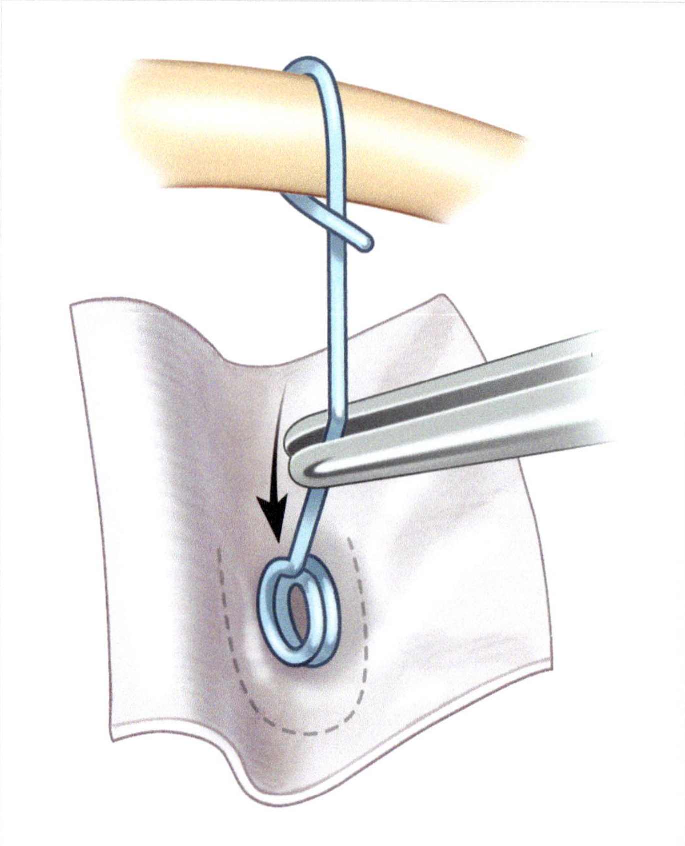

Fig. 4.150 The malleus to footplate prosthesis seated into position.

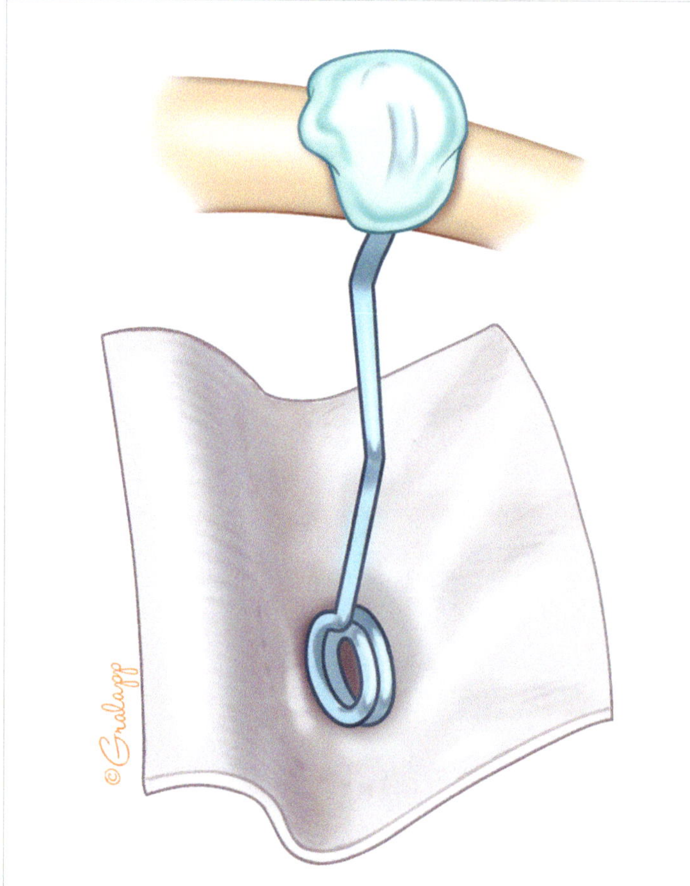

Fig. 4.151 A drop of cement may be placed to reinforce the stability of the malleus crimp.

4.8 Revision Stapes Surgery

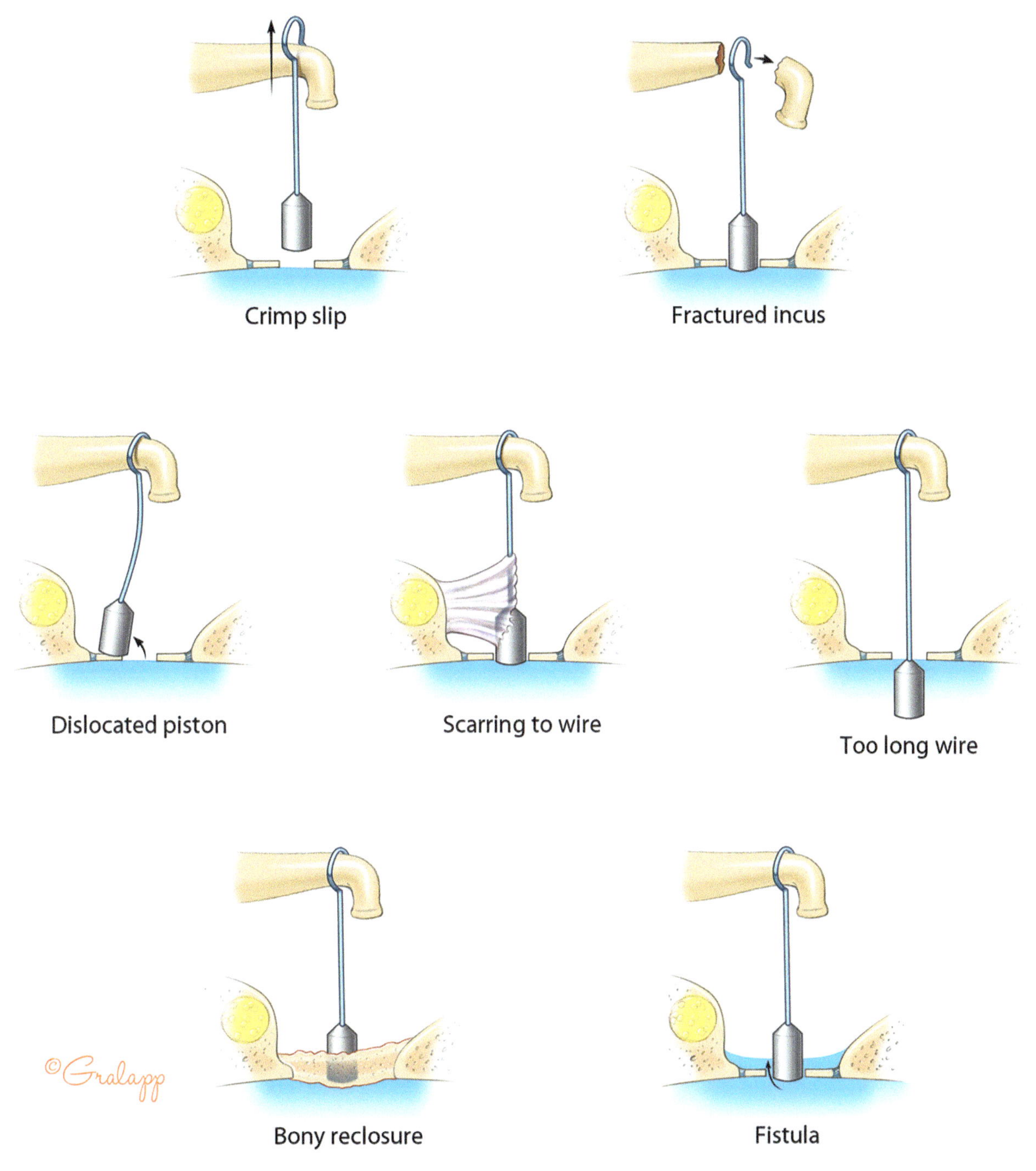

Fig. 4.152 The seven most common findings encountered during revision stapes surgery.

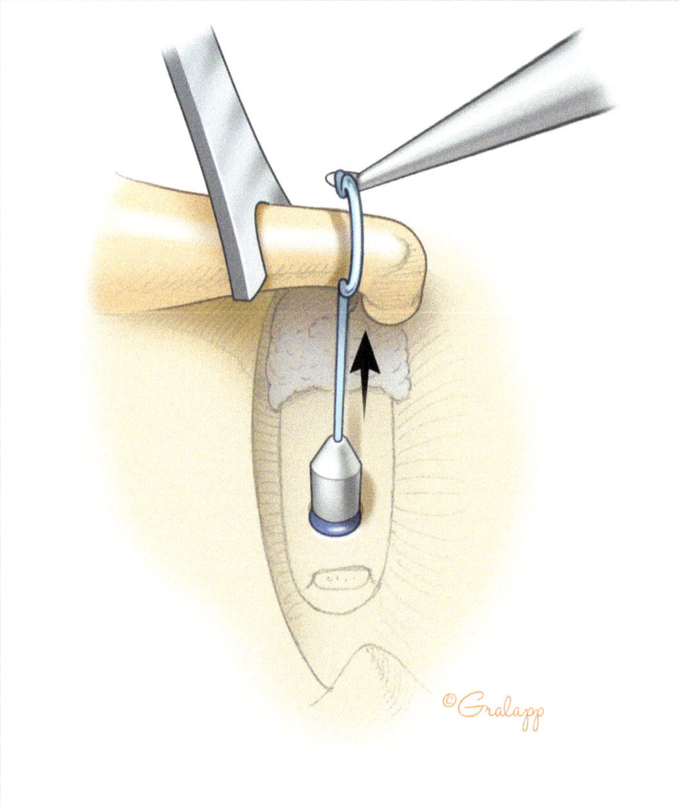

Fig. 4.153 Removing a stapes prosthesis during revision surgery requires a two-handed maneuver with stabilization of the incus (shown here with a notched chisel also known as a strut guide). A hook is used to pry the prosthesis from the stabilized incus.

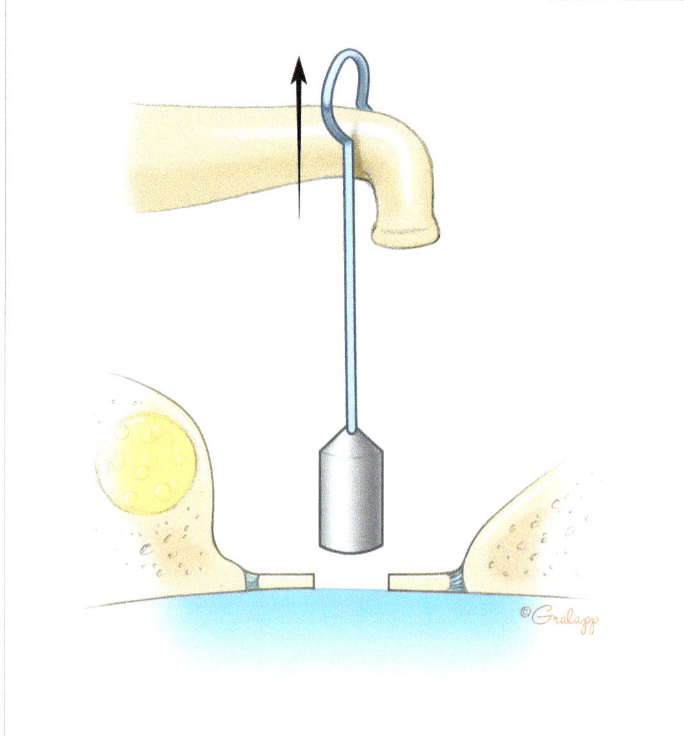

Fig. 4.154 Displacement of the prosthesis due to loosening of the crimp from the incus. A fully slipped crimp will cause major conductive hearing loss while loose crimp may be associated with variable conductive hearing loss that comes and goes as middle ear pressure varies.

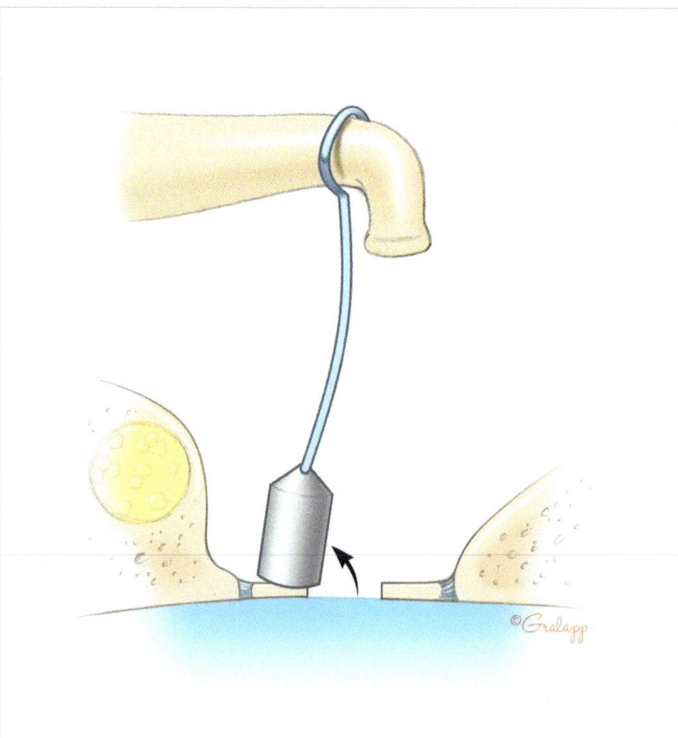

Fig. 4.155 Dislodgement of the prosthesis from the oval window fenestra. Too short of a prosthesis can contribute to this complication. Sometimes it occurs during vigorous autoinflation.

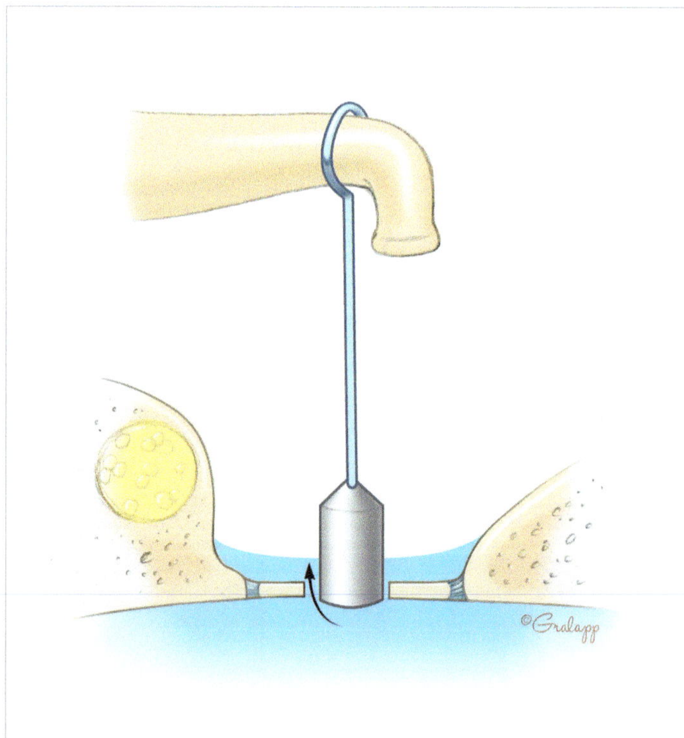

Fig. 4.156 Perilymphatic fistula may be associated with sensory loss and/or vestibular symptoms.

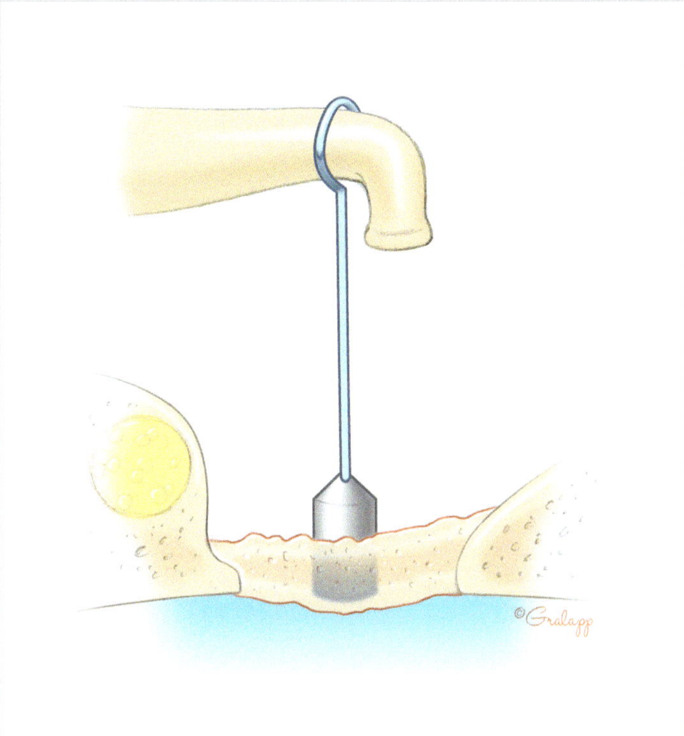

Fig. 4.157 Bony reclosure of the oval window. Because repeat drill out of recurrent obliterative otosclerosis carries a heighted risk of sensory loss, consideration should be given to amplification.

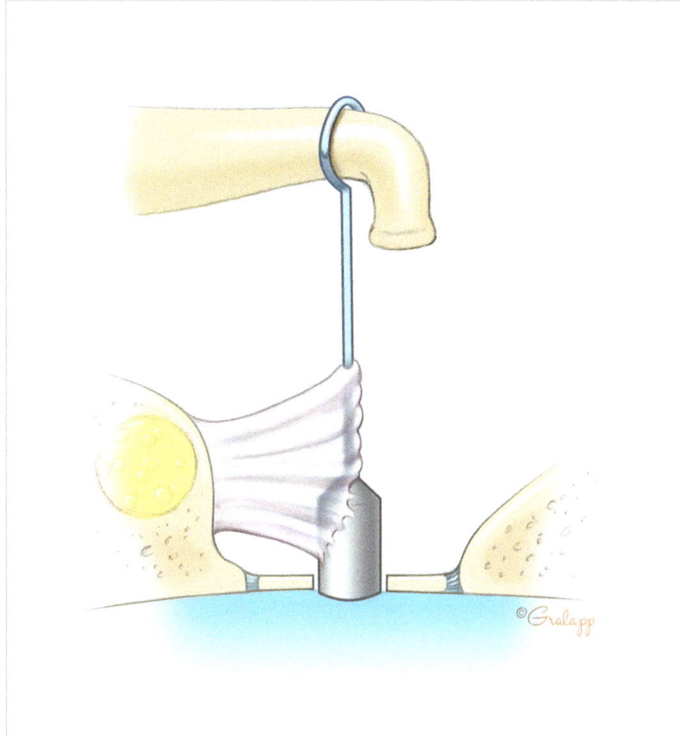

Fig. 4.158 Scarring between the margins of the oval window (especially the facial nerve canal) and the prosthesis can reduce its mobility. Laser removal of the scar bands may be effective, but scarring tends to recur.

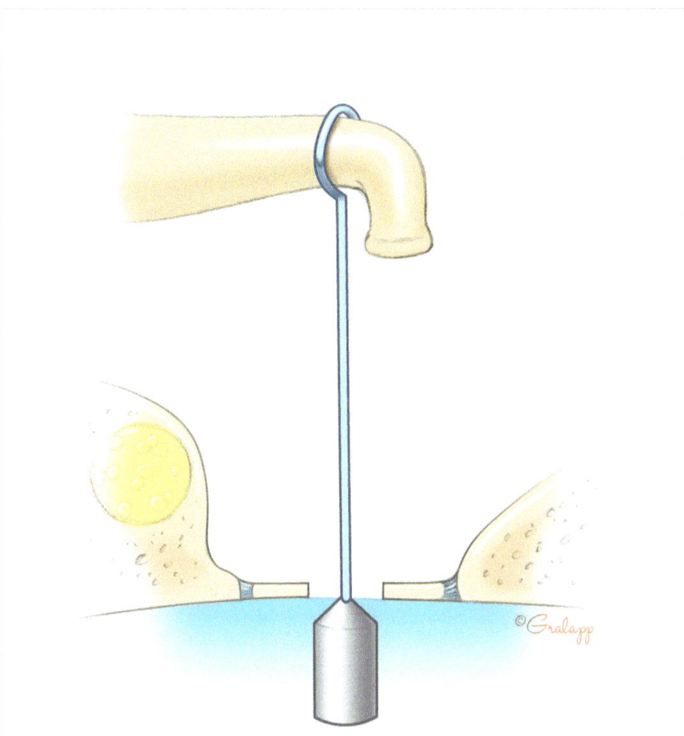

Fig. 4.159 An overly long prosthesis may cause vestibular symptoms, especially vertigo triggered by loud sounds (Tullio's phenomenon).

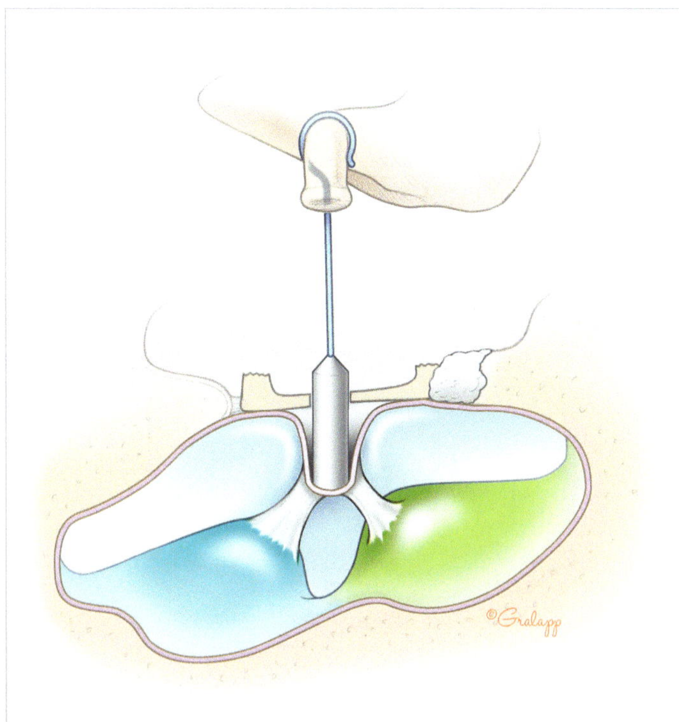

Fig. 4.160 Due to adhesion with the endolymphatic membranes, removing an overly inserted prosthesis carries a risk of inner ear damage.

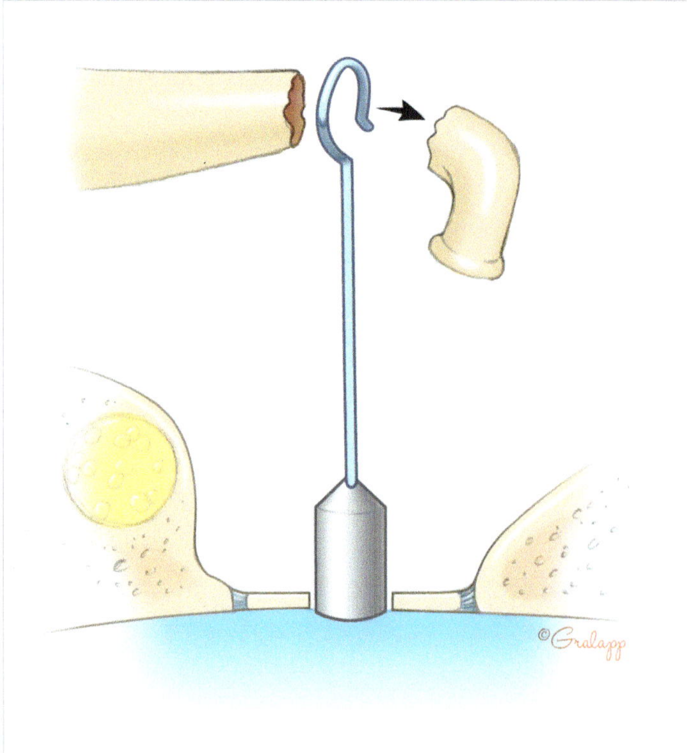

Fig. 4.161 Fracture of the long process of the incus. This may occur due to a movement of a loose prosthesis, an overly hermetic crimp resulting in devascularization of the lenticular process, or fragile incus as in osteogenesis imperfecta.

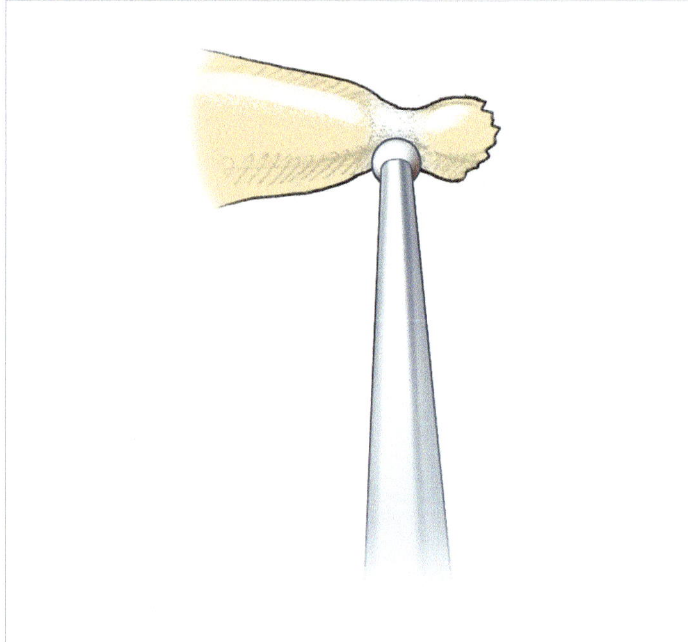

Fig. 4.162 Because a fractured incus will not retain a wire without modification, a groove is created to anchor the crimp.

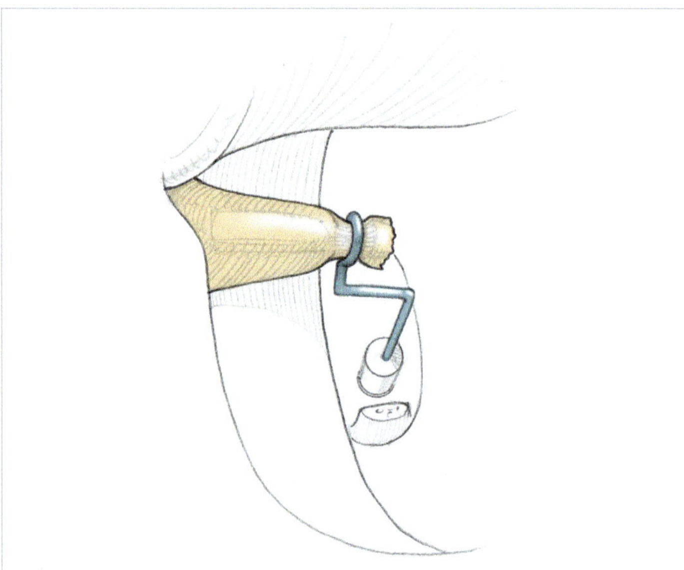

Fig. 4.163 A longer prosthesis using a double-bend technique restores continuity. A malleus to footplate prosthesis is an alternative solution.

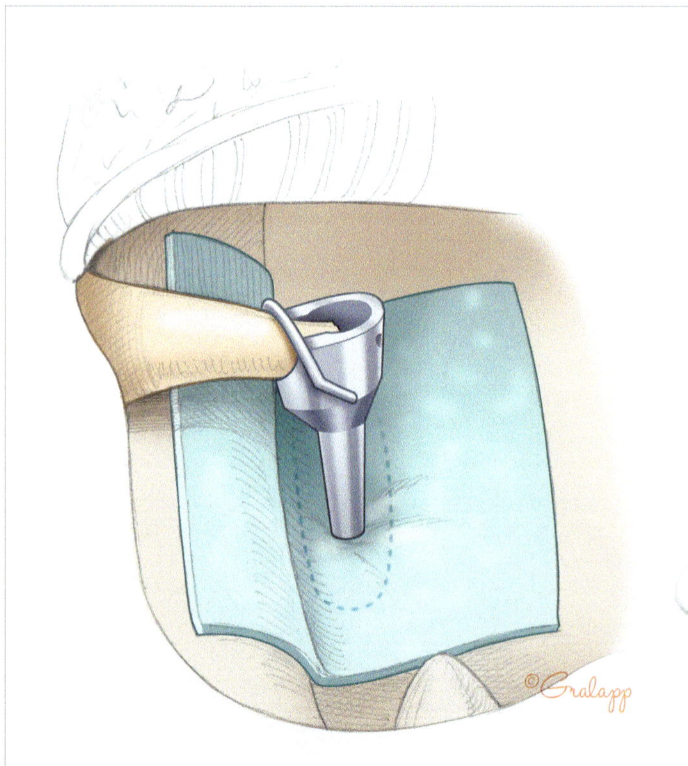

Fig. 4.164 A Lippy modified prosthesis with an elongated bucket is designed to accommodate a deficient incus.

4.9 Tympanosclerotic Stapes Fixation

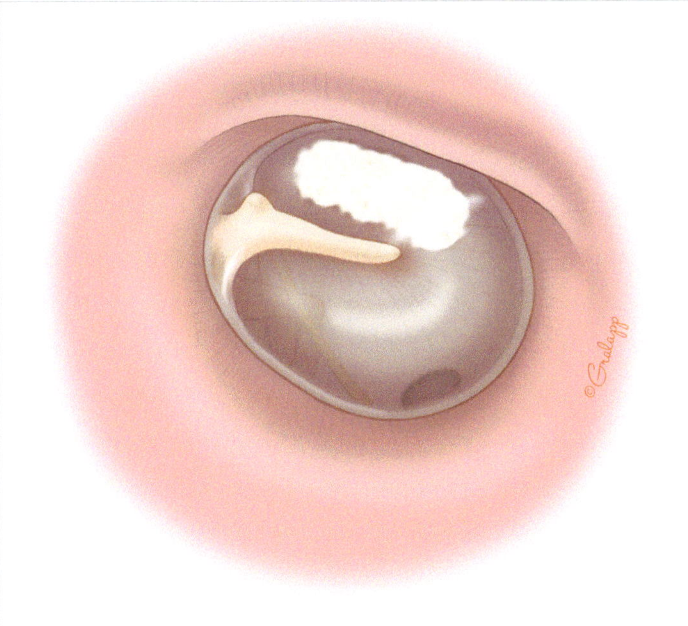

Fig. 4.165 The finding of myringosclerosis should raise suspicion of tympanosclerotic ossicular fixation.

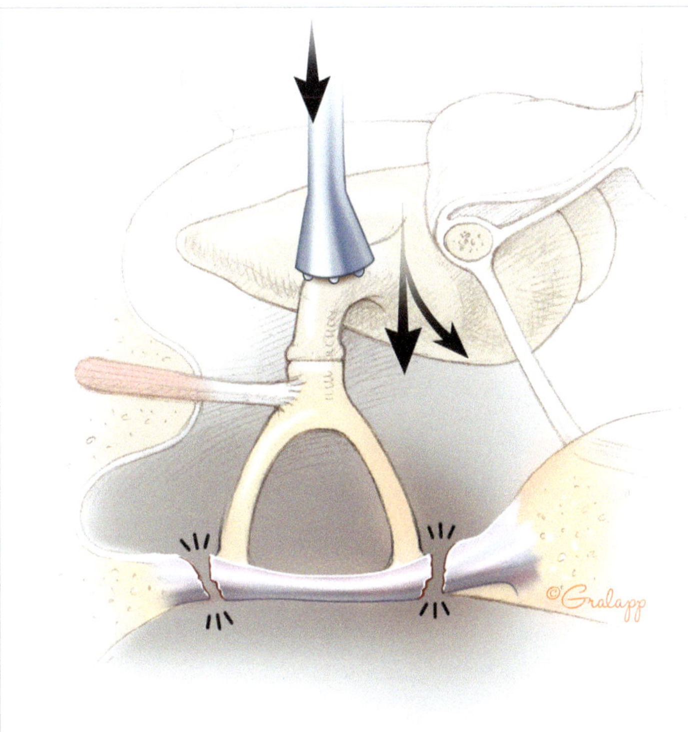

Fig. 4.167 In stapes mobilization, an elephant's foot (the "Derlacki mobilizer") is used to rock the superstructure. Mobilization should always be attempted during surgery for congenital stapes fixation, but is not often successful due to lack of an annular ligament. Should mobilization be achieved, there is no need to proceed with stapedotomy as, in the absence of active bone disease such as otosclerosis, the stapes will not refix.

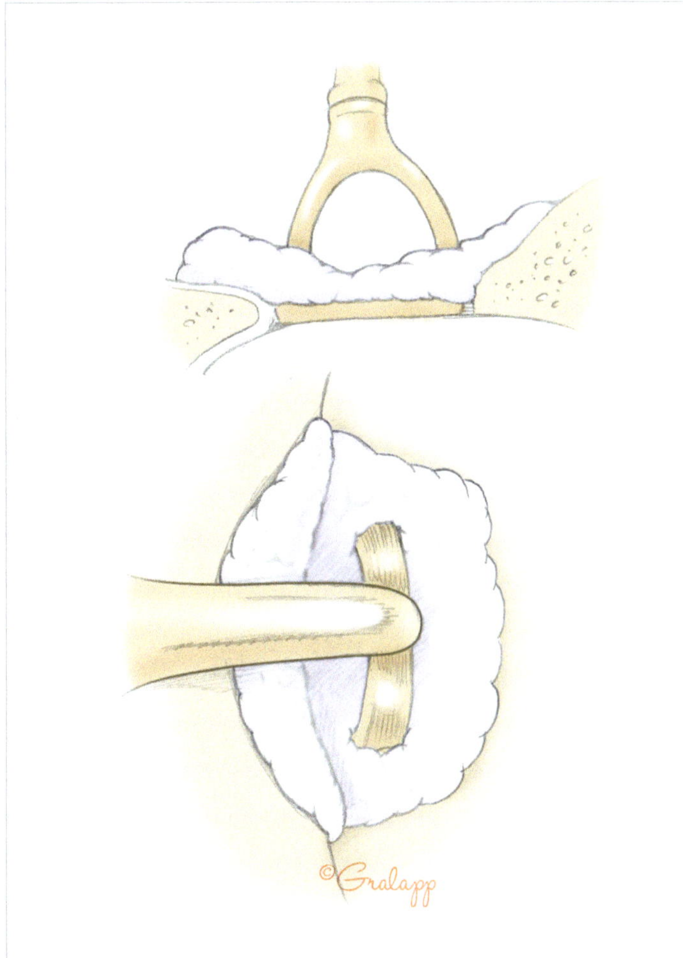

Fig. 4.166 Extensive, circumferential tympanosclerotic stapes fixation. Stapes surgery is generally not effective with such extensive disease.

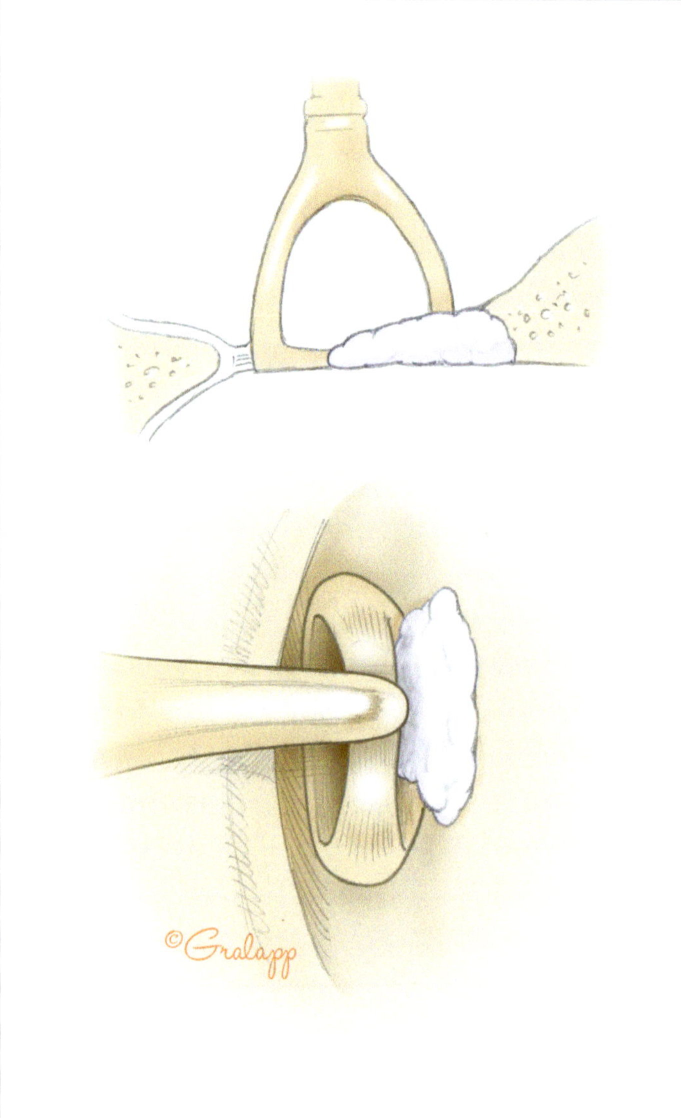

Fig. 4.168 Focal tympanosclerotic stapes fixation is more amenable to surgical correction.

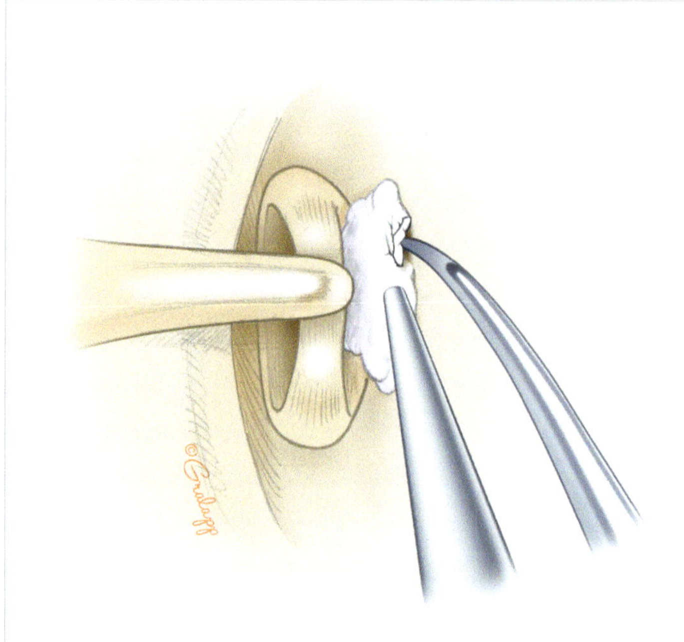

Fig. 4.169 Attempt should be made to chip away the fixing bridge of tympanosclerosis. When thoroughly removed, the stapes has a good chance of retaining mobility.

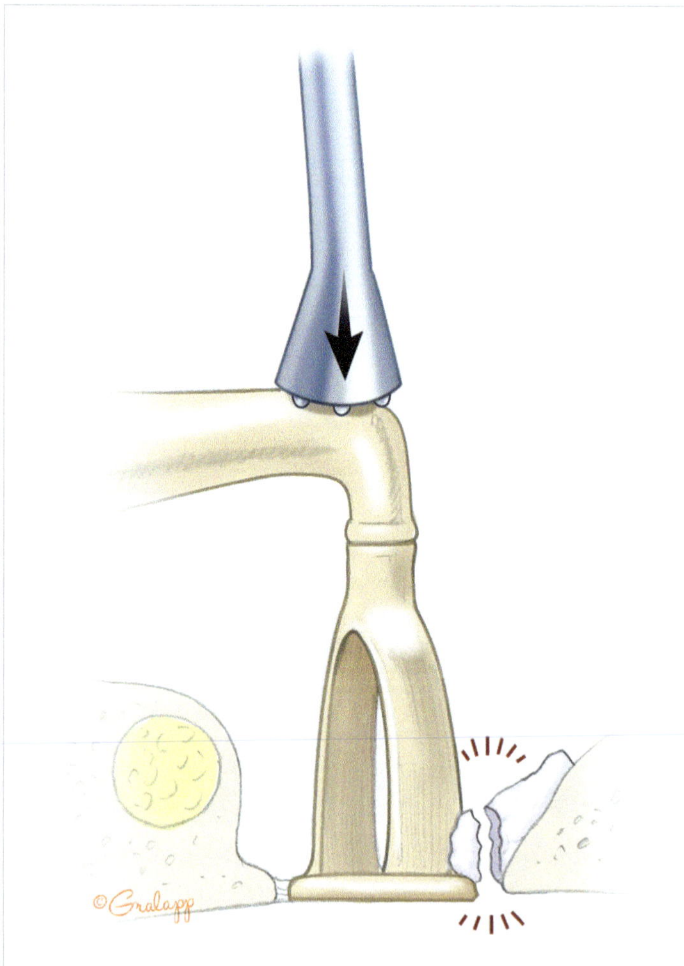

Fig. 4.170 Mobilization is also possible in tympanosclerotic fixation, but the fixation tends to recur. Stapedectomy is usually avoided in tympanosclerotic fixation unless the ear has a long infection-free period, the middle ear mucosa is mostly healthy, and the tympanic membrane is not prone to retraction.

5 Tympanoplasty

Robert K. Jackler

5.1 Introduction to Tympanoplasty

The invention of microsurgical repair of chronic tympanic membrane perforation was one of the great contributions of 20th century otology. With success rates in experienced hands well over 90%, it is also among the most successful of all ear surgeries. As autologous material is readily available (e.g., temporalis fascia, tragal perichondrium), there is little rationale to employ artificial graft material. The recent trend has shown an increasing use of autologous cartilage (e.g., tragal, conchal) both to prepare for ossiculoplasty and because the resulting neomembrane better resists reperforation. Small islands of myringosclerosis may be left in place, but larger areas of calcification are best removed as they may impair vibration of the drum. As a general rule, perforations posterior to the malleus can be handled transcanal, whereas those anterior to the malleus are best approached postauricularly for the superior visualization of the anterior tympanum it affords. Anteriorly situated perforations which extend to the annulus require special techniques lest perforation persist.

While some surgeons routinely rim the margin of the perforation, others (including the author) never do as graft take results are equivalent without rimming. Scratching the mucosa on the medial side of the tympanic membrane remnant is routine to expose subepithelial tissue and to stimulate bleeding which both helps graft adhesion and provides the initial substrates for healing. Today, most surgeons use the technique of placing the graft medial to the tympanic membrane remnant. The lateral graft technique has more complications such as epithelial pearl formation, anterior blunting, and lateralization. The push through or butterfly technique is gaining in popularity, especially for smaller perforations. In the coming years, autologous growth factors may well allow a biologically based, nonsurgical approach to healing tympanic membrane perforations.

Further Reading

1. Alain H, Esmat NH, Ohad H, Yona V, Nageris BI. Butterfly myringoplasty for total, subtotal, and annular perforations. Laryngoscope 2016;126(11):2565–2568 PubMed
2. Anzola JF, Nogueira JF. Endoscopic techniques in tympanoplasty. Otolaryngol Clin North Am 2016;49(5):1253–1264 PubMed
3. Hardman J, Muzaffar J, Nankivell P, Coulson C. Tympanoplasty for chronic tympanic membrane perforation in children: systematic review and meta-analysis. Otol Neurotol 2015;36 (5):796–804 PubMed
4. Hsu YC, Kuo CL, Huang TC. A retrospective comparative study of endoscopic and microscopic tympanoplasty. J Otolaryngol Head Neck Surg 2018;47(1):44 PubMed
5. Jalali MM, Motasaddi M, Kouhi A, Dabiri S, Soleimani R. Comparison of cartilage with temporalis fascia tympanoplasty: a meta-analysis of comparative studies. Laryngoscope 2017;127(9):2139–2148 PubMed
6. Jumaily M, Franco J, Gallogly JA, et al. Butterfly cartilage tympanoplasty outcomes: a single-institution experience and literature review. Am J Otolaryngol 2018;39(4):396–400 PubMed
7. Luukkainen V, Kivekäs I, Silvola J, Jero J, Sinkkonen ST. Balloon eustachian tuboplasty: systematic review of long-term outcomes and proposed indications. J Int Adv Otol 2018;14 (1):112–126 PubMed
8. Mudry A. History of myringoplasty and tympanoplasty type I. Otolaryngol Head Neck Surg 2008;139(5):613–614 PubMed
9. Neudert M, Zahnert T. Tympanoplasty - news and new perspectives. GMS Curr Top Otorhinolaryngol Head Neck Surg 2017;16:Doc07 PubMed
10. Randrup TS, Ovesen T. Balloon eustachian tuboplasty: a systematic review. Otolaryngol Head Neck Surg 2015;152 (3):383–392 PubMed
11. Silvola J, Kivekäs I, Poe DS. Balloon dilation of the cartilaginous portion of the eustachian tube. Otolaryngol Head Neck Surg 2014;151(1):125–130 PubMed
12. Visvanathan V, Vallamkondu V, Bhimrao SK. Achieving a successful closure of an anterior tympanic membrane perforation: evidence-based systematic review. Otolaryngol Head Neck Surg 2018;158(6):1011–1015 PubMed
13. Yang T, Wu X, Peng X, Zhang Y, Xie S, Sun H. Comparison of cartilage graft and fascia in type 1 tympanoplasty: systematic review and meta-analysis. Acta Otolaryngol 2016;136 (11):1085–1090 PubMed

5.2 Tympanic Membrane Perforations

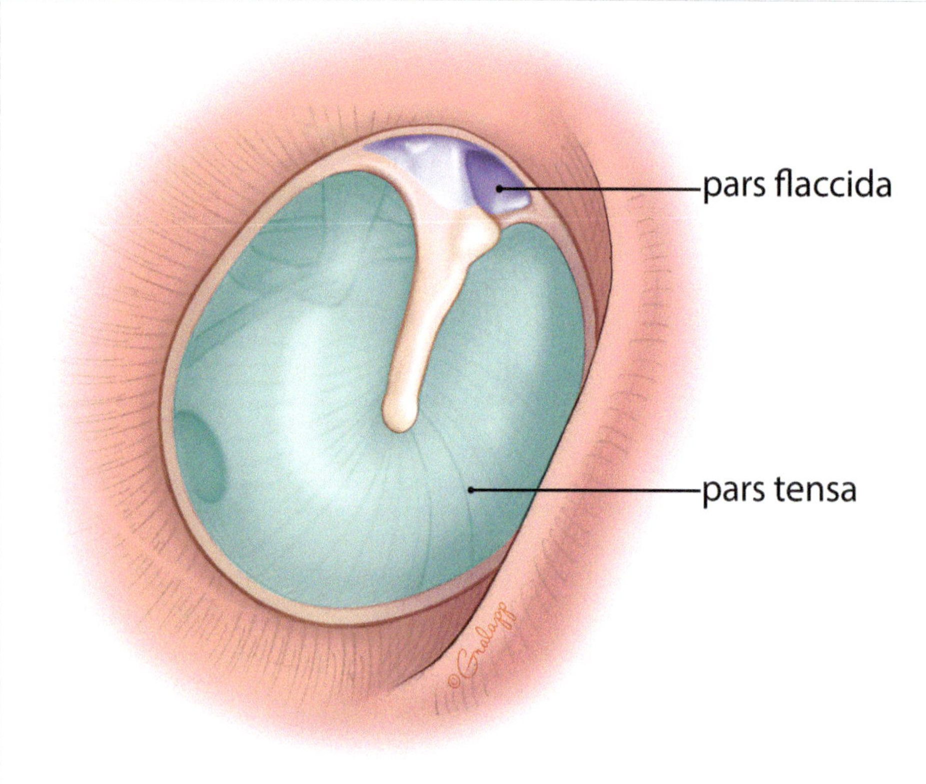

Fig. 5.1 Pars tensa and pars flaccida of the tympanic membrane. The pars tensa has three layers: lateral stratified squamous epithelium, central fibrous layer, and medial low cuboidal mucosal epithelium. The pars flaccida is deficient in its fibrous layer.

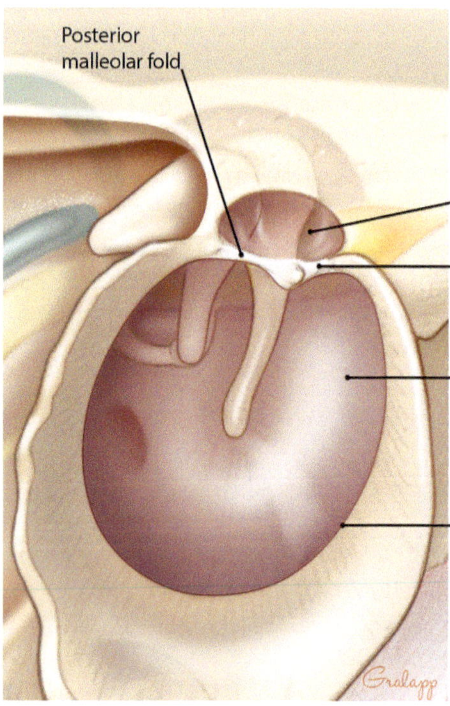

Fig. 5.2 Relationship of the tympanic membrane to the tympanic ring and ossicles.

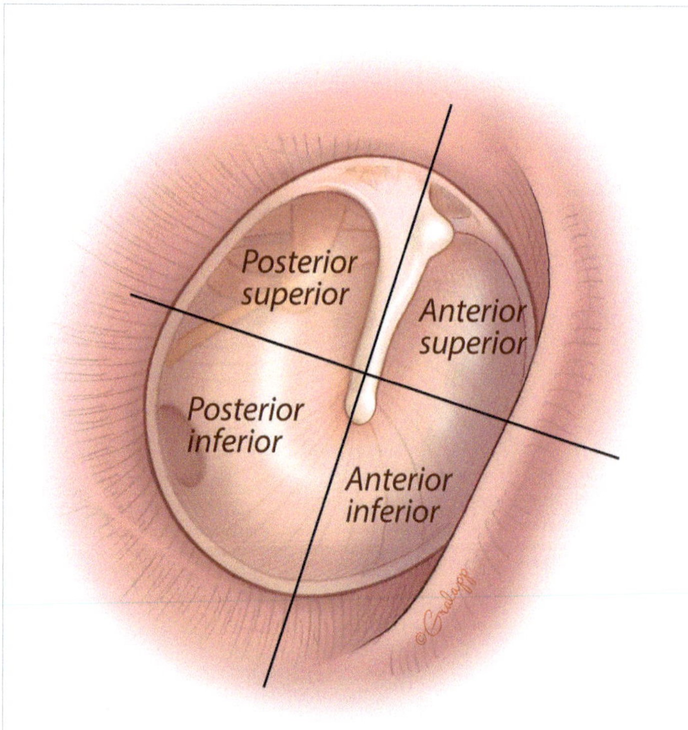

Fig. 5.3 Quadrants of the tympanic membrane.

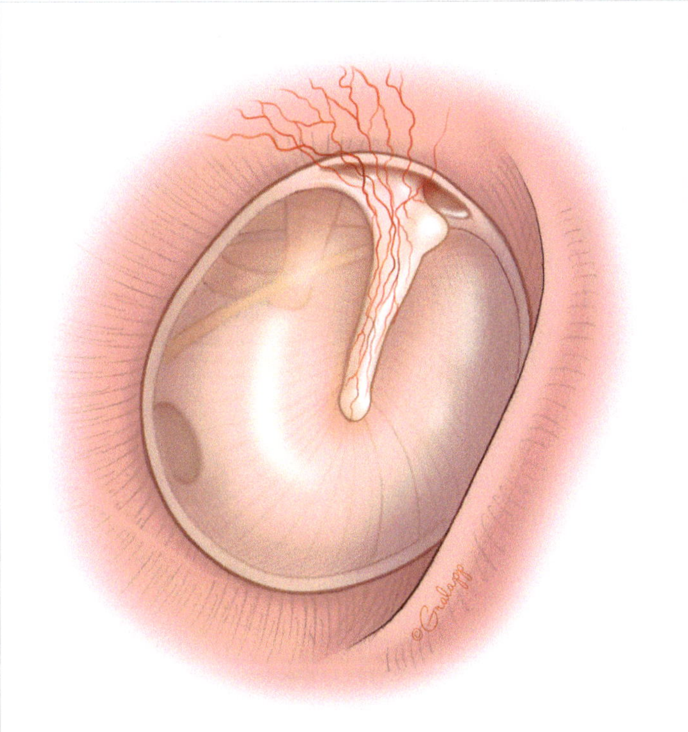

Fig. 5.4 The vascular strip in the posterior-superior ear canal provides blood supply to the central portion of the tympanic membrane.

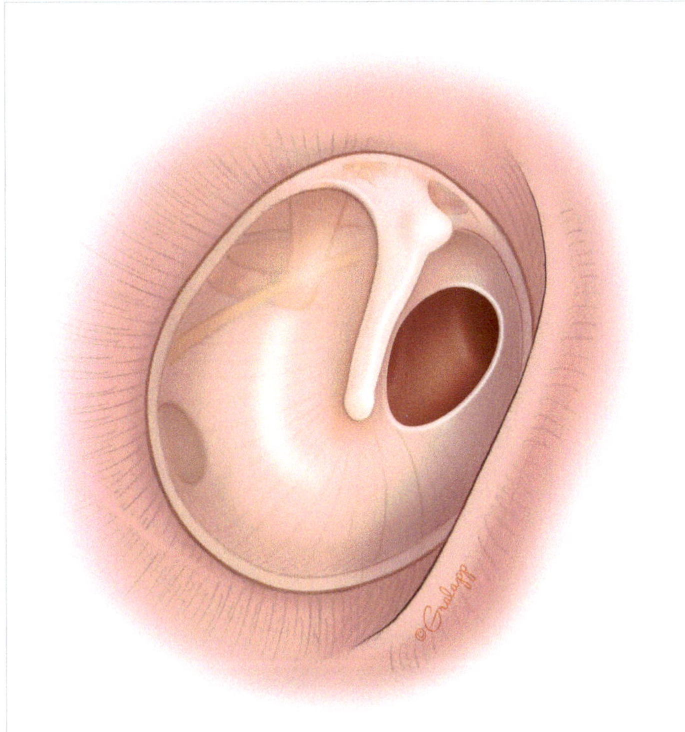

Fig. 5.5 Anterior tympanic membrane perforation with a remaining rim. Note the Eustachian tube orifice in the depth.

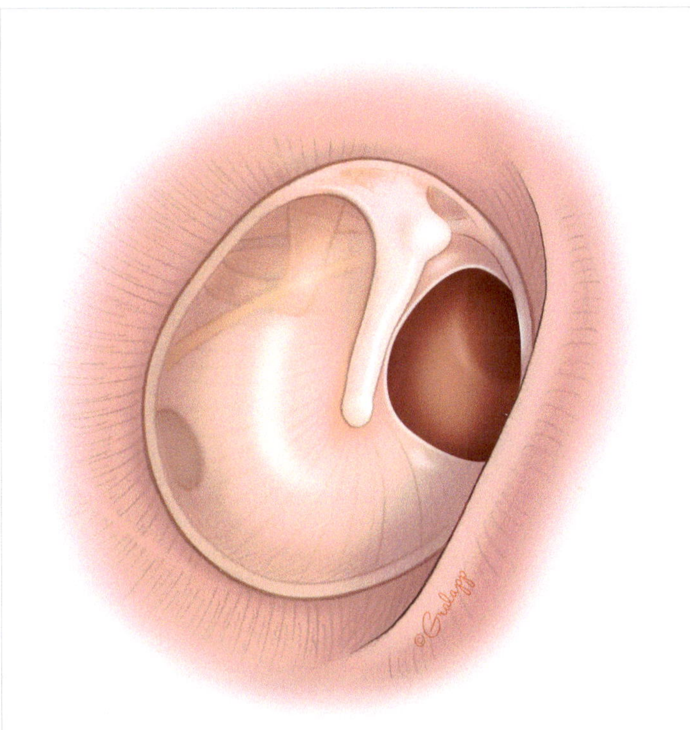

Fig. 5.6 Anterior tympanic membrane perforation without a remaining rim. This type of perforation has a higher reperforation rate unless specialized techniques are used.

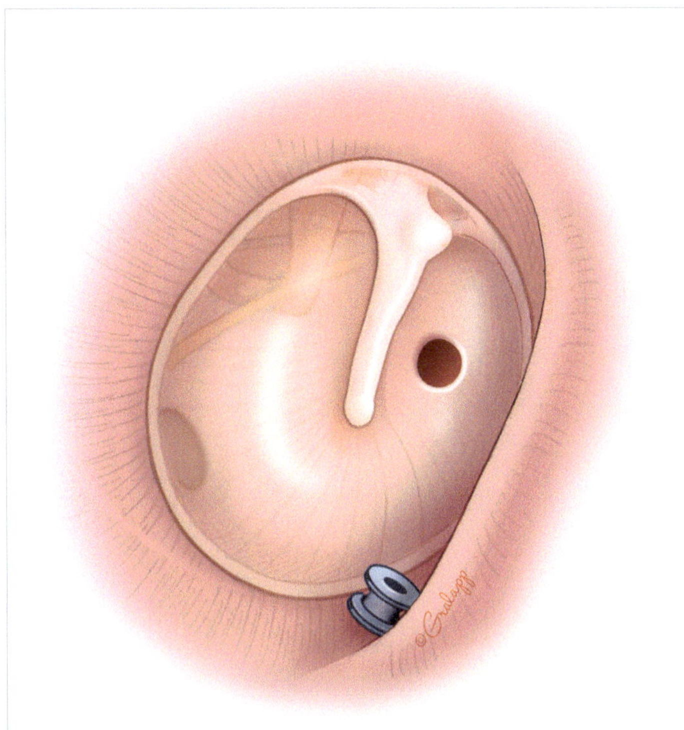

Fig. 5.7 Posttympanostomy tube residual perforation. Often such residual small anterior perforations have little effect on hearing and provide ventilation in the face of Eustachian tube dysfunction.

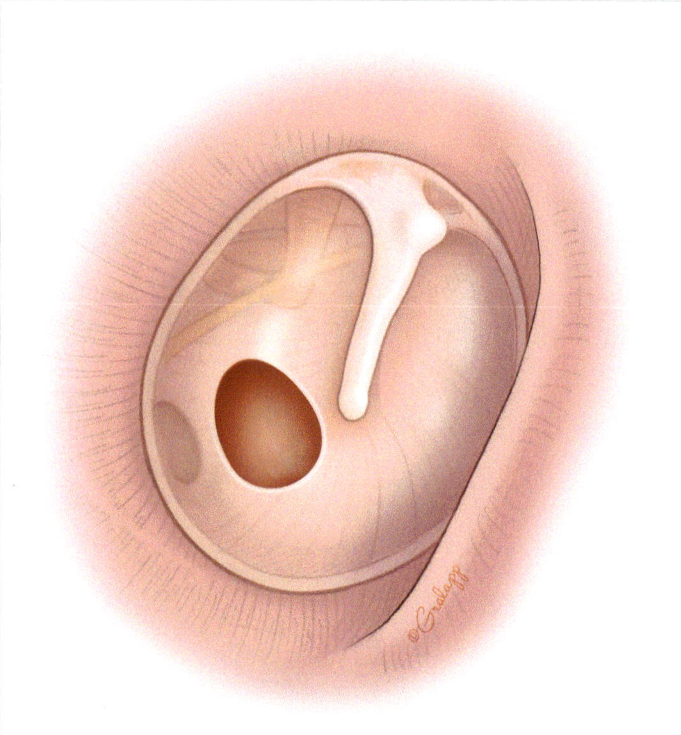

Fig. 5.8 Posterior central tympanic membrane perforation. Perforations such as this one, which lie posterior to the malleus, can be addressed with a transcanal approach to tympanoplasty.

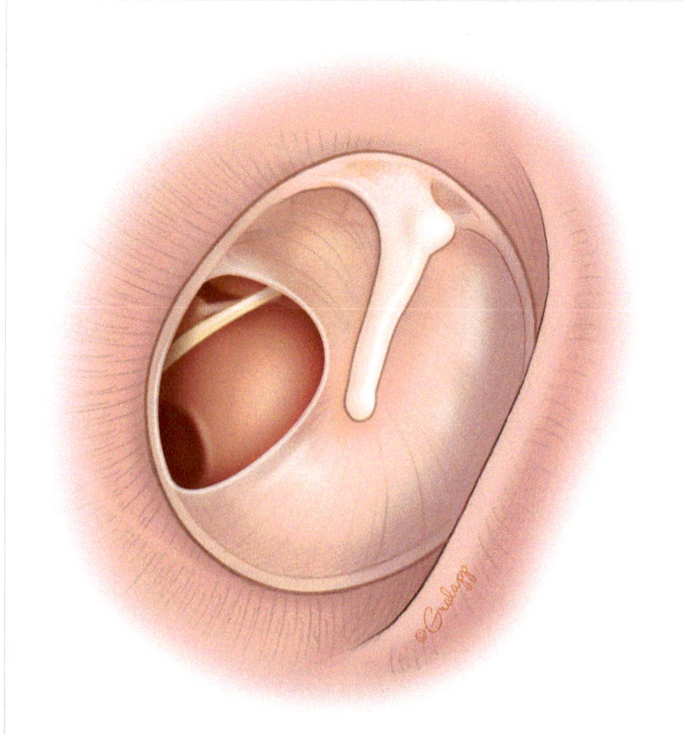

Fig. 5.9 Posterior marginal tympanic membrane perforation. The location over the round window leads to a greater conductive hearing loss due to phase cancellation.

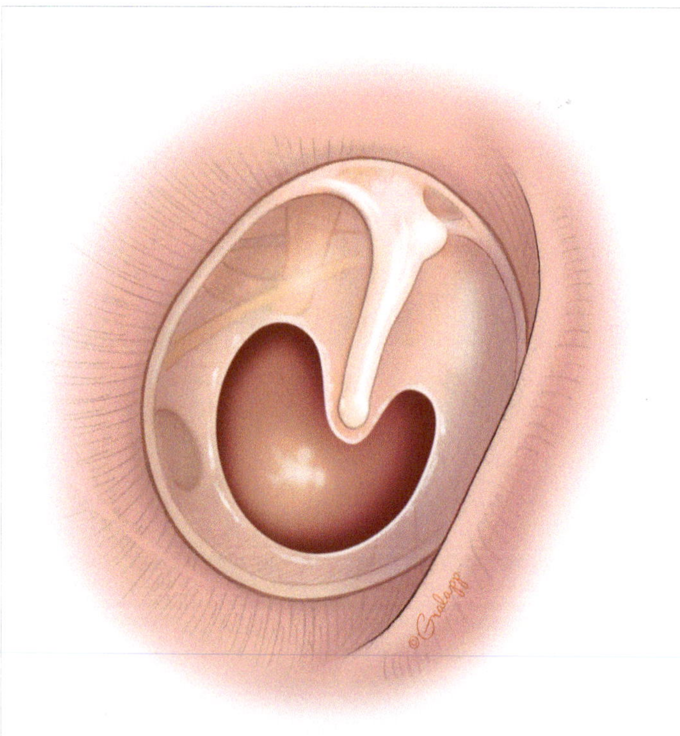

Fig. 5.10 Typical "kidney bean shaped" central tympanic membrane perforation.

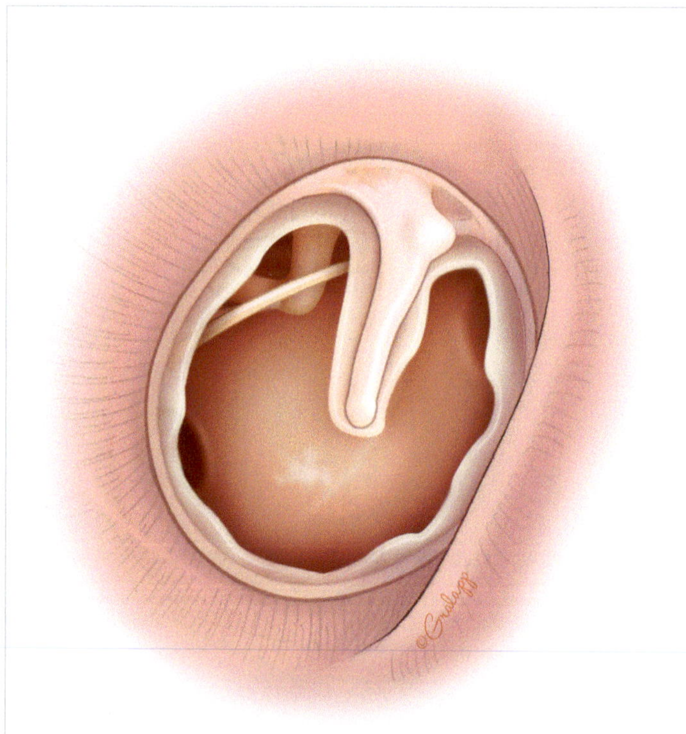

Fig. 5.11 Near-total tympanic membrane perforation with a small remaining rim at the annulus.

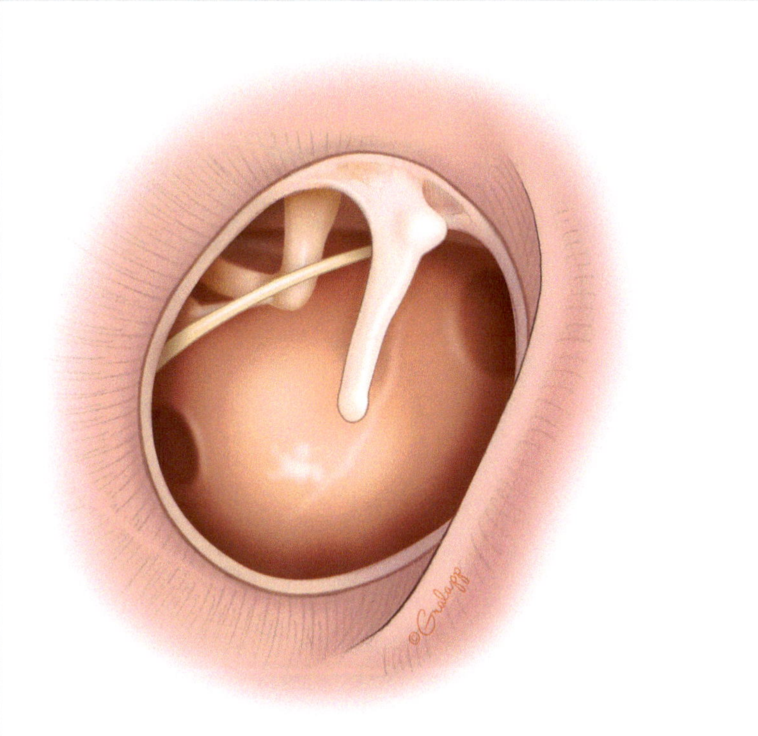

Fig. 5.12 Total tympanic membrane perforation.

5.3 Fascia Harvesting

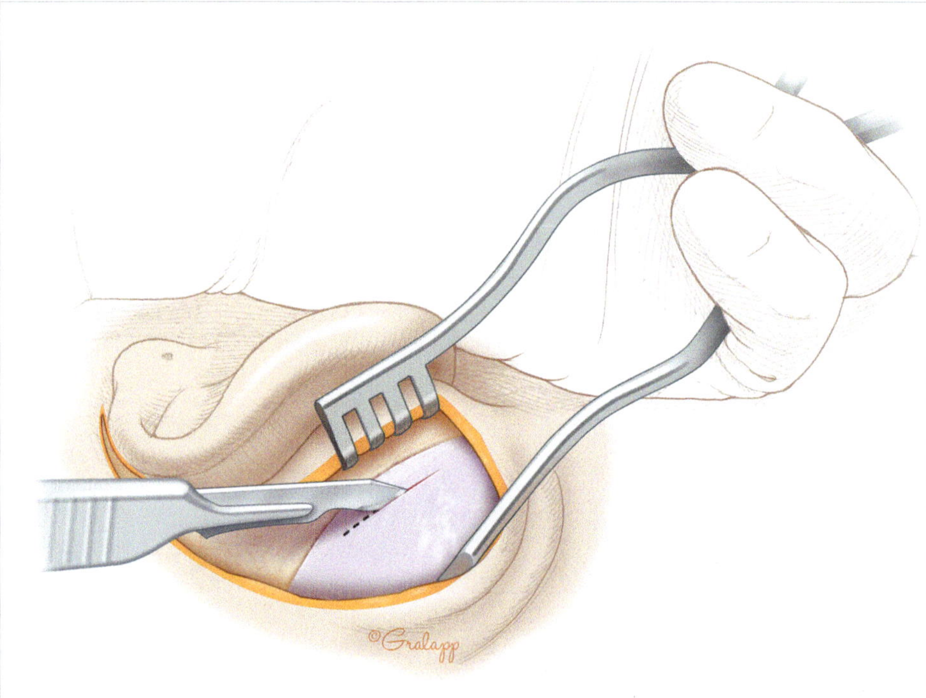

Fig. 5.13 Harvesting fascia for tympanoplasty. An incision is made above the linea temporalis leaving about 1 cm of intact fascia to facilitate closure of the postauricular incision.

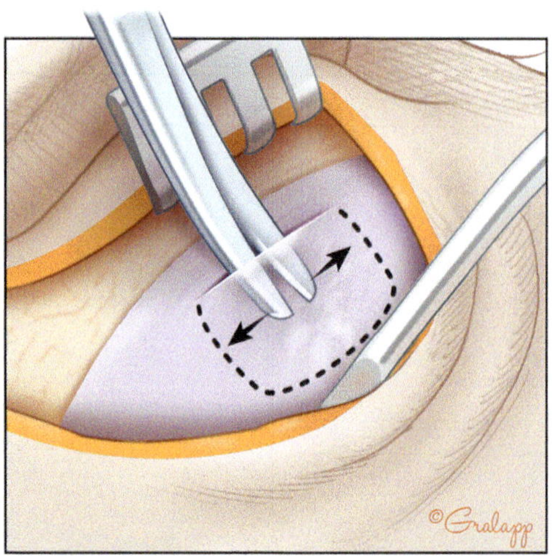

Fig. 5.14 Elevating the fascia off of the underlying temporalis muscle. Getting in the proper plane minimizes bleeding and obtains a cleaner piece of fascia.

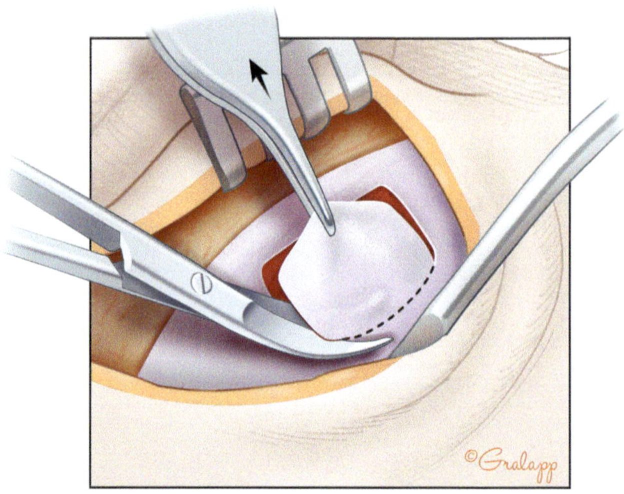

Fig. 5.15 The superior incision is made easier by curved scissors such as Fomon upper lateral cartilage scissors.

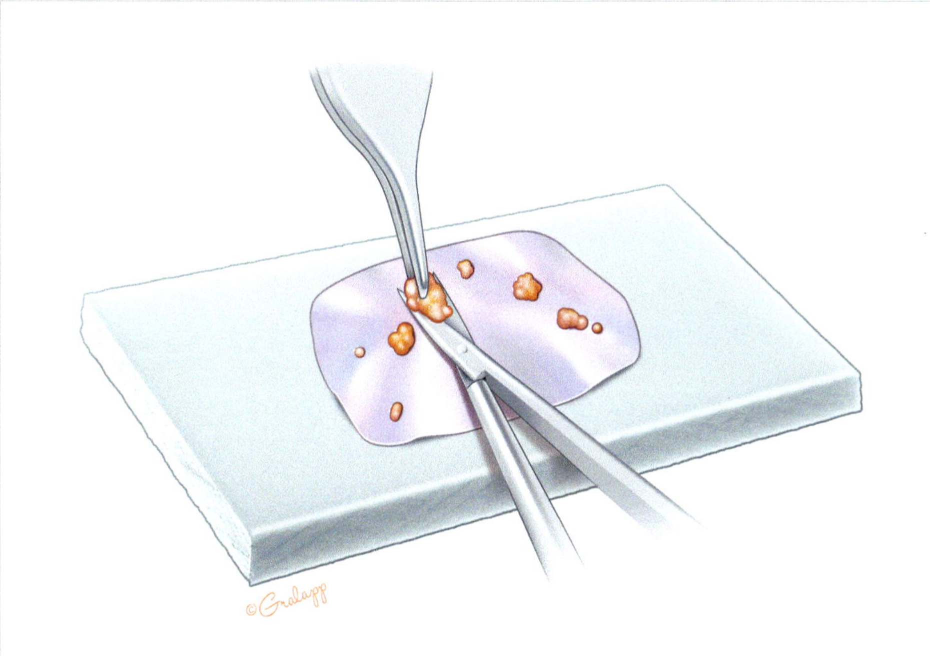

Fig. 5.16 Extra tissue on the fascia can be trimmed on a Teflon block where the fascia is cut to the desired shape.

5.4 Tragal Cartilage Harvesting

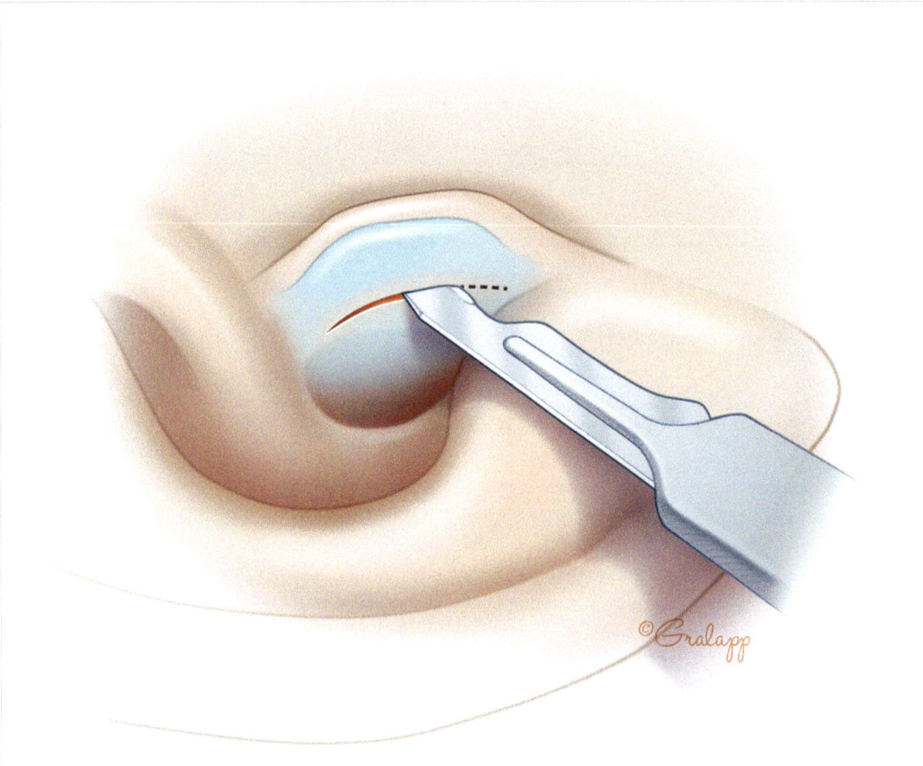

Fig. 5.17 In cartilage and/or perichondrium harvesting, the incision is hidden on the canal side of the tragus.

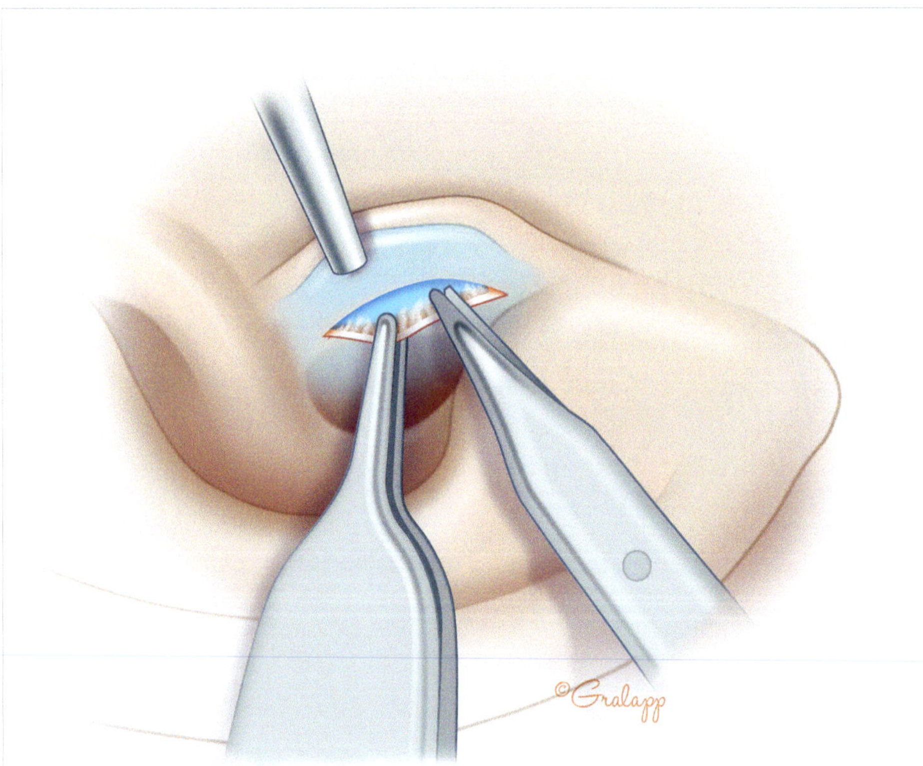

Fig. 5.18 Scissor dissection establishes the plane.

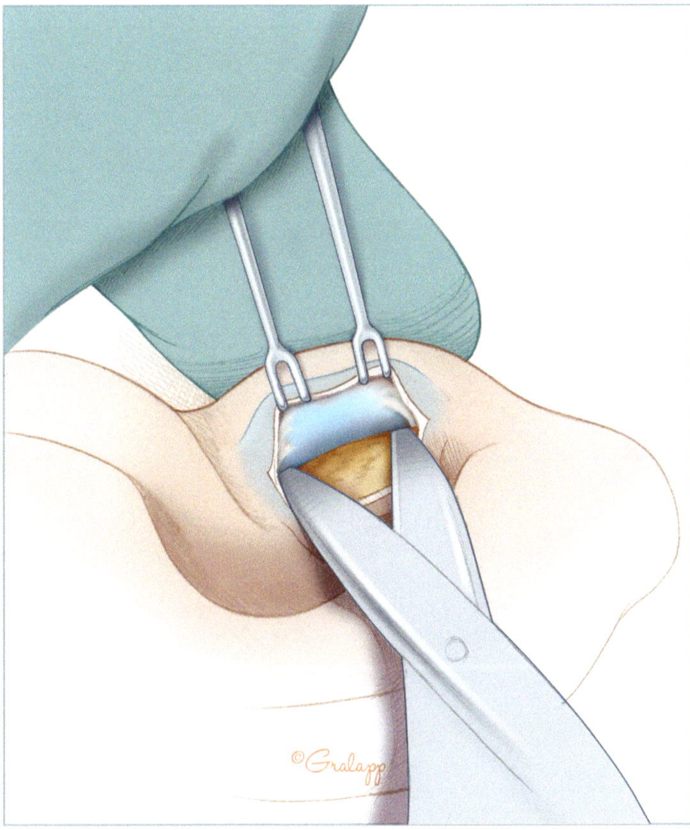

Fig. 5.19 Dissection is carried down the posterior surface of the tragus.

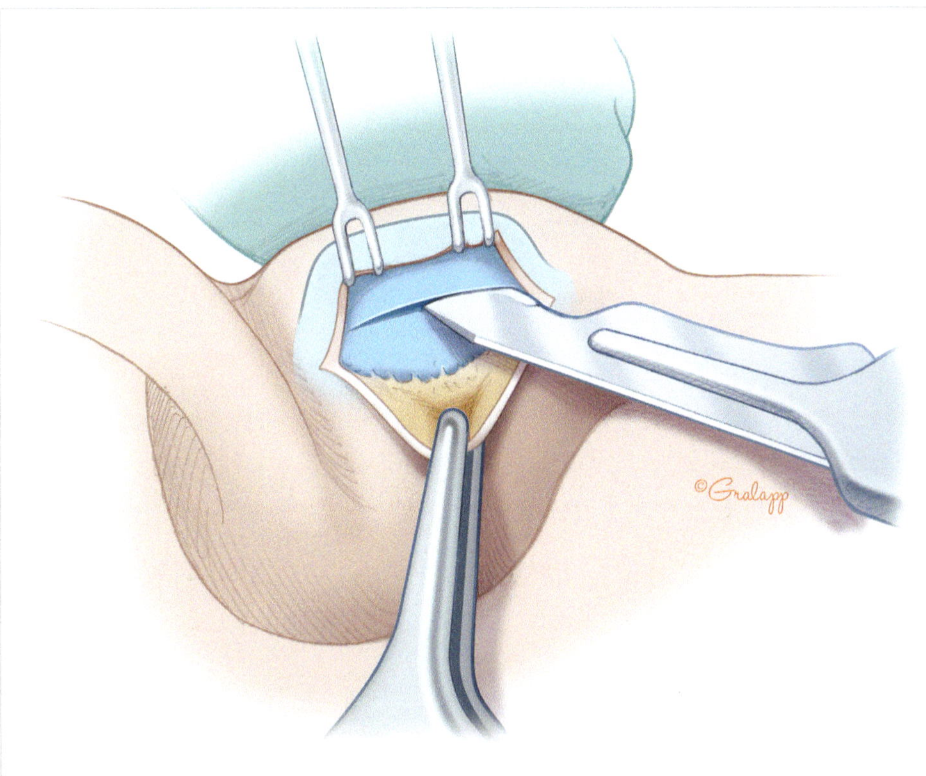

Fig. 5.20 Incision is made through the ipsilateral perichondrium and partial thickness into the cartilage.

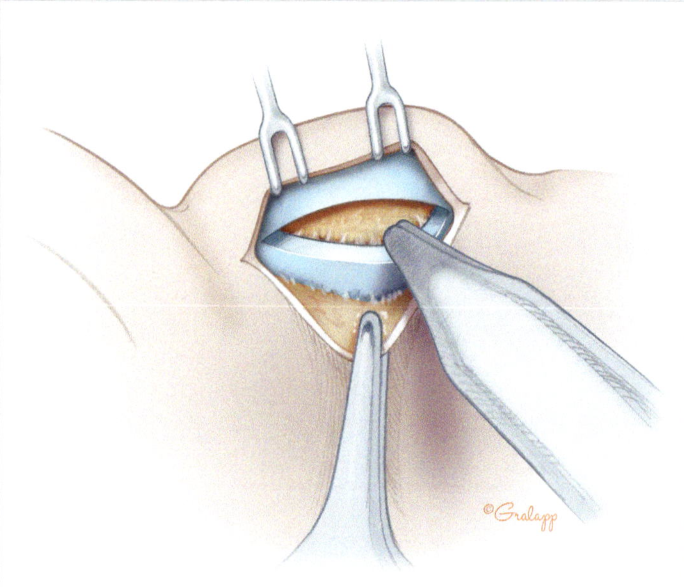

Fig. 5.21 Scissors complete the cartilage incision and establish the plane on the anterior surface.

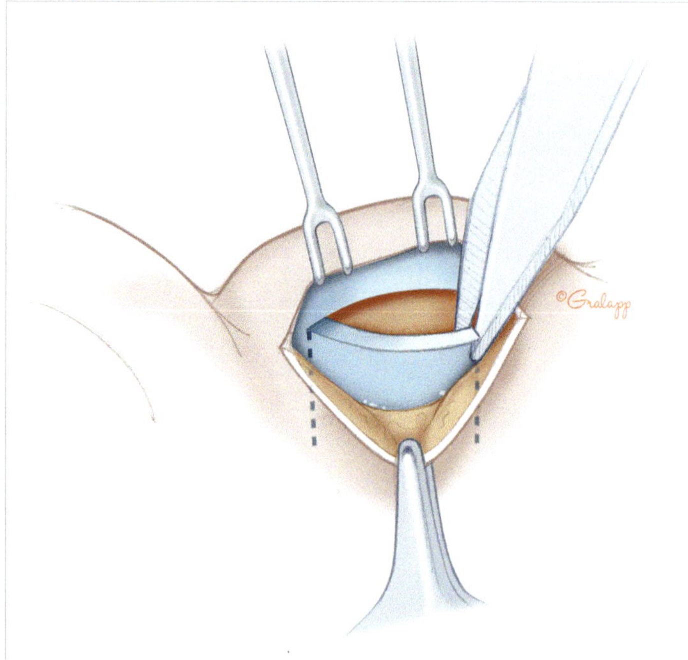

Fig. 5.22 Cuts are made superiorly and inferiorly.

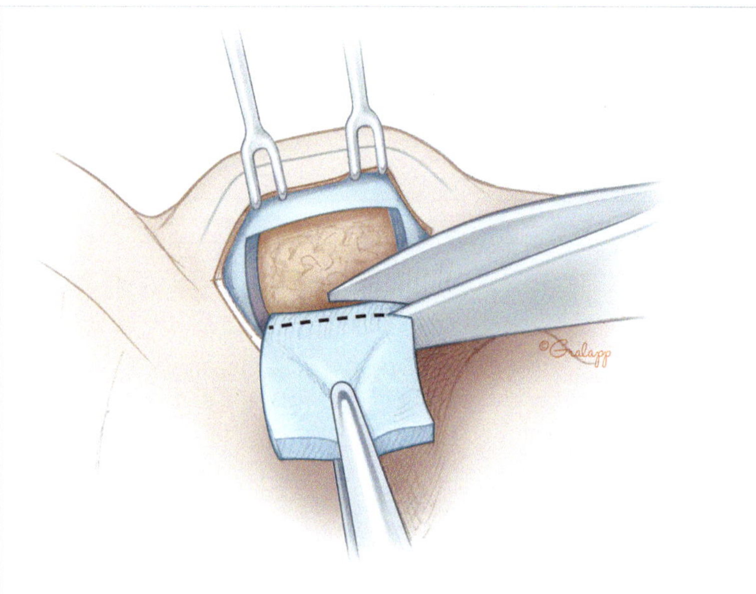

Fig. 5.23 Pulling laterally with Brown-Adson forceps while making the medial cut. Handling cartilage with standard toothed Adson forceps should be avoided, as they tend to lacerate the cartilage.

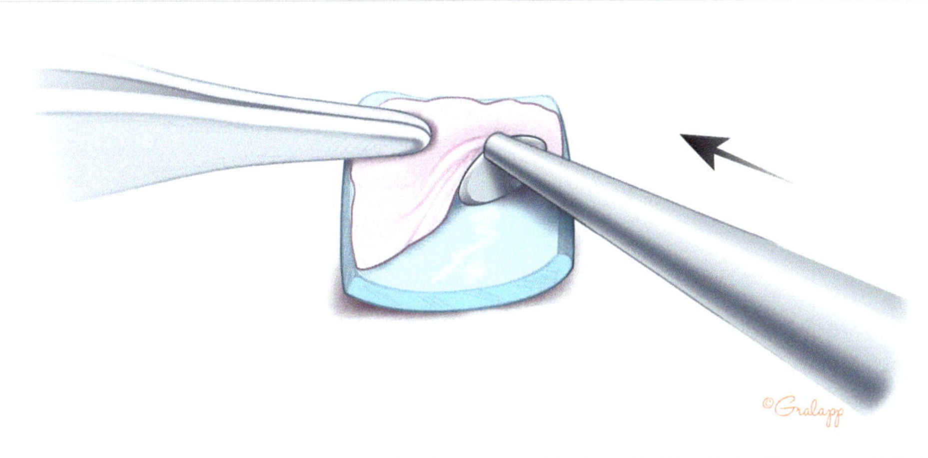

Fig. 5.24 Dissection of perichondrium from the cartilage with a stapes knife.

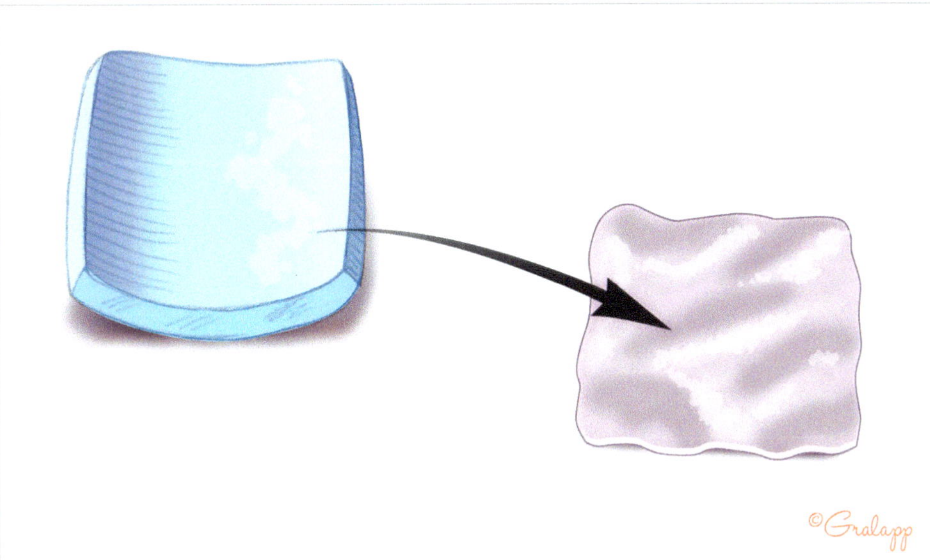

Fig. 5.25 Perichondrial graft is separated.

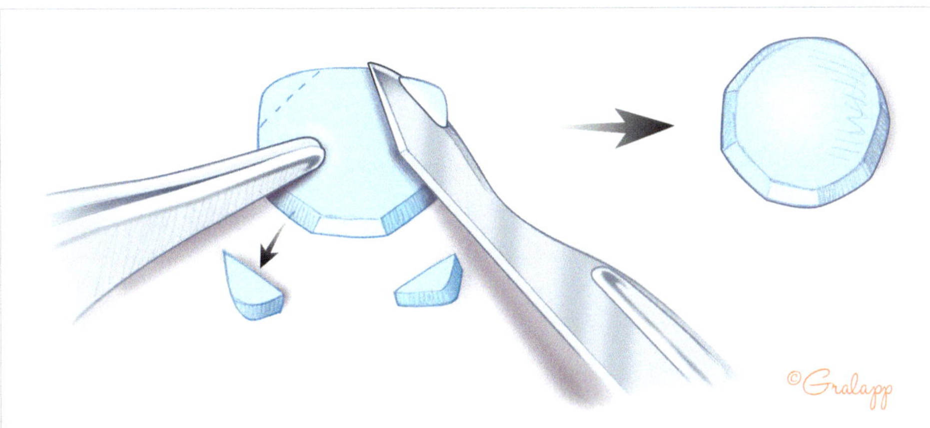

Fig. 5.26 Cartilage disc is shaped for use in tympanic membrane reconstruction, to overlie an ossicular prosthesis, and/or to repair an epitympanic defect. Note the beveling of the cartilage on the surface facing the tympanic membrane.

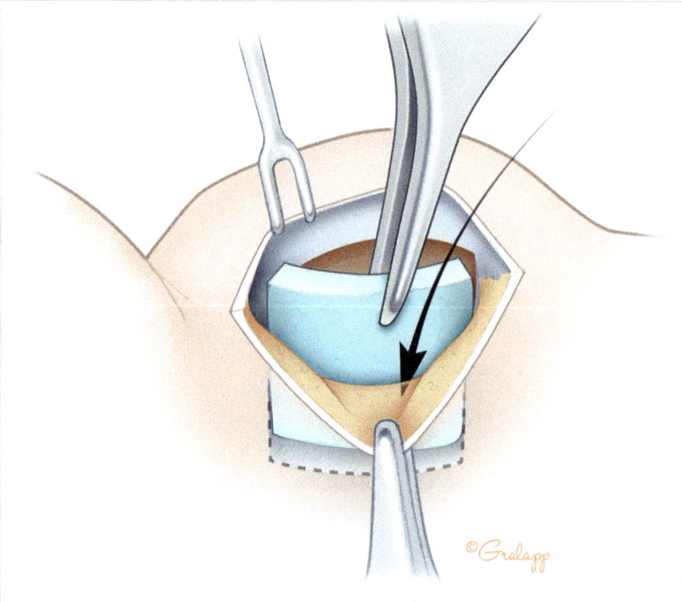

Fig. 5.27 If only perichondrium is needed, the cartilage can be replaced.

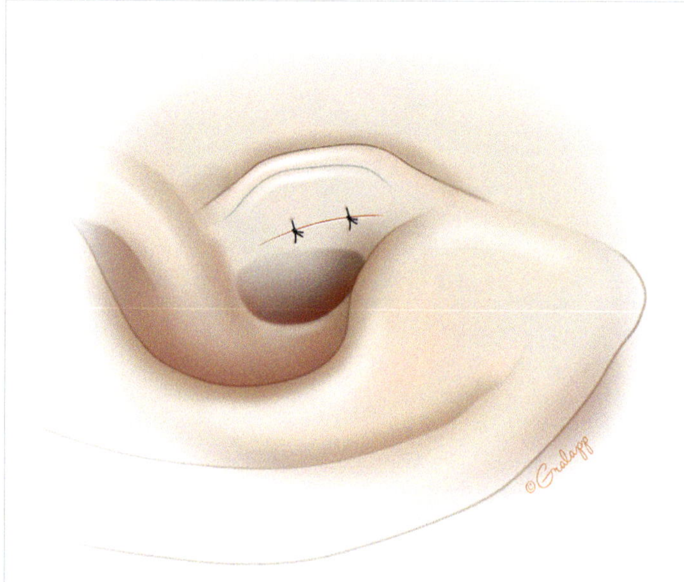

Fig. 5.28 The wound is closed loosely with two absorbable sutures.

5.5 Medial Graft Tympanoplasty

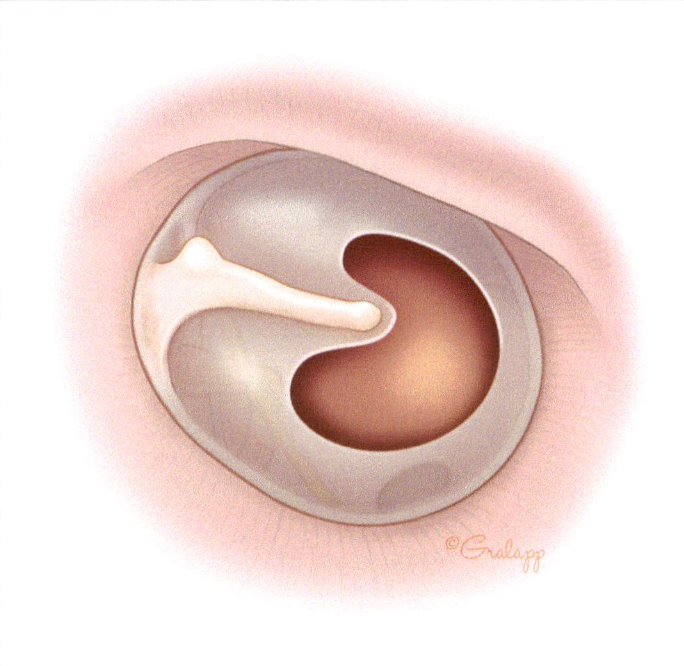

Fig. 5.29 Typical central tympanic membrane perforation. Most microsurgical tympanic membrane perforations are managed via medial grafting.

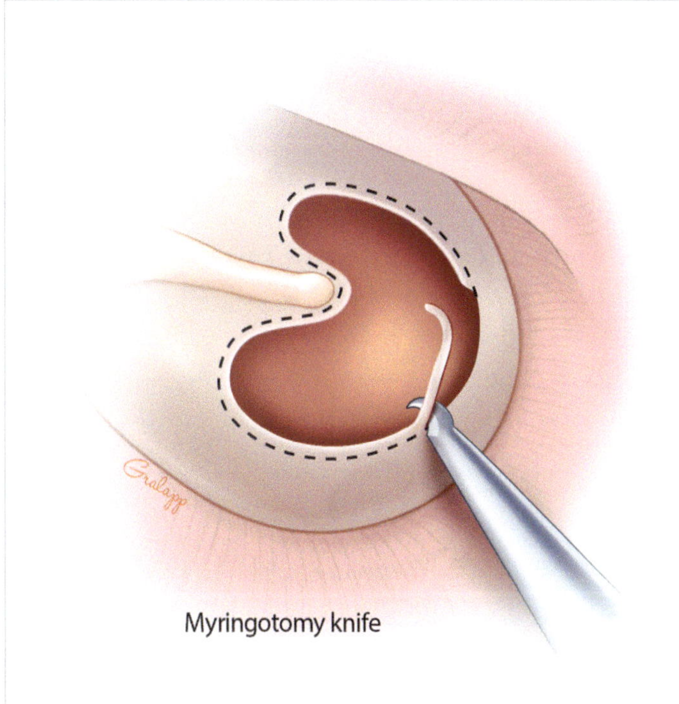

Fig. 5.30 Many surgeons rim the perforation by removing the squamous margin under the theory that an intact margin may inhibit graft healing. Others believe this step is unnecessary. The author stopped doing this maneuver decades ago with equivalent results.

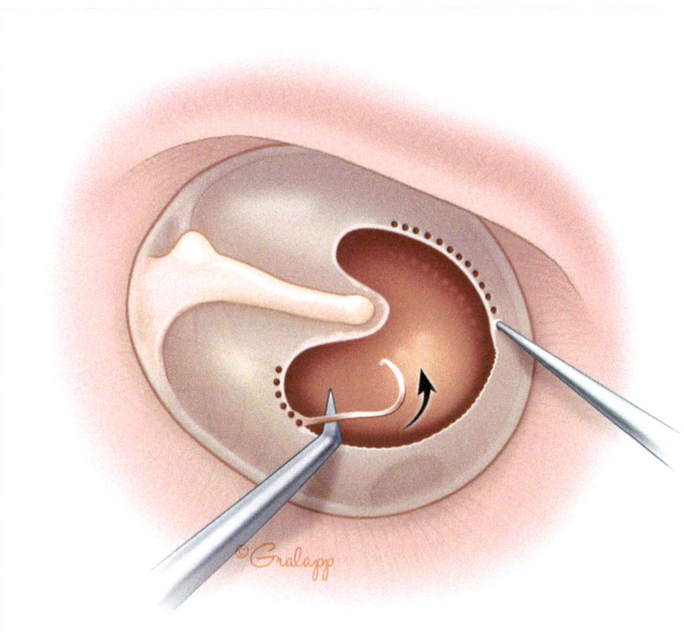

Fig. 5.31 A classical technique of rimming is to create a “pie crust” edge with a needle and then stripping the rimming with a hook or cup forceps.

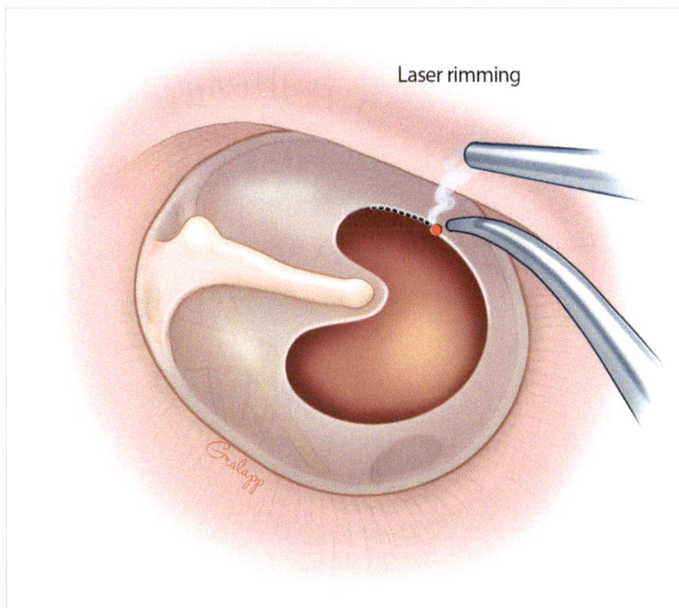

Fig. 5.32 Rimming of the tympanic membrane perforation with a laser.

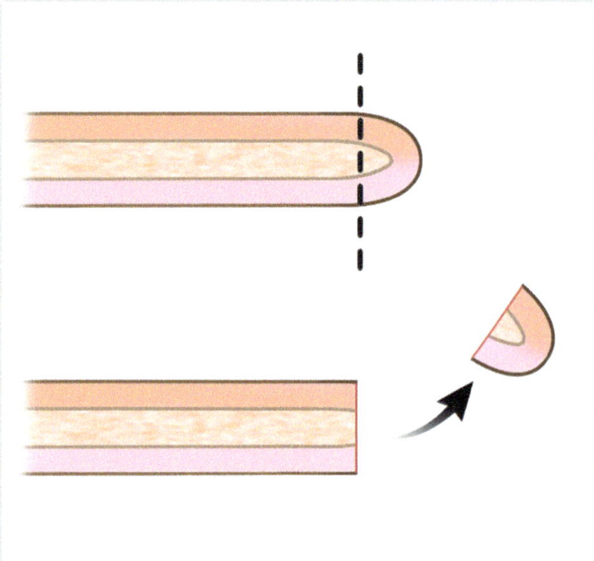

Fig. 5.33 The concept of perforation rimming is to remove the epithelial margin of the perforation.

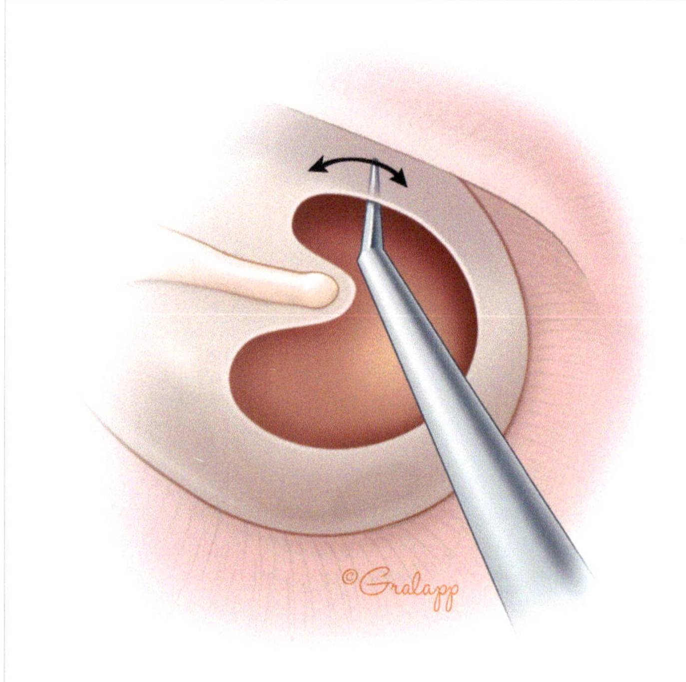

Fig. 5.34 Roughing up the mucosal surface on the medial aspect of the tympanic membrane enhances adhesion of the graft and opens vessels for neovascularization.

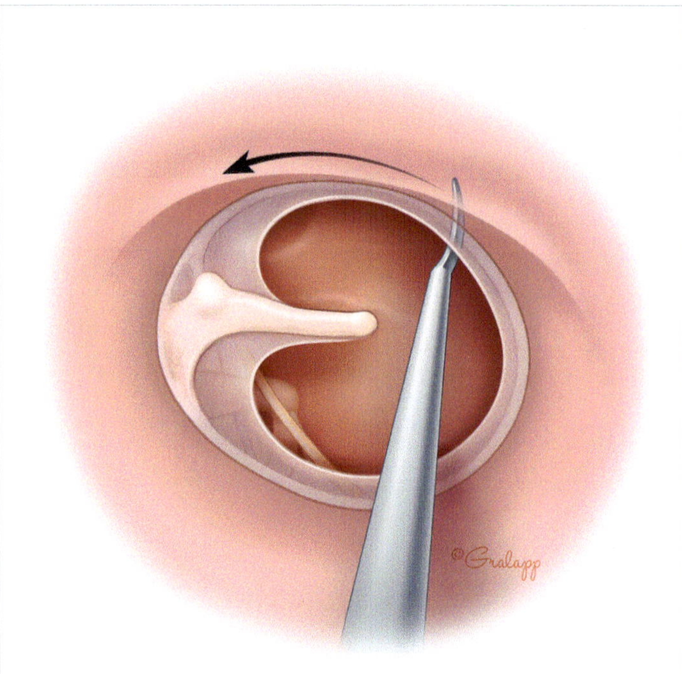

Fig. 5.35 Scoring the mucosa in the protympanum is important for graft adhesion in anterior marginal perforations.

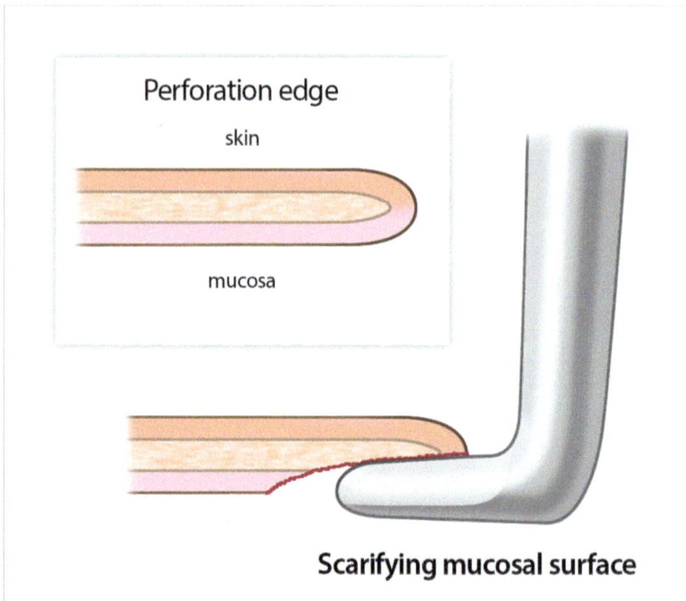

Fig. 5.36 The concept of disrupting the medial mucosal layer of the tympanic membrane is that it encourages vascularization of the graft.

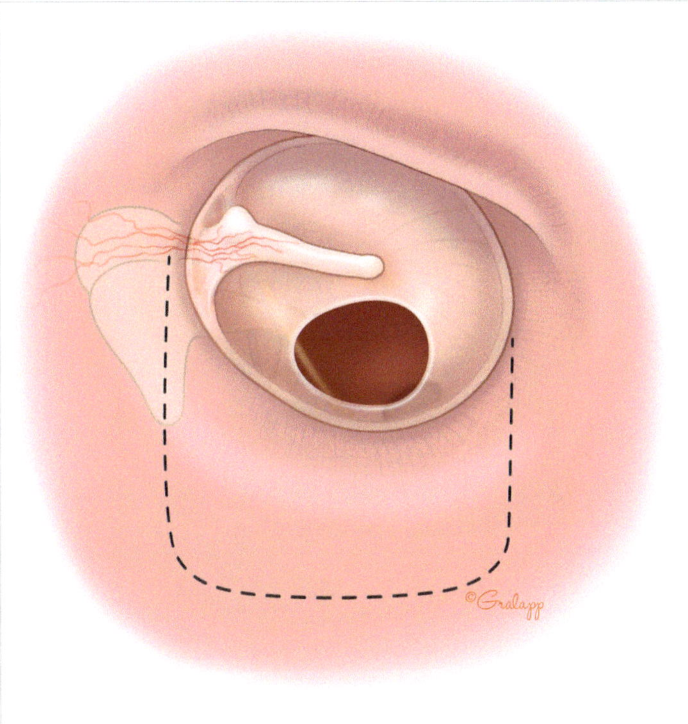

Fig. 5.37 The tympanomeatal flap used in tympanoplasty and ossiculoplasty is longer than that used in stapes surgery.

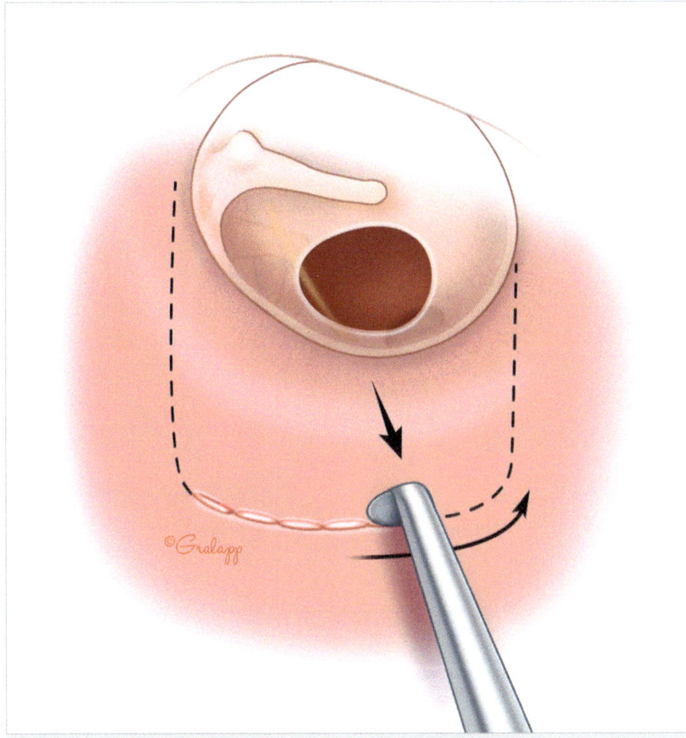

Fig. 5.38 Crushing the tissue along the incision line reduces bleeding and helps obtain a smoothly cut incision.

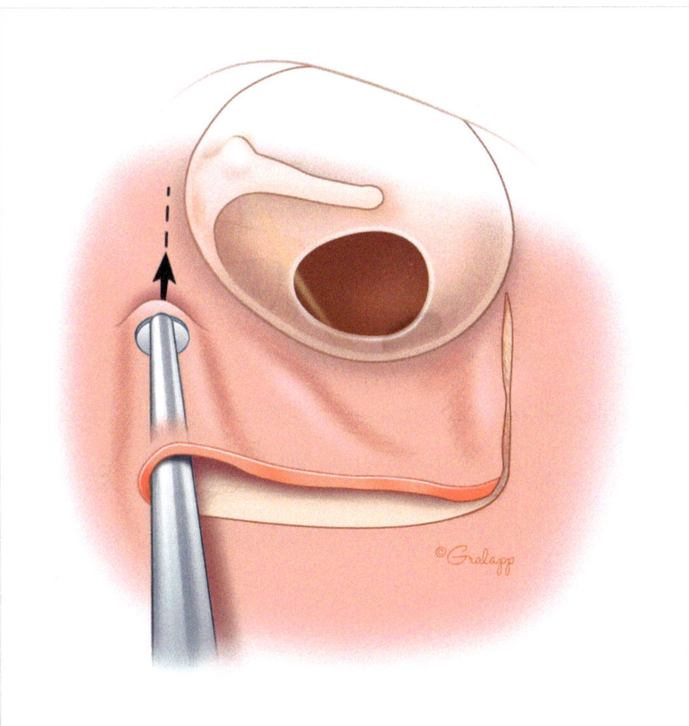

Fig. 5.39 Tunneling superiorly under the vascular strip.

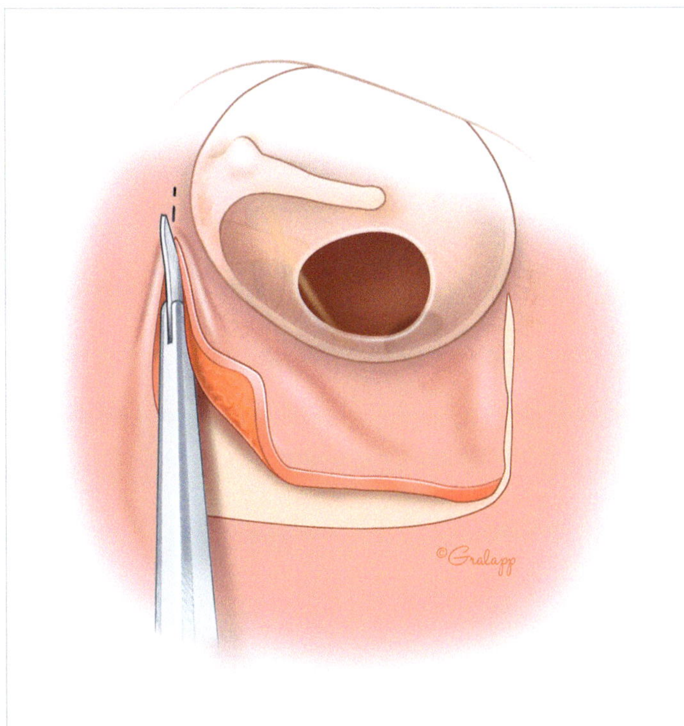

Fig. 5.40 Cutting the vascular strip with microscissors reduces bleeding and achieves a cleaner incision.

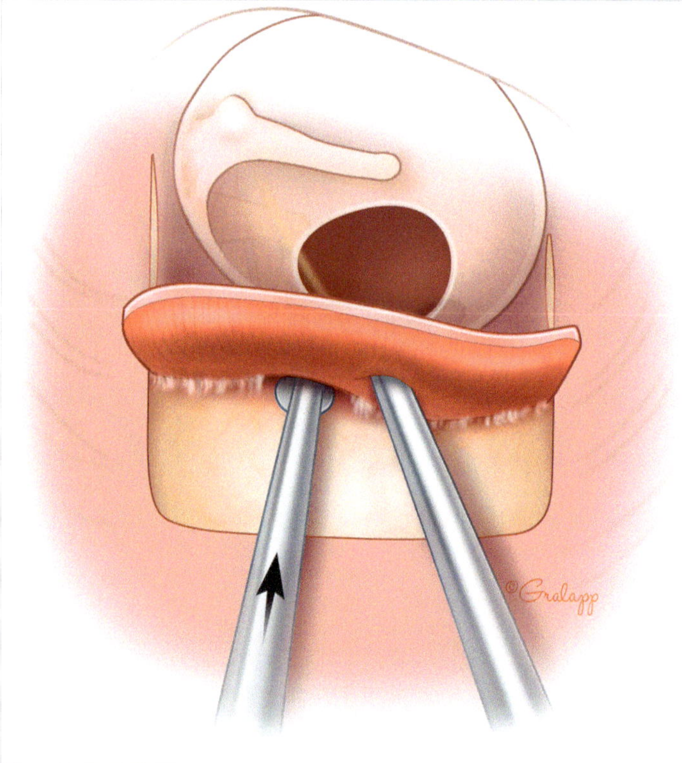

Fig. 5.41 Elevation of the tympanomeatal flap toward the annulus.

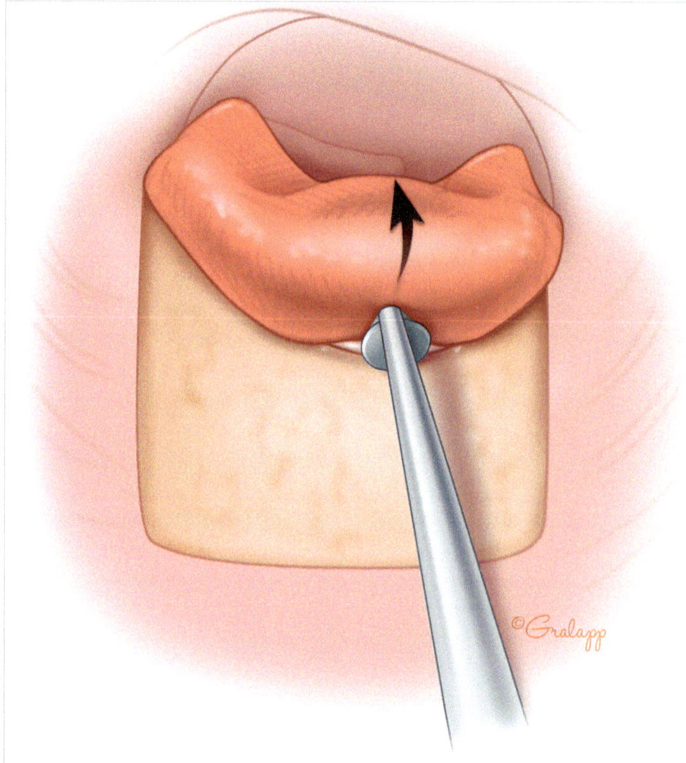

Fig. 5.42 Elevating the tympanic annulus.

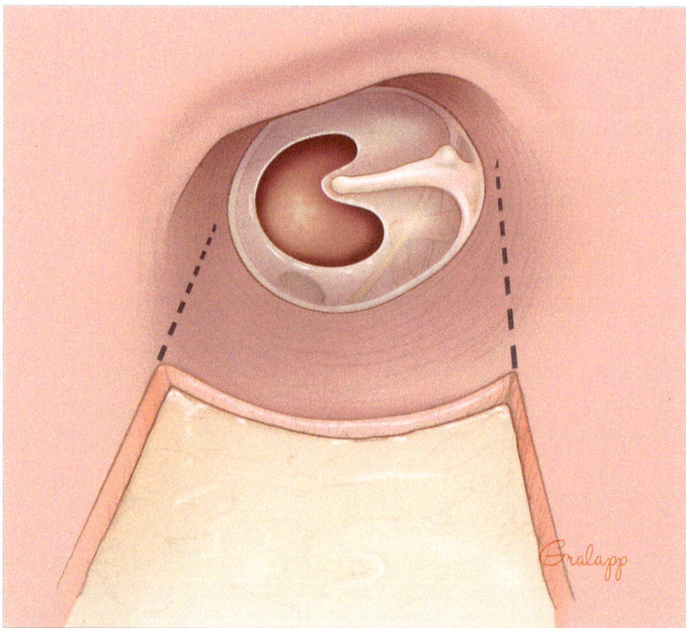

Fig. 5.43 Postauricular approach to tympanoplasty after elevation of a posterior ear canal flap (Koerner's flap).

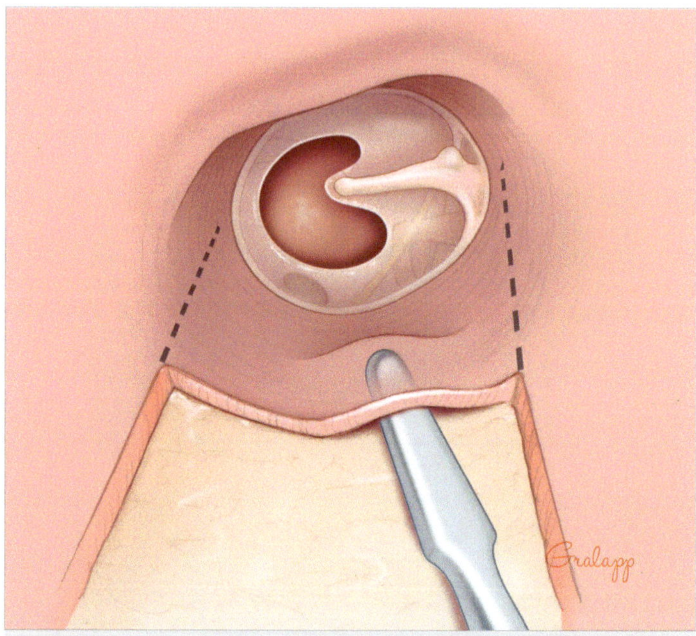

Fig. 5.44 Working via the postauricular approach flap elevation can be done with larger periosteal elevators.

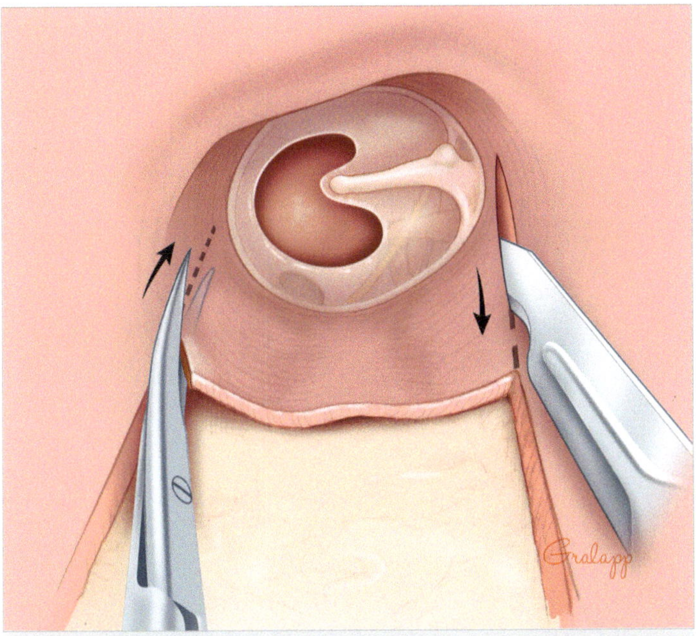

Fig. 5.45 From the postauricular approach, the tympanomeatal flap can be cut rapidly with scissors or a blade rather than microsurgical instruments.

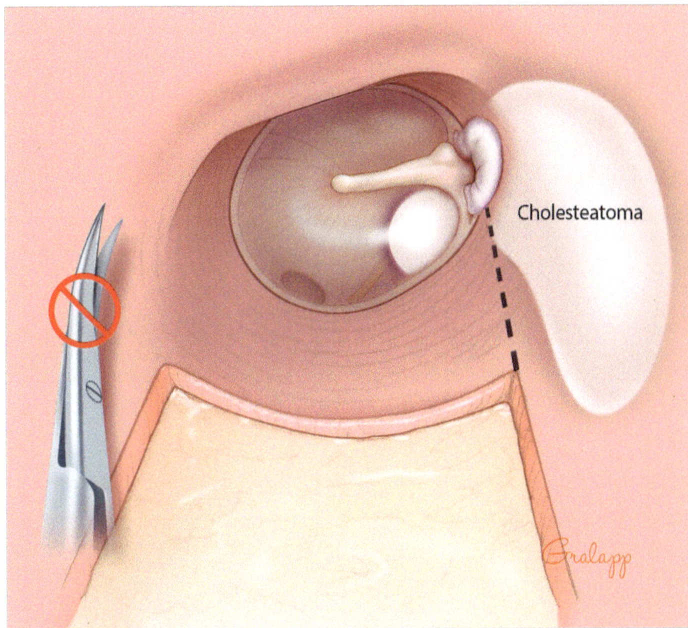

Fig. 5.46 In cholesteatoma, only a superior incision is utilized in tympanoplasty which outlines an inferiorly based meatal skin flap.

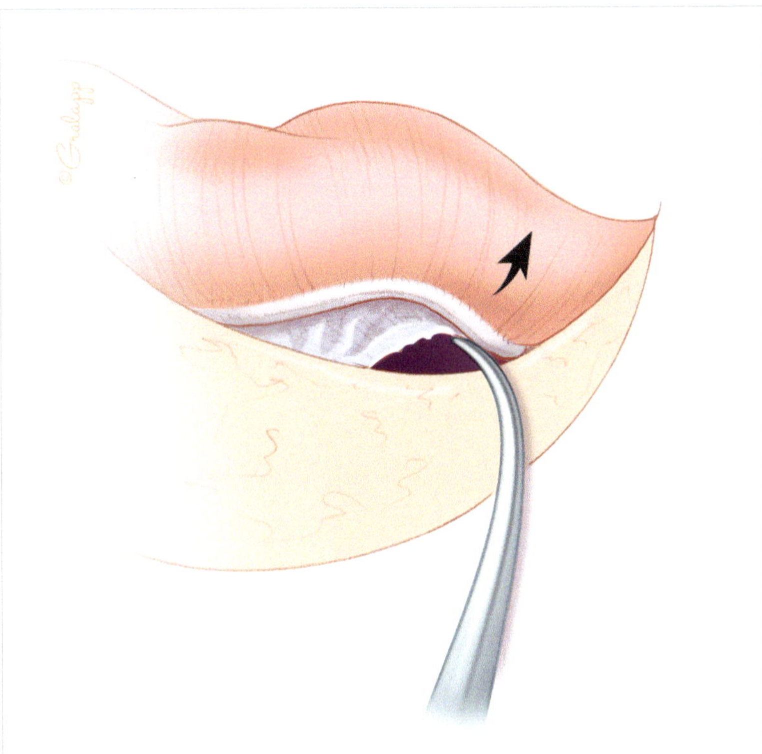

Fig. 5.47 The tympanic mucosa is lysed with a curved needle. When done under local, lidocaine is infused into the middle ear to anesthetize the tympanic mucosa. To avoid anesthetizing the labyrinth with resultant postoperative vertigo, lidocaine should be promptly suctioned from the middle ear, especially from the round window niche where it tends to accumulate.

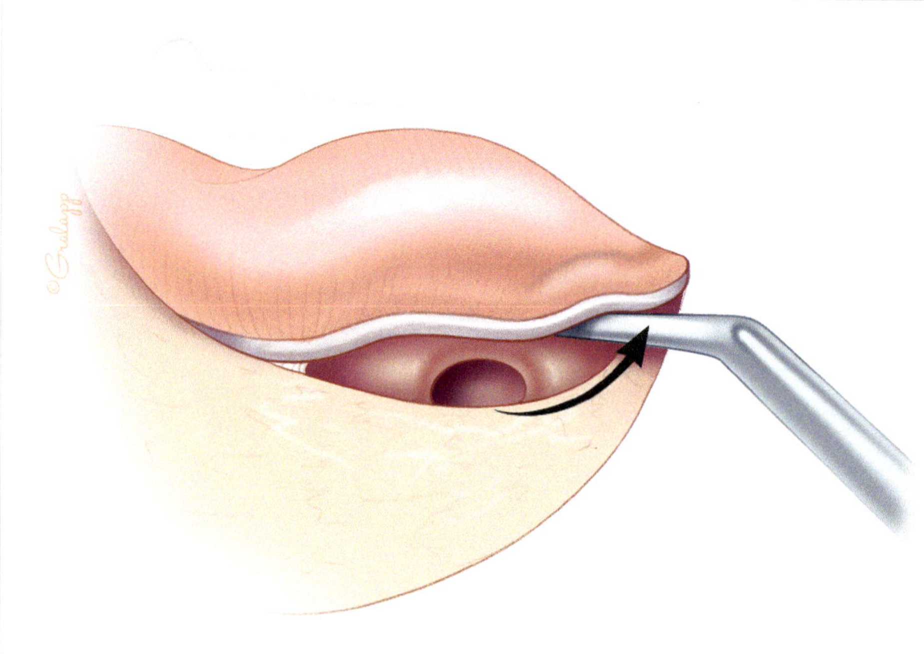

Fig. 5.48 Elevation of the tympanic annulus inferiorly using an annulus elevator. To avoid tearing, it is important to maintain firm pressure against the bone. Elevation is with the side of the shaft, not the tip of the instrument. When under local, this maneuver is often incompletely anesthetized.

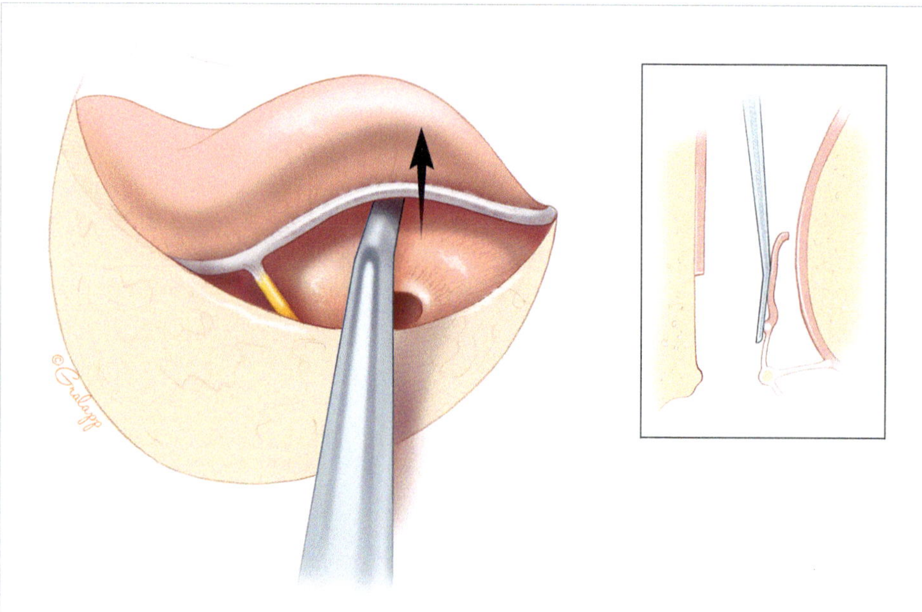

Fig. 5.49 It is important to have the middle ear exposure remain adequately open throughout the surgery. Using the back of the annulus elevator, the flap can be pushed against the anterior canal wall where surface tension will adhere to it.

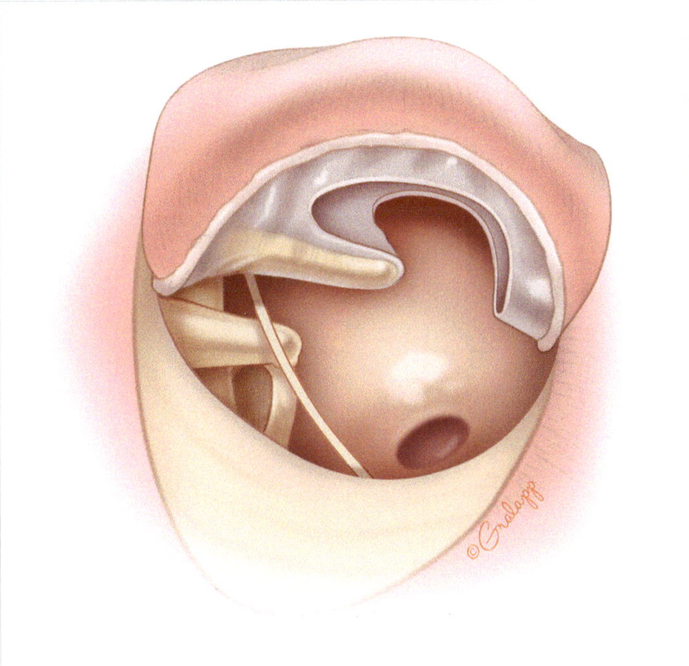

Fig. 5.50 Tympanomeatal flap folded forward revealing the undersurface of the remnant tympanic membrane.

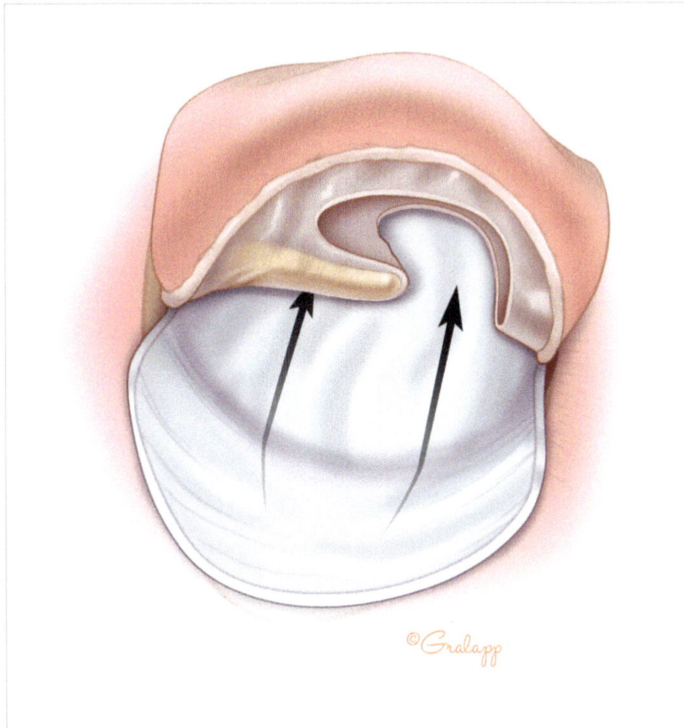

Fig. 5.51 The fascia graft is positioned under the tympanic membrane remnant.

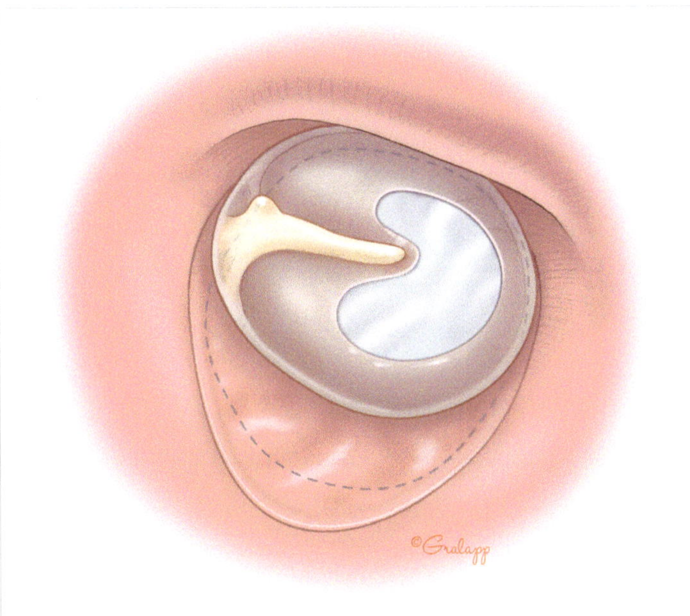

Fig. 5.52 Replacement of the tympanomeatal flap with the graft in place. Dotted line represents the graft on the medial aspect of the tympanic membrane and under the tympanomeatal flap.

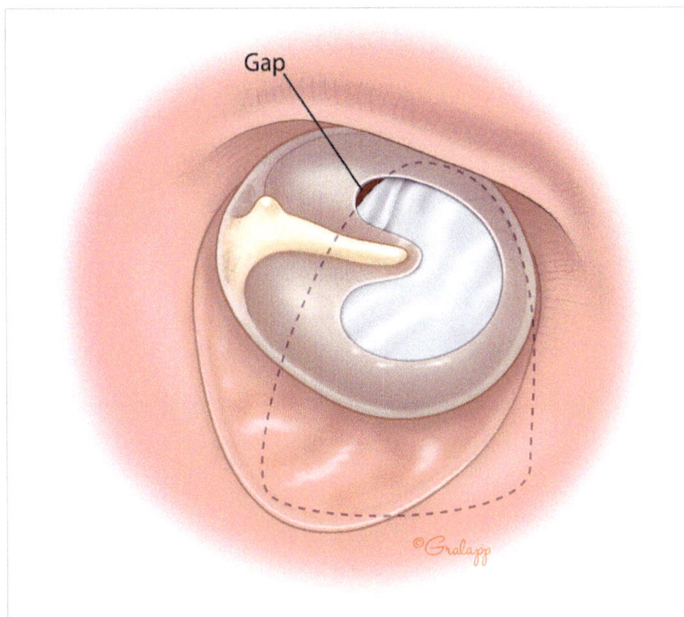

Fig. 5.53 Usually the graft is not optimally adjusted after its initial placement. It is essential in tympanoplasty that the graft underlies the margin of the perforation significantly to foster its vascularization and integration with the tympanic membrane remnant.

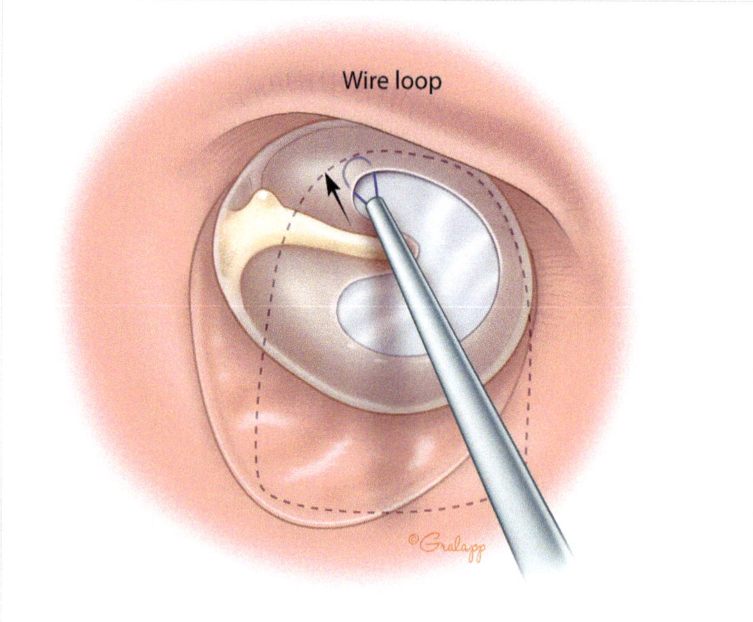

Fig. 5.54 Adjusting the graft into position using a wire loop. If suction is needed, use a small diameter suction (e.g., no. 3 Fr or no. 20 needle) and keep an instrument (e.g., annulus elevator or wire loop) between the suction and graft. When using a suction near a graft in position, it is prudent to request your assistant to be ready to plug the suction so that it can be disengaged without disturbing the graft.

5.6 Anterior Perforation Repair

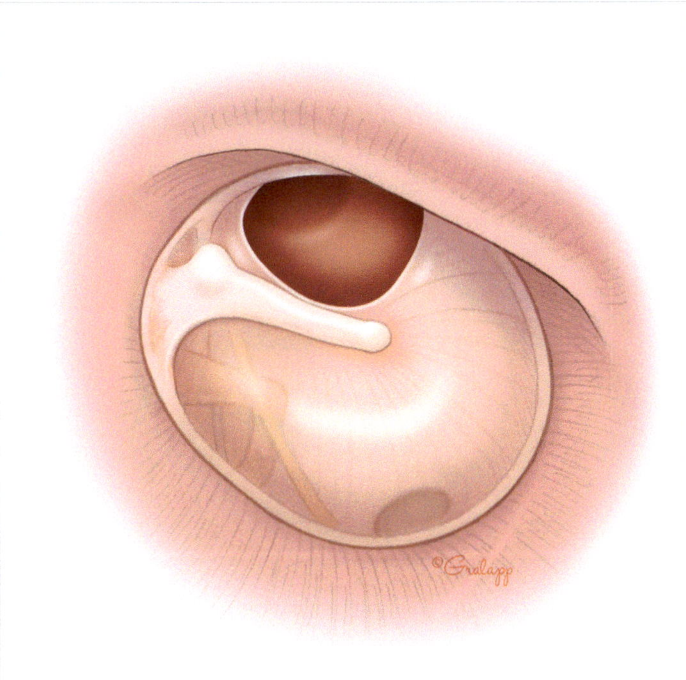

Fig. 5.55 Anterior tympanic membrane perforations are more technically challenging and have a higher reperforation rate unless specialized techniques are utilized. Canaloplasty to remove overhanging anterior canal bulge is commonly needed (see section 3.8 Anterior Canaloplasty in Chapter 3).

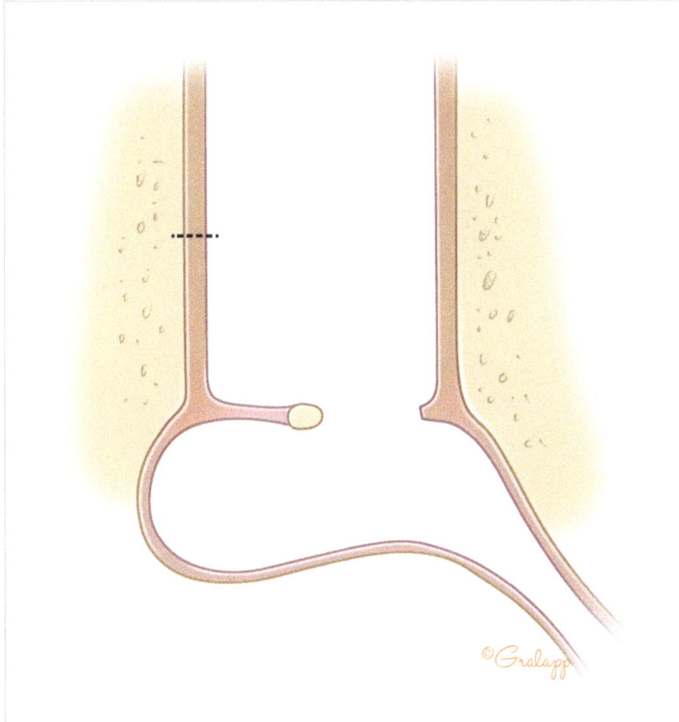

Fig. 5.56 Anterior tympanic membrane perforation. Dotted line represents canal skin = incision.

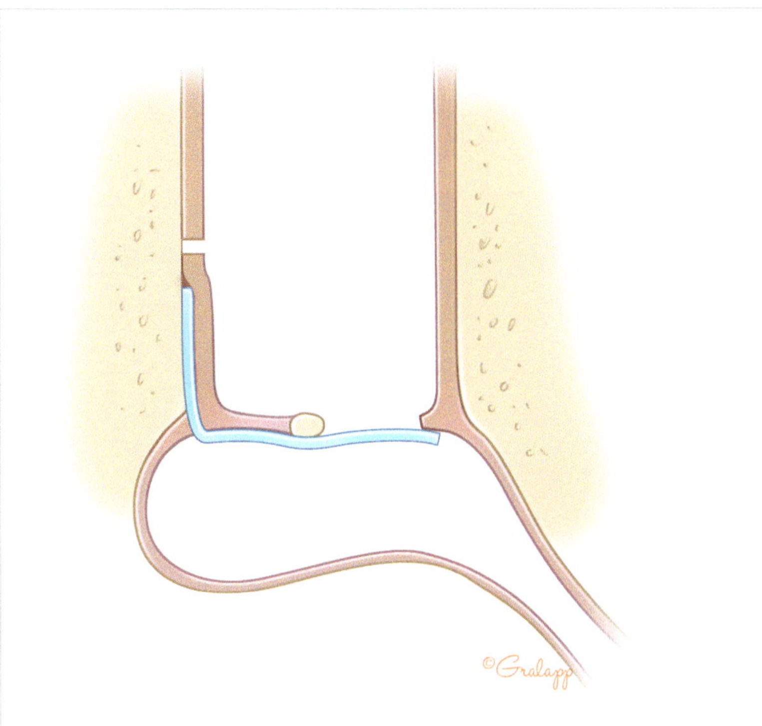

Fig. 5.57 Classical medial fascia graft tympanoplasty with insufficient purchase anteriorly has a higher rate of failure.

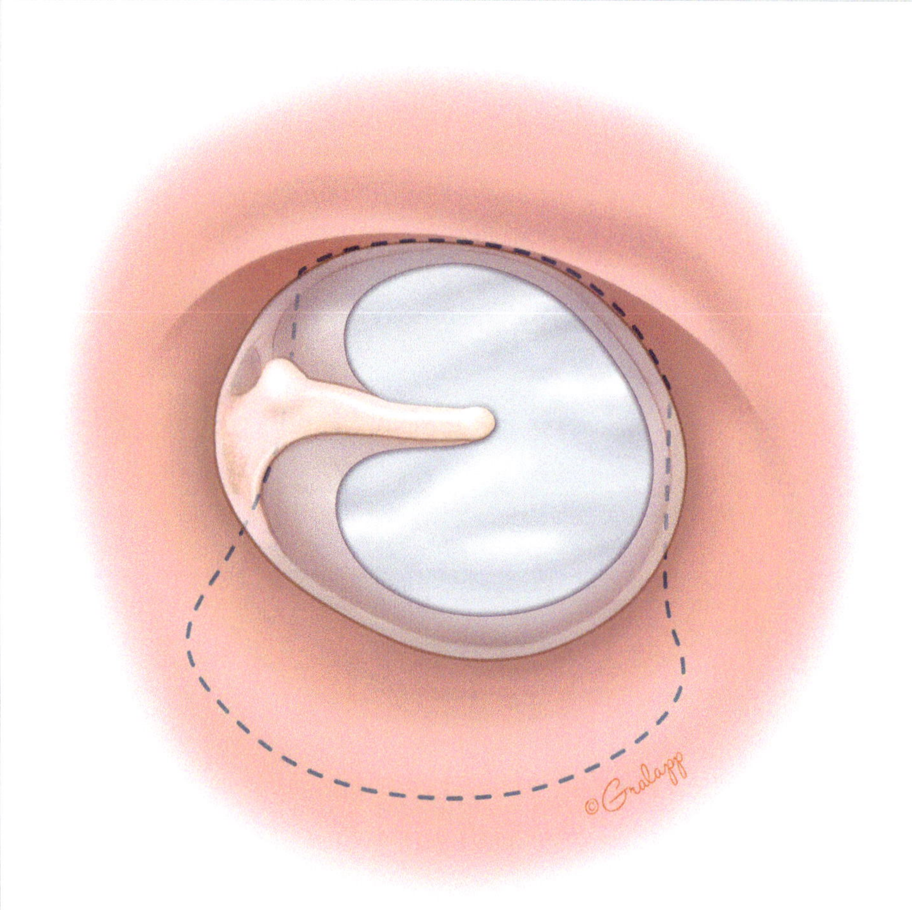

Fig. 5.58 Classical medial fascia graft tympanoplasty with insufficient purchase anteriorly has a higher rate of failure.

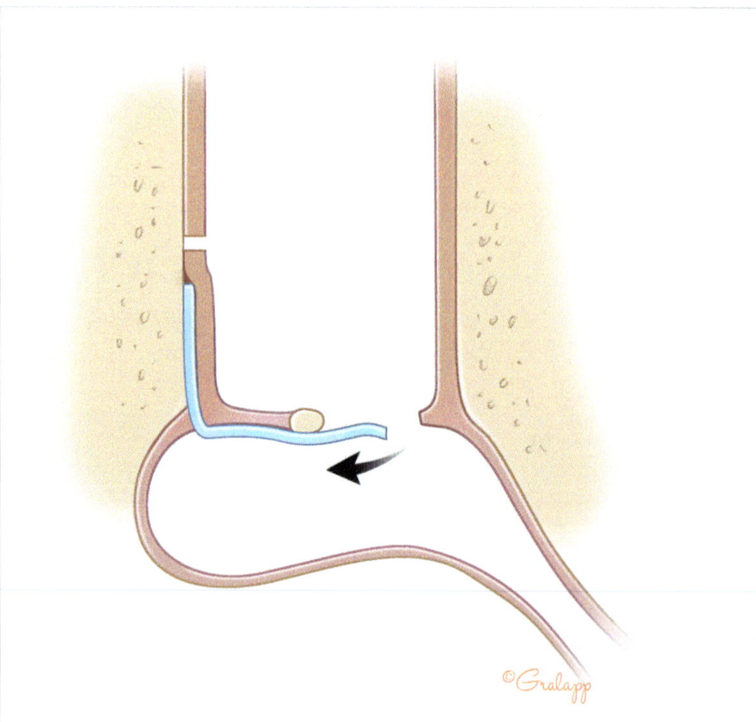

Fig. 5.59 Classical medial fascia graft tympanoplasty failure due to graft retraction during healing.

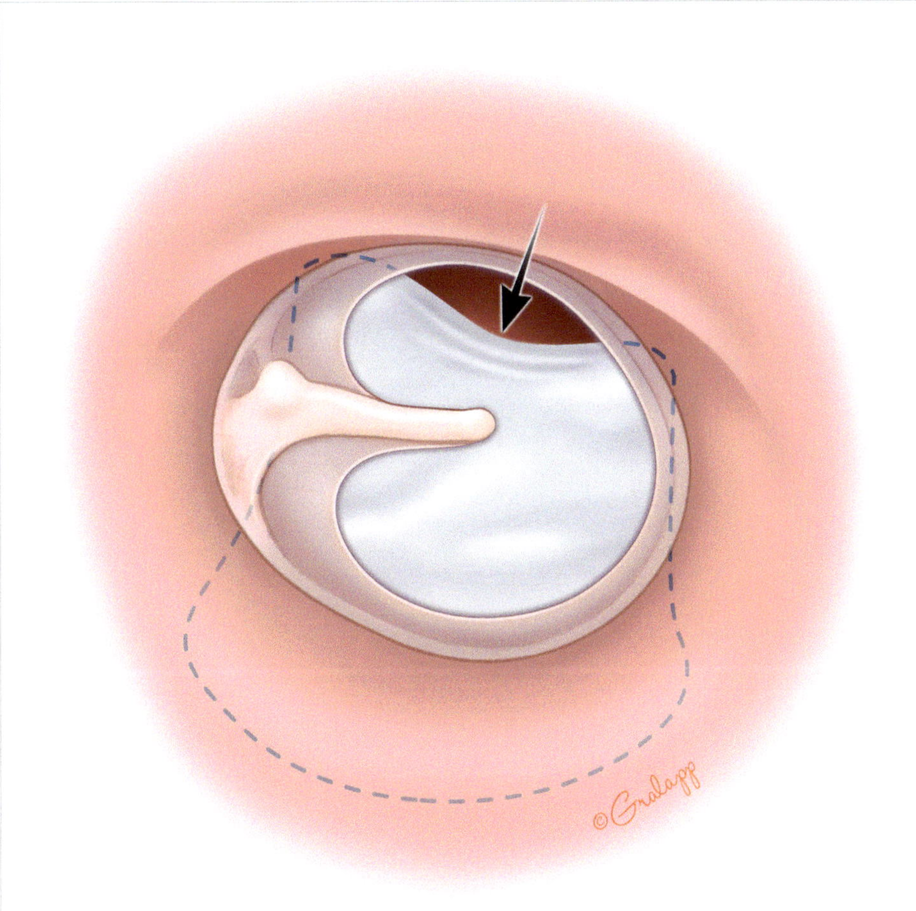

Fig. 5.60 Recurrent perforation due to graft retraction.

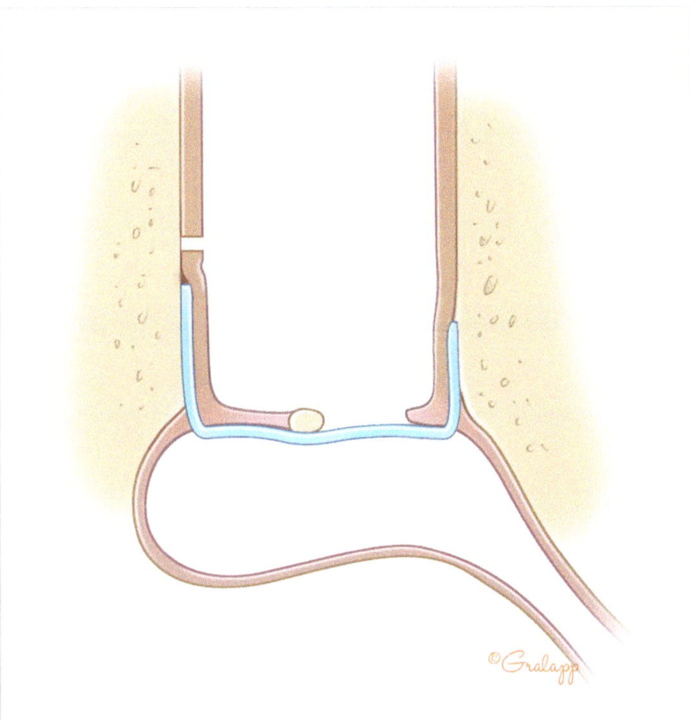

Fig. 5.61 Anterior "window shade" technique.

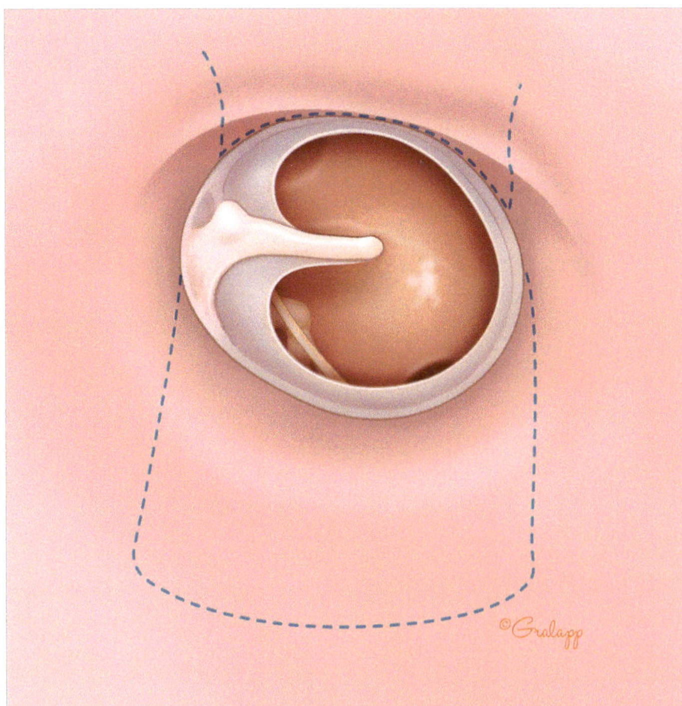

Fig. 5.62 Anterior incisions in "window shade" technique.

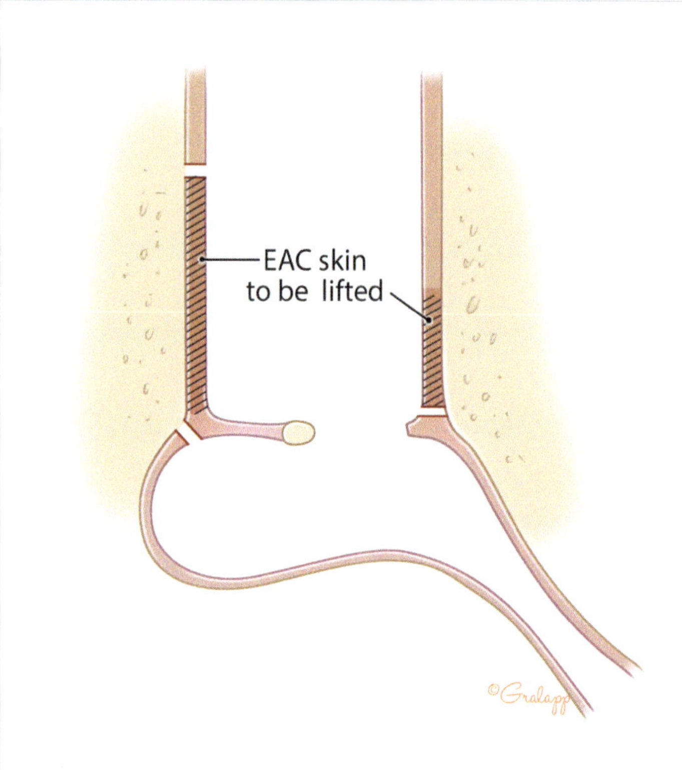

Fig. 5.63 Flap elevation in "window shade" technique.

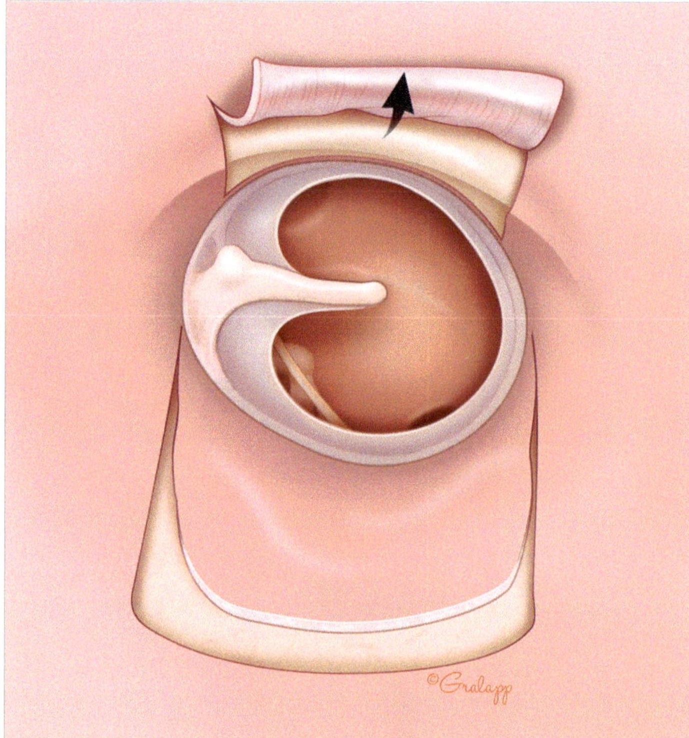

Fig. 5.64 Anterior flap elevation in "window shade" technique.

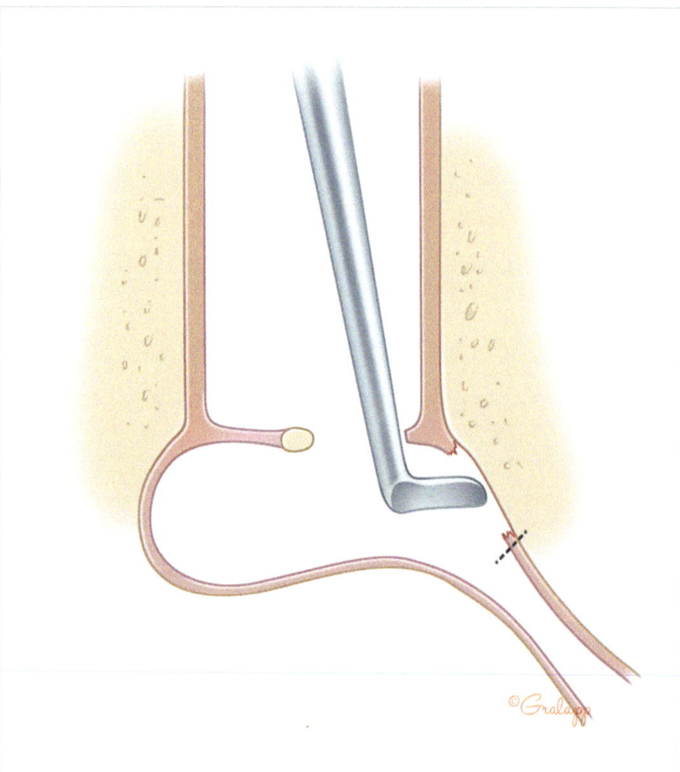

Fig. 5.65 Disrupting protympanic mucosa to facilitate adhesion and vascular ingrowth.

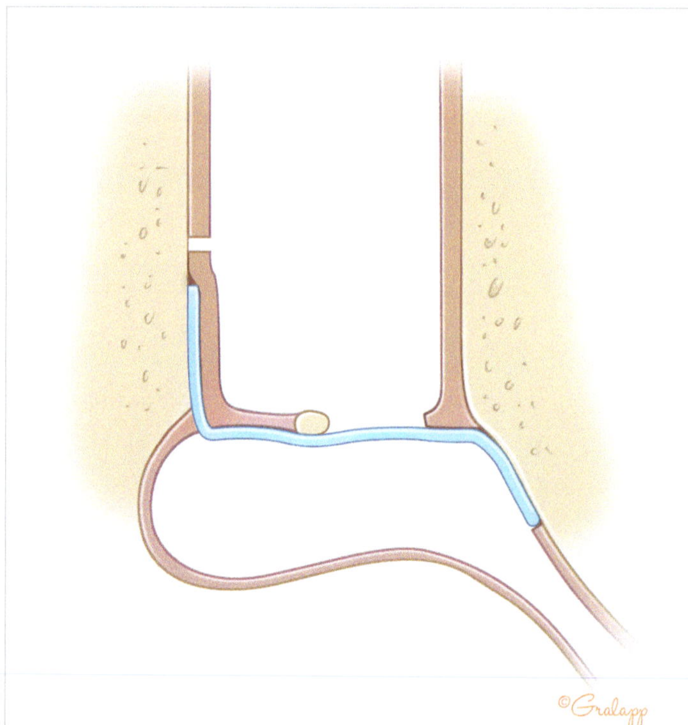

Fig. 5.66 Supplemental graft length in protympanum.

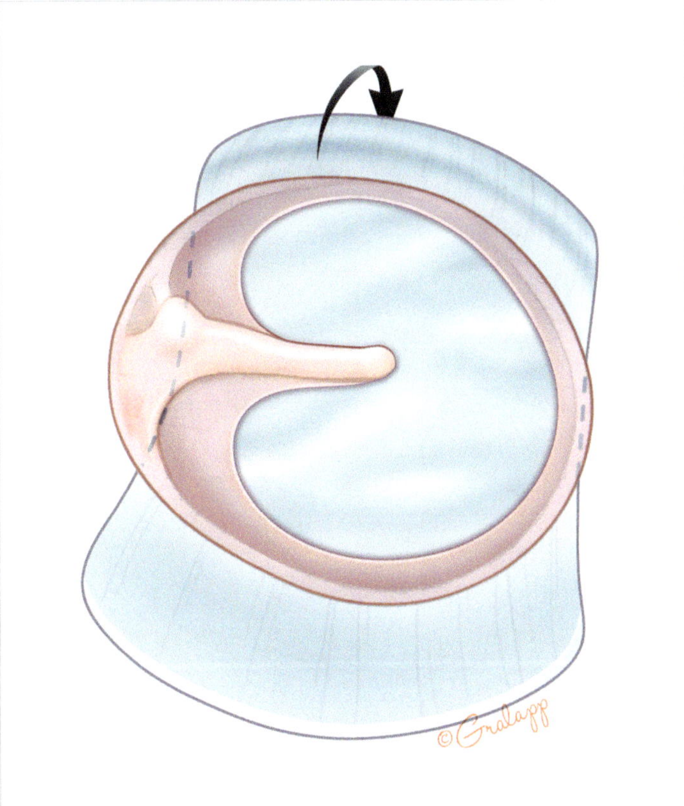

Fig. 5.67 Repair of anterior tympanic membrane perforation with graft extending into the protympanum.

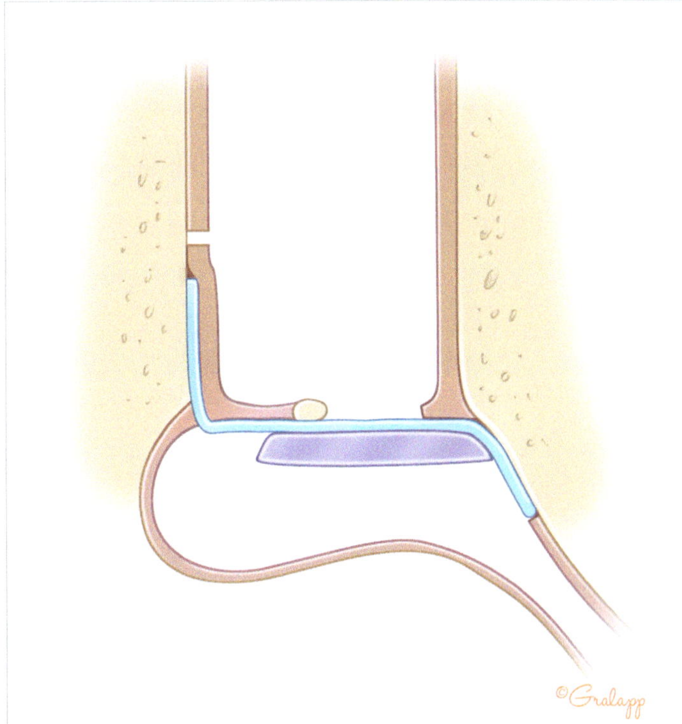

Fig. 5.68 Reinforcing anterior tympanic membrane perforation repair with cartilage. This is the preferred method of the author.

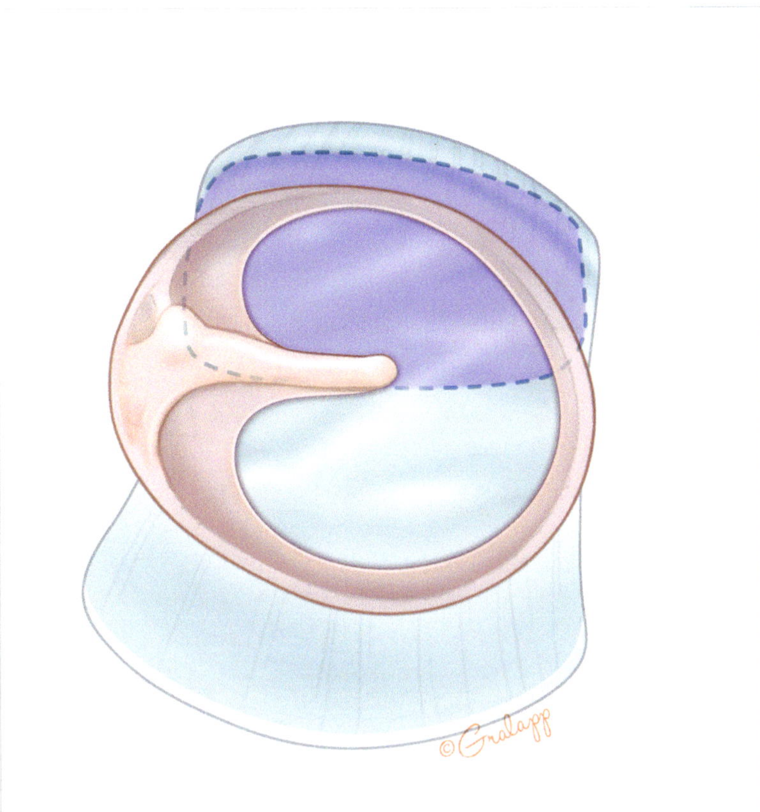

Fig. 5.69 Reinforcing anterior tympanic membrane perforation repair with cartilage.

5.7 Lateral Graft Tympanoplasty

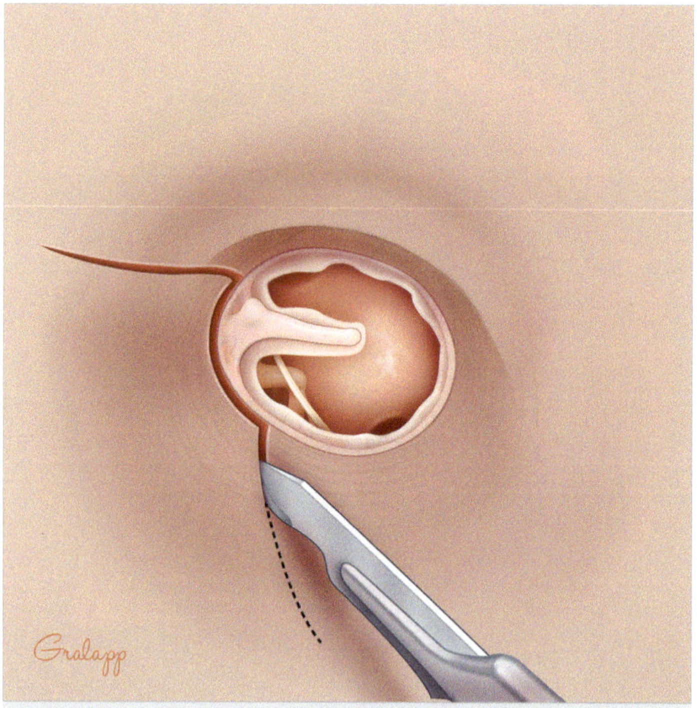

Fig. 5.70 In the lateral graft technique, superior incisions describe a vascular strip flap to be elevated laterally.

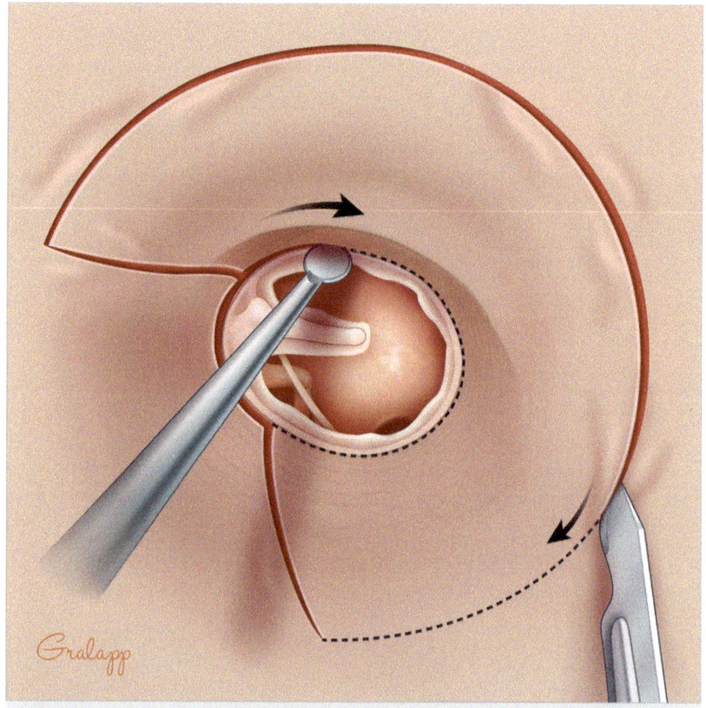

Fig. 5.71 The remaining canal skin and periosteum are dissected from the bony canal and placed aside for later use as a free graft. Note that the medial incision is placed just lateral to the tympanic annulus.

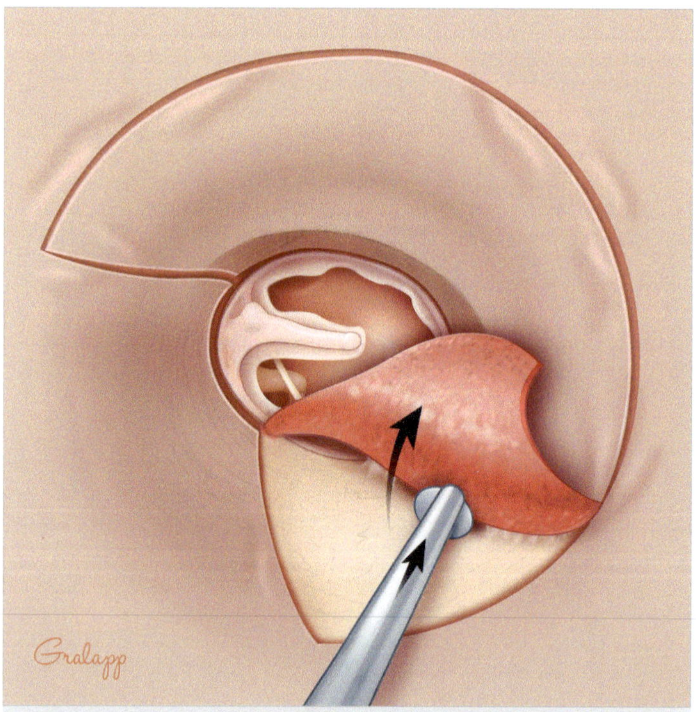

Fig. 5.72 Elevation of the canal skin.

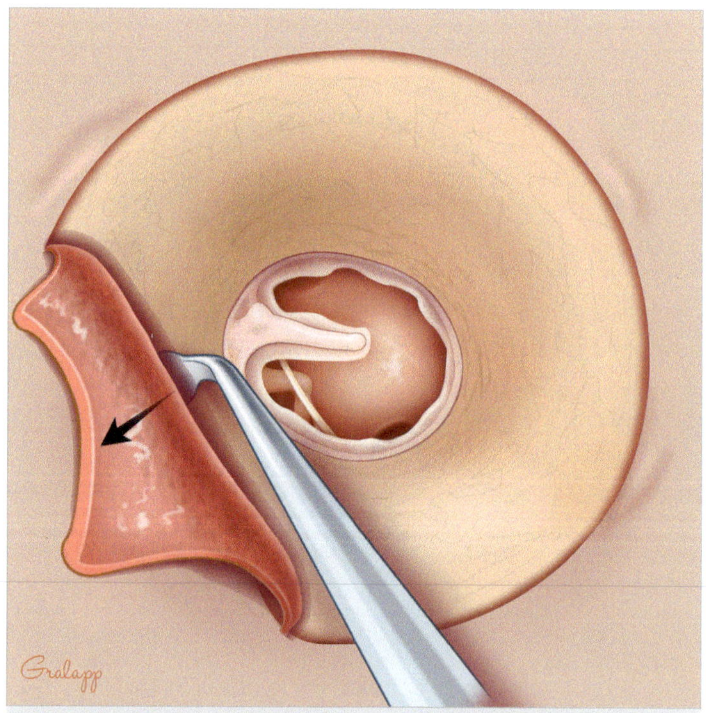

Fig. 5.73 Window shading of vascular strip flap superiorly.

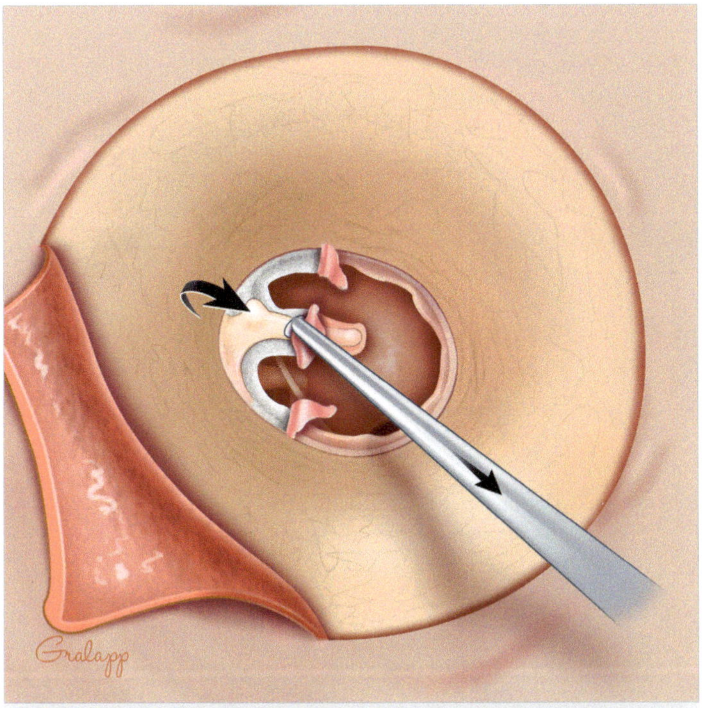

Fig. 5.74 Removing squamous layer for the tympanic membrane remnants leaving the fibrous and mucosal layers in place. It is important that all epithelial elements are removed to prevent epithelial pearls from developing in the future. The skin of the canal and TM remnant can be removed separately, as shown here, or in continuity.

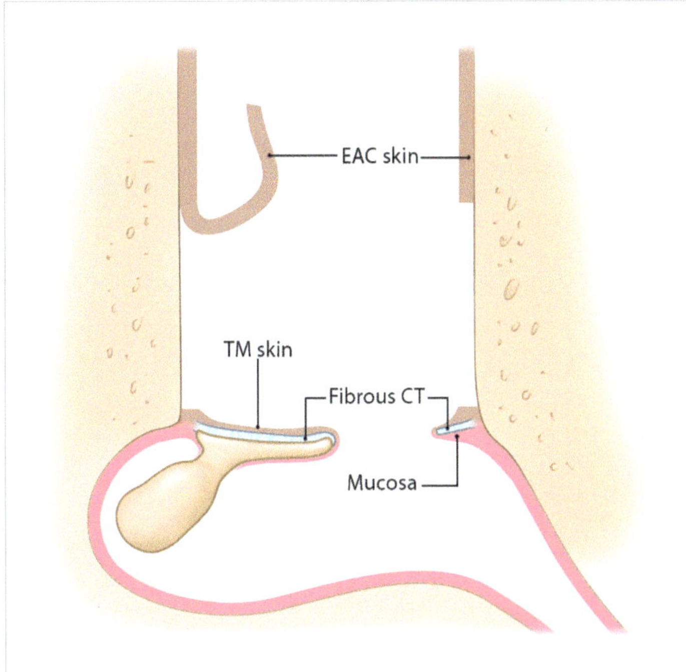

Fig. 5.75 Schematic illustrating the initial stages of the lateral graft technique. EAC, external auditory canal; TM, tympanic membrane; CT, connective tissue.

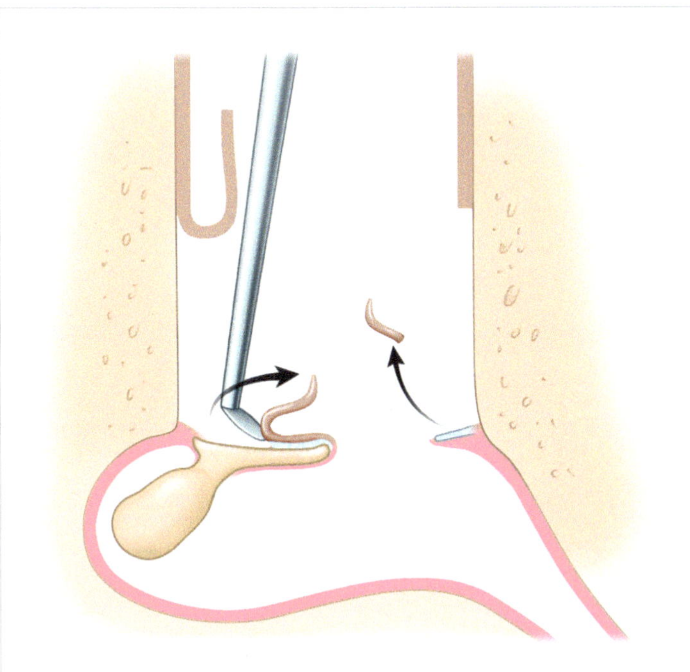

Fig. 5.76 Removing the squamous layer from the tympanic membrane remnant.

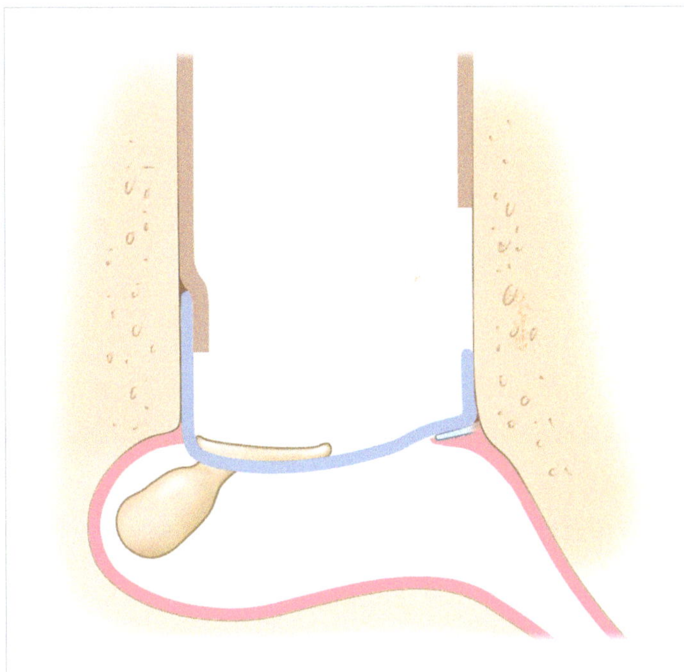

Fig. 5.77 Placement of the fascia graft in the lateral graft technique. Note that the fascia is positioned lateral to the tympanic membrane remnant but medial to the malleus handle.

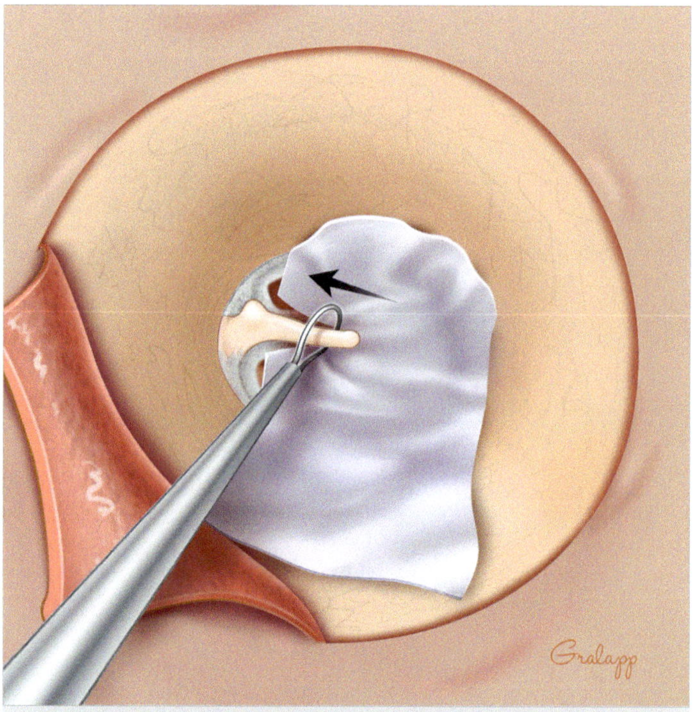

Fig. 5.78 Placement of the fascia graft over the tympanic membrane remnant. A wire loop may be used to position the graft beneath the umbo.

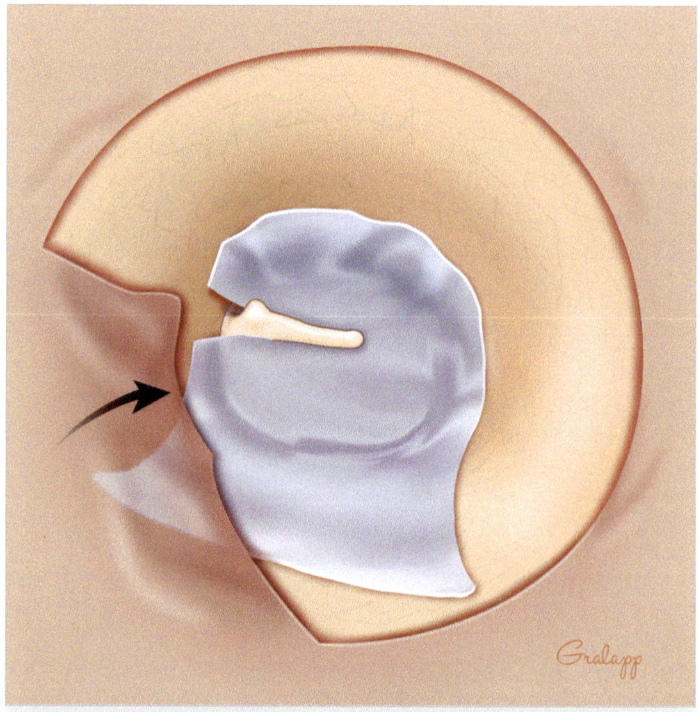

Fig. 5.79 Replacement of the superior flap overlapping the fascia graft.

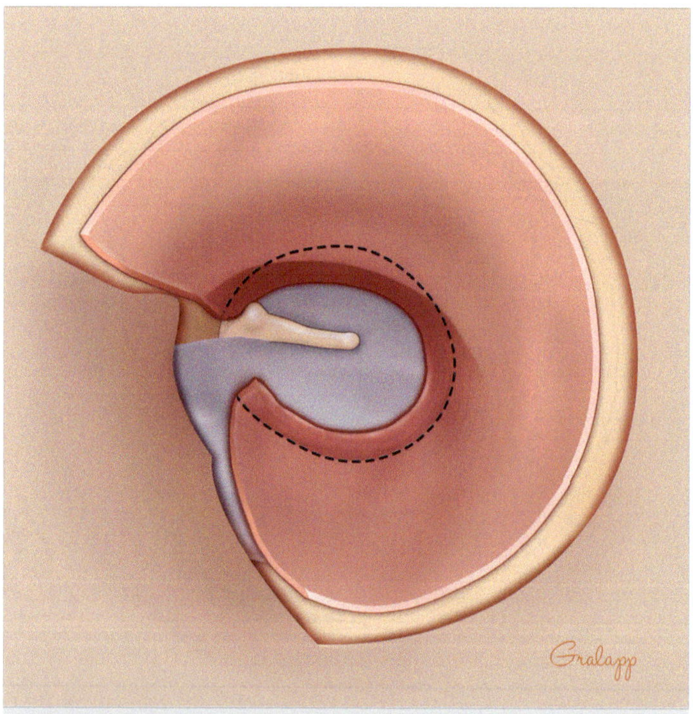

Fig. 5.80 Replacing the free graft which is advanced a few millimeters over the fascia graft.

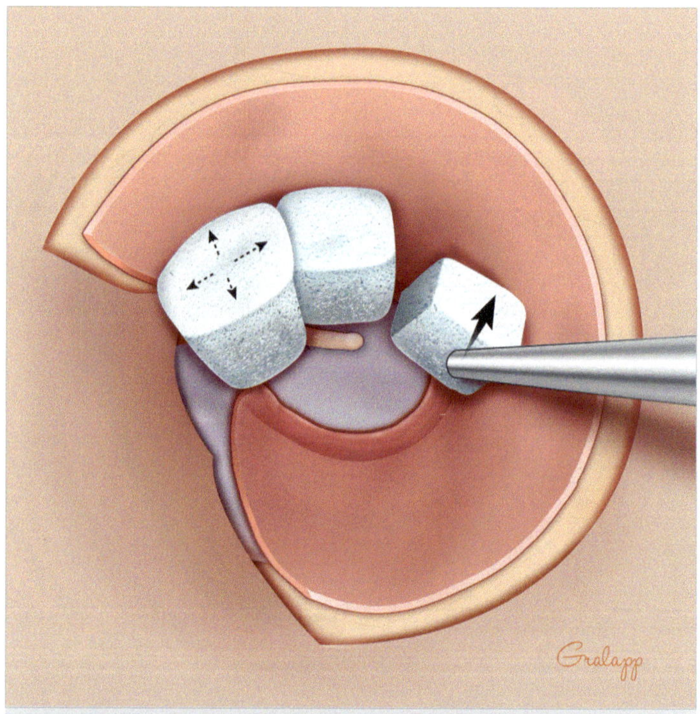

Fig. 5.81 Packing firmly is important to reduce the likelihood of anterior blunting or lateralization.

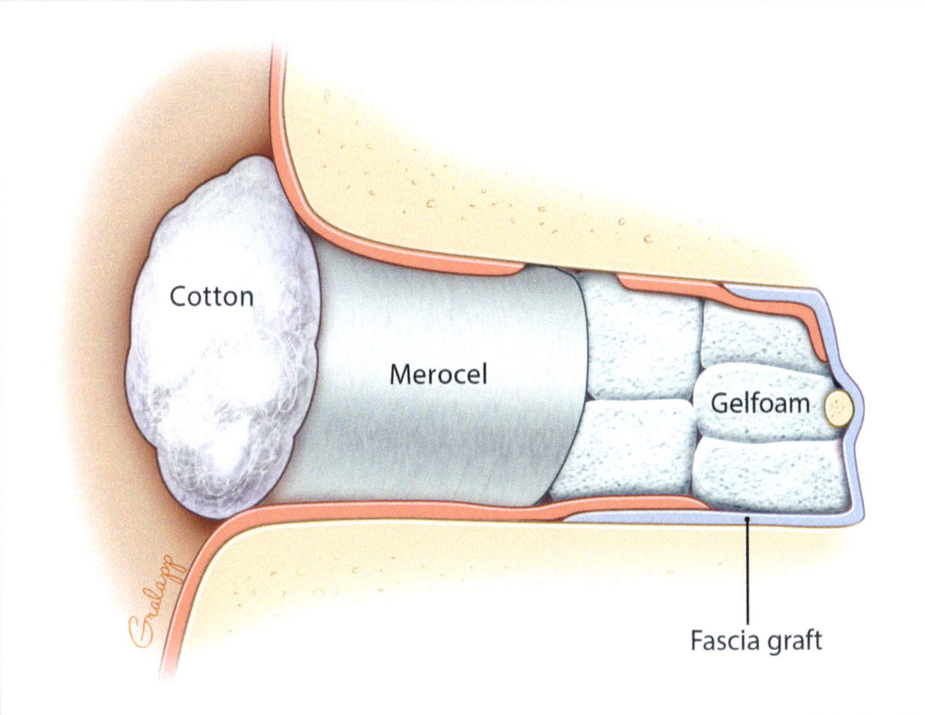

Fig. 5.82 Packing schema.

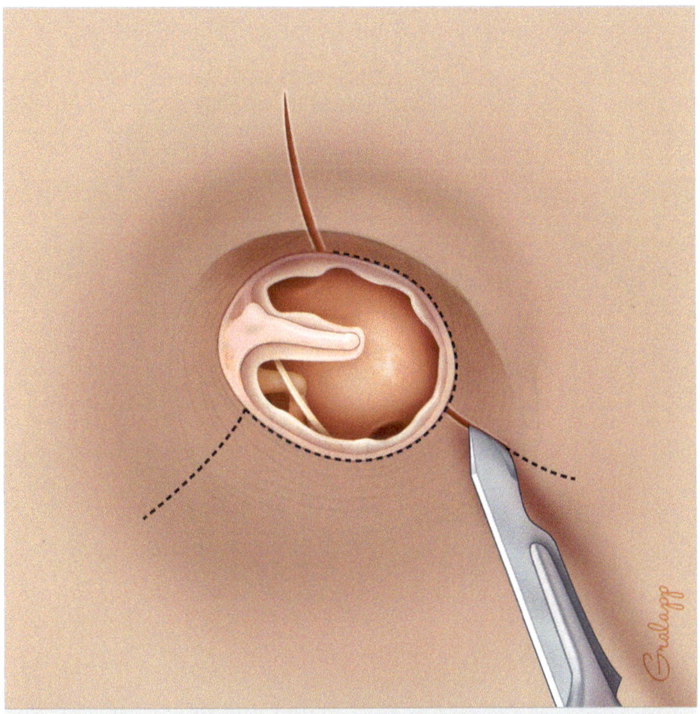

Fig. 5.83 An alternative technique of lateral grafting using three flaps rather than a free skin graft.

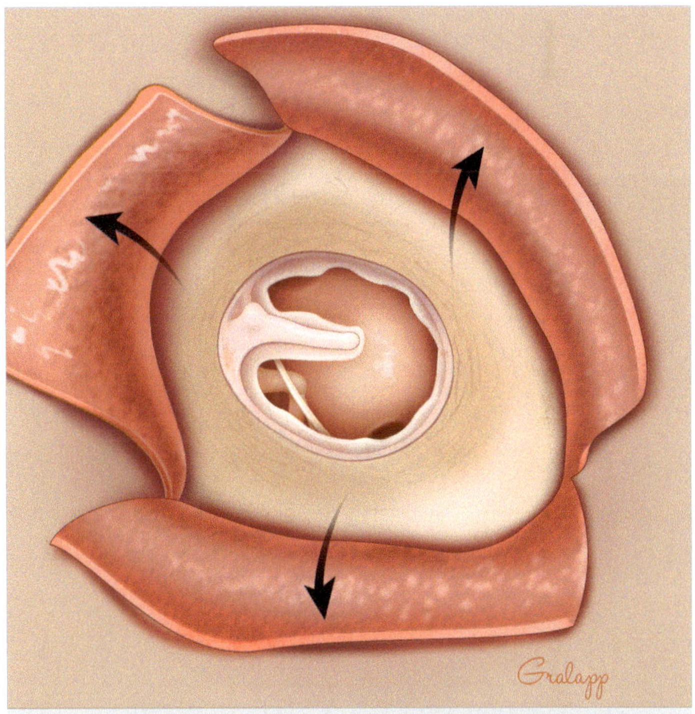

Fig. 5.84 Alternative technique of lateral grafting using three flaps reflected laterally.

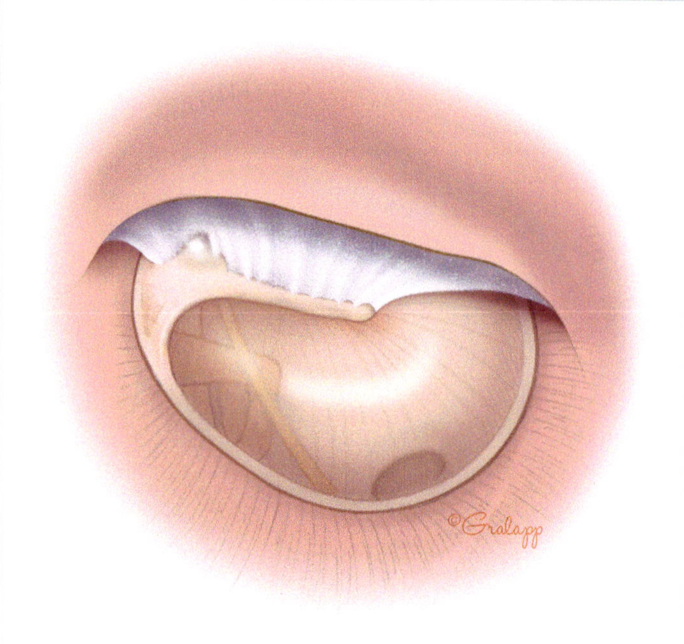

Fig. 5.85 Anterior blunting is a complication of lateral graft technique which results from insufficient contouring of the anterior canal (see section 3.8 Anterior Canaloplasty in Chapter 3).

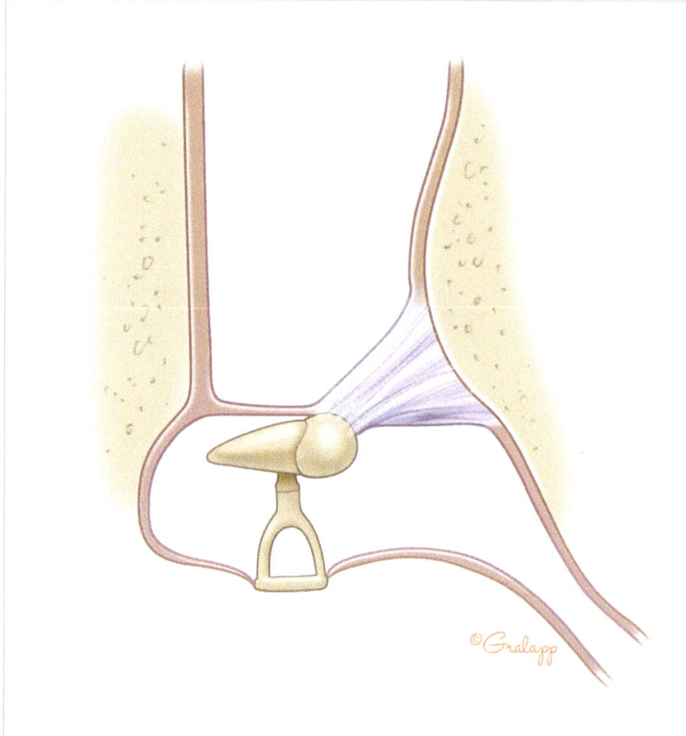

Fig. 5.86 Anterior blunting may result when anterior canal bulge is not corrected. This complication is more common with lateral graft technique.

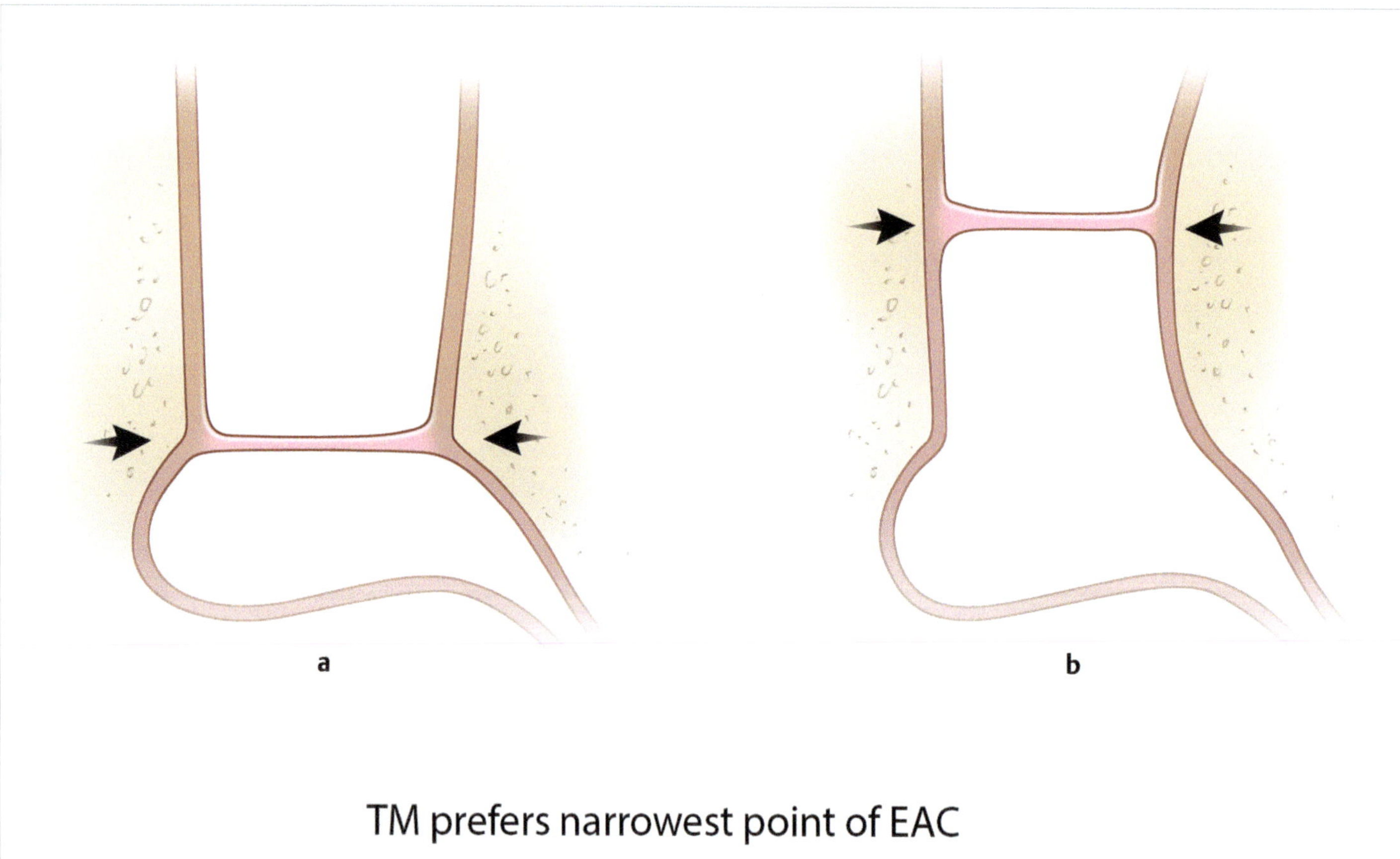

Fig. 5.87 The healing tympanic membrane may favor the narrowest portion of the ear canal. A prominent temporomandibular joint bulge should be corrected by anterior canaloplasty so that the narrowest point is at the tympanic annulus.

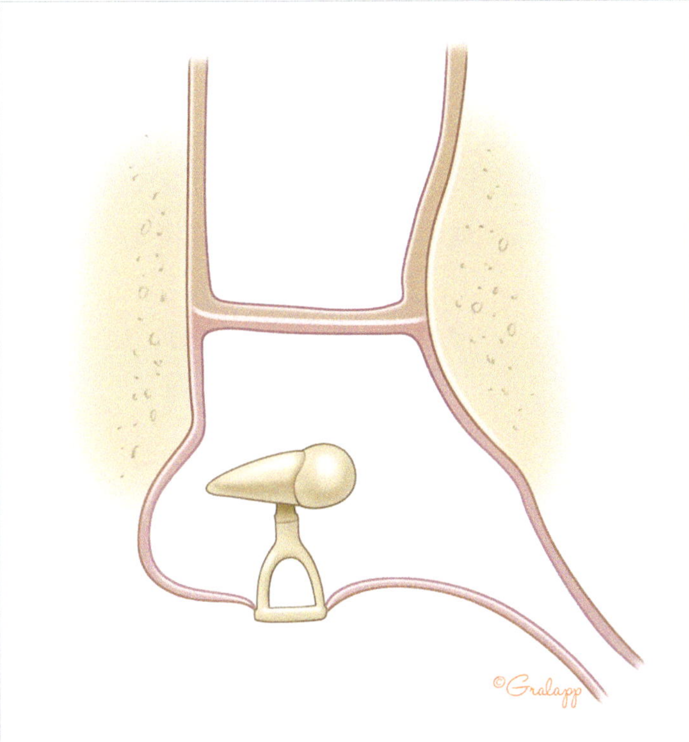

Fig. 5.88 Lateralization of the tympanic membrane leads to a maximal conductive hearing loss. Repairing this defect requires removing the mucosa which lines the medial aspect of the external auditory canal and may require a skin graft to discourage recurrence.

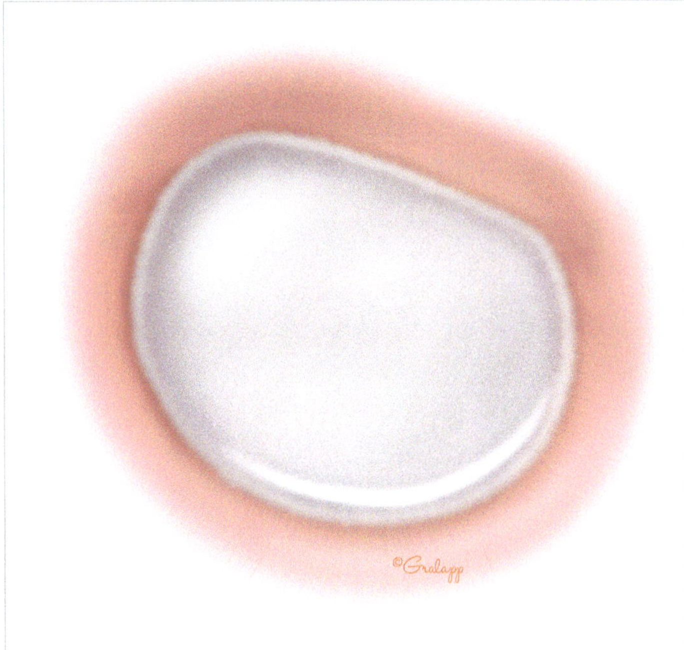

Fig. 5.89 Appearance of the tympanic membrane in lateralization. The ear canal is shortened and the membrane is featureless.

5.8 Butterfly Tympanoplasty

Yona Vaisbuch

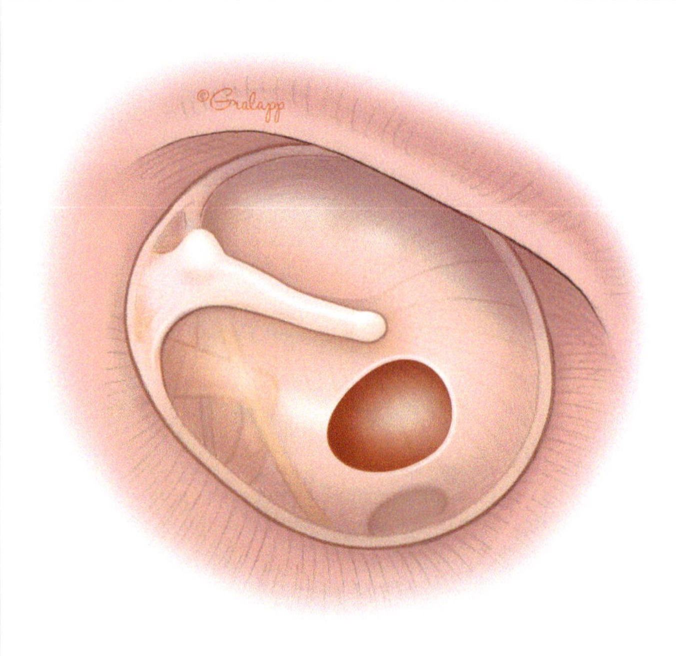

Fig. 5.90 The "butterfly" technique is most suitable for small- and medium-size posterior or central perforations.

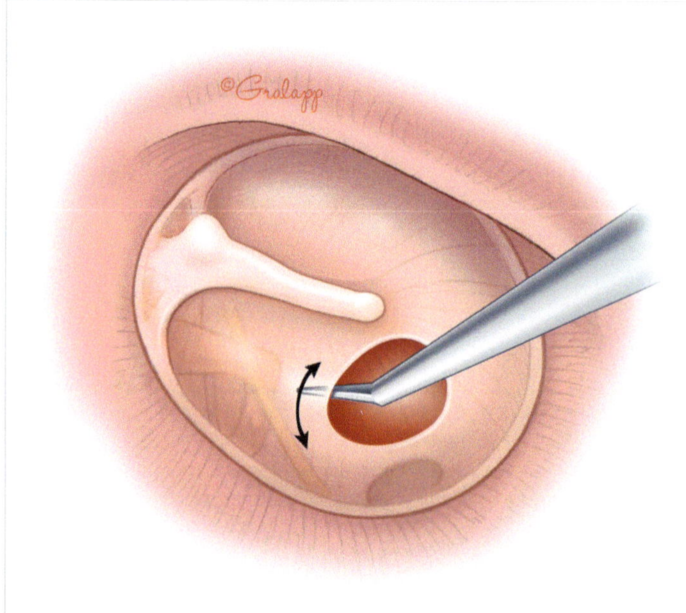

Fig. 5.91 In preparation, disrupting the mucosa on the medial surface of the tympanic membrane.

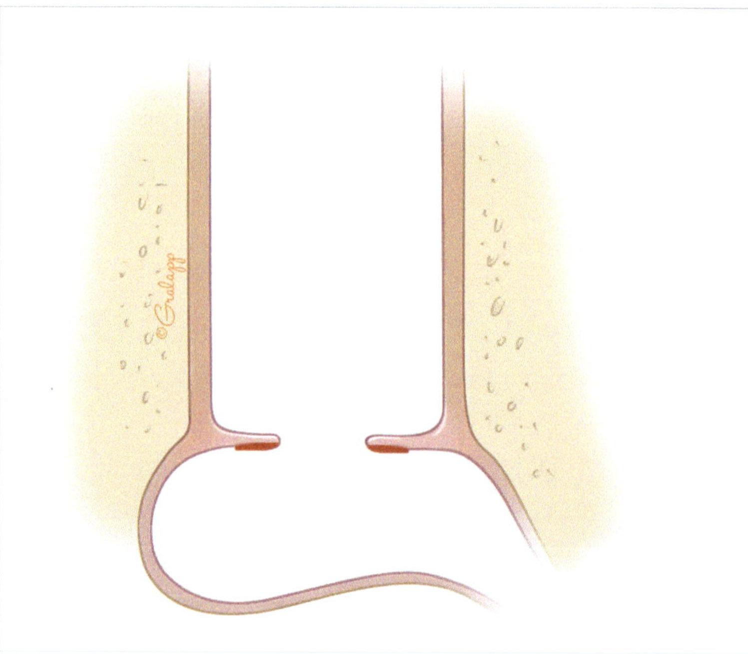

Fig. 5.92 Disrupting the mucosa on the medial surface of the tympanic membrane to encourage vascular ingrowth.

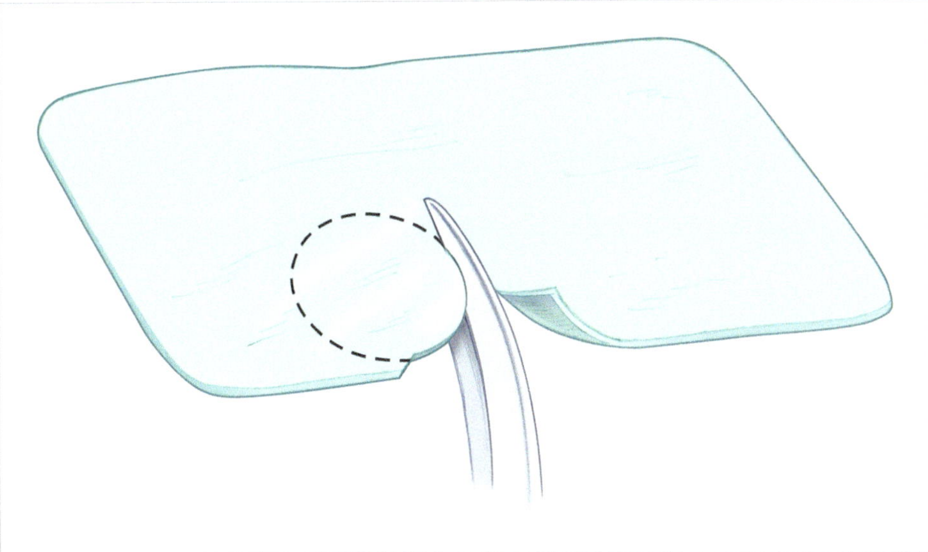

Fig. 5.93 Cut an estimated size template using the cover of a suture pack or other convenient sterile material.

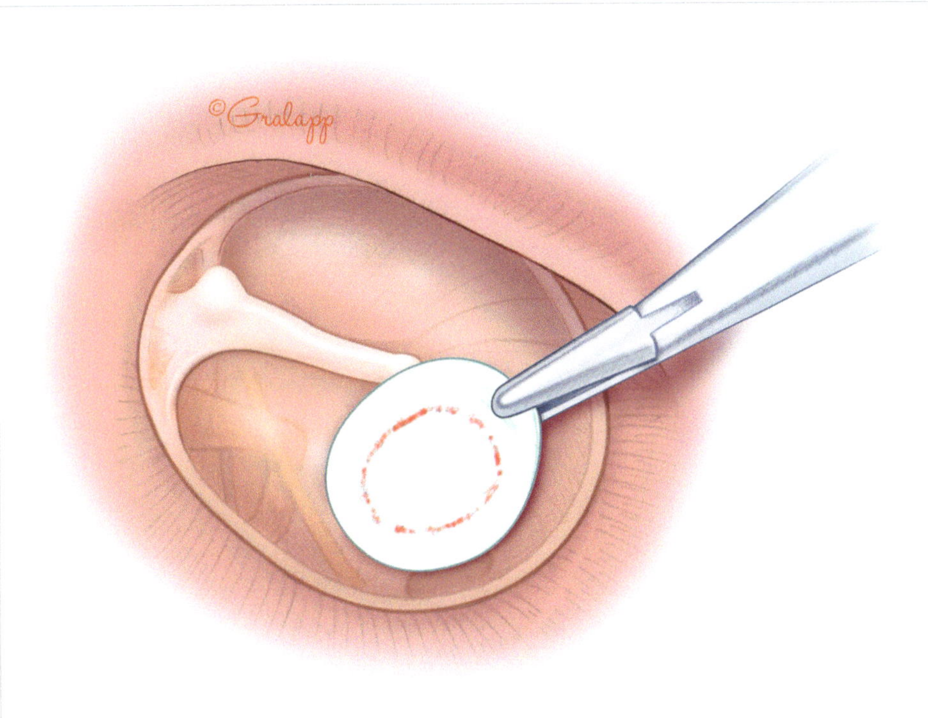

Fig. 5.94 Place the template on the tympanic membrane in order to stain it with some blood from the edges. This enables more accurate shaping, especially for other than round-shape perforations.

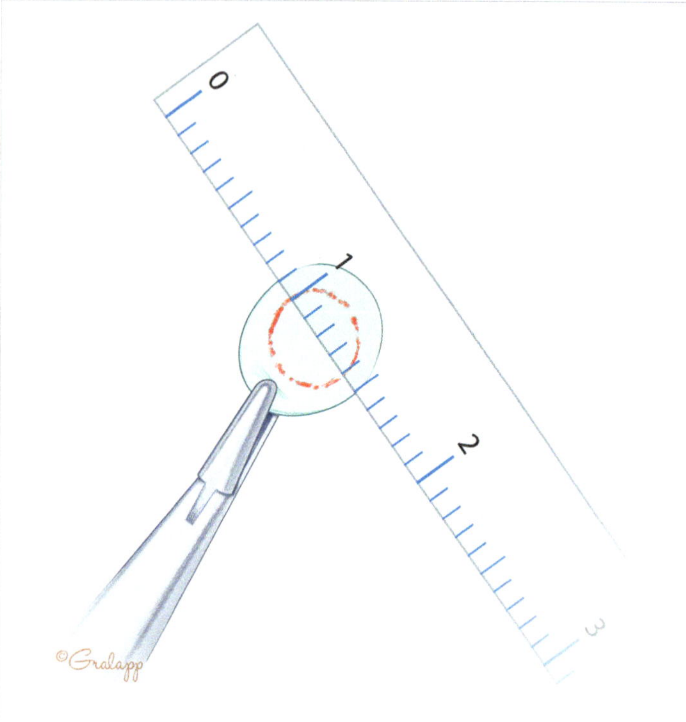

Fig. 5.95 Measure the perforation dimensions. If round, then the diameter is sufficient.

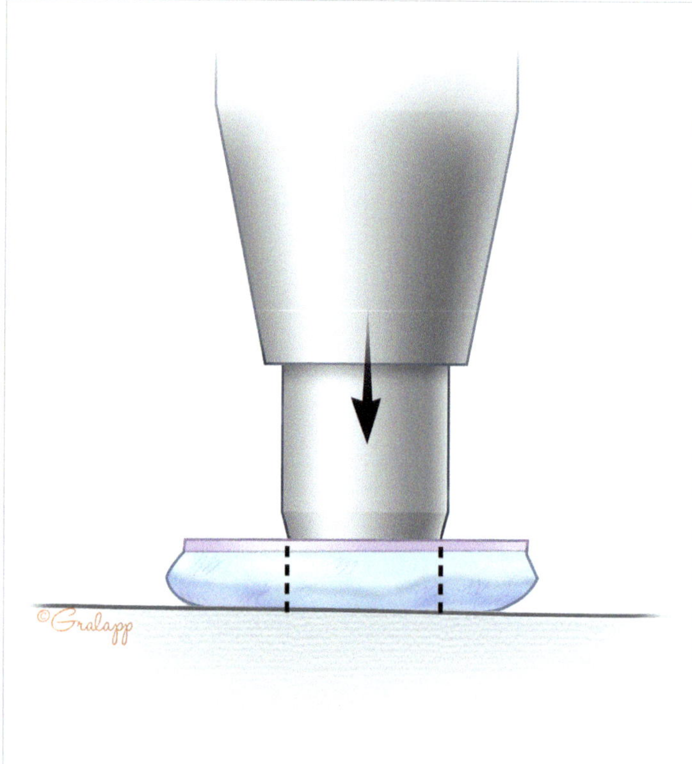

Fig. 5.96 For a round perforation, the cartilage is cut with a dermatological punch 1 mm wider than the measured perforation. If the perforation is irregularly sized, the cartilage is shaped with a scalpel.

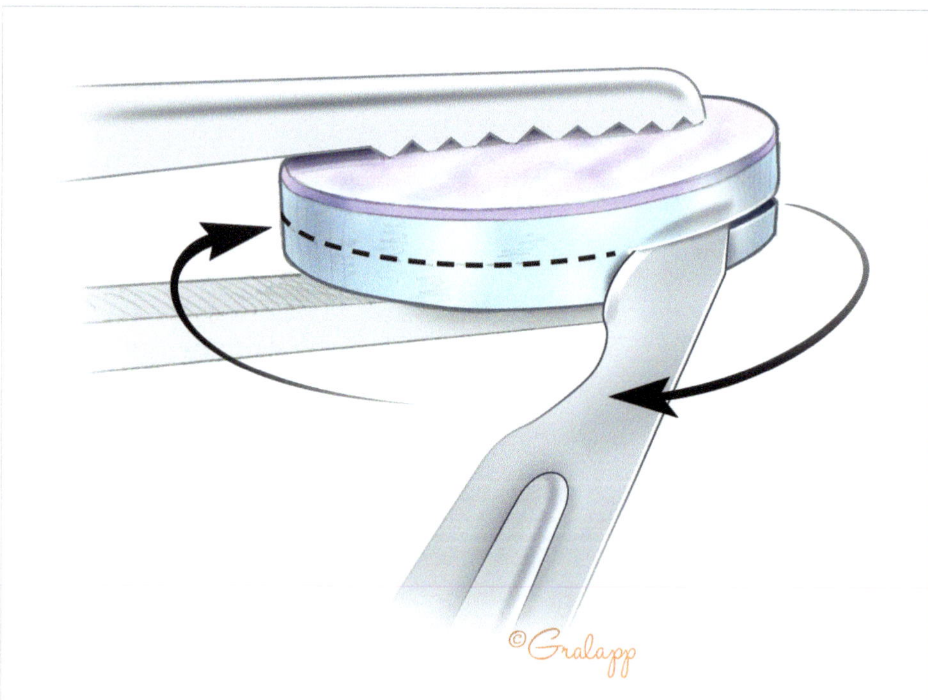

Fig. 5.97 While holding the graft with Adson-Brown forceps, a no. 15 blade is used to create a slit in the cartilage circumferentially. The slit can be deepened if more prominent wings are desired for greater retention. Some surgeons remove the perichondrium while other leave it attached to one (as shown here) or both leaves.

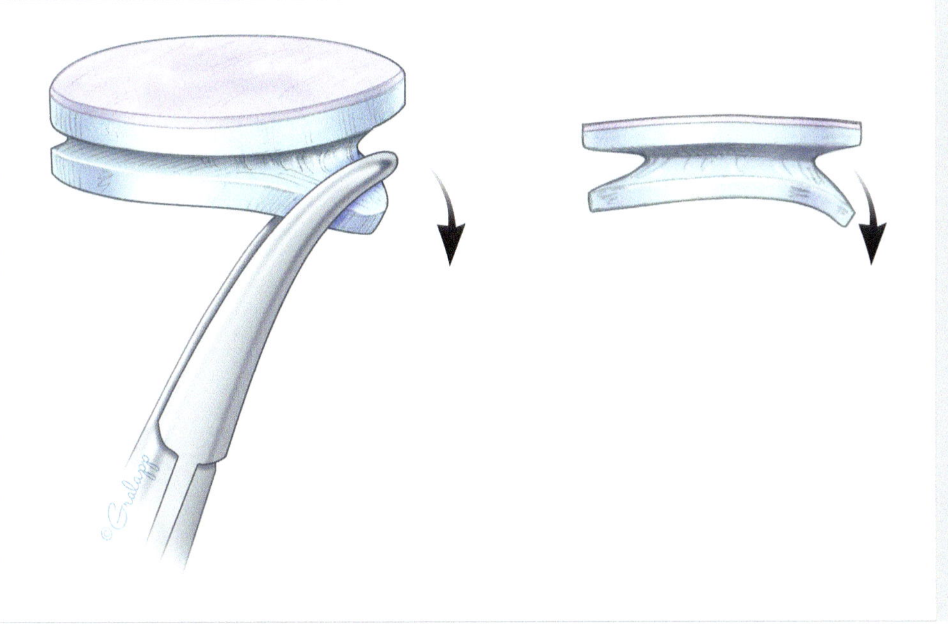

Fig. 5.98 Use a fine-tipped forceps to gently crush the medial wing edges, separating them to create space for the TM perforation edges. The anterior side of the medial wing is bent more prominently to facilitate easier insertion.

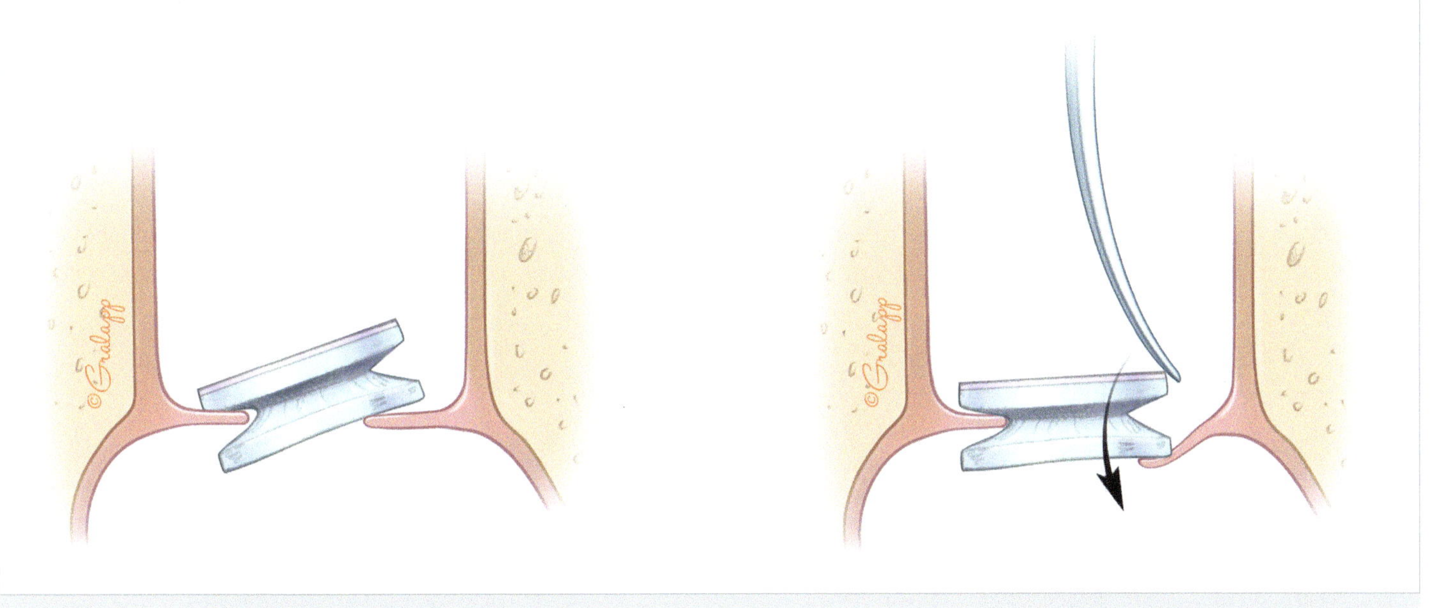

Fig. 5.99 Holding the posterior wing of the butterfly cartilage graft with alligator forceps, the graft is positioned with the perforation (left). Using a curved needle, the graft is rotated into position.

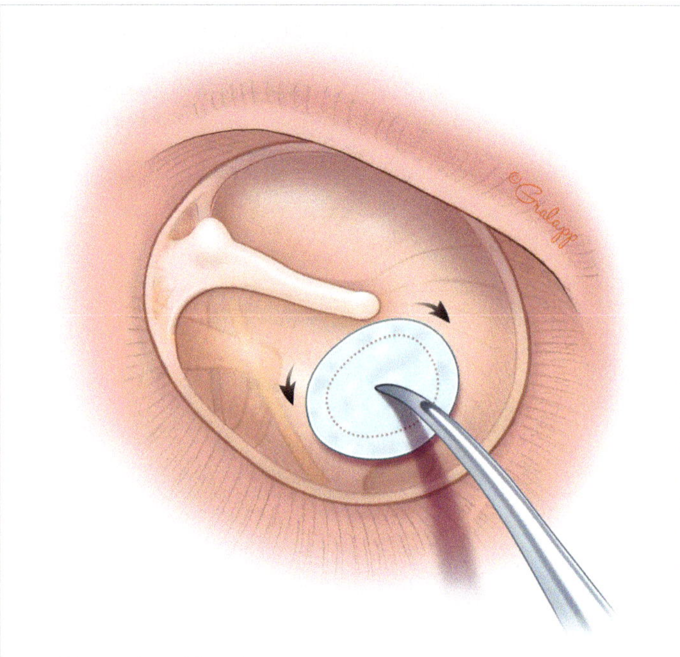

Fig. 5.100 After placement of the graft, a curved needle is used to rotate the graft clockwise and counter clockwise to ensure optimal seating of the wings.

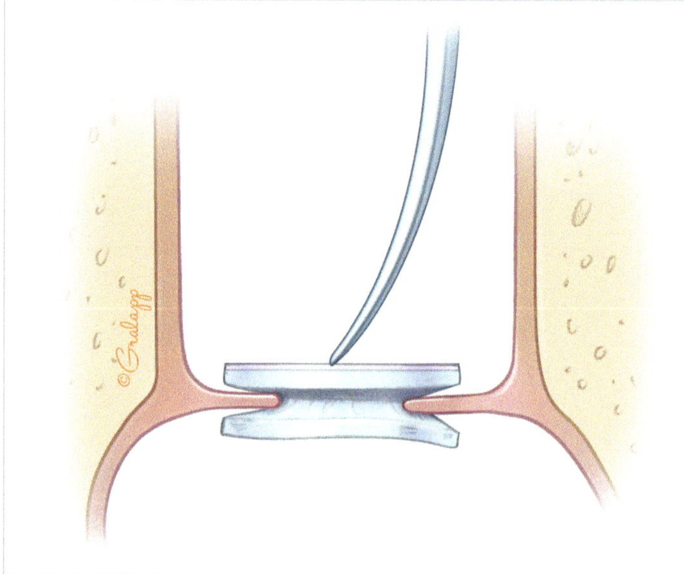

Fig. 5.101 Final position of the butterfly graft into the tympanic membrane perforation.

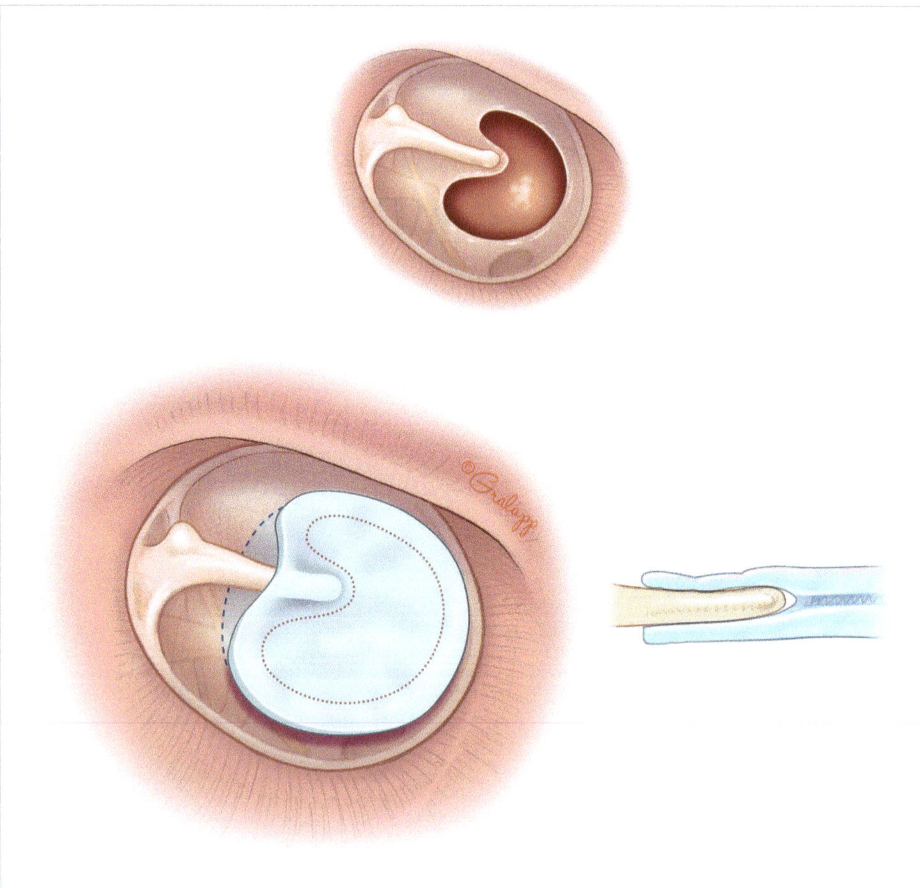

Fig. 5.102 In case of subtotal perforation, the butterfly cartilage graft is designed with a pocket for the malleus handle. This is done by leaving the perichondrium on both sides of the graft and crushing and removing a slit of cartilage to accommodate the malleus handle.

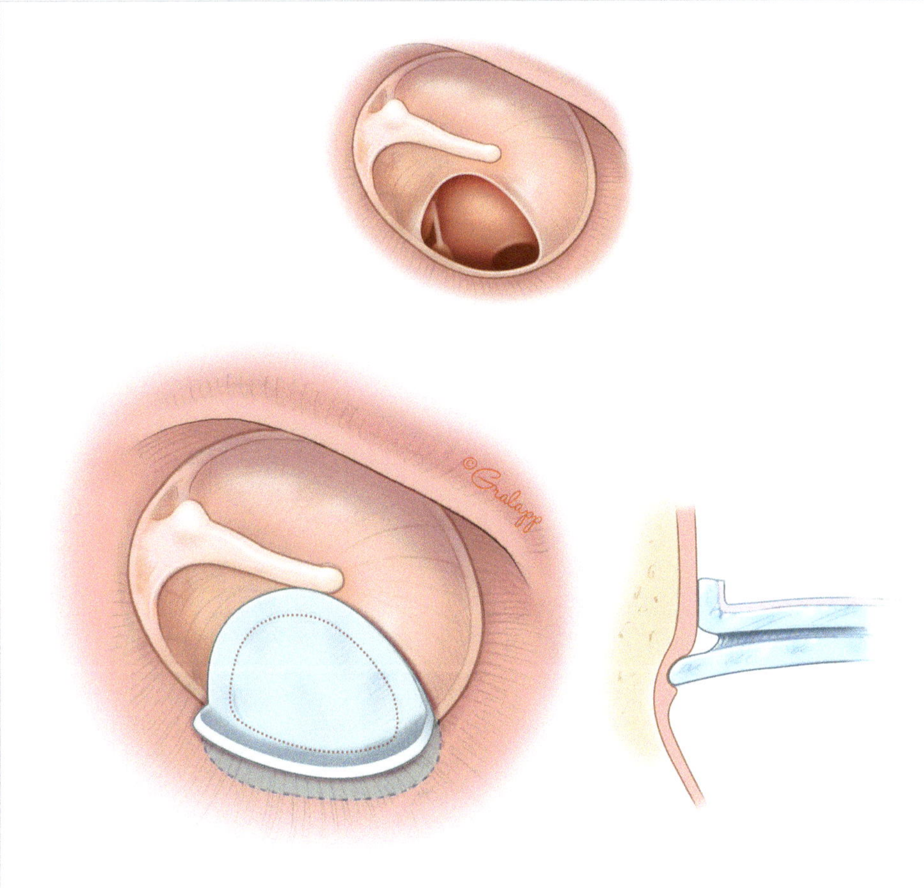

Fig. 5.103 In case of marginal perforation where there is no tympanic membrane remnant, the medial wing of the butterfly cartilage graft is placed inside the annular sulcus.

5.9 Eustachian Tuboplasty

Jennifer Y. Lee

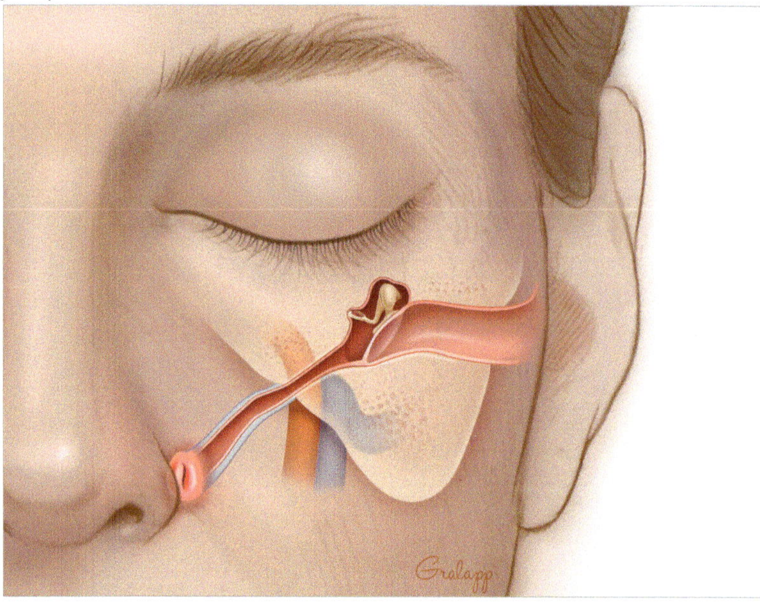

Fig. 5.104 Frontal view of Eustachian tube. Eustachian tube is a curved structure that is usually at a 30-degree angle from the middle ear cavity and curves anteriorly toward the nasopharynx.

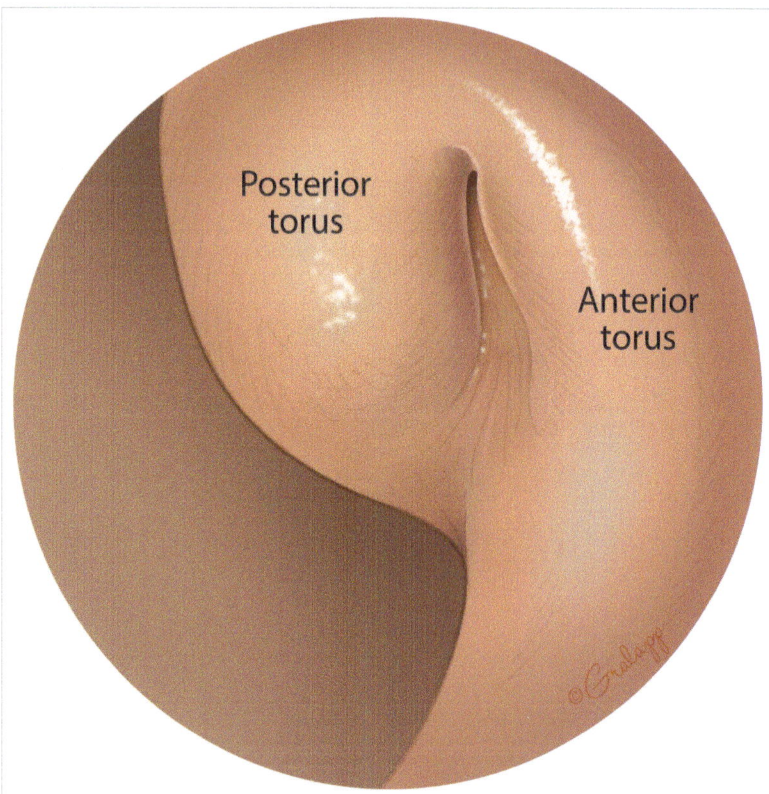

Fig. 5.105 The opening of the Eustachian tube in the nasopharynx has anterior and posterior tori which are closed or can be touching at rest.

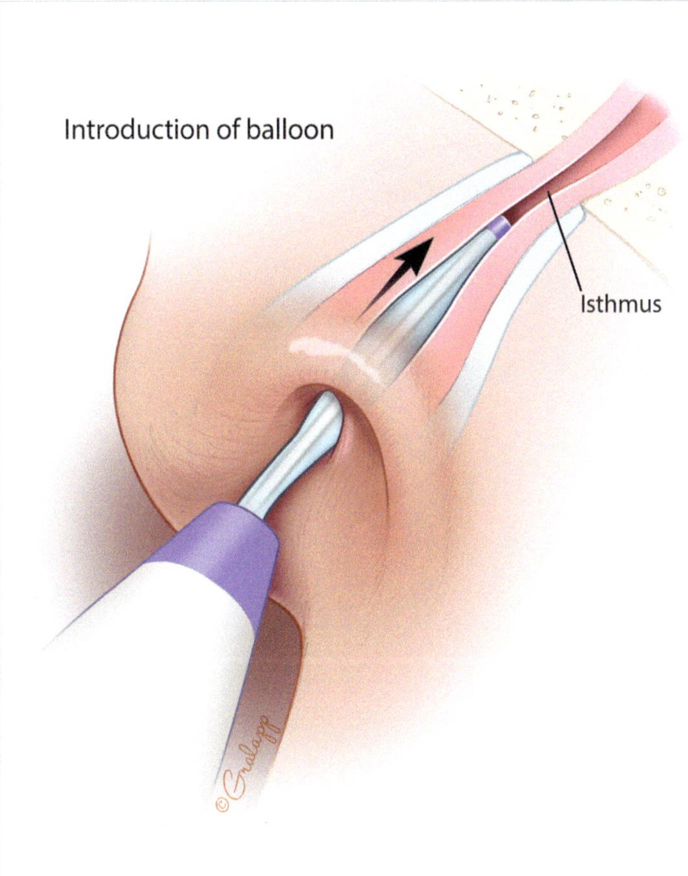

Fig. 5.106 The deflated balloon is inserted into the opening of the Eustachian tube in the nasopharynx. The balloon will slide in without significant resistance if in the native lumen.

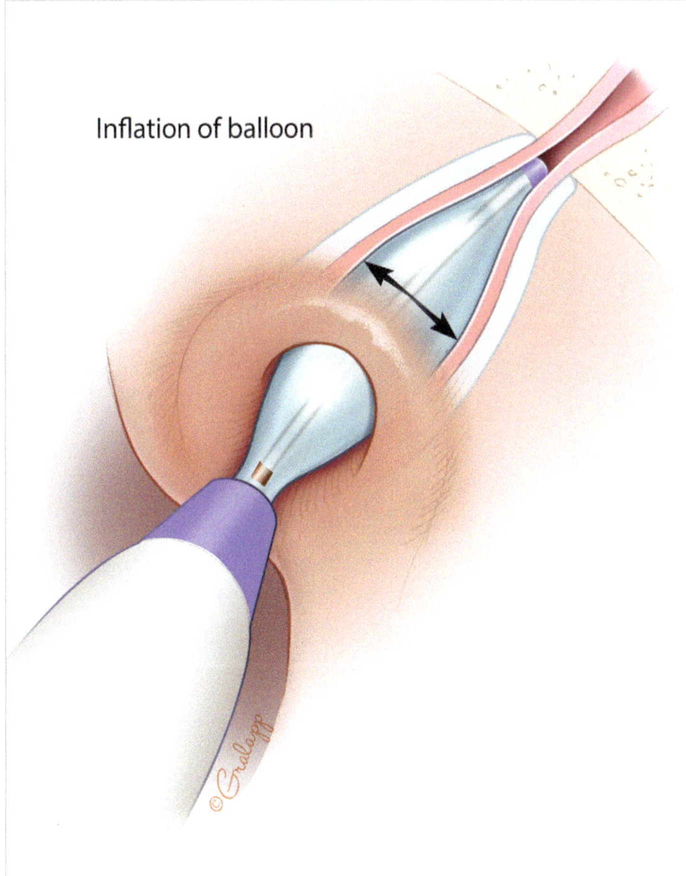

Fig. 5.107 Once balloon has encountered the bony isthmus, resistance will be met and advancement should be stopped. Next the balloon is inflated and kept in place. Then the balloon is deflated and removed.

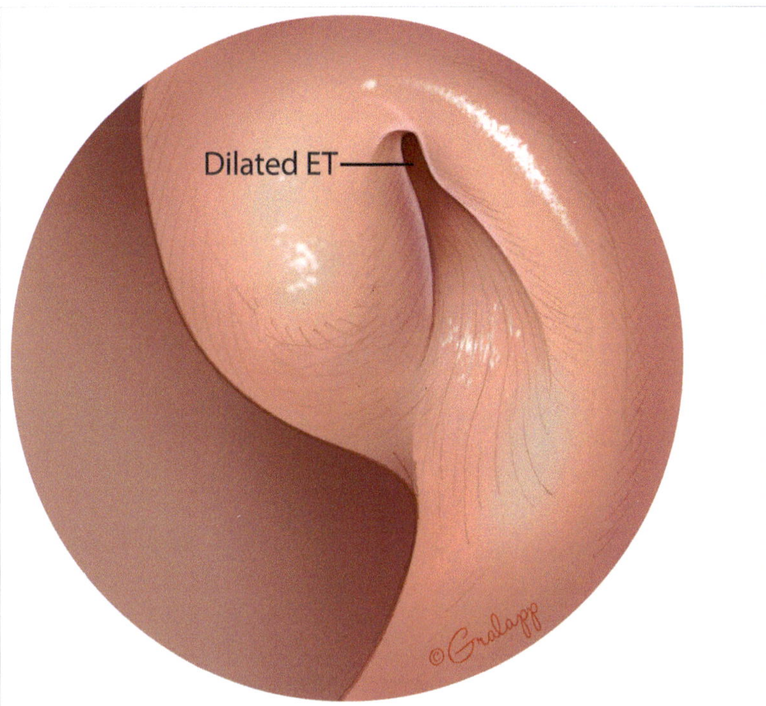

Fig. 5.108 Balloon is removed. The Eustachian tube (ET) post-dilation appears to be enlarged at the superior aspect of the opening.

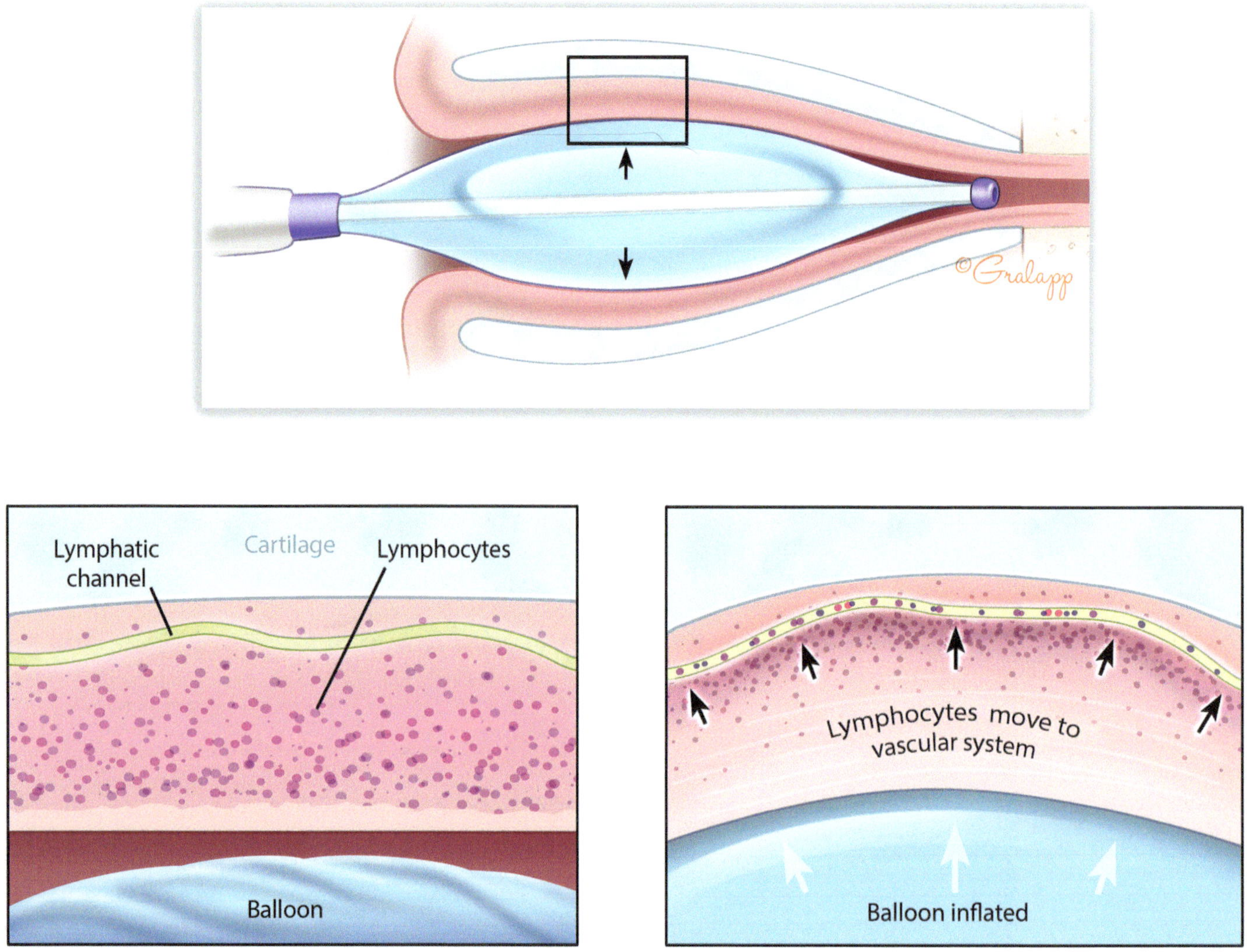

Fig. 5.109 The pathophysiology reported is that the lymphocytes which cause inflammation and swelling of the mucosa are pushed out of the submucosa. The mucosal lining of the Eustachian tube tunnel can return to its native state and there can be less obstruction.

6 Ossiculoplasty

Robert K. Jackler

6.1 Introduction to Ossiculoplasty

Diseases of the ossicular chain most often occur as an aftermath of infection and less commonly due to trauma or tumor. Conductive hearing loss may result from either discontinuity of the chain or its fixation due to fibrosis or dystrophic calcification (tympanosclerosis). In chronic otitis media, with or without cholesteatoma, the portions of the chain most vulnerable to erosion are the long process of the incus followed by the stapedial arch. The stapes footplate is seldom breached by infection, although it may be involved by cholesteatoma, by inflammation (granulation tissue or polypoid mucosa), or both. In chronic otitis media, the umbo is often medially rotated narrowing the tympanic cavity or even compartmentalizing it into anterior and posterior segments. Before ossiculoplasty, the malleus should be forcibly lateralized. Dividing the tensor tympanic tendon helps maintain the lateral position after repair.

Most frequently disrupted in blunt trauma are the incudostapedial joint followed by massive dislocation of the incus (both incudostapedial and incudomalleolar joints) and less commonly stapes arch fracture. The malleus and stapes footplate are not commonly fractured. A rule of thumb is that in both trauma and chronic otitis media, the incus is most vulnerable.

The most common biocompatible materials used in ossiculoplasty today are titanium and hydroxyapatite. Plastics (e.g., porous polyethylene) were popular in the past but are not commonly used today. Autologous bone such as a reshaped incus body or malleus head are generally less stable and give less reliable results than more mechanically stable artificial prostheses. Most surgeons would prefer not to reposition an ossicle which had been involved with cholesteatoma for fear of residual disease. As a general rule to reduce the chance of extrusion, cartilage should be interposed between the tympanic membrane and ossicular replacement prostheses. It is prudent to use a large piece of cartilage designed to completely underlay the posterior-superior quadrant of the tympanic membrane.

There are myriad designs of ossicular replacement prostheses. Thematically, most are either partial (replacing malleus and incus and connecting to the stapes superstructure) or total (replacing all three ossicles and resting on the stapes footplate). Partial prostheses, which clasp onto the capitulum of the stapes, are generally more stable. Total prostheses which sit on top of the oval window are inherently less stable. To enhance stability, some surgeons place a cartilage block in the oval window niche with a hole to seat the prosthesis. Some two-component total systems use a footplate shoe. While the importance of a remaining malleus handle is debated, some use prostheses designed to attach to the umbo which may afford greater stability. However, the malleus handle in chronic otitis media is often medialized and anteriorly rotated to an unfavorable angle. Other prostheses span minimal defects such as the incudostapedial connection, a defect sometimes repaired with glue which hardens into a rigid solid.

In contrast to the high success rates with tympanoplasty, durable hearing improvement with ossicular chain reconstruction is less reliably achieved. Failure may be early or late. Early malfunctions are most often from a lack of mechanical stability. Properly sized and positioned prostheses remain vulnerable displacement from even minor head trauma or forced ear inflation until they are locked into place by an enveloping mucosal membrane which takes several weeks to develop. Late deterioration may result from scar displacement, fixation of the prosthesis by scarring or dystrophic calcification, or further biological impairment of the middle ear cavity due to recurrent infection. While substantial hearing improvement is achieved in approximately 80% of partial and 50% or total reconstructions, early improvements all too often deteriorate over time. Most of the "long-term" outcomes reported are with only 1 or 2 years in follow-up with few studies reporting outcomes of ≥ 5 years.

Ossicular fixation, which may occur with or without concomitant tympanic membrane perforation, is a special problem. Epitympanic fixation of the malleus head and/or incus body due to scarring from infection has a high risk or refixation if it is merely mobilized by breaking its adhesive bands. It is better to remove the lateral ossicles, leaving the umbo in place and reconstructing directly to the stapes. Tympanosclerotic stapes fixation is considered in Chapter 4, section 4.9 Tympanosclerotic Stapes Fixation.

Success with ossiculoplasty is related to the health of the middle ear mucosal envelope. This is why results are superior after traumatic ossicular injuries than those associated with infection, which often has an underlying tendency to recur. When the middle ear mucosal lining is compromised, many surgeons stage the procedure preferring to undertake ossiculoplasty months later when the mucosal envelope has improved.

Further Reading

1. Bartel R, Cruellas F, Hamdan M, et al. Hearing results after type III tympanoplasty: incus transposition versus PORP. A systematic review. Acta Otolaryngol 2018;138(7):617–620 PubMed
2. Blom EF, Gunning MN, Kleinrensink NJ, et al. Influence of ossicular chain damage on hearing after chronic otitis media and cholesteatoma surgery: a systematic review and meta-analysis. JAMA Otolaryngol Head Neck Surg 2015;141 (11):974–982 PubMed
3. Cox MD, Page JC, Trinidade A, Dornhoffer JL. Long-term complications and surgical failures after ossiculoplasty. Otol Neurotol 2017;38(10):1450–1455 PubMed
4. Cox MD, Trinidade A, Russell JS, Dornhoffer JL. Long-term hearing results after ossiculoplasty. Otol Neurotol 2017;38 (4):510–515 PubMed
5. Iñiguez-Cuadra R, Alobid I, Borés-Domenech A, Menéndez-Colino LM, Caballero-Borrego M, Bernal-Sprekelsen M. Type III tympanoplasty with titanium total ossicular replacement prosthesis: anatomic and functional results. Otol Neurotol 2010;31(3):409–414 PubMed
6. Kamrava B, Roehm PC. Systematic review of ossicular chain anatomy: strategic planning for development of novel middle ear prostheses. Otolaryngol Head Neck Surg 2017;157 (2):190–200 PubMed
7. Lee JI, Yoo SH, Lee CW, Song CI, Yoo MH, Park HJ. Short-term hearing results using ossicular replacement prostheses of hydroxyapatite versus titanium. Eur Arch Otorhinolaryngol 2015;272(10):2731–2735 PubMed
8. Mishiro Y, Sakagami M, Kitahara T, Kondoh K, Kubo T. Long-term hearing outcomes after ossiculoplasty in comparison to short-term outcomes. Otol Neurotol 2008;29(3):326–329 PubMed
9. O'Connell BP, Rizk HG, Hutchinson T, Nguyen SA, Lambert PR. Long-term outcomes of titanium ossiculoplasty in chronic otitis media. Otolaryngol Head Neck Surg 2016;154(6):1084–1092 PubMed
10. Şevik Eliçora S, Erdem D, Dinç AE, Damar M, Bişkin S. The effects of surgery type and different ossiculoplasty materials on the hearing results in cholesteatoma surgery. Eur Arch Otorhinolaryngol 2017;274(2):773–780 PubMed
11. Wegner I, van den Berg JW, Smit AL, Grolman W. Systematic review of the use of bone cement in ossicular chain reconstruction and revision stapes surgery. Laryngoscope 2015;125 (1):227–233 PubMed

6.2 Patterns of Ossicular Deficiency

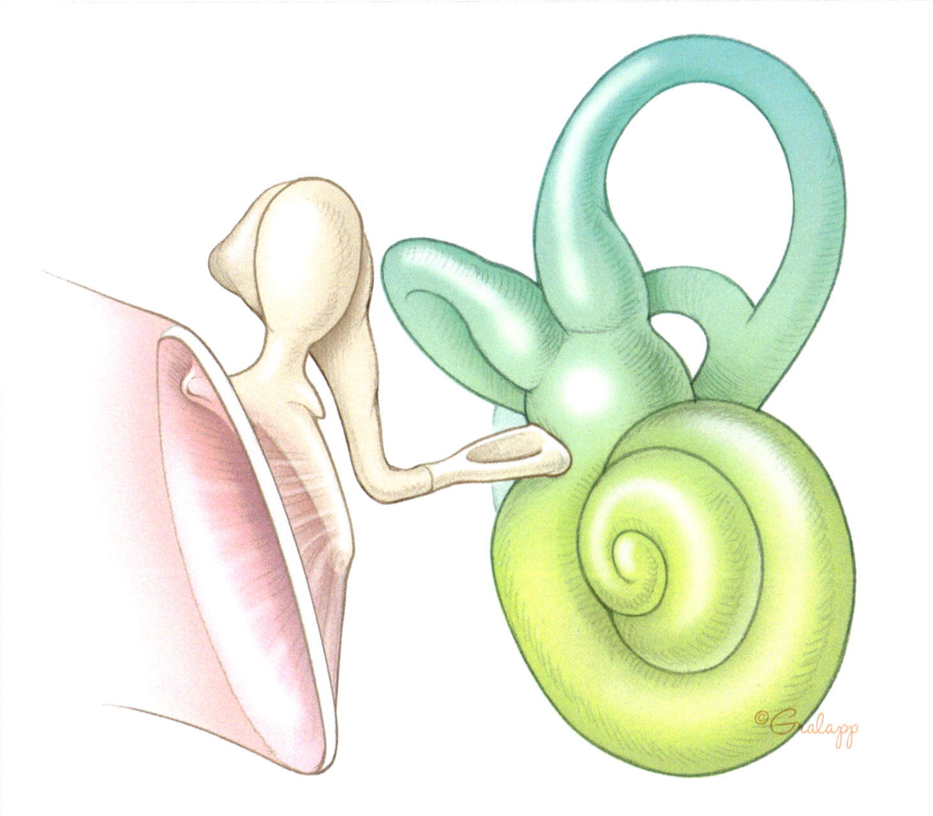

Fig. 6.1 Normal ossicular chain (malleus–incus–stapes) showing the tympanic membrane and inner ear (cochlea and semicircular canals).

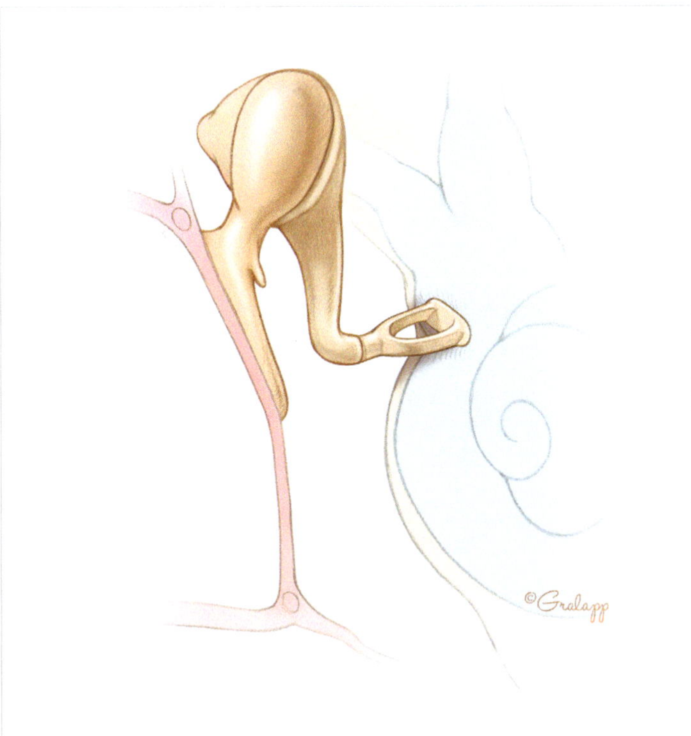

Fig. 6.2 Normal ossicular chain (malleus–incus–stapes).

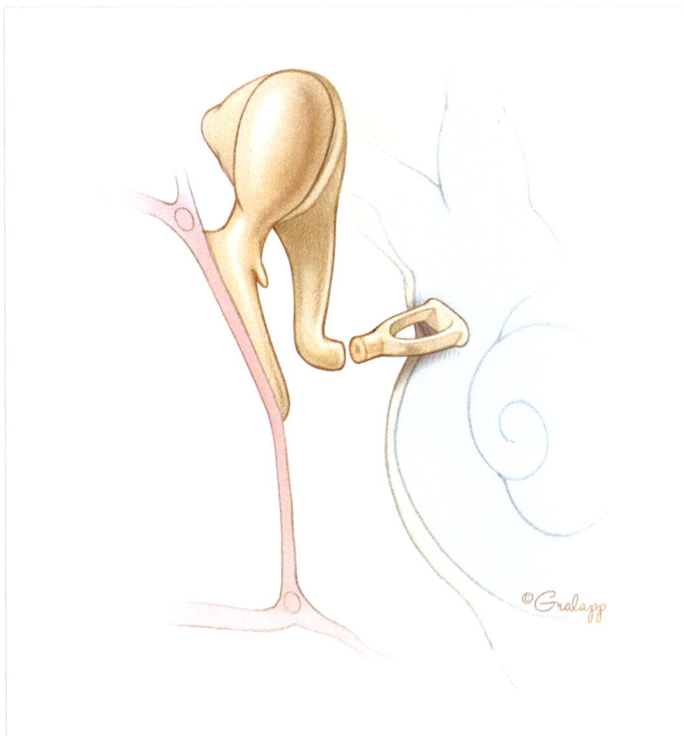

Fig. 6.3 Incudostapedial joint separation most commonly occurs after temporal bone fracture.

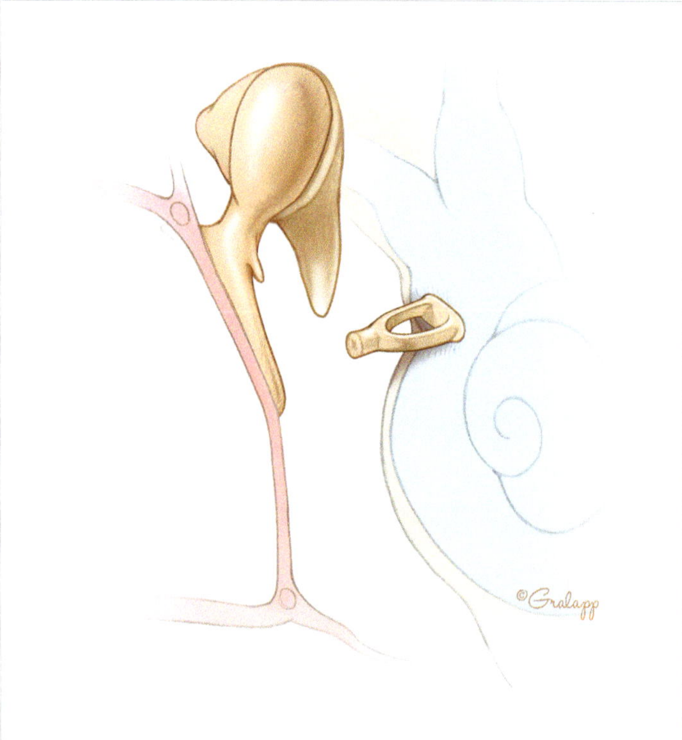

Fig. 6.4 Erosion of the long process of the incus most often occurs as a consequence of chronic otitis media or cholesteatoma. The long process sometimes fractures, especially following stapes surgery or in osteogenesis imperfecta.

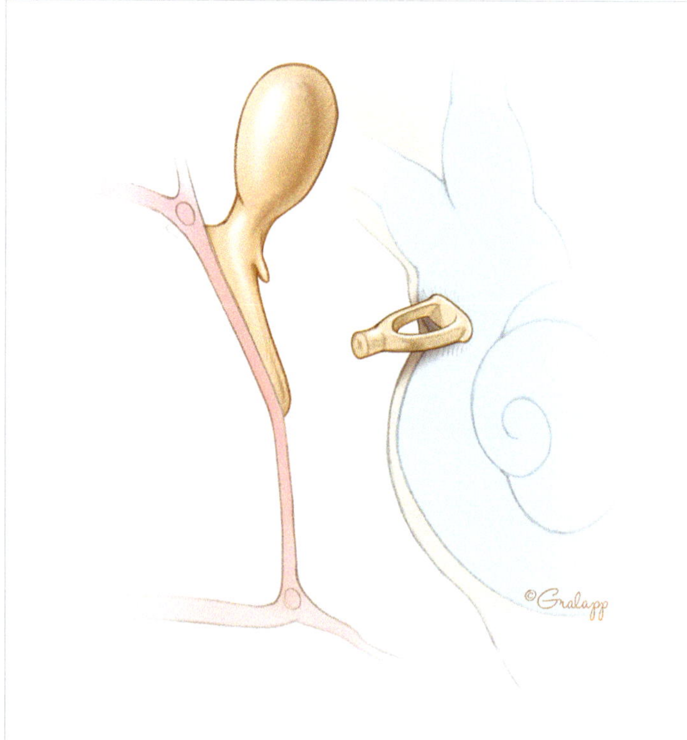

Fig. 6.5 Absence of a functional incus is common in chronic otitis media and cholesteatoma.

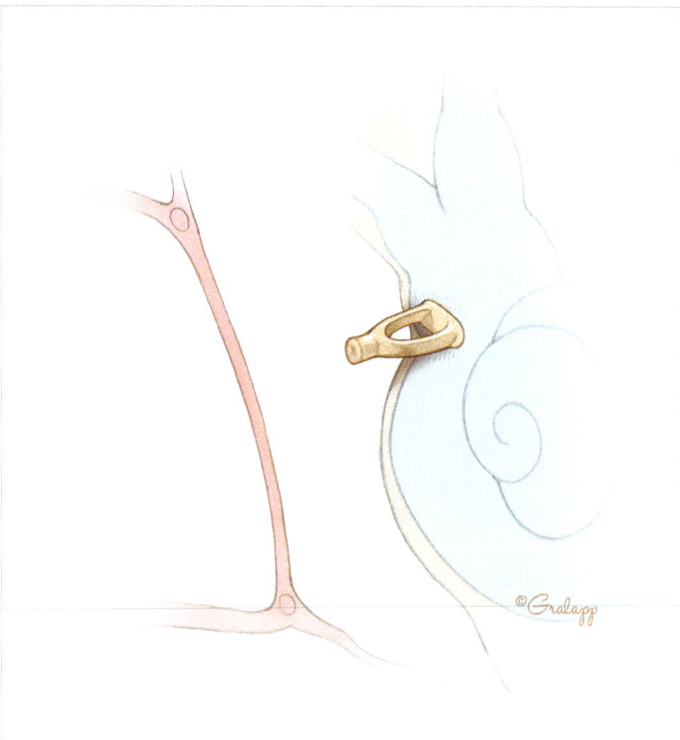

Fig. 6.6 Absence of malleus and incus.

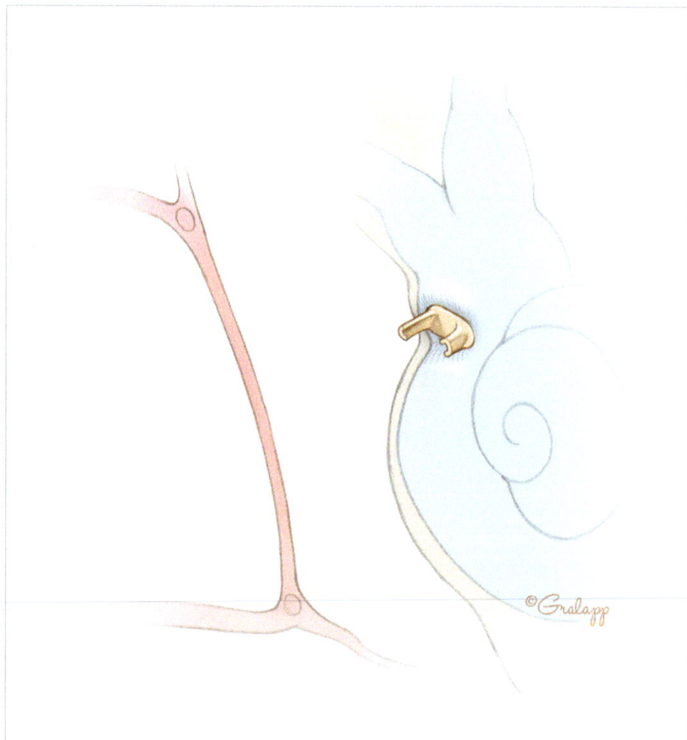

Fig. 6.7 Cholesteatoma often involves the malleus, incus, and stapes arch leaving a crural remnant.

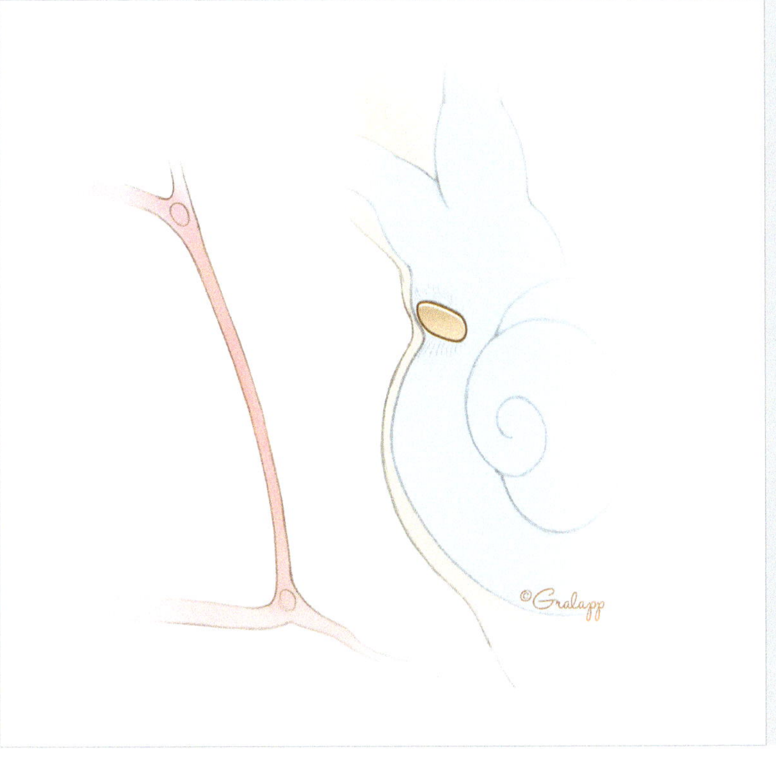

Fig. 6.8 Absence of the entire ossicular chain except for the stapes footplate is common in cholesteatoma.

6.3 Autologous Ossiculoplasty

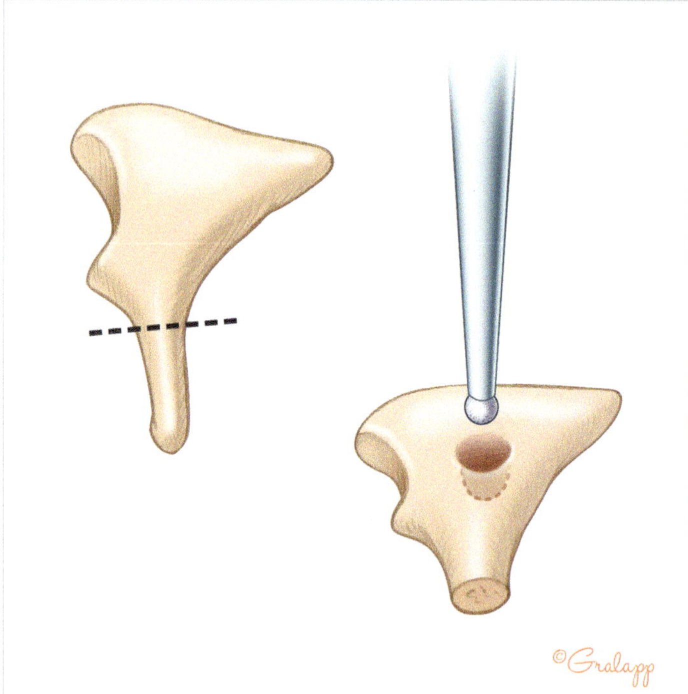

Fig. 6.9 Shaping the incus body to serve as an autologous ossicular reconstruction. The long process is removed and a well for the capitulum is drilled in the incus body.

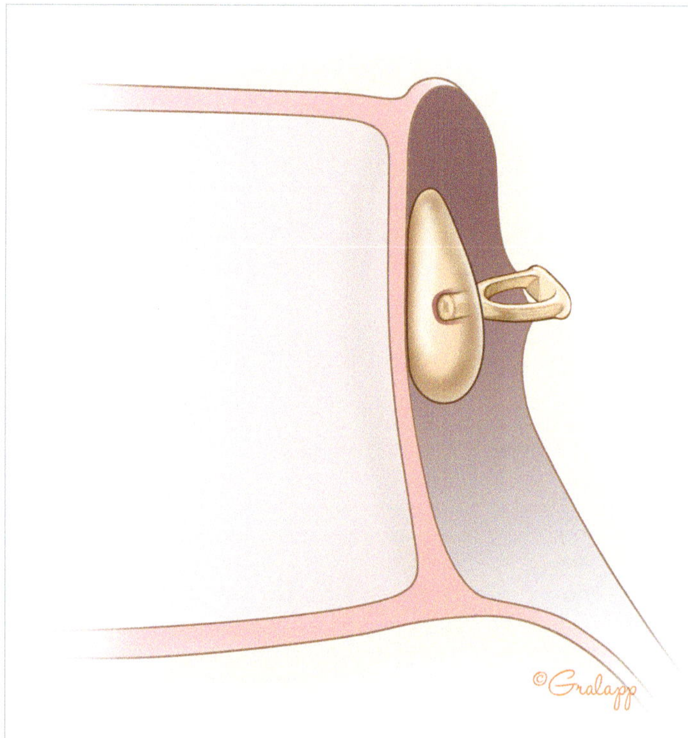

Fig. 6.10 A rotated incus used in reconstruction. This method is employed primarily in canal wall down procedures as, with normal anatomy, the middle space is not sufficiently shallow.

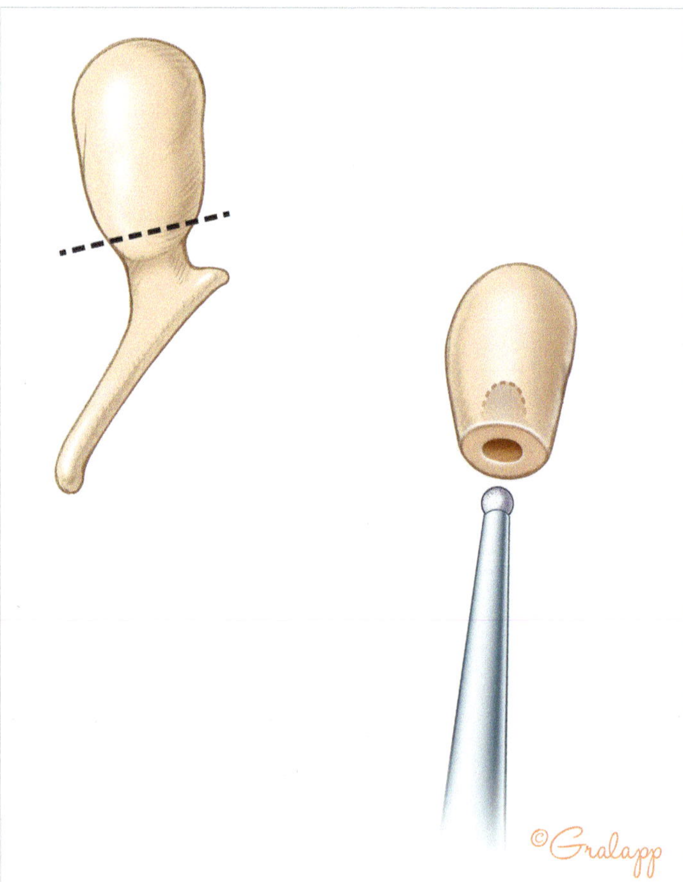

Fig. 6.11 Shaping the malleus head for ossiculoplasty. The long process is separated at the neck and a well is drilled into the malleus head.

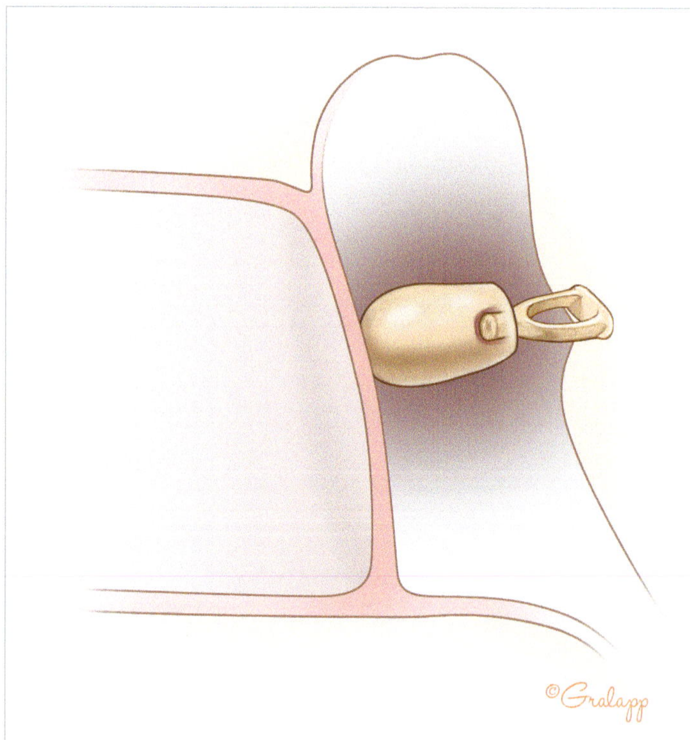

Fig. 6.12 Use of the malleus head in reconstruction on top of the stapes capitulum. Because of the top-heavy nature of this reconstruction, it may be mechanically unstable.

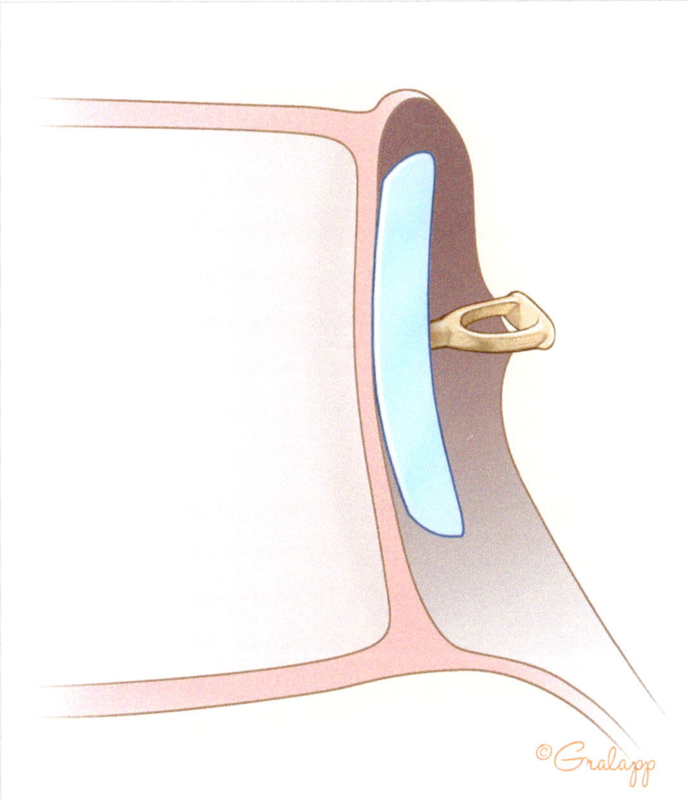

Fig. 6.13 Ossiculoplasty using cartilage alone is sometimes possible following canal wall down mastoidectomy when the middle ear space is narrow. Laying the tympanic membrane directly on the capitulum has a substantial failure rate due to poor contact. A cartilage sheet resting on the capitulum enhances contact with the tympanic membrane.

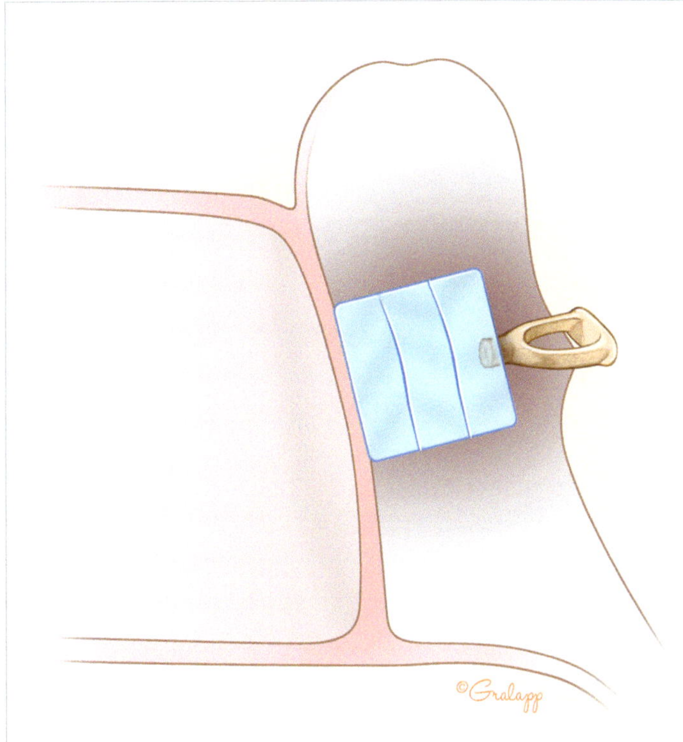

Fig. 6.14 Stacked cartilage spanning a several-millimeter gap between the capitulum and the tympanic membrane. Cohesion of the stack can be facilitated by leaving the perichondrium intact.

6.4 Prosthetic Ossiculoplasty

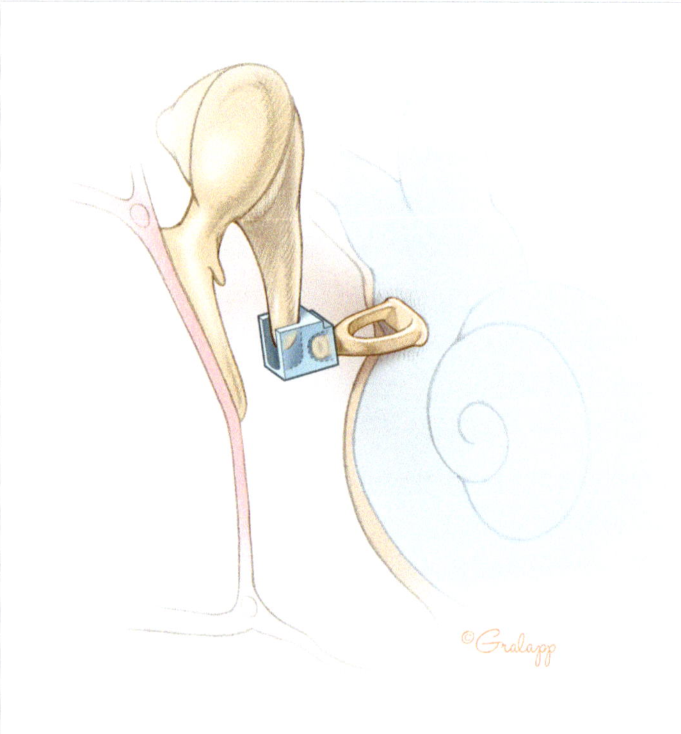

Fig. 6.15 Applebaum ceramic prosthesis spanning a distal long process defect.

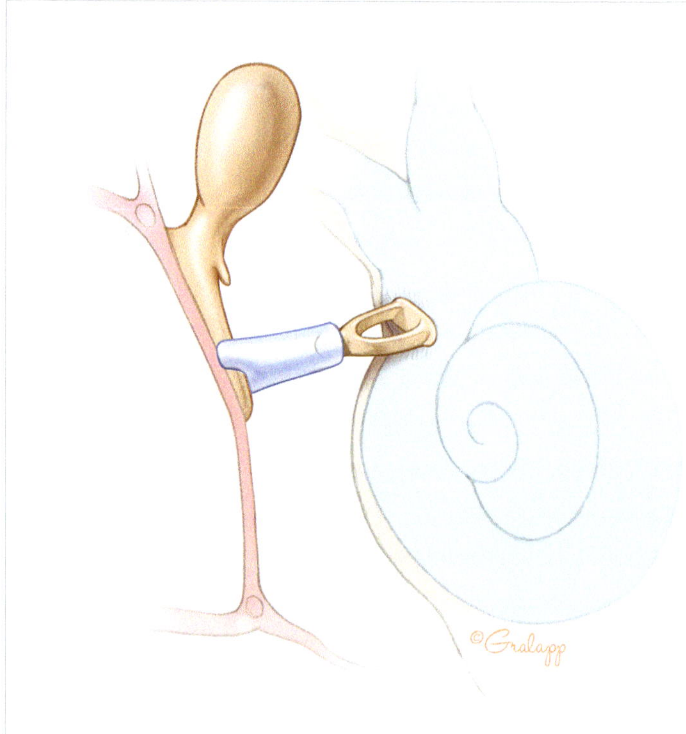

Fig. 6.16 Ceramic crutch and cup-type prosthesis connecting the malleus long process (manubrium) with the capitulum of the stapes. Because the manubrium lies anterior to the stapes, and is often medialized due to retraction and scarring from infection, it is often challenging to achieve stability. Both crutch and cup often need to be modified with a drill to mortise into position.

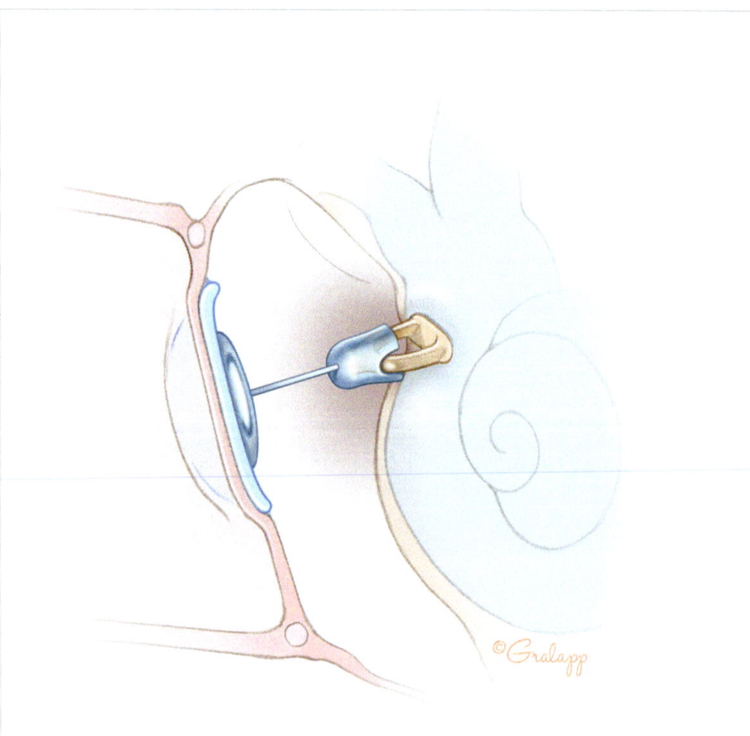

Fig. 6.17 Titanium partial ossicular replacement prosthesis (PORP). To discourage extrusion, autologous cartilage is interposed between the prosthesis and tympanic membrane. Many surgeons use this form of reconstruction whenever the incus is deficient regardless of the status of the malleus.

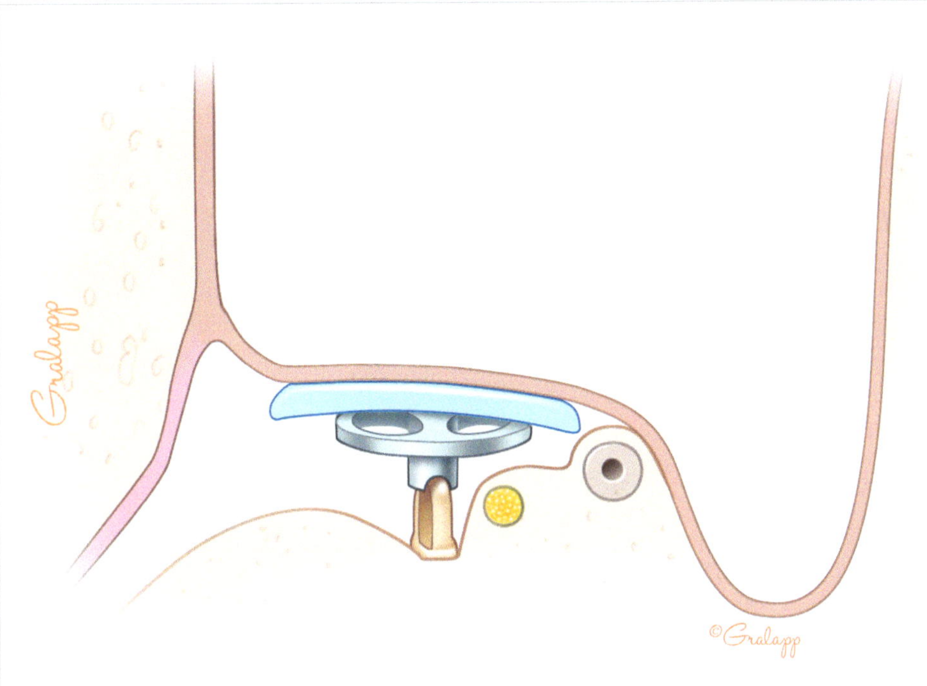

Fig. 6.18 A Frisbee prosthesis is used in canal wall down settings when the middle ear is narrow. Cartilage alone may not develop a satisfactory connection with the capitulum of the stapes. This type of prosthesis widens the surface area of contact.

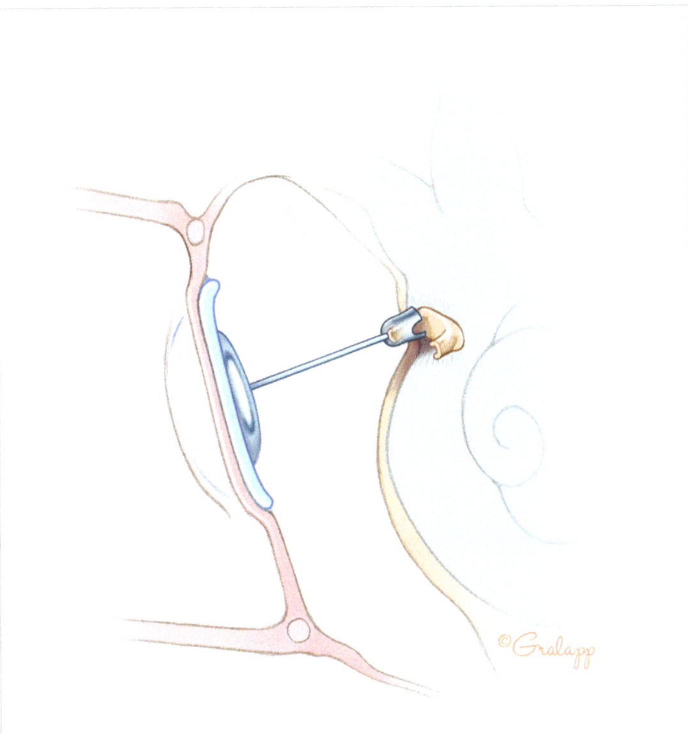

Fig. 6.19 Use of a long titanium partial ossicular replacement prosthesis (PORP) onto an anterior crural remnant sufficient to serve as an anchor.

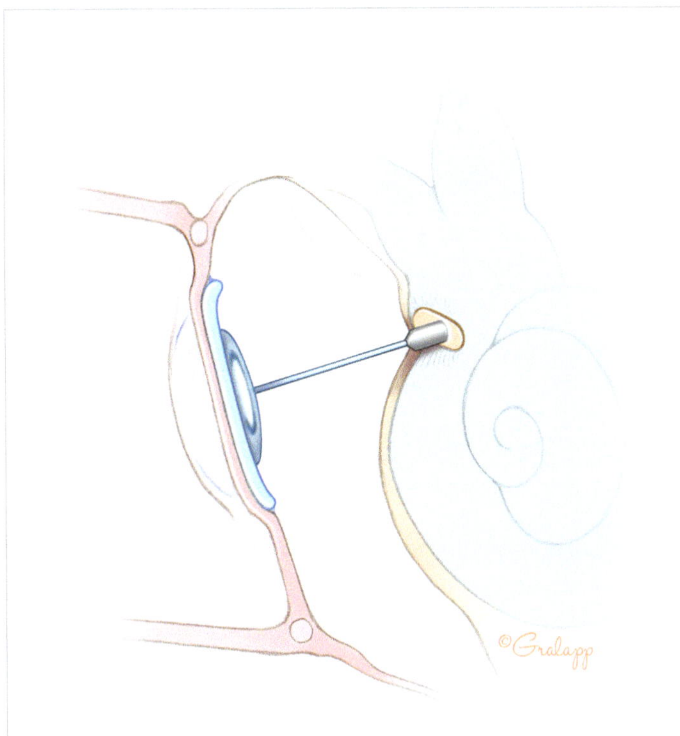

Fig. 6.20 Total ossicular replacement prosthesis (TORP). To discourage extrusion, autologous cartilage is interposed between the prosthesis and the tympanic membrane.

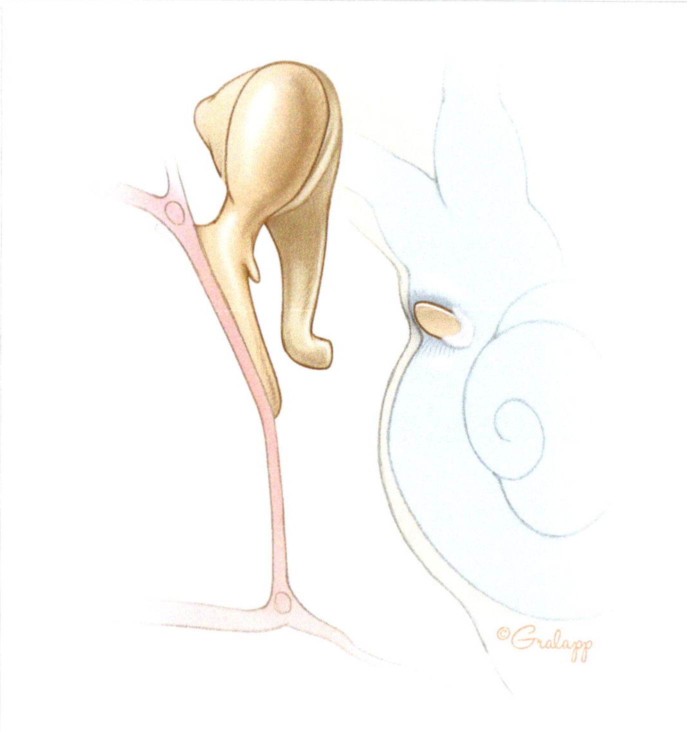

Fig. 6.21 The ossicular defect in otosclerosis which follows removal of the stapes arch. Note the fixation of the stapes footplate.

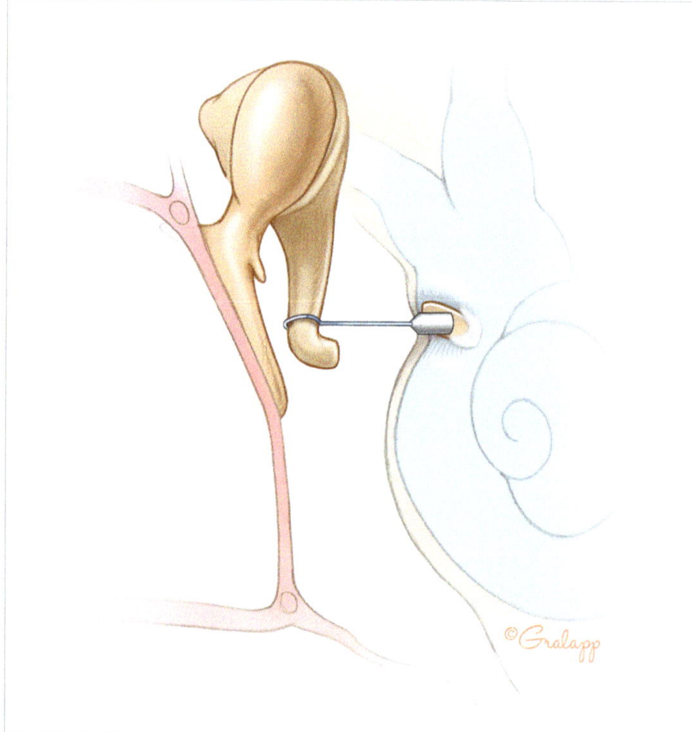

Fig. 6.22 A piston stapes prosthesis crimped onto the long process of the incus and is anchored in surgically created footplate fenestra (stapedotomy).

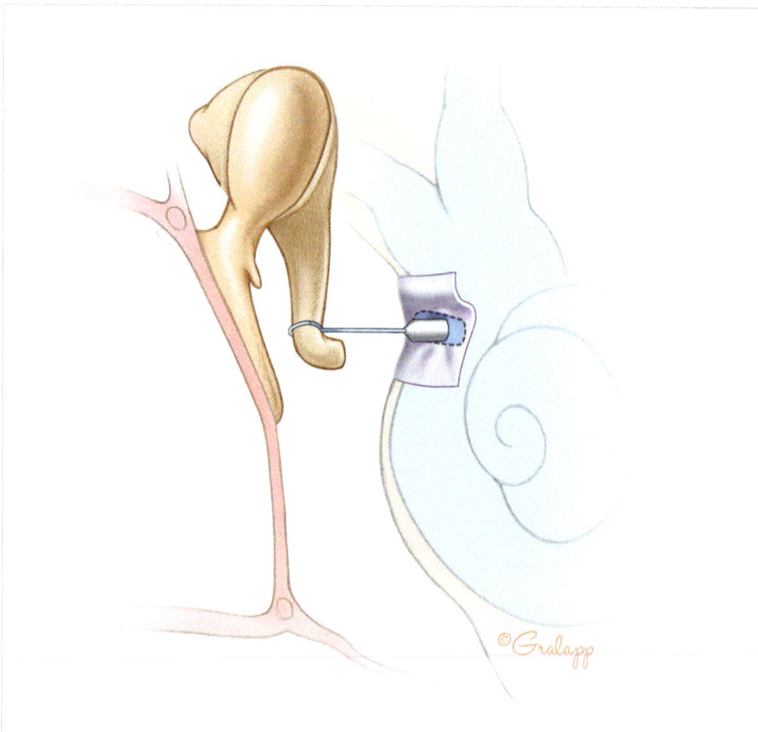

Fig. 6.23 Stapes prosthesis in place following total stapedectomy with tissue grafting covering the oval window.

6.5 Ossiculoplasty Placement Technique

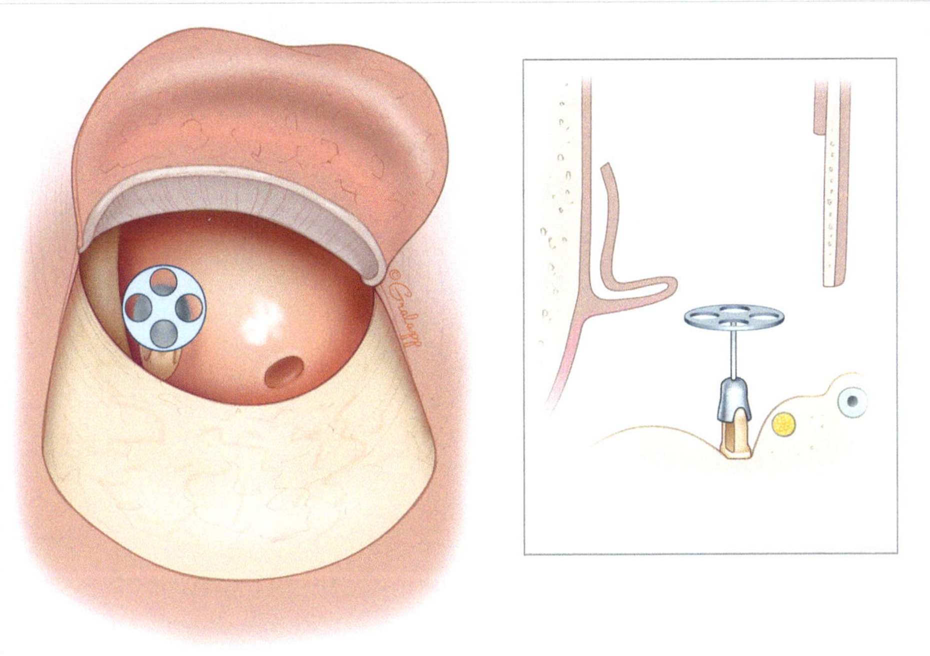

Fig. 6.24 Partial ossicular replacement prosthesis in position prior to placement of cartilage.

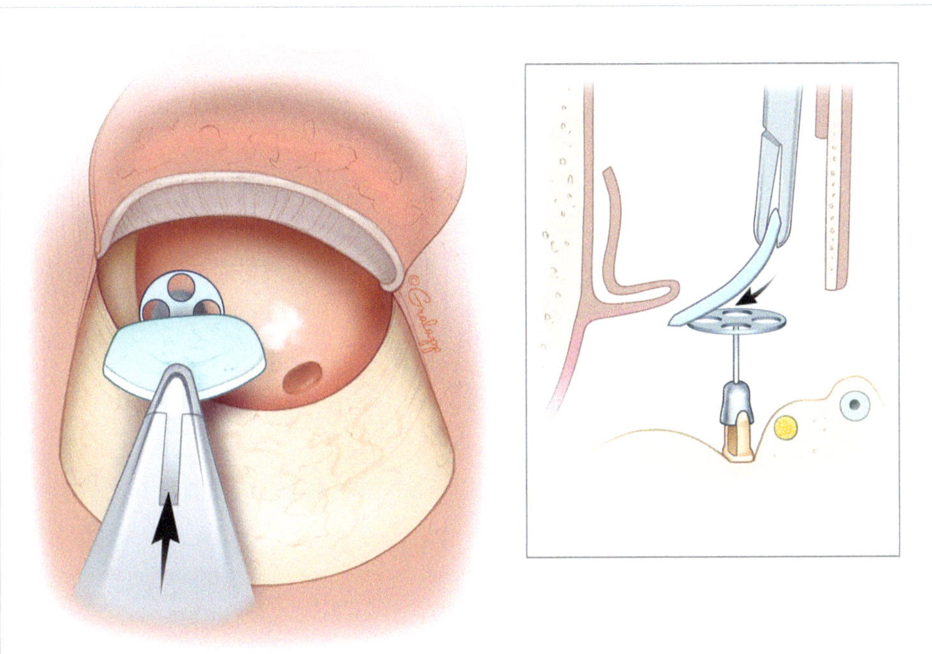

Fig. 6.25 Placement of cartilage graft can displace the prosthesis.

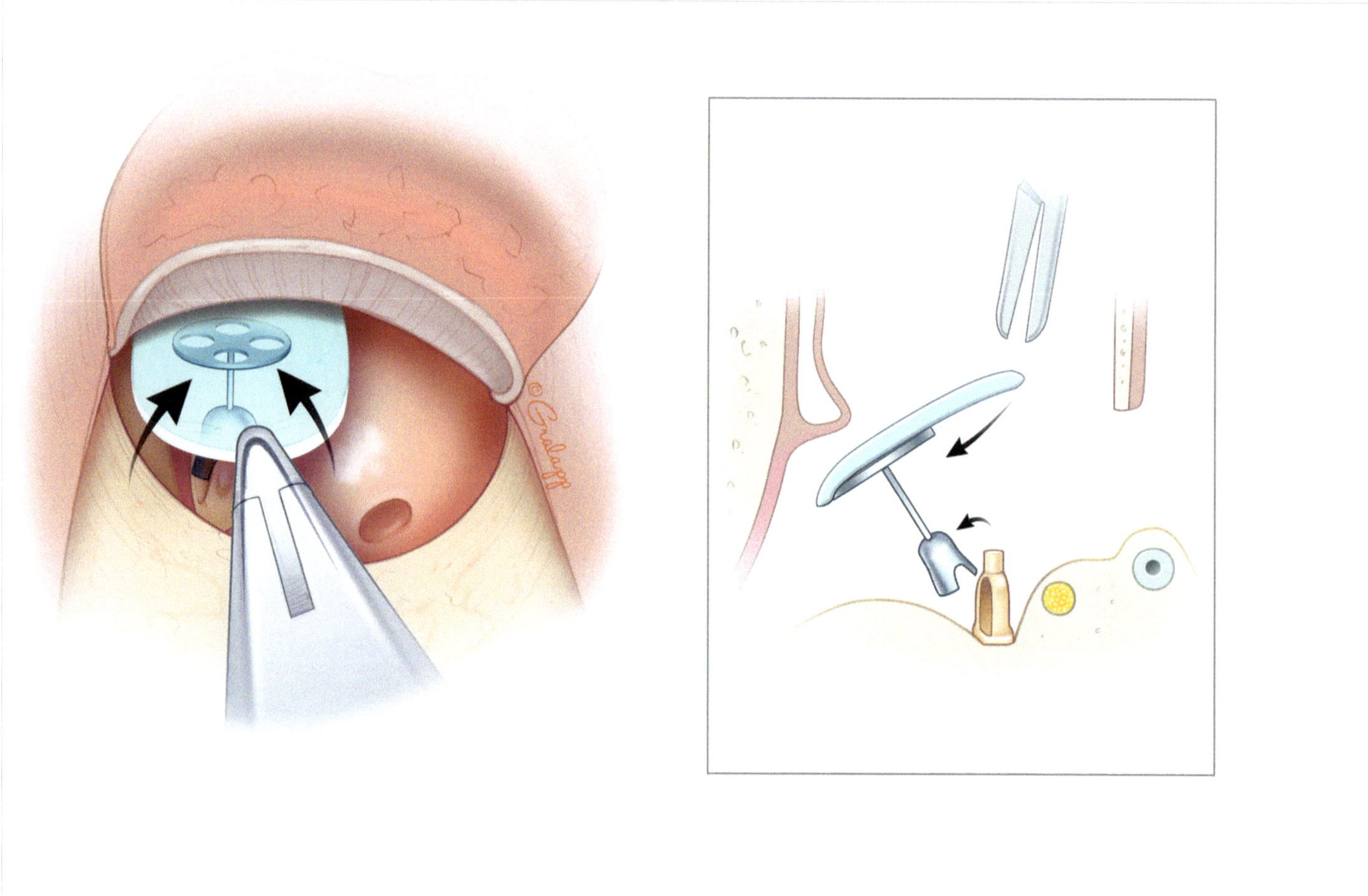

Fig. 6.26 If the cartilage contacts the prosthesis prematurely, it rotates anteriorly.

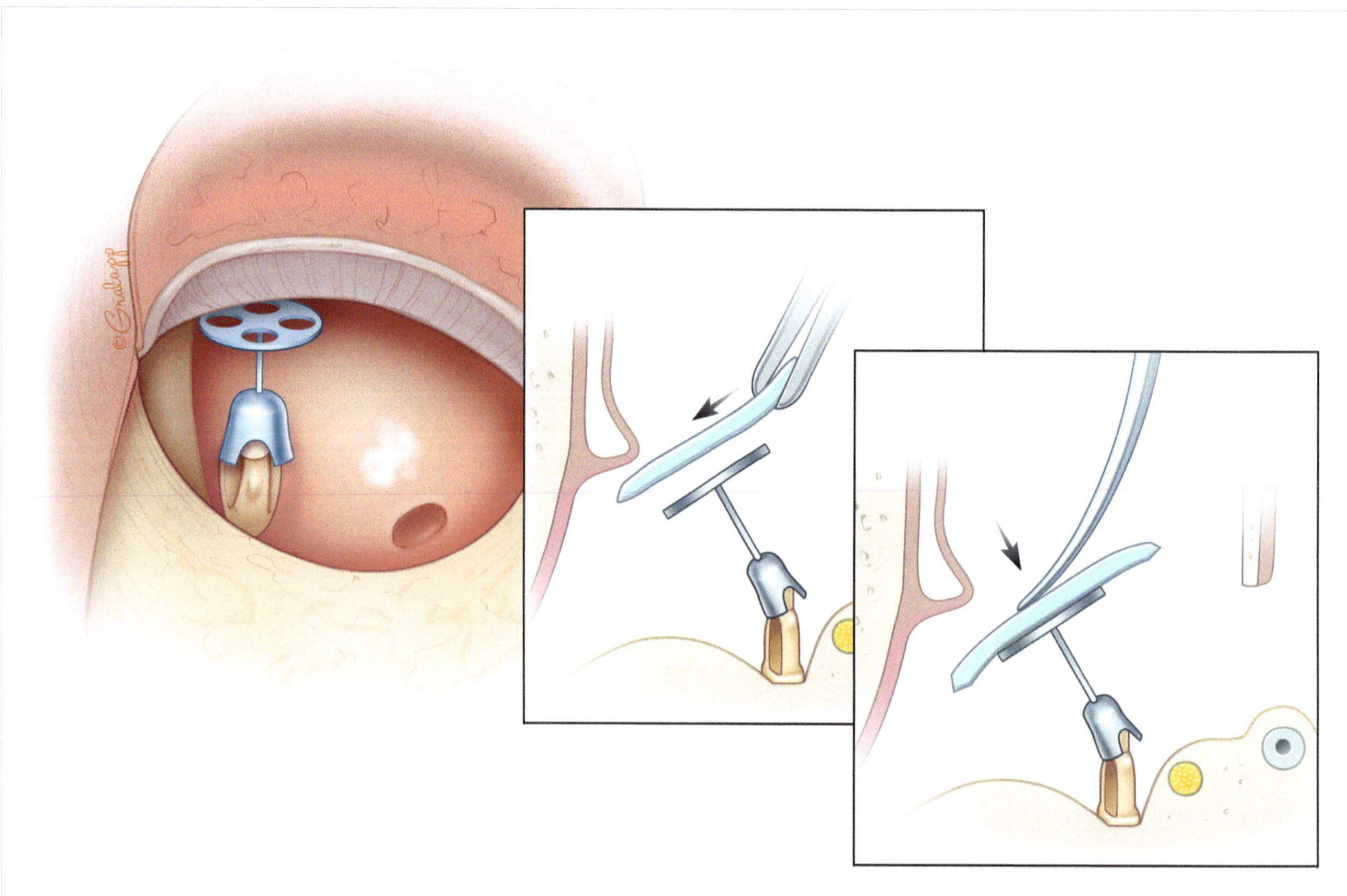

Fig. 6.27 Tilting the prosthesis anteriorly before contacting the cartilage.

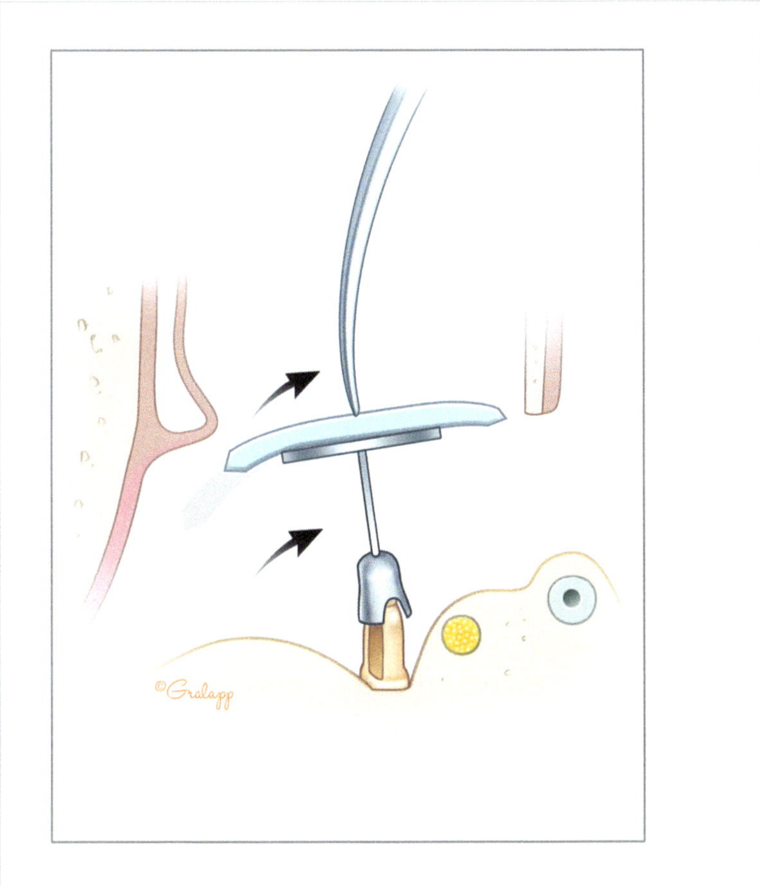

Fig. 6.28 Pulling the cartilage back toward the scutum edge restores upright position.

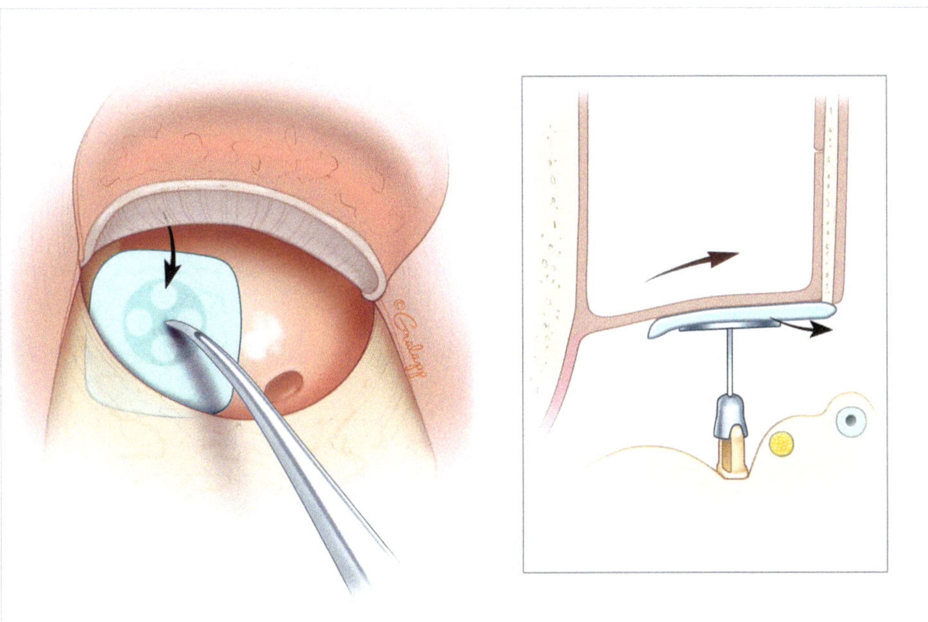

Fig. 6.29 Sliding the cartilage beneath the scutal edge helps stabilize the prosthesis by creating longitudinal tension. It also seals the margin thus discouraging cholesteatoma recurrence.

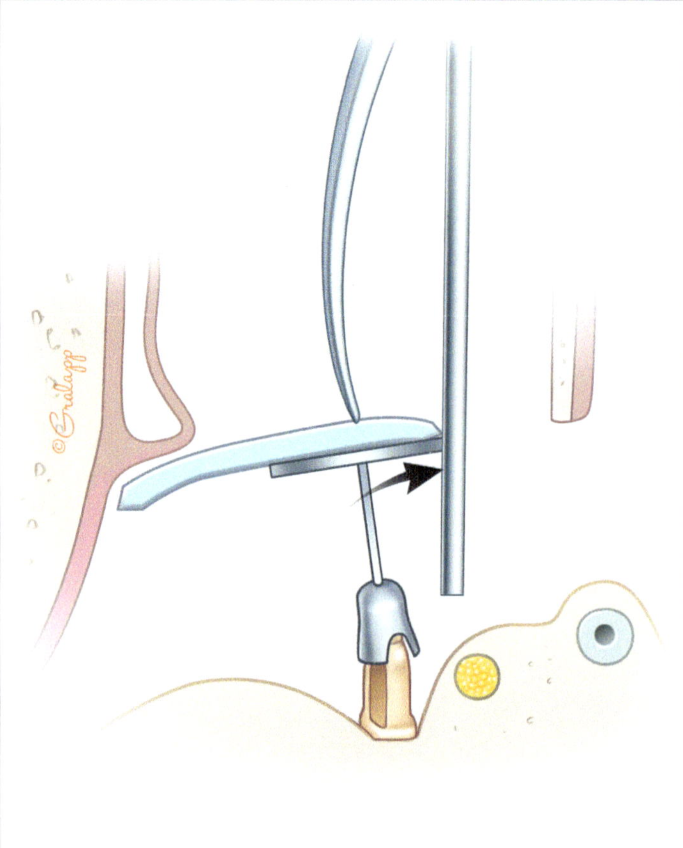

Fig. 6.30 The shaft of a suction can be used to help stabilize the prosthesis during cartilage placement.

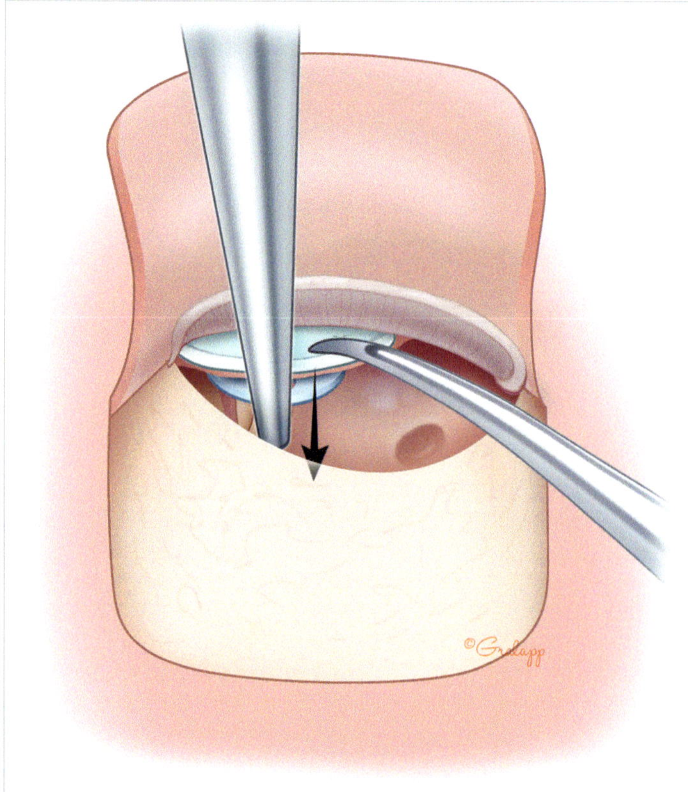

Fig. 6.31 The shaft of a suction can be used to help stabilize the prosthesis during cartilage placement.

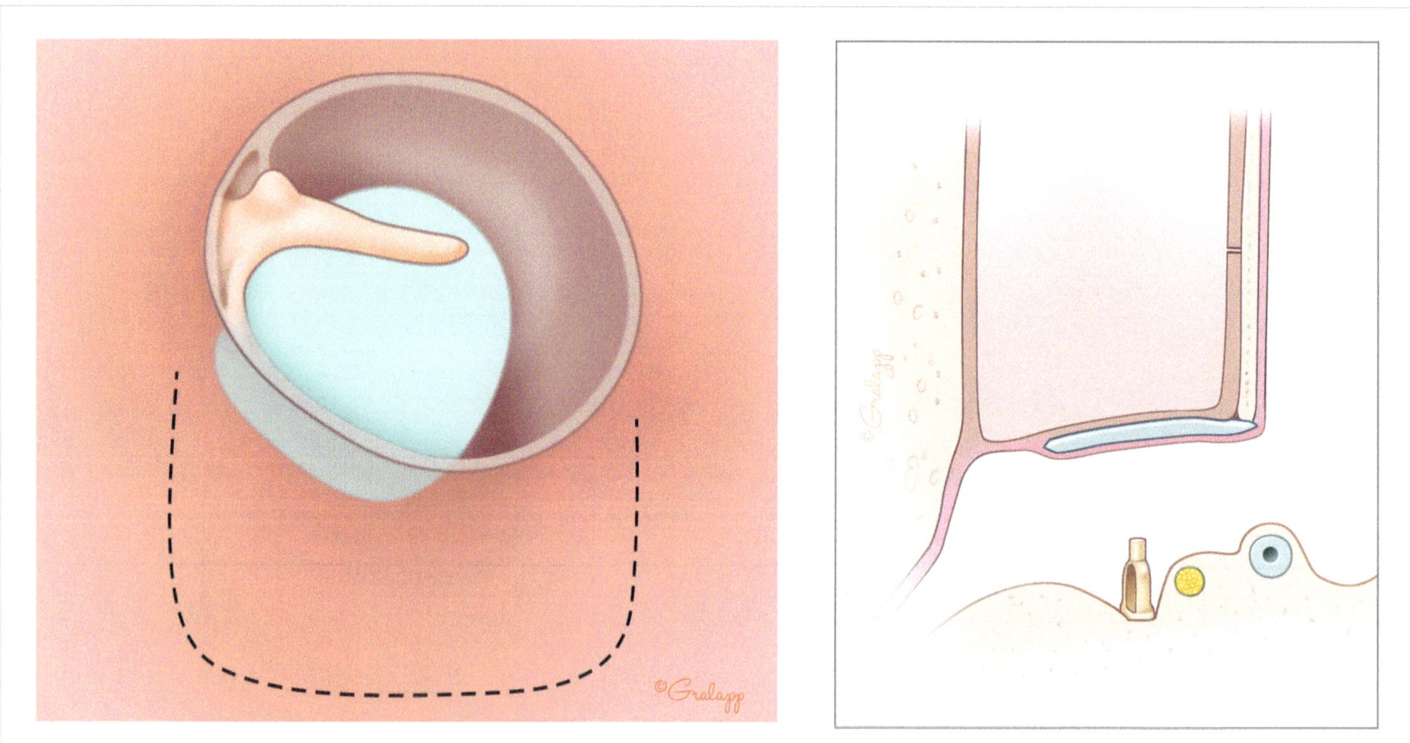

Fig. 6.32 One advantage of staging the procedure is that cartilage placed at the first stage is already integrated with the tympanic membrane. It is important to have a tympanomeatal flap of adequate length as the flap shortens due to tenting of the drum by the prosthesis and an annular dehiscence may result if the flap is of insufficient length. Note that the tympanomeatal flap stops short of the annulus so that the tympanic membrane remains under tension to help support the prosthesis in position.

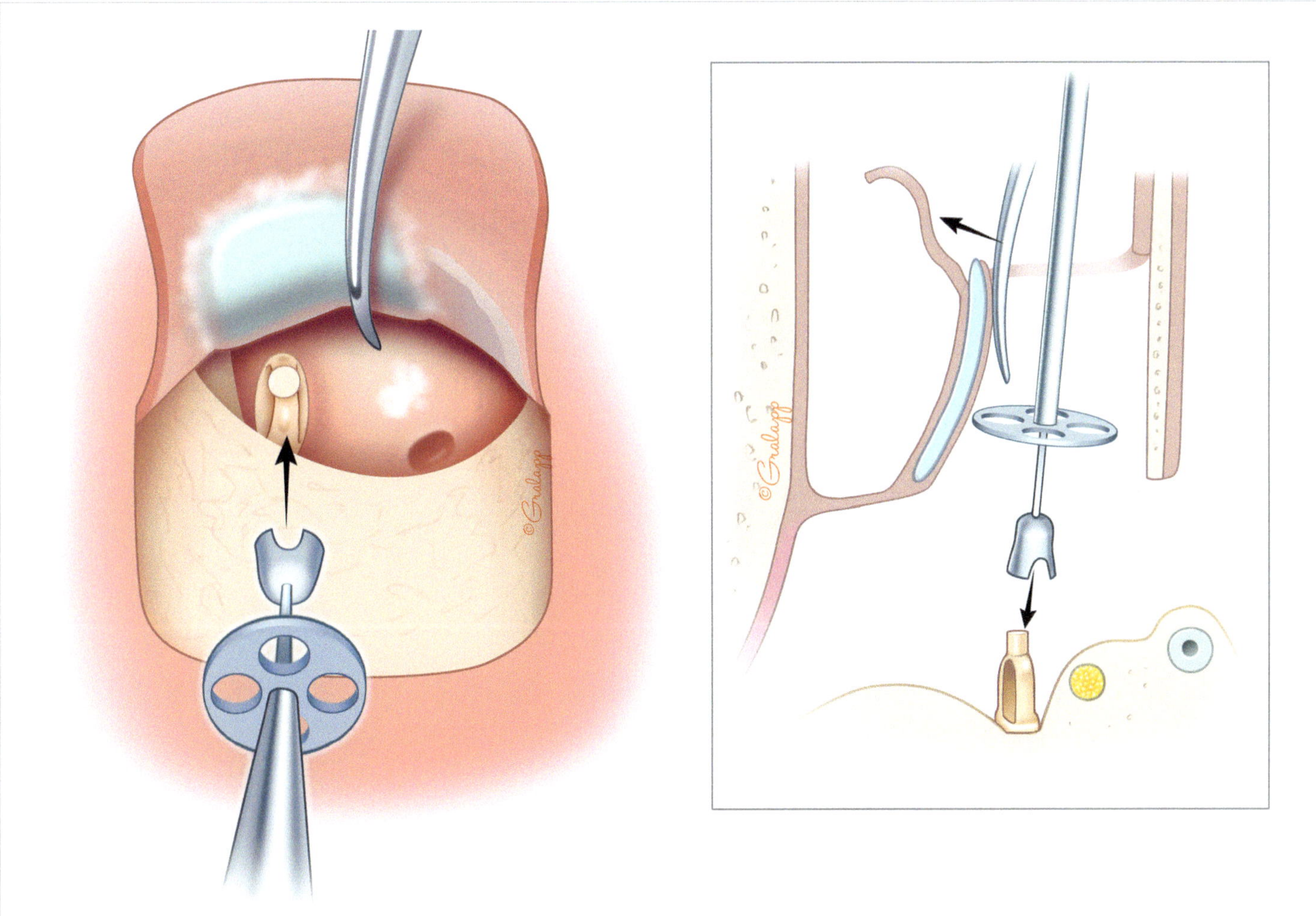

Fig. 6.33 An instrument forcibly holds up the cartilage embedded in the tympanic membrane while the prosthesis is positioned.

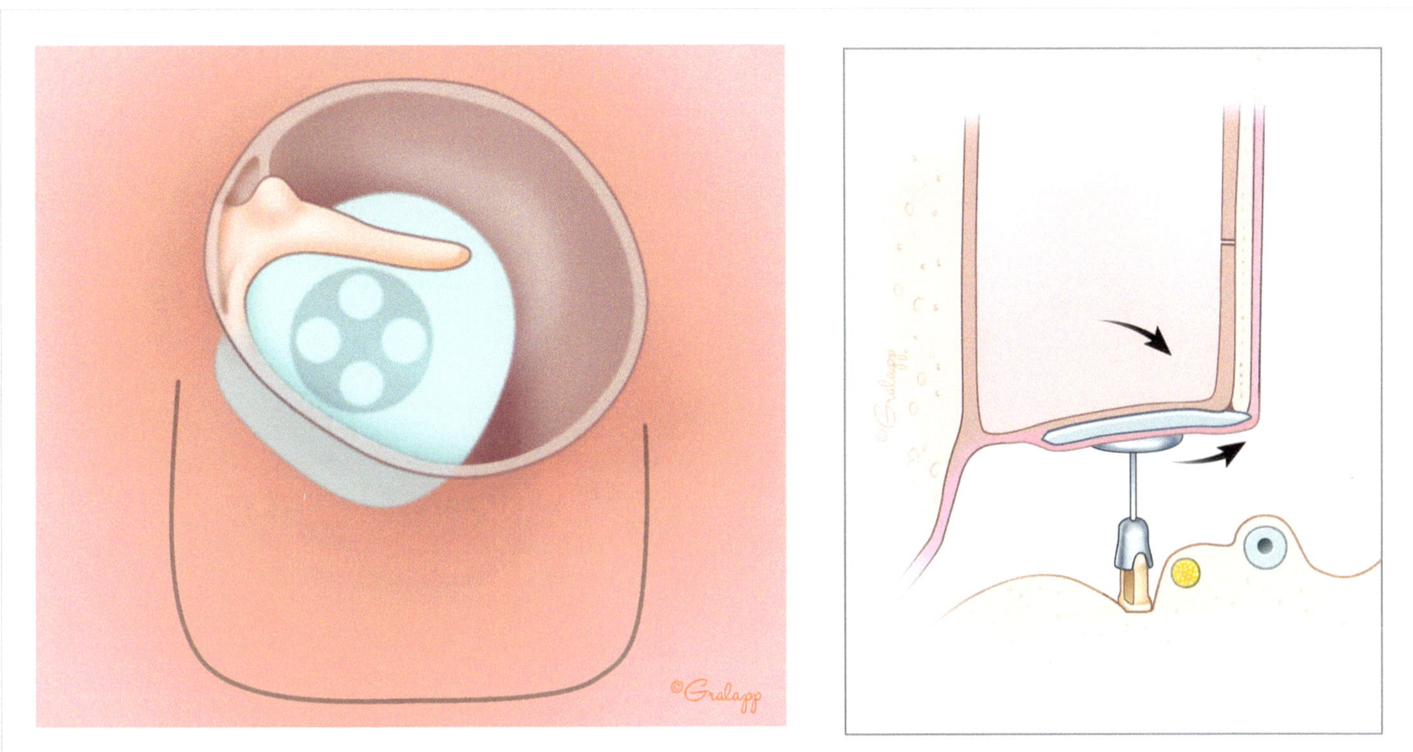

Fig. 6.34 Releasing the cartilage allows it to snap back thus holding the prosthesis in position.

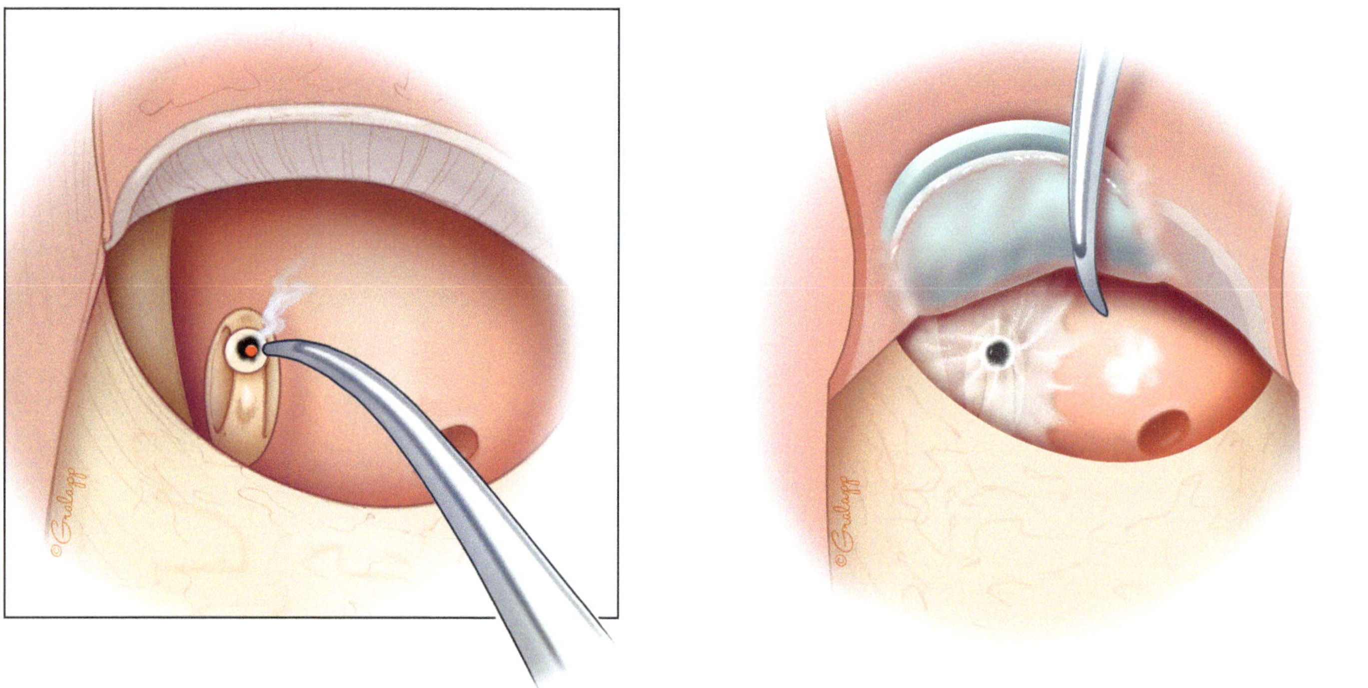

Fig. 6.35 During the first stage of a two-stage procedure in which cholesteatoma and/or scarring has affected the stapes, placing a laser mark on the capitulum is a helpful guide to identification of the stapes during the second stage.

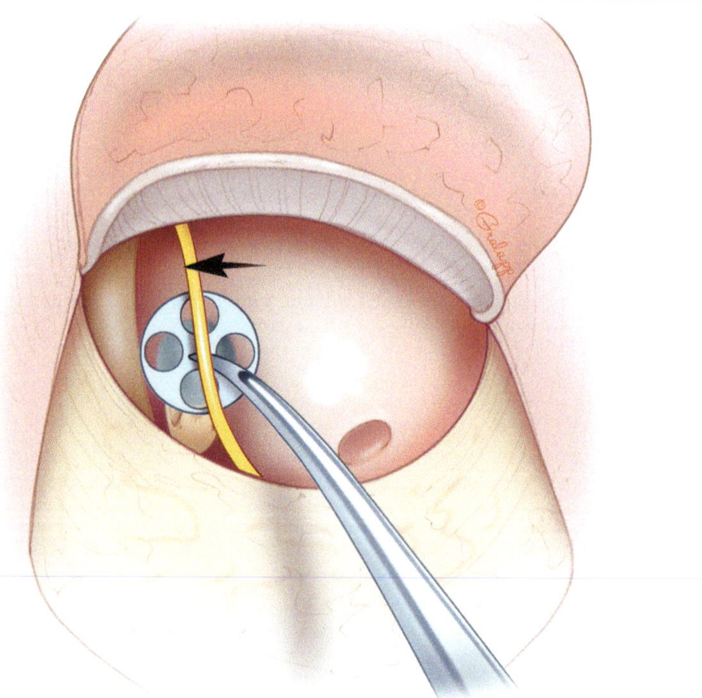

Fig. 6.36 When the chorda tympani is intact, using it as a sling to establish longitudinal tension is helpful in stabilizing the prosthesis.

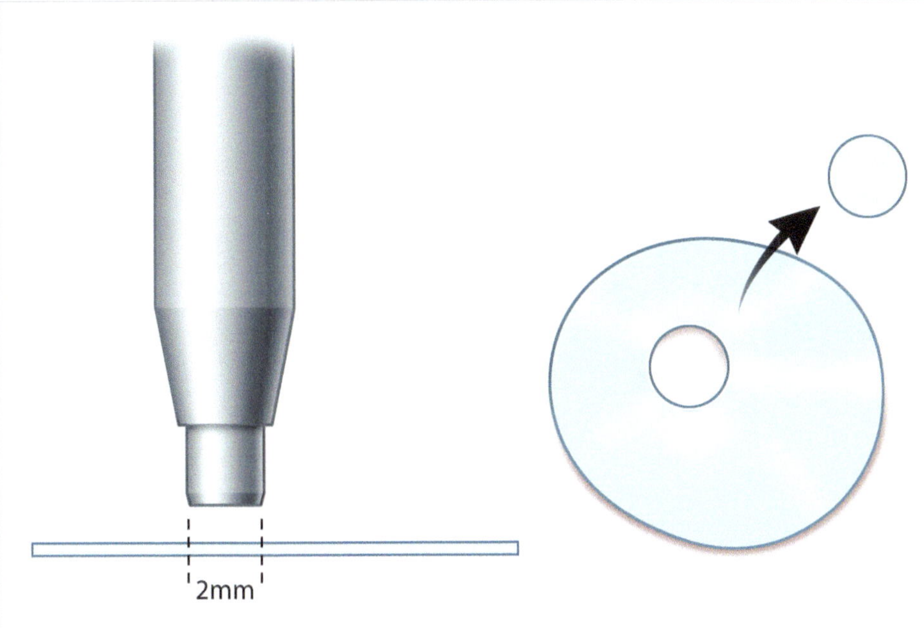

Fig. 6.37 A disc of Gelfilm can help stabilize the prosthesis and discourage scar formation. After trimming to size, a dermatological punch is used to create a small aperture for the capitulum.

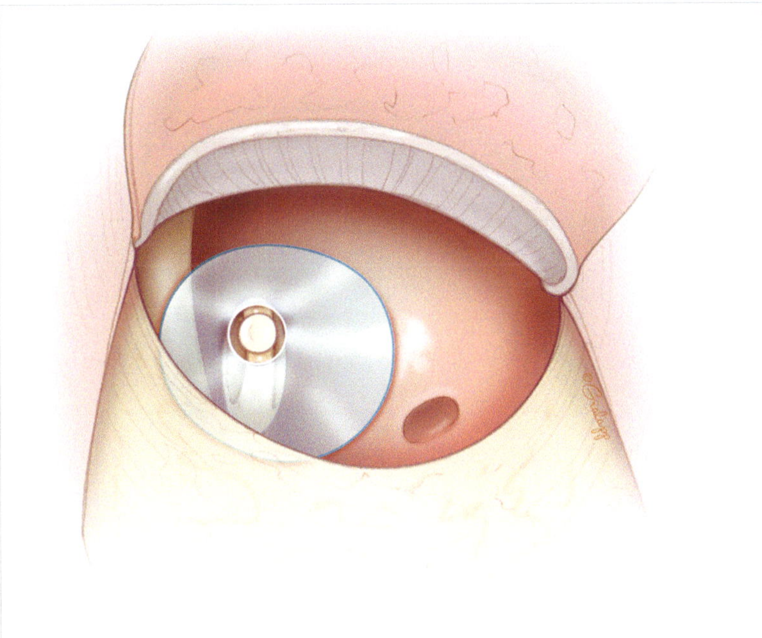

Fig. 6.38 Placement of the disc over the capitulum.

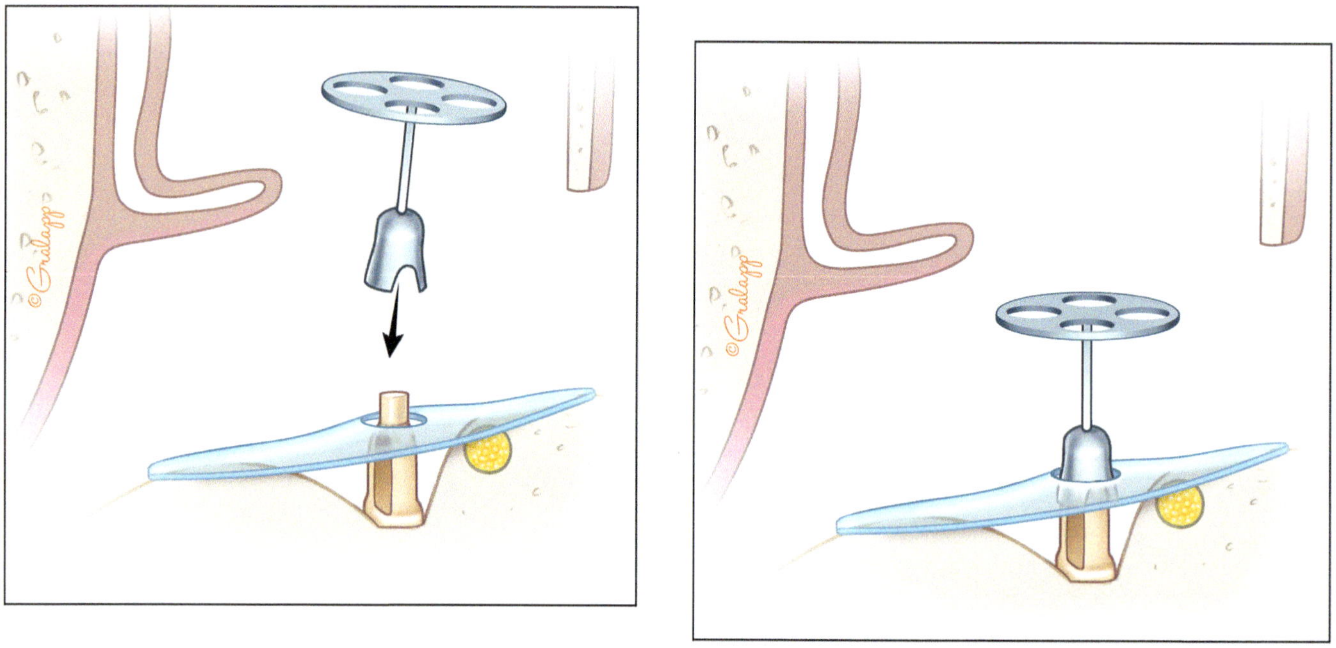

Fig. 6.39 Insertion of the prosthesis.

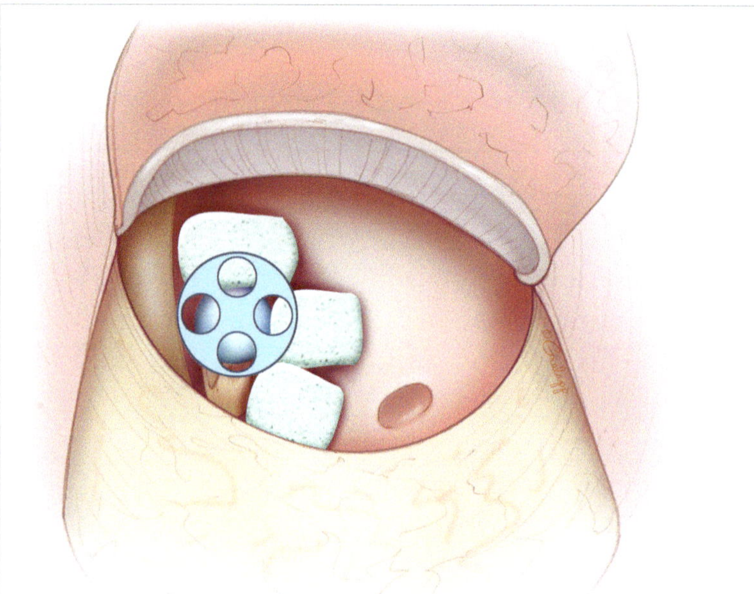

Fig. 6.40 Prostheses tend to be less stable inferiorly and anteriorly and are more likely to displace in those directions. Packing is used to counter this tendency.

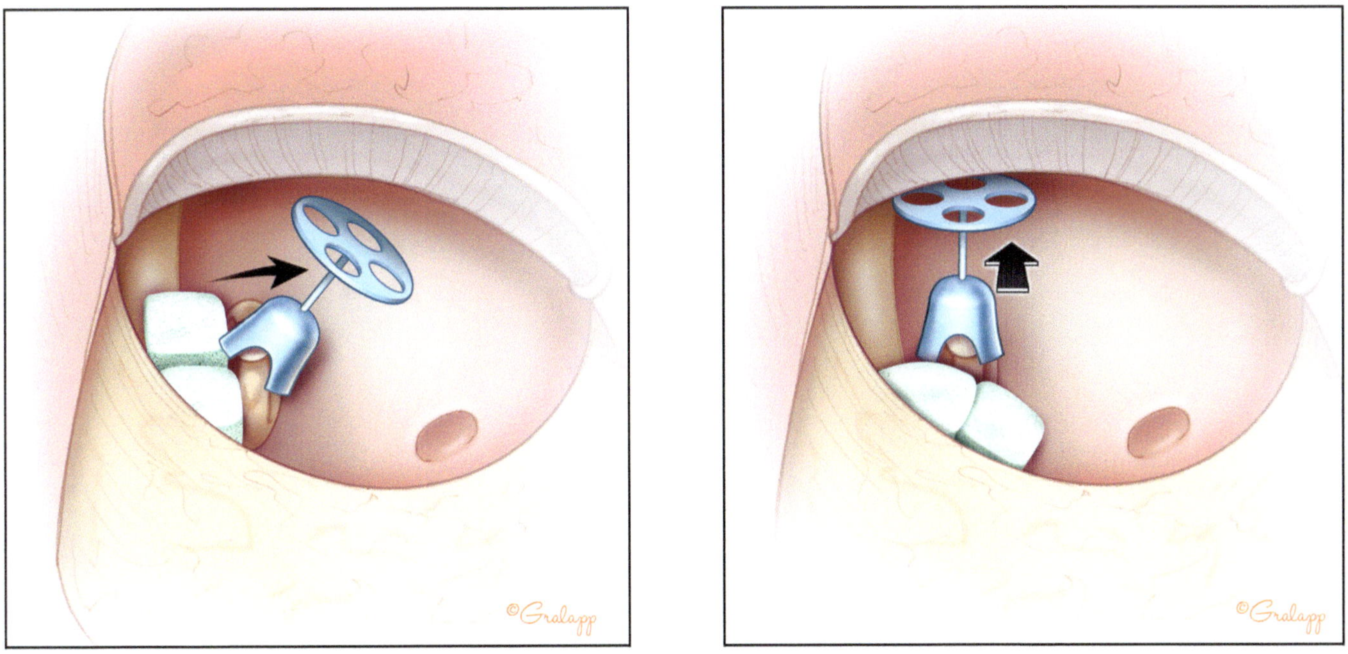

Fig. 6.41 Packing placed superiorly over the facial nerve or posteriorly can actually destabilize the prosthesis.

6.6 Transfacial Recess Ossiculoplasty

Nikolas H. Blevins

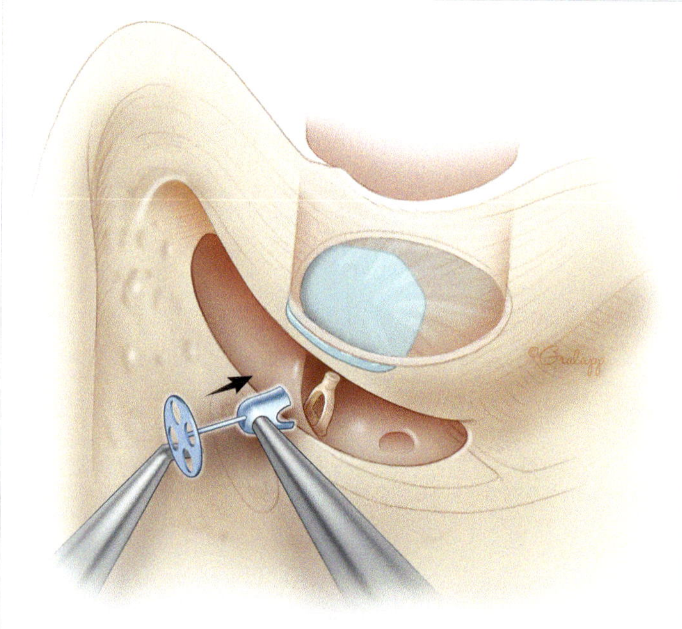

Fig. 6.42 During a planned second-stage procedure in which the facial recess had been opened during the first stage, it is possible to insert an ossicular prosthesis through the mastoid via the facial recess.

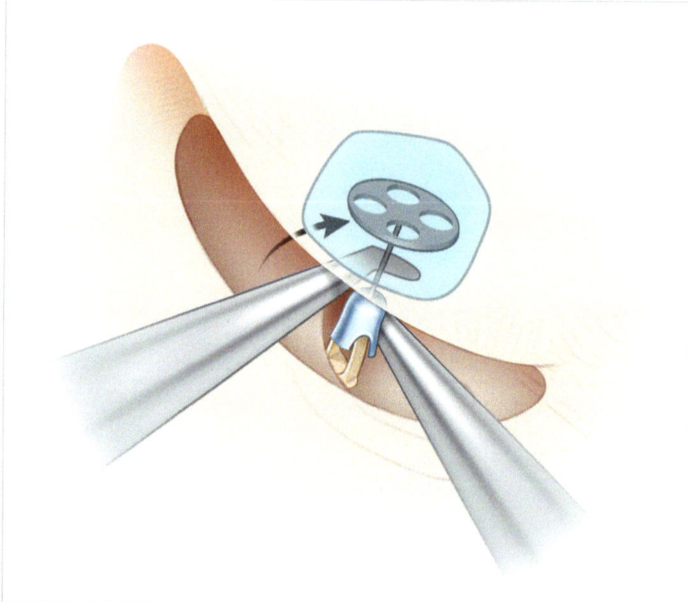

Fig. 6.43 Using a suction to stabilize and a hook to position, the prosthesis is rotated into position.

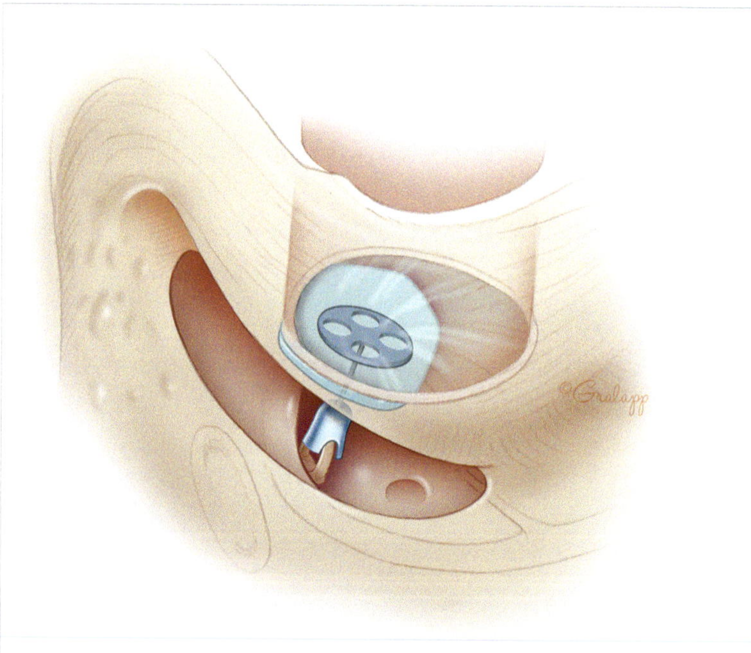

Fig. 6.44 Prosthesis in position.

6.7 Medialized Malleus

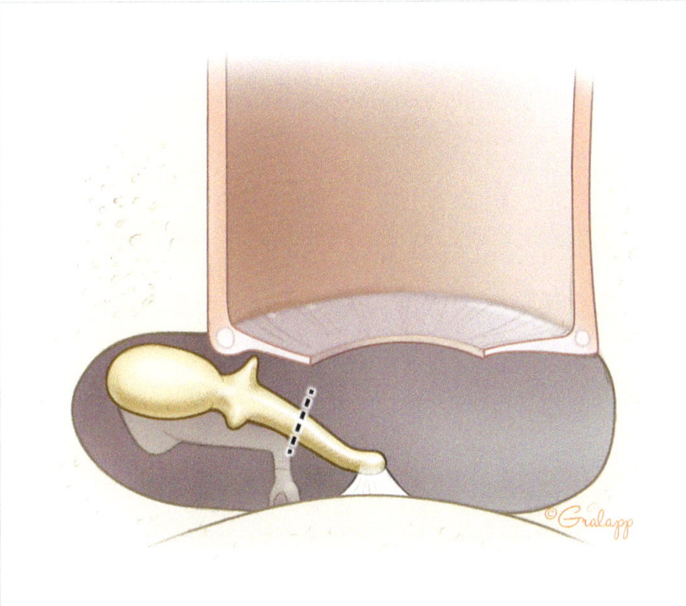

Fig. 6.45 Medialized umbo attached to the promontory in presence of an intact ossicular chain. Without correcting the medial rotation, grafting of the tympanic membrane is technically difficult and results in a slit-like middle ear cavity. Pulling the umbo laterally with an intact chain traumatizes the cochlea. The classical answer to this situation is to cut the incudostapedial joint, forcibly lateralize the malleus, cut the tensor tympani tendon, and then attempt to reattach the incudostapedial joint. The difficulty is that the joint does not always reattach sufficiently.

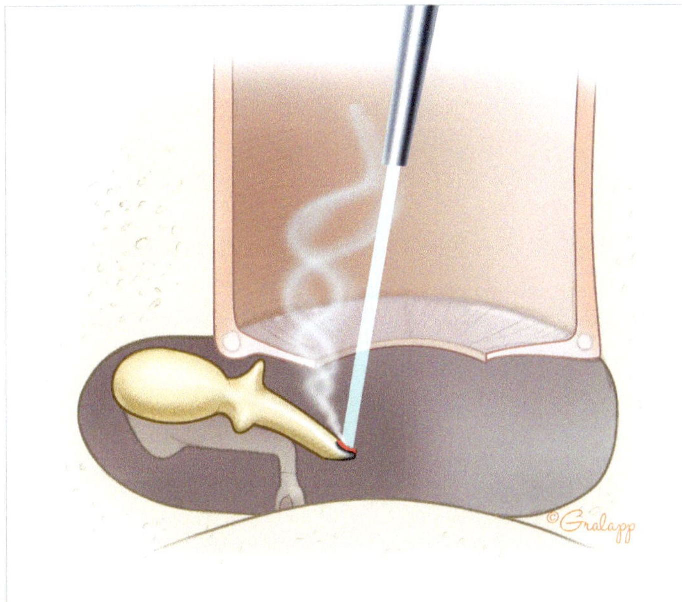

Fig. 6.46 Laser resection of the distal segment of the umbo enables placement of the graft without need for interrupting the ossicular chain. The laser chars bone rather than vaporizing it, necessitating sequentially picking away the char while the bone thins. Placing moist-absorbable gelatin sponge beneath the umbo lessens the injury to the promontory mucosa due to overshoot.

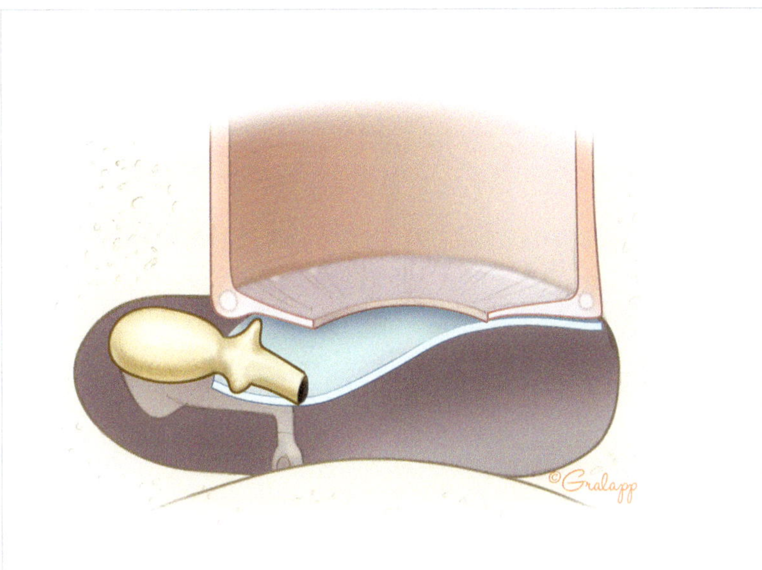

Fig. 6.47 Placement of the graft medial to the umbo remnant.

6.8 Staging Ossiculoplasty

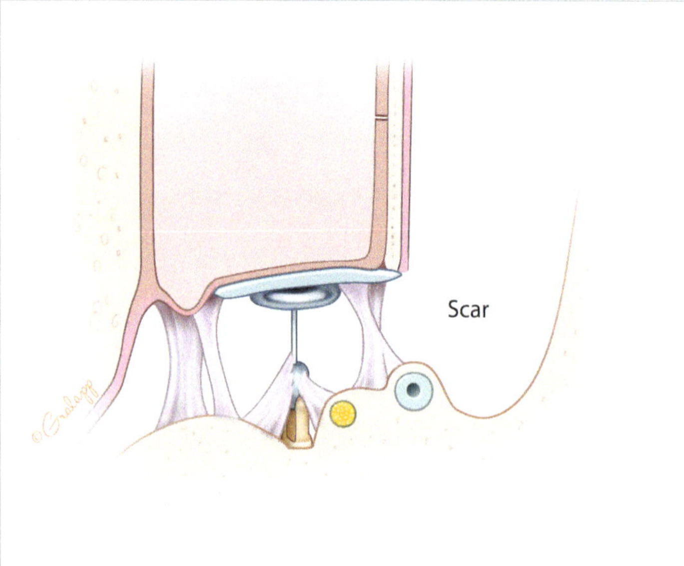

Fig. 6.48 Ossiculoplasty performed in a single stage with poor middle ear mucosa may result in scarring with either displacement or impaired vibration of the prosthesis.

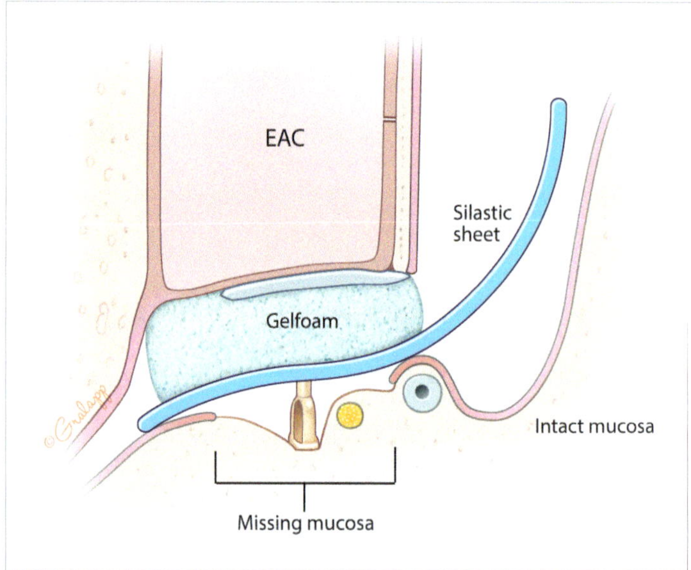

Fig. 6.49 Staging ossiculoplasty may be best when a sizable portion of the middle ear mucosa is diseased or absent. During the first stage, the cartilage graft is placed and silicon rubber sheet inserted to discourage scarring.

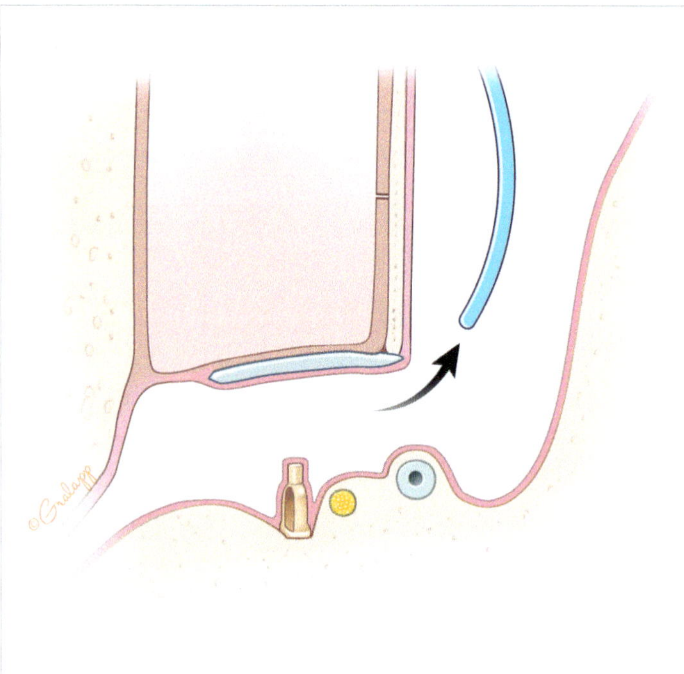

Fig. 6.50 Removal of silicon rubber sheet at second stage. Note the healthy middle ear mucosal envelope.

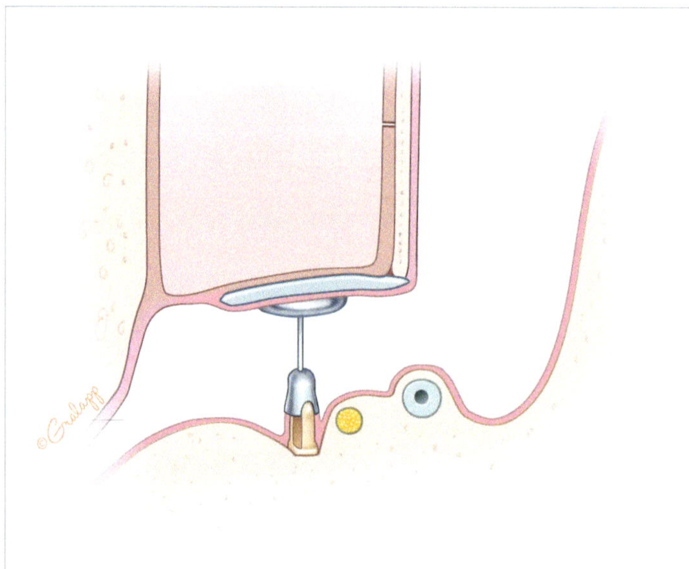

Fig. 6.51 Placement of partial ossicular chain prosthesis into a middle ear with a healthy mucosal envelope is a key factor in obtaining favorable hearing outcomes.

7 Mastoidectomy

Robert K. Jackler

7.1 Introduction to Mastoidectomy

While most mastoid surgery is conducted for infection, mastoidectomy is also performed to create a pathway to the deeper recesses of the temporal bone. These include surgery for neoplasia, vestibular procedures, and access to the dural interfaces for repair of CSF leakage and encephalocele. Mastoidectomy can be "complete" with exenteration of all mastoid pneumatization or limited as in the case of antrotomy sometimes also called "simple" mastoidectomy.

Acute and chronic ear infections are not typically limited to the middle ear; they involve the entire pneumatized spaces of the temporal bone. The mastoid consists of a large cell medially, called the antrum, which connects to the epitympanum via the aditus-ad-antrum. A variable extent of peripheral air cells may be present. Most mastoid surgery done for infection occurs in older children and adults and is in the setting of chronic otitis media in which entrapped infection has led to formation of granulation tissue and polyps. Acute mastoiditis is uncommon in the antibiotic era. When antibiotics have proven ineffective and/or when the air cells have become coalescent due to breakdown of their septa, mastoidectomy for abscess drainage is indicated. Special care is needed with postauricular incision in the first few years of life due to incomplete development of the mastoid tip which places the facial nerve in jeopardy in the lower limb of the incision. In infants and toddlers, it is best to make a more transverse incision above the ear rather than the traditional C-shaped incision curving behind the postauricular sulcus.

The mastoid anatomy has both consistent aspects and considerable variability. While the antrum is a consistent feature and the facial nerve and semicircular canals are consistently located, the extent of peripheral pneumatization and the size of the mastoid are highly variable. In poorly pneumatized temporal bones, only an antrum may remain. In such cases, the mastoid is said to be "contracted" and the temporal dura is low and the sigmoid sinus is forwardly placed.

When the mastoid is exteriorized and made confluent with the ear canal, a cavity of variable size is created (see section 8.3 Canal Wall Down Mastoidectomy in Chapter 8). When the mastoid is extensively pneumatized, a large cavity results that can accumulate debris and is more likely to discharge. In such cases, an effort is made to reduce the size of the cavity by mastoid obliteration. This can be done with autologous bone paté alone or in combination with various designs of soft-tissue rotational flaps.

Further Reading

1. Aslan A, Goktan C, Okumus M, Tarhan S, Unlu H. Morphometric analysis of anatomical relationships of the facial nerve for mastoid surgery. J Laryngol Otol 2001;115(6):447–449 PubMed
2. Cinamon U. The growth rate and size of the mastoid air cell system and mastoid bone: a review and reference. Eur Arch Otorhinolaryngol 2009;266(6):781–786 PubMed
3. Göksu N, Kemaloğlu YK, Köybaşioğlu A, Ileri F, Ozbilen S, Akyildiz N. Clinical importance of the Korner's septum. Am J Otol 1997;18(3):304–306 PubMed
4. Green JD Jr, Shelton C, Brackmann DE. Iatrogenic facial nerve injury during otologic surgery. Laryngoscope 1994;104(8, Pt 1):922–926 PubMed
5. Harun A, Clark J, Semenov YR, Francis HW. The role of obliteration in the achievement of a dry mastoid bowl. Otol Neurotol 2015;36(9):1510–1517 PubMed
6. Kullman GL, Dyck PJ, Cody DT. Anatomy of the mastoid portion of the facial nerve. Arch Otolaryngol 1971;93(1):29–33 PubMed
7. Loh R, Phua M, Shaw CL. Management of paediatric acute mastoiditis: systematic review. J Laryngol Otol 2018;132 (2):96–104 PubMed
8. Makki FM, Amoodi HA, van Wijhe RG, Bance M. Anatomic analysis of the mastoid tegmen: slopes and tegmen shape variances. Otol Neurotol 2011;32(4):581–588 PubMed
9. Ryu NG, Kim J. How to avoid facial nerve injury in mastoidectomy? J Audiol Otol 2016;20(2):68–72 PubMed
10. Sethia R, Kerwin TF, Wiet GJ. Performance assessment for mastoidectomy. Otolaryngol Head Neck Surg 2017;156 (1):61–69 PubMed
11. Sunder S, Jackler RK, Blevins NH. Virtuosity with the Mallet and Gouge: the brilliant triumph of the "modern" mastoid operation. Otolaryngol Clin North Am 2006;39(6):1191–1210 PubMed

7.2 Intact Canal Wall Mastoidectomy

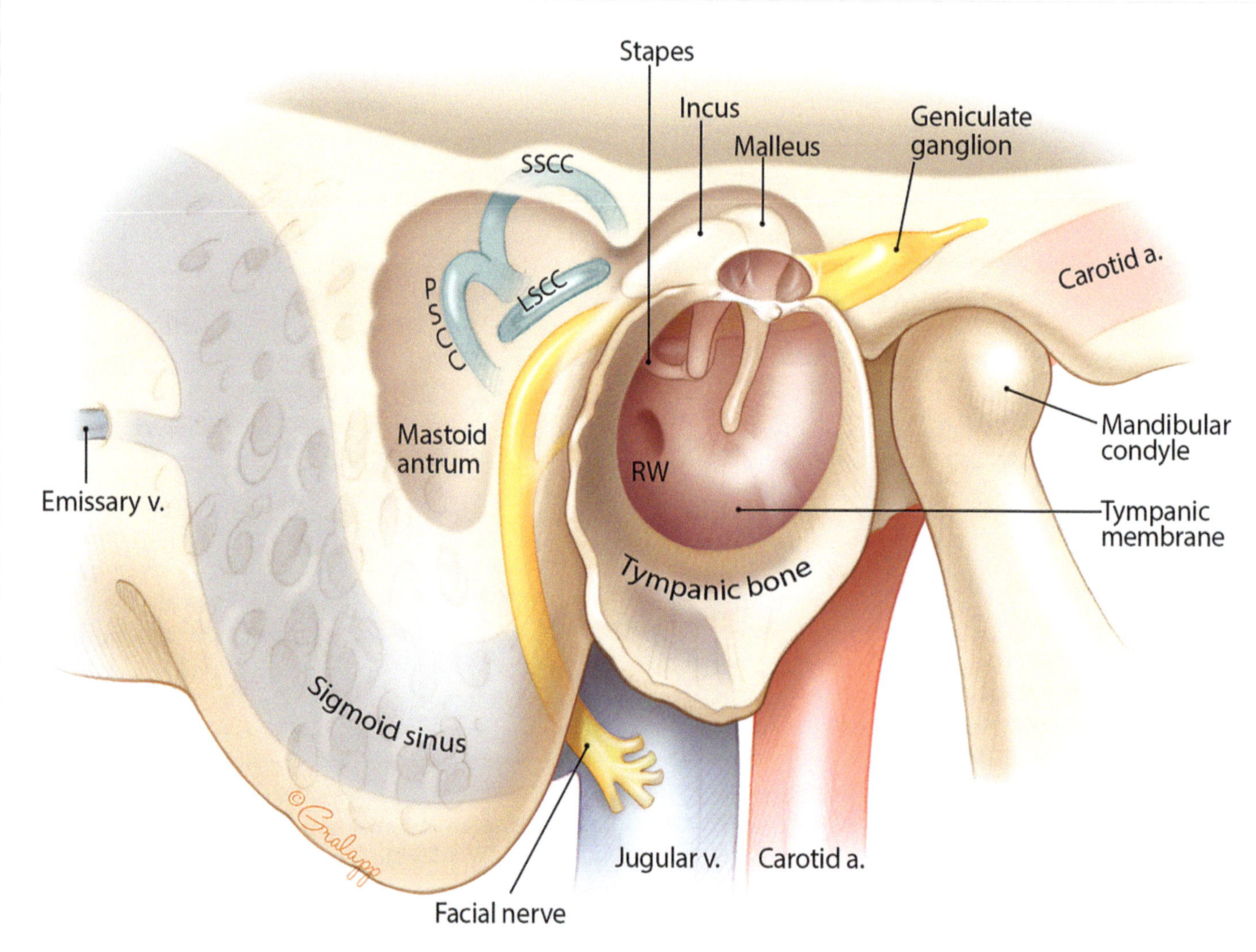

Fig. 7.1 Anatomical relationships of the mastoid antrum and air cells: lateral view. LSCC, lateral semicircular canal; PSCC, posterior semicircular canal; SSCC, superior semicircular canal.

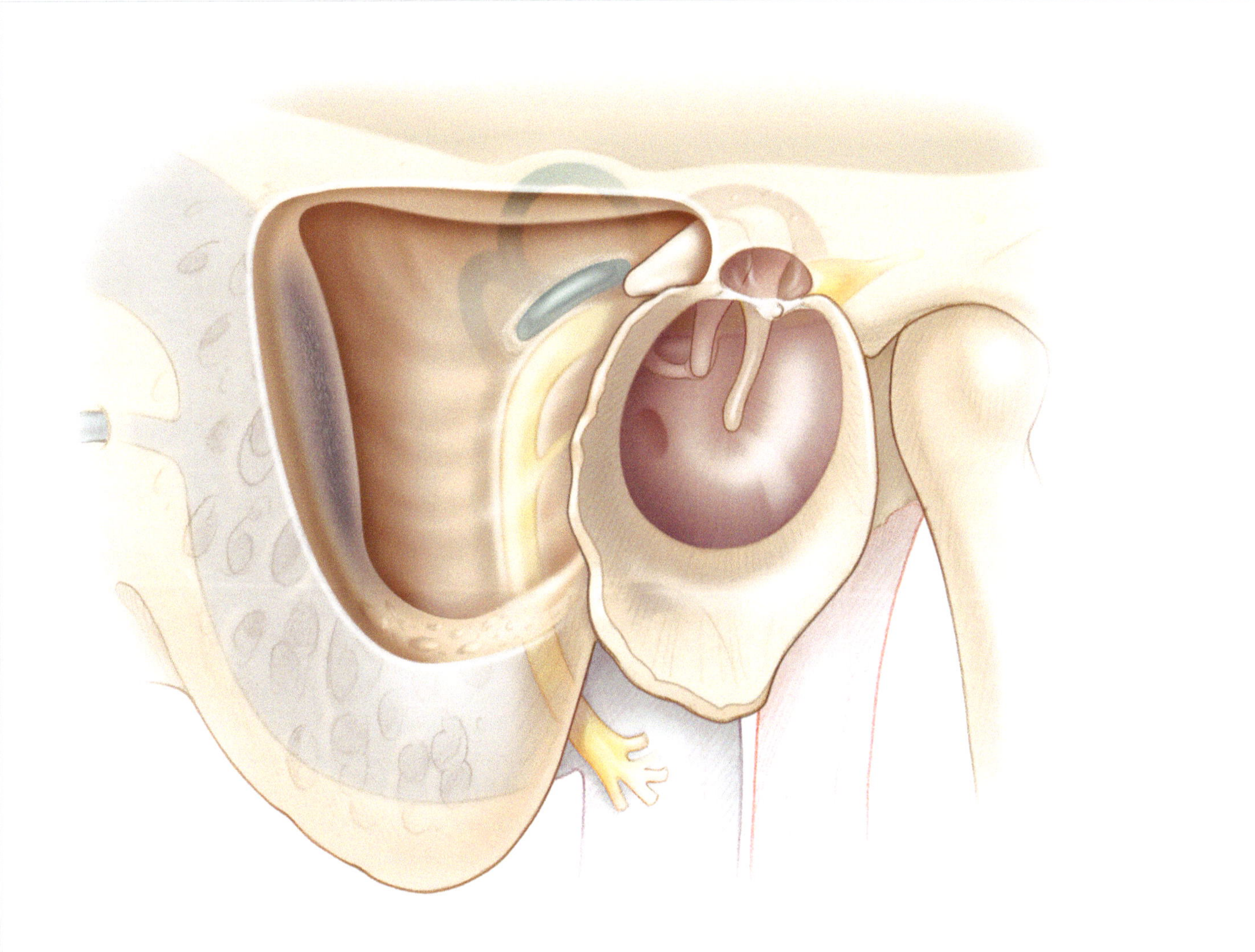

Fig. 7.2 Intact canal wall mastoidectomy bounded superiorly by the tegmen, posteriorly by the sigmoid sinus, and anteriorly by the ear canal.

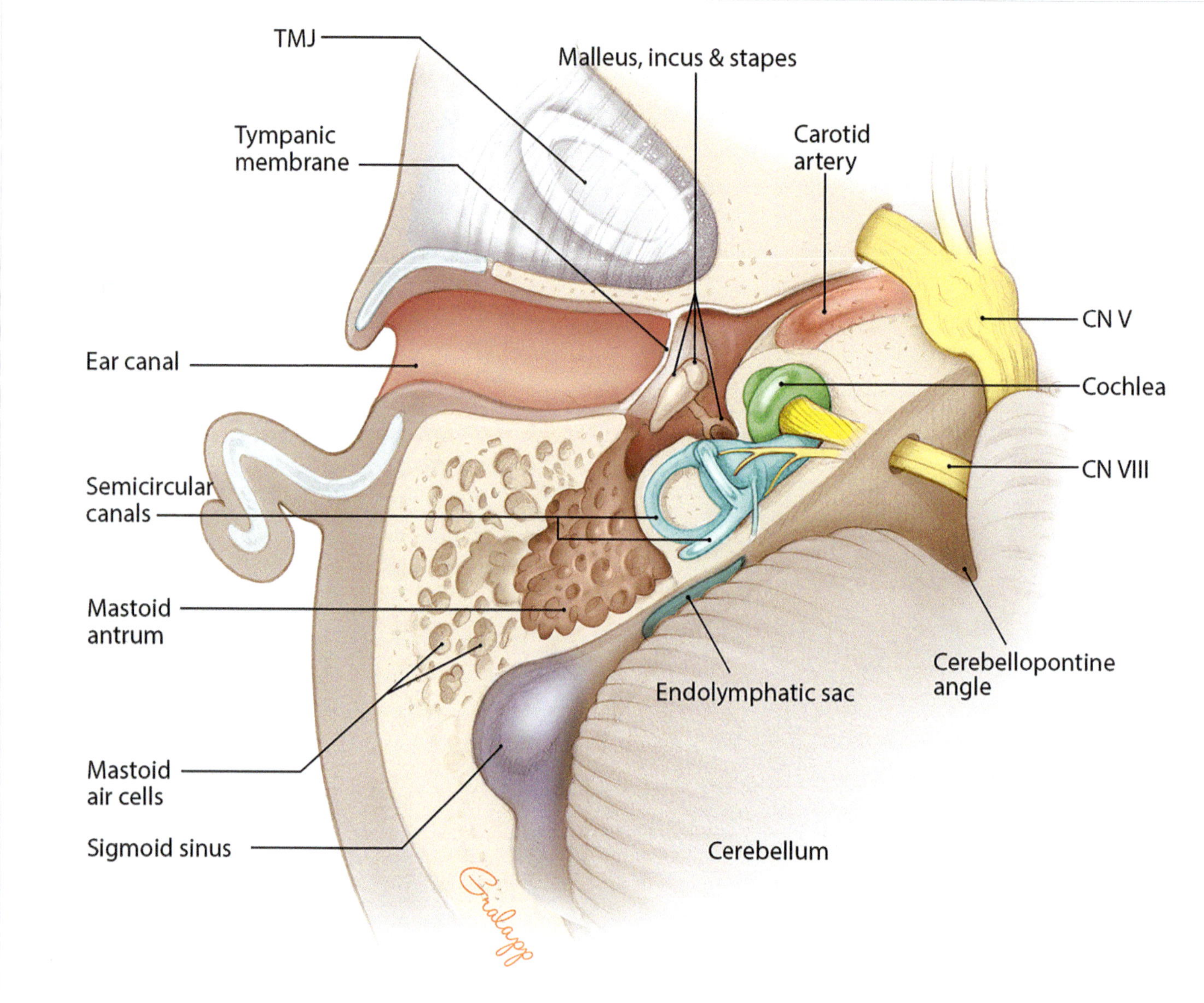

Fig. 7.3 Anatomical relationships of the mastoid antrum and air cells: axial view. CN V, trigeminal nerve; CN VII, facial nerve.

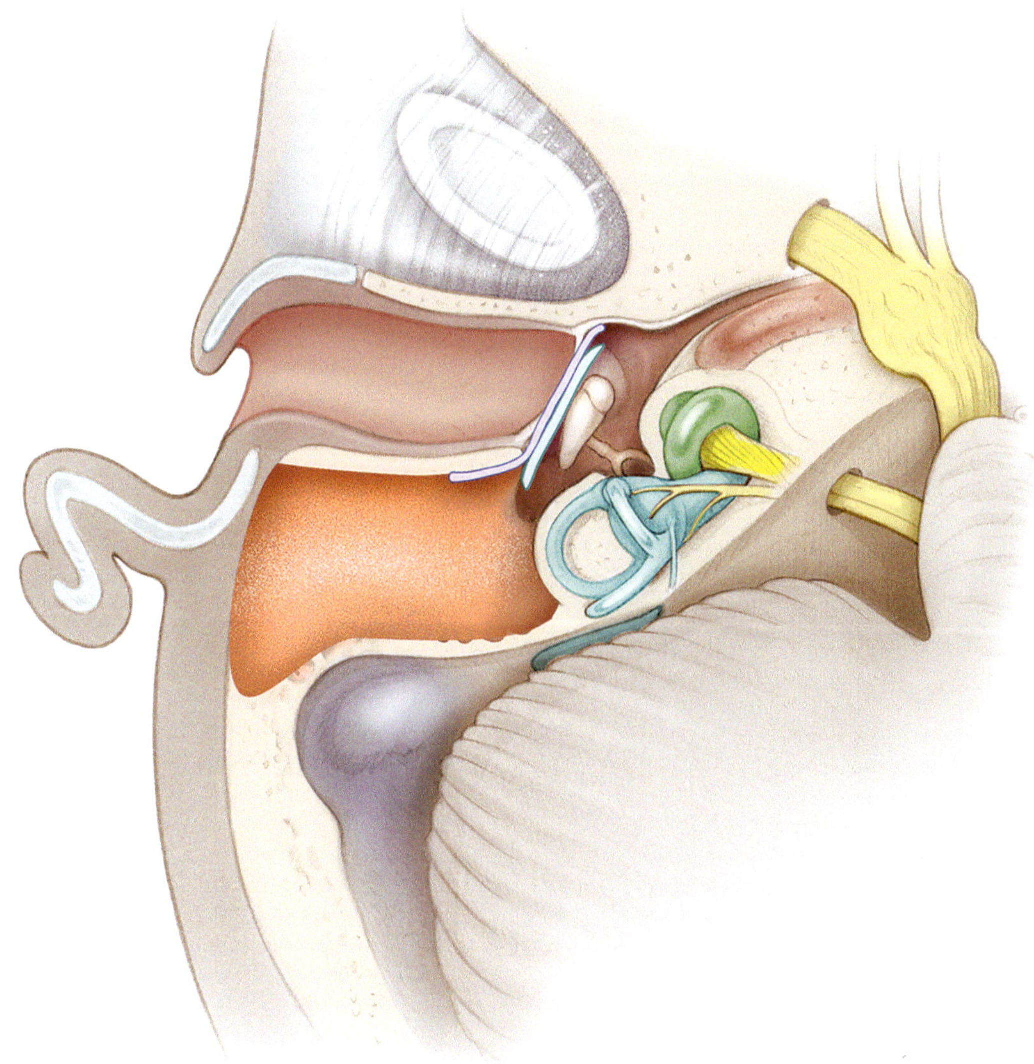

Fig. 7.4 Intact canal wall mastoidectomy connecting to the middle ear via the aditus-ad-antrum.

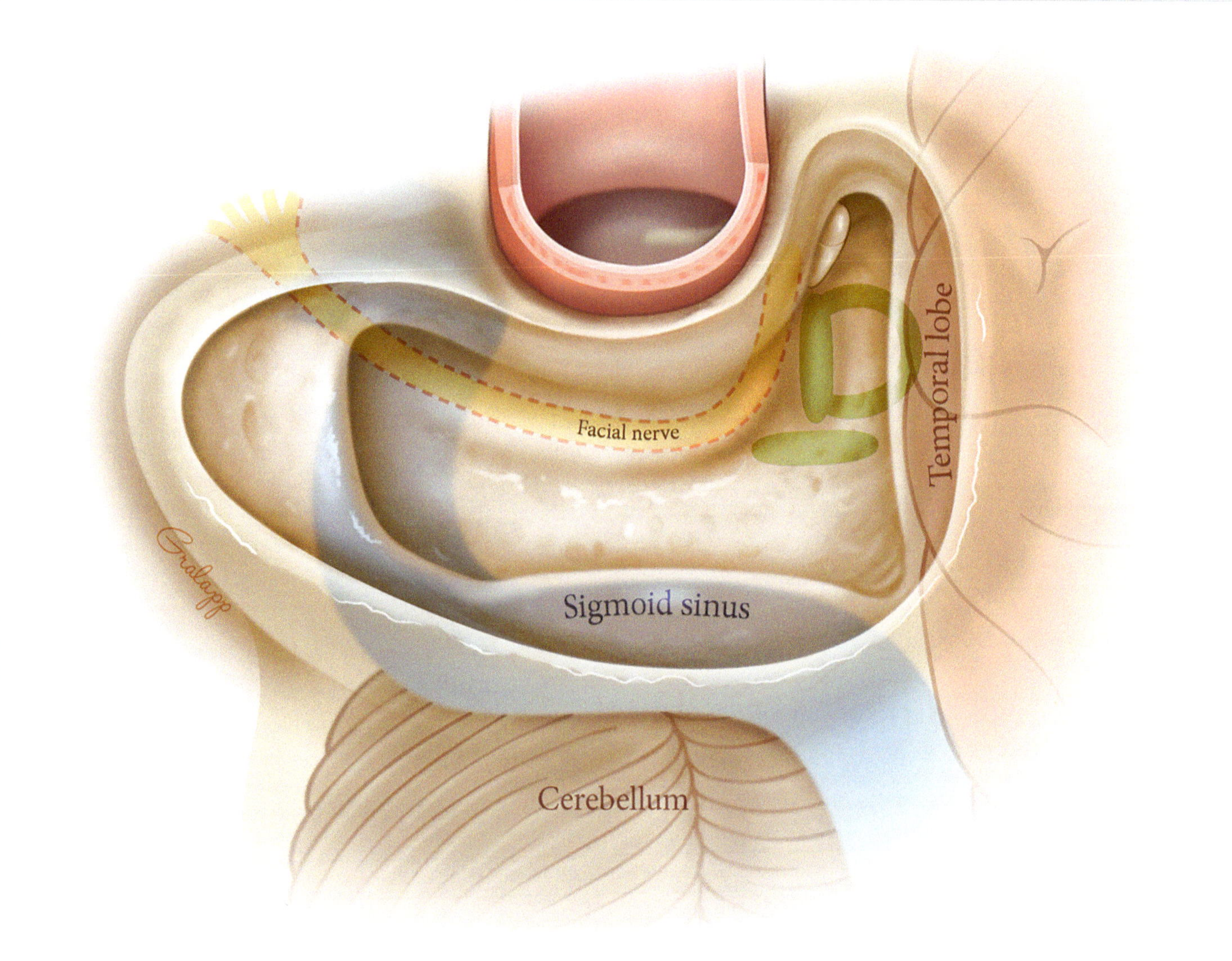

Fig. 7.5 Mastoidectomy and its relationships. Note the temporal lobe above the tegmen and cerebellum behind the sigmoid sinus. The second genu, vertical segment, and stylomastoid foramen of the facial nerve are situated in the floor of the mastoid as are the three semicircular canals.

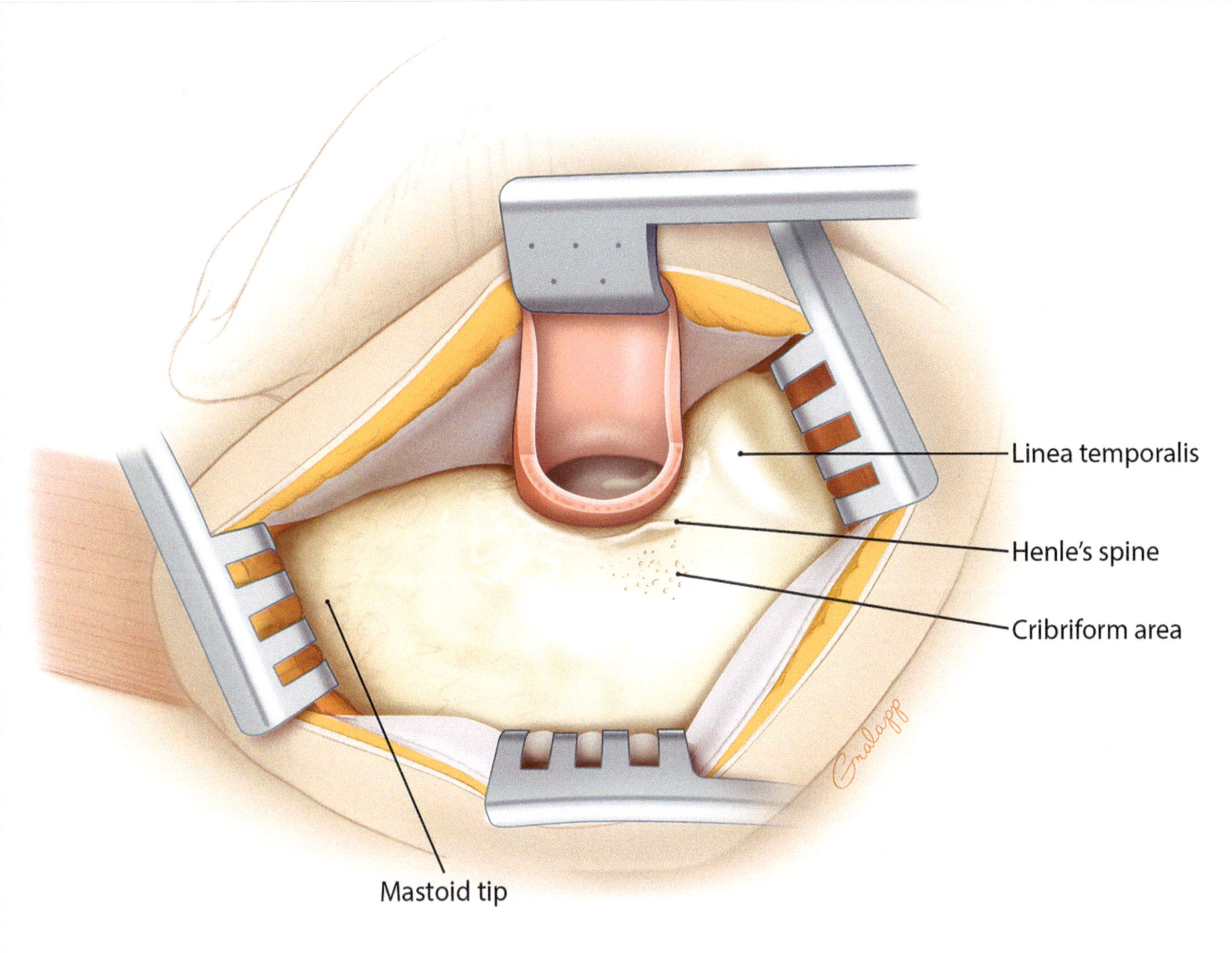

Fig. 7.6 Exposure of the mastoid in preparation for mastoidectomy. Note the surface landmarks.

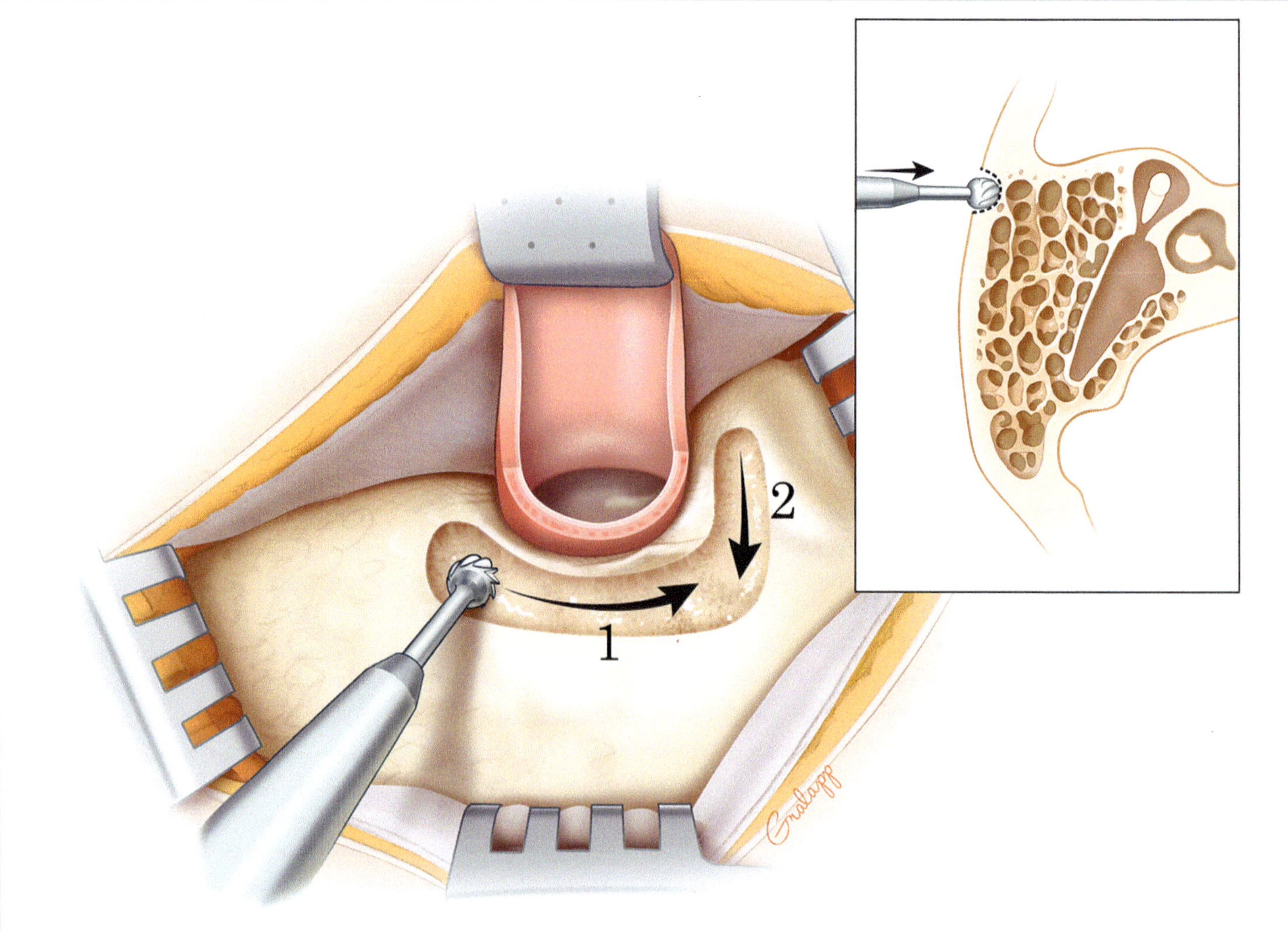

Fig. 7.7 Initial removal of the mastoid cortex behind and above the ear canal is conducted with a cutting burr.

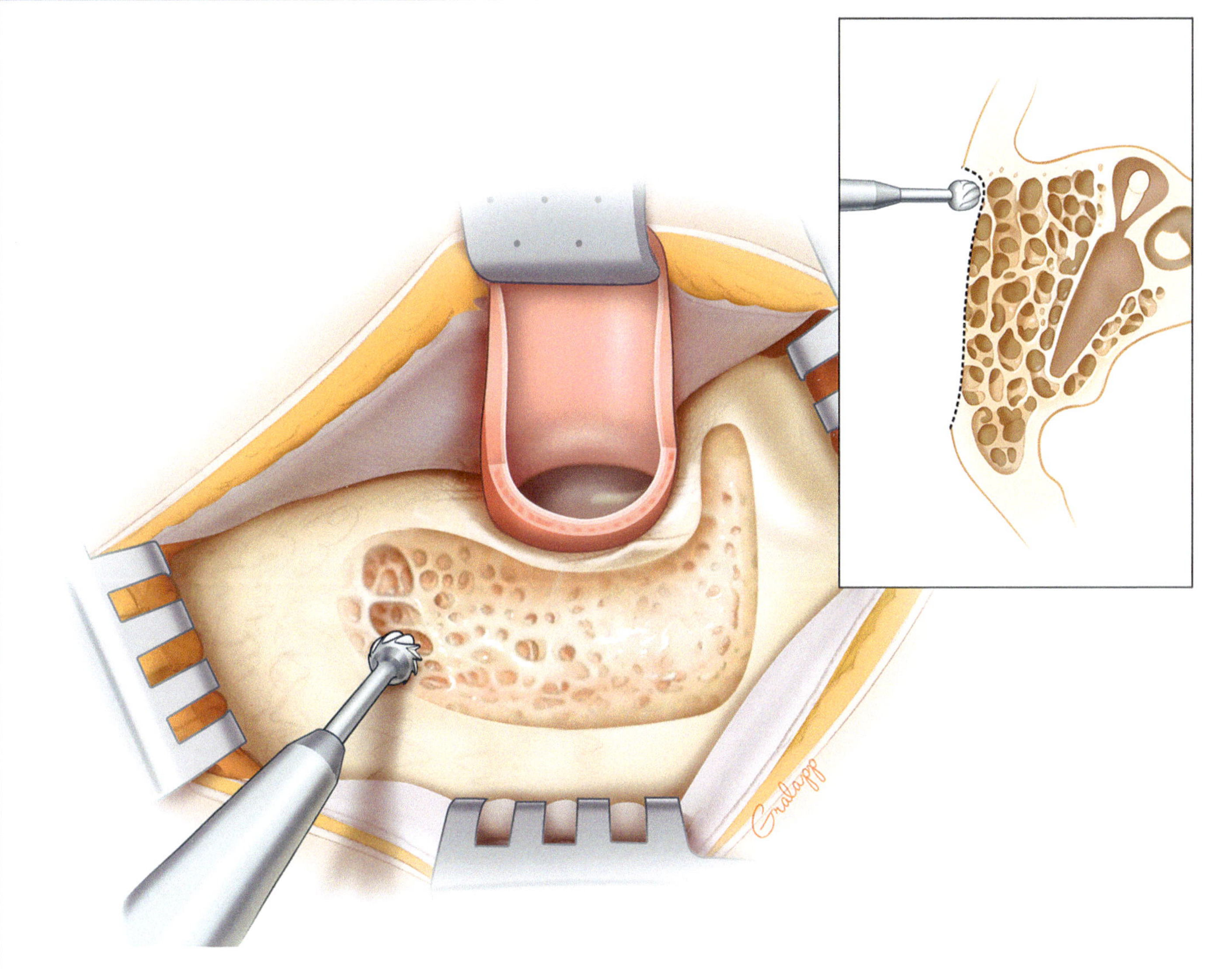

Fig. 7.8 Removal of the outer cortex reveals the peripheral air cell system in the well pneumatized temporal bone.

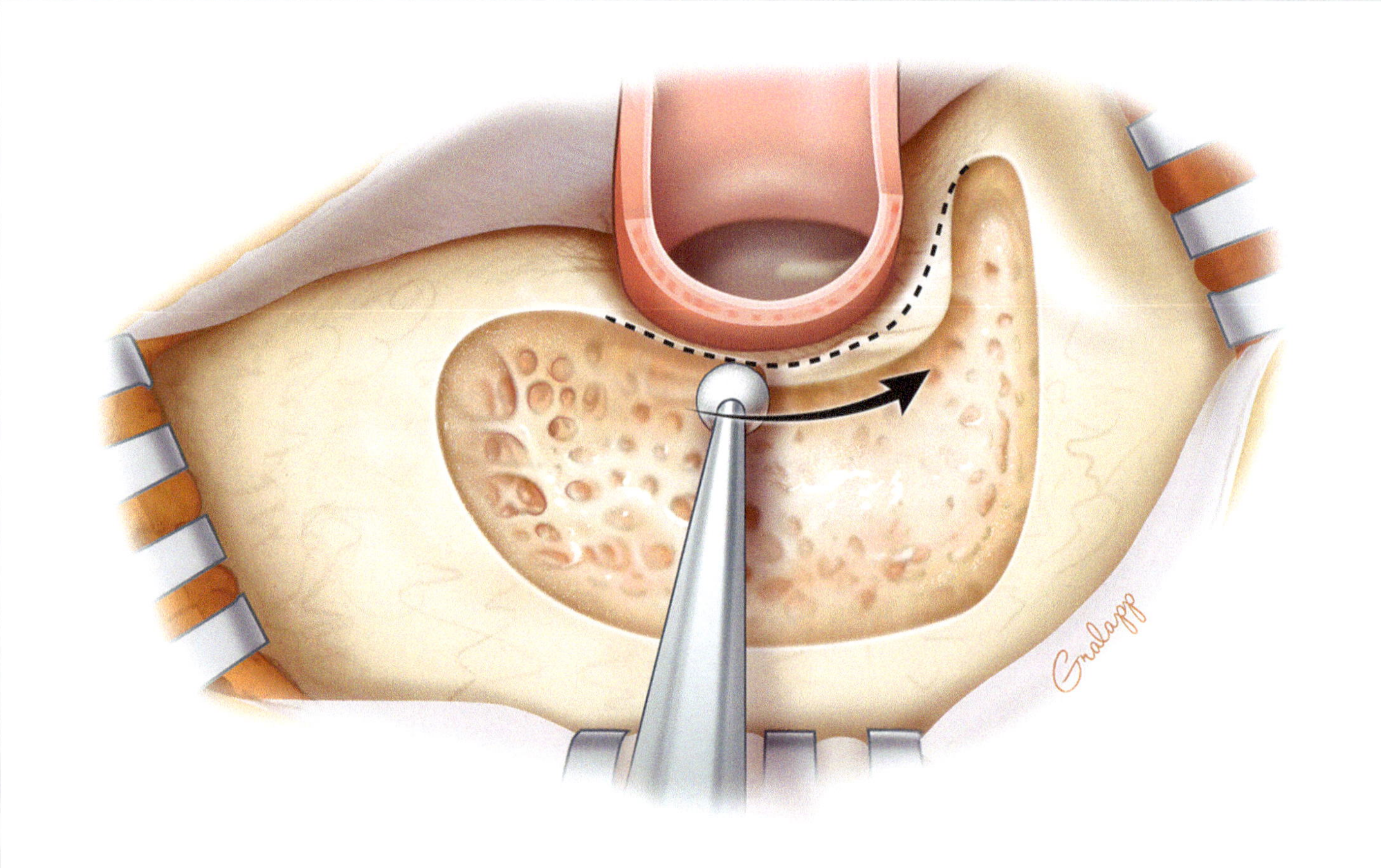

Fig. 7.9 Thinning of the bony ear canal by removing air cells.

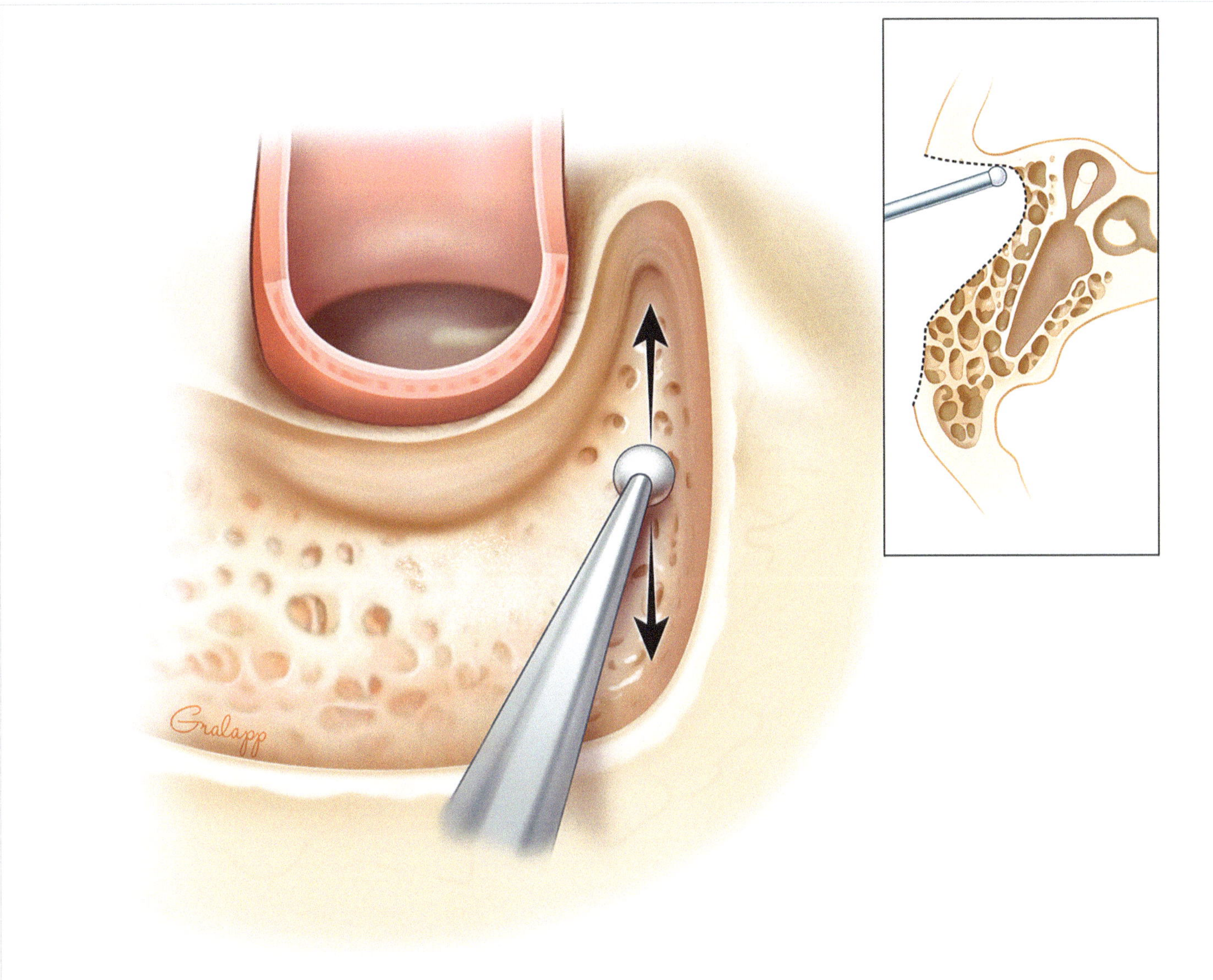

Fig. 7.10 As a general principle, the deepest bone excavation is always kept high and forward approaching the tegmen mastoideum and toward the epitympanum. This is the surest way of encountering the antrum and avoiding possible injury to the facial nerve at its second genu.

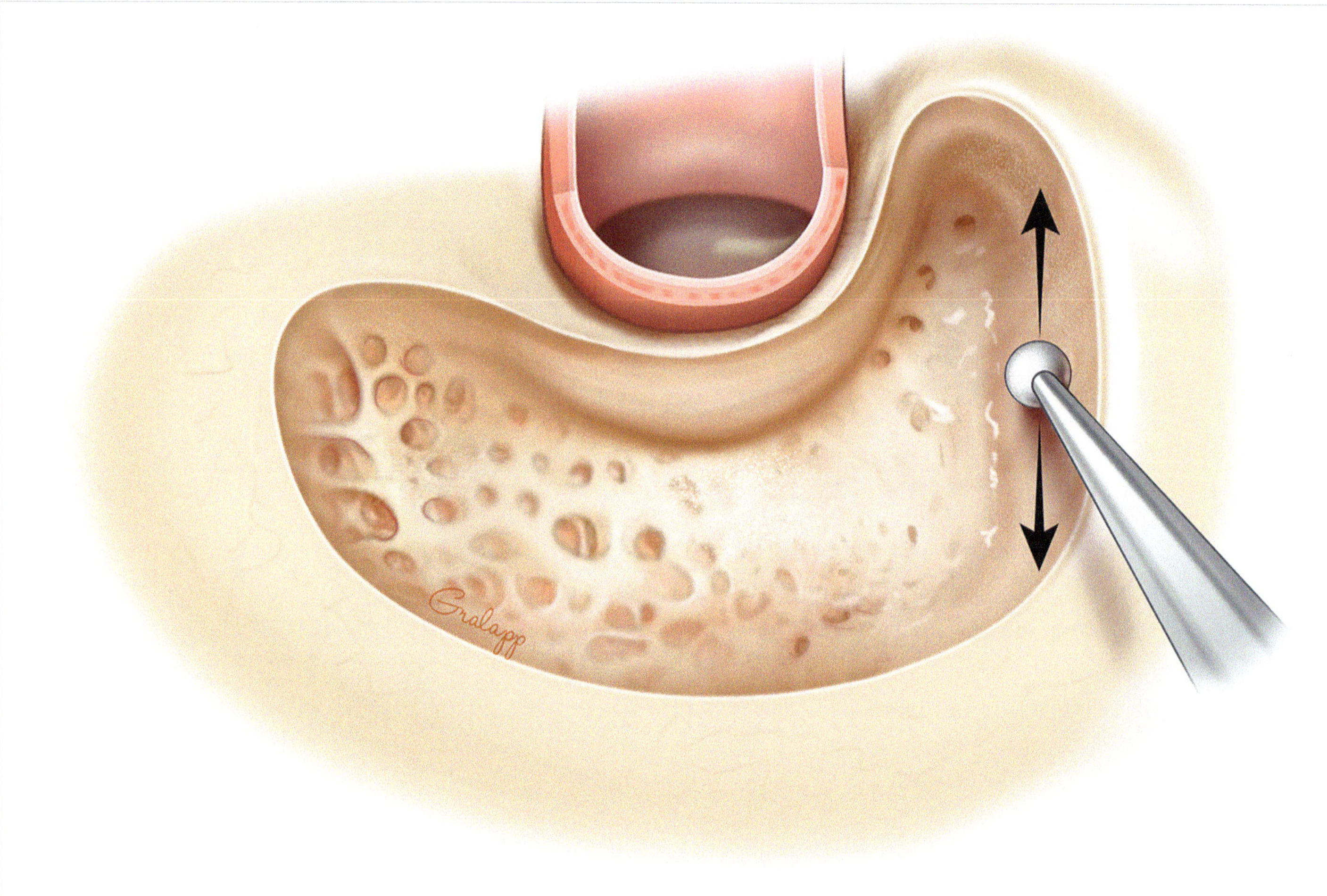

Fig. 7.11 Identifying the tegmen mastoideum: note the smooth sheet of bone. The drill noise may become higher pitched as the tegmen is approached.

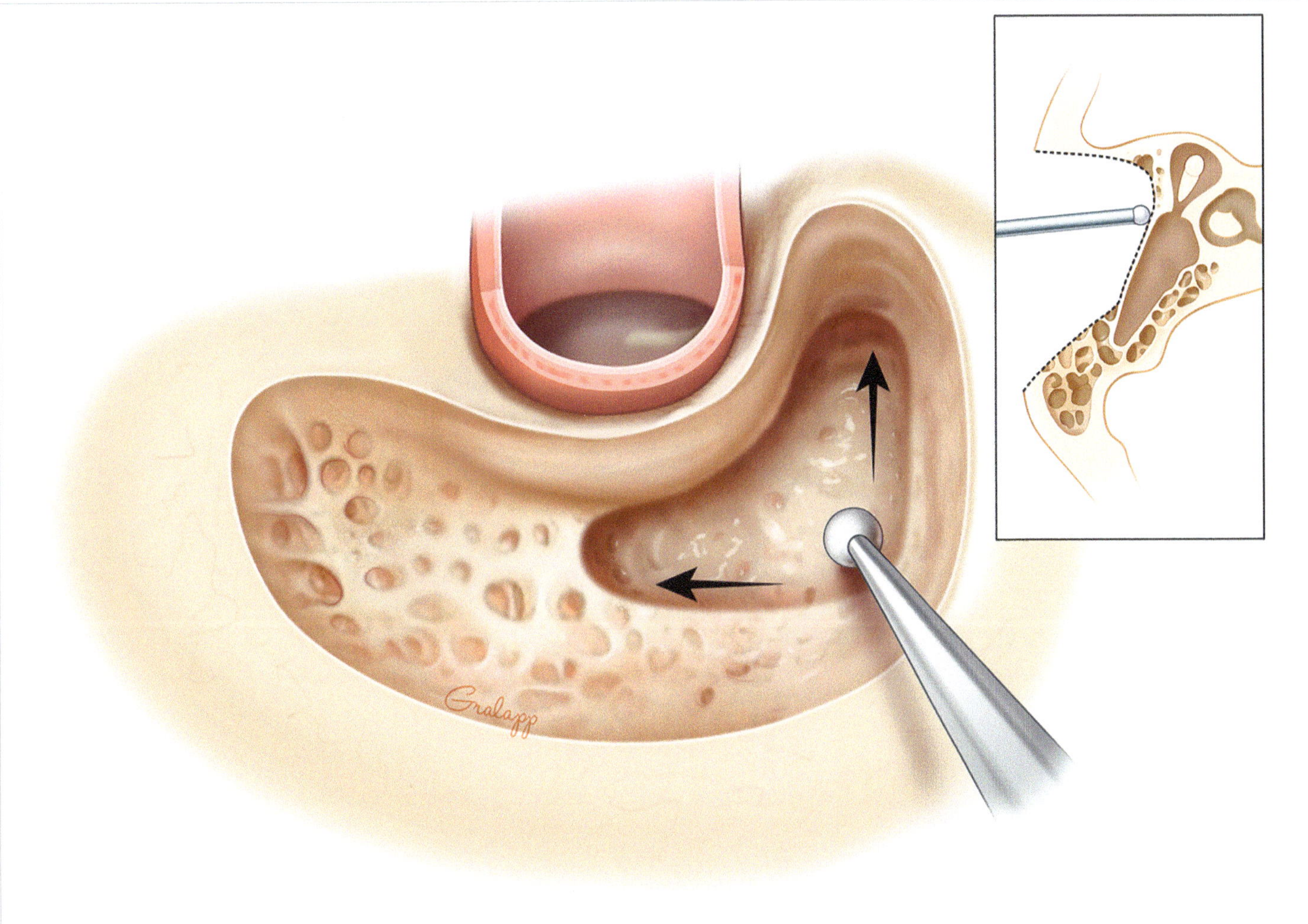

Fig. 7.12 The safest way to approach the antrum is high up along the tegmen and forward toward the epitympanum. The floor of the opening at this stage sometimes is a flat sheet of bone, called Koerner's septum, which is a false bottom and not the actual floor of the antrum.

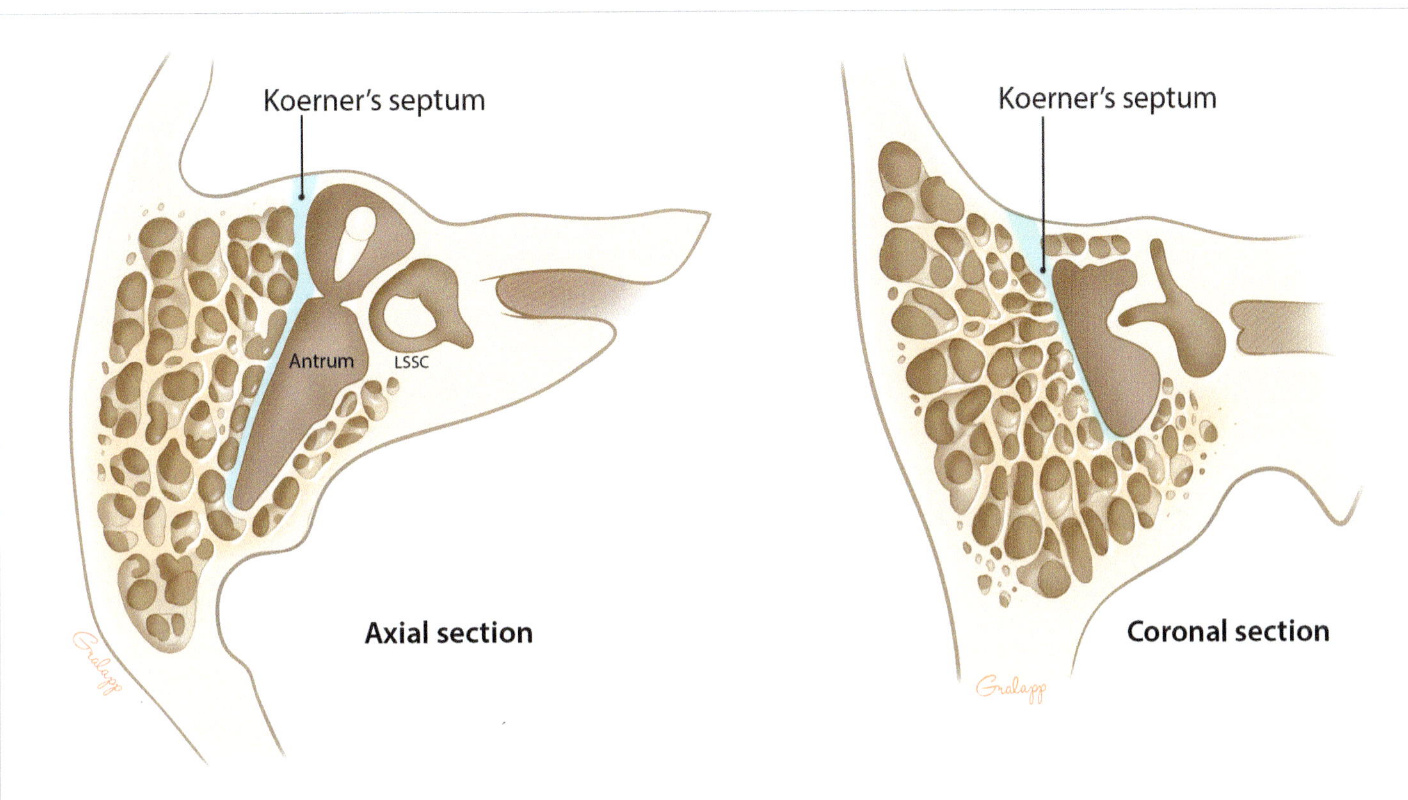

Fig. 7.13 Koerner's septum needs to be penetrated to enter the antrum.

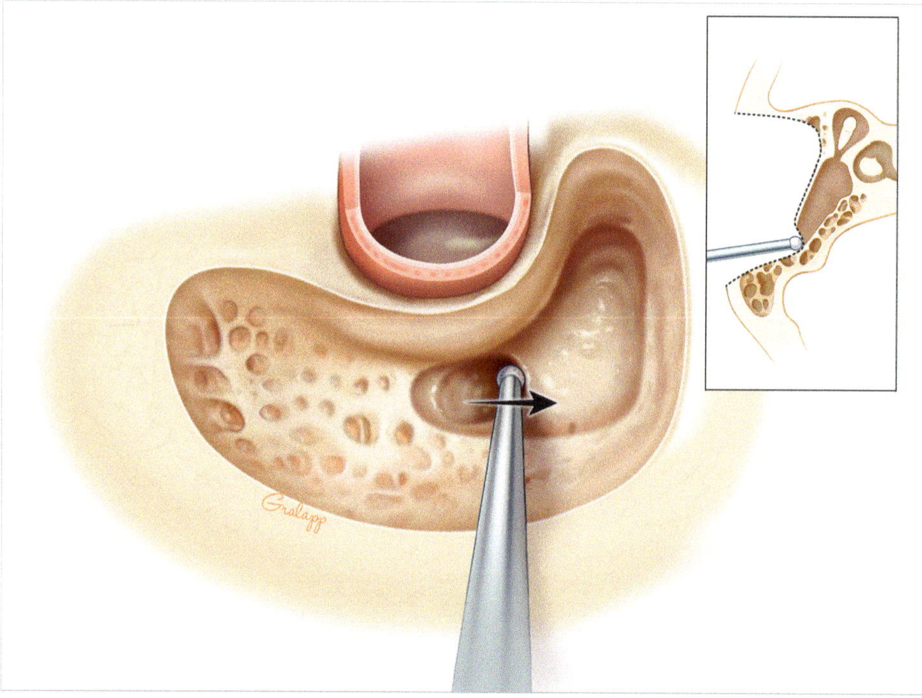

Fig. 7.14 Initial entry into the mastoid antrum.

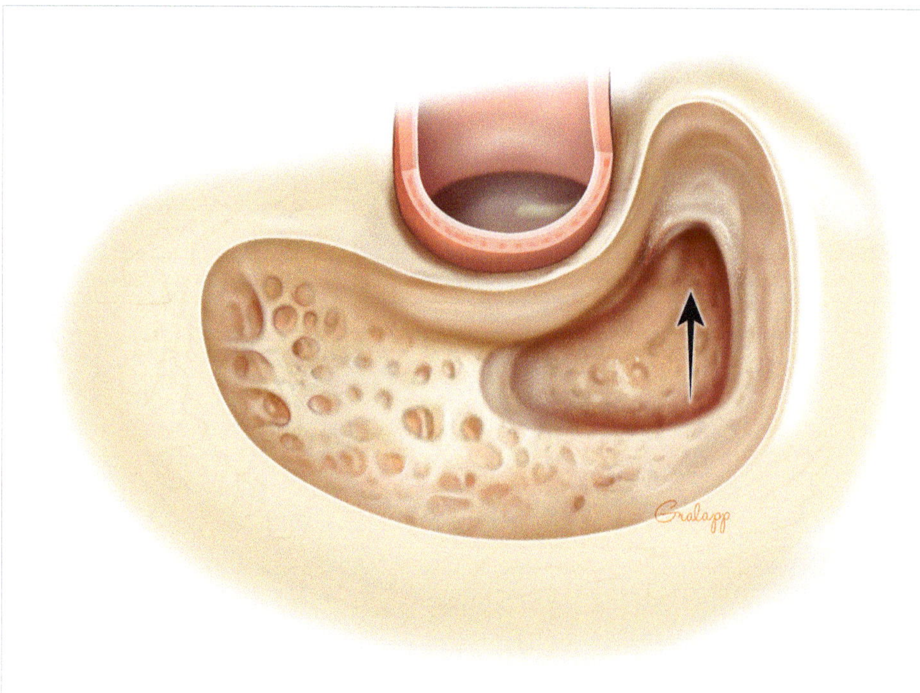

Fig. 7.15 Further opening of the antrum brings the lateral semicircular canal into view.

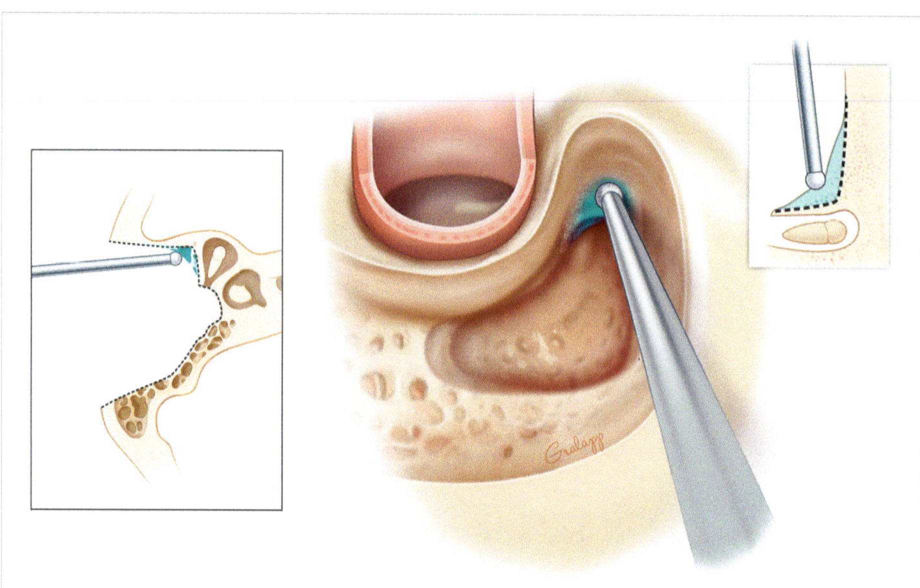

Fig. 7.16 Thinning of the bony shelf over the ossicles in the epitympanum.

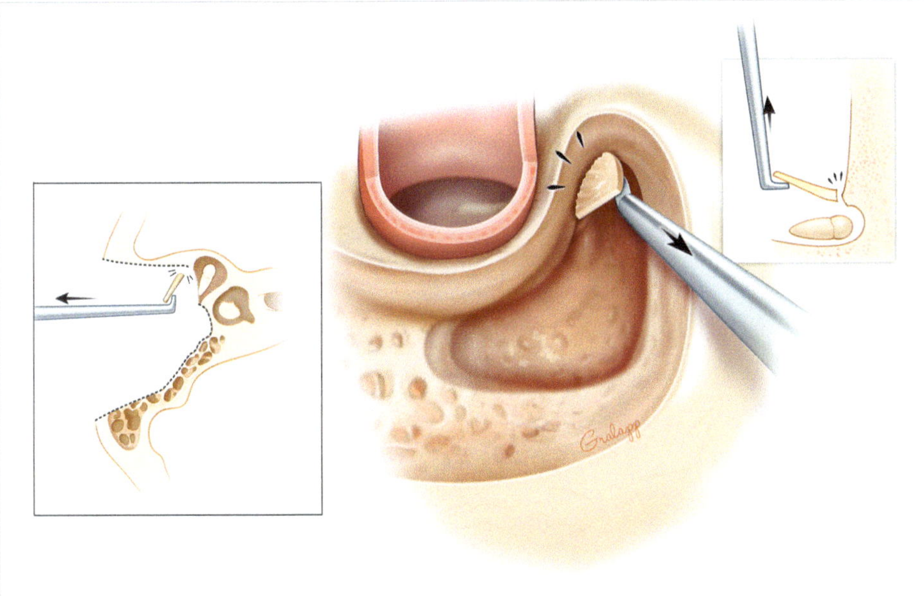

Fig. 7.17 Flaking off the last thin sheet of bone over the incus and malleus with a stapes knife or curette protects the ossicles from contact with the drill which could cause cochlear injury.

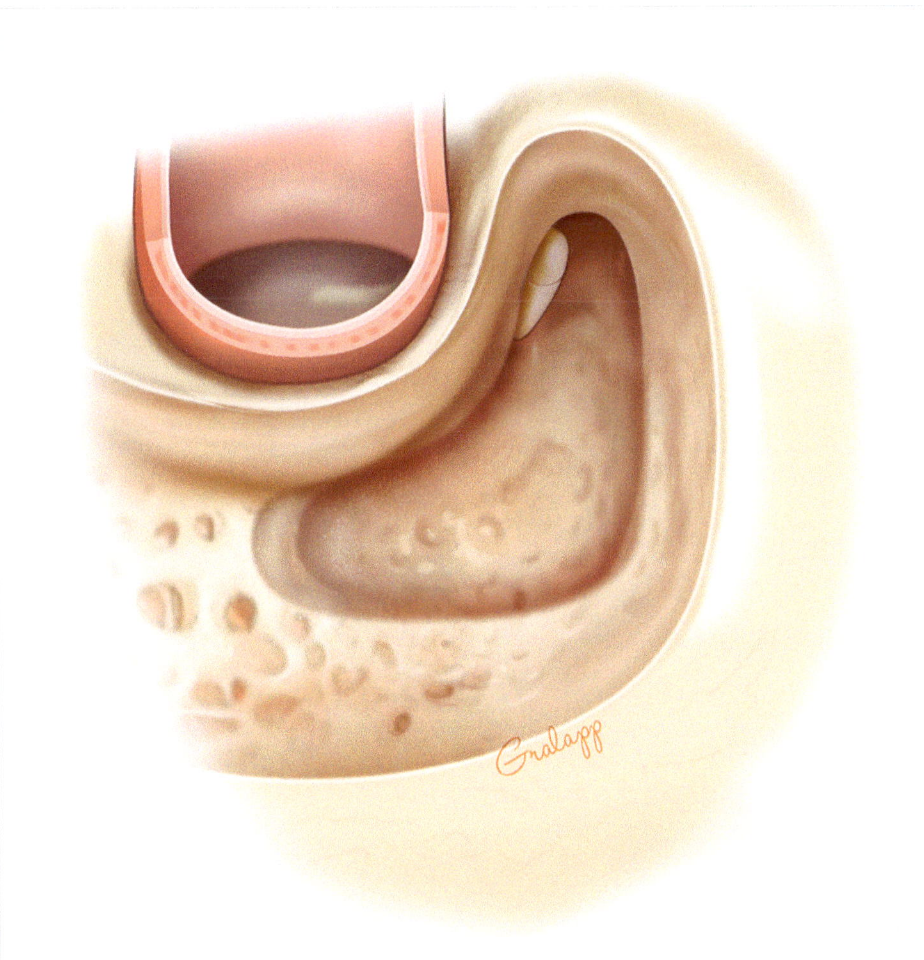

Fig. 7.18 Completion of the antrotomy and exposure of the epitympanum including the body of the incus and the head of the malleus. Note that the opening anteriorly fully exposes the head of the malleus and the anterior epitympanum.

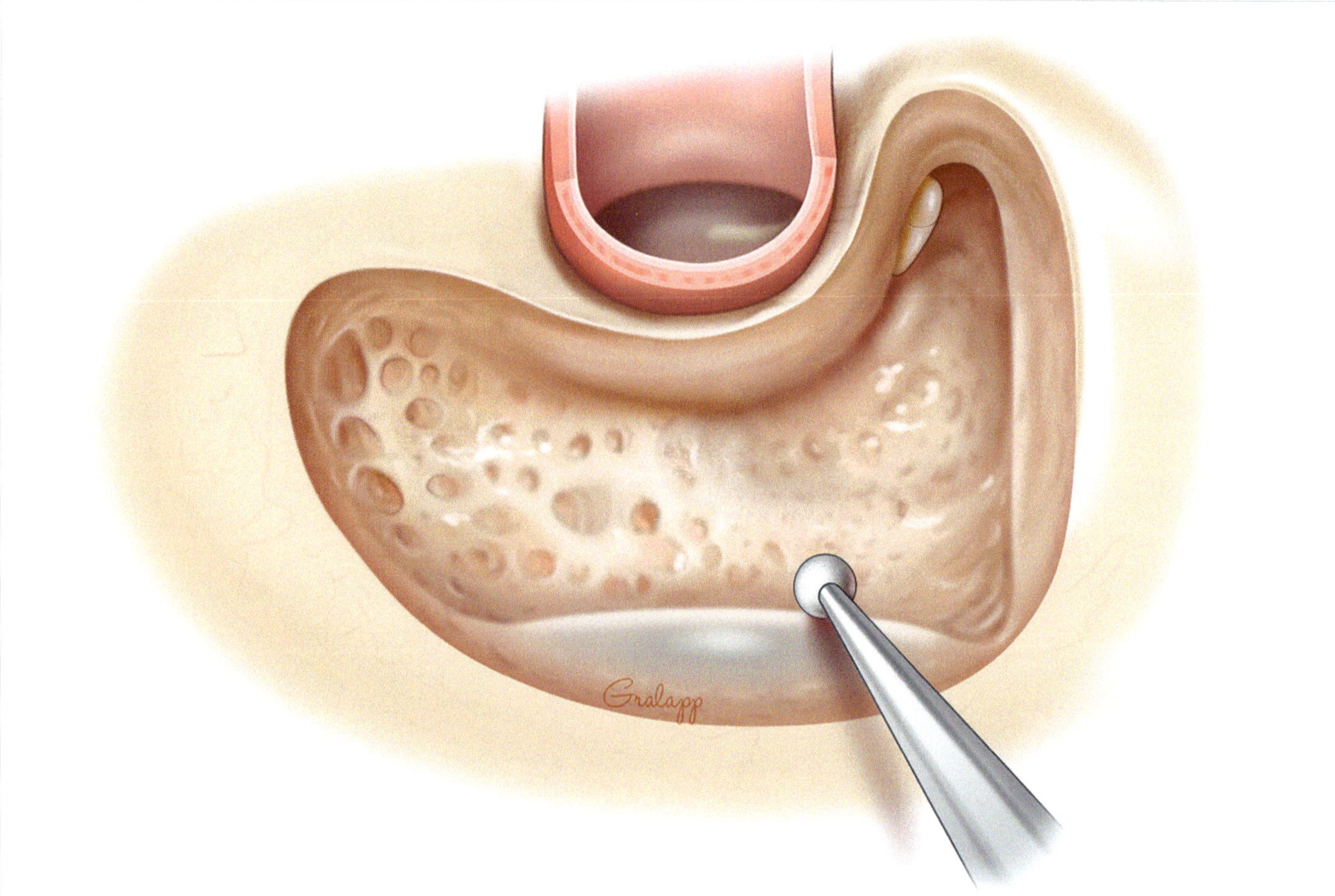

Fig. 7.19 Thinning of air cells over the sigmoid sinus and the sinodural angle (also known as Citelli's angle).

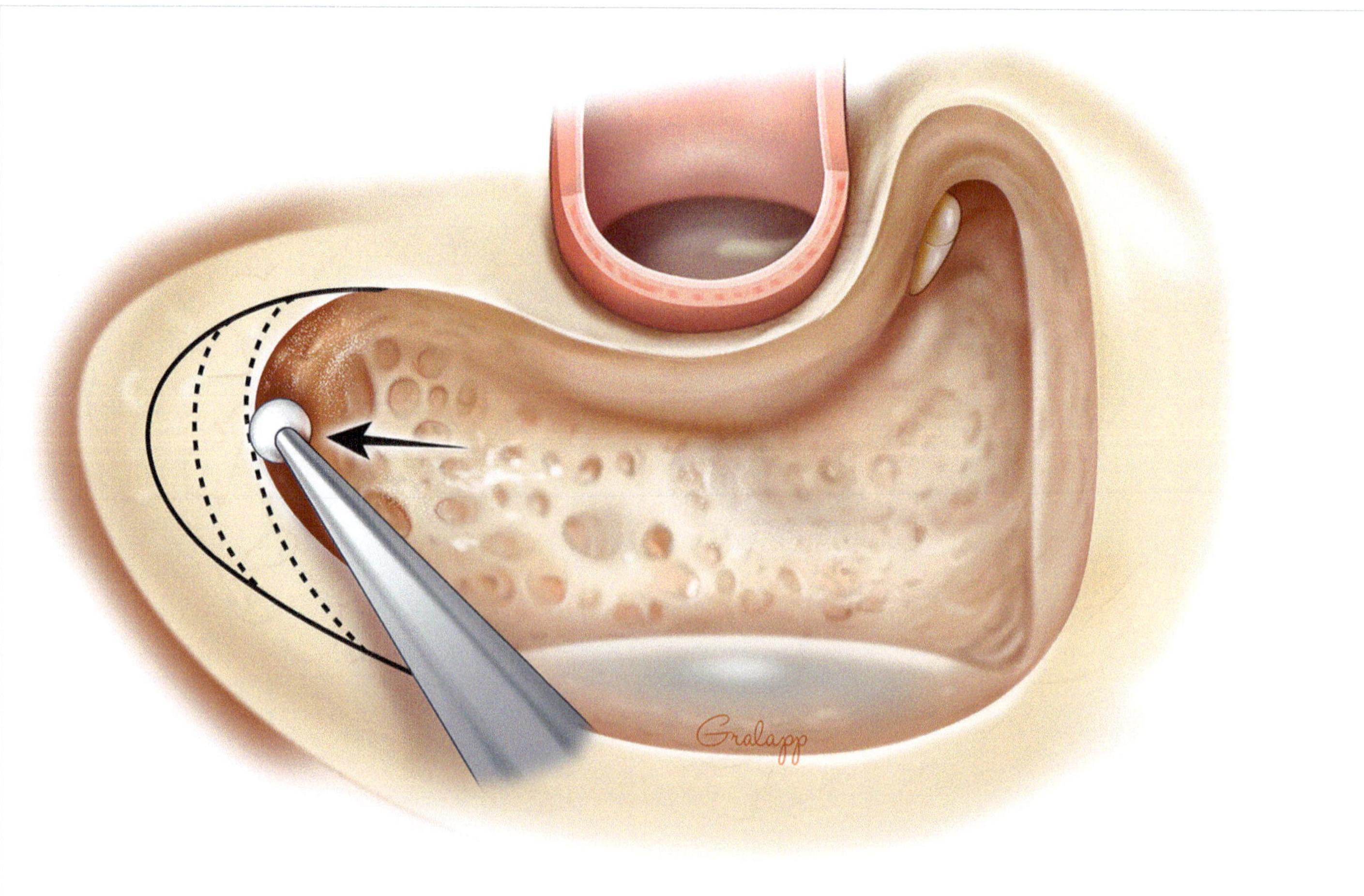

Fig. 7.20 Tip cells are opened as necessitated by the extent of pneumatization.

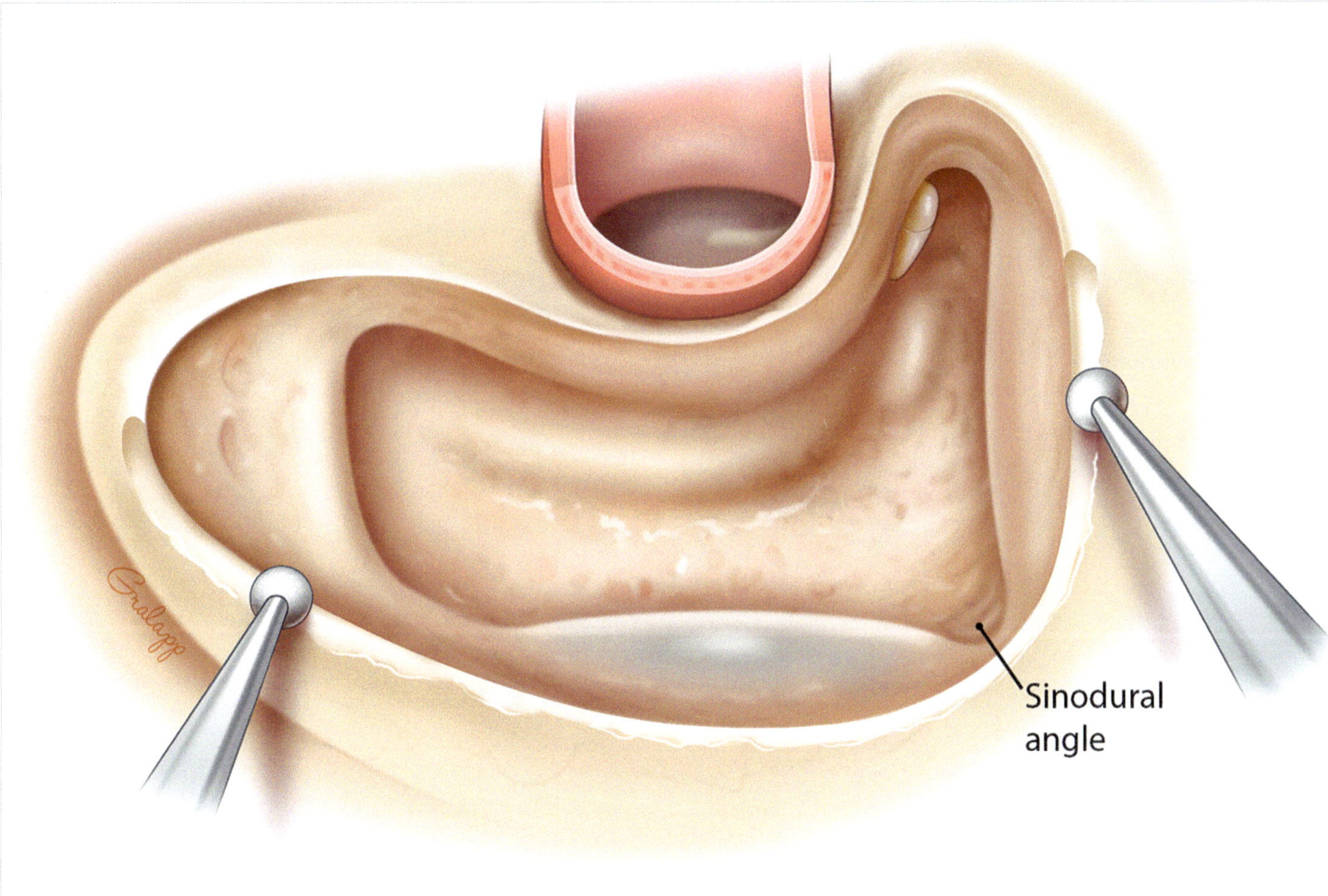

Fig. 7.21 Beveling of the edges of the mastoid is important to avoid sharp edges which may cause discomfort, especially in eyeglass wearers.

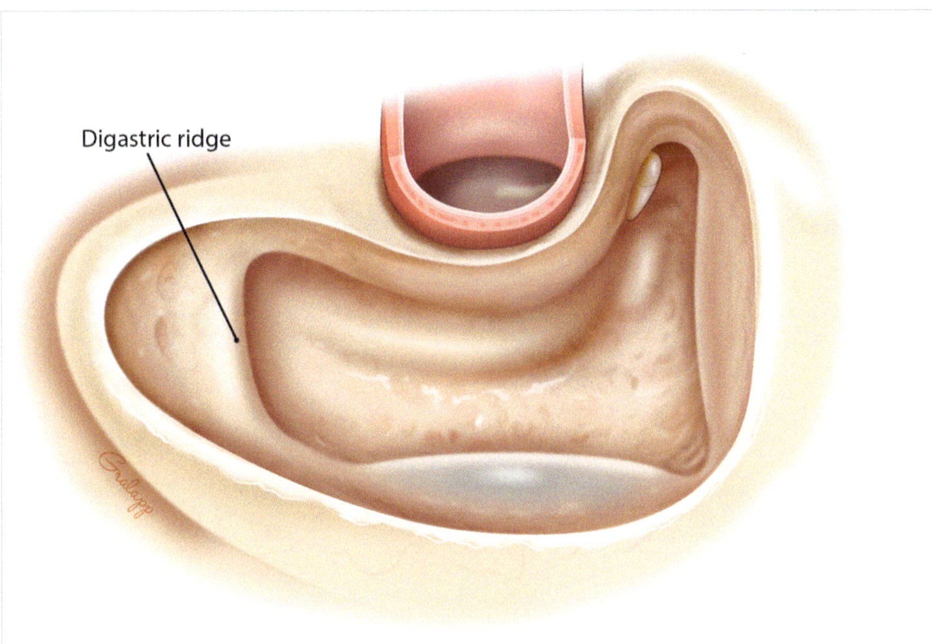

Fig. 7.22 Completed mastoidectomy. Completion of the tip cell removal has exposed the digastric ridge.

7.3 Anatomical Variations in Mastoidectomy

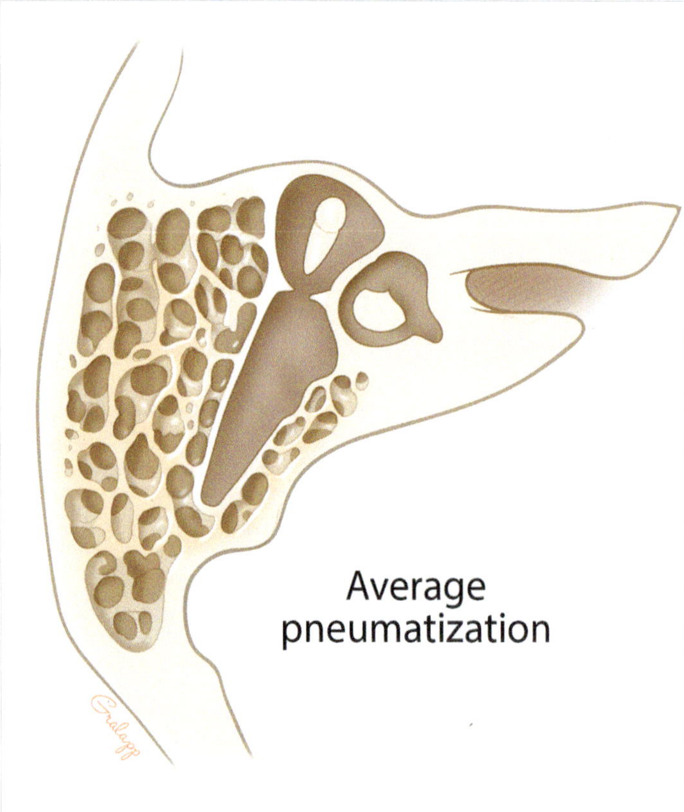

Fig. 7.23 While the mastoid antrum is consistent, much variation exists in the pattern and extent of the peripheral air cell system. This is the average degree of pneumatization.

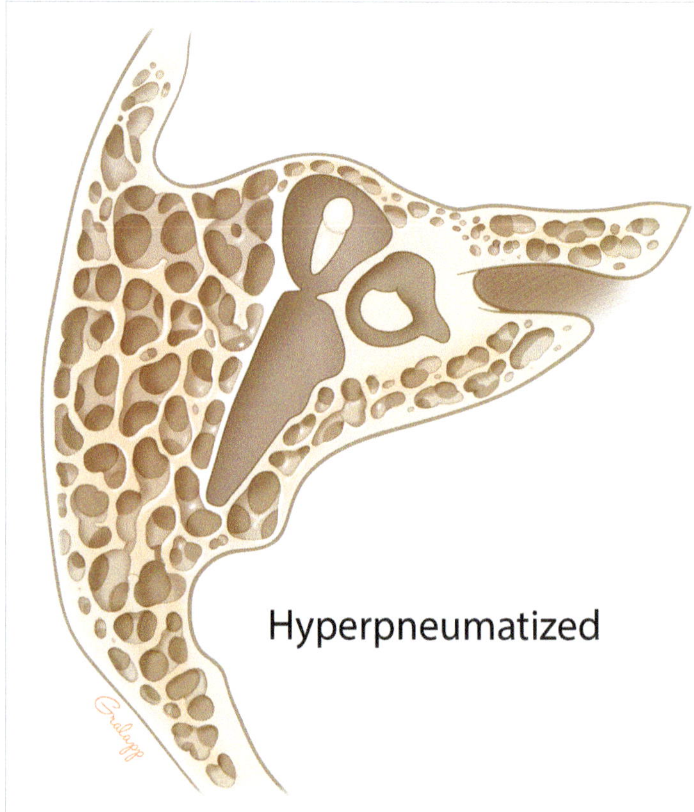

Fig. 7.24 An extensively pneumatized temporal bone with cells extending into the root of the zygoma and retrosigmoid regions. Note the pneumatization of the petrous apex deep to the inner ear.

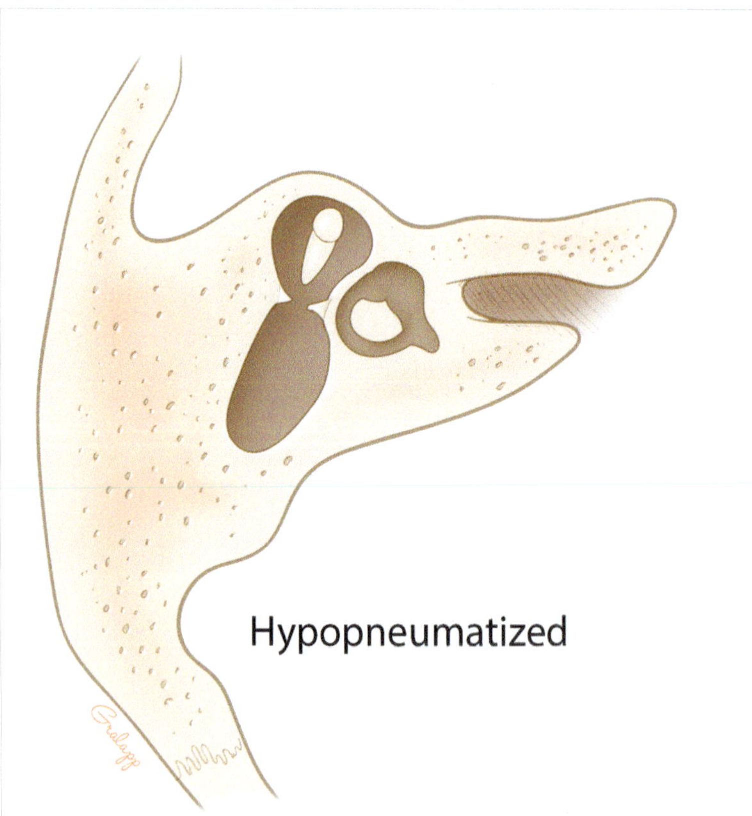

Fig. 7.25 A severely hypopneumatic temporal bone of the type often seen in chronic otitis media. Note the preservation of the antrum.

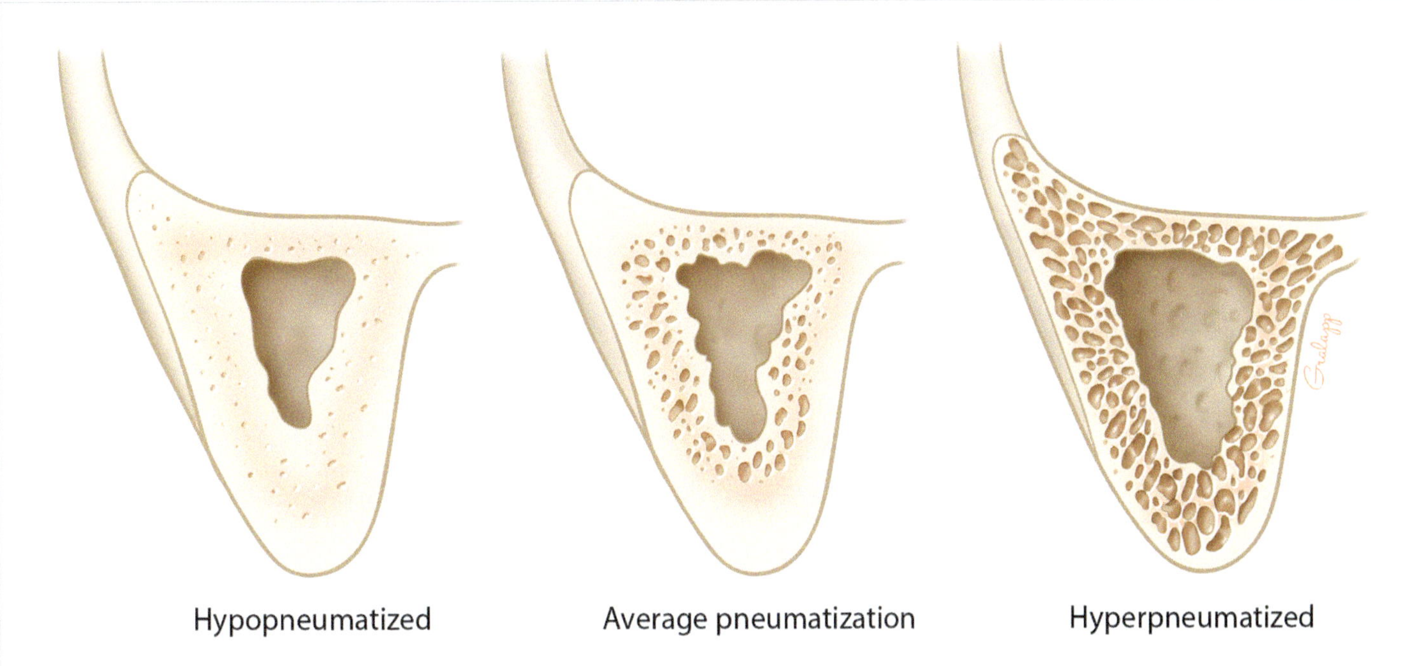

Fig. 7.26 Coronal illustration of variability of mastoid air cells.

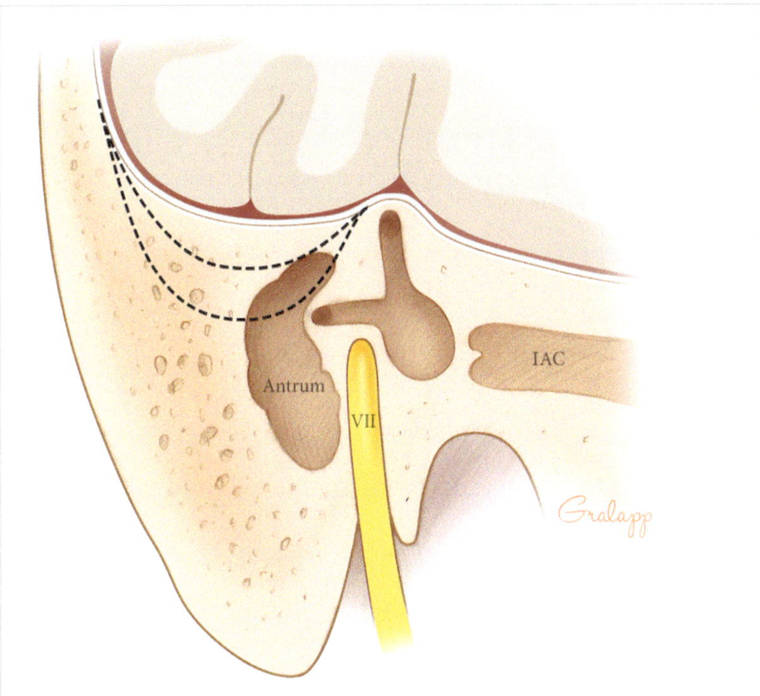

Fig. 7.27 Variation of the tegmen mastoideum from normal to low position. VII, facial nerve; IAC, internal auditory canal.

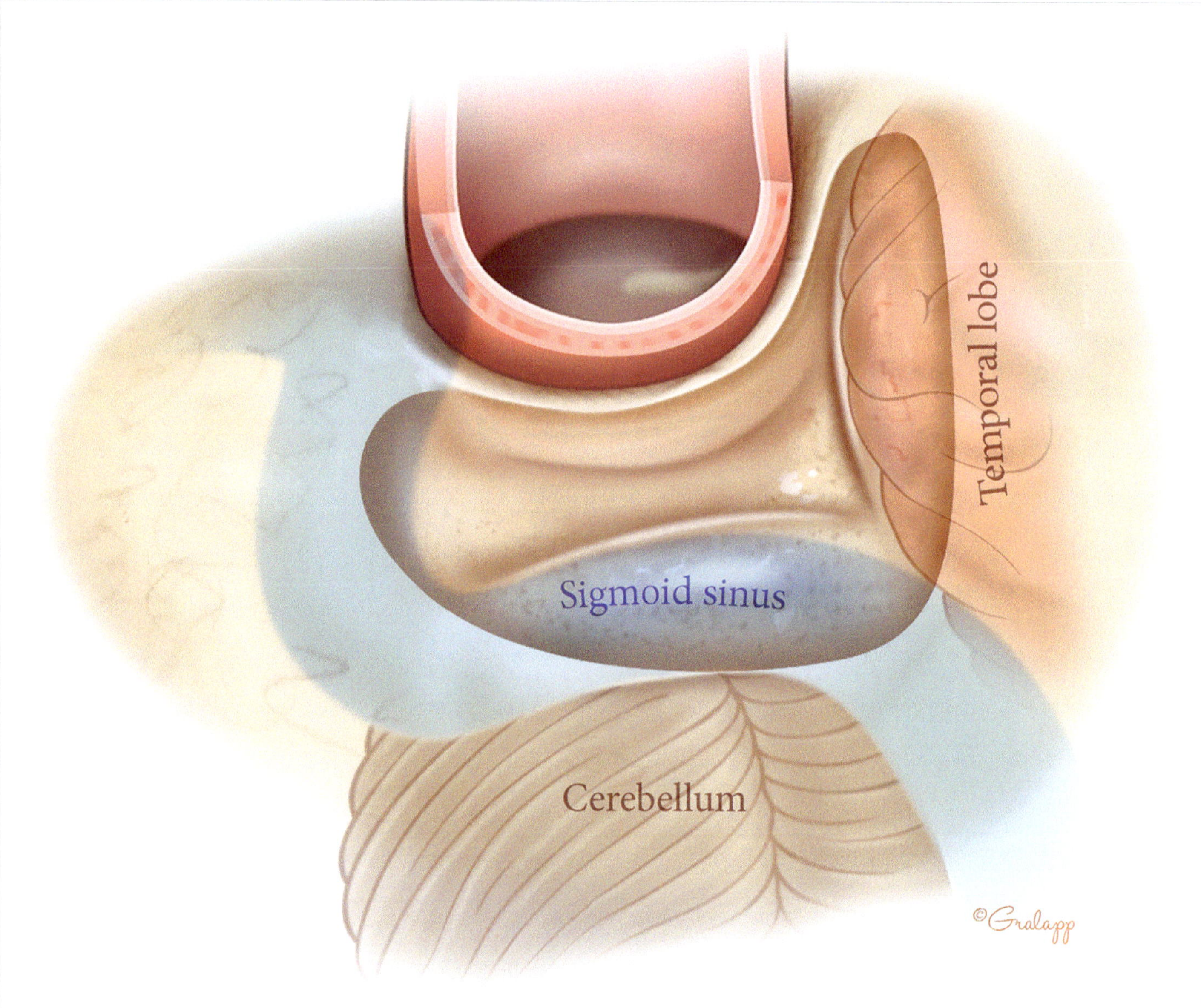

Fig. 7.28 Poorly pneumatized mastoid with low temporal dura and forward sigmoid sinus. This constrains the size of the mastoid cavity.

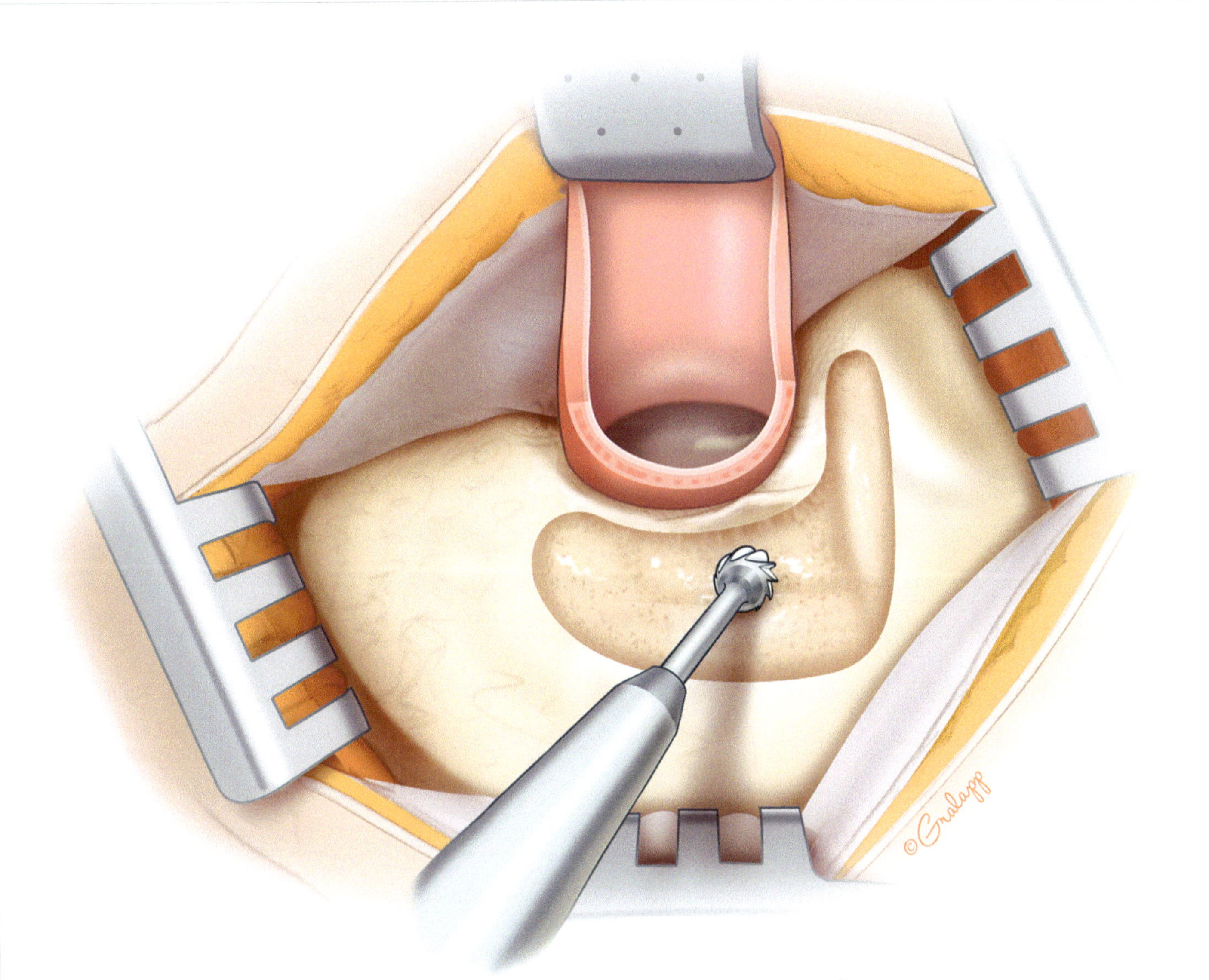

Fig. 7.29 Mastoidectomy in a hypopneumatic mastoid. Note that the tegmen may be so low as to preclude the superior extension above the ear canal.

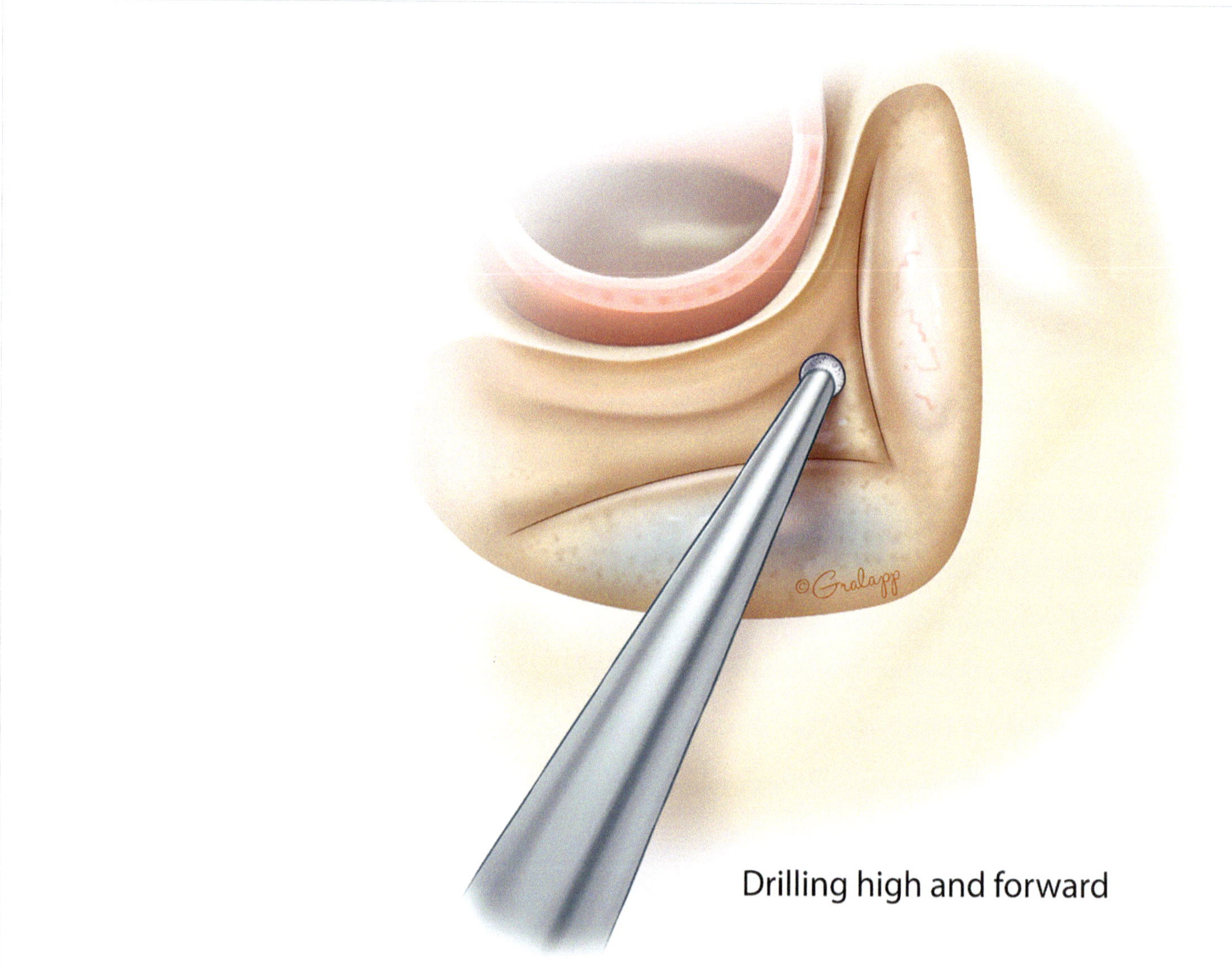

Fig. 7.30 The deepest point of drilling should be kept high and forward along the dura. As the dura forces the excavation inferiorly, care must be taken to identify the lateral semicircular canal and second genu of the facial nerve.

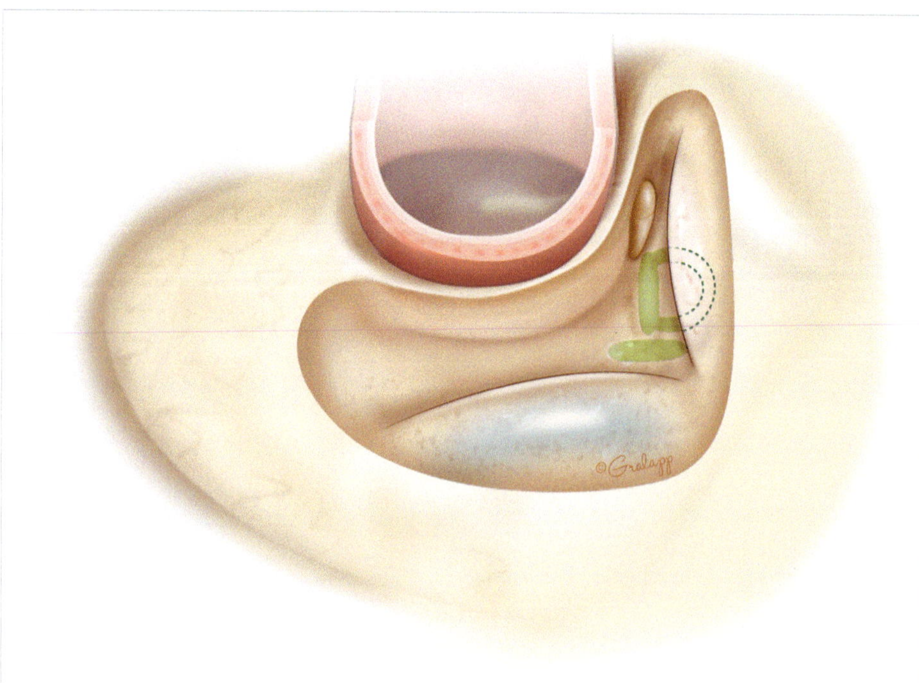

Fig. 7.31 Completed mastoidectomy in a hypopneumatic temporal bone.

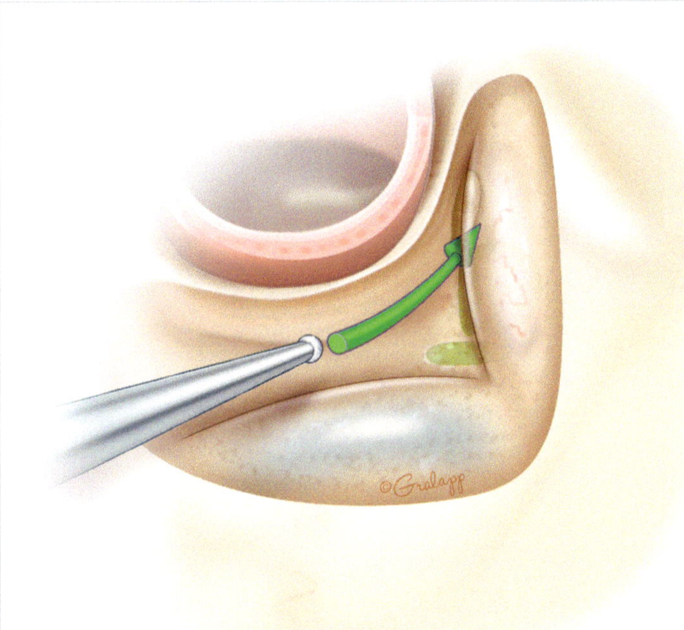

Fig. 7.32 Angle of view toward the epitympanum and ossicles in a hypopneumatic mastoid.

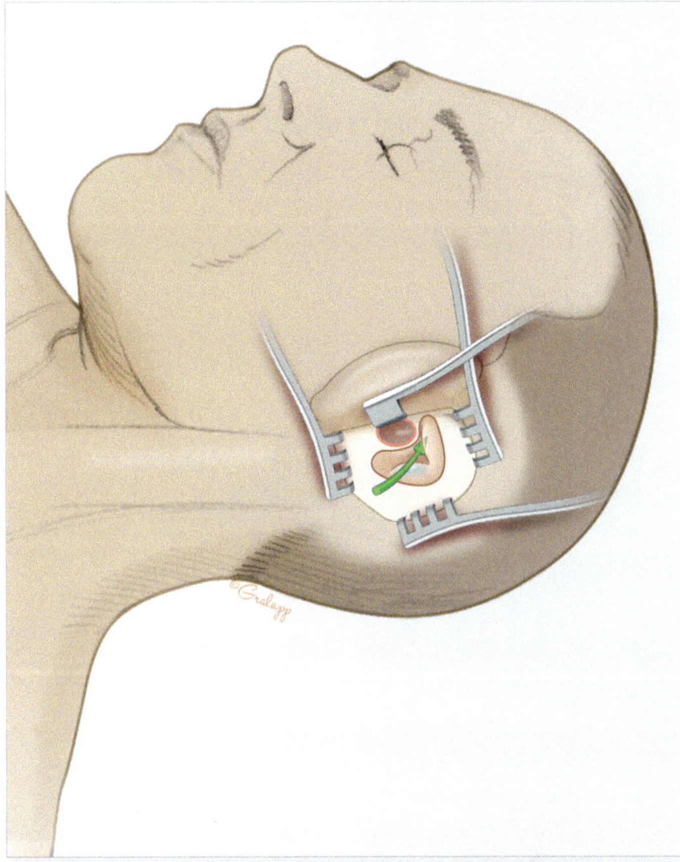

Fig. 7.33 View toward the epitympanum and ossicles in a hypopneumatic mastoid.

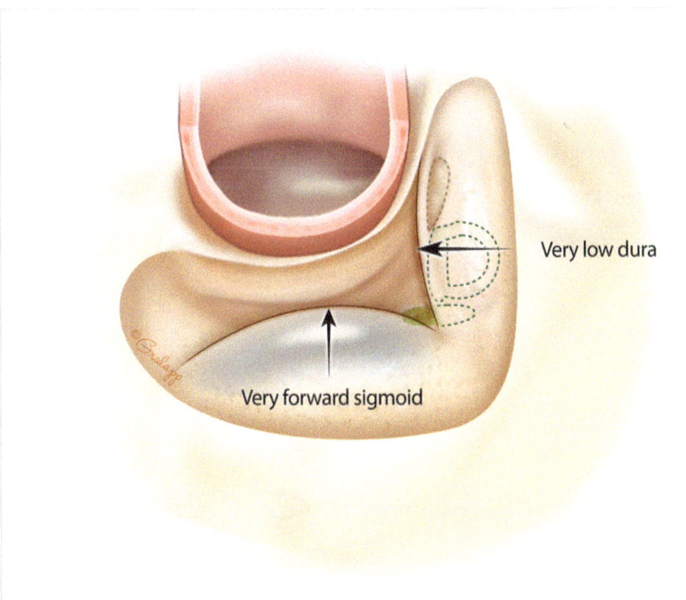

Fig. 7.34 Severe hypopneumatization with a very forward sigmoid sinus and low dura. In this case, there is insufficient room between the middle fossa dura and the ear canal to enable transmastoid exposure of the malleus head and incus body.

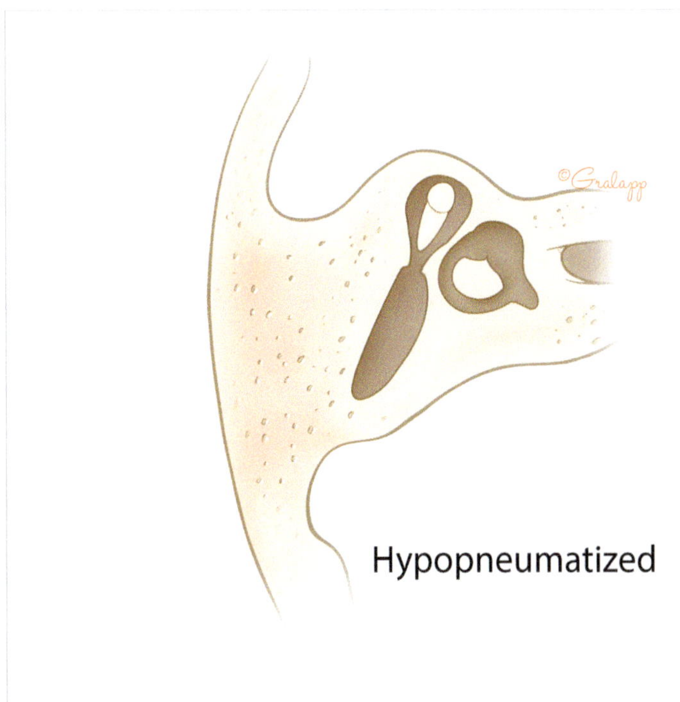

Fig. 7.35 Hypopneumatized mastoid: axial view.

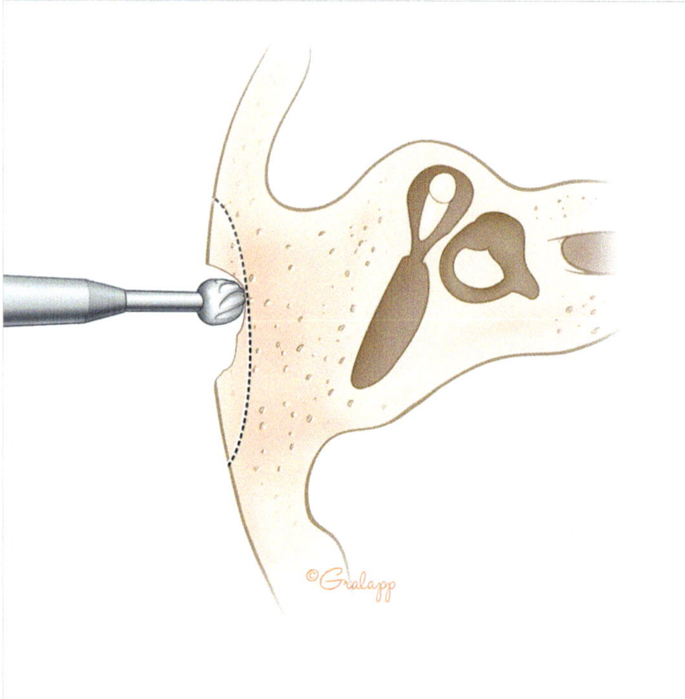

Fig. 7.36 Commencing mastoidectomy in hypopneumatized mastoid. Unlike in pneumatized temporal bones, there is not an outer cortex followed by air cells, but rather solid bone from the surface all the way to the antrum.

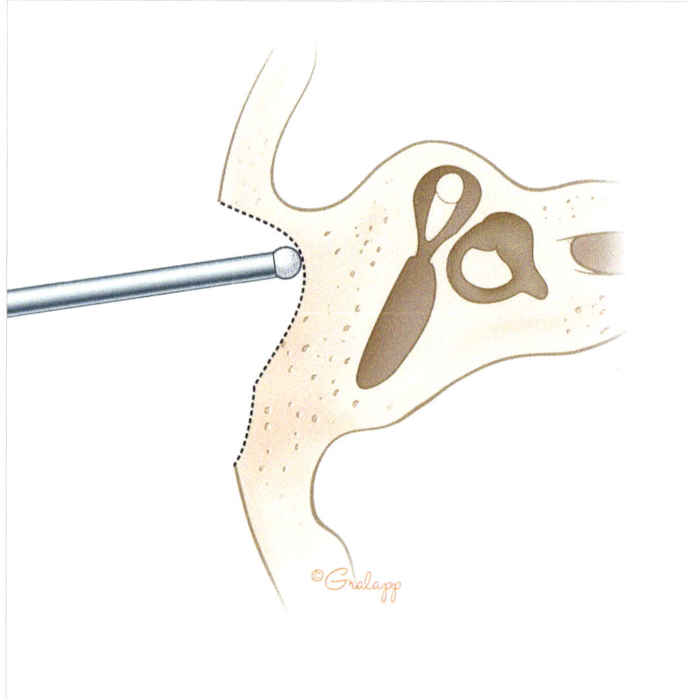

Fig. 7.37 Deepening the excavation proceeds superiorly and anteriorly.

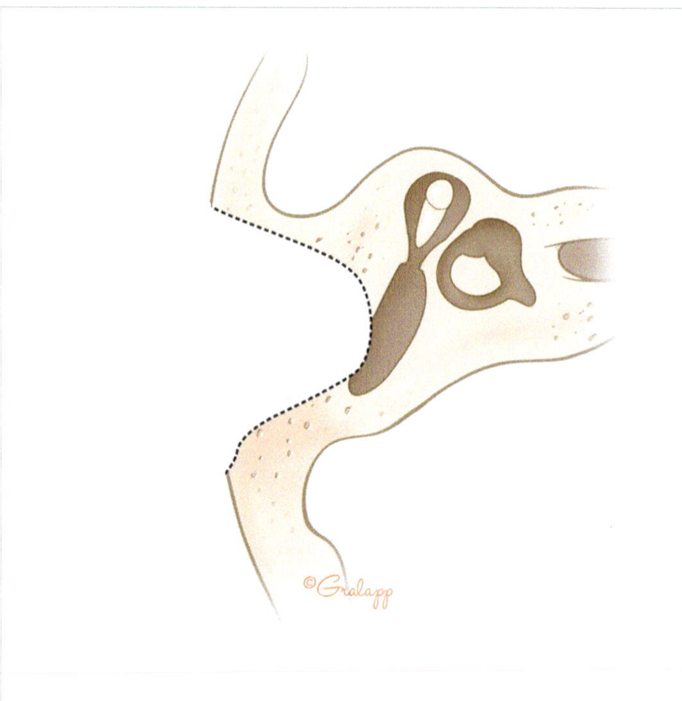

Fig. 7.38 Entering the antrum.

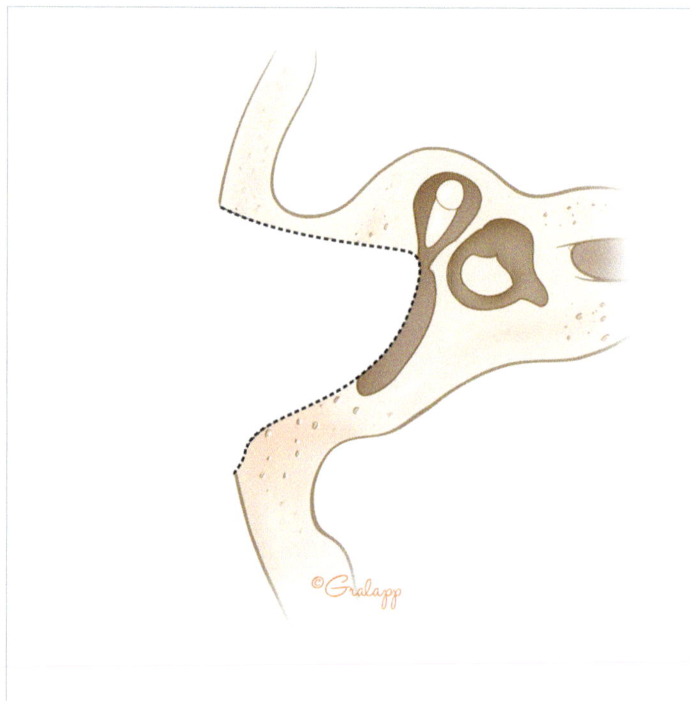

Fig. 7.39 Extending the antral opening.

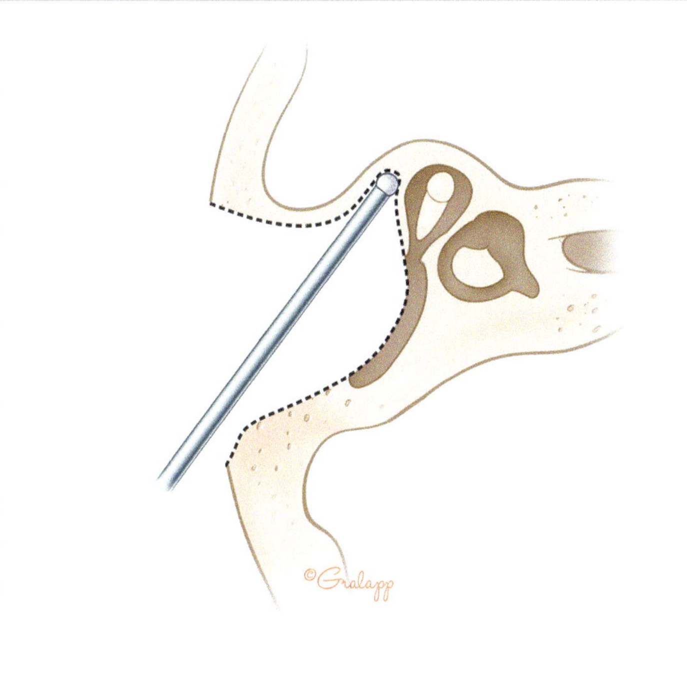

Fig. 7.40 Thinning bone over epitympanum.

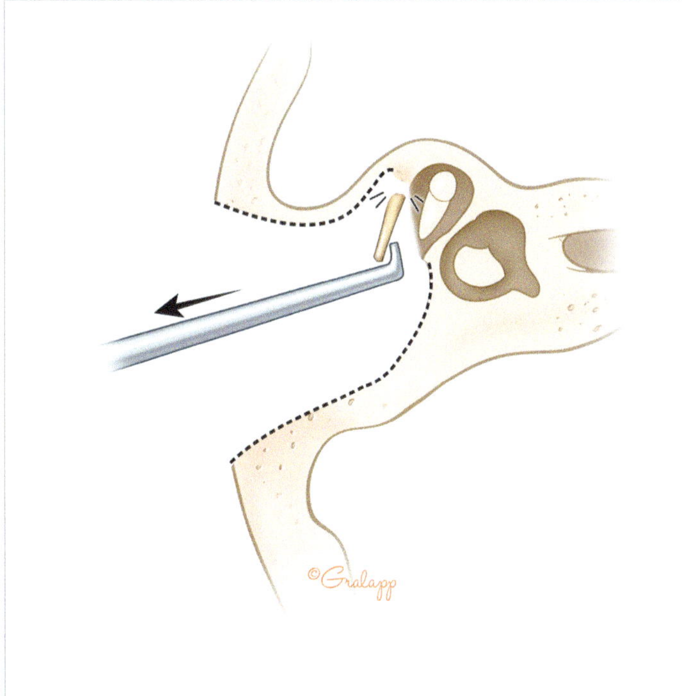

Fig. 7.41 Flaking bone overlying the ossicles.

7.4 Complications of Mastoidectomy

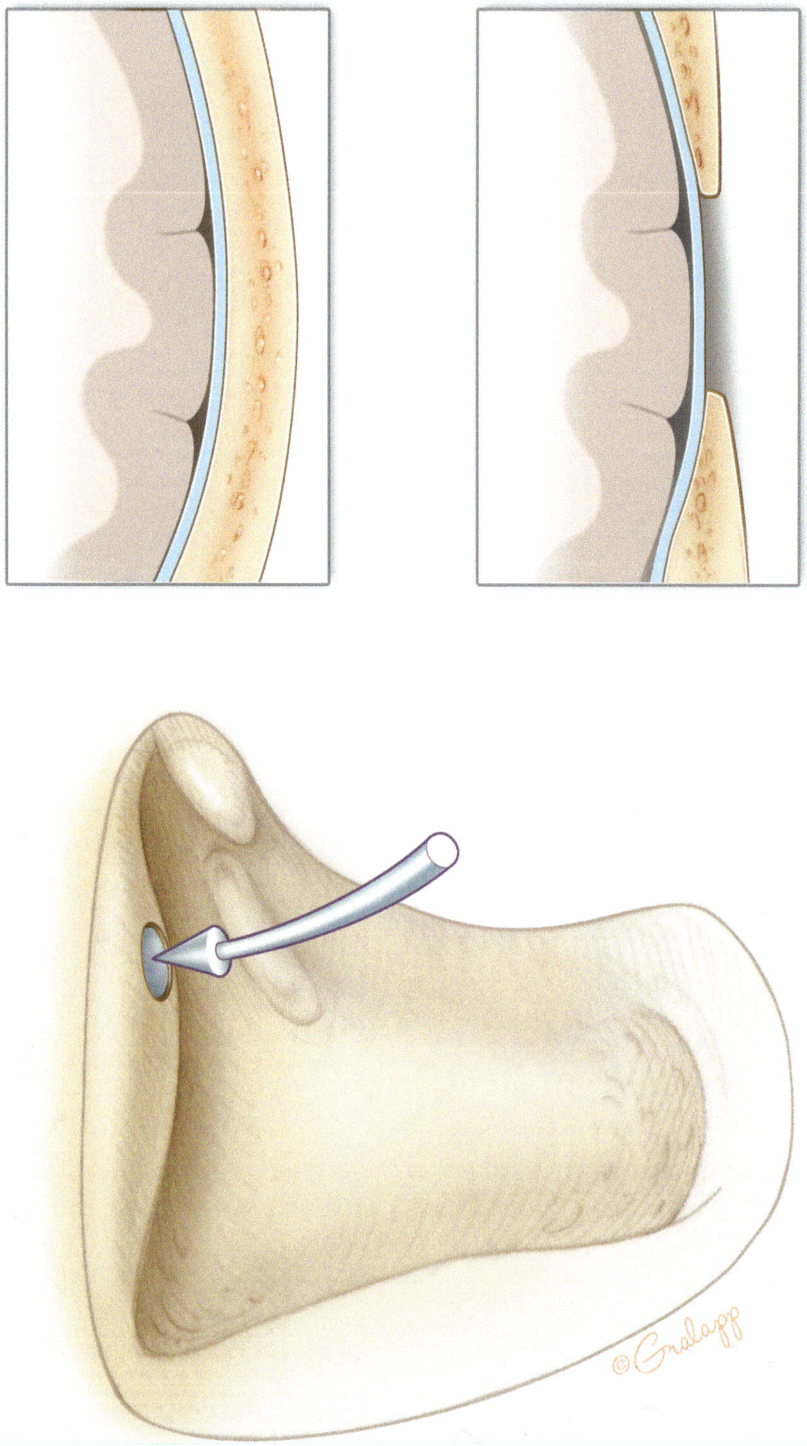

Fig. 7.42 Exposure of tegmen dura is common in cholesteatoma surgery due to either disease erosion or drill exposure. In the vast majority of cases, the dura remains intact. If bleeding occurs, it is best to use absorbable gelatin sponge adrenalin and avoid electrocautery which might disrupt the dura. CSF leakage necessitates repair.

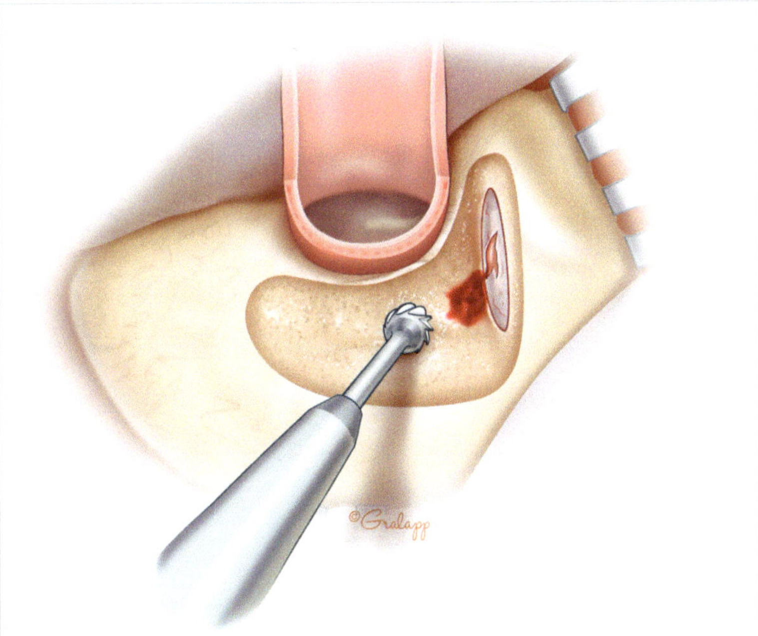

Fig. 7.43 Dural injury due to use of a cutting burr. A rough-cut diamond burr works well in exposing the tegmen and is less likely to cause dural injury.

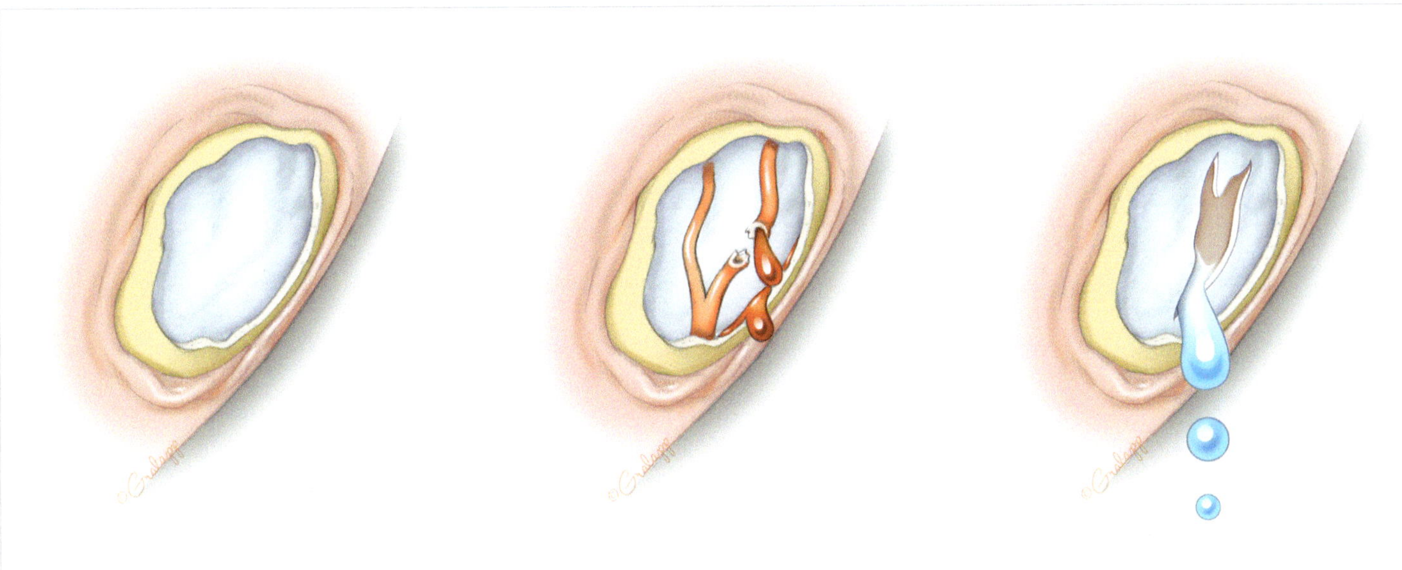

Fig. 7.44 If bleeding occurs from exposed dura, it is best to control with an absorbable gelatin sponge–adrenalin pledget and avoid electrocautery which might disrupt the dura. Cerebrospinal fluid leakage necessitates repair. This can be achieved from below if minor and easily controlled or from above (extradural middle fossa craniotomy) if the injury is large or leakage is difficult to control from below.

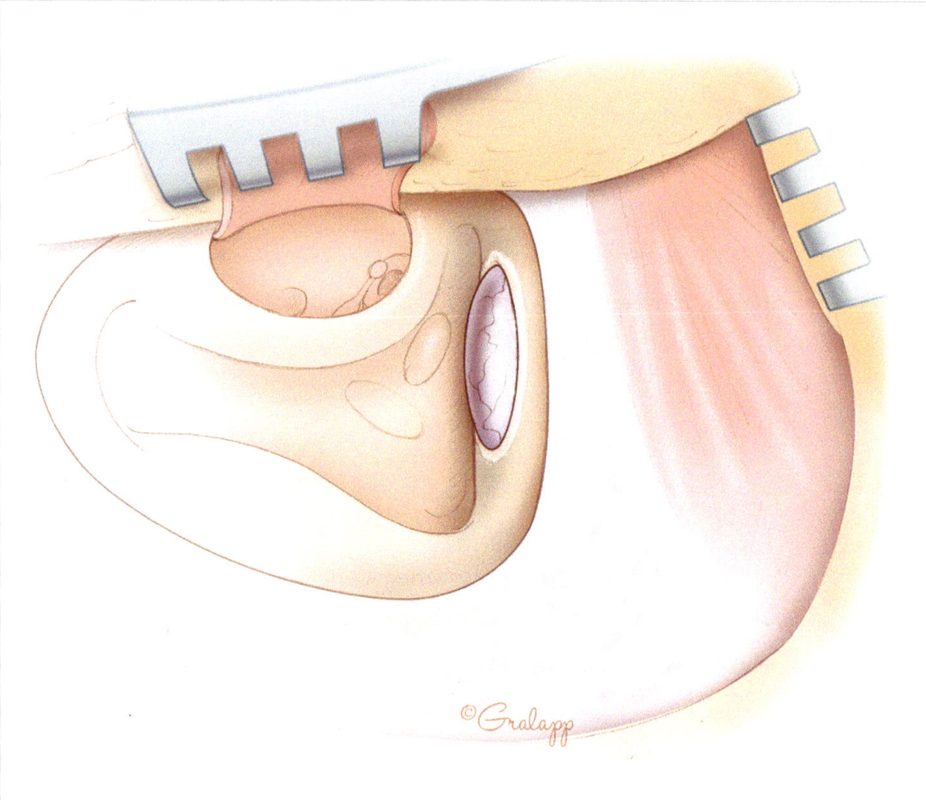

Fig. 7.45 Extensive dural exposure is best repaired to reduce the risk of developing an encephalocoele. After canal wall down procedures, extensively exposed dura could theoretically be injured during routine office cleaning, although this is fortunately rare.

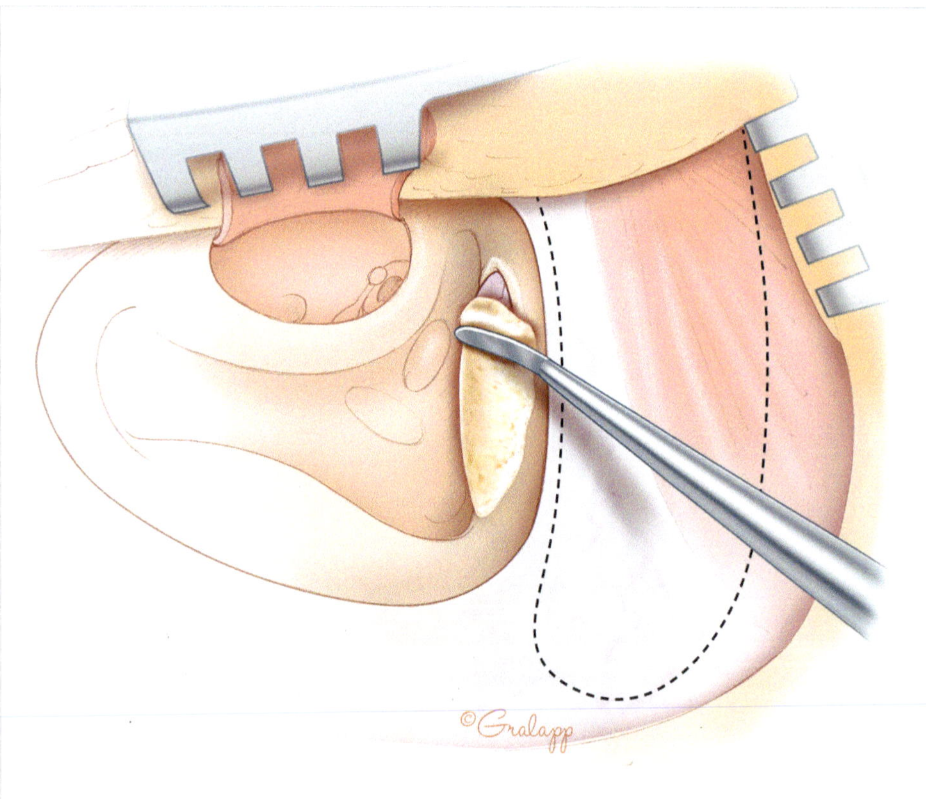

Fig. 7.46 Repair of tegmen dehiscence with autologous bone dust covering the dural defect. In small defects, bone dust covered by a piece of fascia is usually sufficient. In larger defects, reinforcement with a rotation flap may be needed. Note the outline of the temporal periosteal flap.

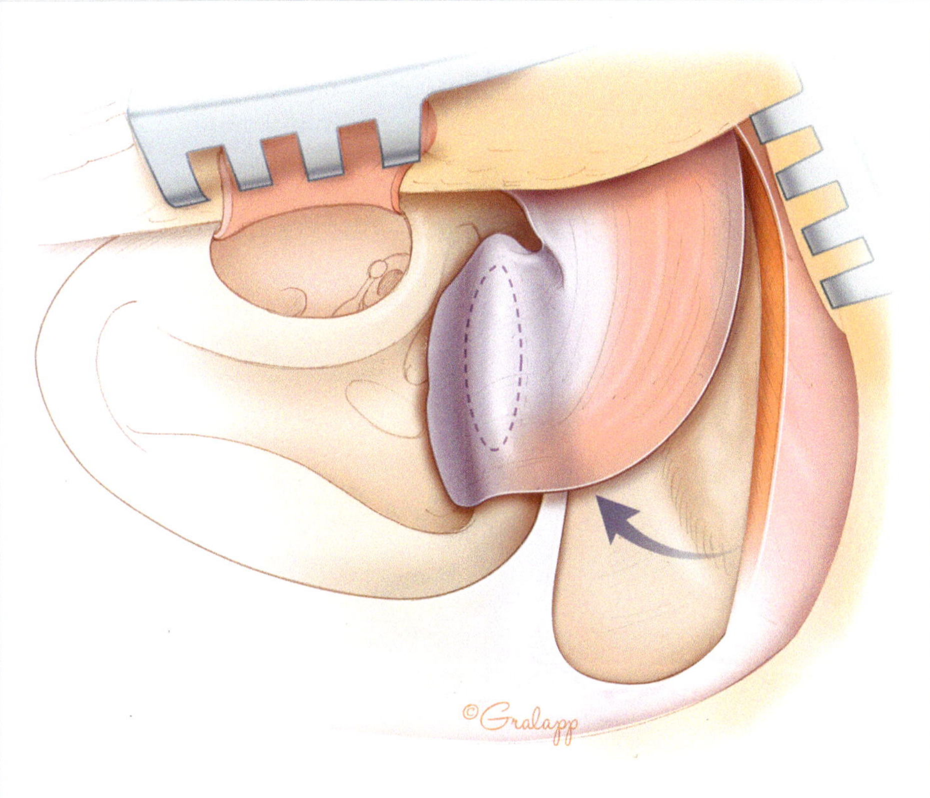

Fig. 7.47 Temporal periosteal flap rotated to cover the middle fossa floor dural exposure.

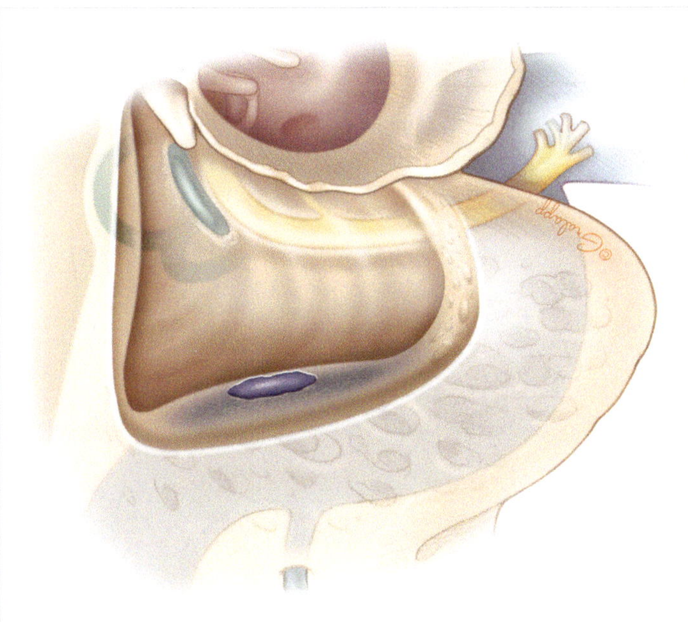

Fig. 7.48 Exposure of the sigmoid sinus during mastoid surgery is common.

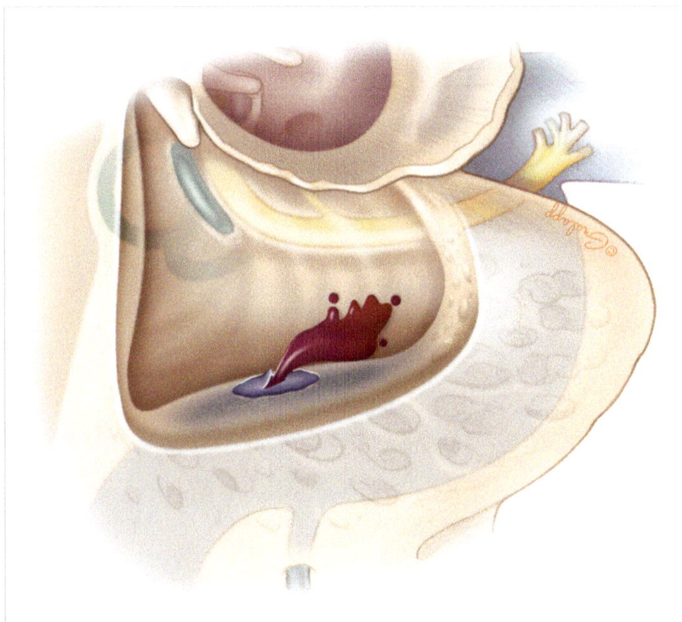

Fig. 7.49 Sigmoid sinus hemorrhage in mastoid surgery is not common, but the otological surgeon must know how to manage it.

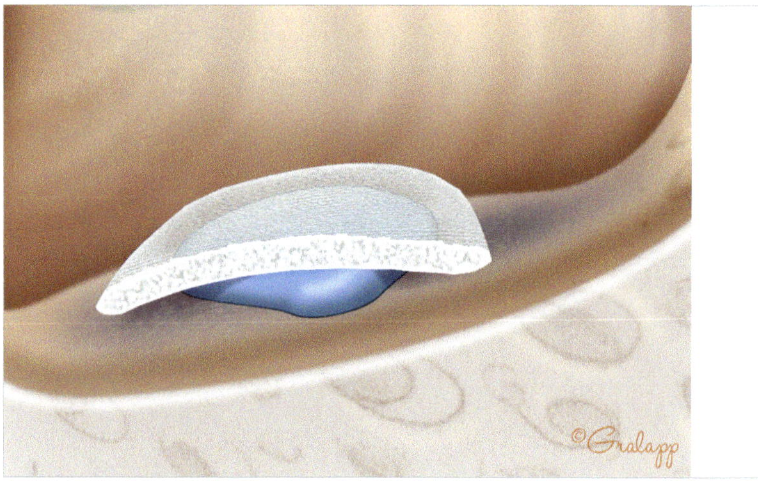

Fig. 7.50 Sigmoid sinus hemorrhage is readily controllable with hemostatic packing. The author uses Floseal covered by Surgicel, which are held firmly under a cottonoid patty over the rent for a few minutes while hemostasis is obtained. This is a routine procedure in operative neurotology, but is seldom necessary in routine otological surgery.

7.5 Facial Recess Approach

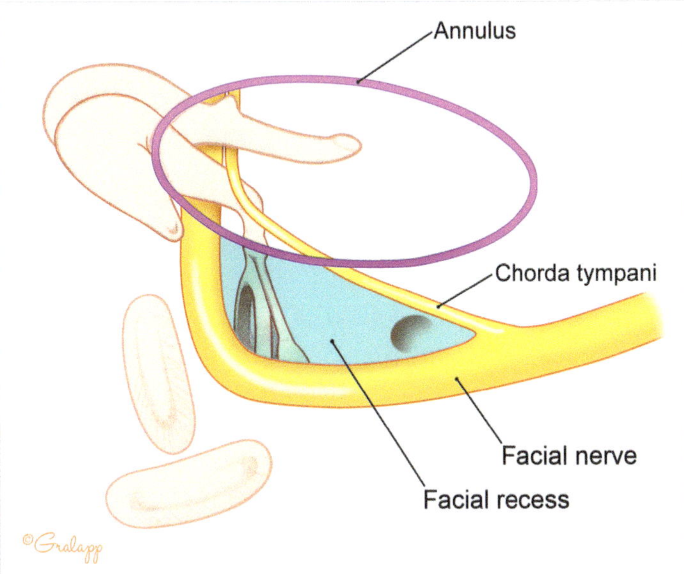

Fig. 7.51 Schematic representation of the relationships of the facial recess and the middle ear exposure afforded by its opening (*blue*).

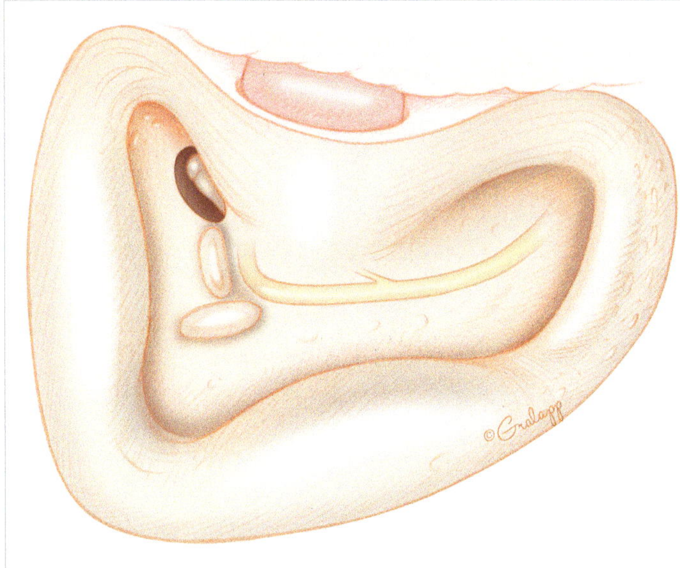

Fig. 7.52 The relationships of the facial recess seen from the mastoid perspective.

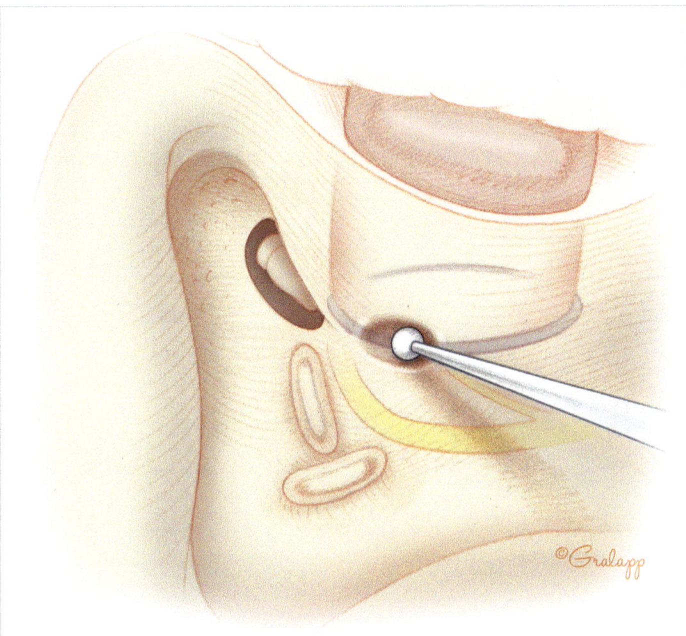

Fig. 7.53 Surgeons overly concerned about the facial nerve may make too lateral of an approach, risking injury to the tympanic annulus.

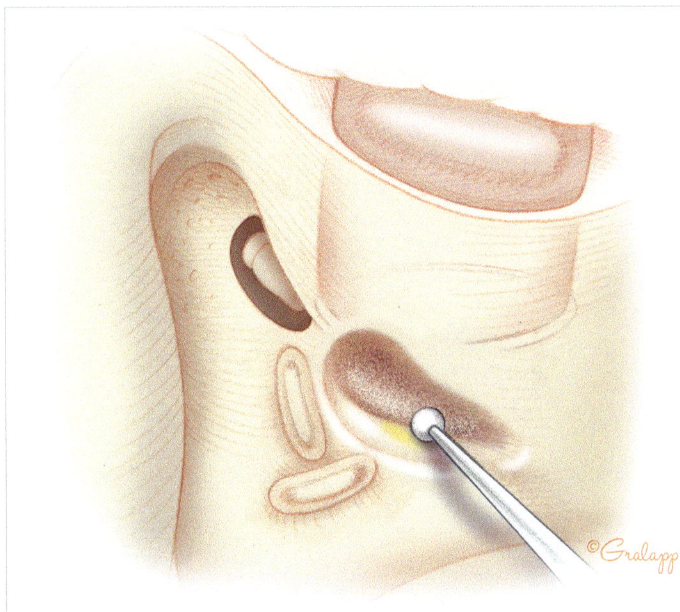

Fig. 7.54 Opening of the facial recess is conducted with a diamond burr using copious irrigation to avoid heat buildup which might injure the facial nerve. Many surgeons routinely identify the facial nerve, preferably leaving it under a thin bony covering.

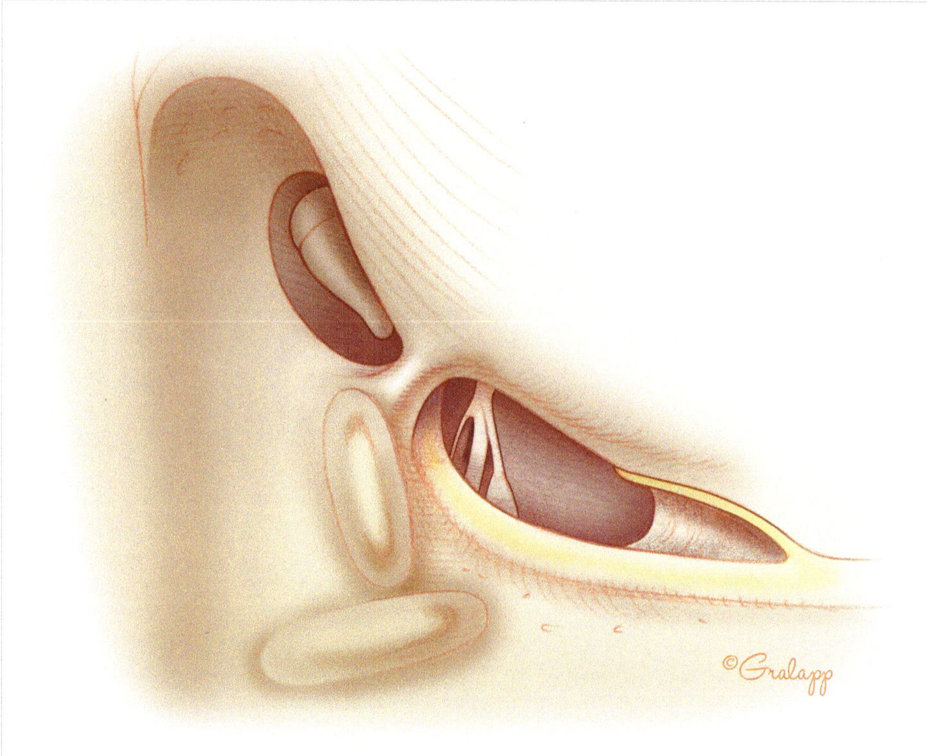

Fig. 7.55 Completed facial recess exposure revealing the stapes and stapedial pyramid.

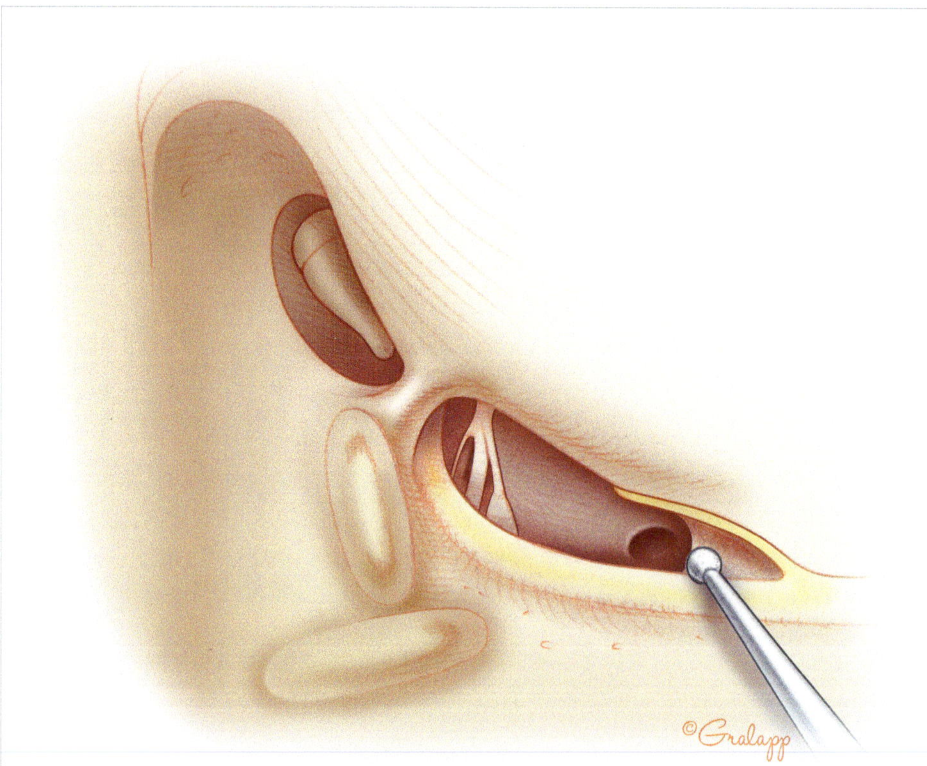

Fig. 7.56 Inferior extension of the facial recess approach, as used in cochlear implantation, to expose the round window.

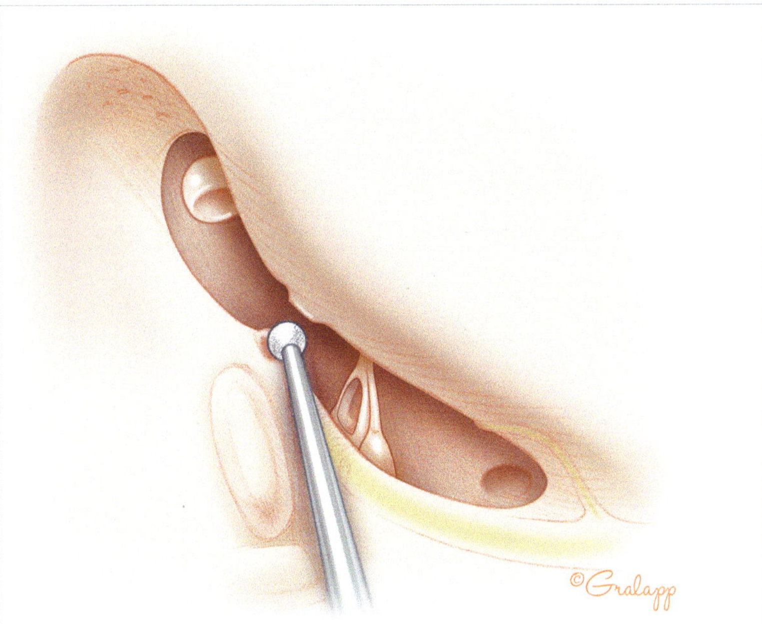

Fig. 7.57 When the incus is absent, the remaining buttress can be removed. Making the space confluent is desirable, as it enhances the communication between the mastoid and the middle ear thus reducing the risk of aditus block.

7.6 The Facial Nerve in Mastoidectomy

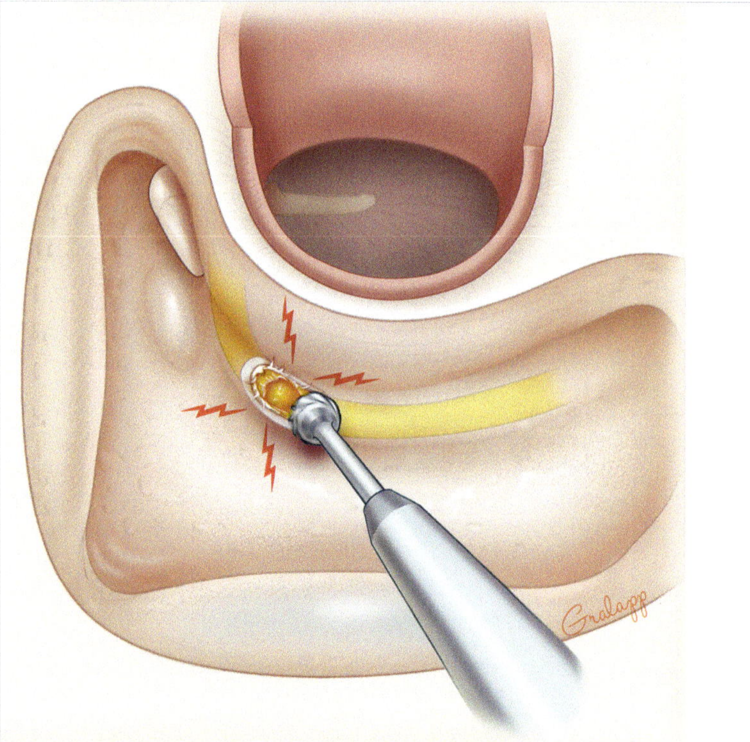

Fig. 7.58 Swipe injury of the facial nerve at the second genu with a cutting burr. This is the classic location of injury sustained during mastoid surgery.

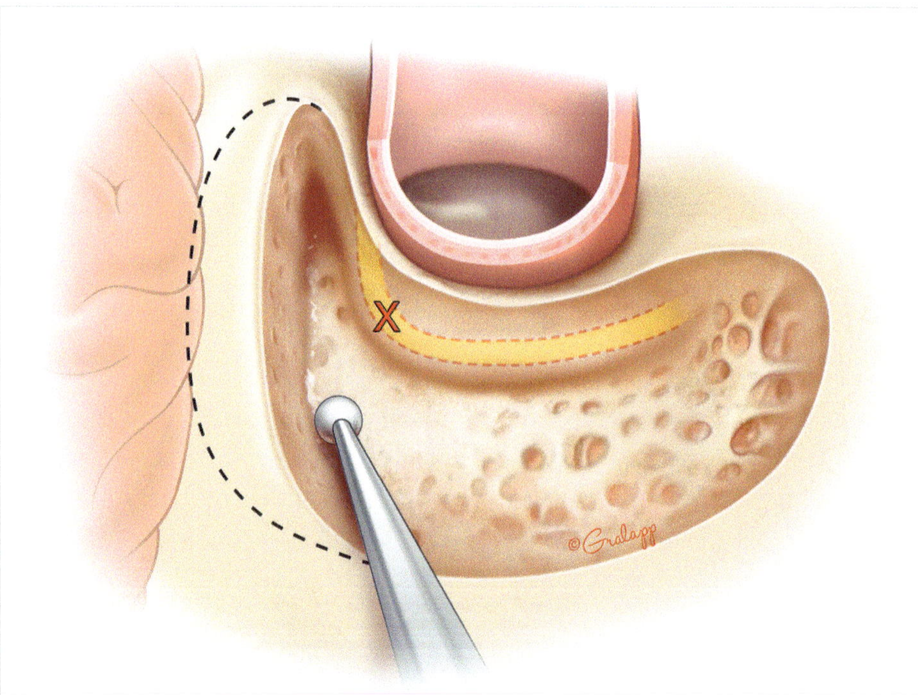

Fig. 7.59 Failing to locate the tegmen can lead to drilling too inferior, thus placing the second genu of the facial nerve at risk.

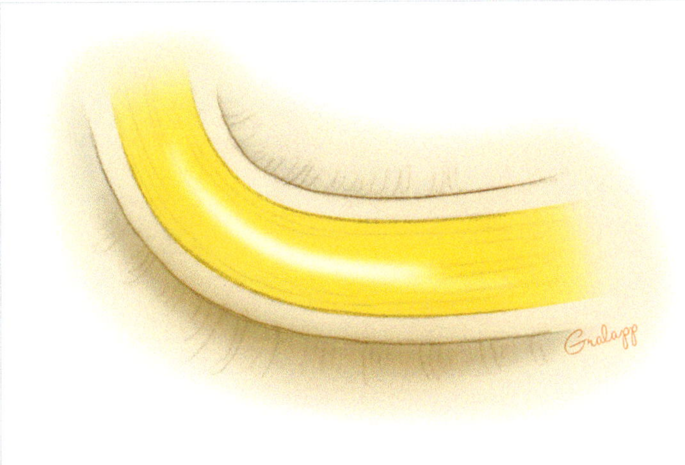

Fig. 7.60 Normal second genu.

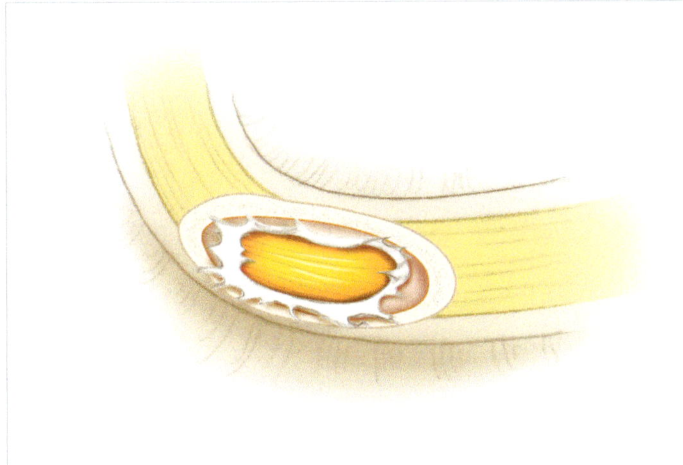

Fig. 7.61 A drill injury which disrupts the epineurium, but leaves the nerve fibers intact.

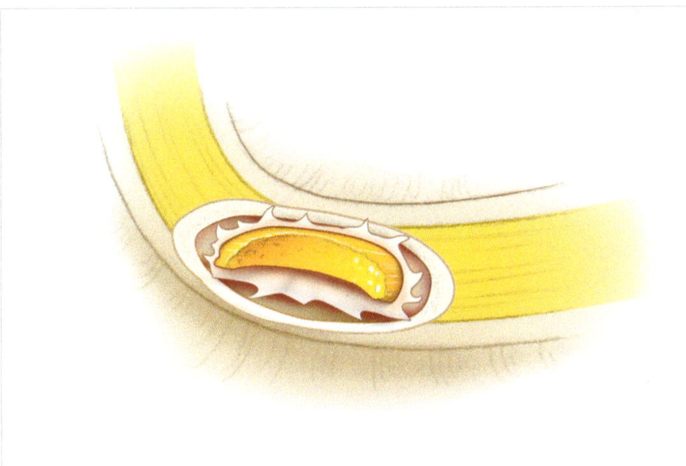

Fig. 7.62 A partial injury due to swipe with a cutting burr.

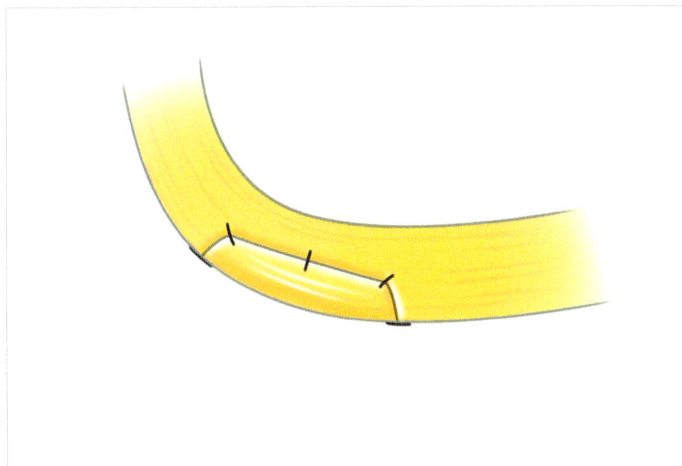

Fig. 7.63 Grafting of a partial injury.

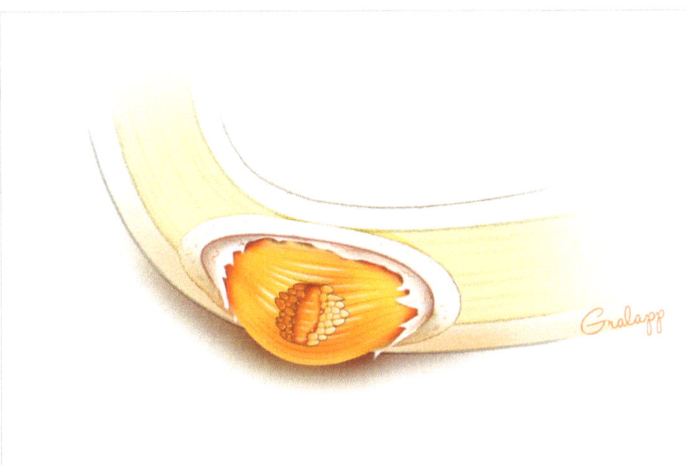

Fig. 7.64 Swelling of the nerve in response to a partial injury.

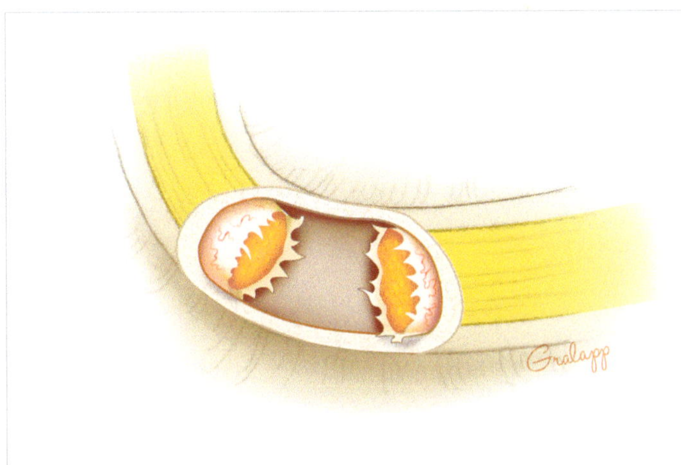

Fig. 7.65 Transection injury.

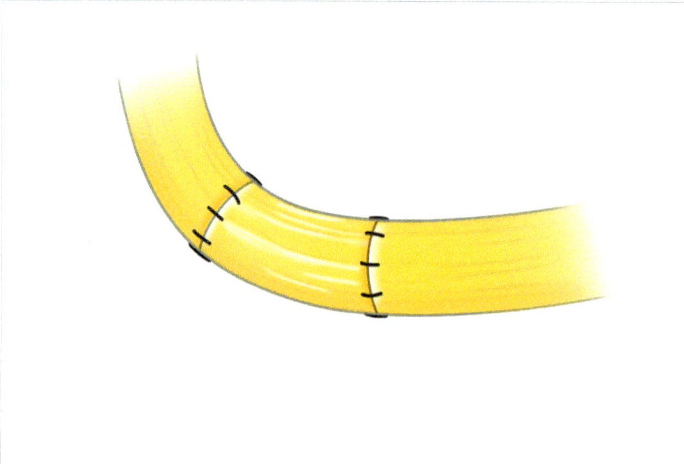

Fig. 7.66 Cable grafting of a transection injury. When the nerve is laid into the fallopian canal, only a couple of epineurial stitches are needed. Some would repair with tissue glue rather than sutures.

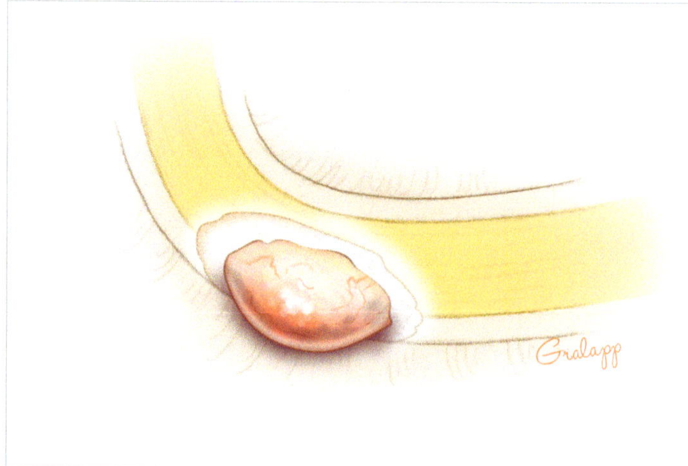

Fig. 7.67 A swollen, herniated nerve following drill injury.

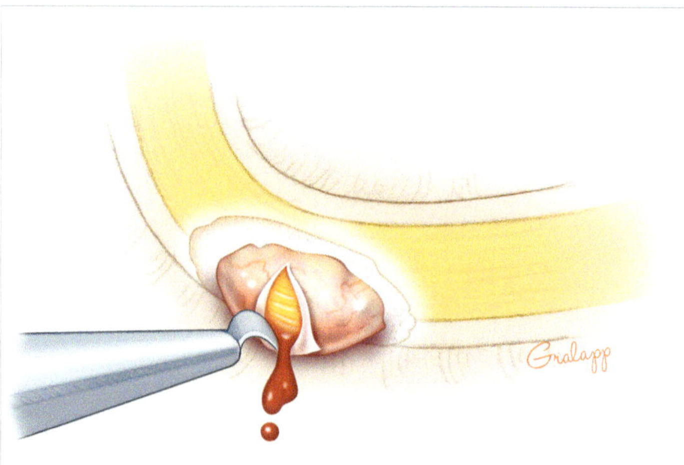

Fig. 7.68 Incising epineurium to release intraneural hematoma.

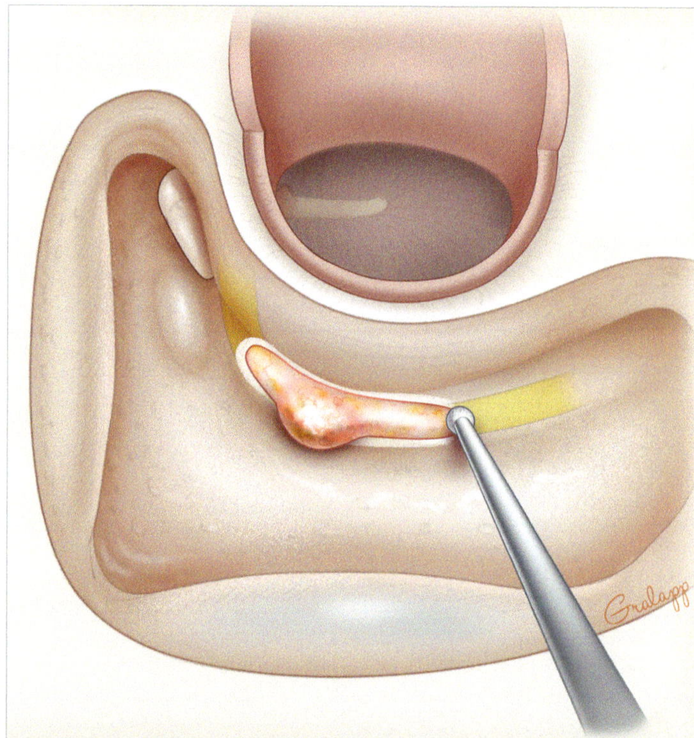

Fig. 7.69 Decompression of the fallopian canal proximal and distal to a swollen nerve at the site of injury.

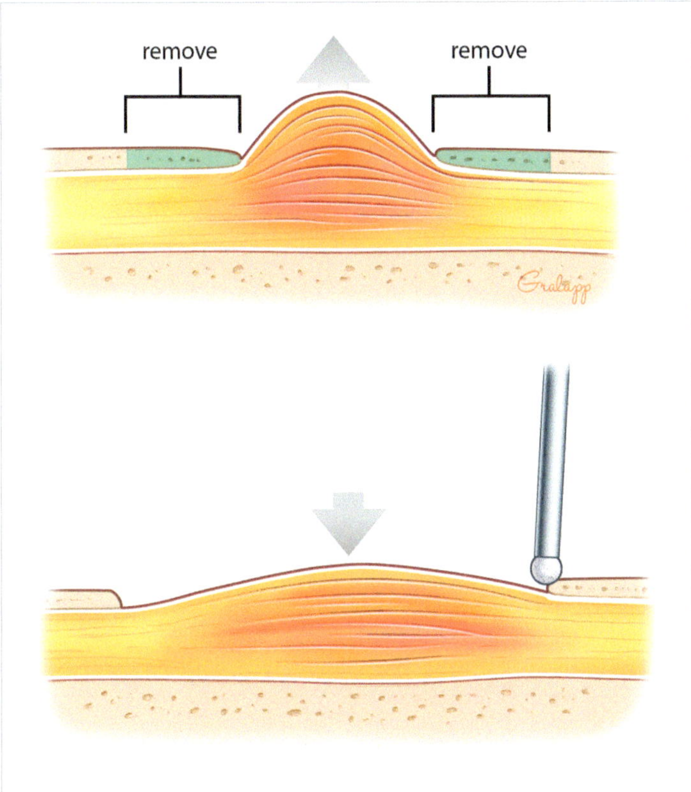

Fig. 7.70 Decompression of an injured nerve.

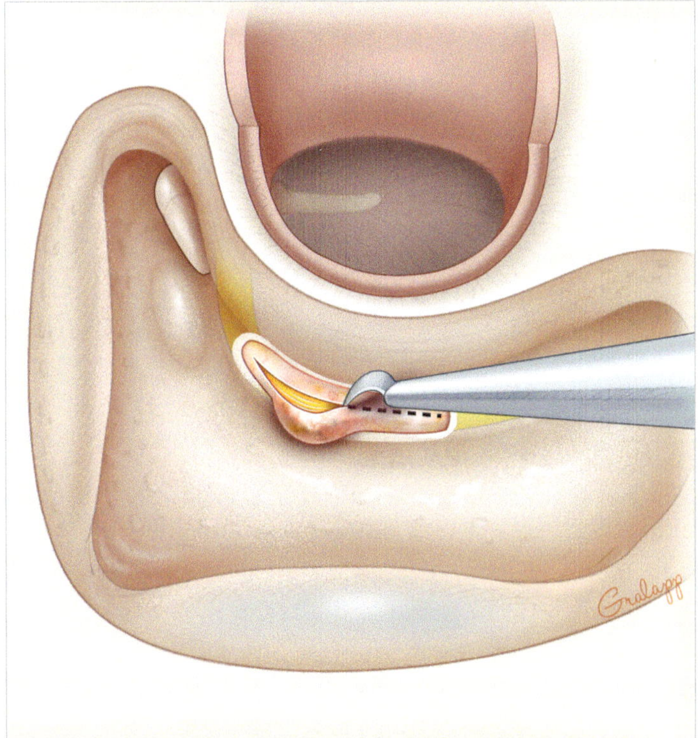

Fig. 7.71 Incising the sheath to relieve compression is controversial and many prefer to leave epineurium intact to preserve vascular supply to the nerve.

7.7 Mastoid Obliteration

Robert K. Jackler, Nikolas H. Blevins, and Jennifer Alyono

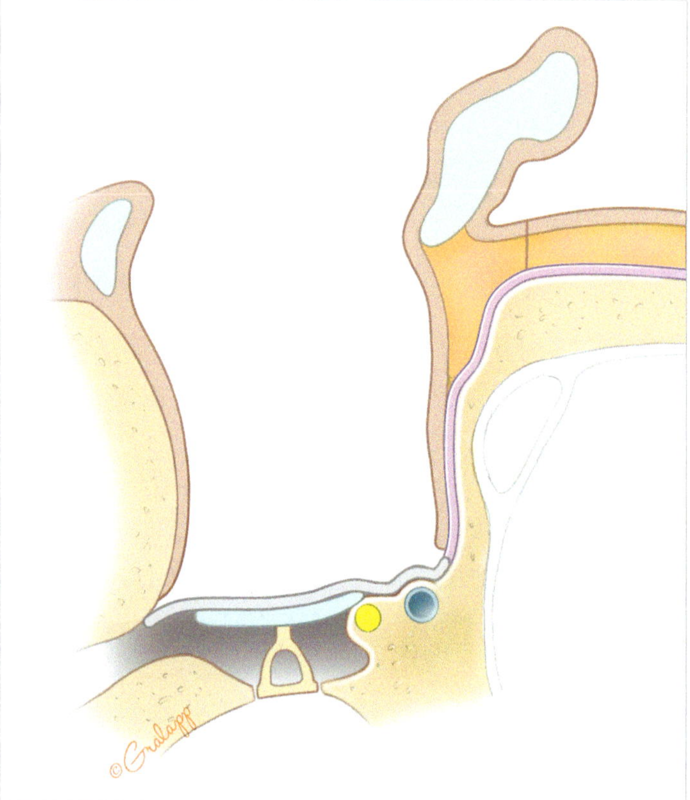

Fig. 7.72 Canal wall down mastoidectomy creates a cavity of varying size depending on the size of the mastoid. A large cavity can accumulate debris and is more likely to discharge.

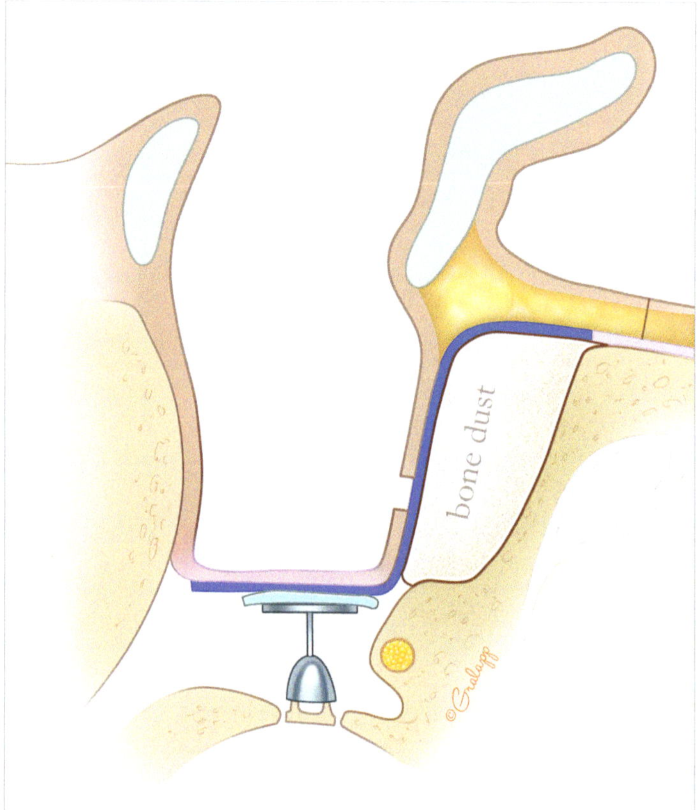

Fig. 7.73 Cross-sectional view of autologous bone dust obliteration of the mastoid to reduce the size of the cavity. Note the large piece of fascia completely covering the bone paté (dust).

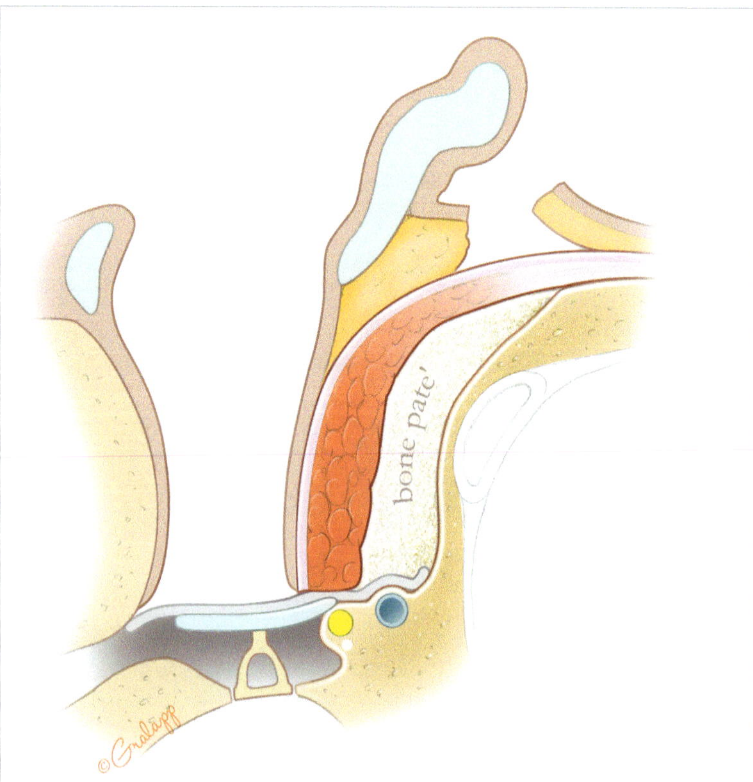

Fig. 7.74 Mastoid obliteration with a combination of musculofascial flap overlying bone paté.

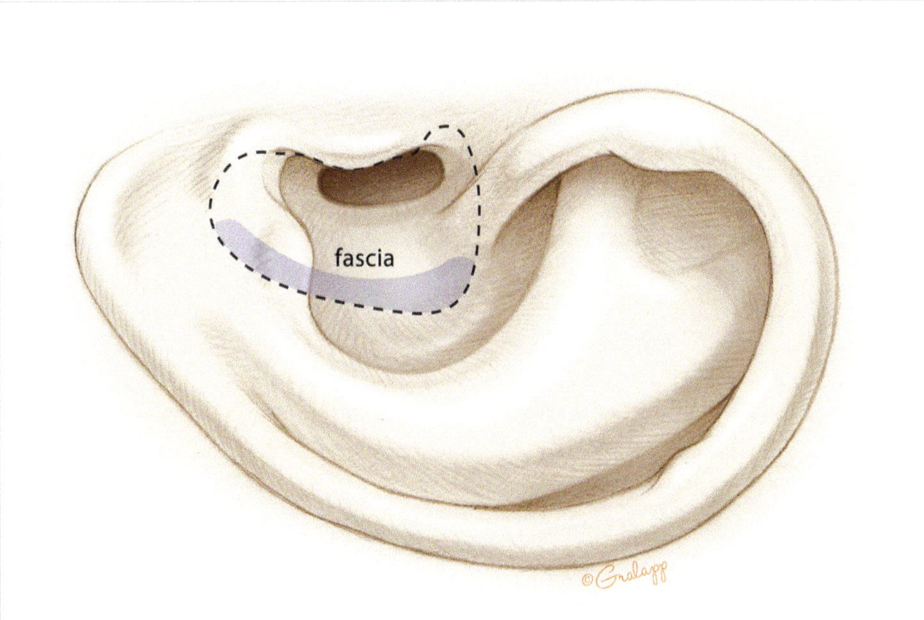

Fig. 7.75 In a small cavity, a fascia or periosteal flap may be sufficient.

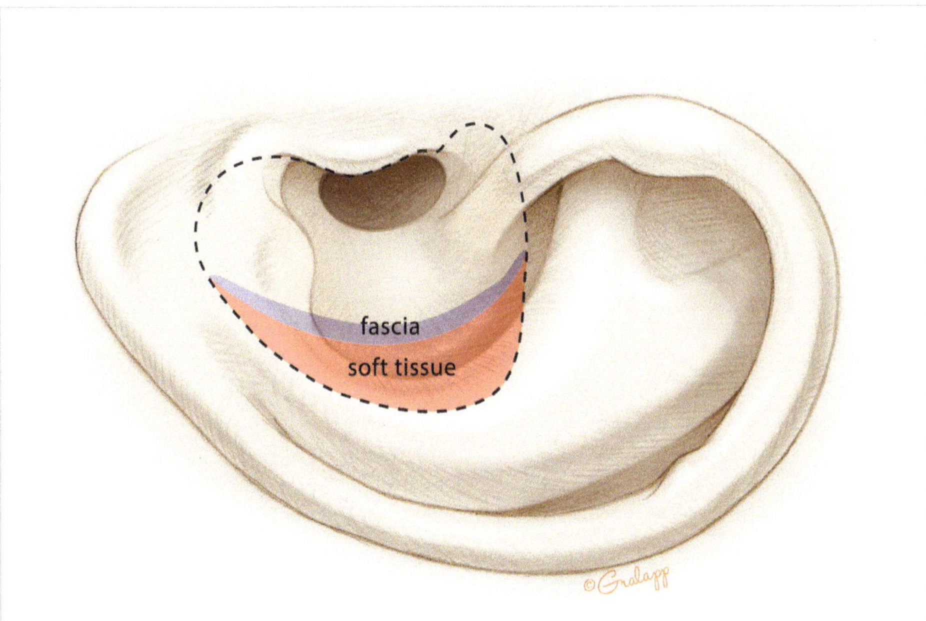

Fig. 7.76 In a larger cavity, fascia and muscle flap provide additional bulk.

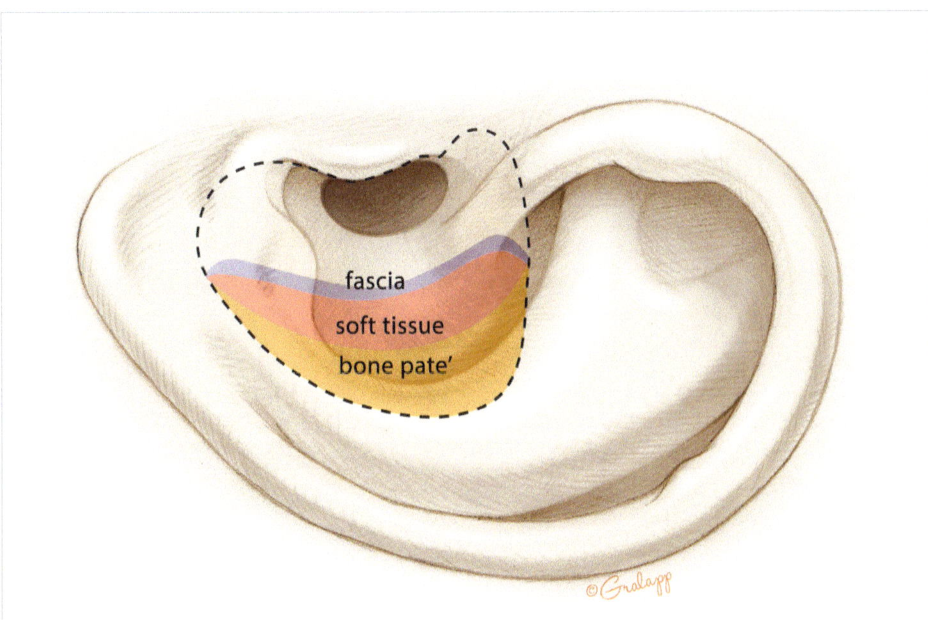

Fig. 7.77 Autologous bone paté may be added to increase the bulk of obliteration.

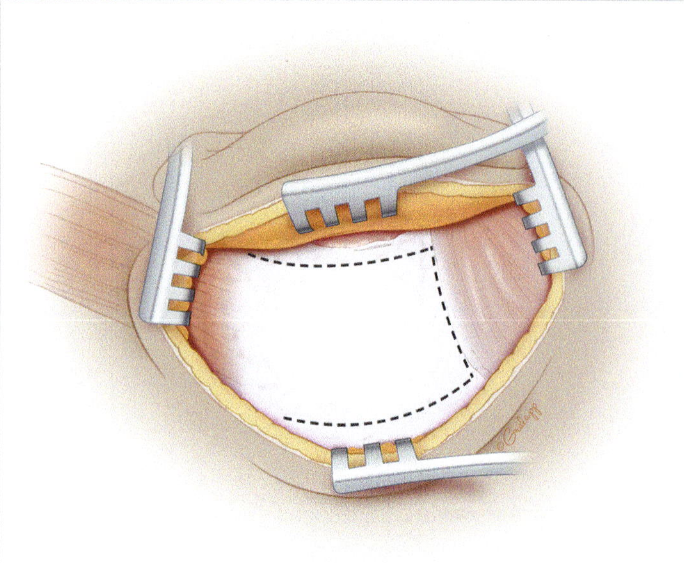

Fig. 7.78 An inferiorly based periosteal flap is fashioned in preparation for mastoid obliteration with autologous bone dust.

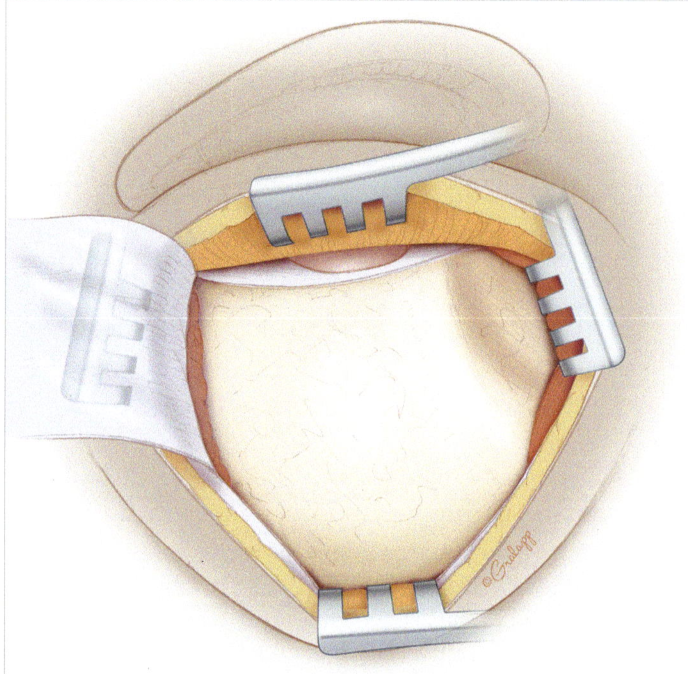

Fig. 7.79 Periosteal flap is reflected inferiorly and the temporalis muscle retracted superiorly.

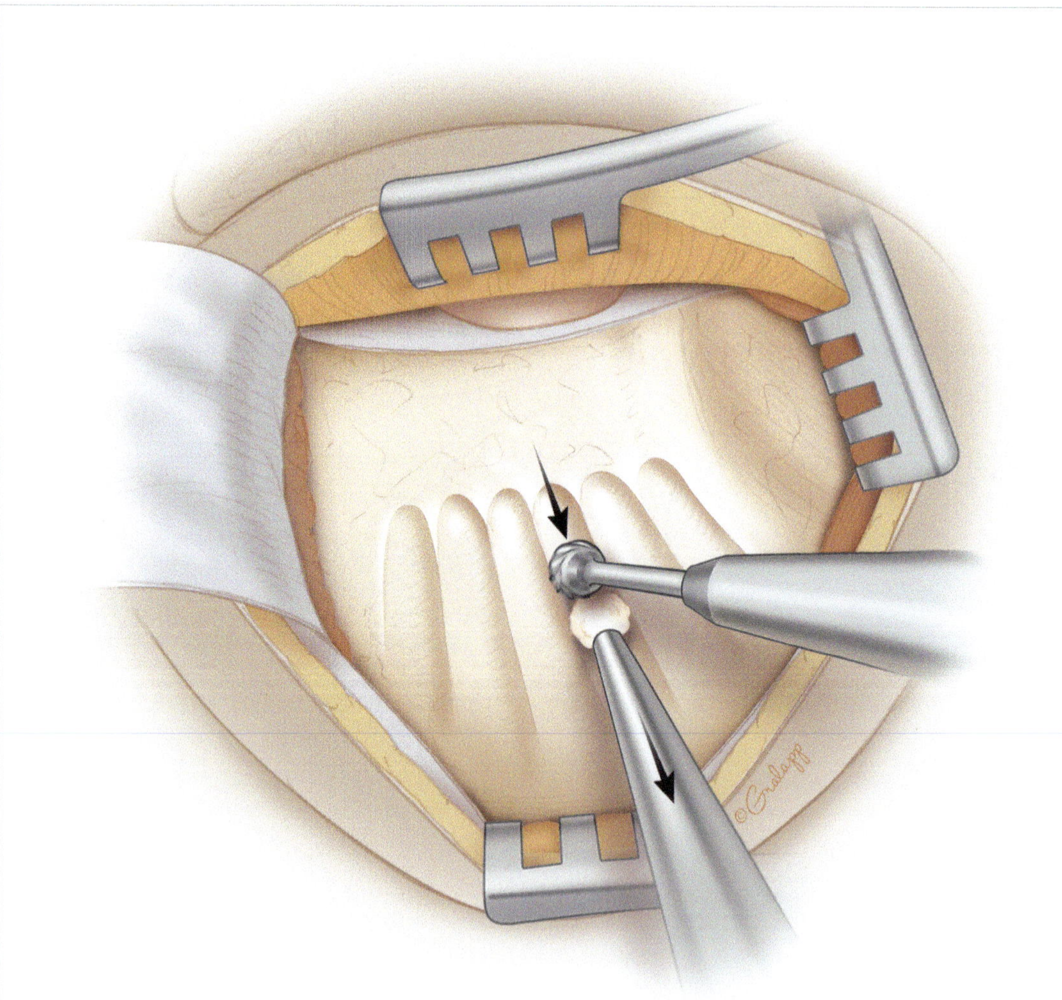

Fig. 7.80 Bone dust is produced with a large cutting burr. Using the burr at slower speed while applying increased tangential pressure to the cortex produces larger, more uniform bone dust particles, which are easily collected. Bone dust collection is typically performed prior to entering the middle ear, and care is taken to avoid entering air cells in order to minimize the risk of collecting epithelial cells or pathogenic bacteria.

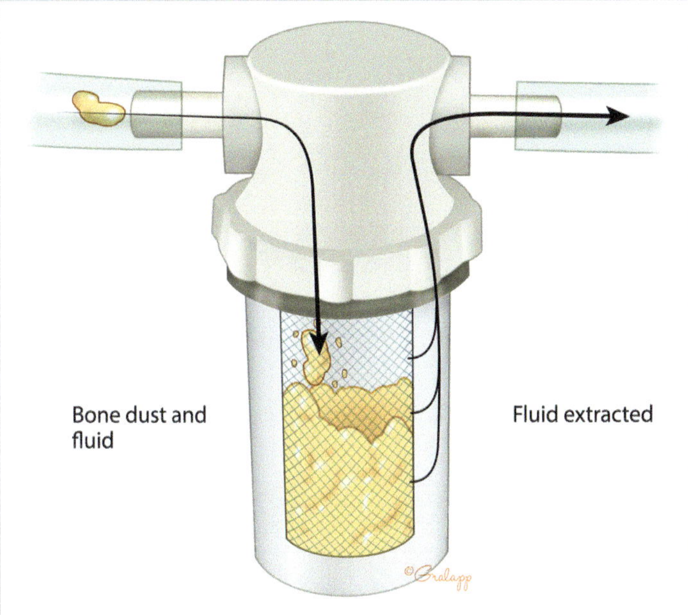

Fig. 7.81 Bone dust is gathered using a collector placed in line with the suction (e.g., Sheehy Bone Duct Collector). A wire-mesh sieve collects particulate matter while allowing irrigant to pass through. Some surgeons mix the harvest bone paté with the patient's blood.

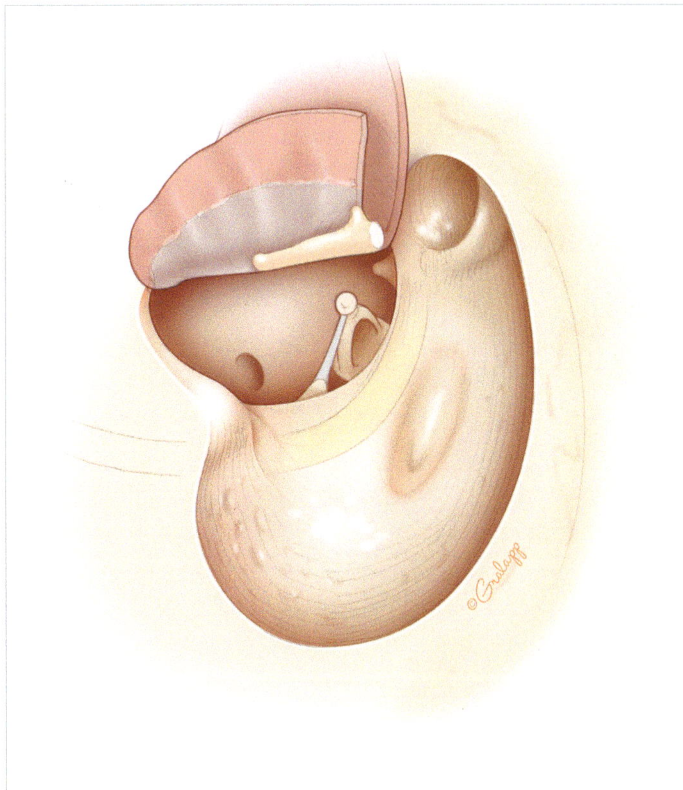

Fig. 7.82 Completed canal wall down mastoidectomy leaving non-pneumatized solid bone in situ.

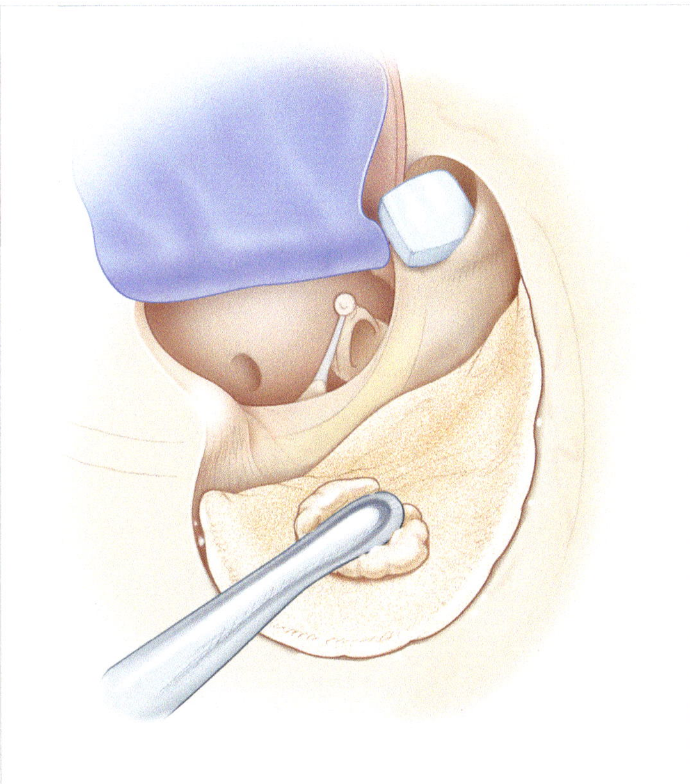

Fig. 7.83 The fascia graft (*blue*) and tympanomeatal flap are retracted anteriorly. The epitympanum may be obliterated with cartilage (as shown here) or bone dust.

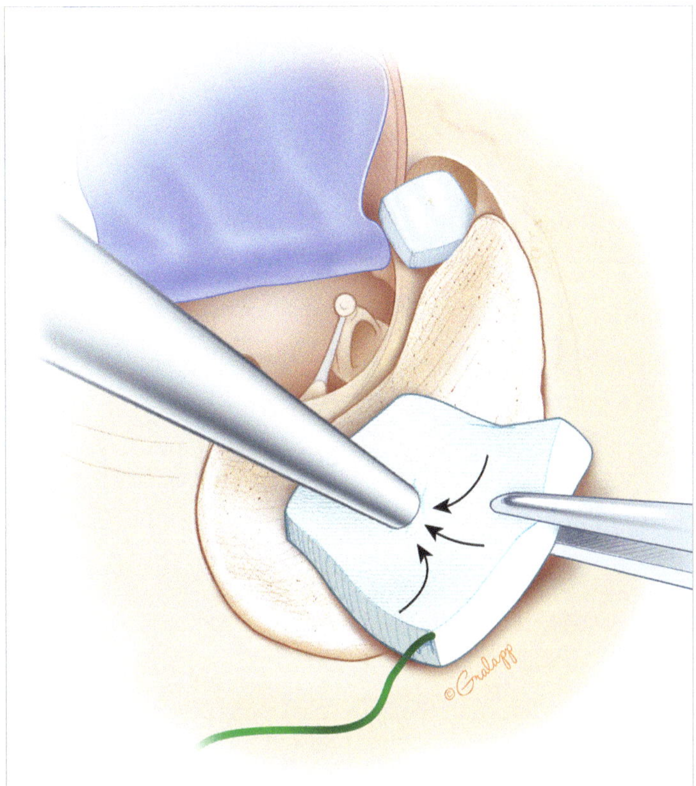

Fig. 7.84 The bone dust is packed tightly by suctioning excess fluid through a cottonoid pledget.

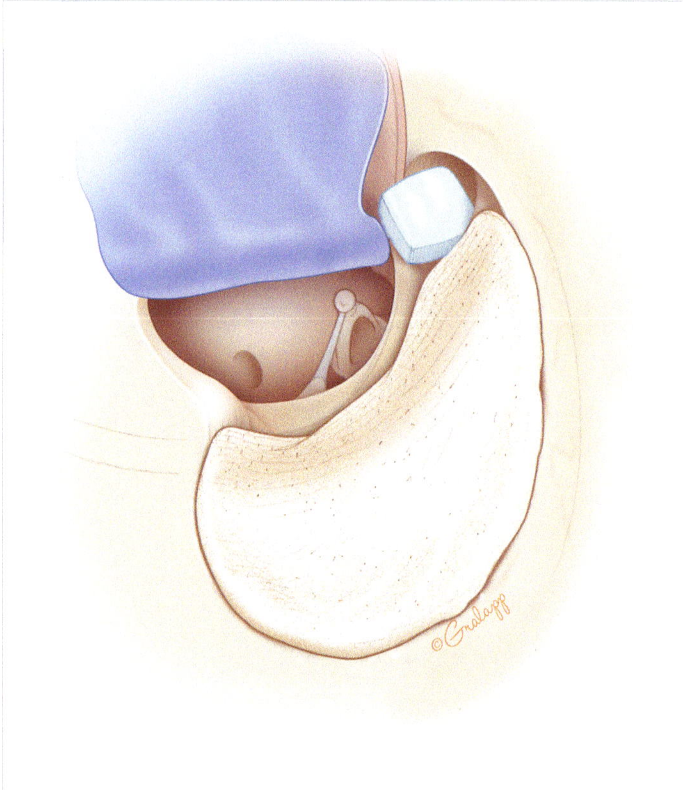

Fig. 7.85 Completed mastoid obliteration using autologous bone dust.

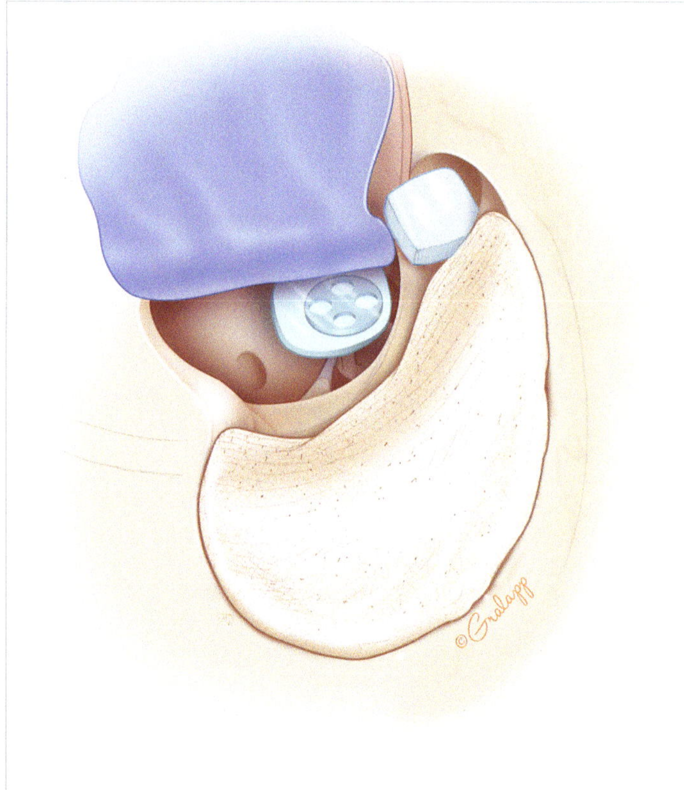

Fig. 7.86 Ossicular reconstruction can be performed following mastoid obliteration as needed.

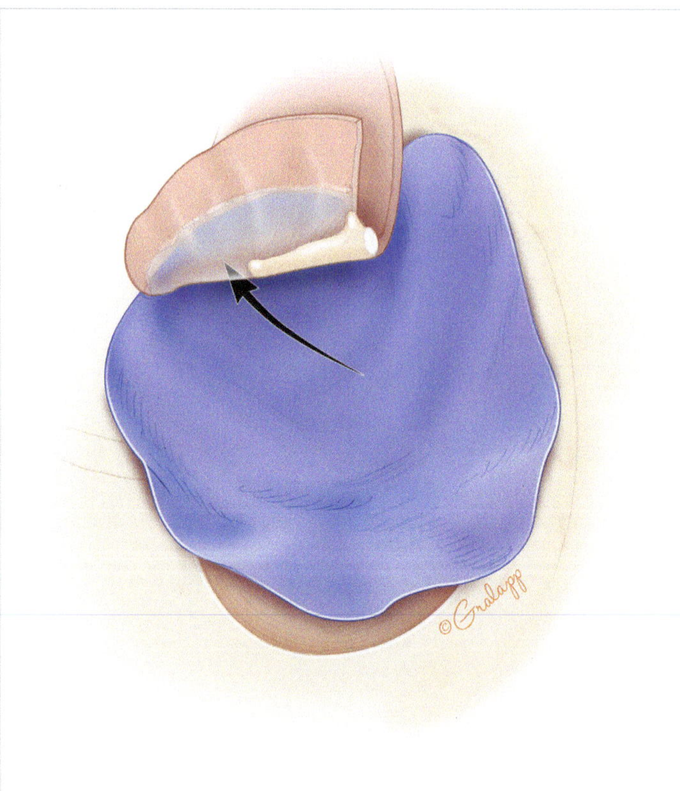

Fig. 7.87 A large temporalis fascia graft both reconstructs any tympanic membrane defect and covers the bone paté.

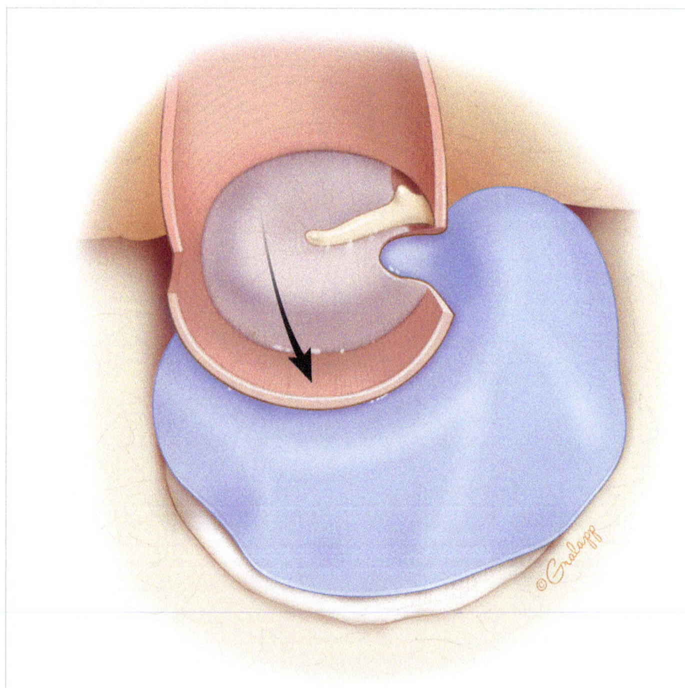

Fig. 7.88 The tympanomeatal flap is laid back down into anatomical position, allowing the underlying fascia graft to cover the exposed bone dust.

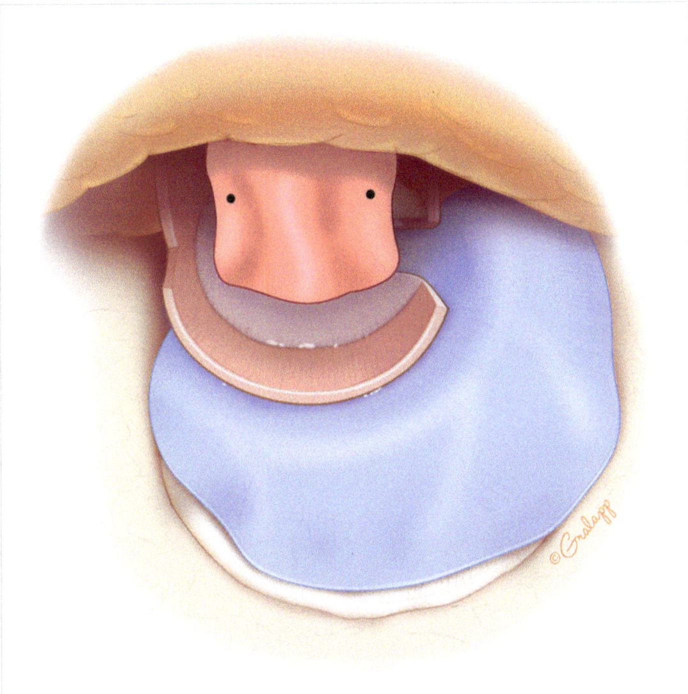

Fig. 7.89 The lateral ear canal skin (Koerner's flap) is then placed back into position and secured posteriorly using two absorbable sutures (indicated by black dots).

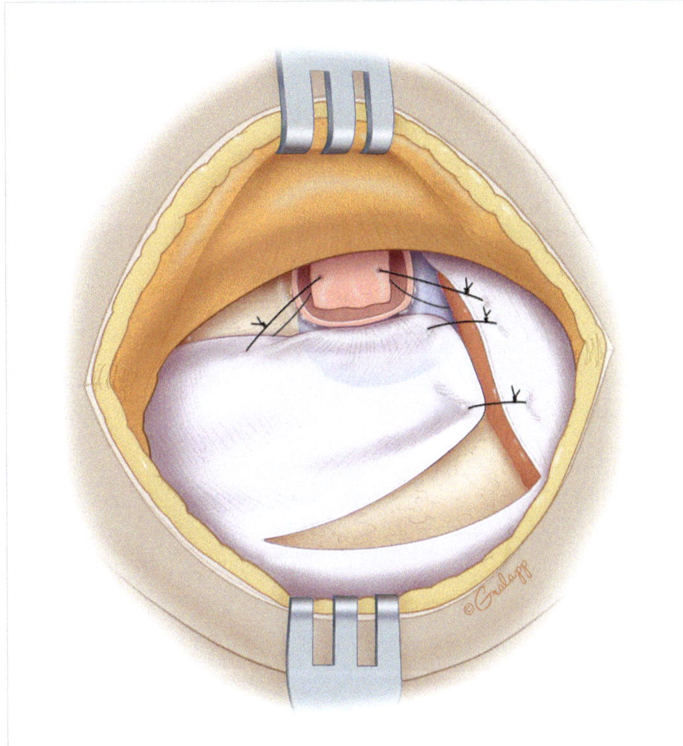

Fig. 7.90 The periosteal flap is reapproximated while advancing anteriorly to cover any bone dust that remains exposed along the lateral aspect of the mastoid.

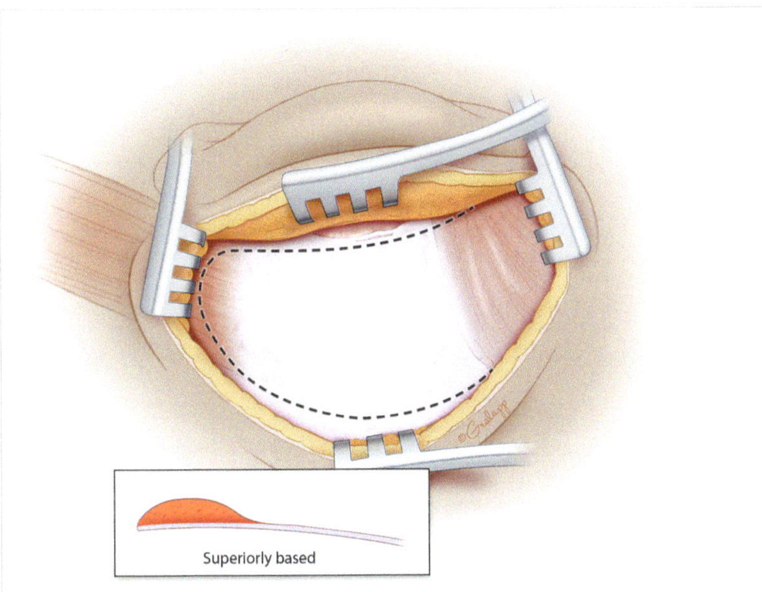

Fig. 7.91 Superiorly based mastoid obliteration flap may be created with only periosteum and fascia only or may incorporate muscle.

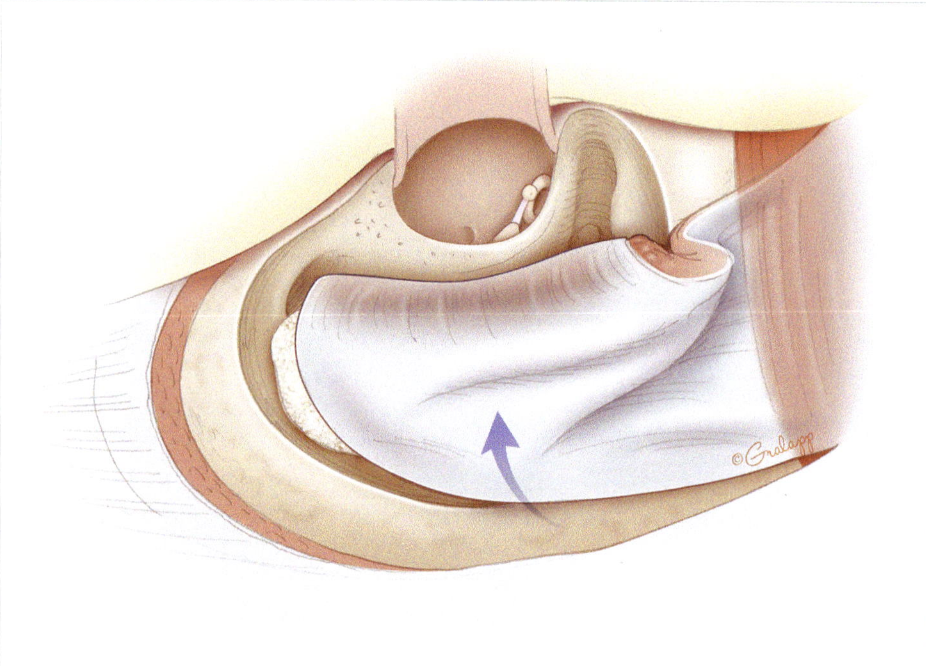

Fig. 7.92 Superiorly based mastoid obliteration flap in place covering underlying bone paté.

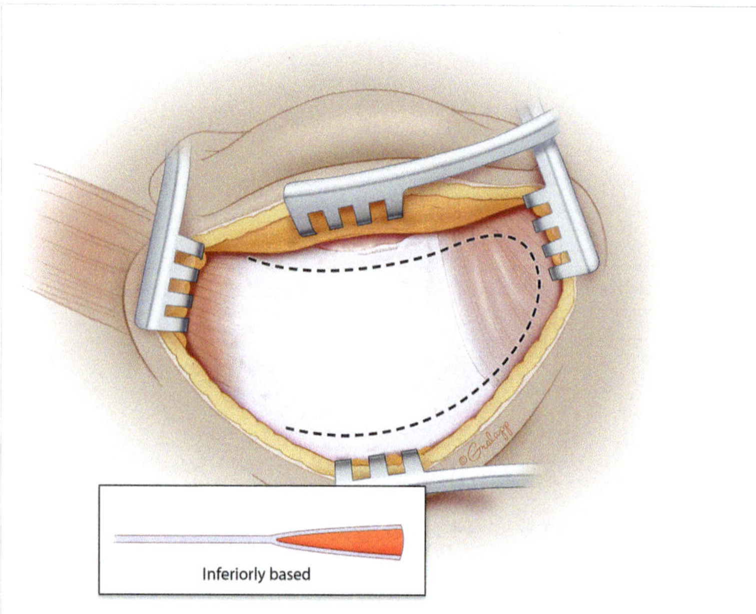

Fig. 7.93 Inferiorly based mastoid obliteration flap may be created with only periosteum and fascia only or may incorporate muscle.

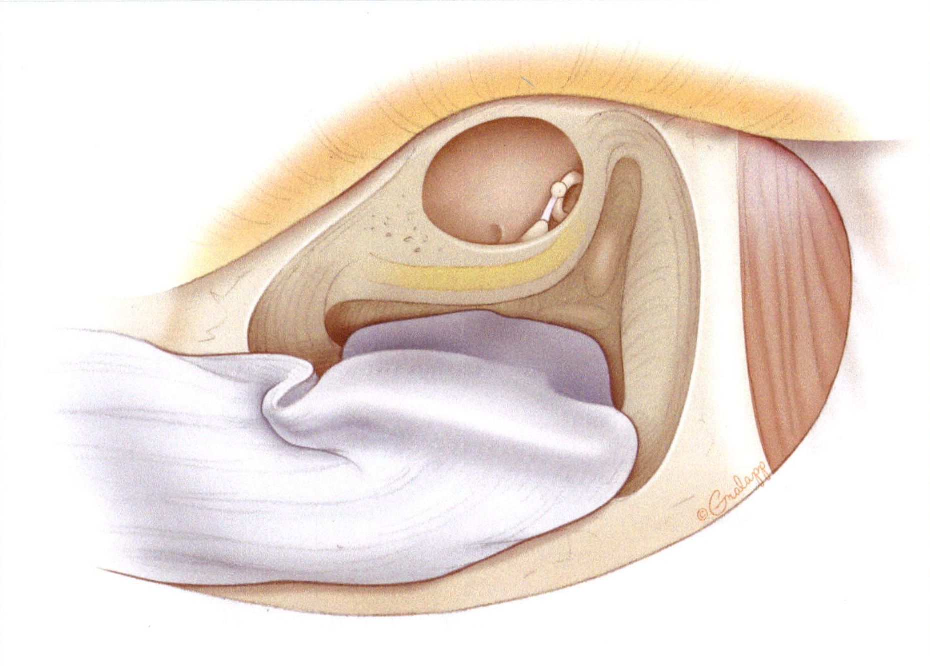

Fig. 7.94 Inferiorly based mastoid obliteration flap with only periosteum.

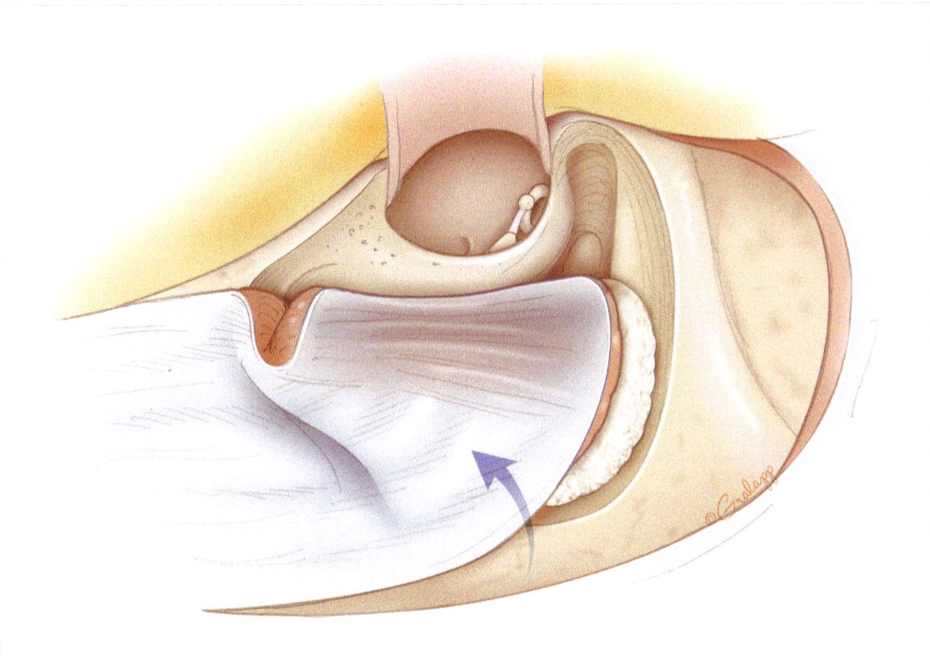

Fig. 7.95 Inferiorly based mastoid obliteration flap with both periosteum and muscle covering bone paté.

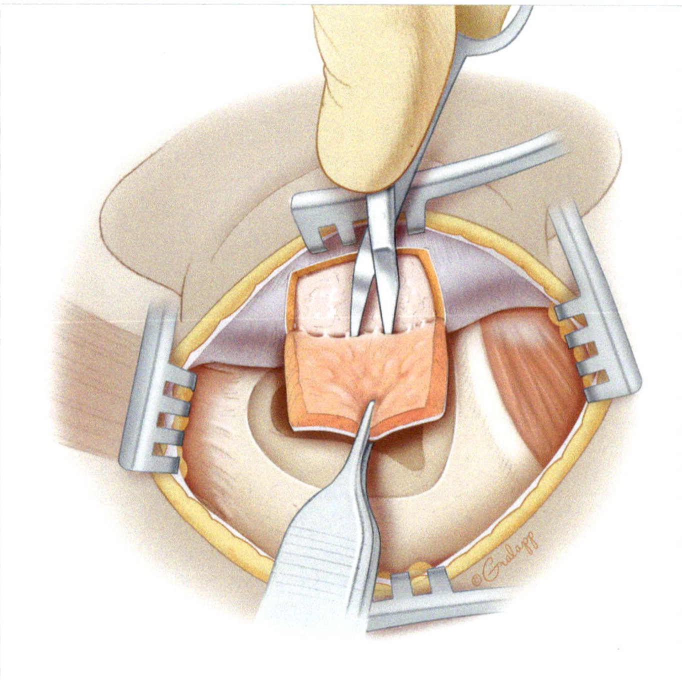

Fig. 7.96 Creation of a meatally based mastoid obliteration flap (also known as a Palva flap).

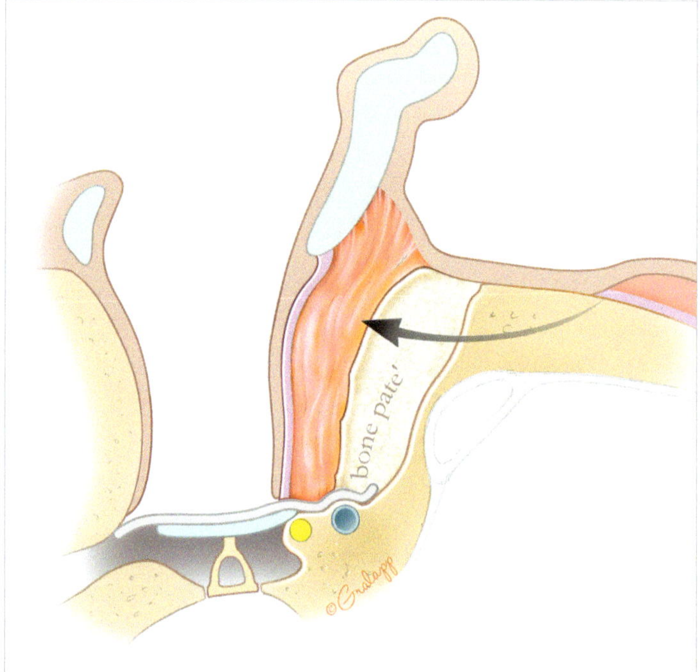

Fig. 7.97 Rotation of a meatally based mastoid obliteration flap covering bone paté to fill the defect.

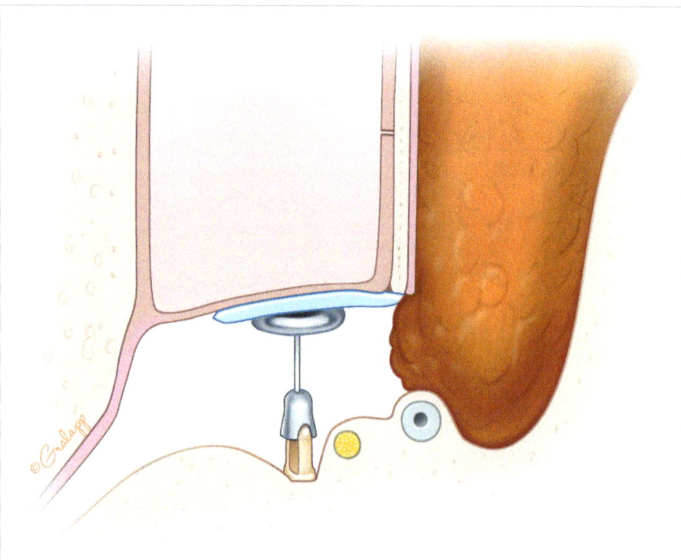

Fig. 7.98 Schematic of a mastoid obliteration flap following intact canal wall mastoidectomy.

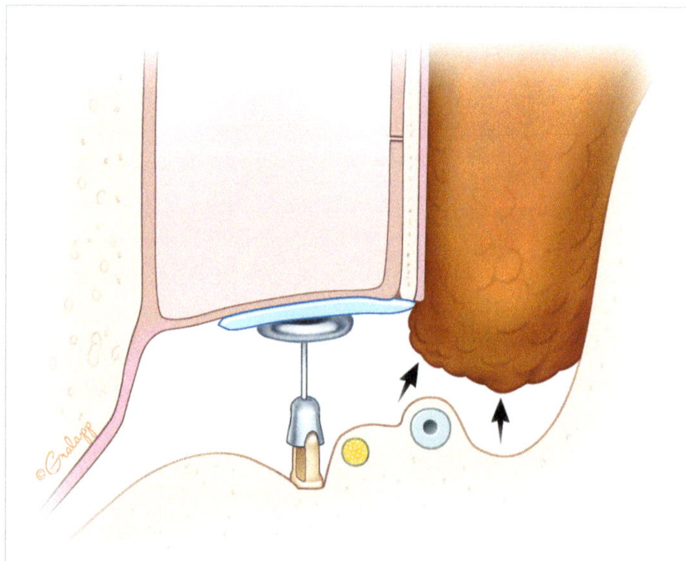

Fig. 7.99 Mastoid obliteration flap retraction.

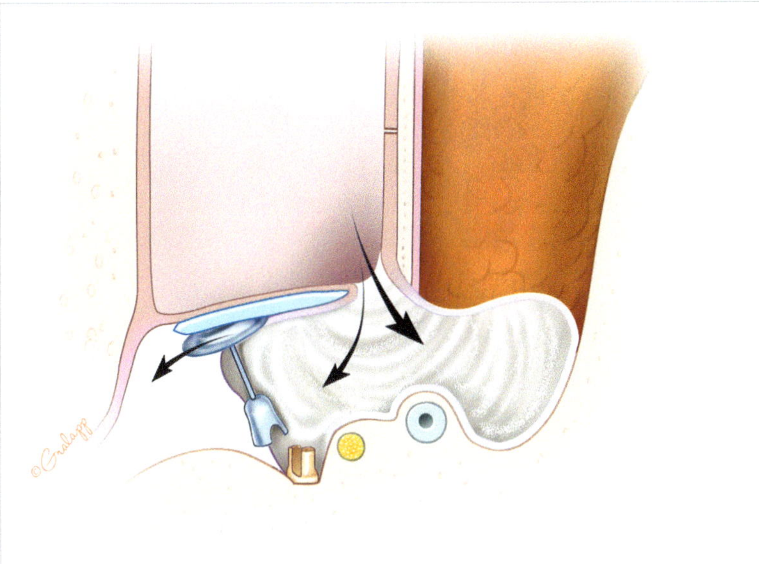

Fig. 7.100 Mastoid obliteration flap retraction with recurrent cholesteatoma. Because of the risk of recurrent cholesteatoma, most surgeons use obliteration techniques only in cases of canal wall down mastoidectomy.

8 Cholesteatoma

Robert K. Jackler

8.1 Introduction to Cholesteatoma

Primary acquired cholesteatoma is an invagination of the tympanic membrane, of variable aggressiveness, with accumulation of desquamated keratin and a notable tendency to destroy bone. It is controversial whether cholesteatoma progression is driven by proliferative activity of the squamous layer or mucosal factors drawing the pouch from its medial aspect. Cholesteatoma has a strong association with mastoid hypopneumatization, is frequently associated with purulent discharge, and has a tendency to be bilateral.

While small cholesteatomas may be managed medically with periodic cleaning, especially in cooperative adults, most cholesteatomas ultimately come to surgery. There are two fundamental strategies in dealing with cholesteatoma: resection and exteriorization. Resection usually involves an intact canal wall tympanomastoidectomy with tympanic membrane repair with reinforcement using cartilage. Exteriorization in small and relatively indolent cases may be achieved via conservative atticotomy. Exteriorization of more advanced cholesteatoma involves canal wall down tympanomastoidectomy with creation of a cavity necessitating ongoing care facilitated by creation of a meatoplasty calibrated to the size of the mastoid bowl. Some advocate a retrograde approach removing only that portion of the mastoid overlying the cholesteatoma as an alternative to thorough removal of mastoid cellularity. Severe hypopneumatization tends to favor the exteriorization approach as the resulting cavity is small. By contrast, cholesteatoma invading a highly pneumatic mastoid is usually managed initially with an intact canal wall procedure. Radical mastoidectomy, removal of all middle ear contents and exteriorization of the tympanum, is not depicted in this atlas because it is largely a historical procedure. In contemporary practice, an effort is made to avoid exteriorization of tympanic mucosa, which can become a source of chronic discharge, by reconstruction of the tympanic membrane.

Unfortunately, cholesteatoma is frequently recidivistic. Recurrence refers to repeat invagination of the tympanic membrane, often via a narrow slit adjacent to the cartilage placed at the initial surgery. Recurrence is not rare following an intact canal wall procedure, especially when the disease is bilateral. The status of the opposite ear is an important determinant in the choice of exteriorization versus resection. The second mechanism is regrowth of residual cholesteatoma matrix left behind, most often in an inaccessible recess of the middle ear, at the initial stage. When cholesteatoma is situated in difficult-to-visualize area (e.g., sinus tympani, oval window, under the facial nerve, or in perilabyrinthine cells), staging is indicated. At second inspection, approximately 6 months later, inconspicuous microscopic fragments become identifiable as small white pearls which can often to be completely excised with confidence.

Congenital cholesteatoma most often originates from an ectopic squamous nest on the promontory. If detected in the first few years of life, it remains confined to the protympanum and can readily be removed *in toto*. If discovered in older childhood, it comes to involve the ossicular chain and anterior epitympanic space and requires more extensive surgery often including a staged procedure for excision validation and ossiculoplasty.

Further Reading

1. Britze A, Møller ML, Ovesen T. Incidence, 10-year recidivism rate and prognostic factors for cholesteatoma. J Laryngol Otol 2017;131(4):319–328 PubMed
2. Calli C, Pinar E, Oncel S, Tatar B, Tuncbilek MA. Measurements of the facial recess anatomy: implications for sparing the facial nerve and chorda tympani during posterior tympanotomy. Ear Nose Throat J 2010;89(10):490–494 PubMed
3. Castle JT. Cholesteatoma pearls: practical points and update. Head Neck Pathol 2018;12(3):419–429 PubMed
4. Dornhoffer JL. Retrograde mastoidectomy. Otolaryngol Clin North Am 2006;39(6):1115–1127 PubMed
5. Jackler RK, Santa Maria PL, Varsak YK, Nguyen A, Blevins NH. A new theory on the pathogenesis of acquired cholesteatoma: mucosal traction. Laryngoscope 2015;125(Suppl 4): S1–S14 PubMed
6. Jackler RK. The surgical anatomy of cholesteatoma. Otolaryngol Clin North Am 1989;22(5):883–896 PubMed
7. Kerckhoffs KG, Kommer MB, van Strien TH, et al. The disease recurrence rate after the canal wall up or canal wall down technique in adults. Laryngoscope 2016;126(4):980–987 PubMed
8. Kuo CL, Liao WH, Shiao AS. A review of current progress in acquired cholesteatoma management. Eur Arch Otorhinolaryngol 2015;272(12):3601–3609 PubMed
9. Lim J, Gangal A, Gluth MB. Surgery for cholesteatomatous labyrinthine fistula. Ann Otol Rhinol Laryngol 2017;126 (3):205–215 PubMed
10. Magliulo G, Iannella G. Endoscopic versus microscopic approach in attic cholesteatoma surgery. Am J Otolaryngol 2018;39(1):25–30 PubMed
11. Mostafa BE, El Fiky L. Congenital cholesteatoma: the silent pathology. ORL J Otorhinolaryngol Relat Spec 2018;80 (2):108–116 PubMed
12. Soldati D, Mudry A. Knowledge about cholesteatoma, from the first description to the modern histopathology. Otol Neurotol 2001;22(6):723–730 PubMed
13. Westerberg J, Mäki-Torkko E, Harder H. Cholesteatoma surgery with the canal wall up technique combined with mastoid obliteration: results from primary surgery in 230 consecutive cases. Acta Otolaryngol 2018;138(5):452–457 PubMed

8.2 Growth Patterns of Cholesteatoma

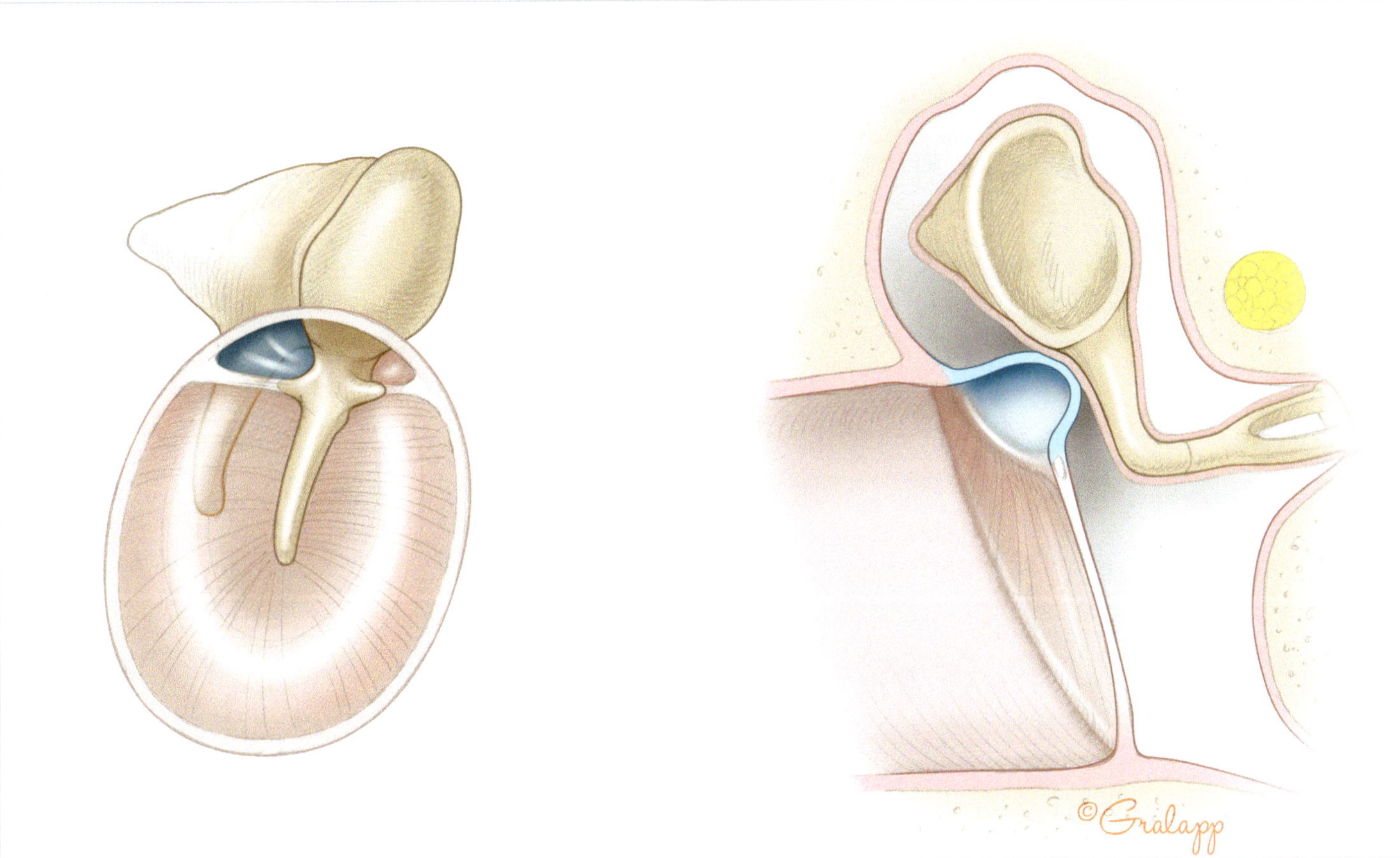

Fig. 8.1 Acquired cholesteatoma begins as a retraction pocket in the tympanic membrane, most often in the pars flaccida.

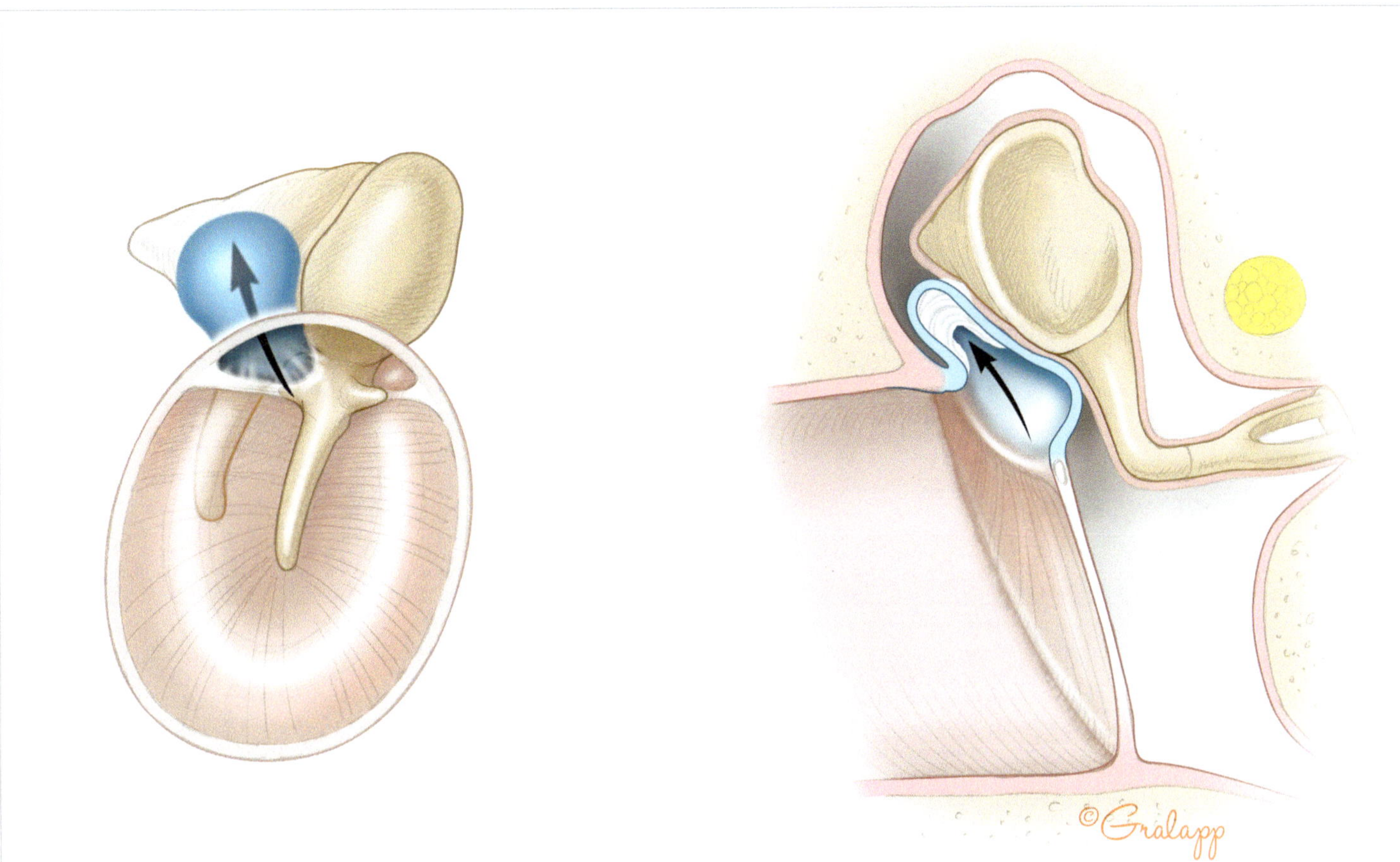

Fig. 8.2 Cholesteatoma draws into the epitympanum along the incus body and malleus head and begins to accumulate keratin.

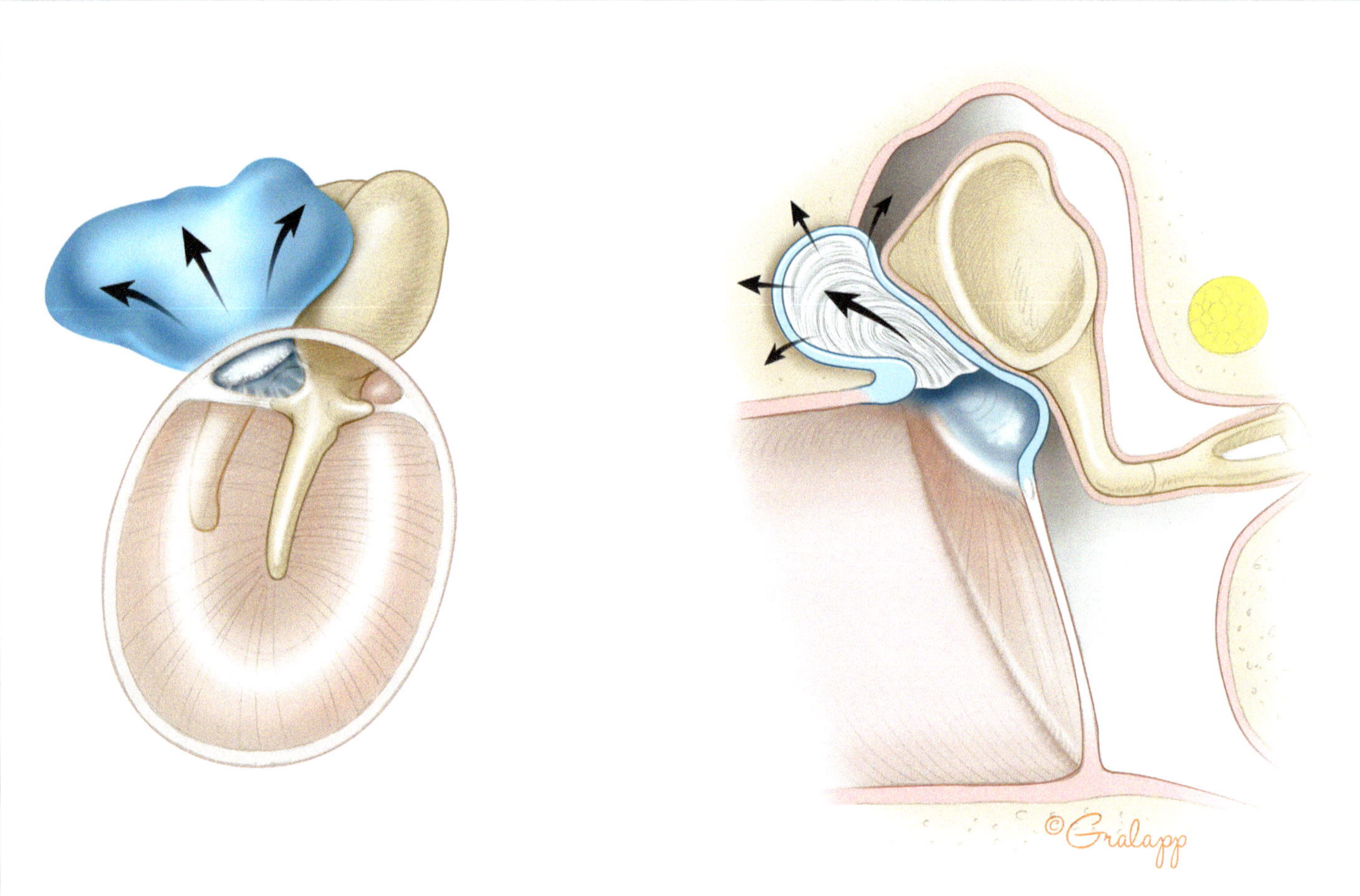

Fig. 8.3 With further growth, the cholesteatoma continues to accumulate keratin as it expands toward the aditus-ad-antrum.

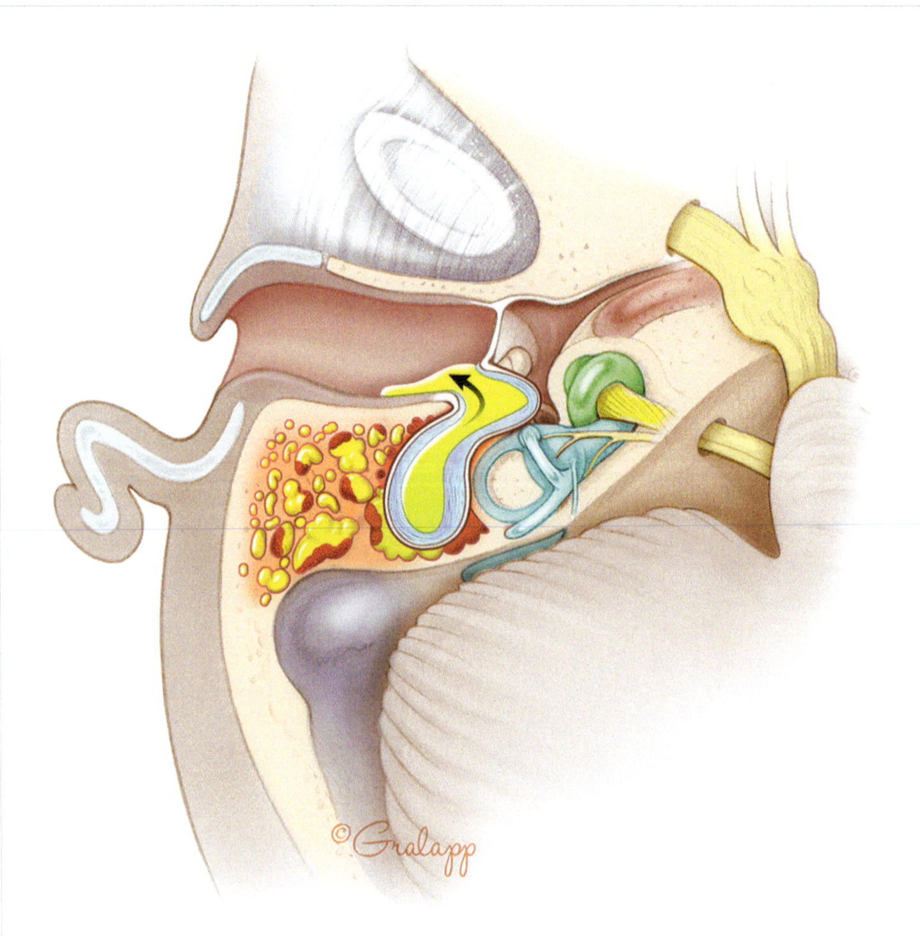

Fig. 8.4 Infected cholesteatoma penetrating the mastoid via the aditus-ad-antrum. The excluded air cells contain purulence and granulation tissue.

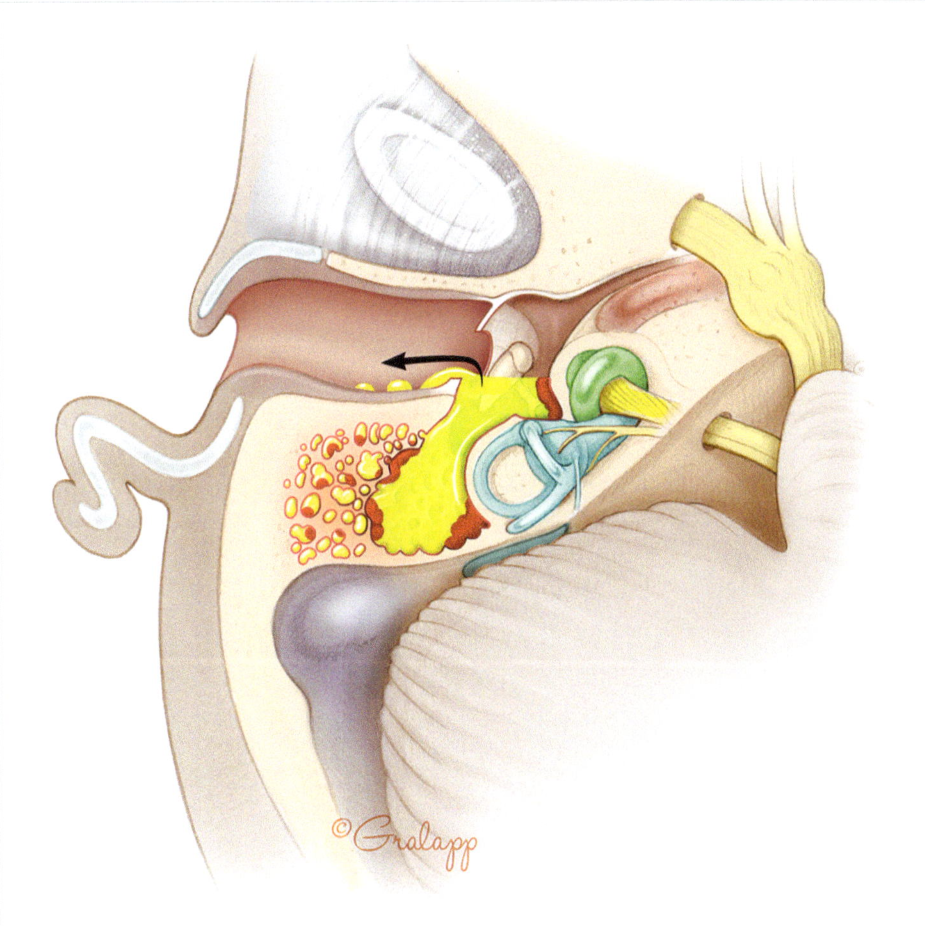

Fig. 8.5 Chronic otitis media without cholesteatoma.

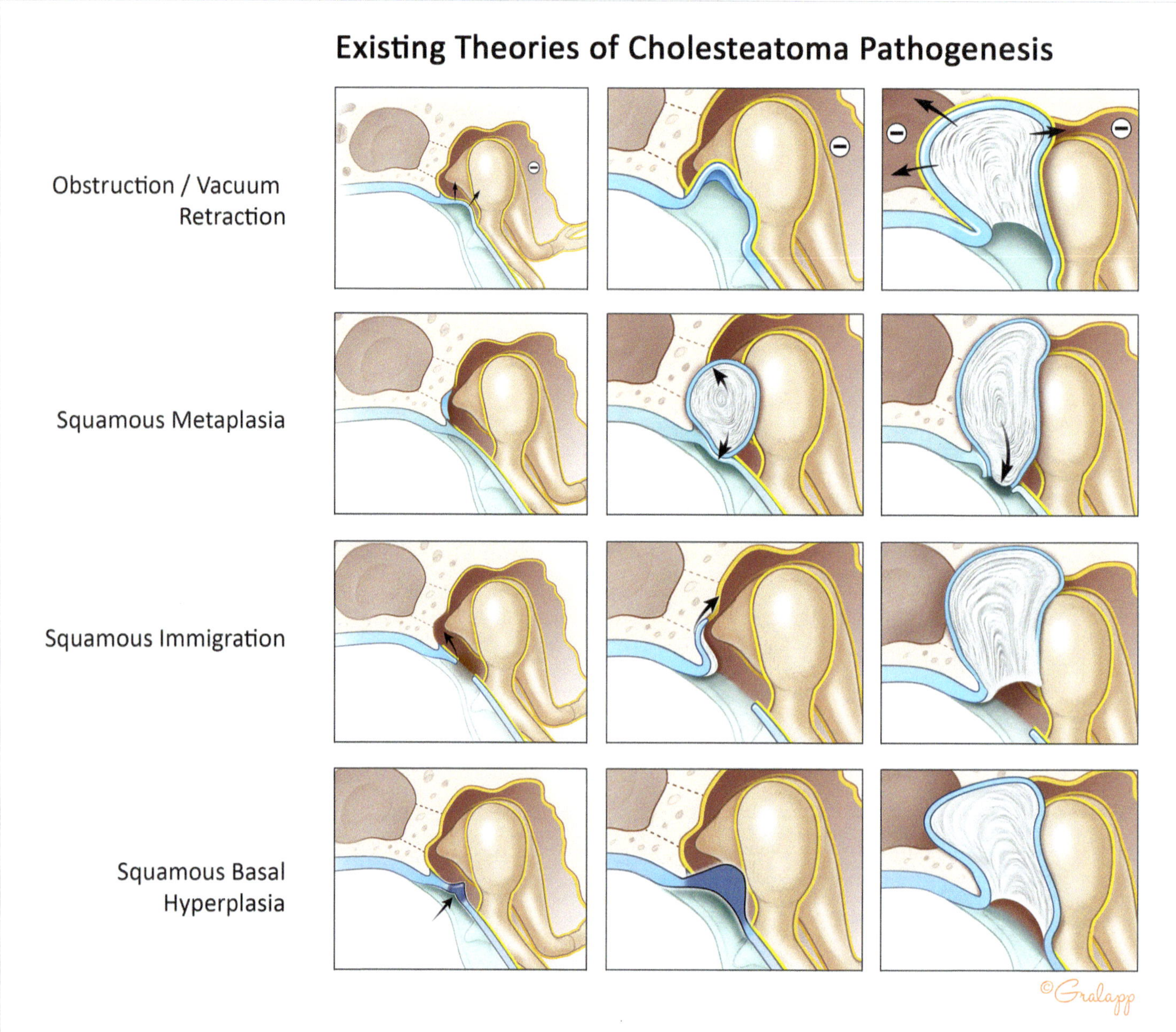

Fig. 8.6 Existing theories of cholesteatoma formation. (Used with permission from Jackler RK, Santa Maria PL, Varav KY, Gguyen A, Blevins NB. A new theory on the pathogenesis of acquired cholesteatoma: mucosal traction. *Laryngoscope* 2015;125(Suppl 4):S1–S14.)

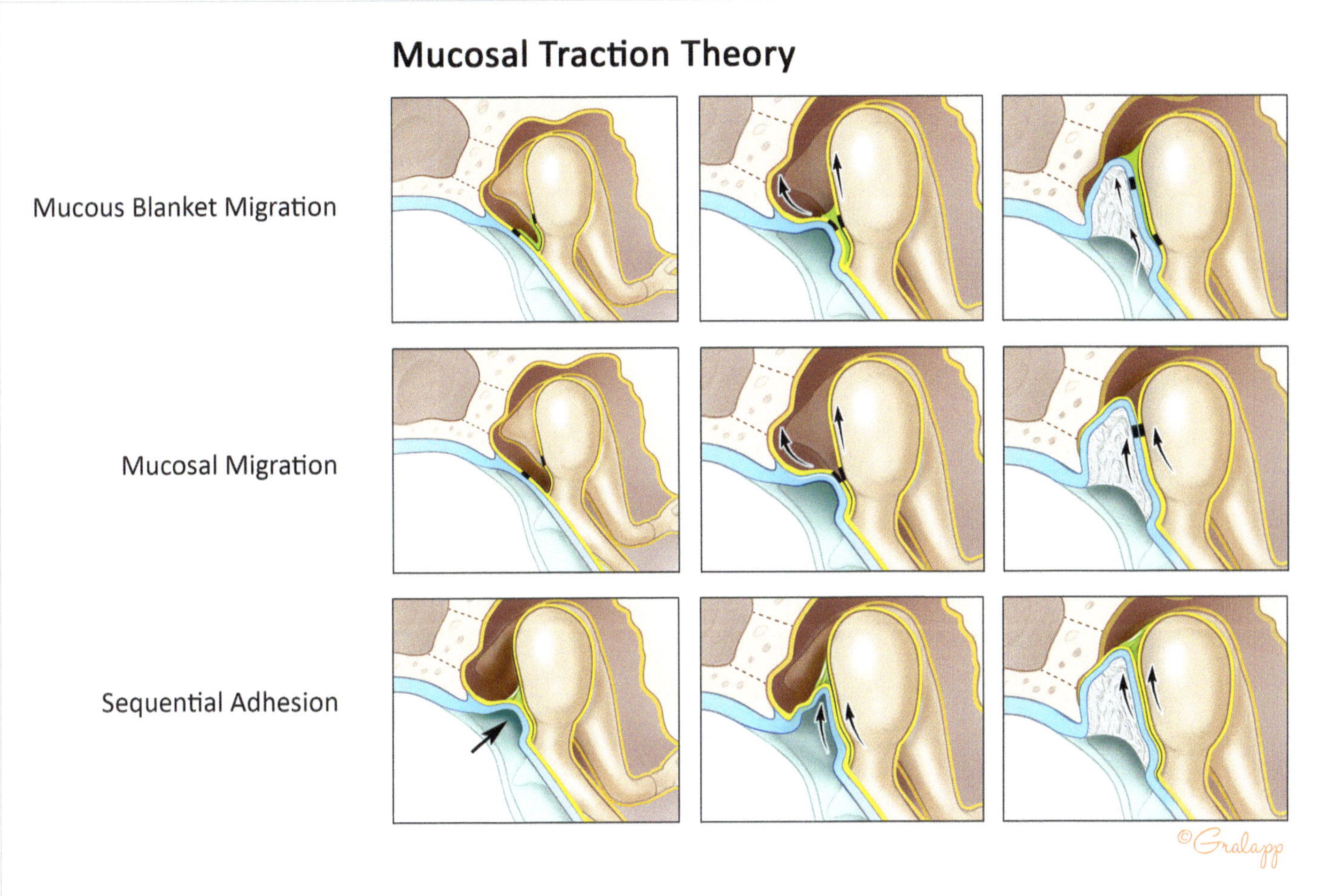

Fig. 8.7 Mucosal traction theory of cholesteatoma formation. (Used with permission from Jackler RK, Santa Maria PL, Varav KY, Gguyen A, Blevins NB. A new theory on the pathogenesis of acquired cholesteatoma: mucosal traction. *Laryngoscope* 2015;125(Suppl 4):S1–S14.)

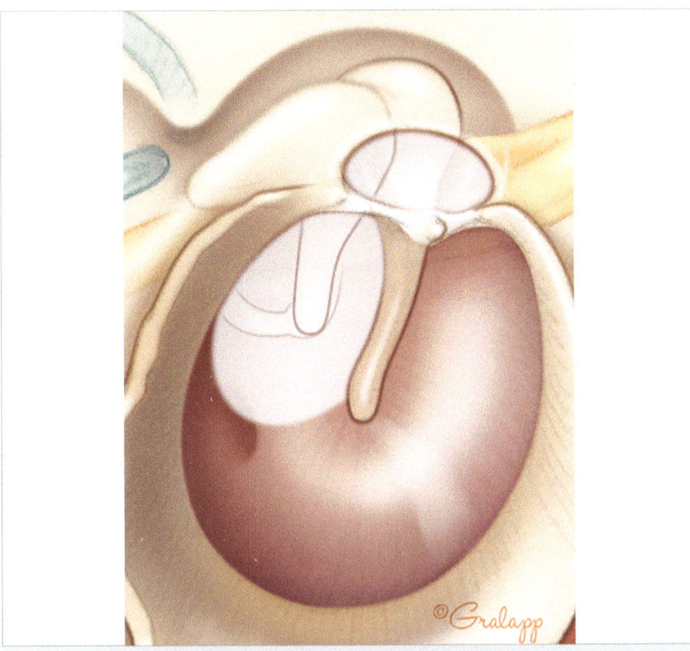

Fig. 8.8 Primary acquired cholesteatoma arises from the epitympanum, posterior mesotympanum, or both, but almost never from the anterior or inferior aspects of the tympanic membrane. This means that primary acquired cholesteatomas almost universally are intimately involved with the ossicles.

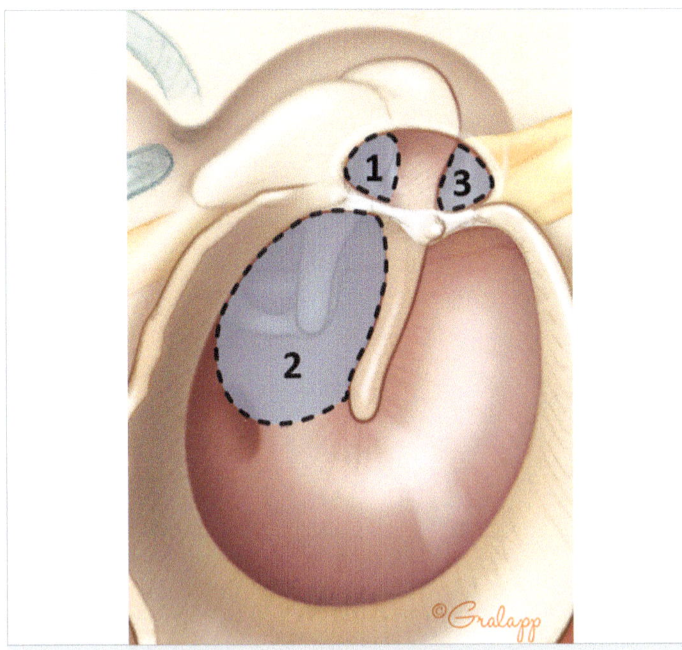

Fig. 8.9 The origin of cholesteatoma is from the posterior epitympanum (1) most commonly, followed by posterior mesotympanum (2), and then anterior epitympanum (3). Sometimes pockets occur in combinations such as posterior epitympanic with posterior mesotympanic or both posterior and anterior epitympanic together.

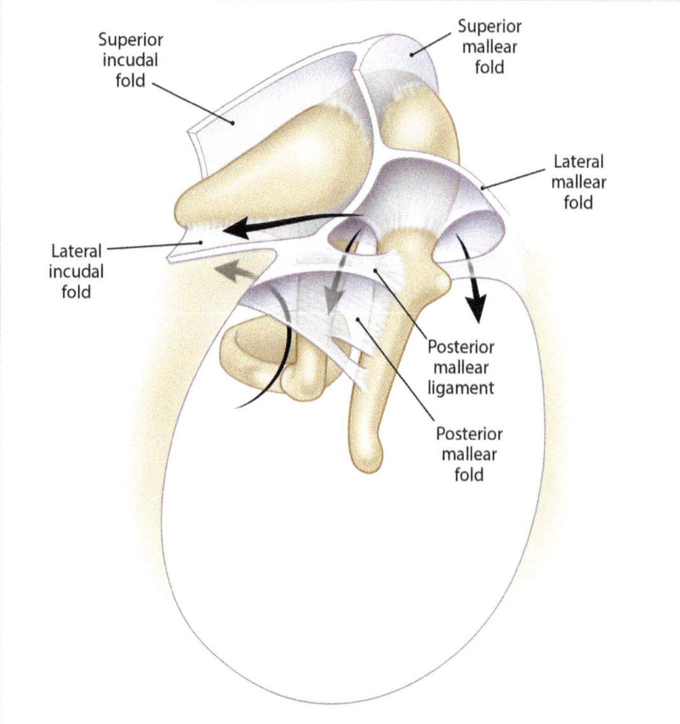

Fig. 8.10 Cholesteatomas invade the middle ear and mastoid along fairly predictable pathways. Their growth is constrained by ligaments and mesenteries which are embryological remnants of the first branchial arch pouches which form the tympanic cavity. (Used with permission from Jackler RK. The surgical anatomy of cholesteatoma. *Otolaryngol Clin NA* 1989;22:883–896.)

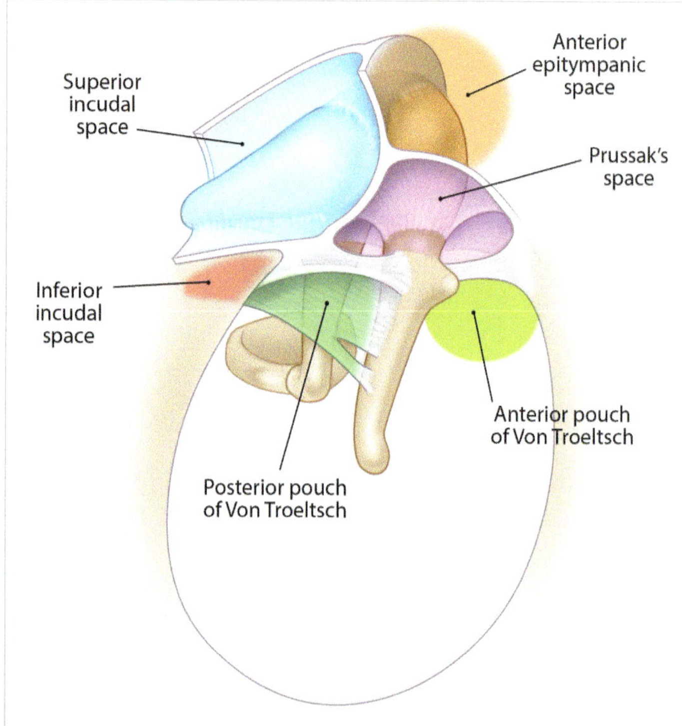

Fig. 8.11 Cholesteatoma growth tends to follow spaces defined by ligaments and mesenteries which compartmentalize the middle ear. (Used with permission from Jackler RK. The surgical anatomy of cholesteatoma. *Otolaryngol Clin NA* 1989;22:883–896.)

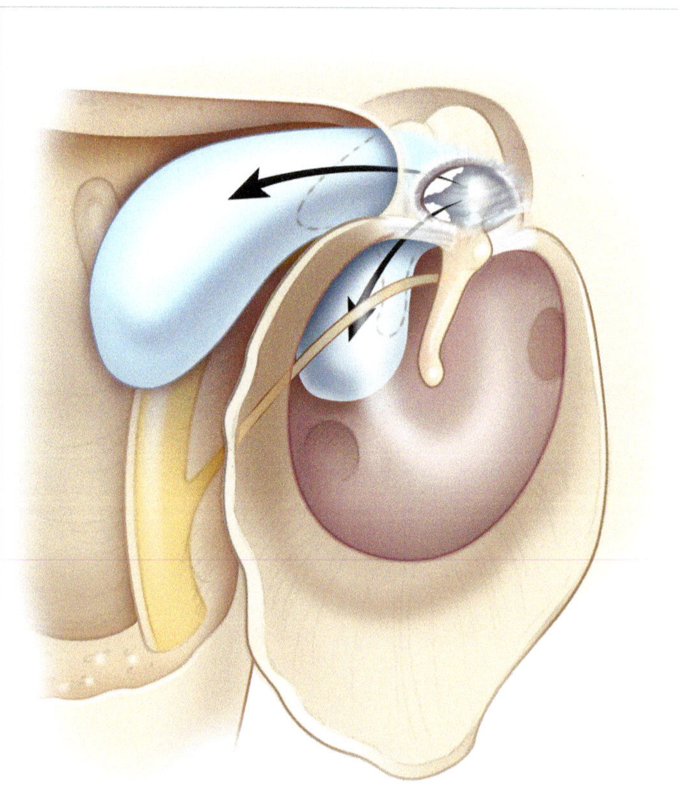

Fig. 8.12 Posterior epitympanic cholesteatoma penetrates the epitympanum and posterior mesotympanum lateral to the ossicles. (Used with permission from Jackler RK. The surgical anatomy of cholesteatoma. *Otolaryngol Clin NA* 1989;22:883–896)

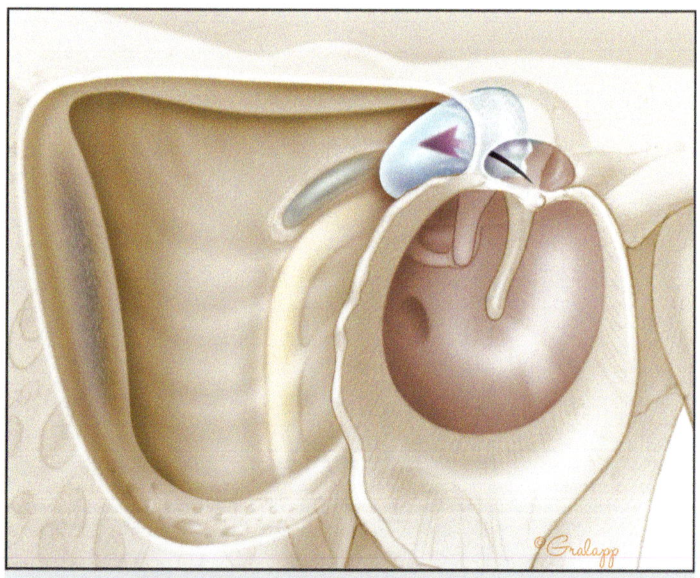

Fig. 8.13 Posterior epitympanic cholesteatoma penetrating the aditus-ad-antrum.

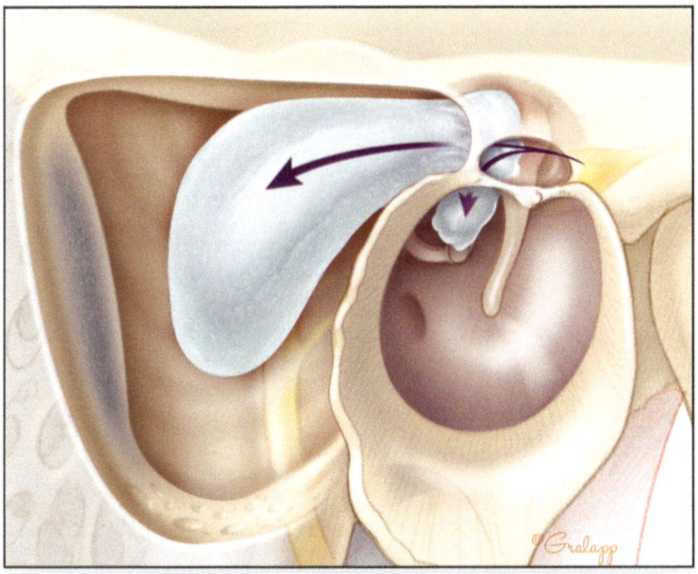

Fig. 8.14 Posterior epitympanic cholesteatoma involving the mastoid which penetrated the epitympanum and posterior mesotympanum lateral to the ossicles.

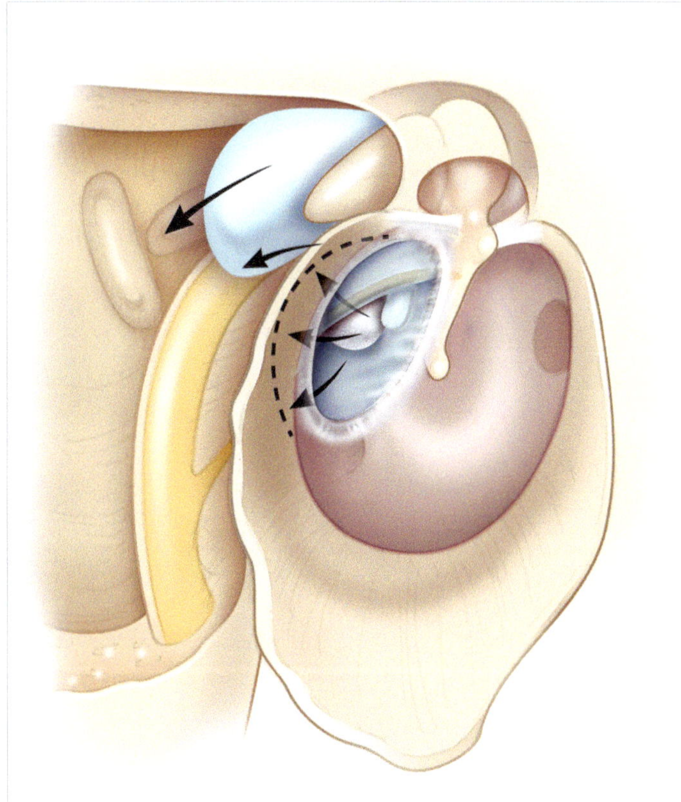

Fig. 8.15 Posterior mesotympanic cholesteatoma illustrating the pathways to the mastoid and middle ear. Note that the penetration to the mastoid is medial to the ossicles. Posterior mesotympanic cholesteatoma tends to involve the posterior tympanic spaces: the sinus tympani and facial recess (see section 8.8 Sinus Tympani and Facial Recess in Cholesteatoma). (Used with permission from Jackler RK. The surgical anatomy of cholesteatoma. *Otolaryngol Clin NA* 1989;22:883–896.)

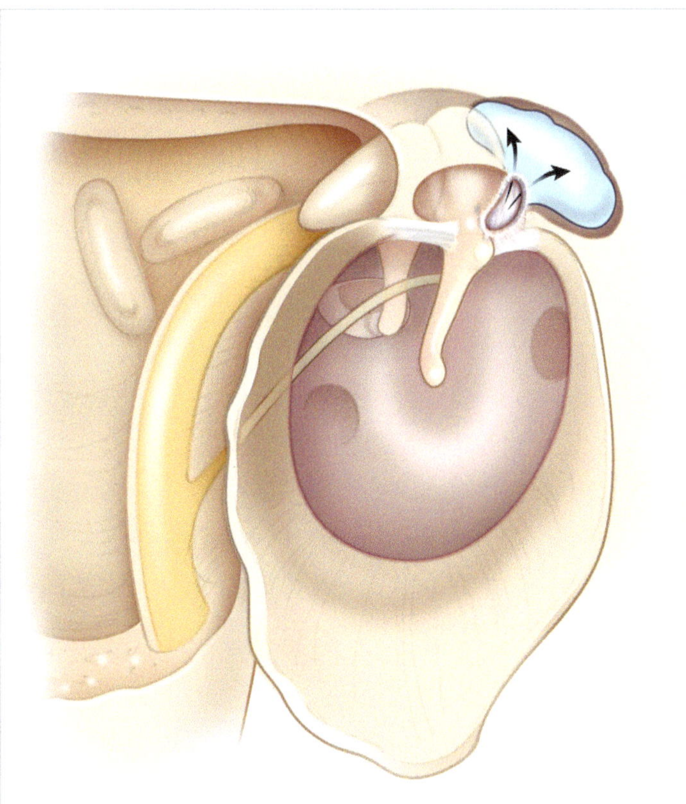

Fig. 8.16 Anterior epitympanic cholesteatoma penetrates the supratubal recess and can involve the geniculate ganglion of the facial nerve (see section 8.9 Anterior Epitympanic Cholesteatoma). (Used with permission from Jackler RK. The surgical anatomy of cholesteatoma. *Otolaryngol Clin NA* 1989;22:883–896.)

8.3 Canal Wall Down Mastoidectomy

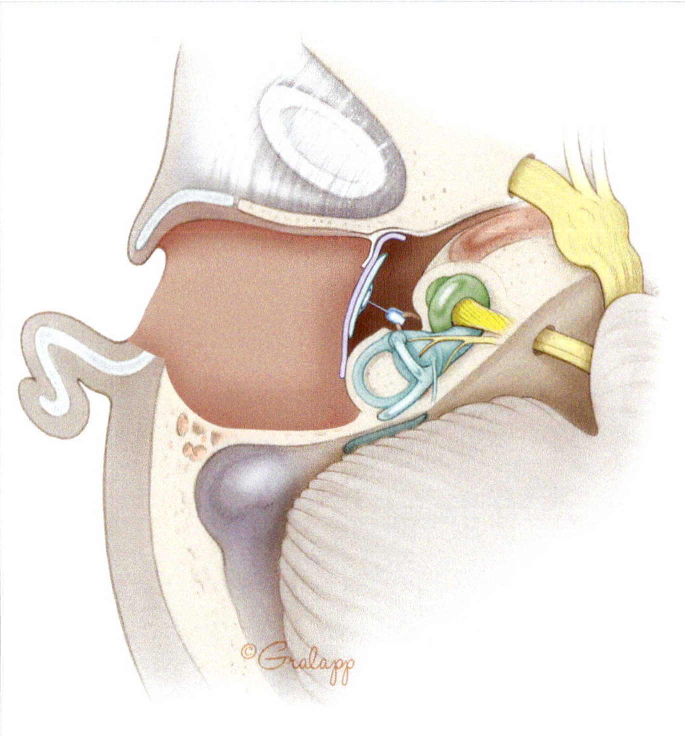

Fig. 8.17 Canal wall down tympanomastoidectomy cavity with fascia tympanoplasty, cartilage graft, and partial ossicular replacement prosthesis.

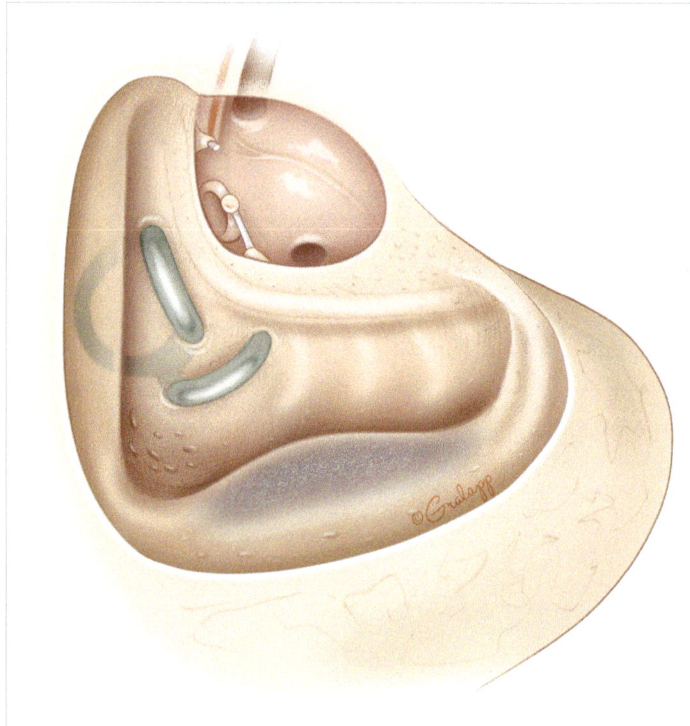

Fig. 8.18 Completed canal wall down mastoidectomy before middle ear reconstruction.

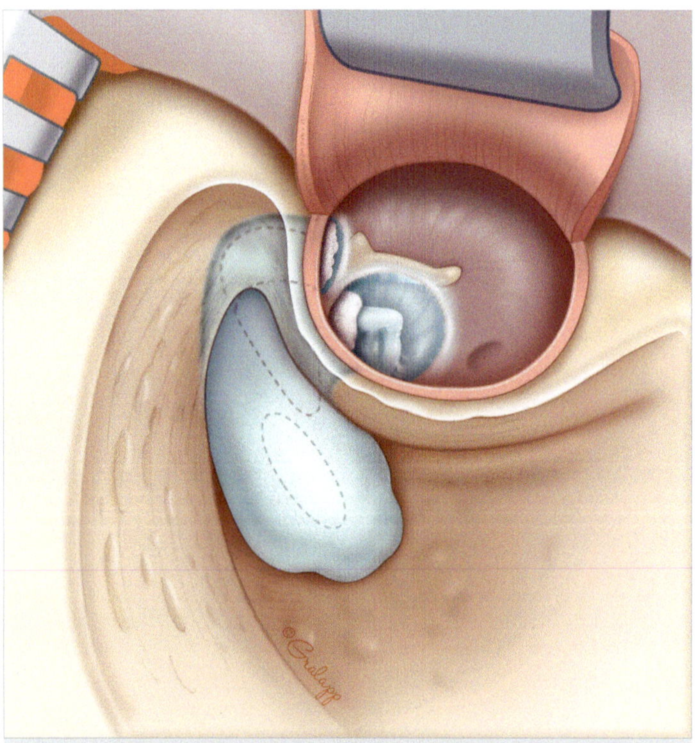

Fig. 8.19 Epitympanic cholesteatoma with involvement of the mastoid.

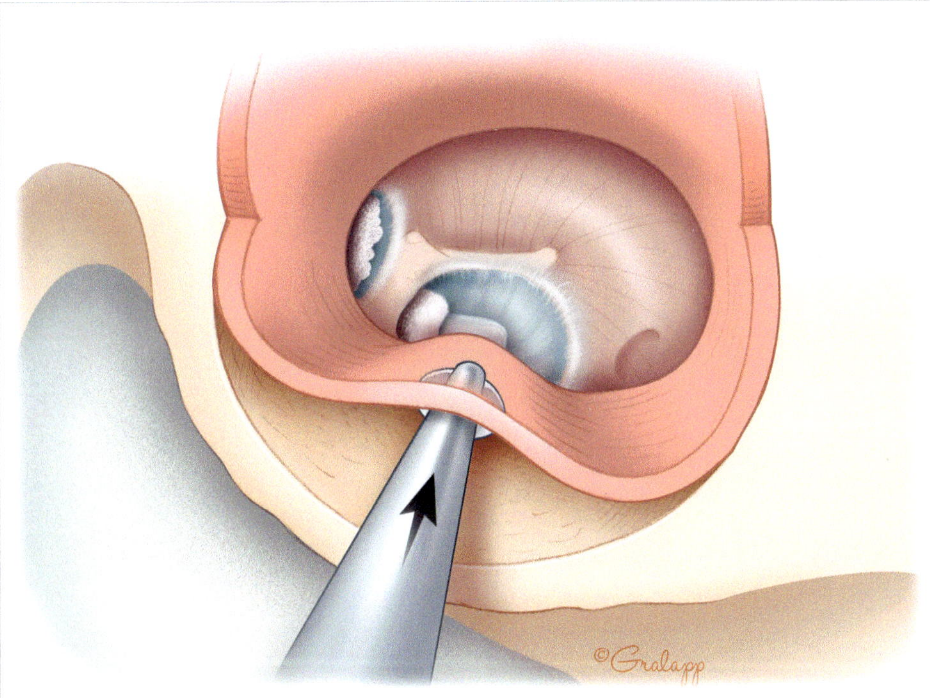

Fig. 8.20 Raising tympanomeatal flap.

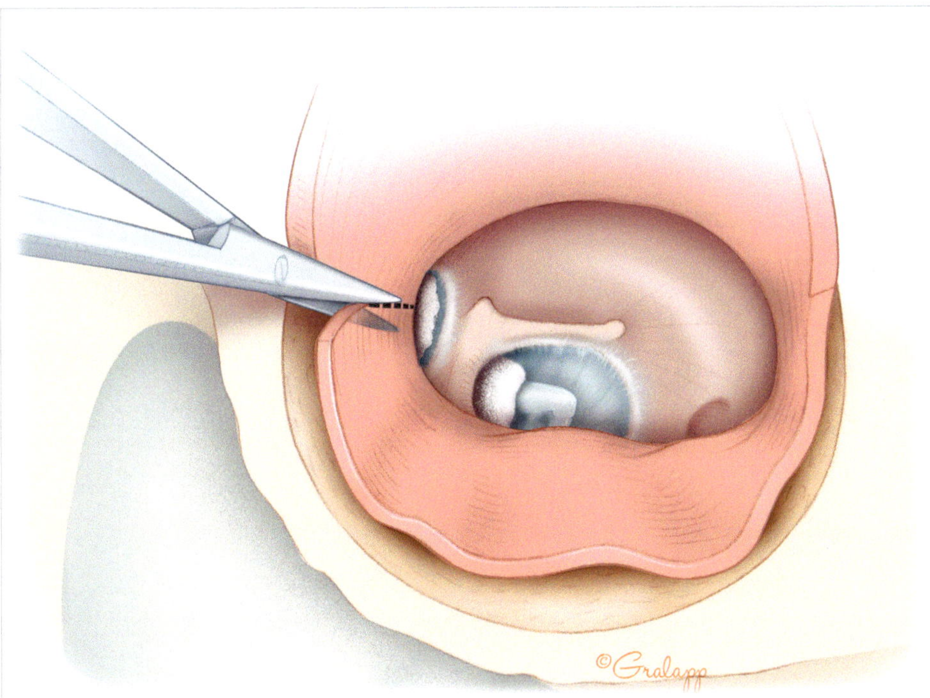

Fig. 8.21 Incision is placed superiorly and carried into the cholesteatoma pocket. No inferior incision is made.

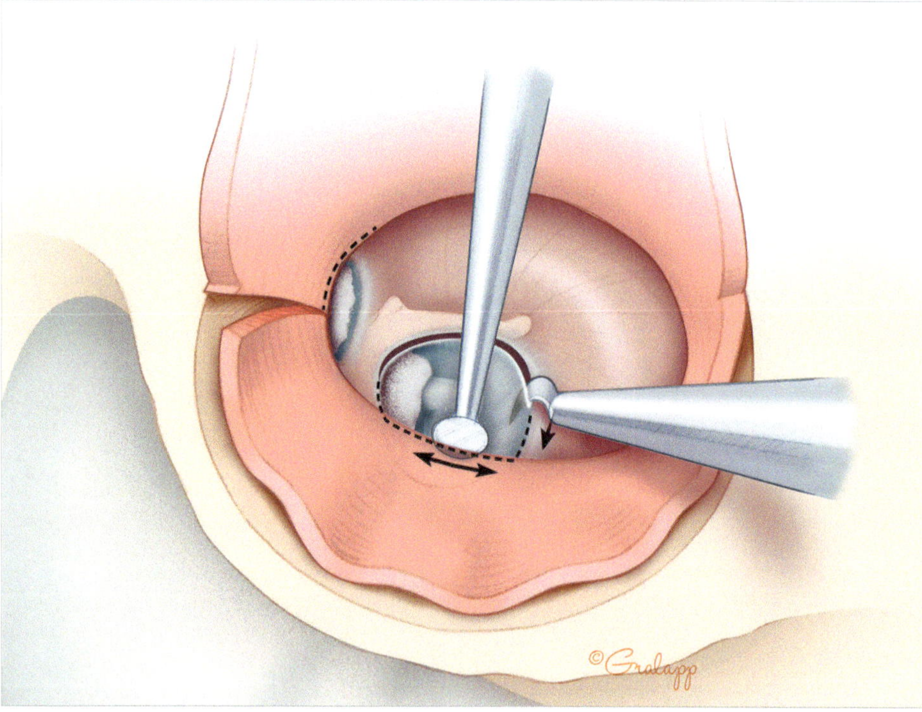

Fig. 8.22 Incising the margin of the cholesteatoma sac.

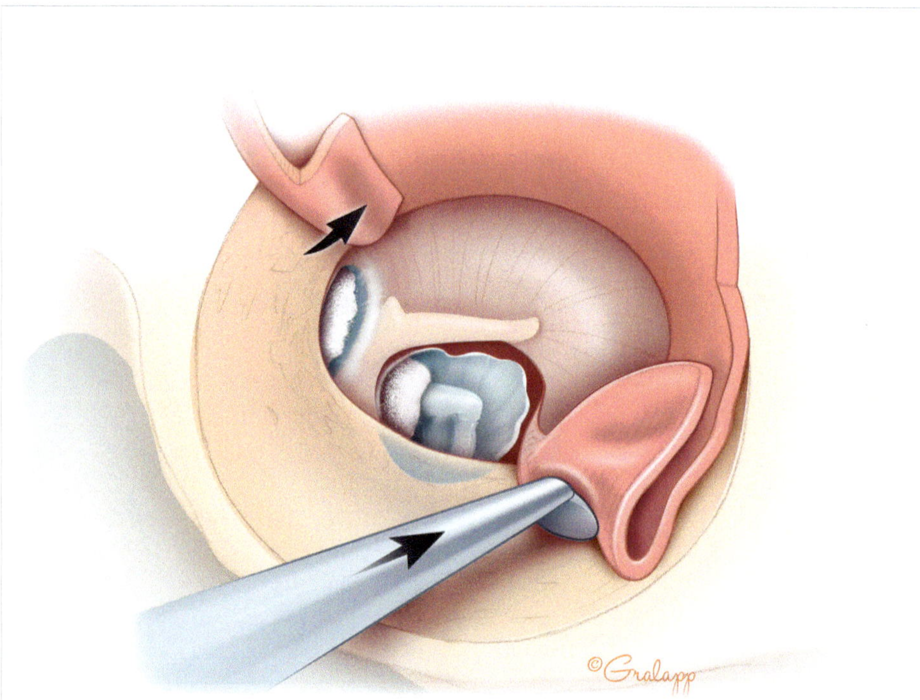

Fig. 8.23 Raising the inferiorly based tympanomeatal flap.

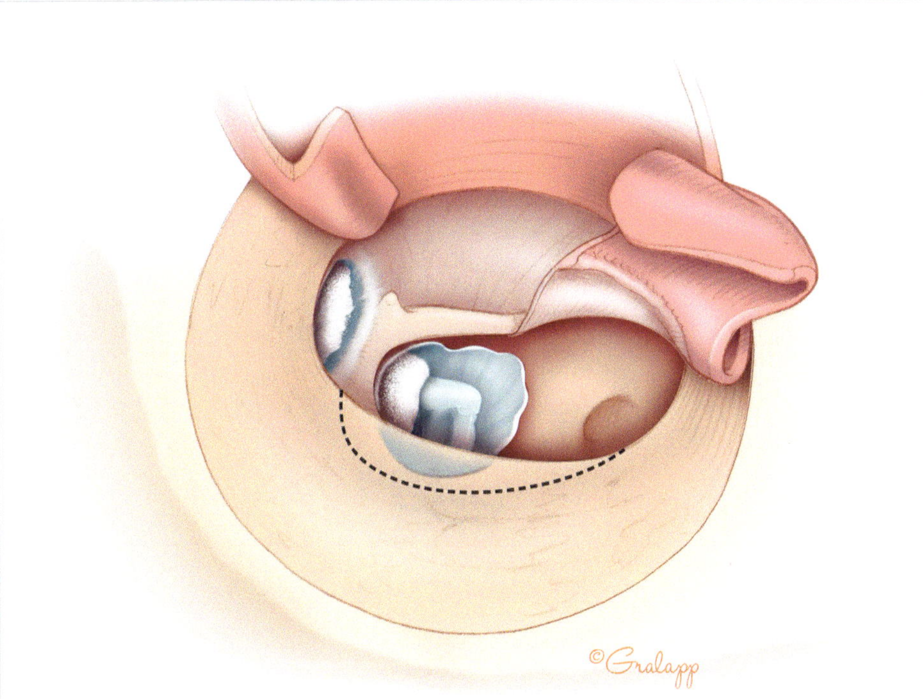

Fig. 8.24 Scutum removal to expose the oval window region. This is done early to determine whether or not the ossicular chain is intact.

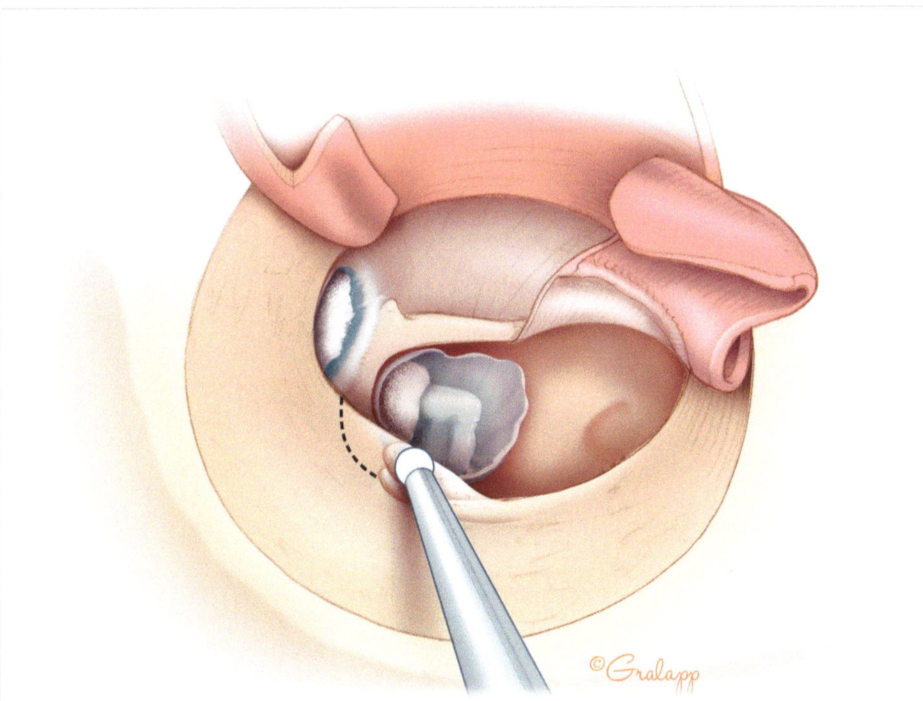

Fig. 8.25 Removal of the scutum (posterior superior ear canal).

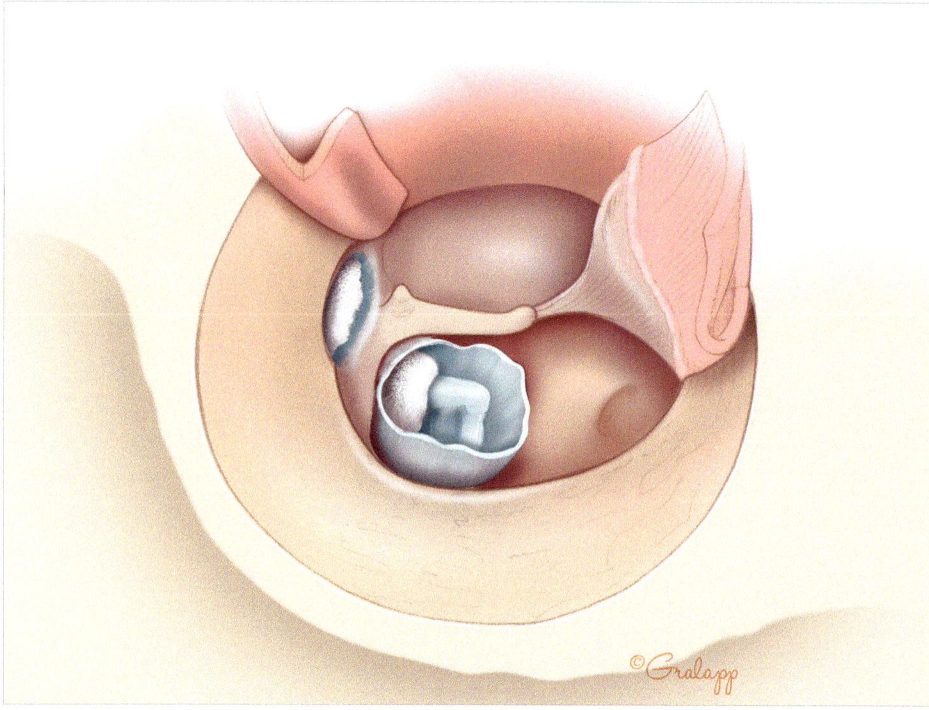

Fig. 8.26 Completed exposure of the incus and stapes which are intact in this drawing, but are often eroded.

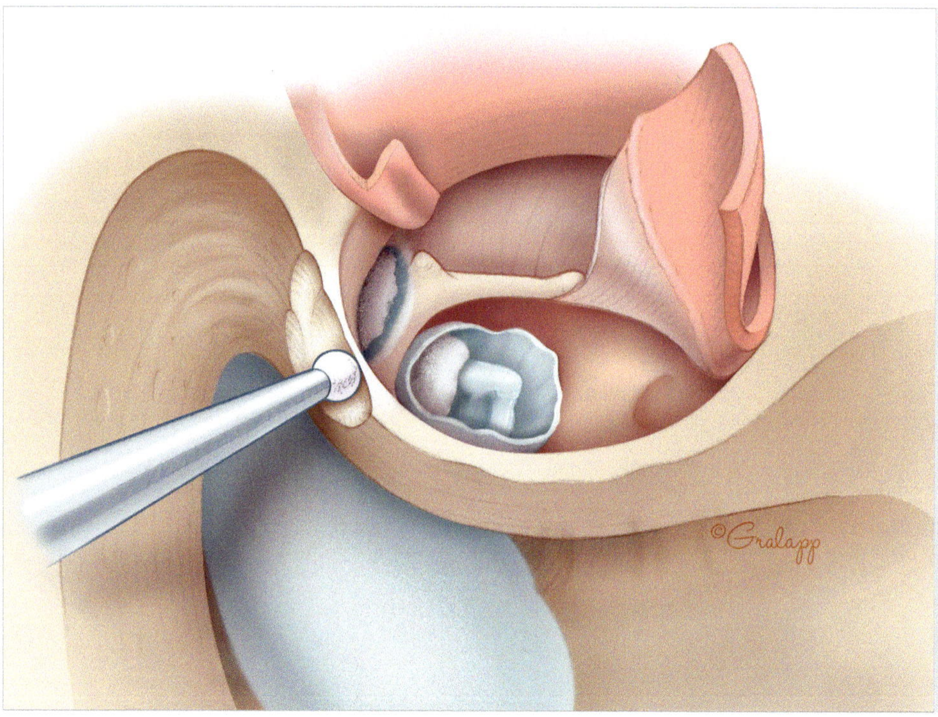

Fig. 8.27 Beginning removal of the posterior ear canal wall.

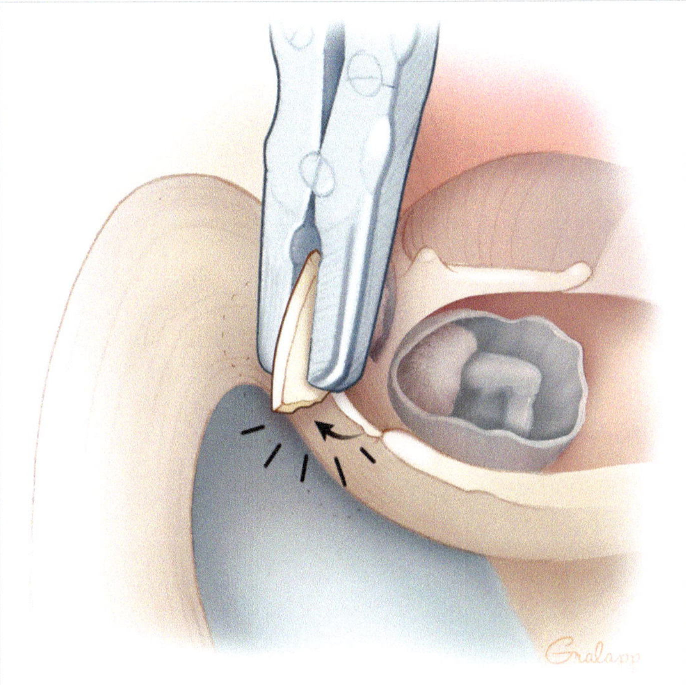

Fig. 8.28 Removing the ear canal wall with a rongeur.

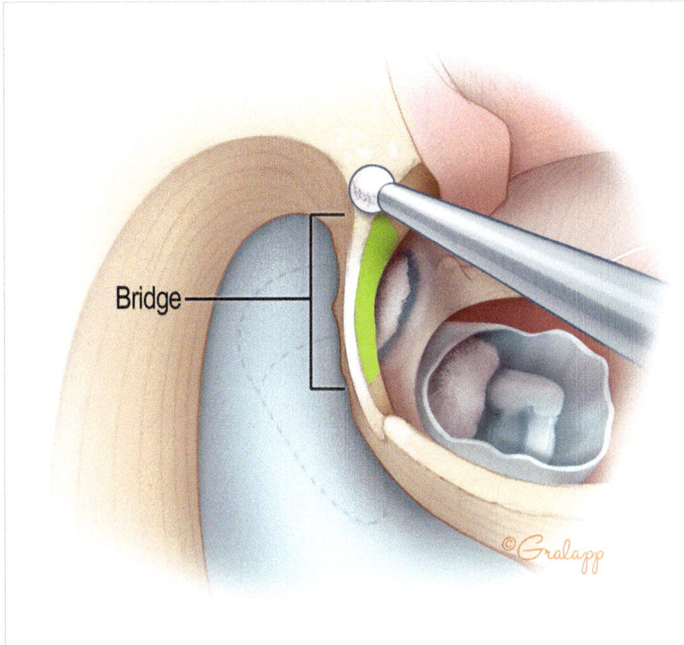

Fig. 8.29 The bridge is the arch of bone over the epitympanum.

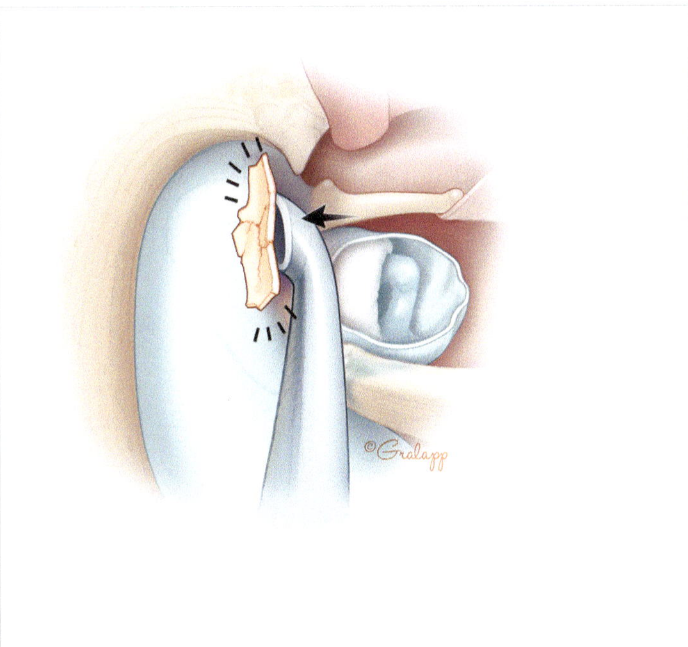

Fig. 8.30 Curetting away the last remnant of the bridge brings the cholesteatoma into view. Switching from a drill to curette is especially important in cases of an intact ossicular chain.

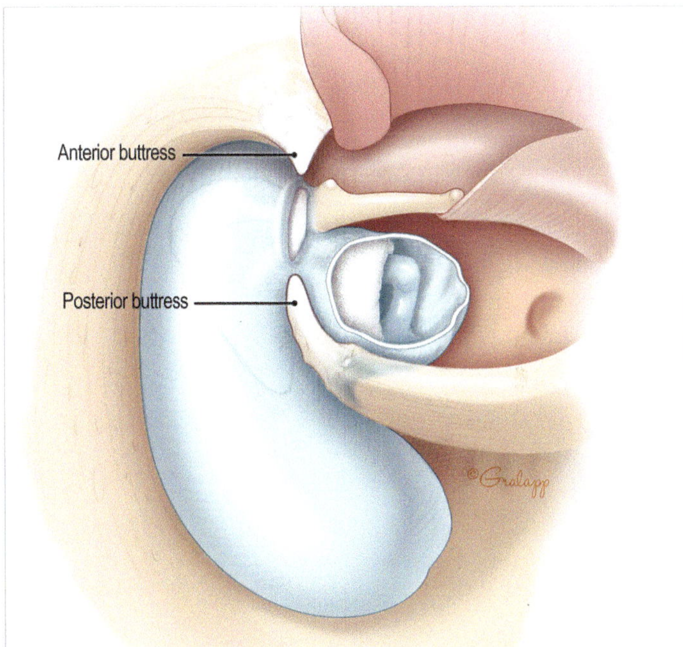

Fig. 8.31 The anterior and posterior buttresses need to be removed.

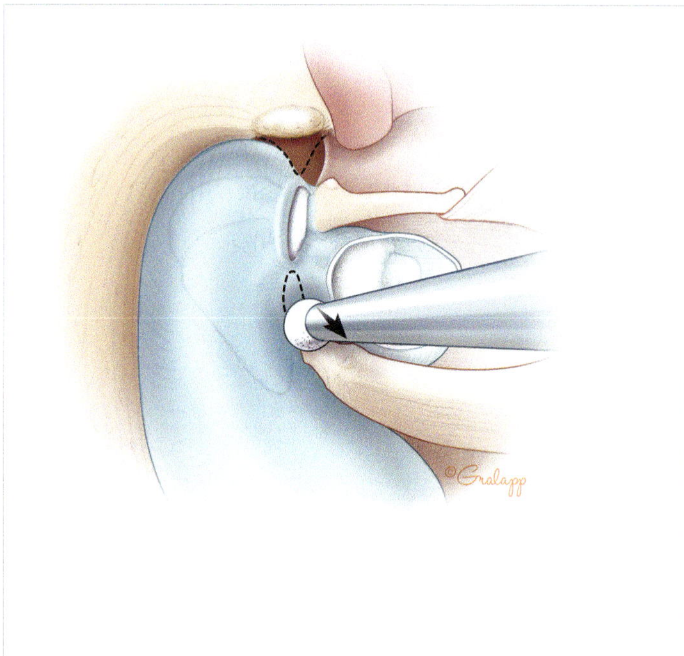

Fig. 8.32 Removal of the anterior and posterior buttresses.

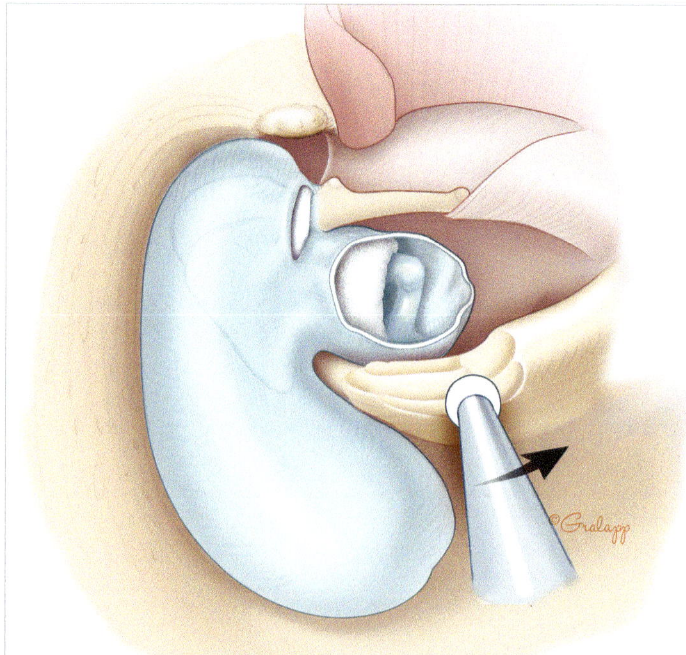

Fig. 8.33 Lowering of the canal wall, also known as the facial ridge because the facial nerve lies in its base.

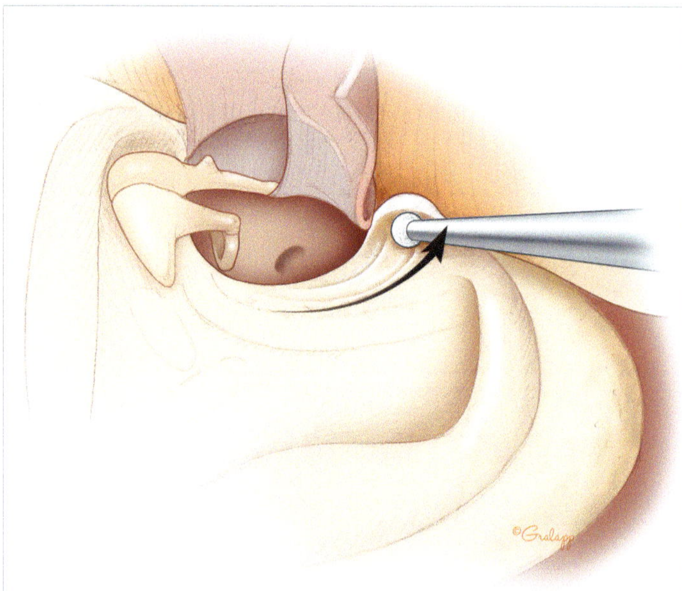

Fig. 8.34 Lowering facial ridge does not require exposure of the facial nerve. It is best to leave 2 to 3 mm of bone over the nerve to maintain a middle ear space.

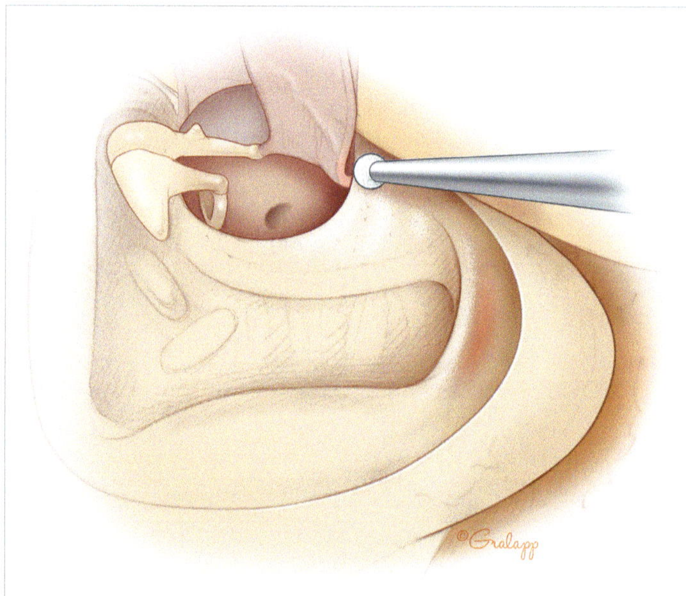

Fig. 8.35 Lowering the floor of the middle ear to the level of the facial ridge (base of the ear canal).

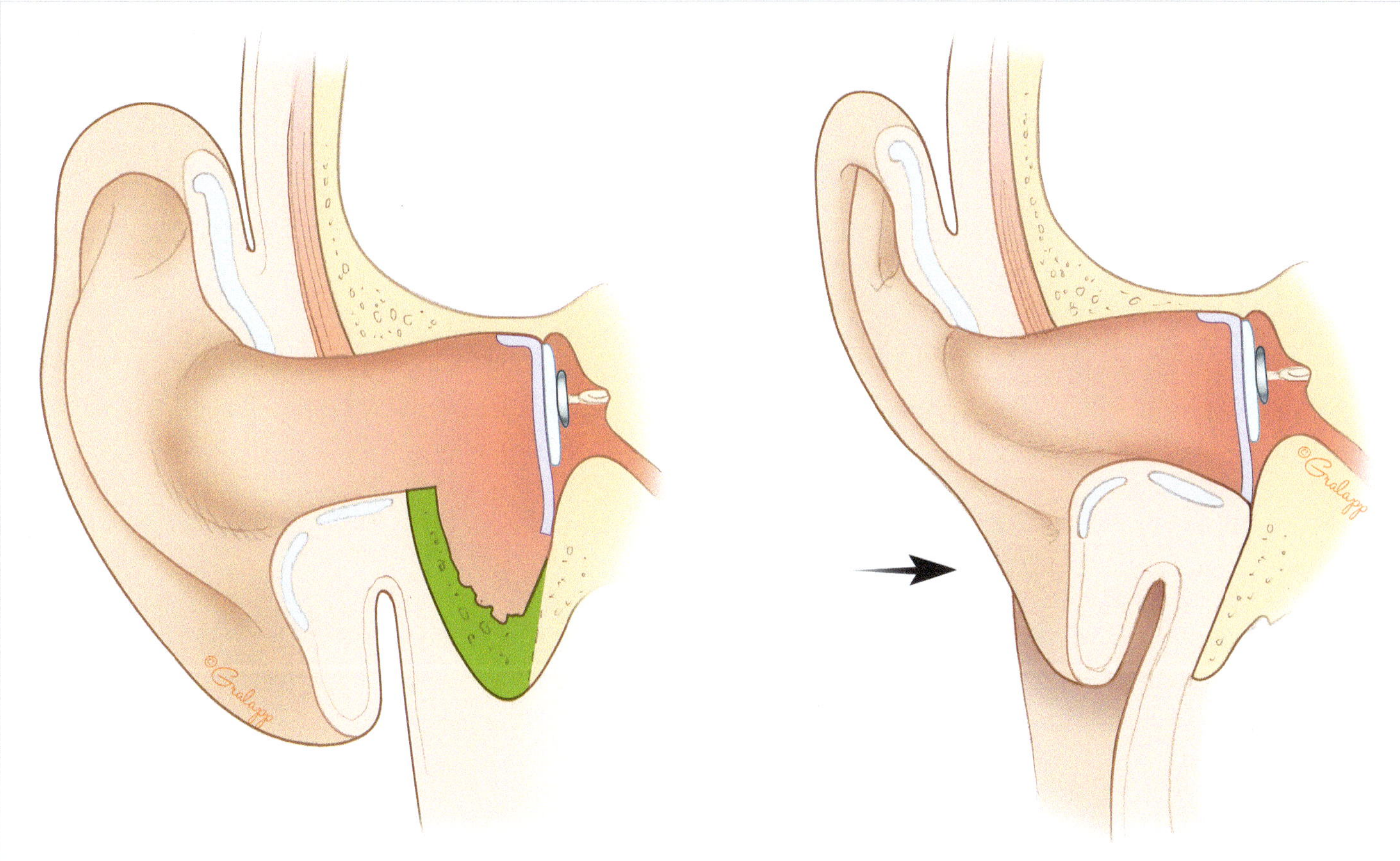

Fig. 8.36 Removal of the mastoid tip creates a smaller cavity. This is indicated in canal wall down surgery in an extensively pneumatized temporal bone.

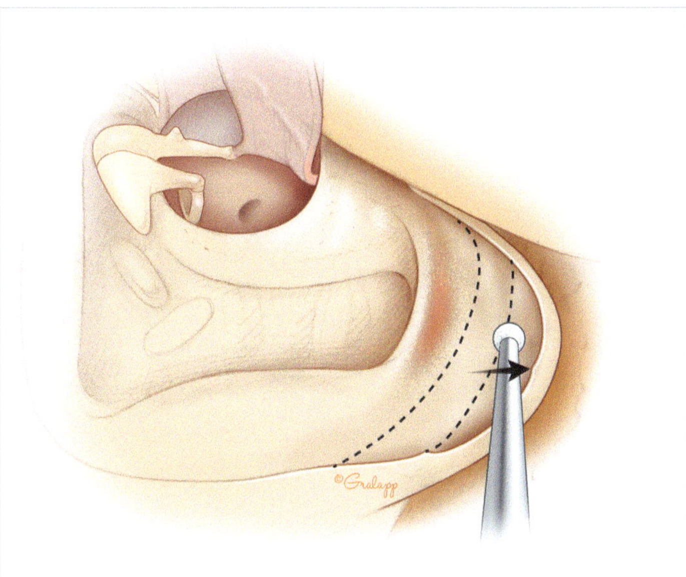

Fig. 8.37 Removal of the mastoid tip. The facial nerve is not related to the tip itself: it exits the mastoid bone anteriorly beneath the digastric ridge.

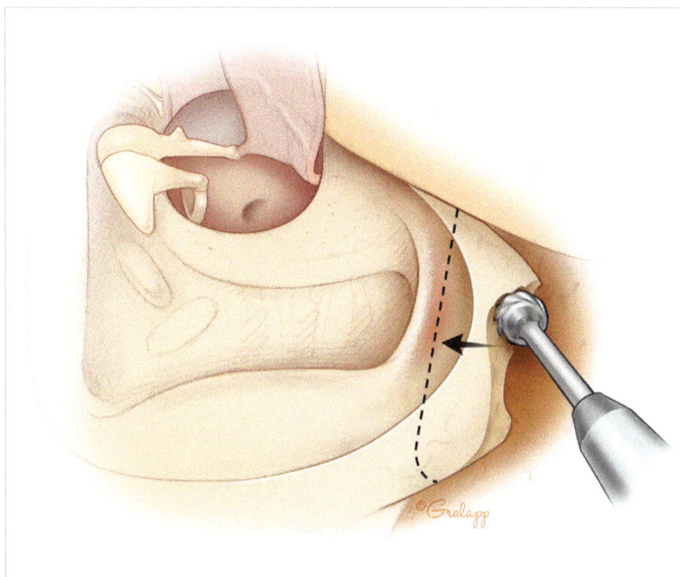

Fig. 8.38 Completing removal of the mastoid tip.

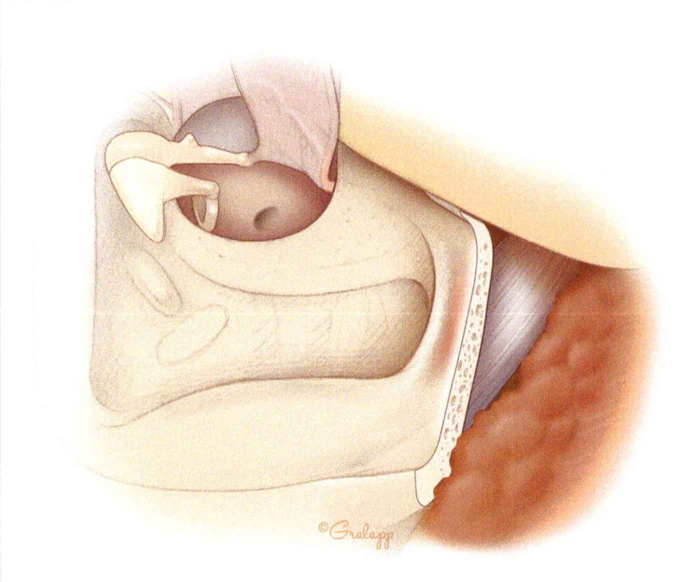

Fig. 8.39 After removal of the mastoid tip.

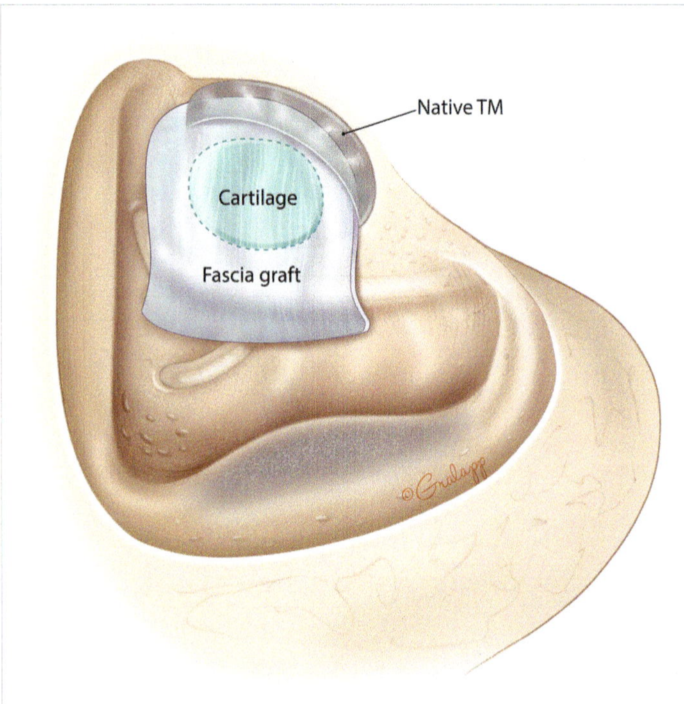

Fig. 8.41 Typical cartilage and fascia reconstruction in a canal wall down mastoidectomy. The skin flaps are not shown.

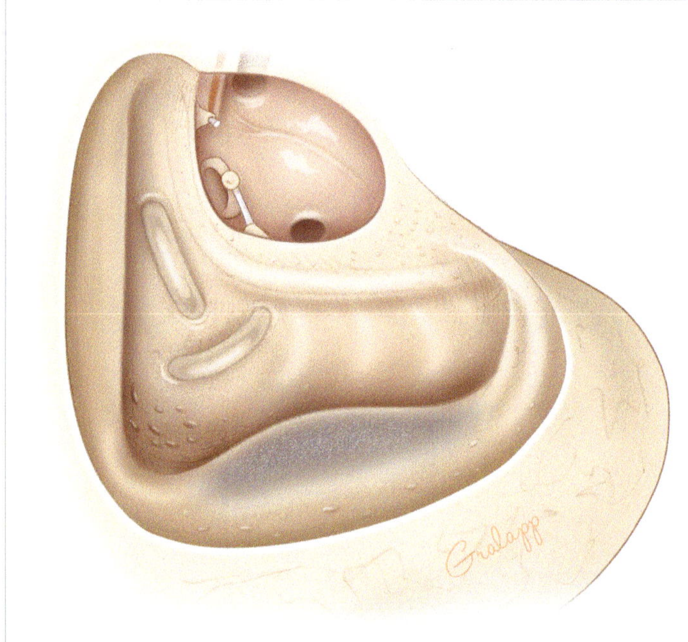

Fig. 8.40 Osseous anatomy of a completed canal wall down mastoidectomy. In modern times, middle ear reconstruction is almost always performed creating a modified radial mastoidectomy. A true radial mastoidectomy, leaving the middle ear open, is seldom used today but may be necessary when the cholesteatoma adheres tenaciously to the tympanic section of the facial nerve and/or stapes footplate, especially when matrix prolapses into the mouth of the Eustachian tube.

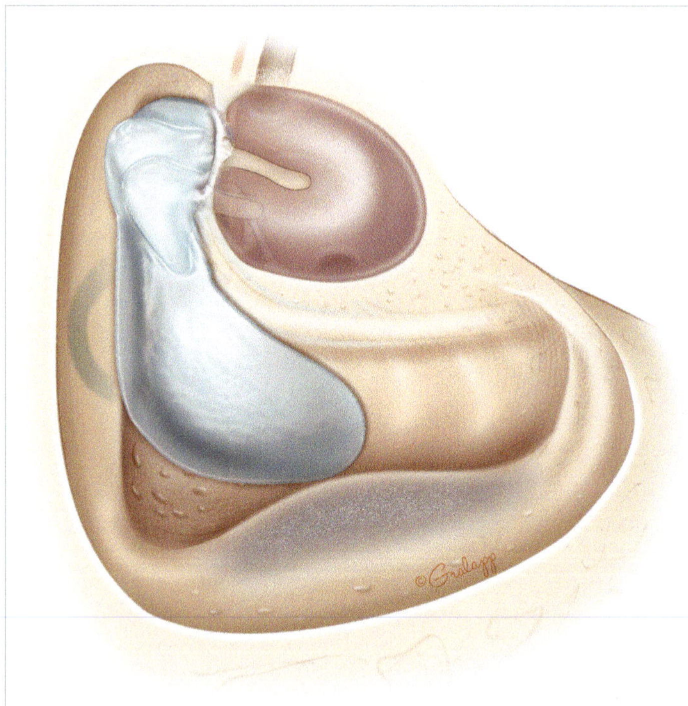

Fig. 8.42 Bondy type of modified radical mastoidectomy. Cholesteatoma matrix is left on the ossicular heads and the middle ear is not explored. This is suitable when the hearing is good and the middle ear is not involved with disease.

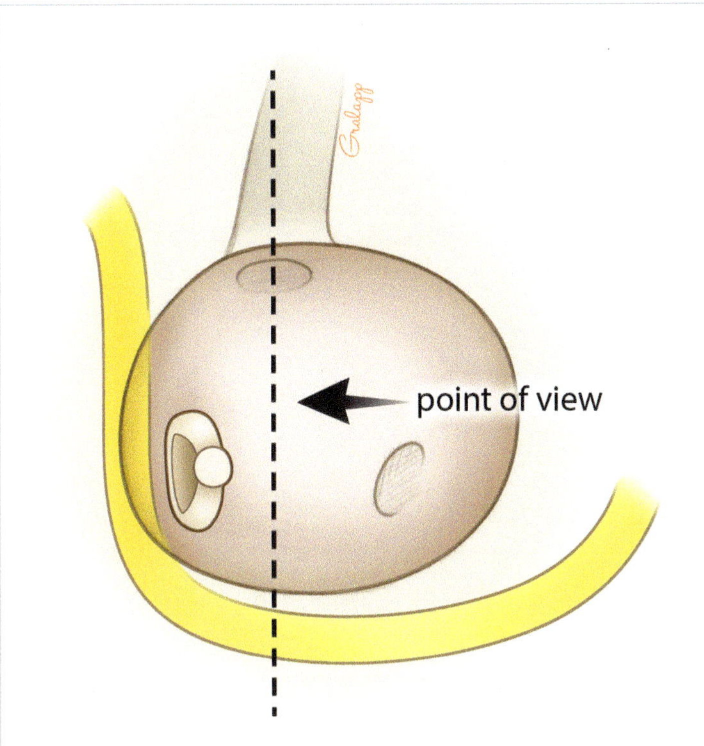

Fig. 8.43 Scout view indicating plane of the following illustrations concerning canal wall height.

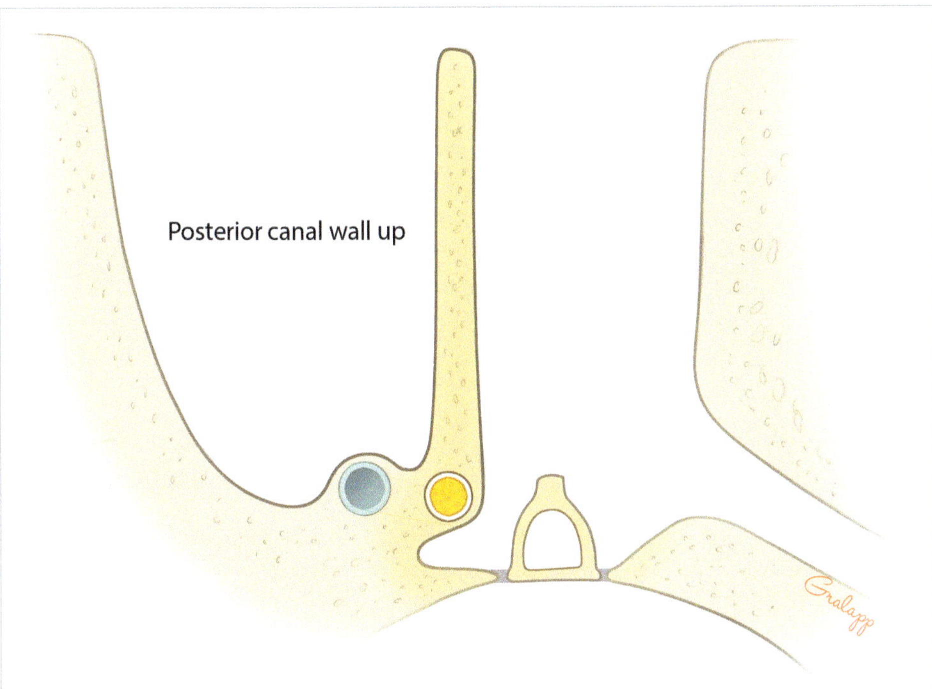

Fig. 8.44 Intact canal wall mastoidectomy.

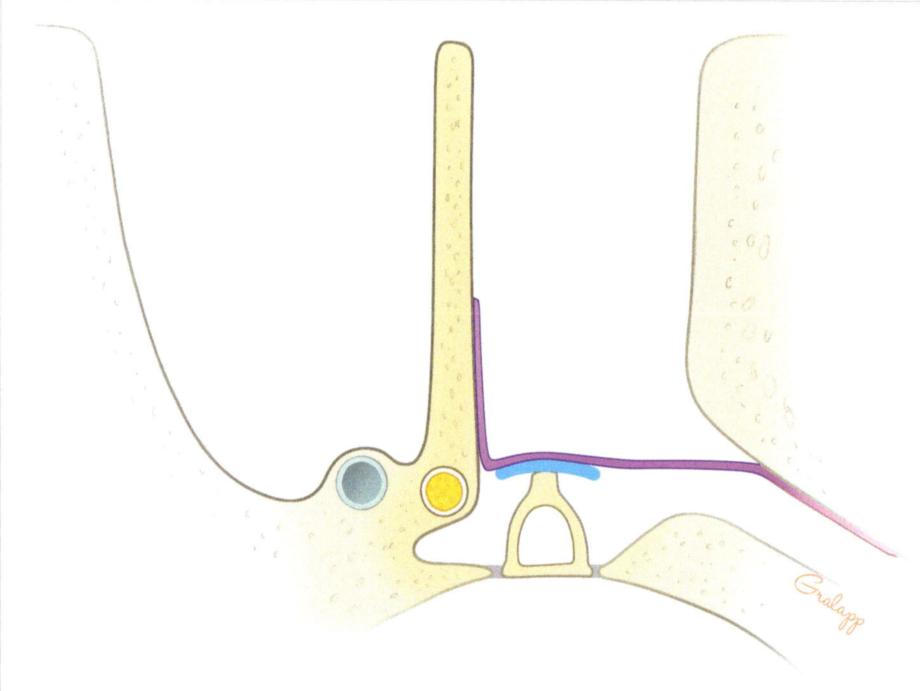

Fig. 8.45 Schematic view of tympanic membrane reconstruction in intact canal wall tympanomastoidectomy.

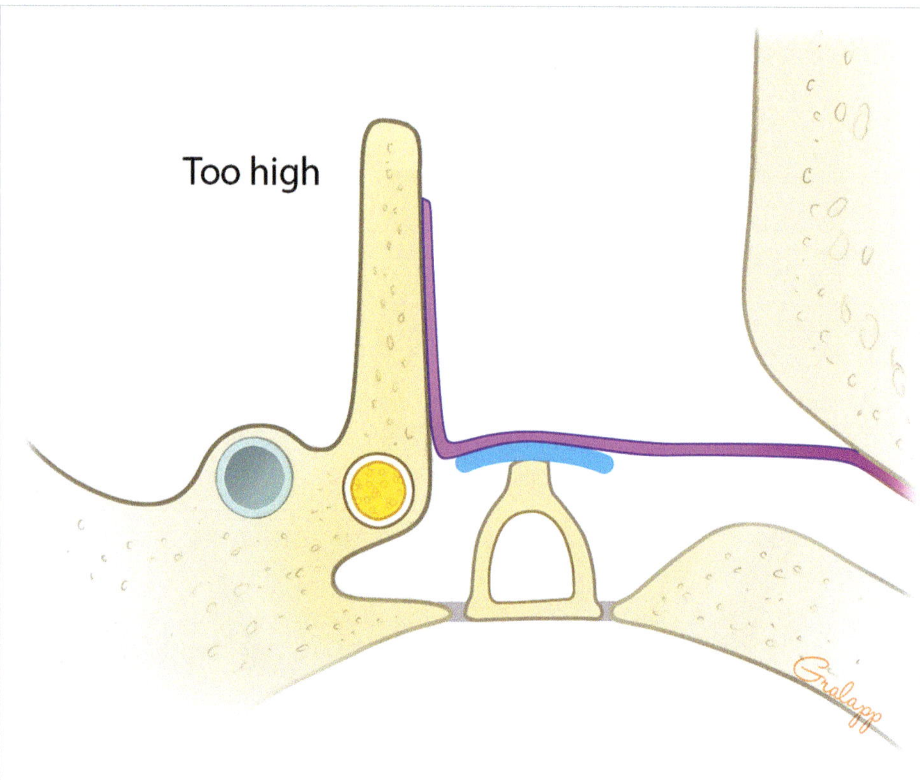

Fig. 8.46 Excessive height in the lowered canal wall ("high facial ridge") makes management of the mastoid cavity difficult.

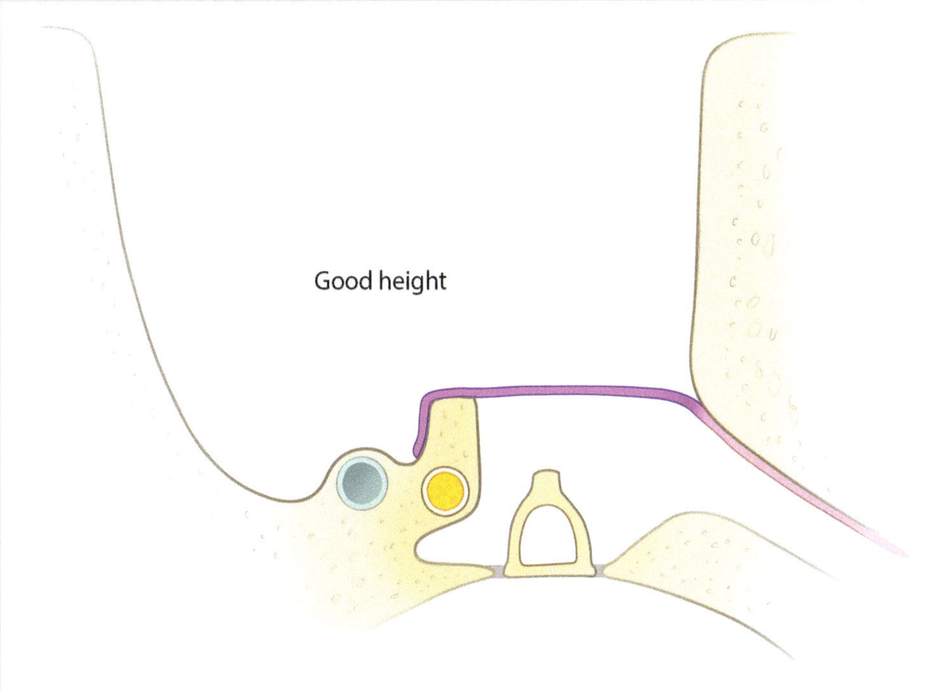

Fig. 8.47 Leaving some bone on the descending facial nerve retains a depth to the middle ear space.

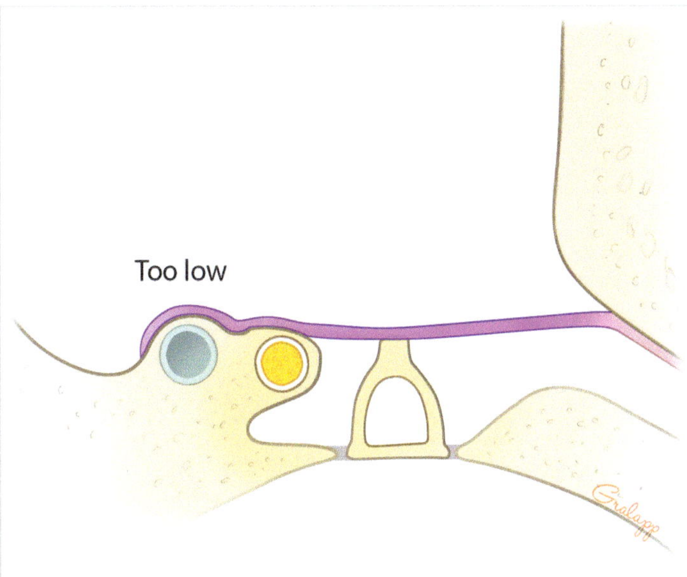

Fig. 8.48 Lowering the ridge to the facial nerve gives a slit-like middle ear cavity which is prone to scarring.

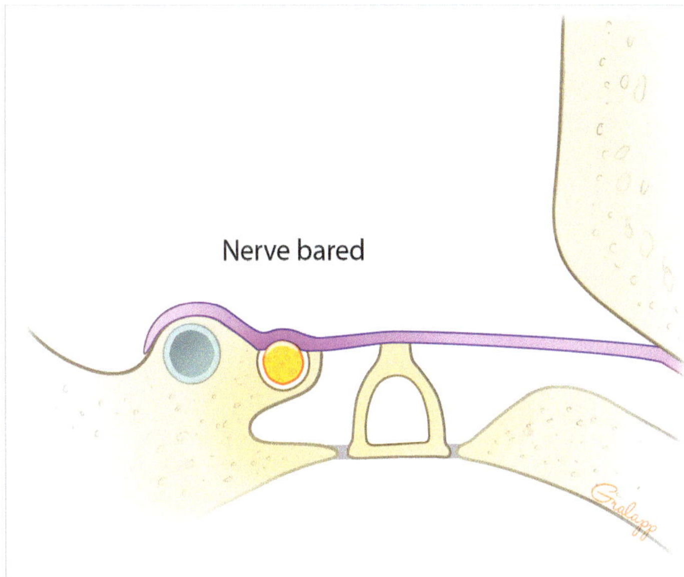

Fig. 8.49 Baring the facial nerve places it at risk raising a flap off the floor of the cavity during subsequent revision surgeries for ossiculoplasty.

8.4 Microdissection of Cholesteatoma

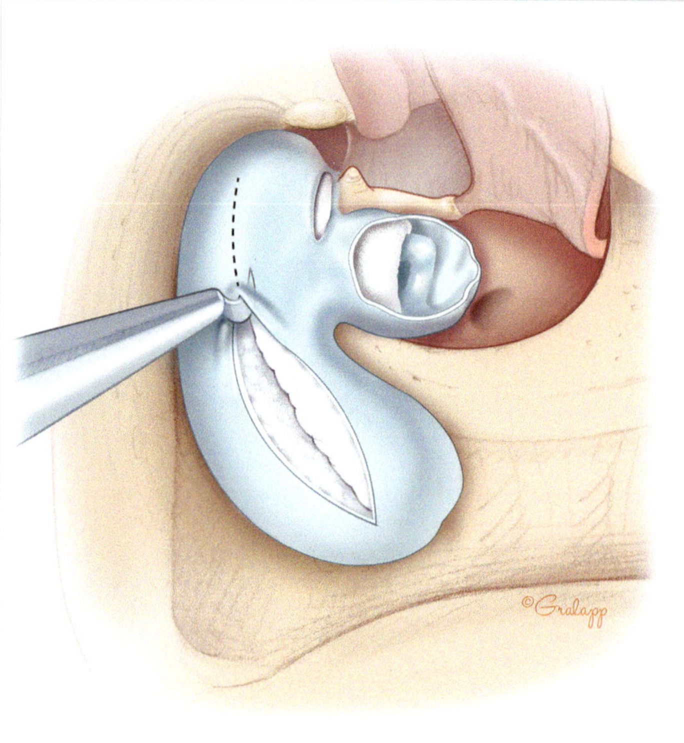

Fig. 8.50 Opening the cholesteatoma matrix to expose the entrapped keratin.

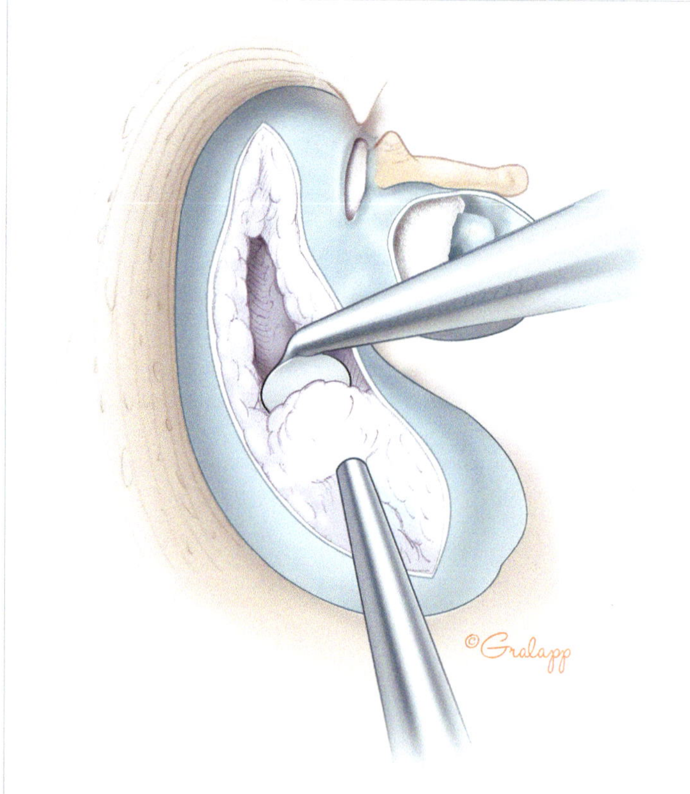

Fig. 8.51 Keratin is fed into a suction.

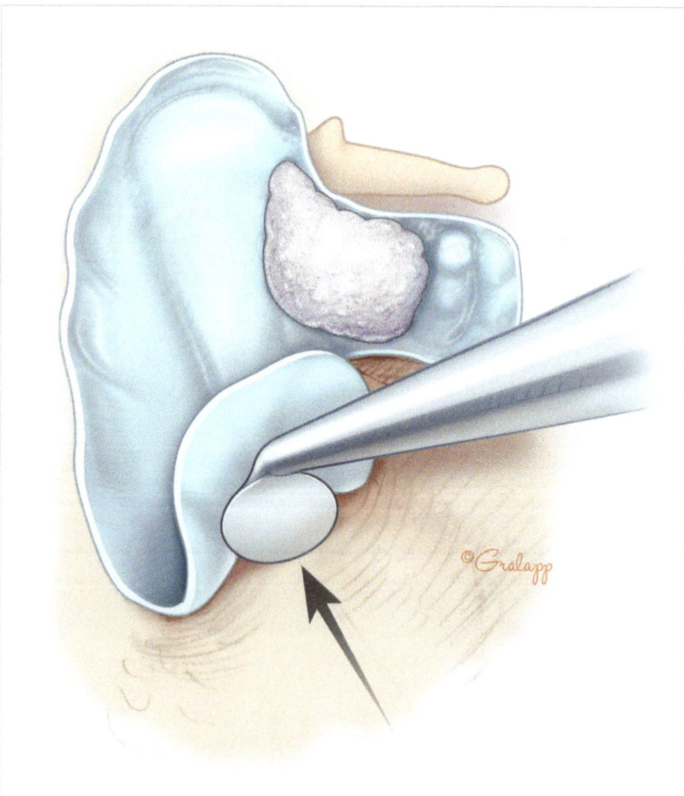

Fig. 8.52 Dissection of the matrix off the floor of the mastoid. The facial nerve is seldom involved in the mastoid segment, but care must be taken in observing from possible lateral semicircular canal fistula.

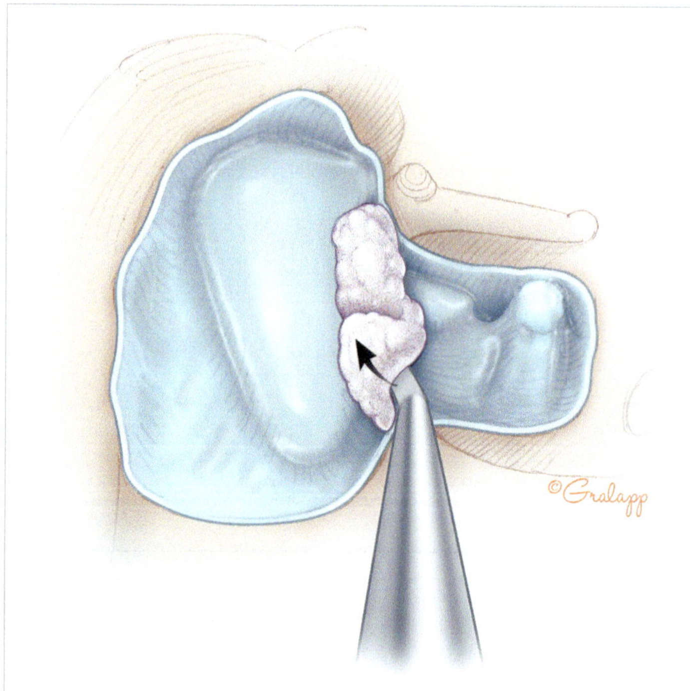

Fig. 8.53 Removing keratin off the matrix adherent to the ossicles.

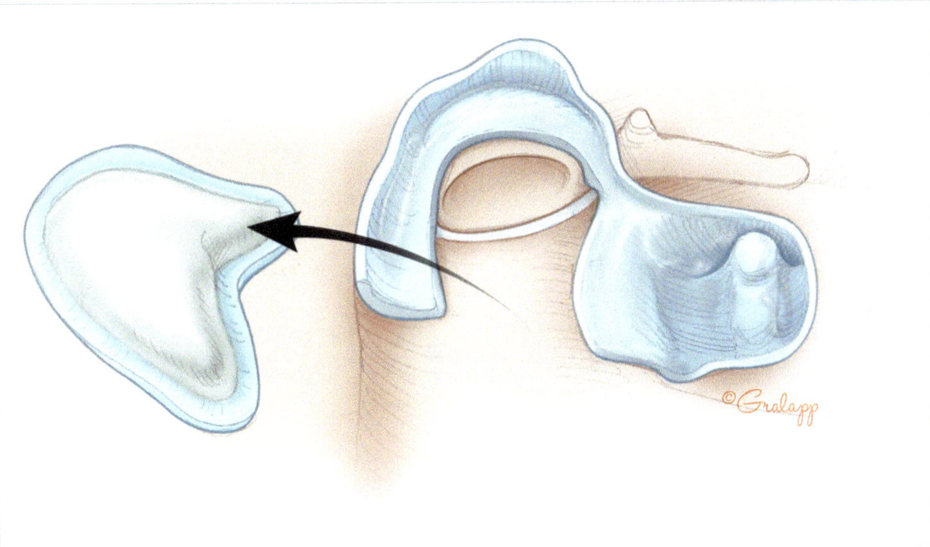

Fig. 8.54 As the long process of the incus is eroded in this case, the remaining incus can be removed. If the chain was intact, it would have been necessary to cut the incudostapedial joint. With the canal wall down, this can be done with a disposable myringotomy knife which is much sharper than an incudostapedial joint knife used in stapes surgery when the stapes is fixed. Severance of the joint with a sharp knife is preferable when the stapes is mobile.

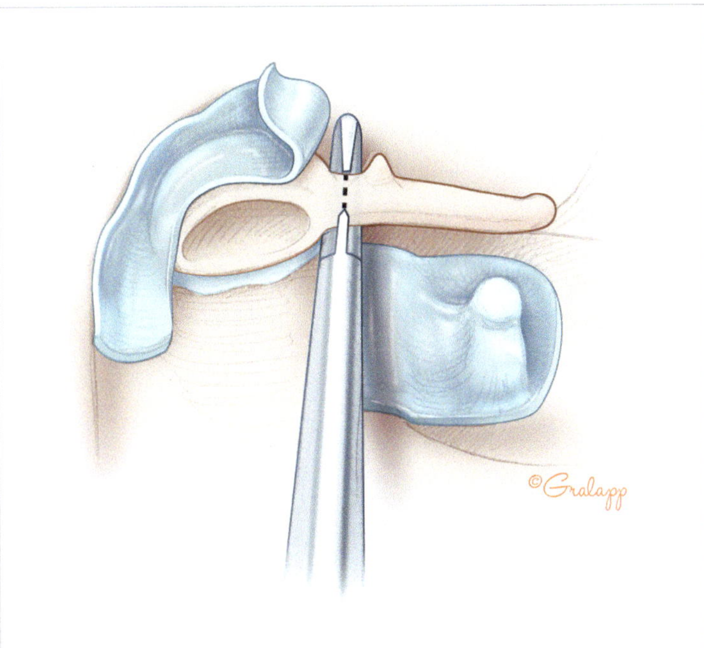

Fig. 8.55 Matrix is dissected off the lateral aspect of the malleus head. A malleus nipper is preparing to sever the malleus neck. If this segment of bone is stout, then it can be thinned with a 1-mm diamond drill before nipping.

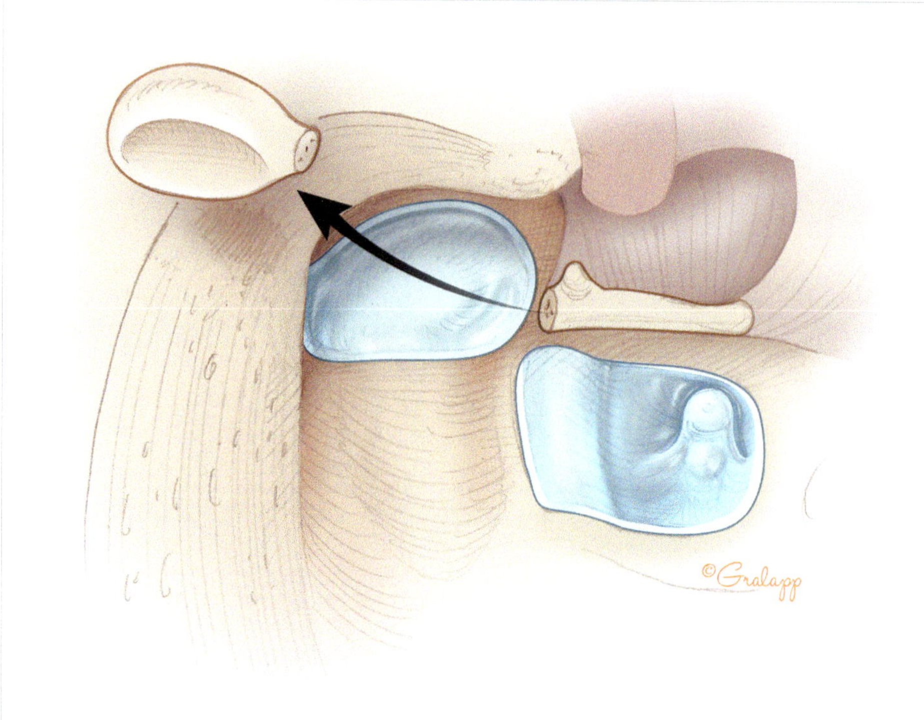

Fig. 8.56 Removal of the malleus head leaving the umbo in the tympanic membrane remnant. See section 8.11 Ossicles in Cholesteatoma for technique of removal of the matrix from the stapes.

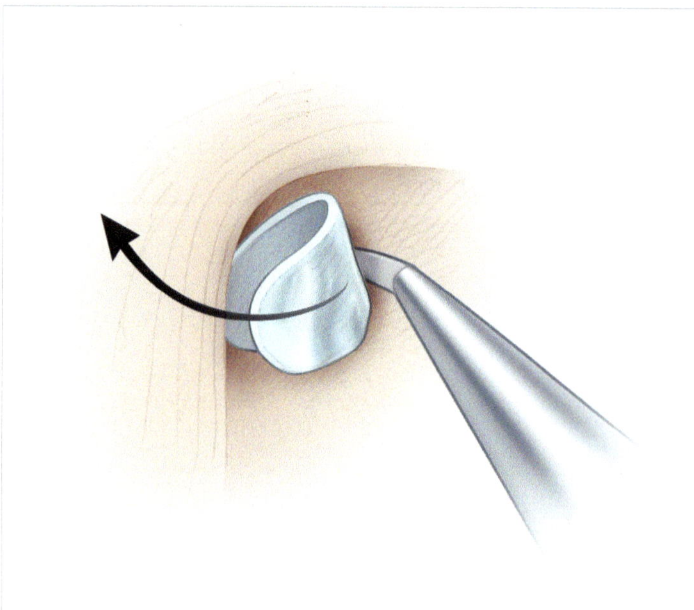

Fig. 8.57 Dissection of the cholesteatoma from the anterior epitympanic space deep to the malleus head.

8.5 Retrograde Technique

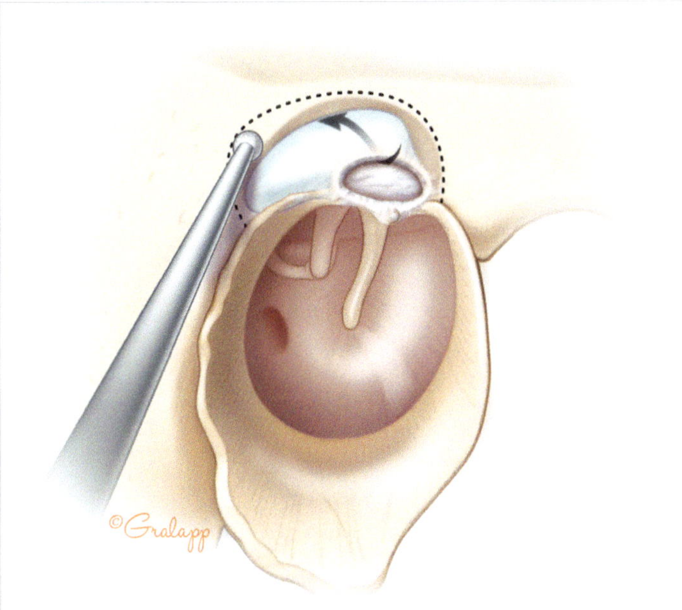

Fig. 8.58 Limited epitympanic disease can be handled by an atticotomy.

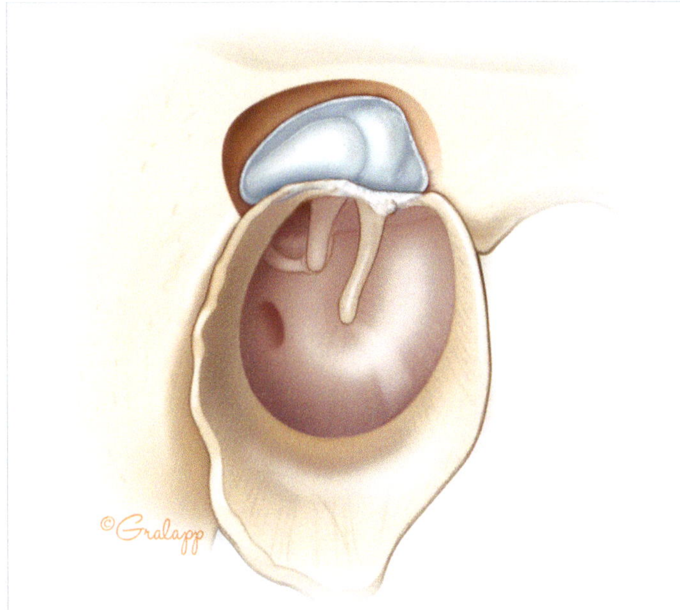

Fig. 8.59 Small epitympanic cholesteatoma exteriorized by an atticotomy.

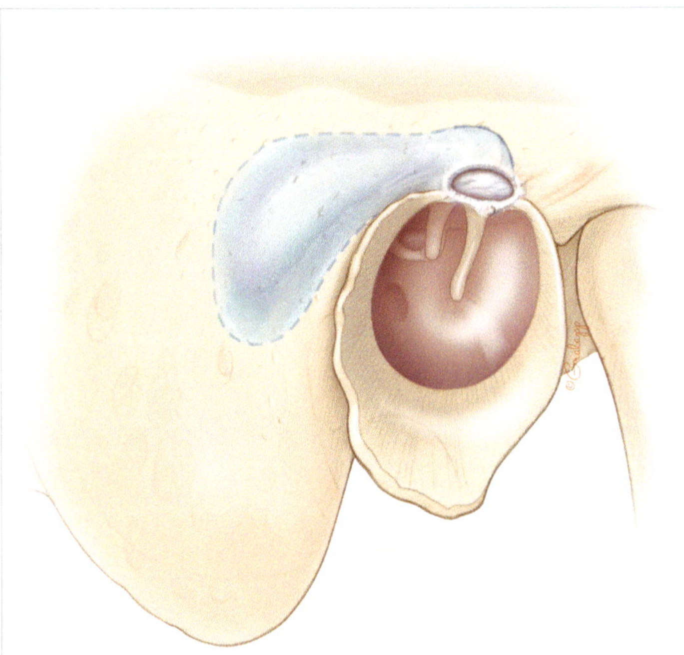

Fig. 8.60 Retrograde approach removing only that portion of the mastoid overlying the cholesteatoma as an alternative to thorough removal of mastoid cellularity.

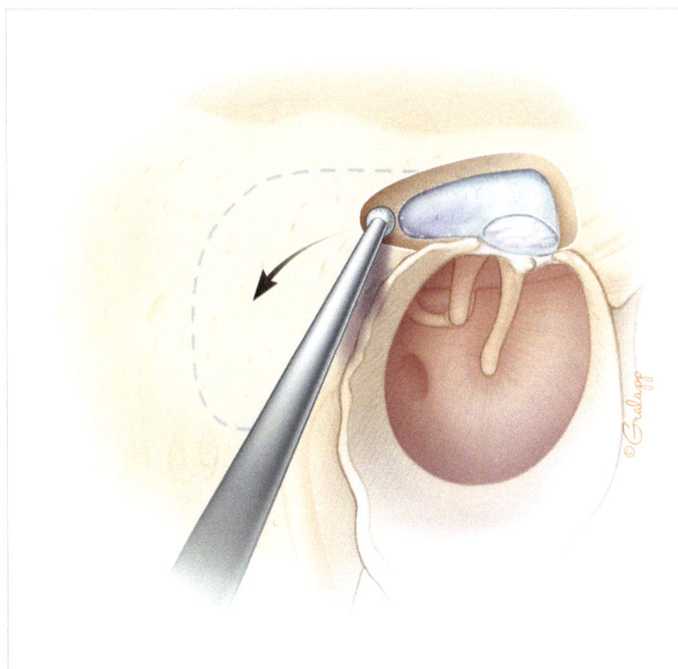

Fig. 8.61 Retrograde mastoidectomy; the so-called inside-out approach.

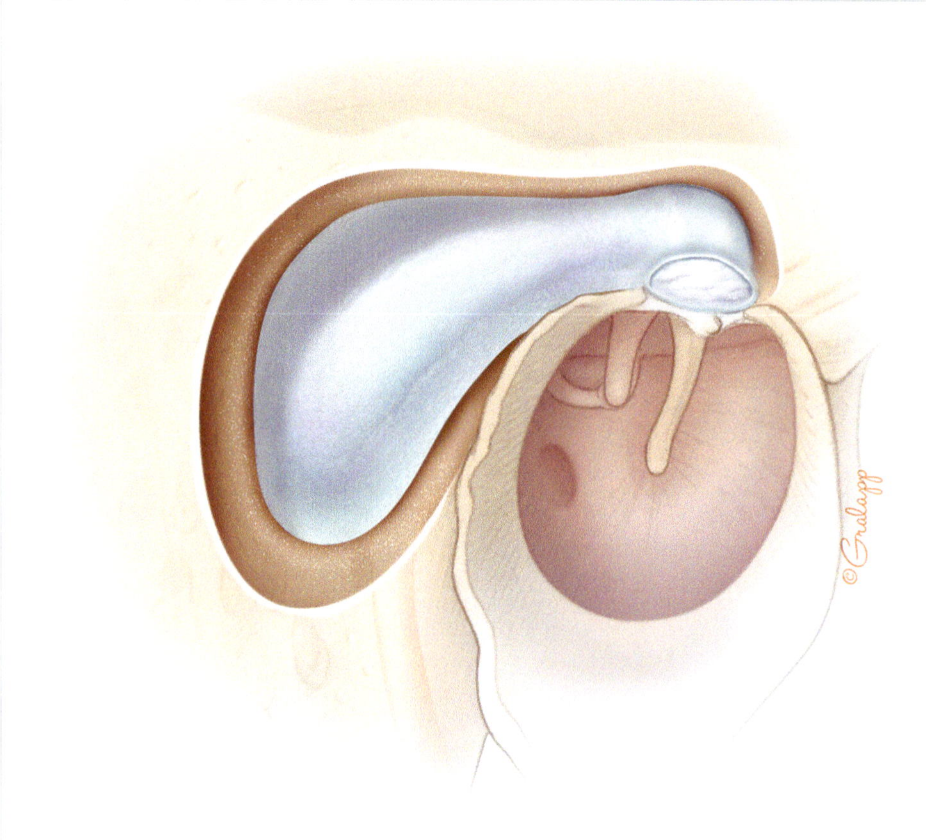

Fig. 8.62 Exposed cholesteatoma.

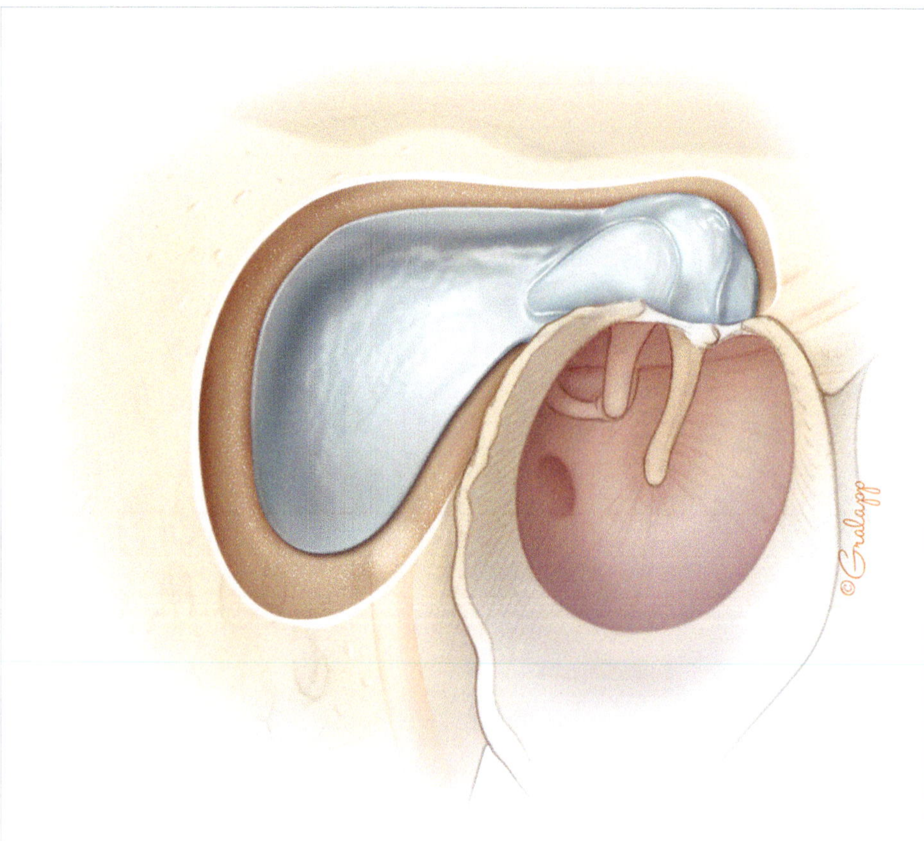

Fig. 8.63 Outer matrix and keratin removed completing a retrograde mastoidectomy. This differs from a Bondy modified radical mastoidectomy as the uninvolved mastoid is not disturbed.

8.6 Epitympanum Repair

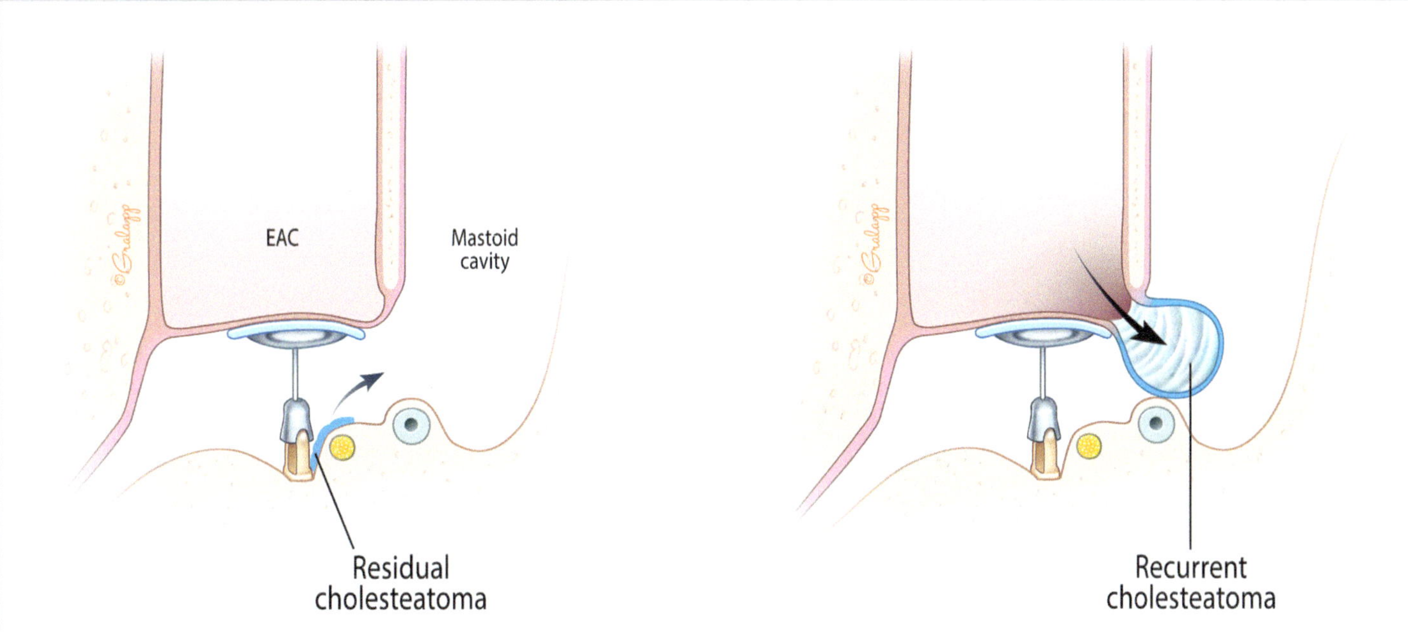

Fig. 8.64 Two varieties of cholesteatoma recidivism: residual and recurrent forms. In residual, a fragment of squamous epithelium was left during surgery. In recurrent, a new pouch forms *de novo*. EAC, external auditory canal.

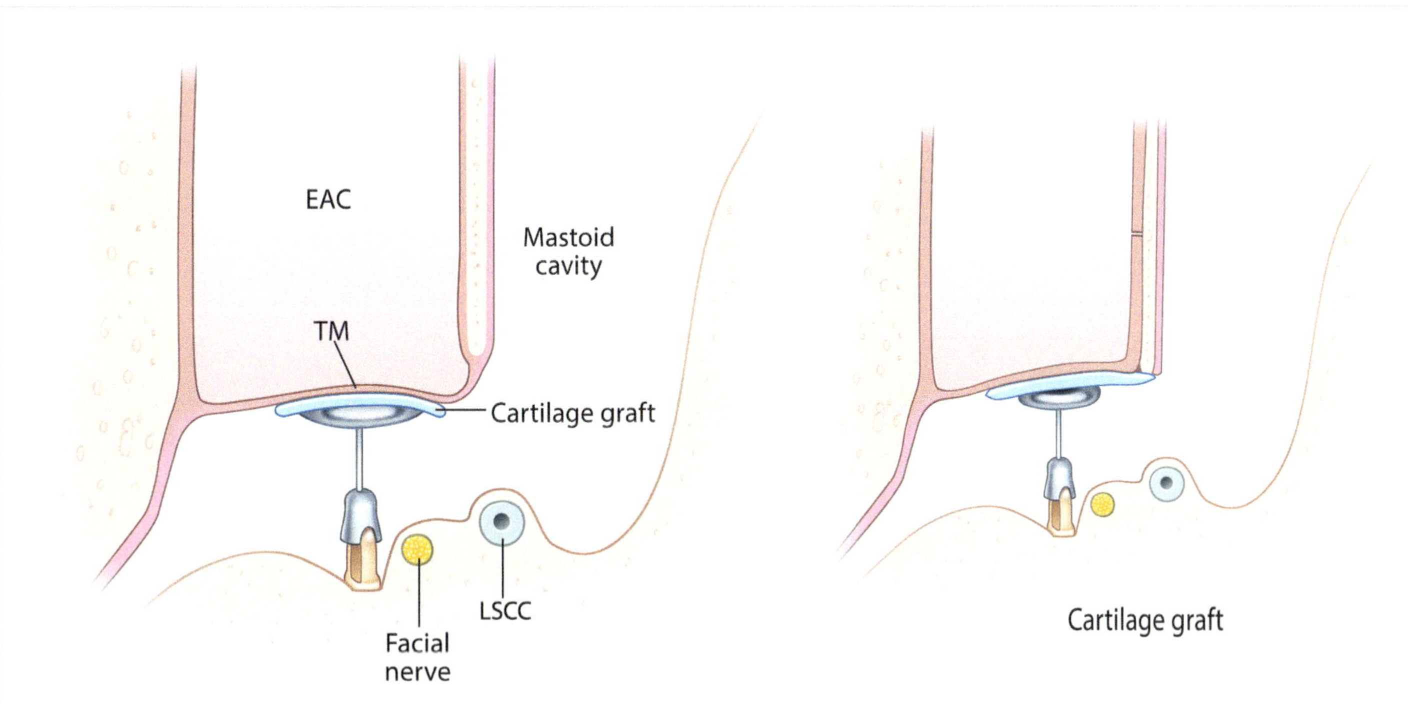

Fig. 8.65 Cartilage placed leaving a space at the scutum (*left*) and abutting the scutum (*right*). Close approximation of the cartilage with the ear canal edge is preferred to discourage cholesteatoma recurrence. EAC, external auditory canal; TM, tympanic membrane; LSCC, lateral semicircular canal.

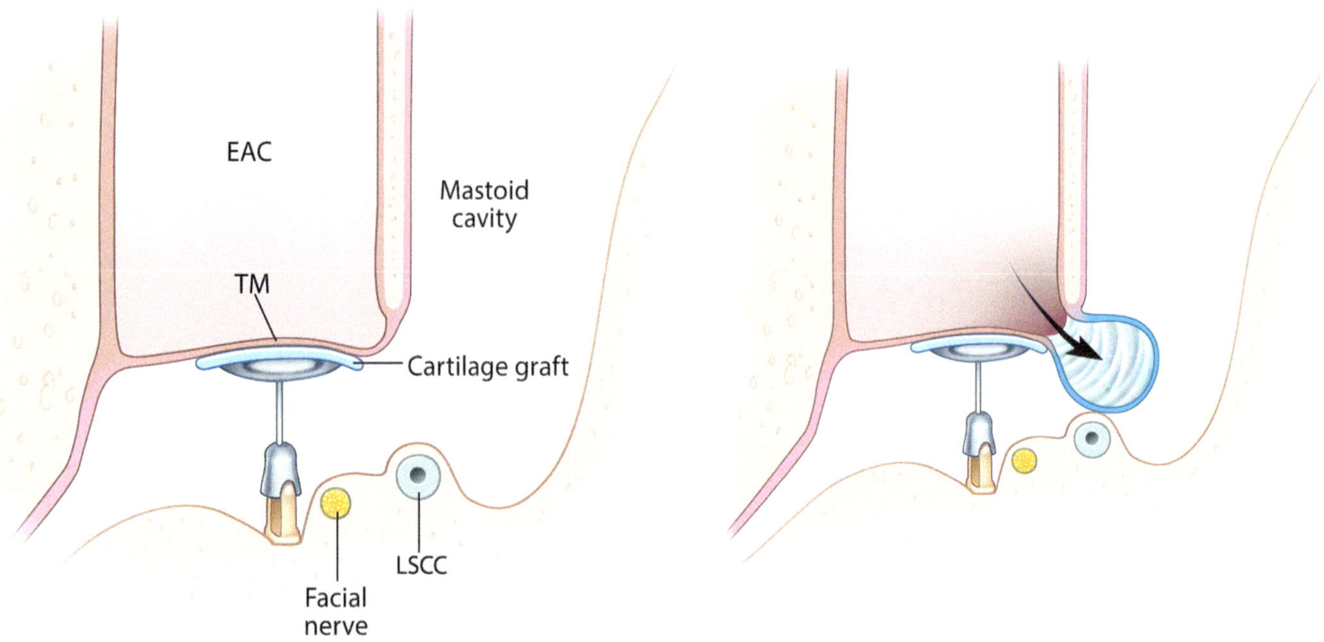

Fig. 8.66 Recurrent cholesteatoma with retraction between the scutum and a cartilage graft which did not fully seal the epitympanum. EAC, external auditory canal; TM, tympanic membrane; LSCC, lateral semicircular canal.

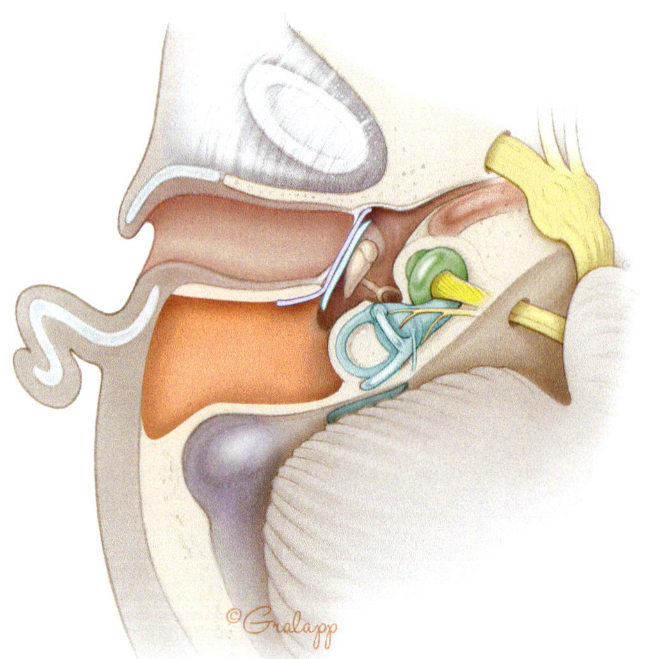

Fig. 8.67 Intact canal wall tympanomastoidectomy with fascia tympanoplasty and cartilage graft.

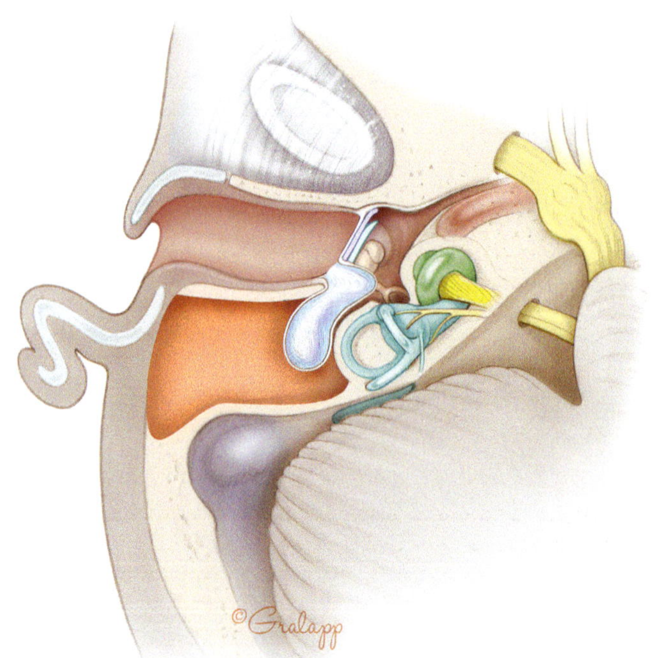

Fig. 8.68 Recurrent cholesteatoma following an intact canal wall tympanomastoidectomy. While a well-placed cartilage graft reduces the risk, recurrent cholesteatoma may occur even in a narrow slit between the cartilage and scutum. This type of recurrence is especially probable when the opposite ear also has a cholesteatoma. Because of the high risk of recurrence with intact canal wall procedures in patients with bilateral disease, consideration should be given for a primary canal wall down approach in these patients.

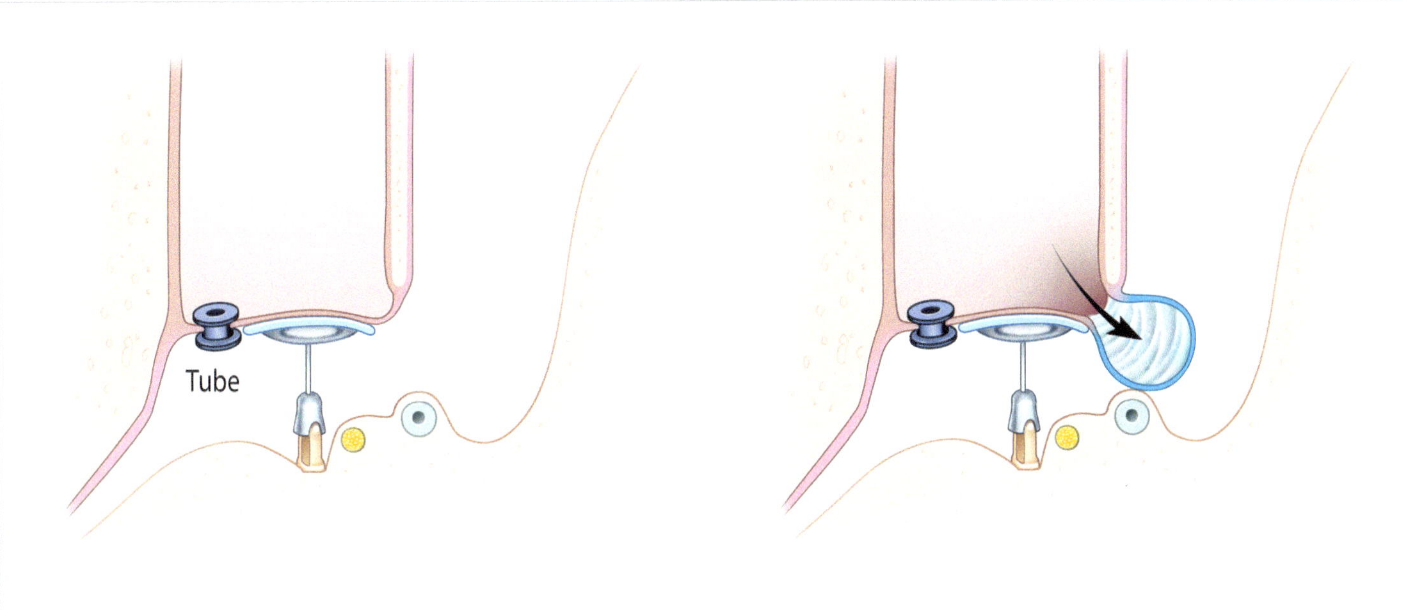

Fig. 8.69 Cholesteatoma recurrence may occur despite adequate middle ear ventilation.

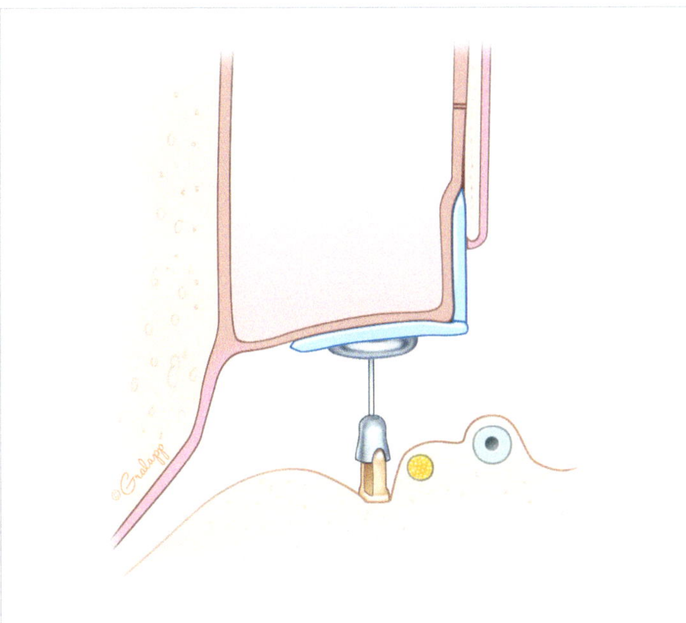

Fig. 8.70 Two pieces of cartilage to both reinforce the tympanic membrane and also to repair an epitympanic defect.

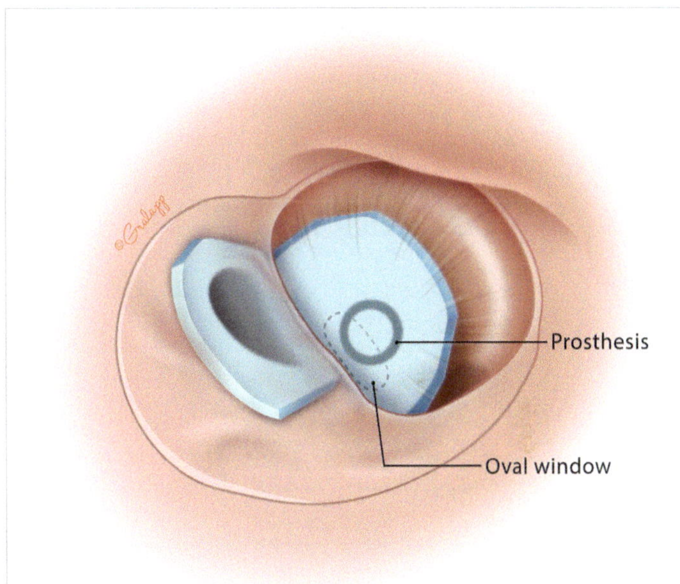

Fig. 8.71 Two pieces of cartilage to both reinforce the tympanic membrane and repair a scutal defect.

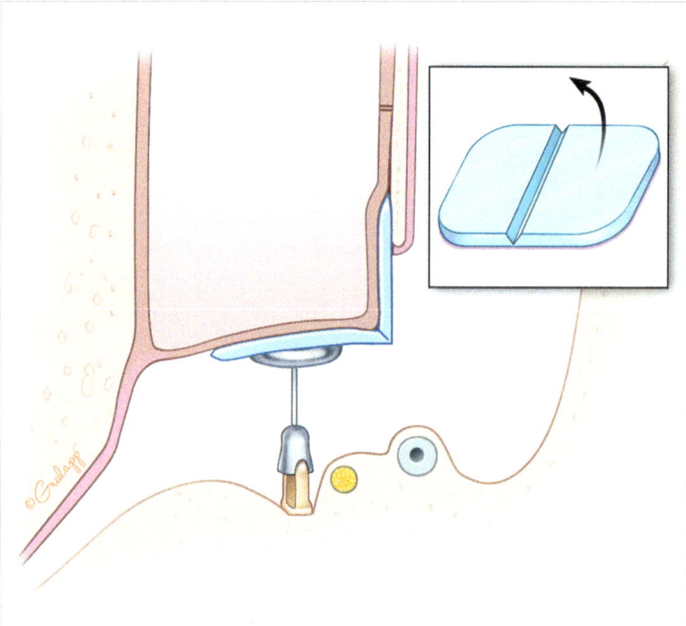

Fig. 8.72 A scored piece of cartilage with perichondrium intact spanning the tympanic membrane and repairing a scutal defect.

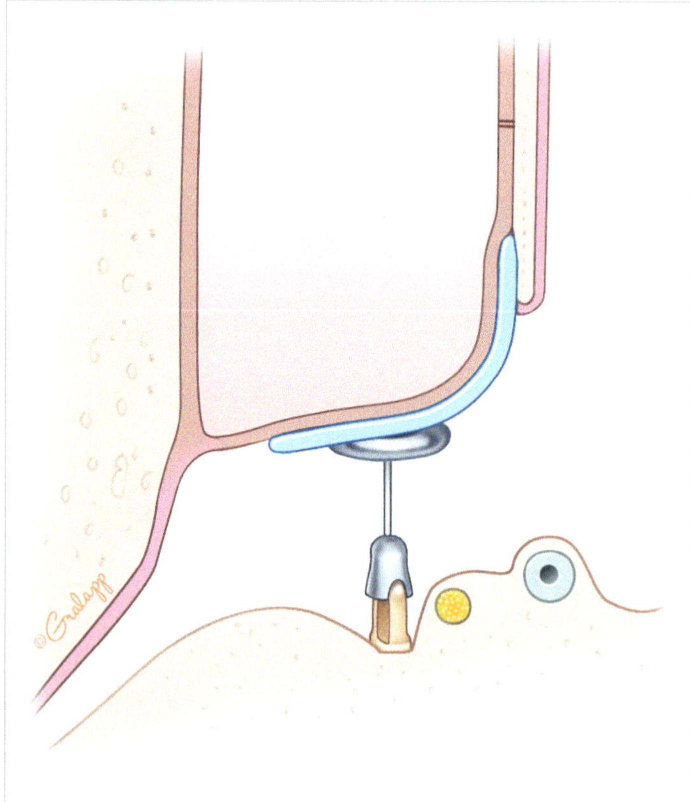

Fig. 8.73 A single piece of cartilage spanning the tympanic membrane and repairing a scutal defect. Note that the cartilage is placed on the ear canal side. Cartilage placed on the mastoid side is less effective in discouraging recurrence.

8.7 The Facial Nerve in Cholesteatoma

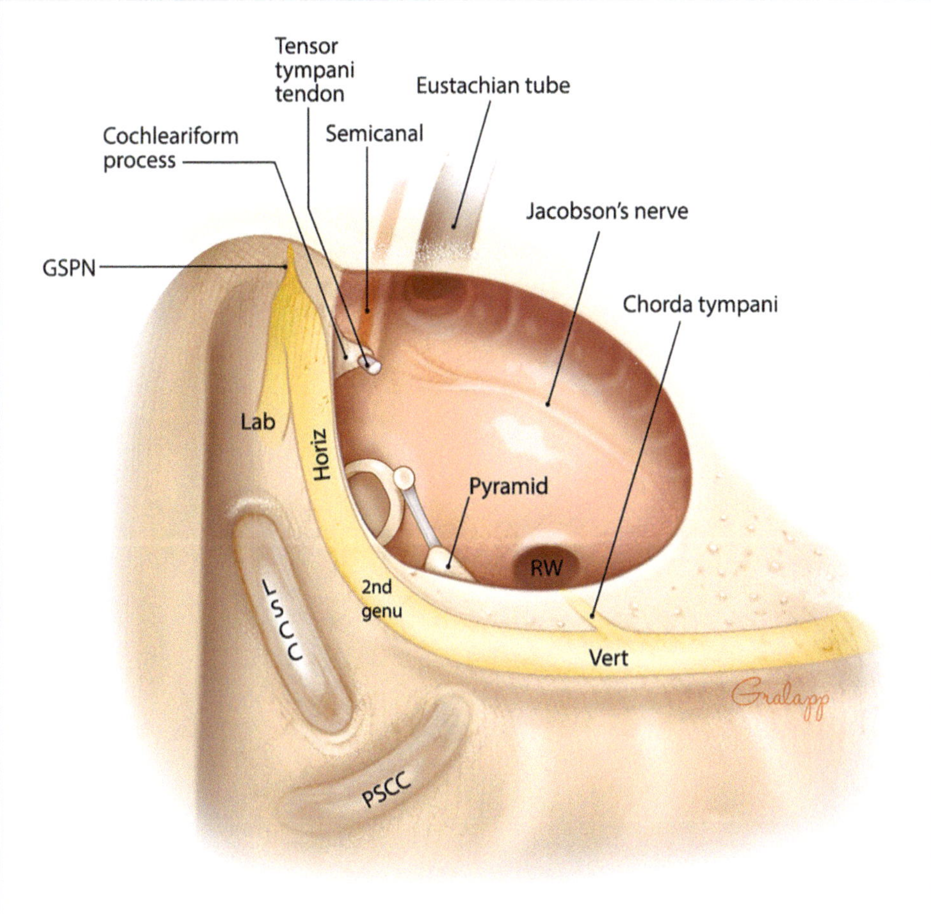

Fig. 8.74 Anatomical detail of the course of the facial nerve on the medial wall of the middle ear and floor of the mastoid. Understanding this anatomy is key to safe and effective ear microsurgery. Note the intimate relationship of the stapes and oval window to the horizontal (tympanic) segment of the nerve. The lateral semicircular canal parallels the facial nerve's horizontal segment. Anteriorly in the middle ear, the cochleariform process lies immediately inferior to the nerve. These landmarks are important in the identification of the nerve when the anatomy is obscured by disease. Lab, labyrinthine segment; Vert, vertical (mastoid) segment; GSPN, greater superficial petrosal nerve; RW, round window; LSCC, lateral semicircular canal; PSCC, posterior semicircular canal.

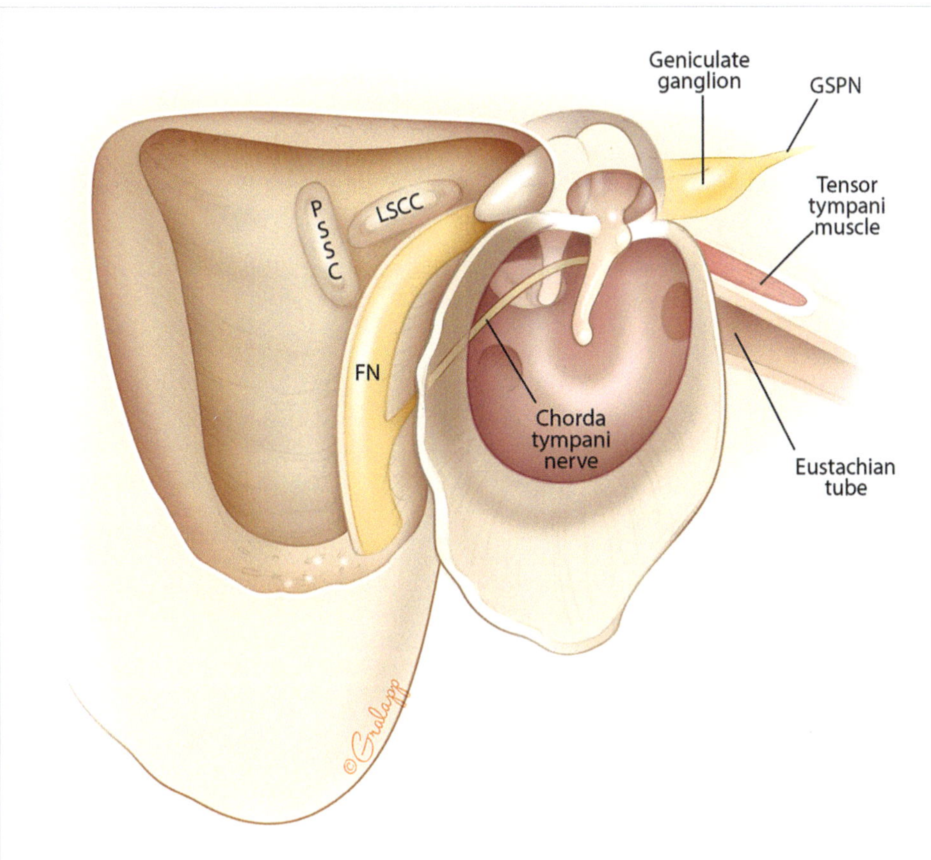

Fig. 8.75 Relationship of the tympanic segment of the facial nerve to the ossicles. FN, facial nerve; GSPN, greater superficial petrosal nerve; LSCC, lateral semicircular canal; PSCC, posterior semicircular canal.

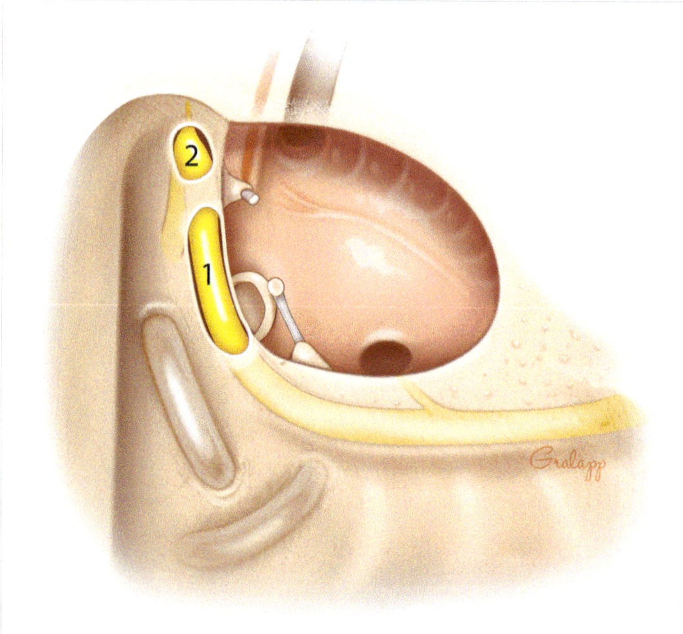

Fig. 8.76 Characteristically, posterior epitympanic cholesteatoma erodes the fallopian canal just superior to the stapes (1). Anterior epitympanic cholesteatoma erodes the nerve anteriorly as it approaches the geniculate ganglion (2). Note that cholesteatoma seldom erodes the bony covering of the nerve in the mastoid.

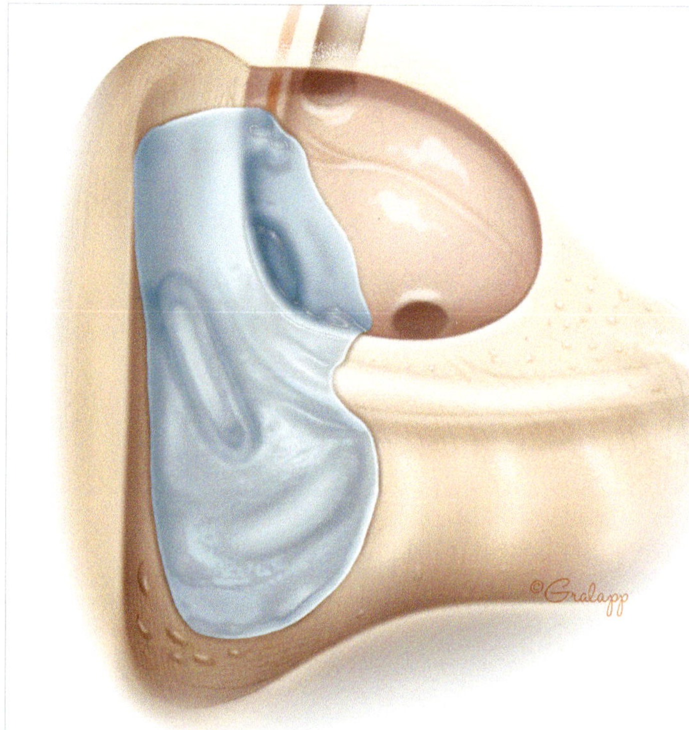

Fig. 8.77 Typical appearance of cholesteatoma matrix on the stapes footplate, facial nerve, and lateral and posterior semicircular canals.

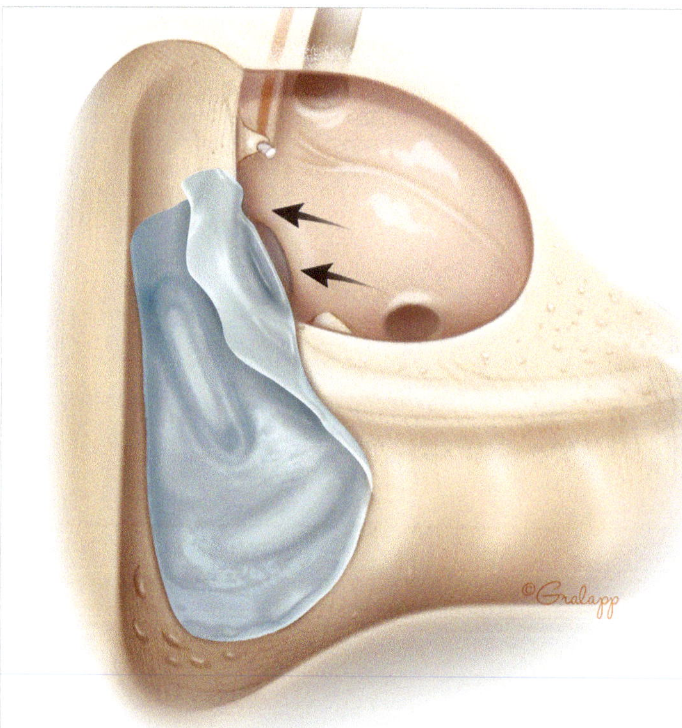

Fig. 8.78 Achieving orientation by dissecting superiorly to find the oval window (or stapes) which is a consistent and reliable landmark for the tympanic segment of the nerve.

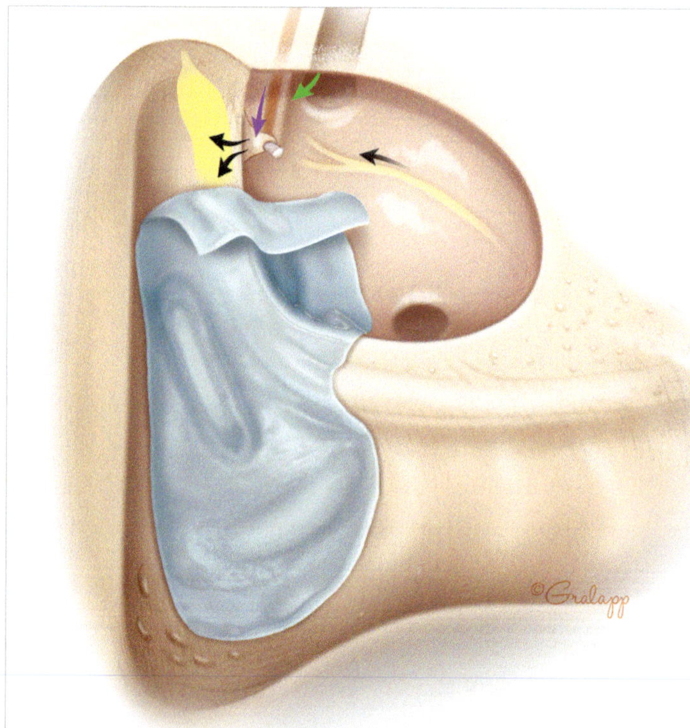

Fig. 8.79 When the oval window area is obscured by disease, the tympanic segment of the facial nerve can be identified by following the tympanic plexus (*black arrow*) to the cochleariform process (*purple arrow*) which hangs from the anterior tympanic segment of the nerve. The Eustachian tube orifice is a helpful landmark in locating the cochleariform process (*green arrow*).

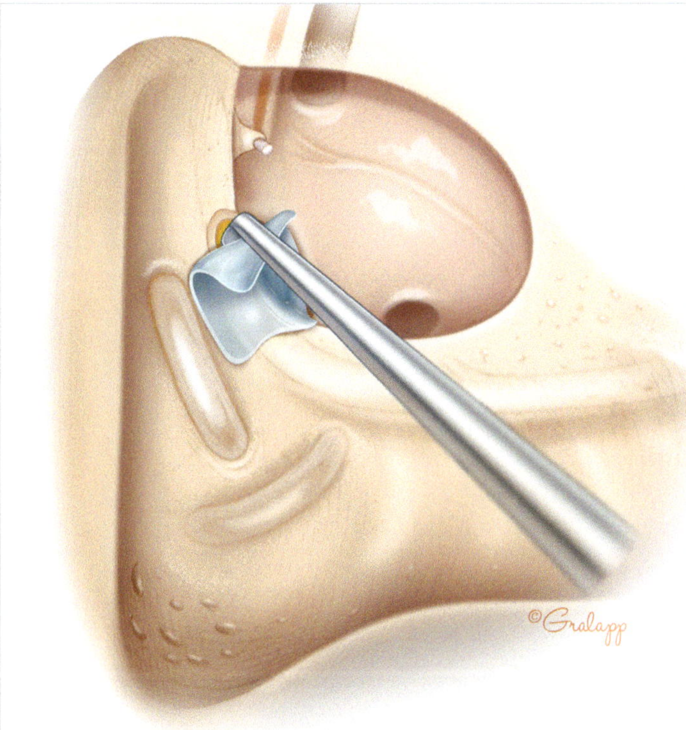

Fig. 8.80 Removal of the cholesteatoma matrix from the facial nerve with an intact fallopian canal.

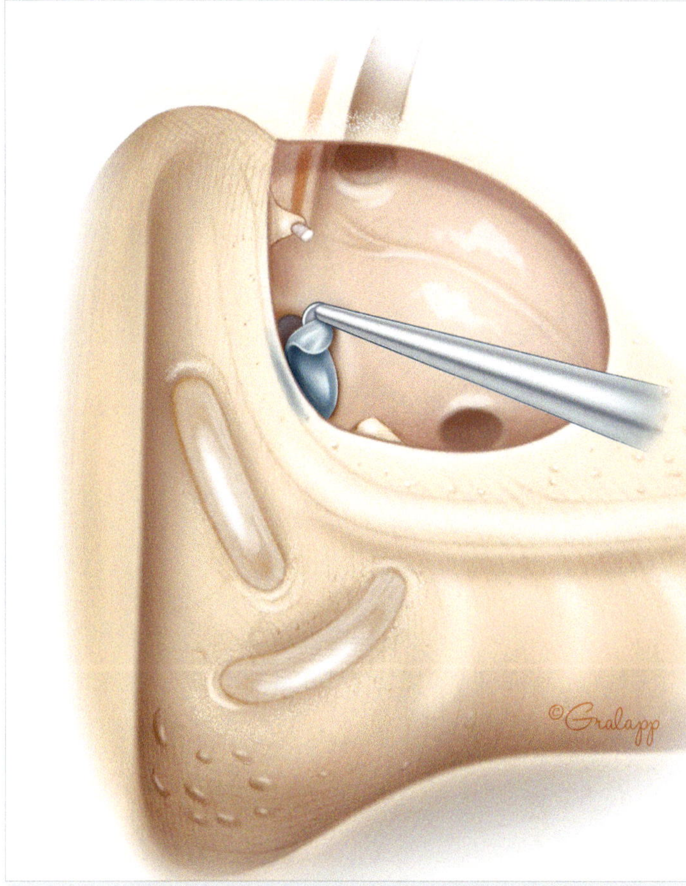

Fig. 8.81 Removal of the cholesteatoma matrix from the oval window is done gently to avoid dislocation of the footplate. An incudostapedial joint knife is a helpful instrument in this maneuver.

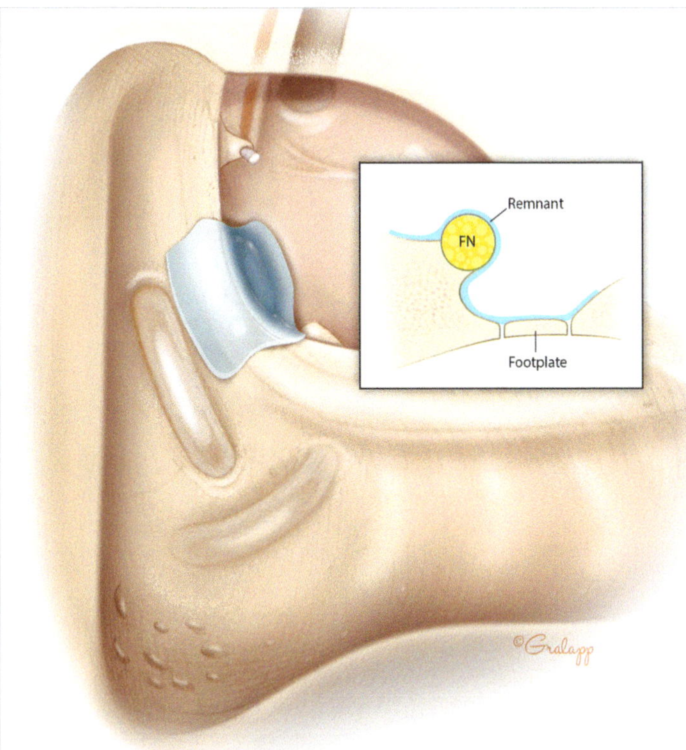

Fig. 8.82 Cholesteatoma erosion of the fallopian canal overlying the intratympanic segment of the facial nerve.

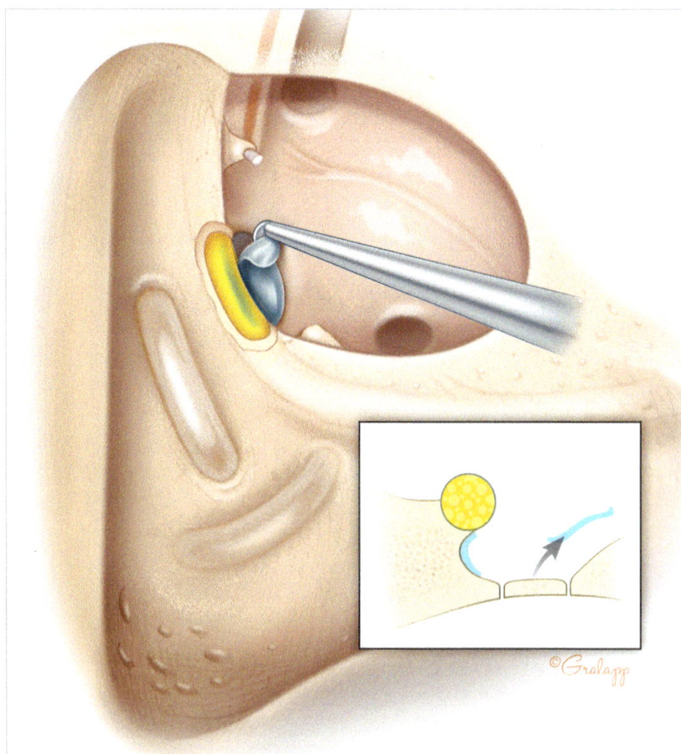

Fig. 8.83 Dissection of cholesteatoma from the stapes footplate using an incudostapedial joint knife. Note that matrix persists under the facial nerve where it is frequently dehiscent.

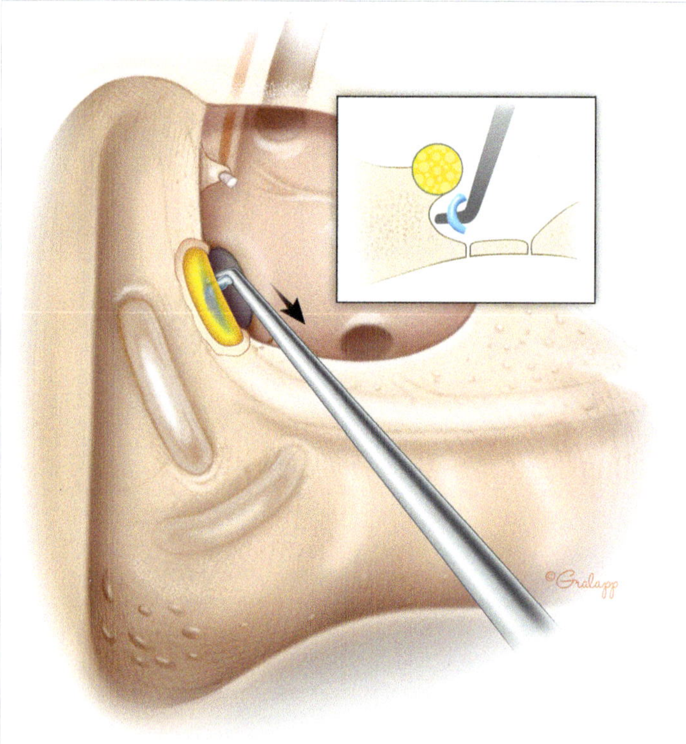

Fig. 8.84 Dissection of cholesteatoma from beneath a dehiscent facial nerve. This is a blind dissection which must be done delicately. The author uses a Crabtree dissector for this maneuver.

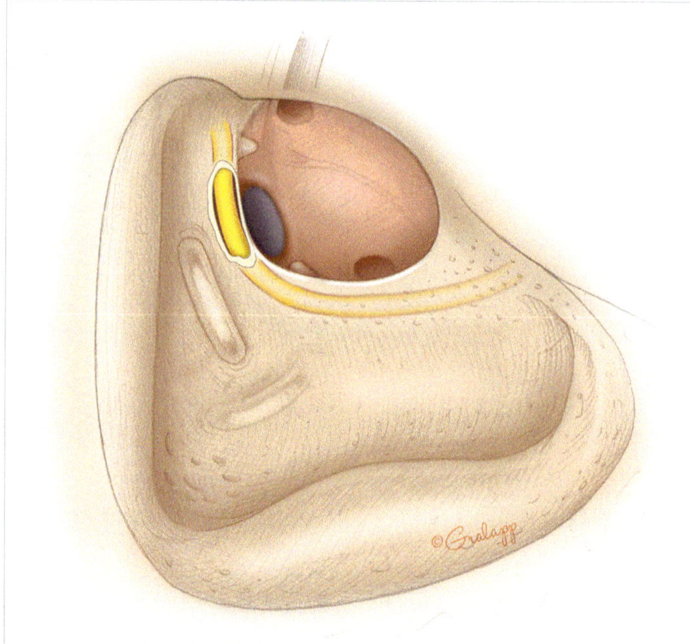

Fig. 8.85 Stapes footplate and dehiscent tympanic segment facial nerve following cholesteatoma removal.

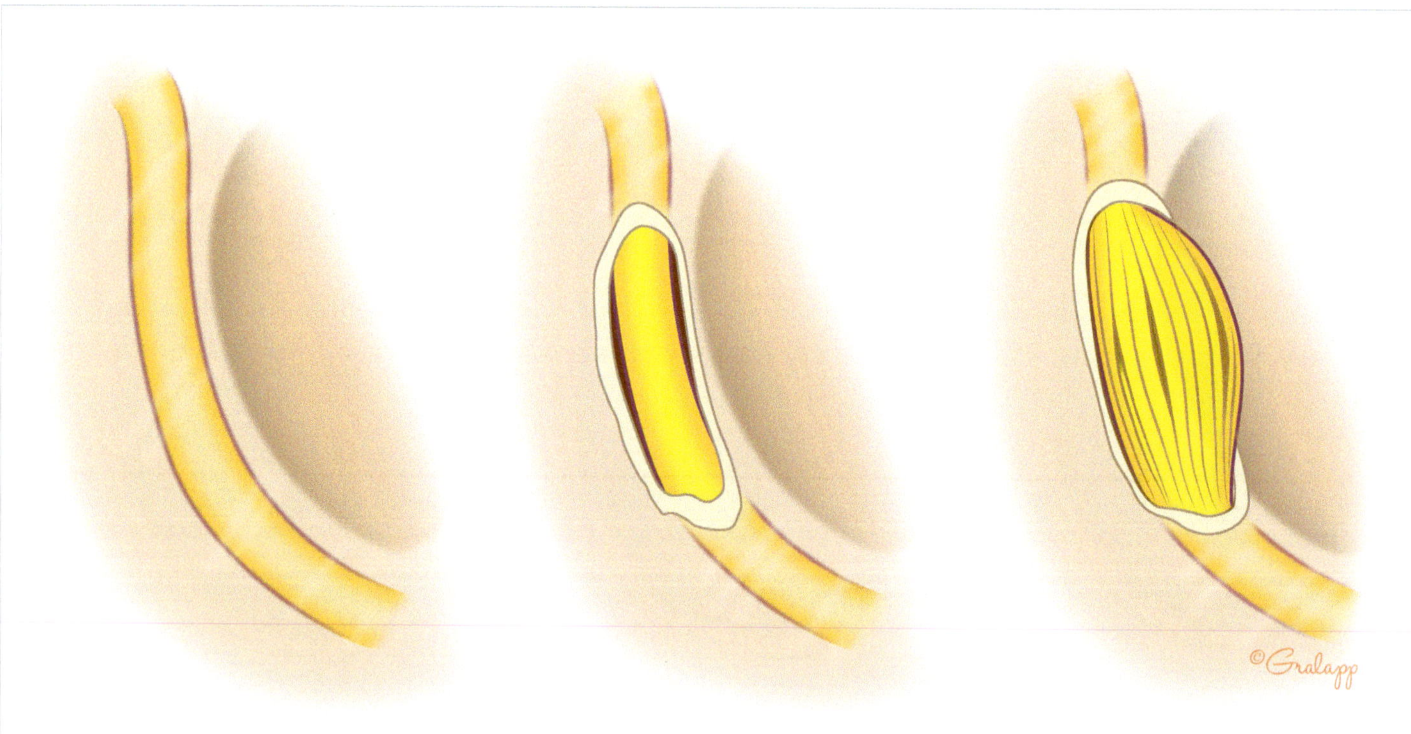

Fig. 8.86 In cholesteatoma, the facial nerve may lie under bone, be dehiscent (either congenitally or acquired due to cholesteatoma erosion) or protuberant. Great caution must be exercised in removing cholesteatoma from an extensively eroded facial nerve, especially when protuberant and/ or inflamed.

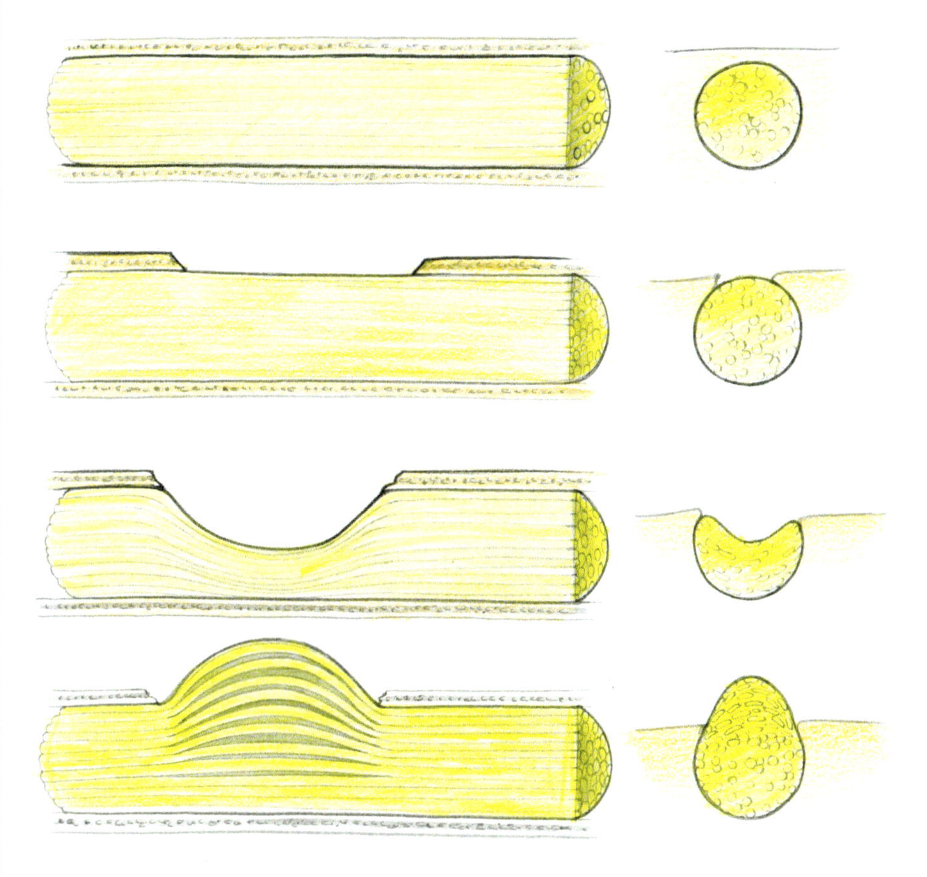

Fig. 8.87 In cholesteatoma, the facial nerve may lie under bone, be dehiscent (either congenitally or acquired due to cholesteatoma erosion), compressed, or protuberant.

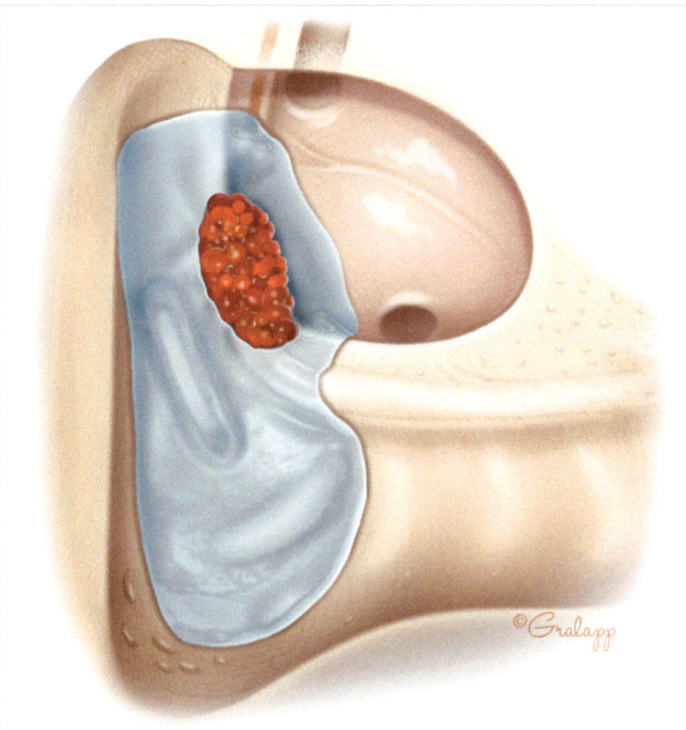

Fig. 8.88 Inflamed granulation tissue associated with cholesteatoma obscuring the oval window and facial nerve.

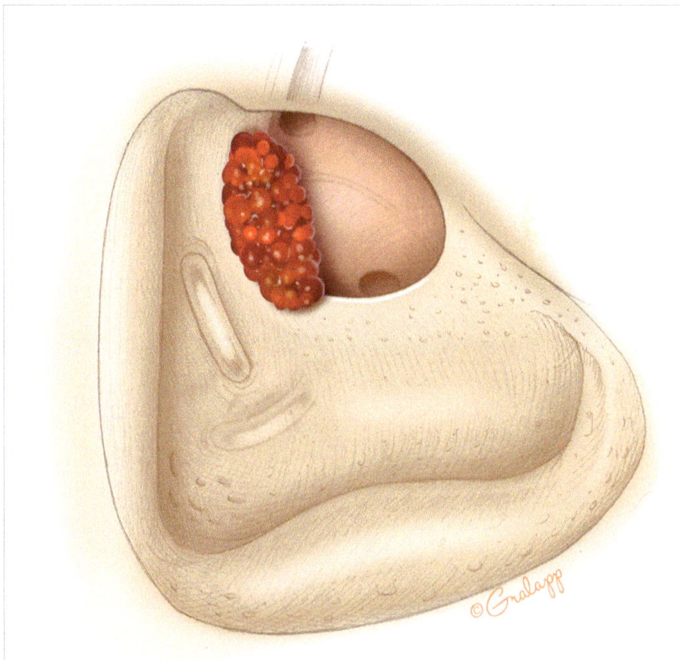

Fig. 8.89 Inflamed granulation tissue in noncholesteatoma chronic otitis media obscuring the oval window and facial nerve.

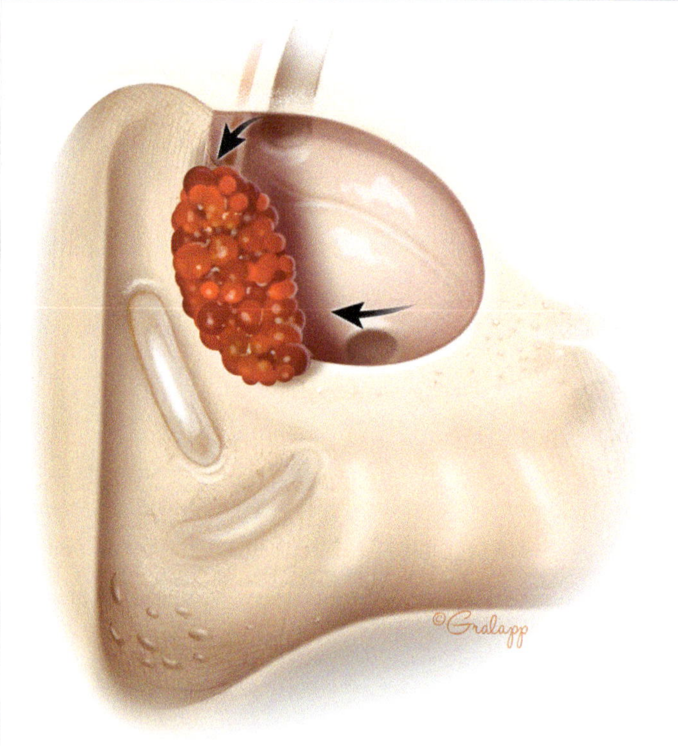

Fig. 8.90 Achieving orientation to the facial nerve by approaching the oval window from inferior to superior and the cochleariform process from anteriorly.

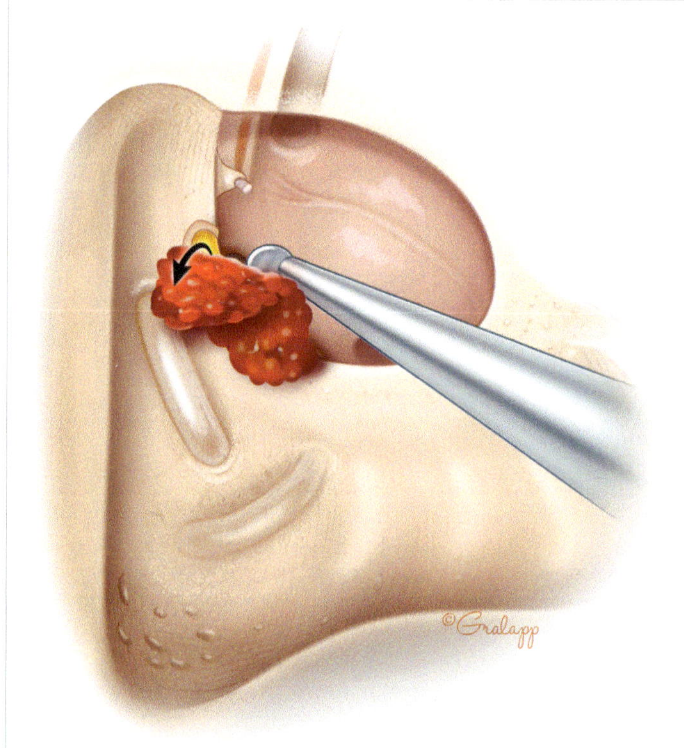

Fig. 8.91 Cautiously removing granulation tissue from an exposed facial nerve. If the dissection proves difficult or complex, it is better to stage the procedure and return once the inflammation has abated.

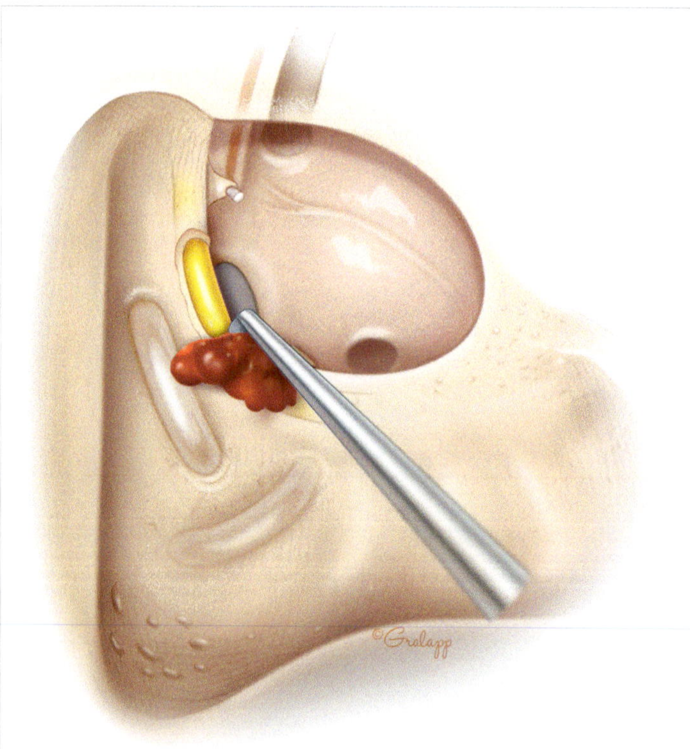

Fig. 8.92 If the plane between the epineurium and granulation tissue is obscure, best not to proceed. Granulation tissue often regresses when the disease has been ameliorated. Similarly, if the nerve appears swollen and protuberant, best to stage the procedure.

8.8 Sinus Tympani and Facial Recess in Cholesteatoma

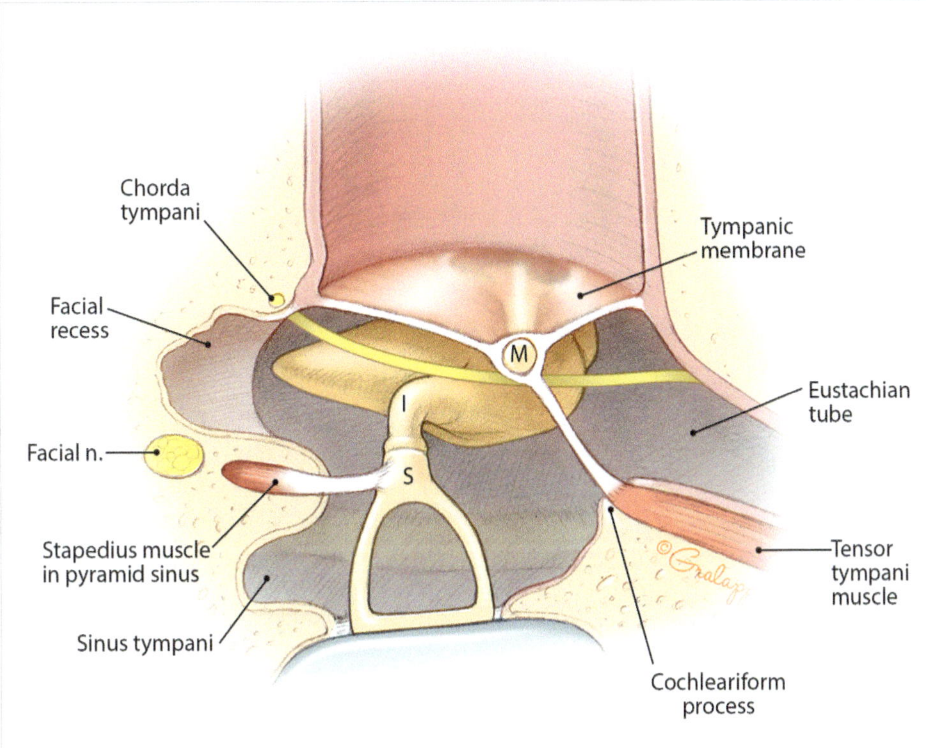

Fig. 8.93 Details of the posterior mesotympanic spaces (facial recess and sinus tympani). (Used with permission from Jackler RK. The surgical anatomy of cholesteatoma. *Otolaryngol Clin NA* 1989;22:883–896.)

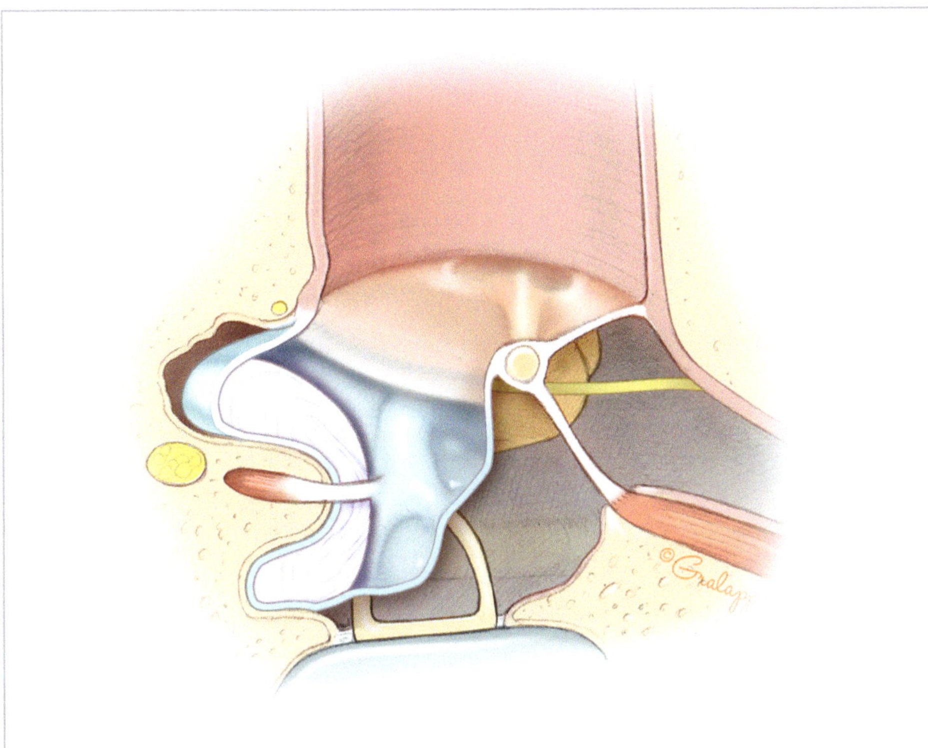

Fig. 8.94 Cholesteatoma involving the posterior mesotympanic spaces (facial recess and sinus tympani). The long process of the incus and stapes superstructure is frequently eroded. (Used with permission from Jackler RK. The surgical anatomy of cholesteatoma. *Otolaryngol Clin NA* 1989;22:883–896.)

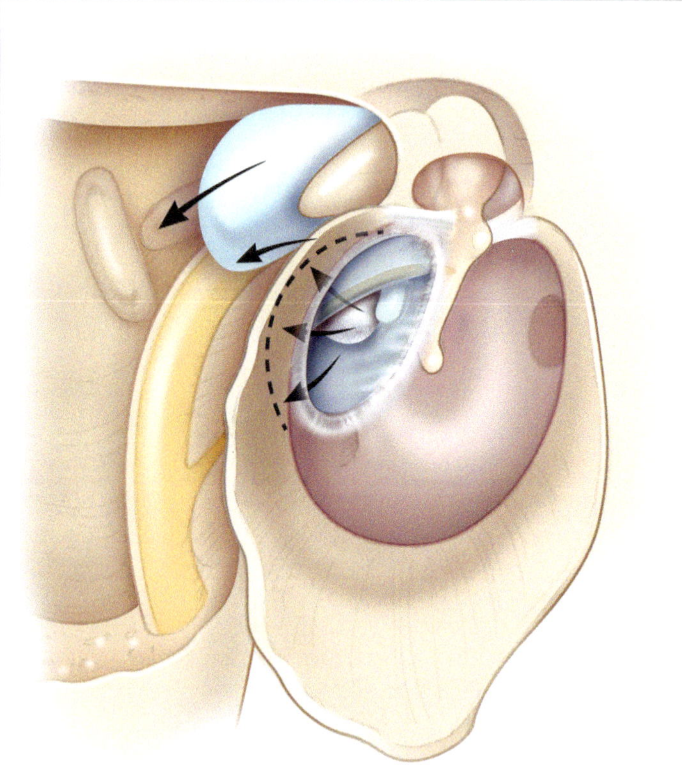

Fig. 8.95 Posterior mesotympanic cholesteatoma illustrating the pathways to the mastoid and middle ear. The three arrows in the posterior middle ear illustrate penetration of the facial recess and sinus tympani. (Used with permission from Jackler RK. The surgical anatomy of cholesteatoma. *Otolaryngol Clin NA* 1989;22:883–896.)

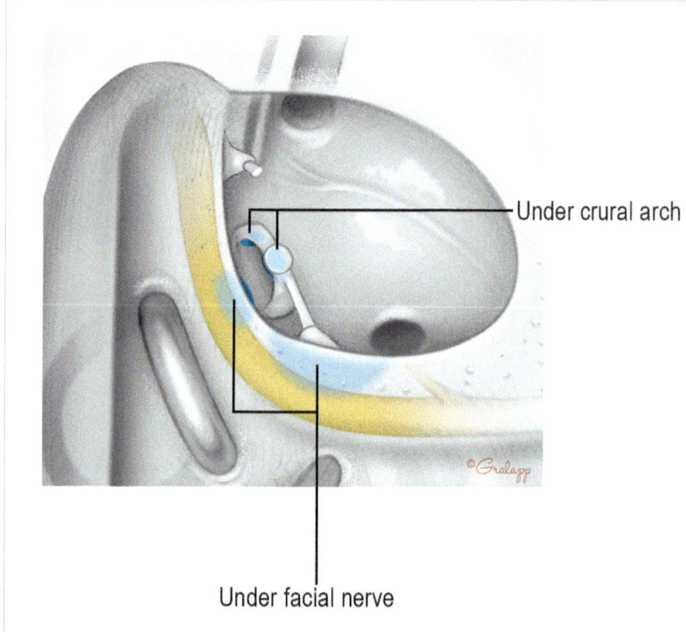

Fig. 8.96 The most common sites of residual cholesteatoma following surgery are under the tympanic segment of the facial nerve, in relation to the stapes and oval window, and in the posterior middle ear spaces (facial recess and sinus tympani).

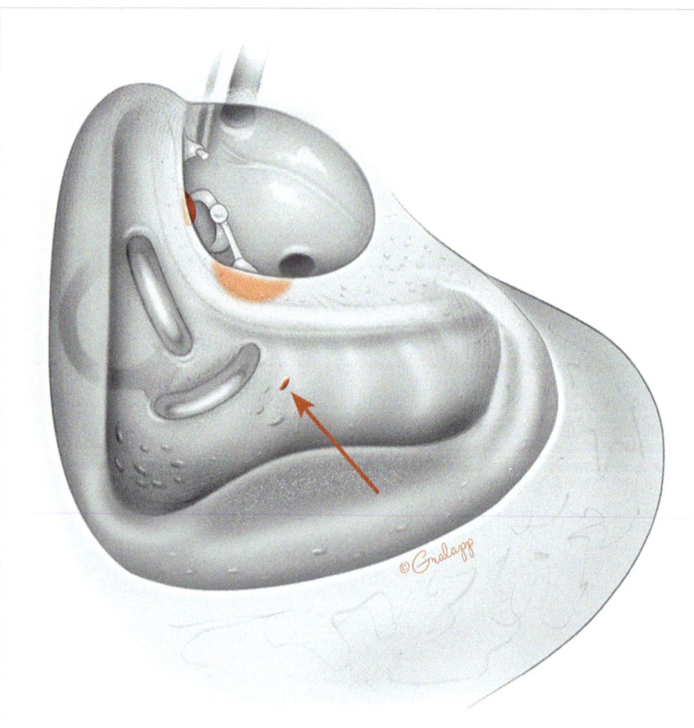

Fig. 8.97 Residual cholesteatoma in a perilabyrinthine cell tract. This is generally present when cholesteatoma invades a well-pneumatized mastoid. As most cholesteatomas occur in poorly pneumatized mastoids, this location for residual is not common.

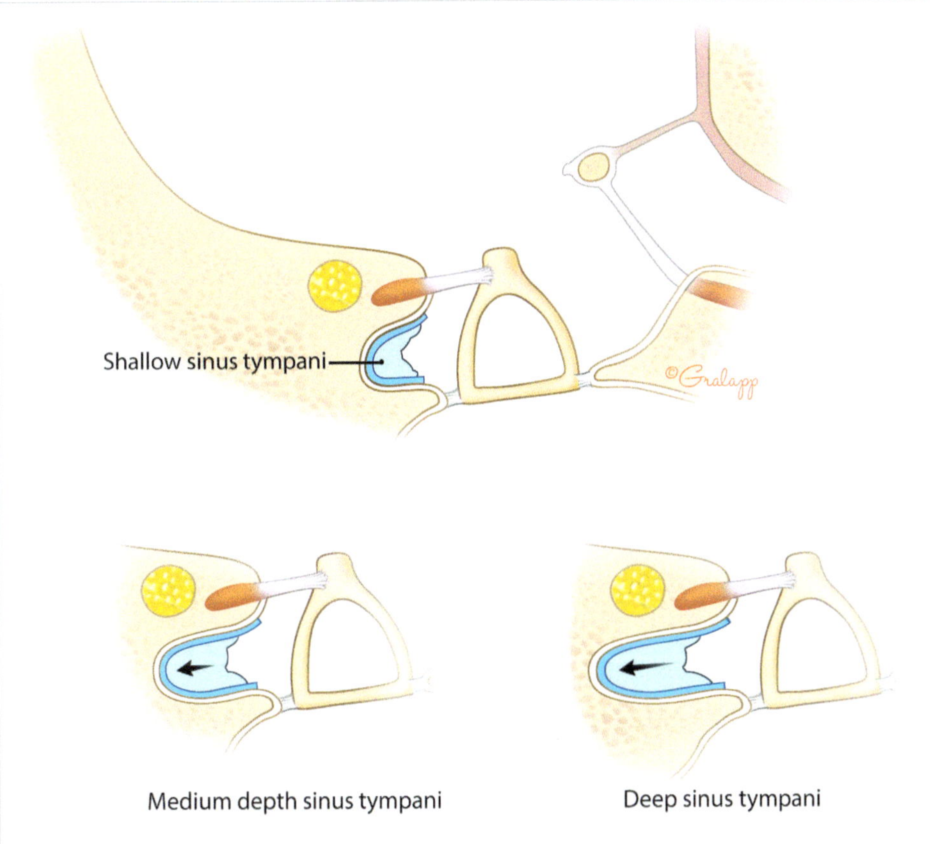

Fig. 8.98 The sinus tympani is of variable depth; it may be shallow or extend posterior to the facial nerve.

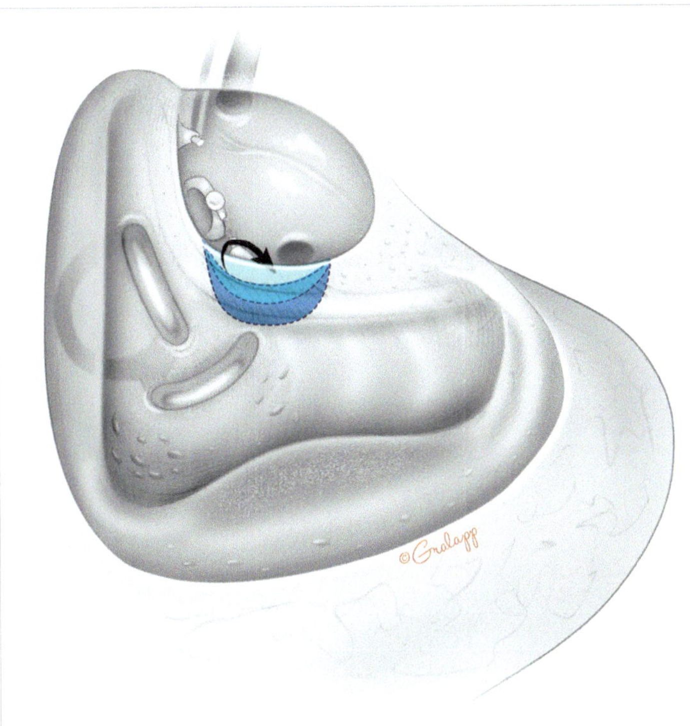

Fig. 8.99 The sinus tympani is of variable depth; it may be shallow or extend posterior to the facial nerve. Note that the recess spans roughly from the oval to the round window.

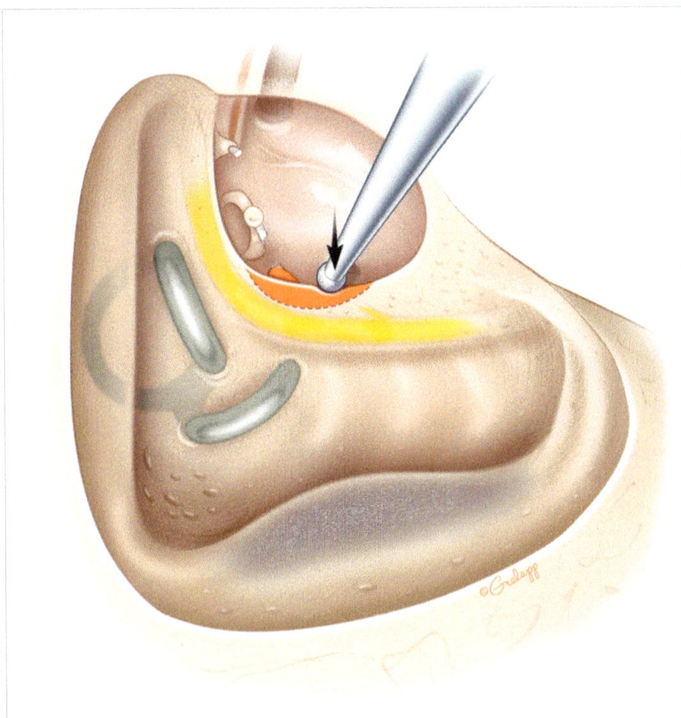

Fig. 8.100 Removing the bone from the posterior annular groove and pyramid (origin of the stapedius muscle) can shallow the sinus tympani and improve access for disease removal.

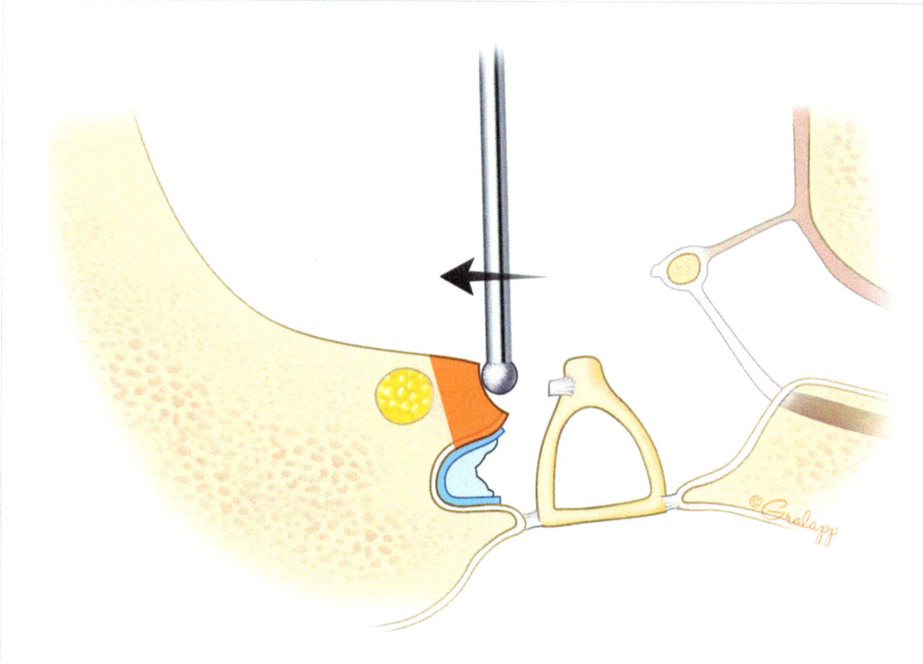

Fig. 8.101 Removing the bone from the posterior annular groove can shallow the sinus tympani and improve access for disease removal.

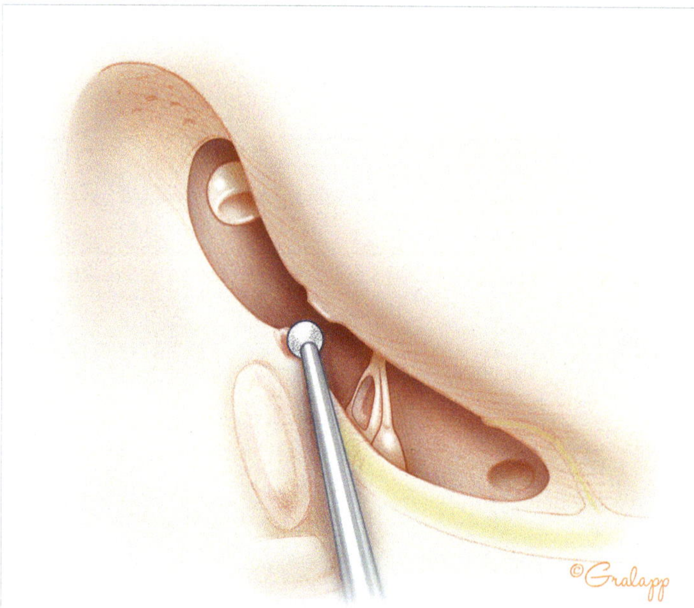

Fig. 8.102 In intact canal wall procedures, cholesteatoma in the facial recess can be removed via the mastoid using a facial recess approach. In canal wall down procedures, the facial recess lateral wall is removed and thus is it readily accessible.

8.9 Anterior Epitympanic Cholesteatoma

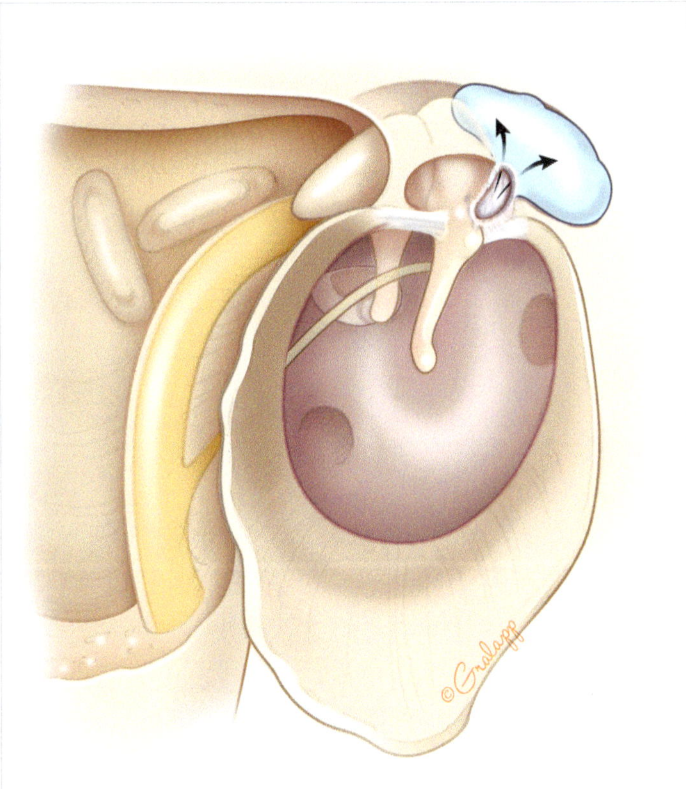

Fig. 8.103 Anterior epitympanic cholesteatoma penetrates anterior to the malleus head and can involve the anterior tympanic segment of the facial nerve. (Used with permission from Jackler RK. The surgical anatomy of cholesteatoma. *Otolaryngol Clin NA* 1989;22:883–896.)

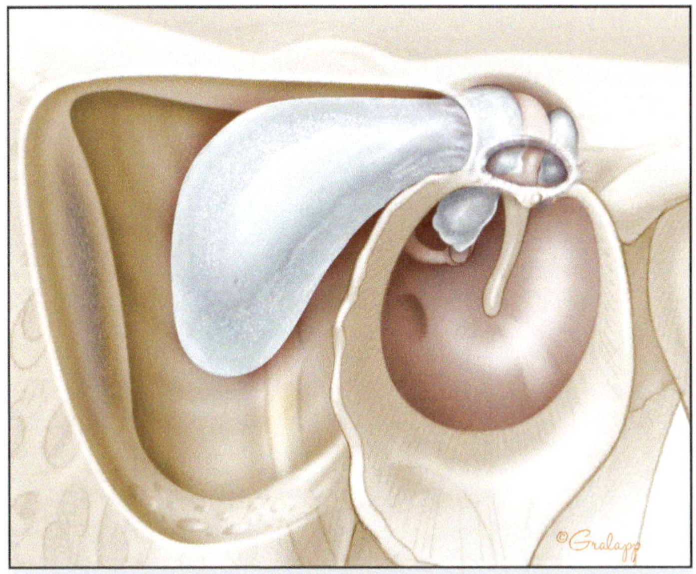

Fig. 8.104 Anterior epitympanic cholesteatoma may occur in isolation, but often occurs concurrently with a posterior epitympanic cholesteatoma.

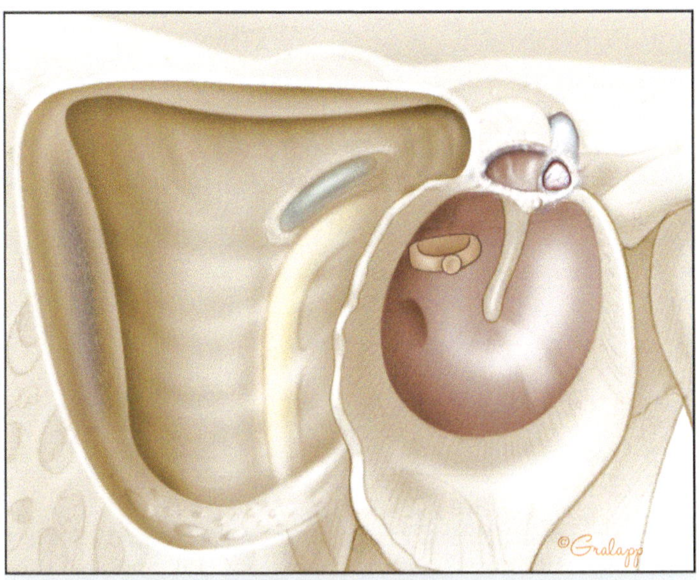

Fig. 8.105 Following resection of the posterior epitympanic cholesteatoma, it is important to open the epitympanum fully to afford visibility anterior to the malleus head to identify potential anterior epitympanic cholesteatoma.

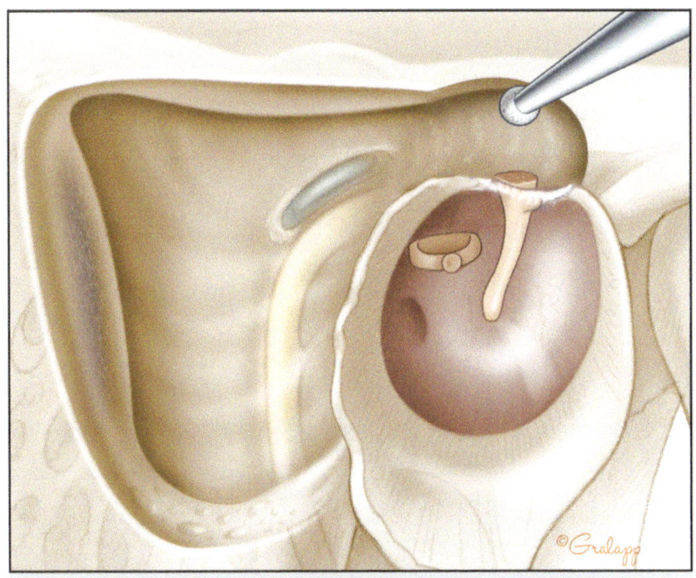

Fig. 8.106 Exposing anterior to the malleus head to identify and remove anterior epitympanic cholesteatoma. Note that the malleus head has been resected. The cog, a bony septum suspended from the tegmen tympani separating the anterior from posterior epitympanum, is also removed.

8.10 Semicircular Canal Fistula in Cholesteatoma

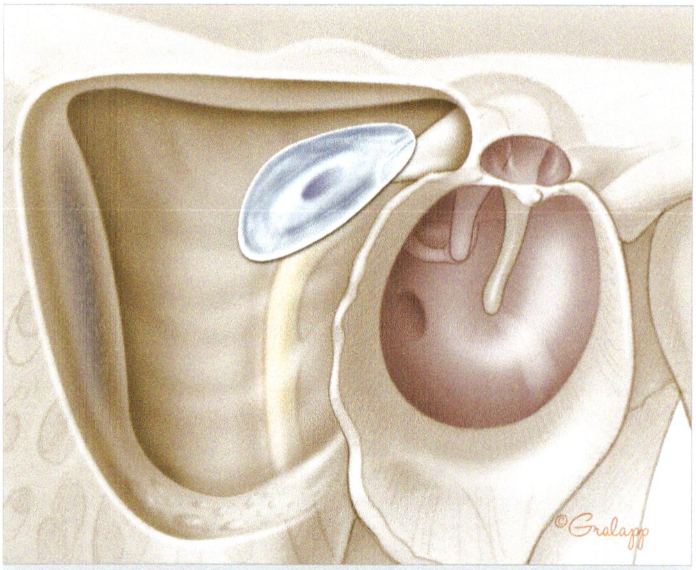

Fig. 8.107 Cholesteatoma matrix on a lateral semicircular canal fistula. Management options include resection of the matrix or exteriorization via canal wall down procedure.

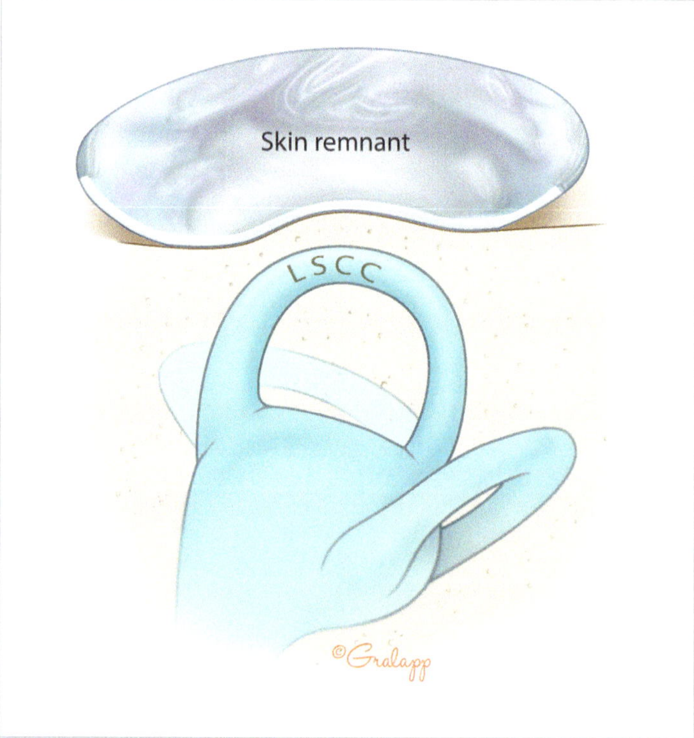

Fig. 8.108 Cholesteatoma overlying the lateral semicircular canal without erosion. As the otic capsule is the hardest bone in the body, semicircular canal erosion occurs only in advanced cholesteatoma with substantial bone erosion expanding the mastoid antrum. Fistulas are more common in poorly pneumatized temporal bones, as the dense lateral bone directs force medially to the otic capsule. LSCC, lateral semicircular canal.

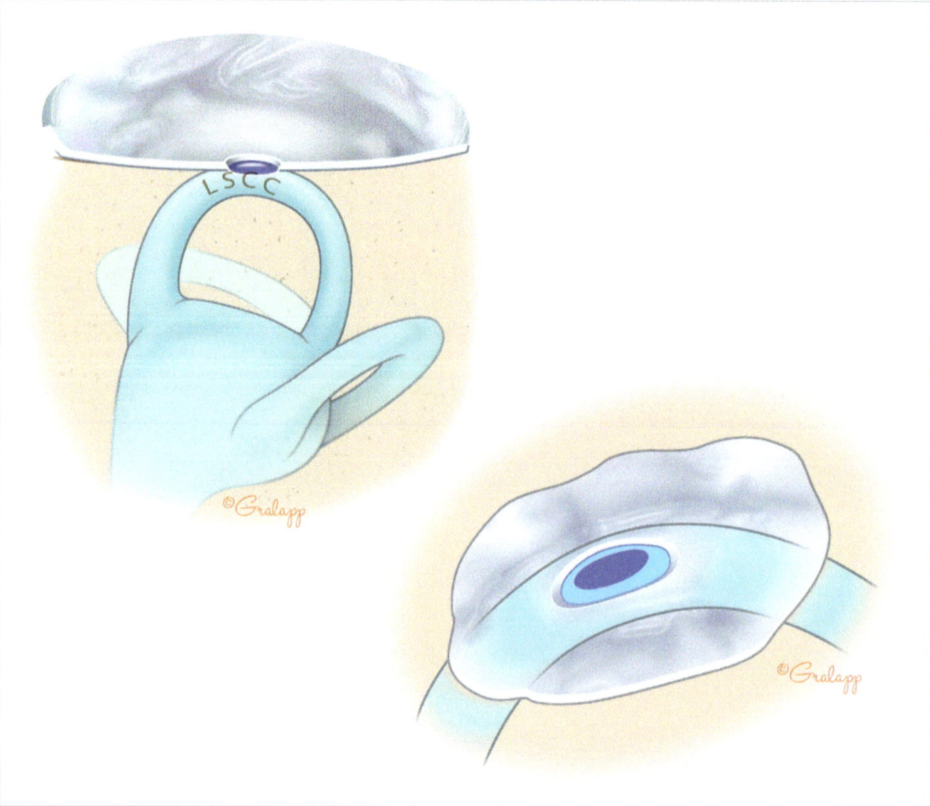

Fig. 8.109 When cholesteatoma erodes the lateral semicircular canal, a small fistula is most commonly encountered and the canal's endosteum remains intact. Whenever a semicircular canal fistula occurs, extra care should be taken in addressing the tympanic segment of the facial nerve, as its bony wall is also often eroded. LSCC, lateral semicircular canal.

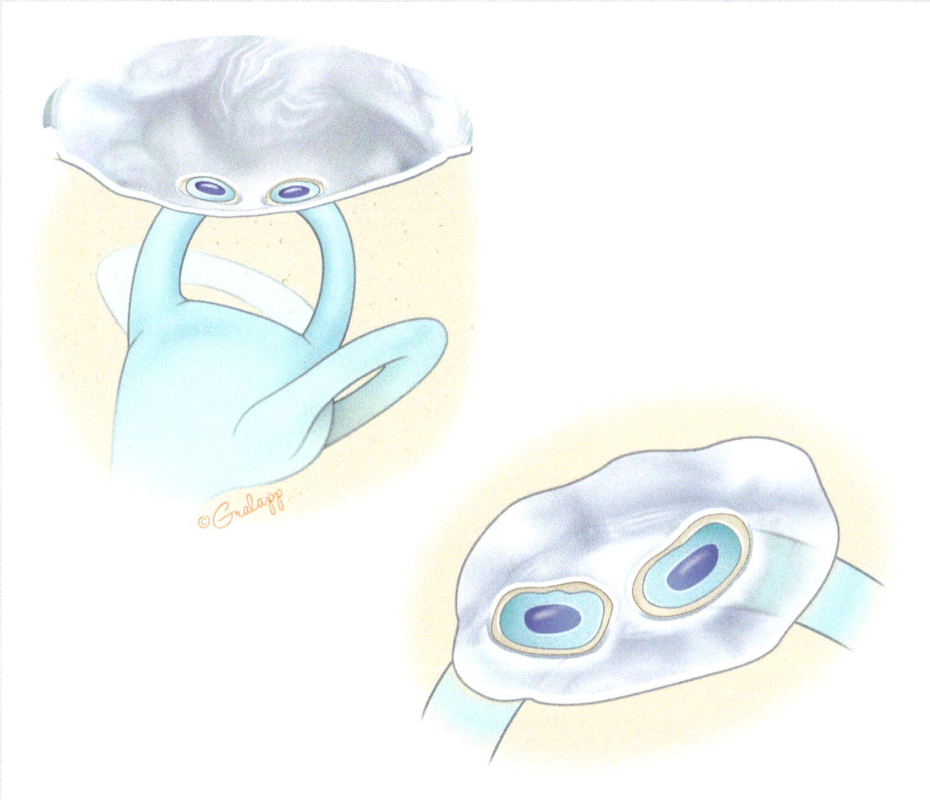

Fig. 8.110 In cholesteatoma erosion of a semicircular canal with a large fistula, the lumen may be entered upon resection of the matrix with increased risk of vertigo and sensory hearing loss. When the endosteum is breached, the lumen must be carefully sealed.

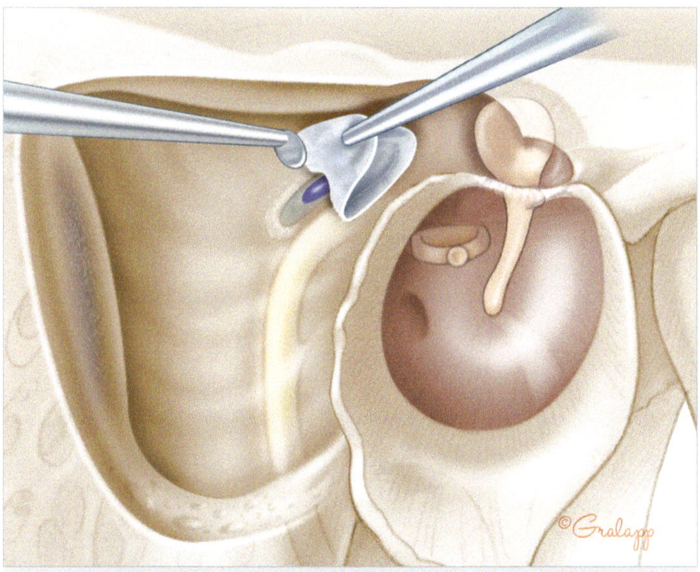

Fig. 8.111 Removing cholesteatoma matrix on a lateral semicircular canal fistula. If the overlying matrix is not inflamed, then usually it can be removed from the intact semicircular canal endosteum with gentle dissection.

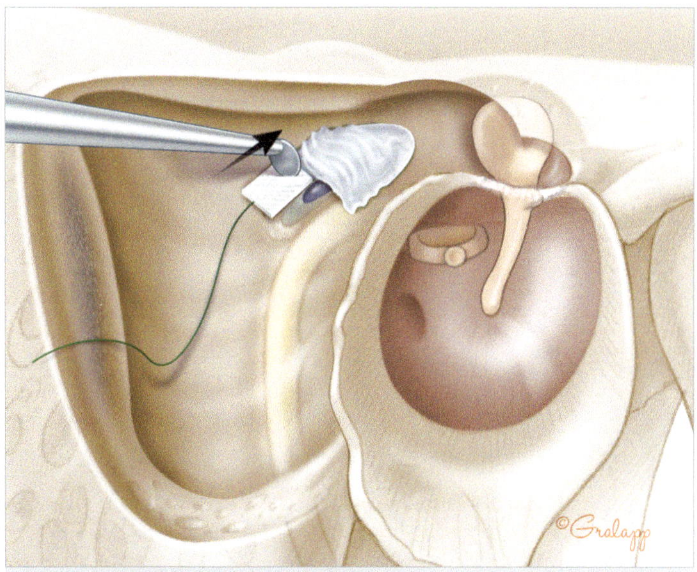

Fig. 8.112 Removing cholesteatoma matrix on a lateral semicircular canal fistula with a cottonoid patty.

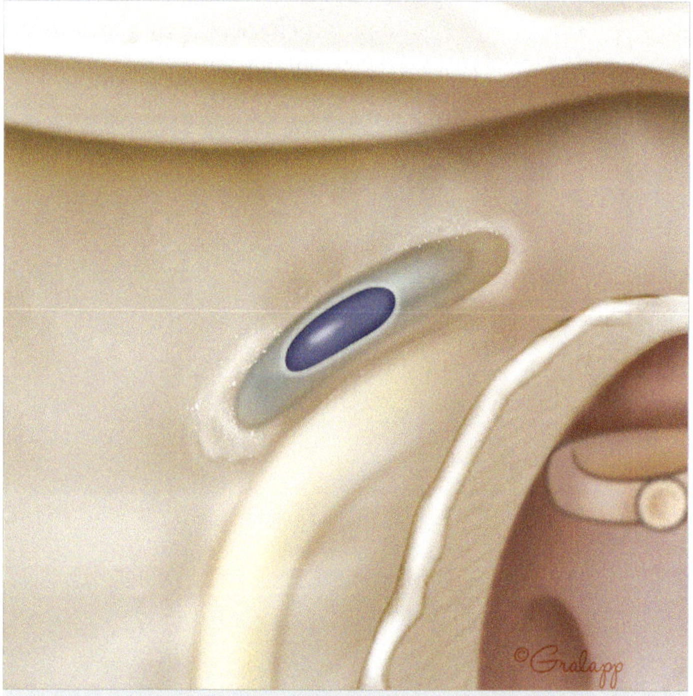

Fig. 8.113 Lateral semicircular canal fistula with intact endosteum.

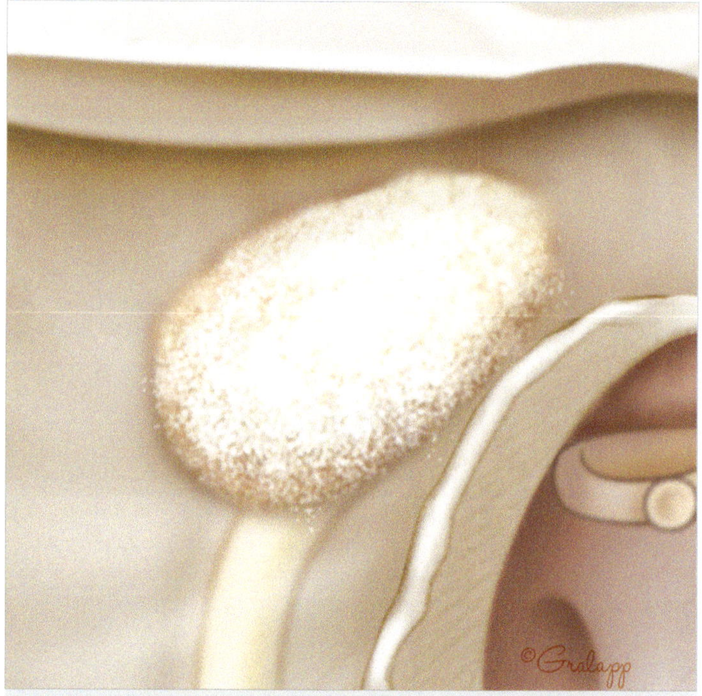

Fig. 8.114 Lateral semicircular canal fistula covered with bone paté.

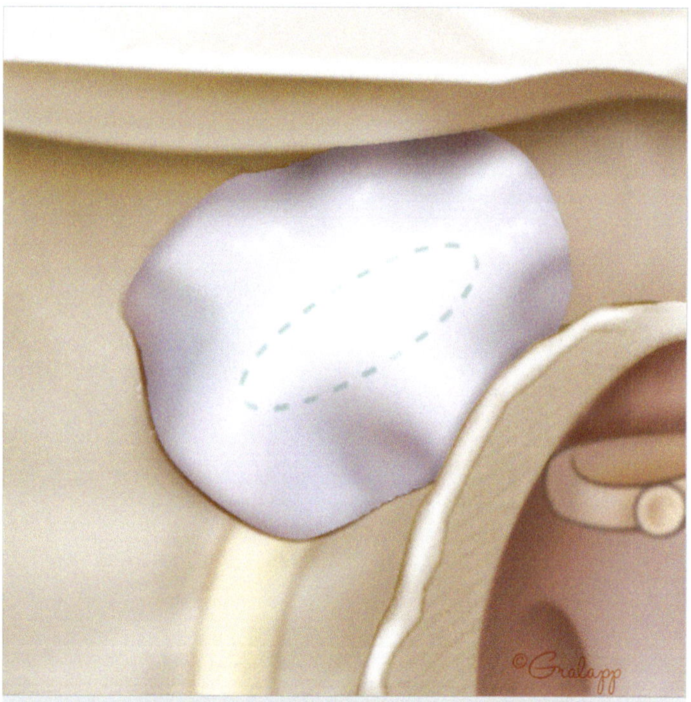

Fig. 8.115 Repair of lateral semicircular canal fistula with bone paté covered with fascia.

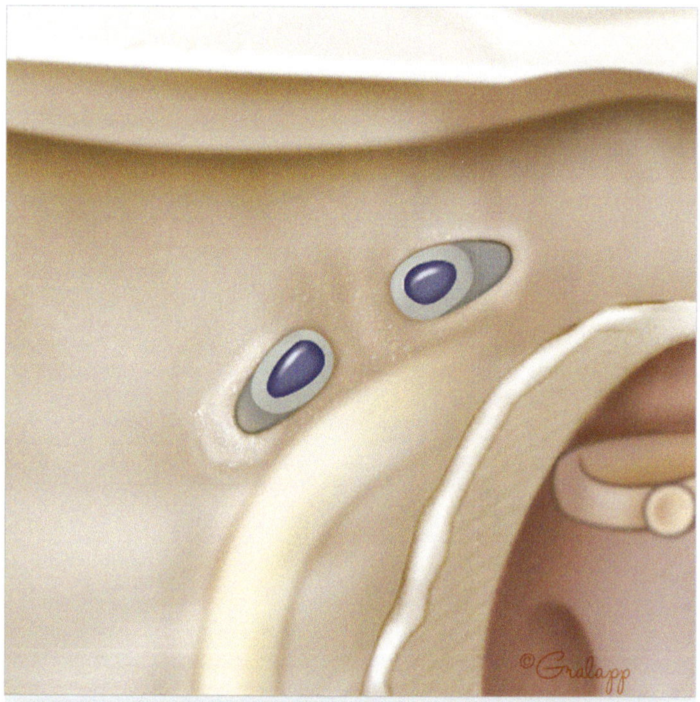

Fig. 8.116 Extensive, lateral, semicircular canal fistula disrupting canal integrity. This may be due to either cholesteatoma or inadvertent drill injury.

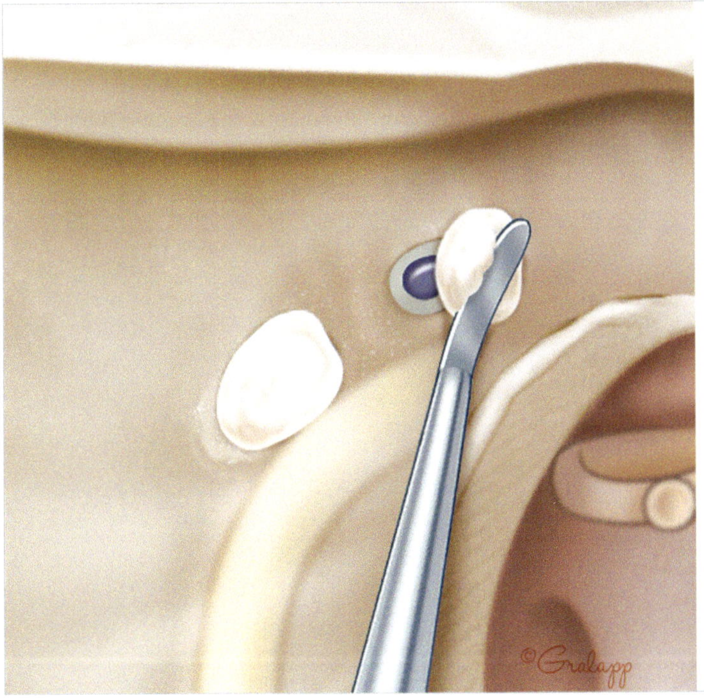

Fig. 8.117 A transected semicircular canal should be sealed. Illustration depicts bone wax plugging. Should the lumen be entered, it is important to avoid use of potentially ototoxic ear drops on the packing.

8.11 Ossicles in Cholesteatoma

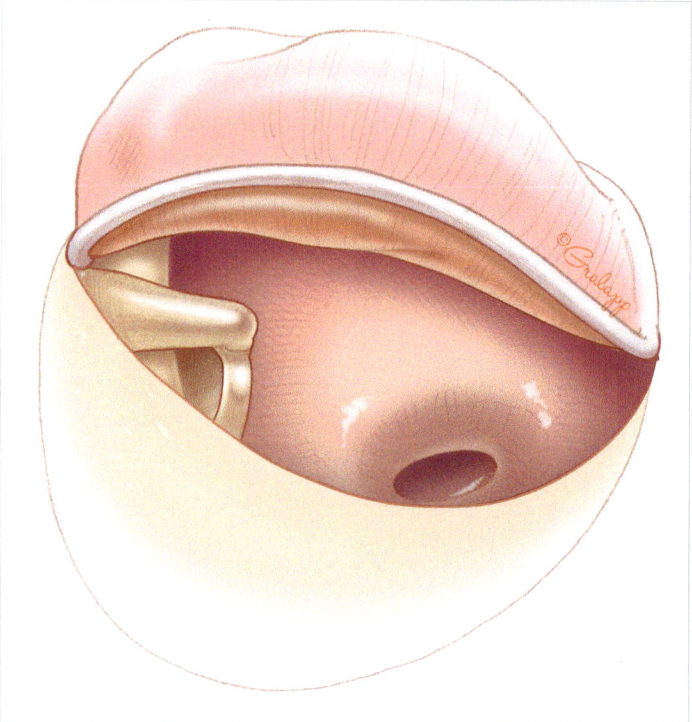

Fig. 8.118 Exposure of the stapes in cholesteatoma surgery often requires removal of a portion of the scutum. As weakening the bony support of the epitympanum by enlarging the epitympanic defect is not desirable in epitympanic cholesteatoma, the smallest amount of bone removal is desirable. This may be facilitated by use of endoscopic assistance.

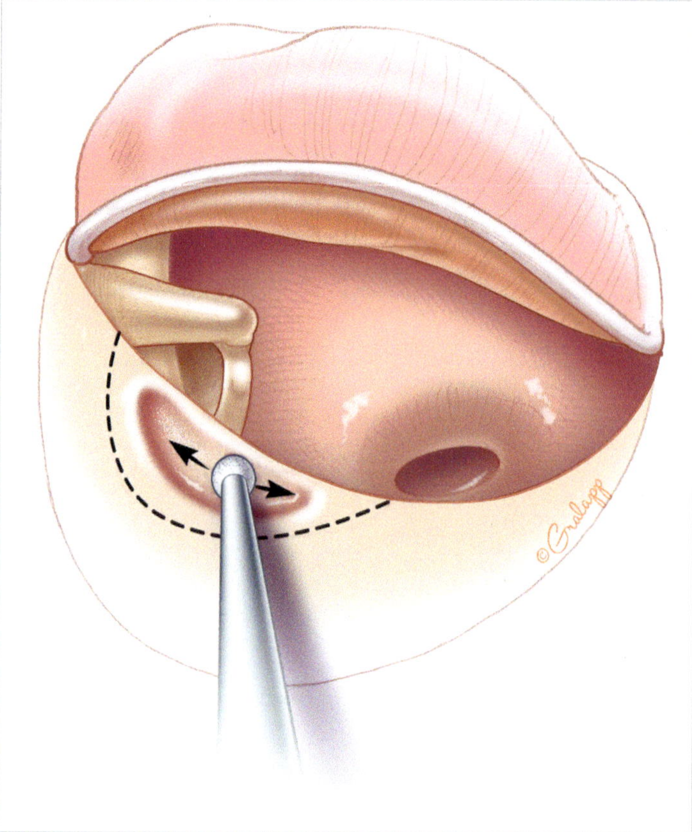

Fig. 8.119 Exposure of the stapes in cholesteatoma surgery often requires removal of a portion of the scutum.

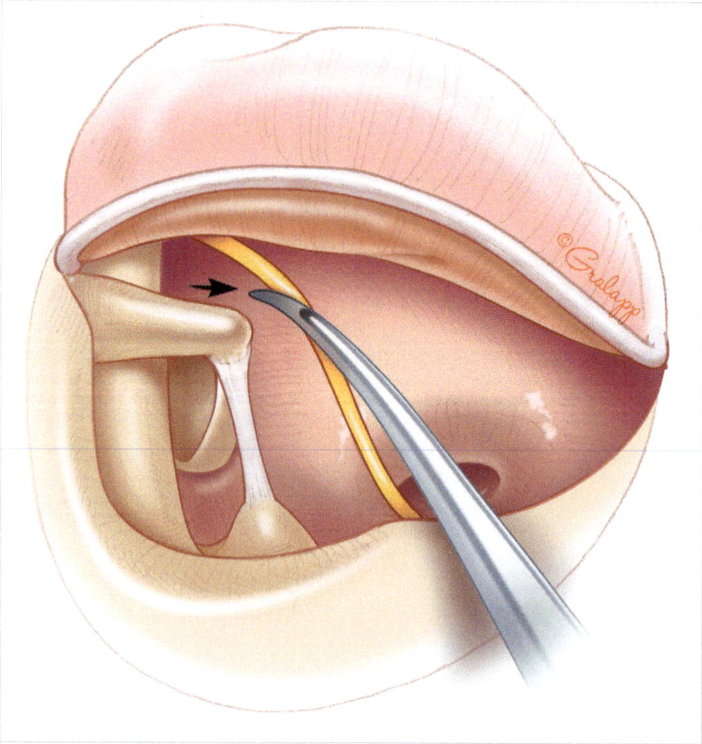

Fig. 8.120 View of the stapes and facial nerve obtained after scutum removal. As removal of disease in this location requires delicacy, obtaining optimal visualization is important.

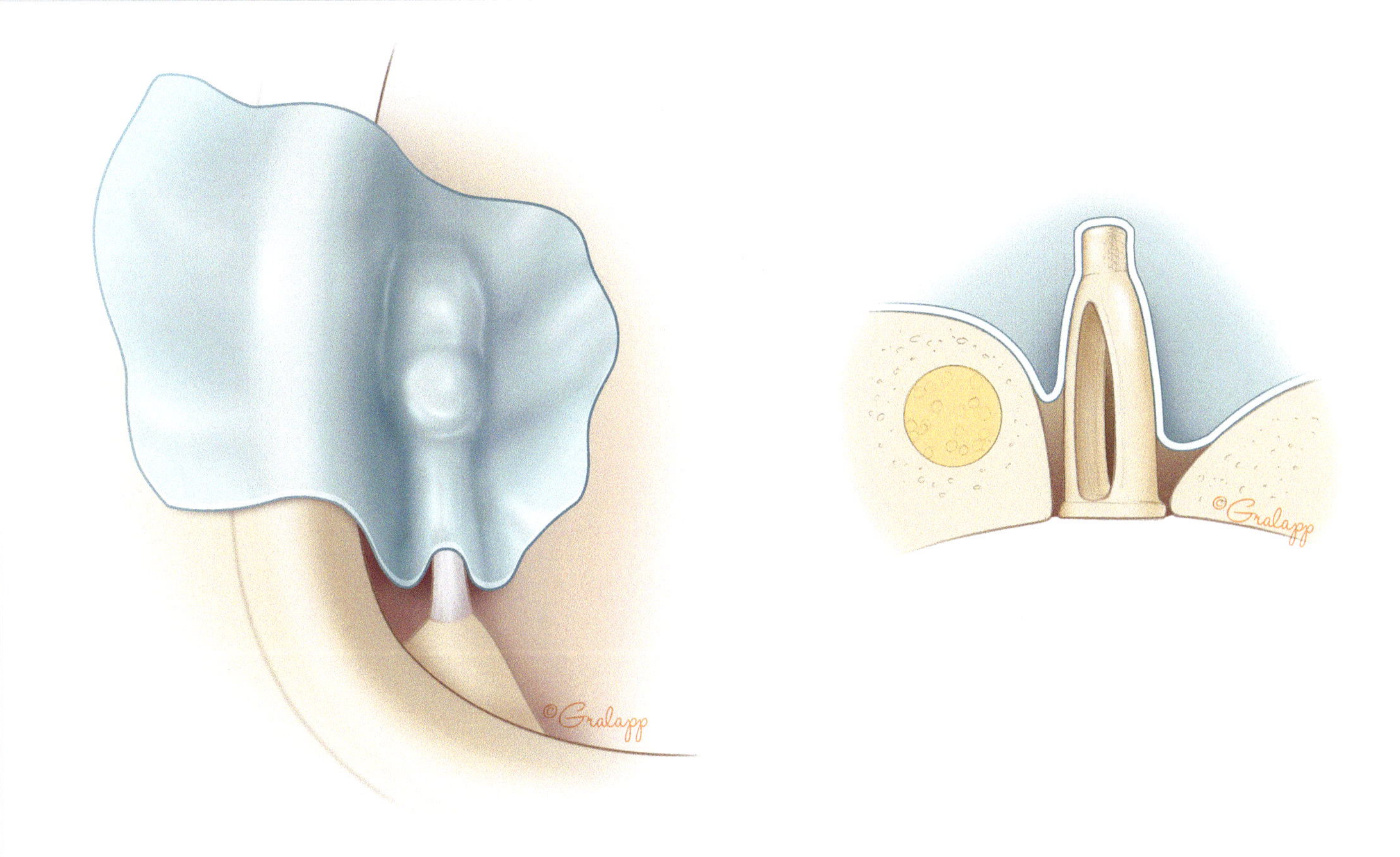

Fig. 8.121 Cholesteatoma matrix wrapping the stapes superstructure and facial nerve is a common finding.

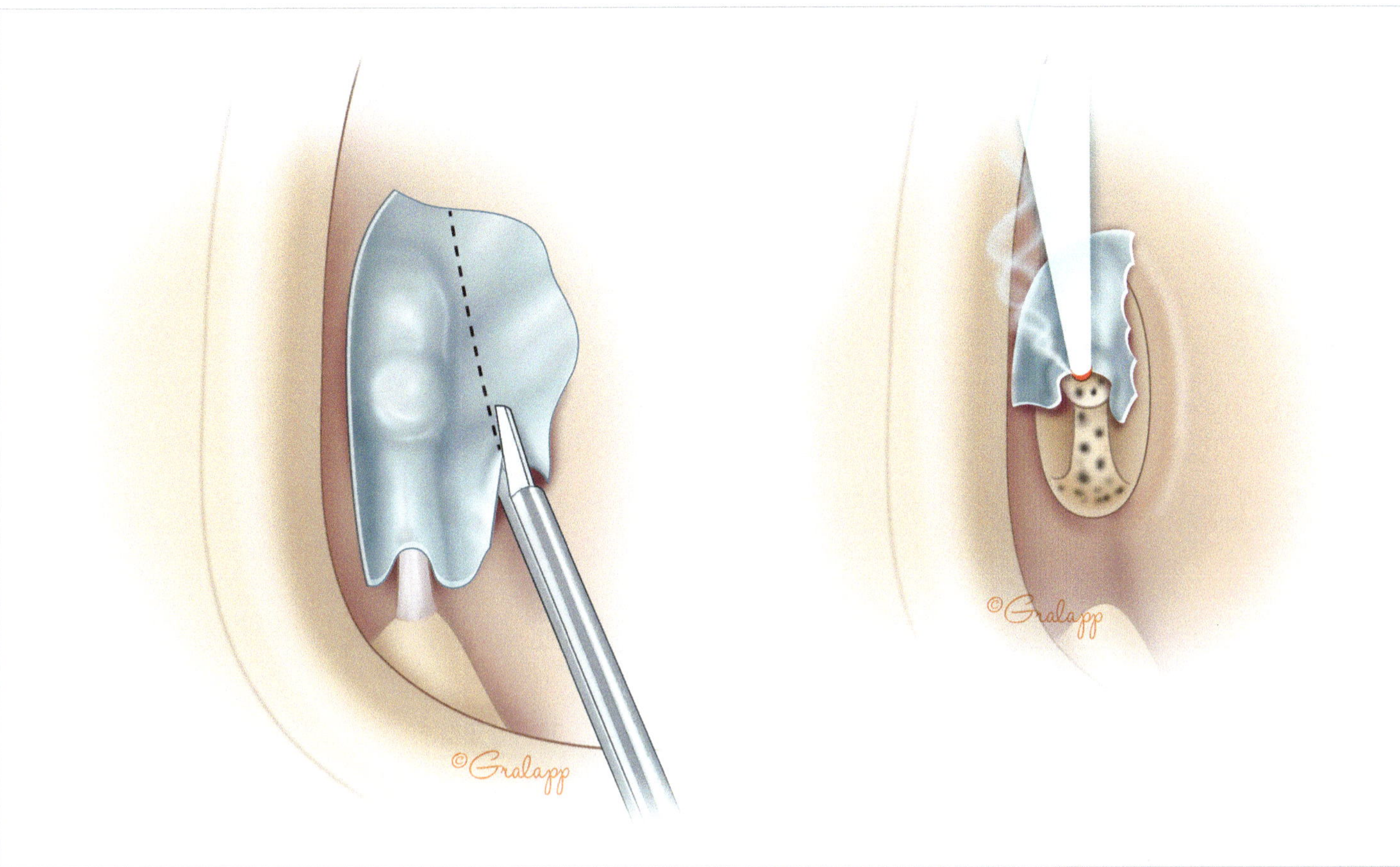

Fig. 8.122 Microsurgical trimming cholesteatoma matrix followed by laser vaporization of the portion adherent to the stapes superstructure. Use of the laser minimizes vibratory trauma to the inner ear. Due to the proximity of the facial nerve, periodic irrigation is important to reduce thermal impact which could injure the nerve.

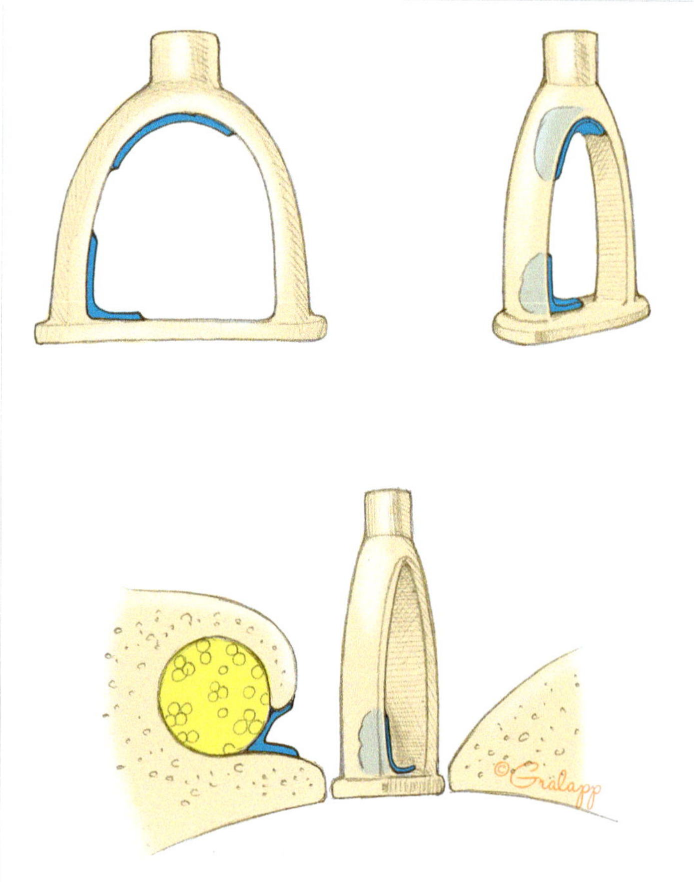

Fig. 8.123 Matrix may adhere under the arch or be tucked into the crural feet of the stapes.

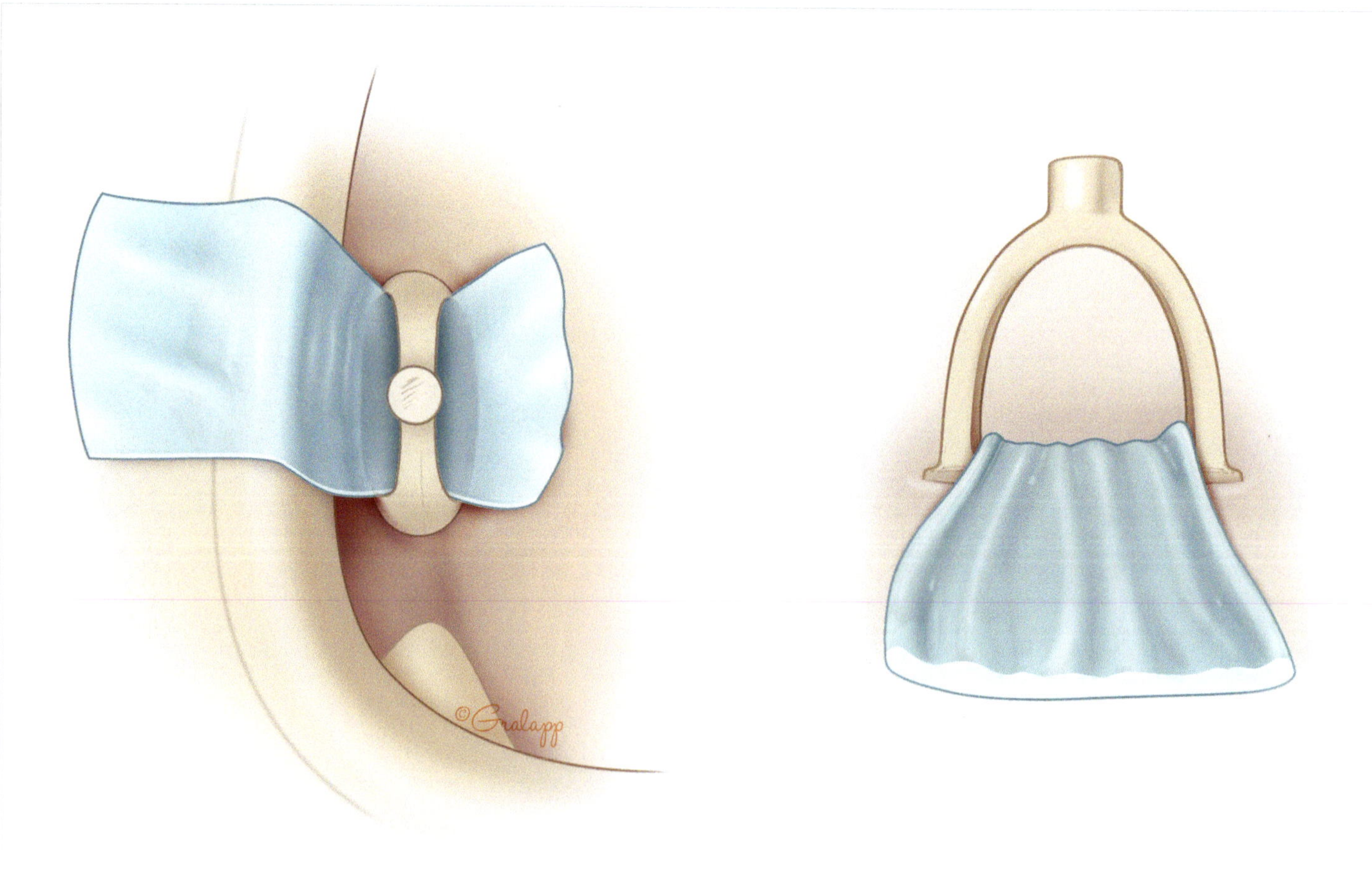

Fig. 8.124 Cholesteatoma matrix under an intact stapes arch creates a technical challenge.

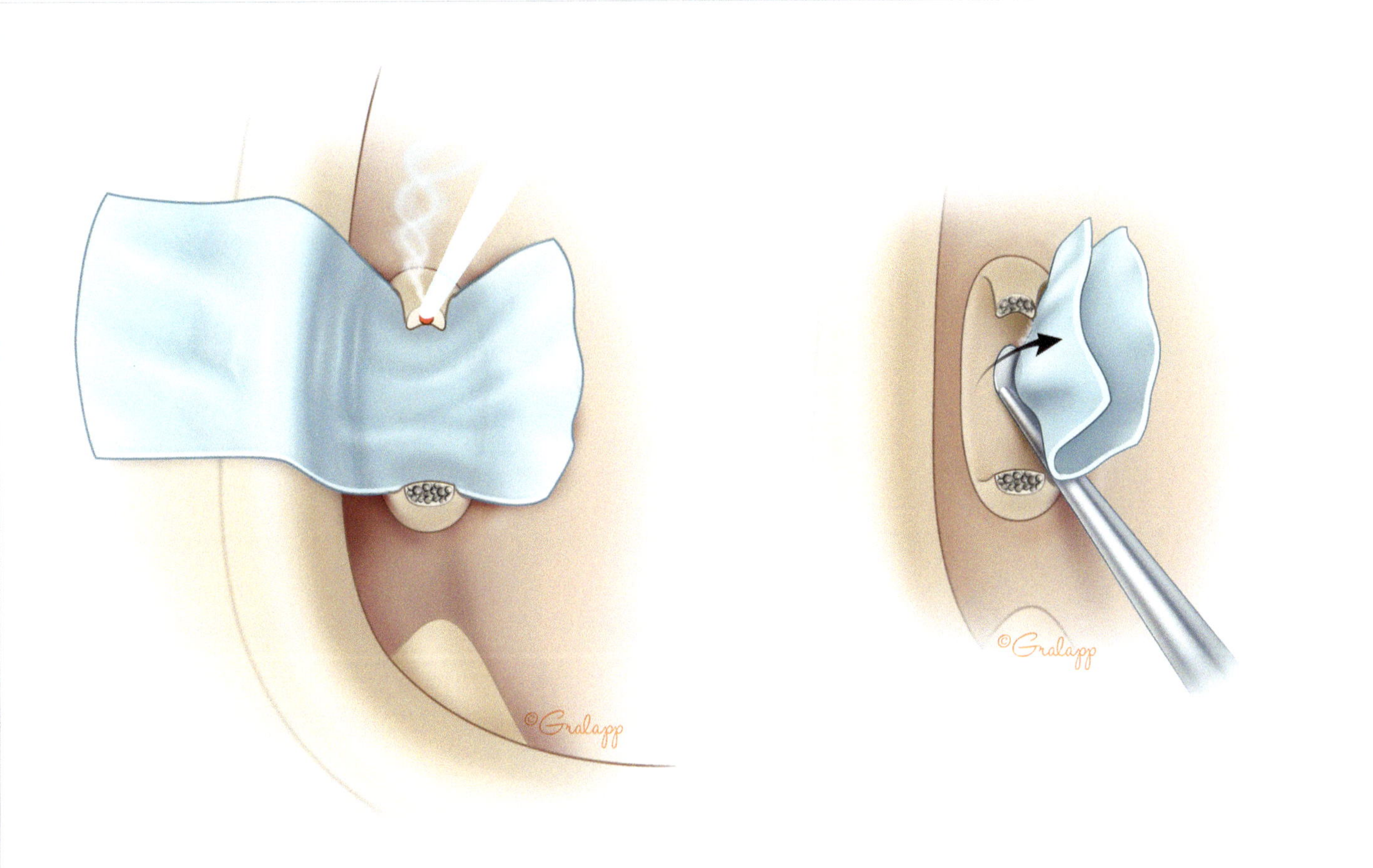

Fig. 8.125 Laser removal of the stapes superstructure, leaving a high anterior crus to employ in ossicular reconstruction, enables microdissection of matrix from the footplate.

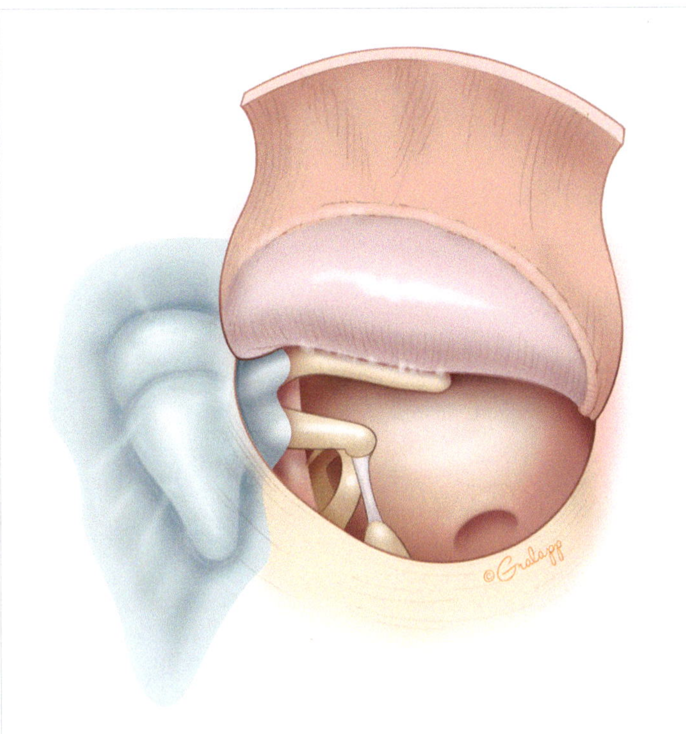

Fig. 8.126 Cholesteatoma encasing the malleus head and incus body with an intact ossicular chain. Ears with this pattern of disease often have good hearing.

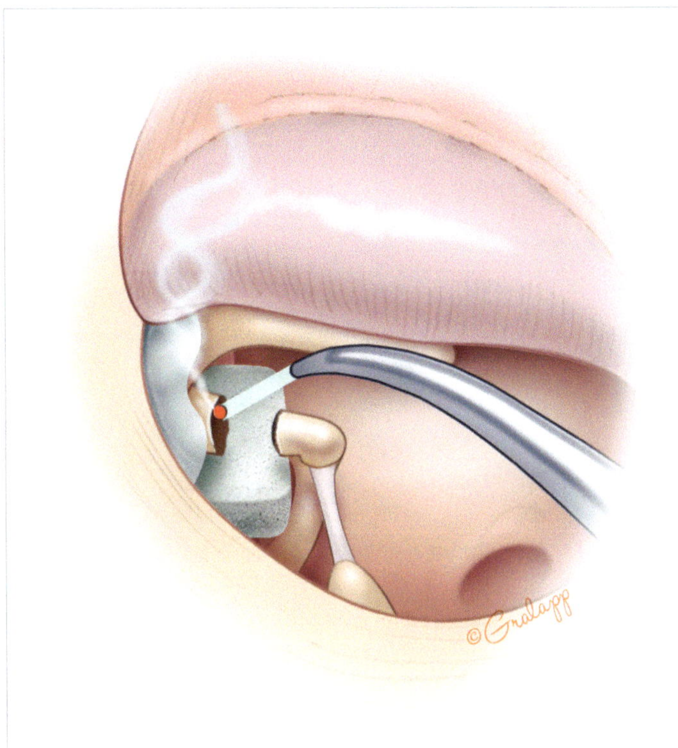

Fig. 8.127 Laser disruption of the ossicular chain in preparation for resection of the cholesteatoma. Note the absorbable gelatin sponge pledget protecting the facial nerve.

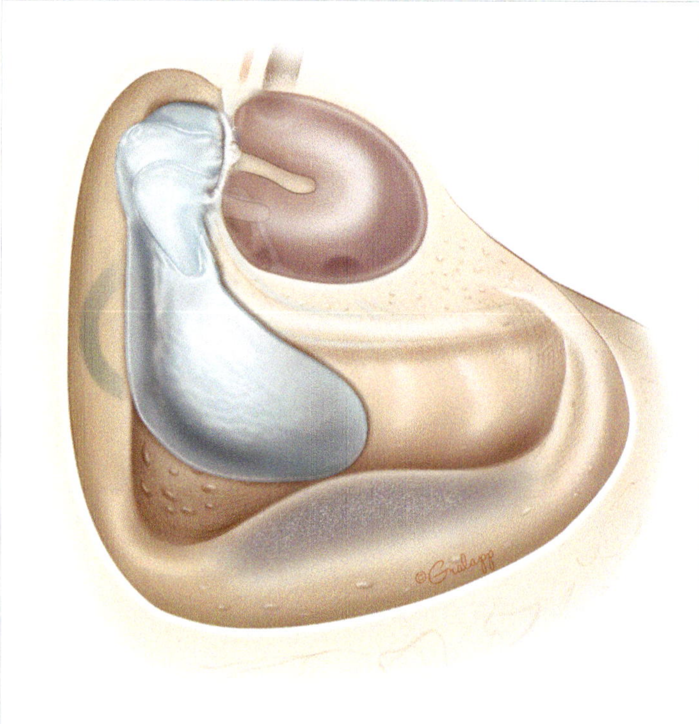

Fig. 8.128 Bondy type of modified radical mastoidectomy exteriorizes the matrix-covered ossicular chain. This is a suitable option when the hearing is good and the middle ear is free of disease.

8.12 Congenital Cholesteatoma

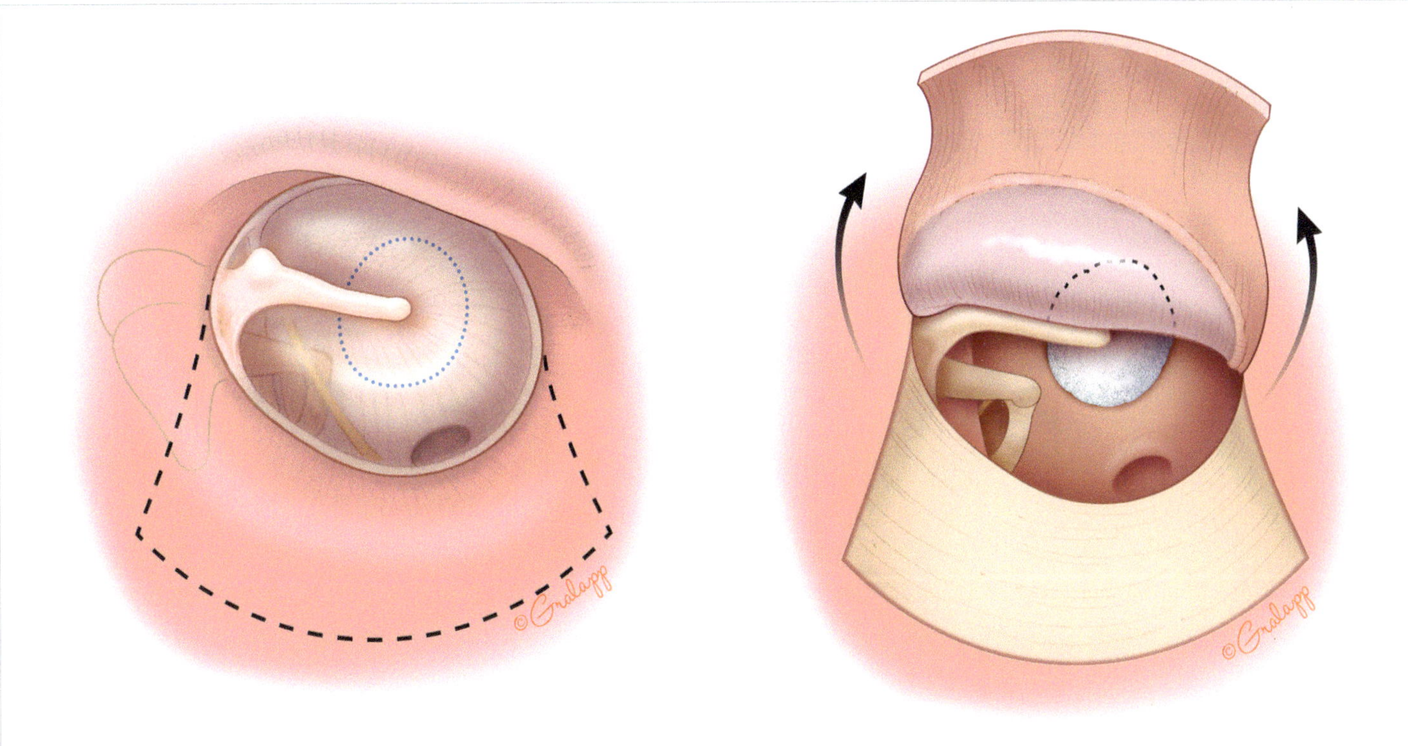

Fig. 8.129 Congenital cholesteatoma characteristically arises from an embryological remnant on the promontory wall anterior to the malleus. Standard posterior tympanotomy is insufficient to expose the anterior aspect of the tympanum.

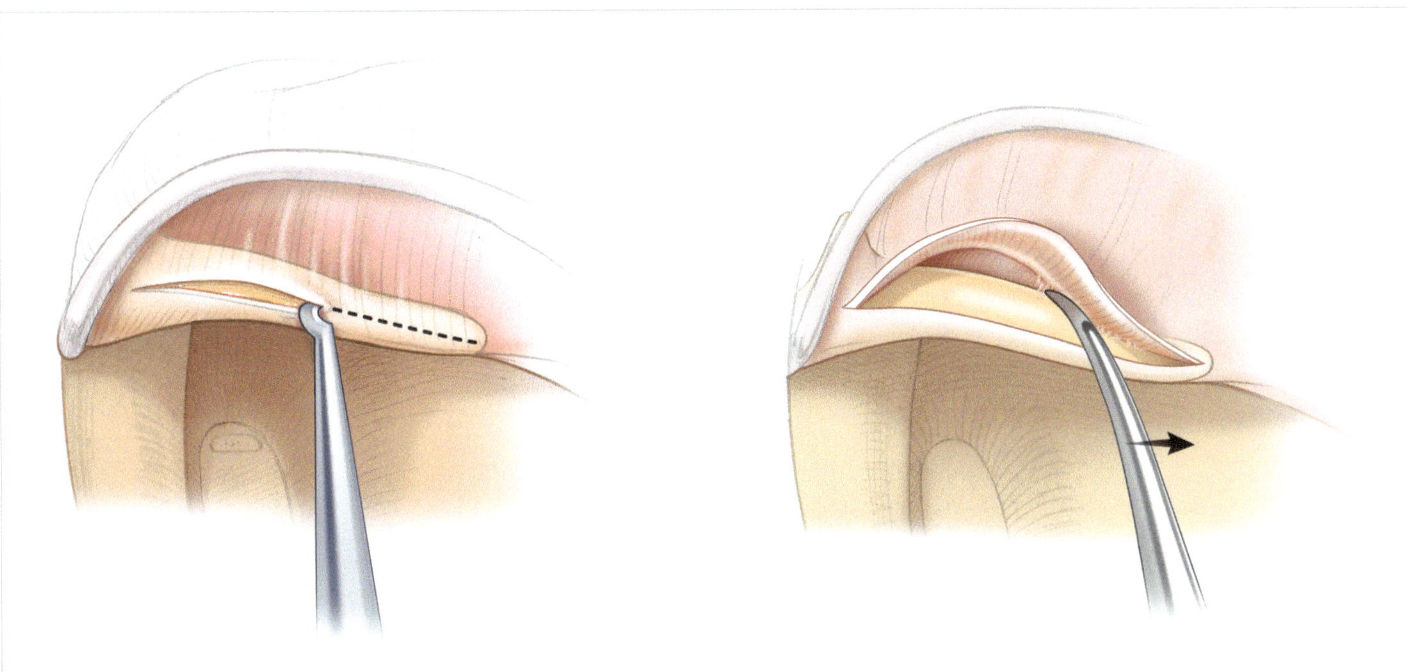

Fig. 8.130 Elevation of the tympanic membrane from the malleus. The membrane adheres at the short process and the tip of the umbo. These attachments need to be severed sharply.

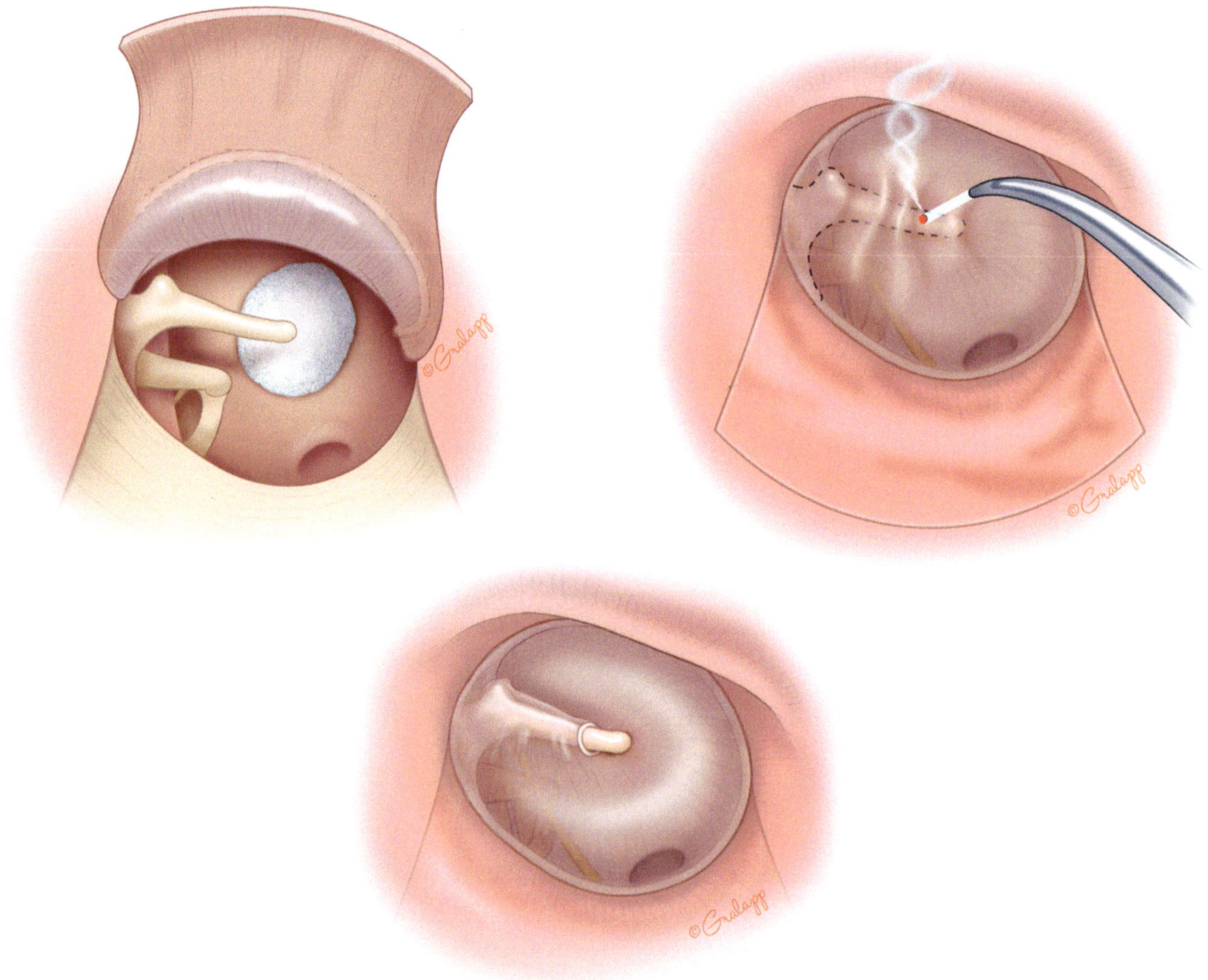

Fig. 8.131 Exposure of a congenital cholesteatoma. If the malleus is not to be reattached to the tympanic membrane, then it may migrate medially due to the unopposed action of the tensor tympani muscle. A laser myringotomy can be created as shown.

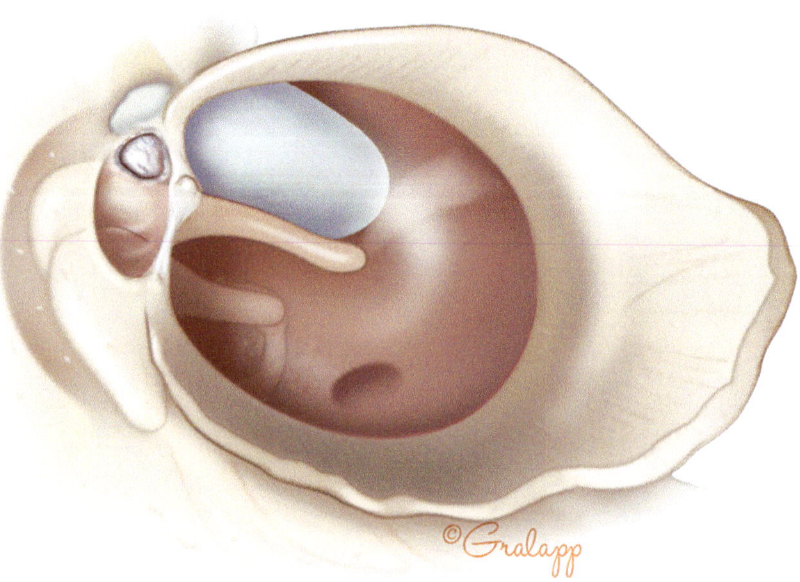

Fig. 8.132 Congenital cholesteatoma sometimes penetrates the anterior epitympanum.

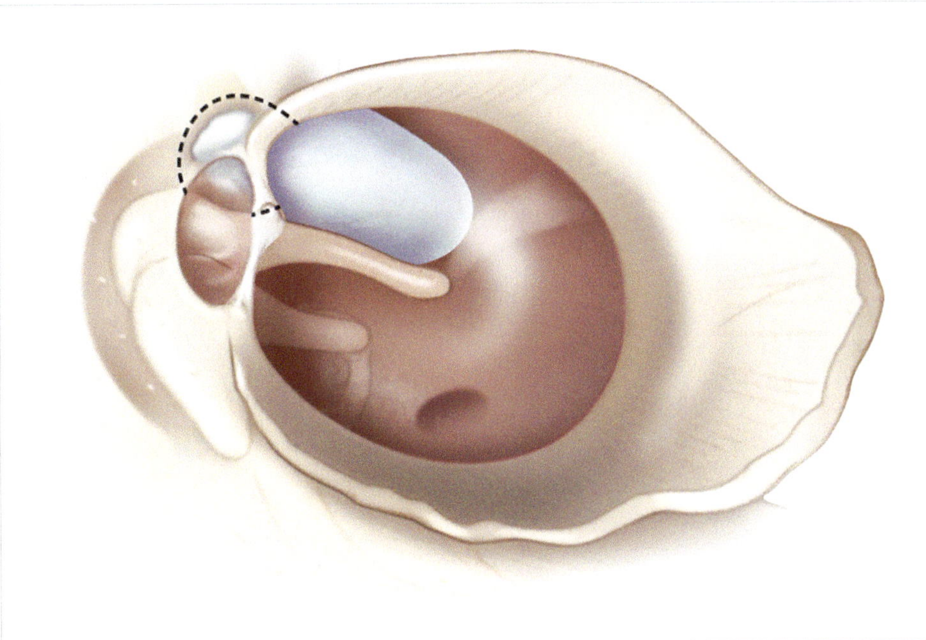

Fig. 8.133 Bone removed to expose the anterior epitympanum.

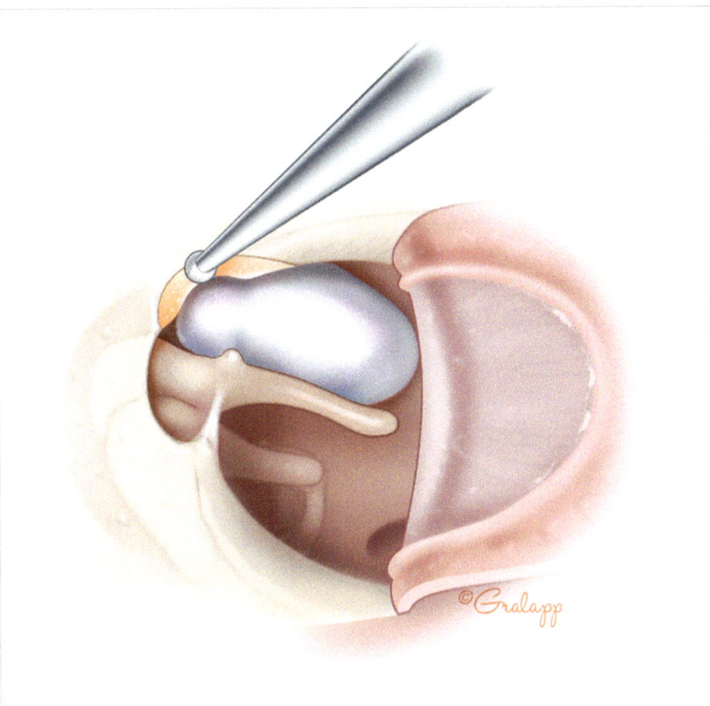

Fig. 8.134 Epitympanic exposure. Note the inferiorly based tympanomeatal flap that is often used in approaches to congenital cholesteatoma.

9 Facial Nerve

Robert K. Jackler

9.1 Introduction to the Facial Nerve

Facial nerve injury is a risk in virtually all ear procedures and its injury is the most dreaded complication in routine otologic surgery. Historically, it was sometimes said that "*God put the facial nerve in the mastoid to keep the general surgeons out.*" As the facial nerve winds through the temporal bone in its course from the internal auditory canal to the stylomastoid foramen, it lies in close relationship with the cochlea, semicircular canals, ossicles, oval window, and jugular bulb. Detailed knowledge of the normal anatomy of the facial nerve and how it is characteristically involved with ear disease is central to safe otologic surgery. It is also key to the effectiveness of ear procedures, as an inexperienced surgeon who is excessively cautious out of fear of the nerve is likely to be less thorough in addressing the disease process. Avoiding iatrogenic facial nerve injury is assisted by neurophysiological monitoring, but it is no substitute for a detailed knowledge of its anatomical relationships. Learning the techniques needed to locate the facial nerve when it is embedded in disease which has obscured its customary landmarks is a crucial skill. See also section 7.6 The Facial Nerve in Mastoidectomy in Chapter 7 and section 8.7 The Facial Nerve in Cholesteatoma Chapter 8.

Repair of intratemporal facial nerve injury usually involves either direct repair or grafting. Iatrogenic injuries usually involve the tympanic or second genu segments, while tumor may occur anywhere along the length but are most common at the geniculate ganglion. Direct repair is not usually possible in a severed facial nerve within the temporal bone because clean knife injuries are rare. Most injuries leave a gap which can be bridged either by rerouting or interposition grafting. Because of the convoluted course of the intratemporal facial nerve, a defect can be overcome by rerouting across the base of a genu. Interposition grafting is usually with the greater auricular nerve, as it is a good size match, is readily accessible, and leaves only a minor deficit of an anesthetic ear lobe. Long defects, or those that require branching such as for lesions extending beyond the pes anserinus, may require sural nerve grafting.

When repair of the facial nerve is not possible due the lack of a proximal stump to graft, most commonly following resection of a cerebellopontine angle tumor, various strategies exist for reanimating the paralyzed face. The traditional hypoglossal–facial anastomosis gives excellent tone at rest, but much synkinesis during movement. Newer techniques using a portion of the hypoglossal nerve for tone and the masseteric branch of the trigeminal nerve for restoration of smile appear to have superior results. When the facial muscles have atrophied due to longstanding paralysis, or the distal branches have been resected (e.g., parotid malignancy), cross-facial anastomosis with gracilis muscle microvascular transfer offers improvement, but it is a multistage procedure. Static or dynamic (temporalis muscle) slings are alternatives, especially in older patients for whom the microvascular muscle transfer procedure works less well.

Further Reading

1. Balaji SM. Temporalis pull-through vs fascia lata augmentation in facial reanimation for facial paralysis. Ann Maxillofac Surg 2016;6(2):267–271 PubMed
2. Bayrak SB, Kriet JD, Humphrey CD. Masseteric to buccal branch nerve transfer. Curr Opin Otolaryngol Head Neck Surg 2017;25(4):280–285 PubMed
3. Boahene KO, Owusu J, Ishii L, et al. The multivector gracilis free functional muscle flap for facial reanimation. JAMA Facial Plast Surg 2018;20(4):300–306 PubMed
4. Garcia RM, Hadlock TA, Klebuc MJ, Simpson RL, Zenn MR, Marcus JR. Contemporary solutions for the treatment of facial nerve paralysis. Plast Reconstr Surg 2015;135(6): 1025e–1046e PubMed
5. Hu J, Fleck TR, Xu J, Hsu JV, Xu HX. Contemporary changes with the use of facial nerve monitoring in chronic ear surgery. Otolaryngol Head Neck Surg 2014;151(3):473–477 PubMed
6. Ishii LE. Facial Nerve Rehabilitation. Facial Plast Surg Clin North Am 2016;24(4):573–575 PubMed
7. Kim L, Byrne PJ. Controversies in contemporary facial reanimation. Facial Plast Surg Clin North Am 2016;24(3):275–297 PubMed
8. Kochhar A, Albathi M, Sharon JD, Ishii LE, Byrne P, Boahene KD. Transposition of the intratemporal facial to hypoglossal nerve for reanimation of the paralyzed face: the VII to XII transposition technique. JAMA Facial Plast Surg 2016;18 (5):370–378 PubMed
9. Linder T, Mulazimoglu S, El Hadi T, et al. Iatrogenic facial nerve injuries during chronic otitis media surgery: a multicentre retrospective study. Clin Otolaryngol 2017;42(3): 521–527 PubMed
10. Proctor B. The anatomy of the facial nerve. Otolaryngol Clin North Am 1991;24(3):479–504 PubMed
11. Rozen SM. Facial reanimation: basic surgical tools and creation of an effective toolbox for treating patients with facial paralysis: Part B. Nerve transfer combined with cross-facial nerve grafting in the acute facial palsy patient. Plast Reconstr Surg 2017;139(3):725–727 PubMed
12. Ryu NG, Kim J. How to avoid facial nerve injury in mastoidectomy? J Audiol Otol 2016;20(2):68–72 PubMed
13. Slattery WH, Azizzadeh B. The Facial Nerve. New York, NY: Thieme; 2014
14. Socolovsky M, Martins RS, di Masi G, Bonilla G, Siqueira M. Treatment of complete facial palsy in adults: comparative study between direct hemihypoglossal-facial neurorrhaphy, hemihipoglossal-facial neurorrhaphy with grafts, and masseter to facial nerve transfer. Acta Neurochir (Wien) 2016;158 (5):945–957, discussion 957 PubMed
15. Yoshioka N. Differential reanimation of the midface and lower face using the masseteric and hypoglossal nerves for facial paralysis. Oper Neurosurg (Hagerstown) 2018;15(2):174–178 PubMed

9.2 Anatomy of the Facial Nerve

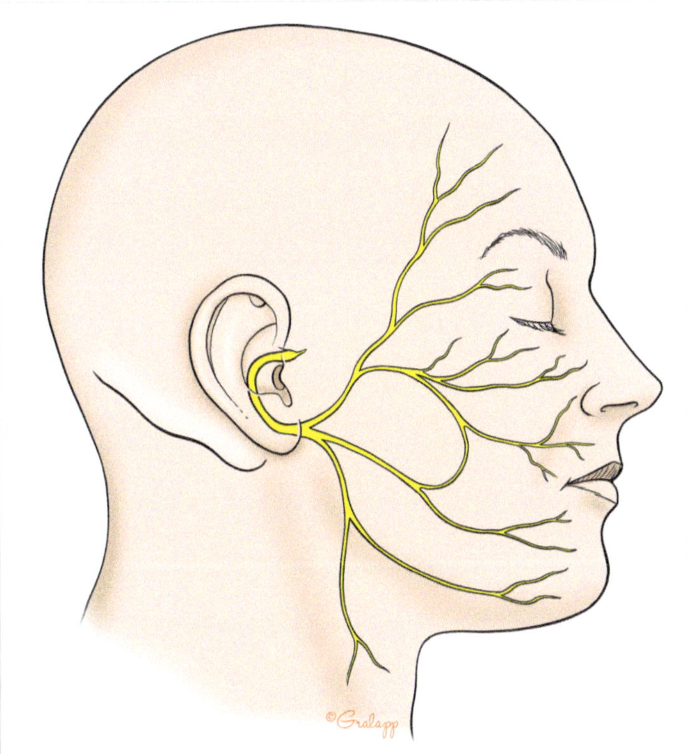

Fig. 9.1 Overview of facial nerve anatomy from the brainstem exit to the terminal branches on the face.

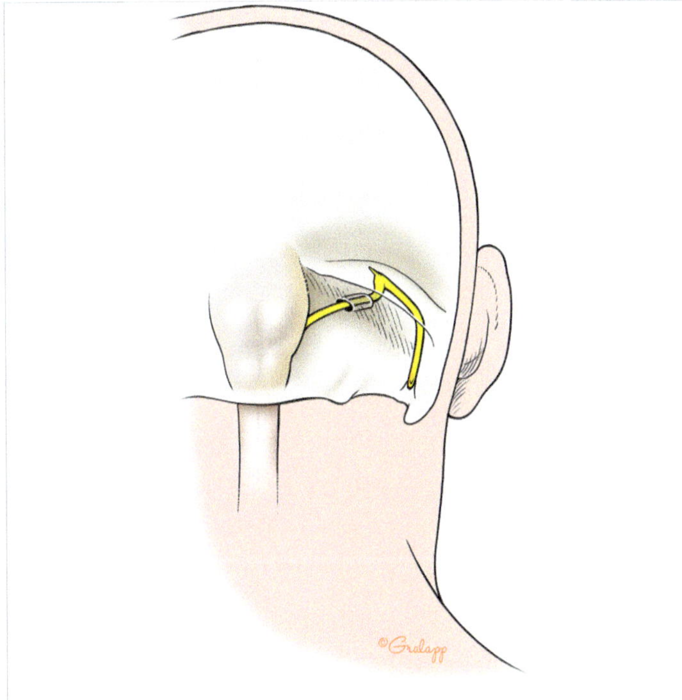

Fig. 9.2 Note the three-dimensional complexity of the bends and turns en route from the brainstem exit to the stylomastoid foramen.

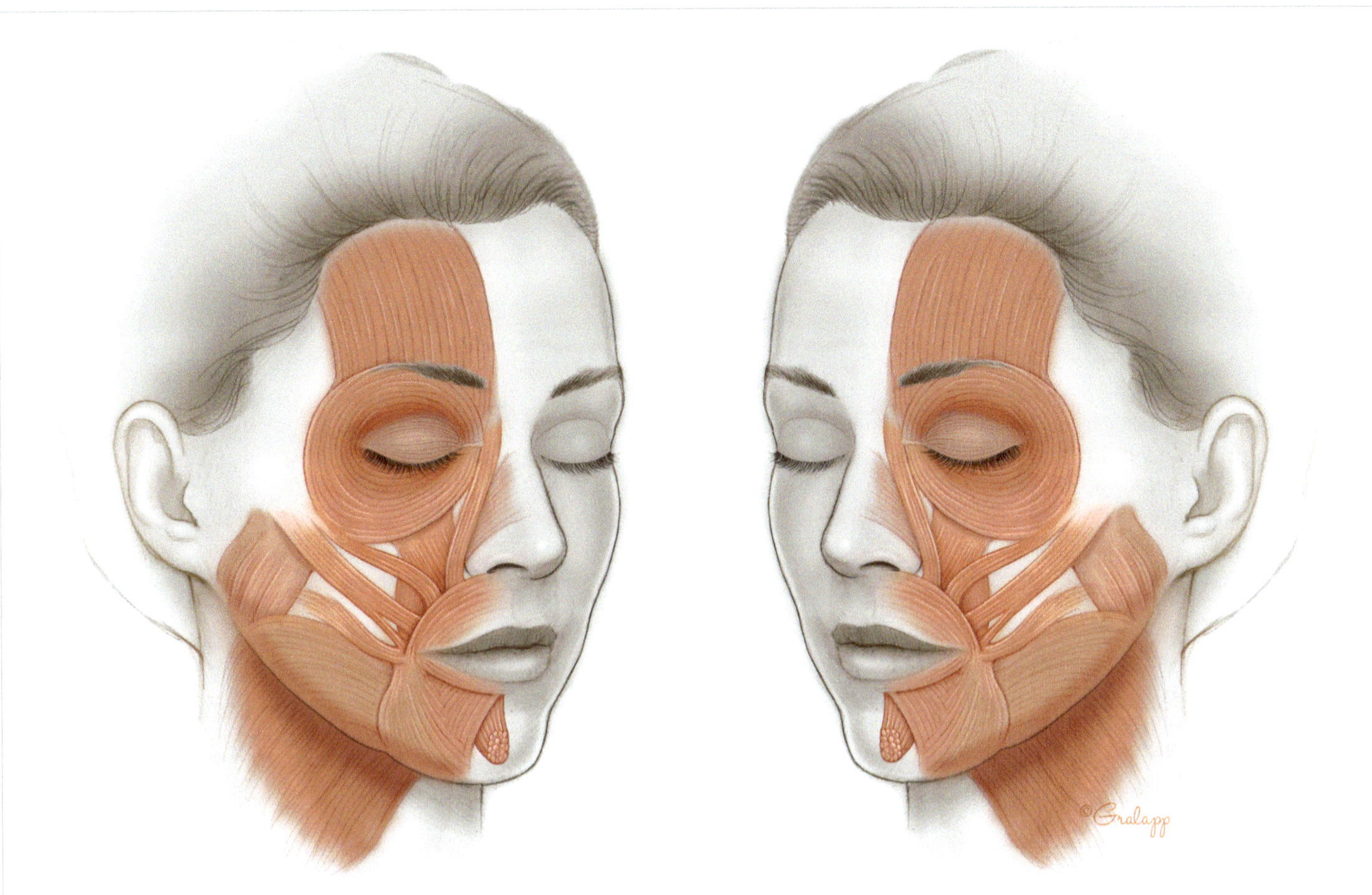

Fig. 9.3 Muscles of facial expression.

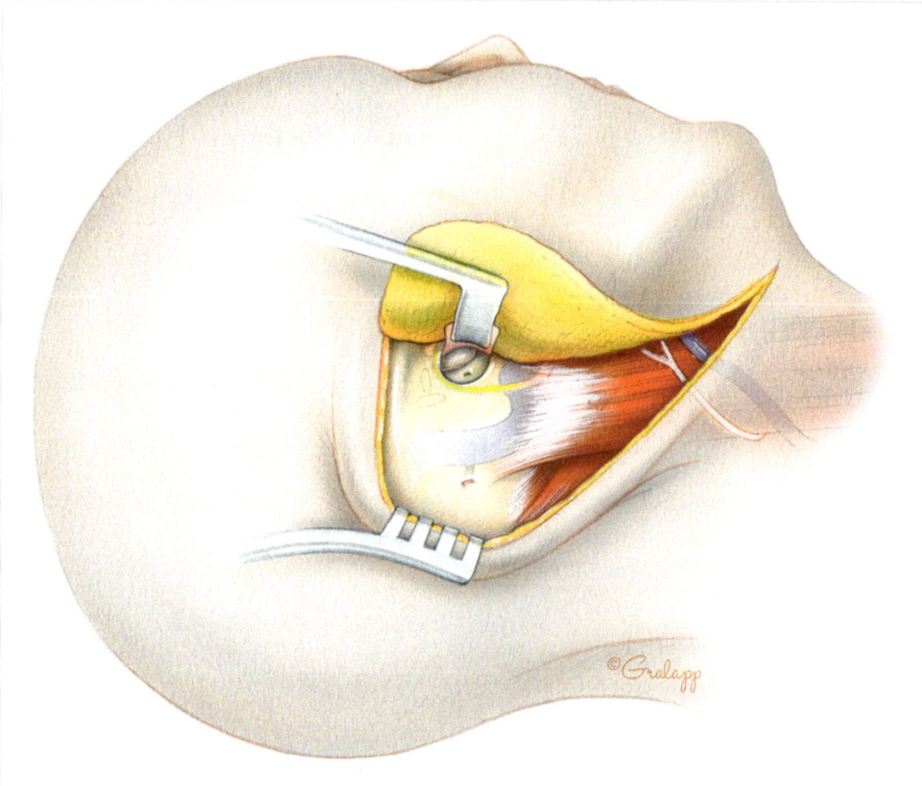

Fig. 9.4 Lateral overview of the facial nerve in the mastoid. Note how the facial nerve crosses lateral to the jugular bulb en route to the stylomastoid foramen.

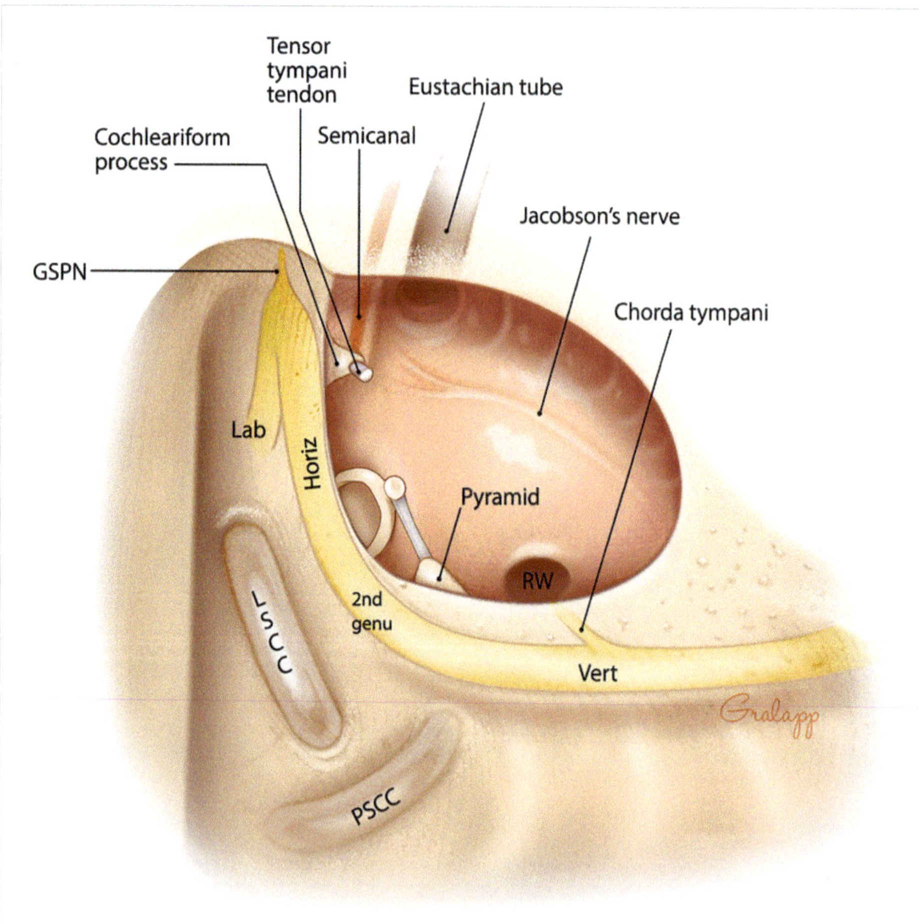

Fig. 9.5 The anatomical relationships of the intratemporal facial nerve. Lab, labyrinthine segment; GG, geniculate ganglion; Horiz, horizontal (tympanic) segment; Vert, vertical (mastoid) segment; RW, round window; PSCC, posterior semicircular canal; LSCC, lateral semicircular canal.

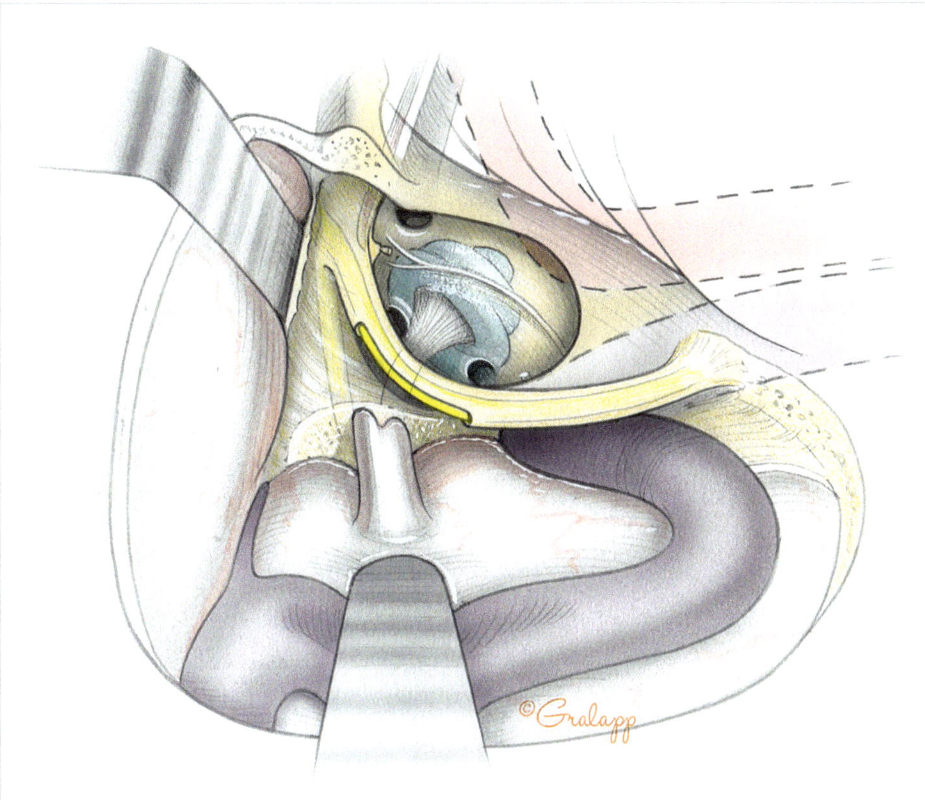

Fig. 9.6 The proximal course of the facial nerve in the temporal bone. Lateral dissection exposing the transparent floor of the middle ear and the internal auditory canal illustrating the proximal course of the nerve between the geniculate ganglion and the internal auditory canal. Note that the semicircular canals have been removed.

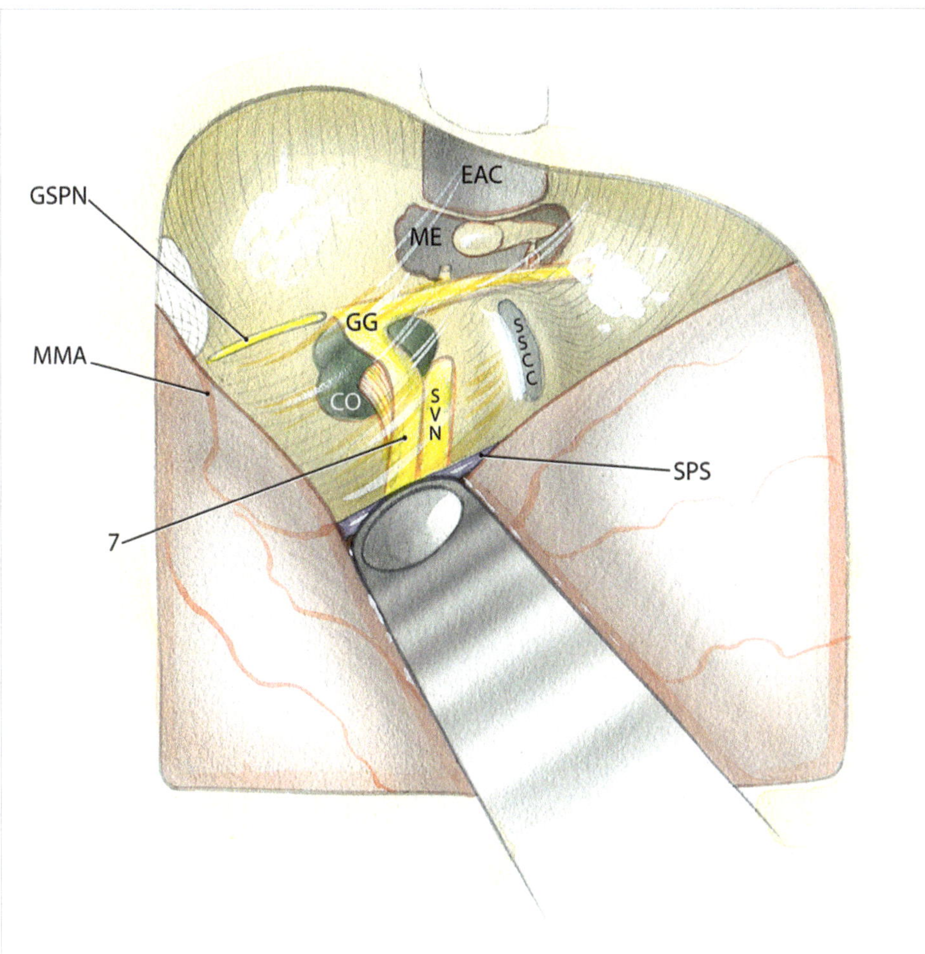

Fig. 9.7 The relationships of the facial nerve as seen from above via the middle fossa approach. Note the intimate relationship of the labyrinthine and upper tympanic sections to the cochlea. The external auditory canal (EAC), middle ear (ME), cochlea (Co), and superior semicircular canal (SSCC) normally lie beneath bone but are made visible as an aid to orientation. GG, geniculate ganglion; GSPN, greater superficial petrosal nerve; 7, facial nerve; SVN, superior vestibular nerve; SPS, superior petrosal sinus; MMA, middle meningeal artery.

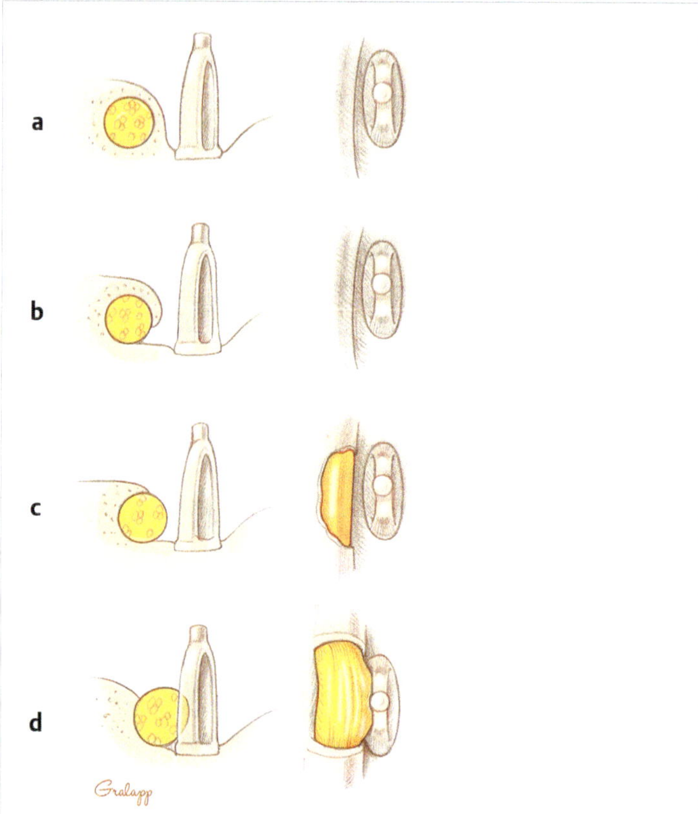

Fig. 9.8 In its tympanic course superior to the stapes, the facial nerve may be fully bony covered (A), dehiscent on its under surface (B)—which is common, fully dehiscent (C), or both dehiscent and protuberant. In rare cases, a protuberant facial nerve will impinge on the stapes and cause conductive hearing loss.

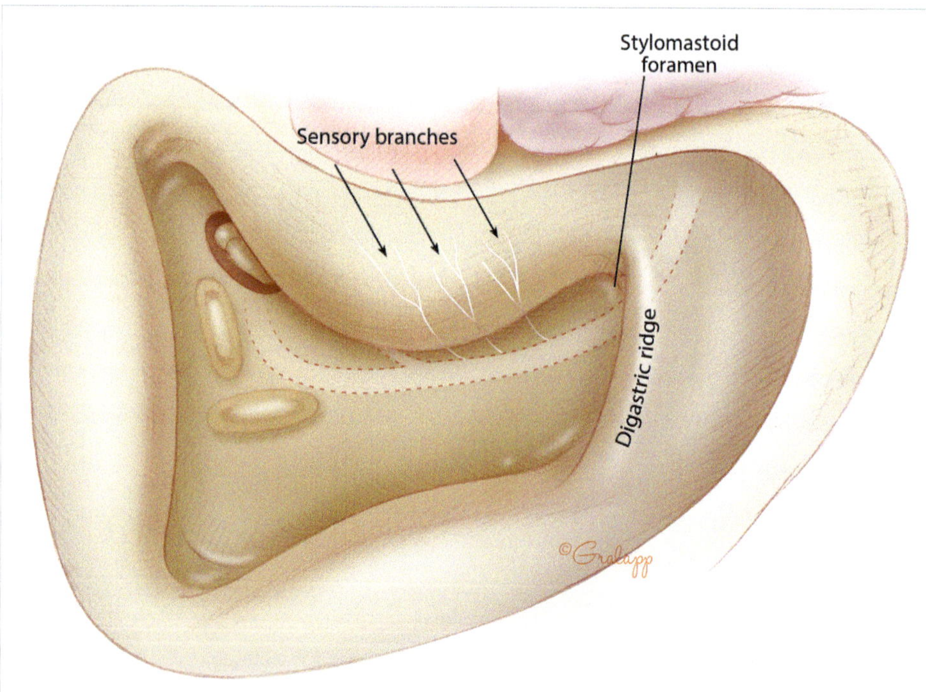

Fig. 9.9 Branches of the facial nerve which provide sensation to the conchal bowl may be seen on the ear canal. The digastric ridge is a useful landmark in identification of the facial nerve at the stylomastoid foramen. The digastric ridge is the bony protuberance crossing the mastoid, just above the mastoid tip, made by the posterior belly of the digastric muscle.

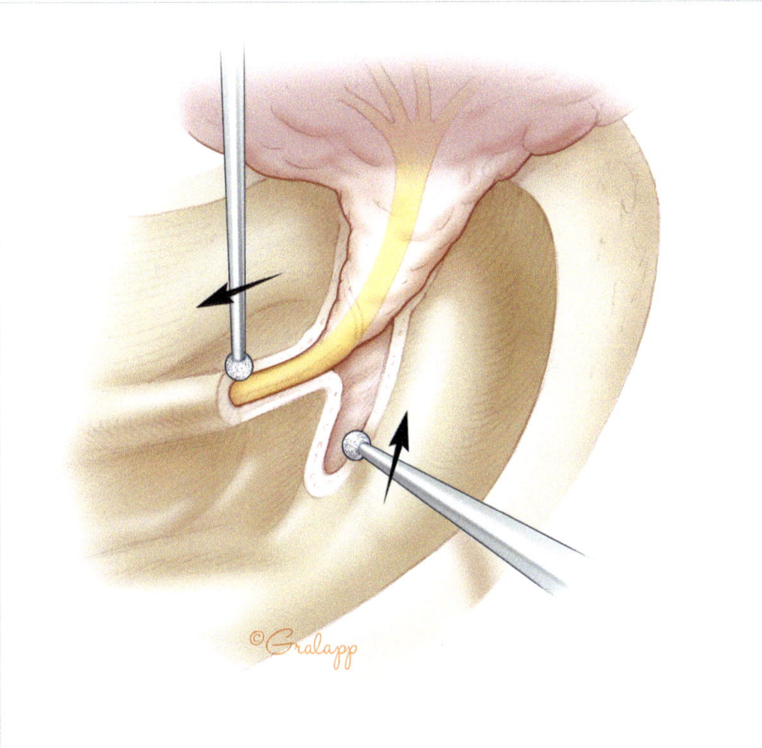

Fig. 9.10 The fascial lining of the superficial surface of the digastric muscle merges with the periosteum lining the stylomastoid foramen. This is a useful method in identifying the distal mastoid segment of the nerve.

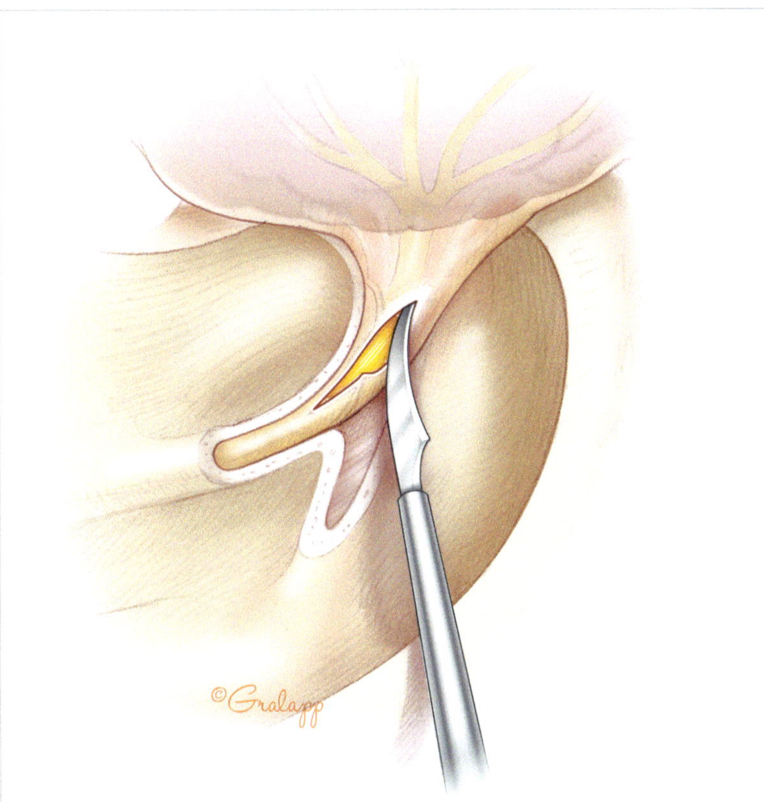

Fig. 9.11 Connecting the mastoid with the parotid segments of the nerve by cutting the tenacious periosteum of the foramen with a no. 12 blade.

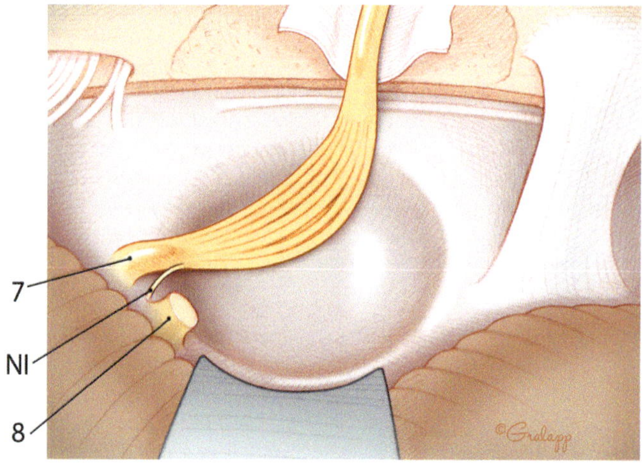

Fig. 9.12 The nervus intermedius (NI) conveys the parasympathetic and sensory components of the facial nerve (7). It exits the pons between the main facial trunk (motor) and the audiovestibular nerve (8). (Used with permission from El Ashram YA, Jackler RK, Pitts LH, Yingling CD. Intraoperative electrophysiologic identification of the nervus intermedius. *Otol Neurotol* 2005;26:274–279.)

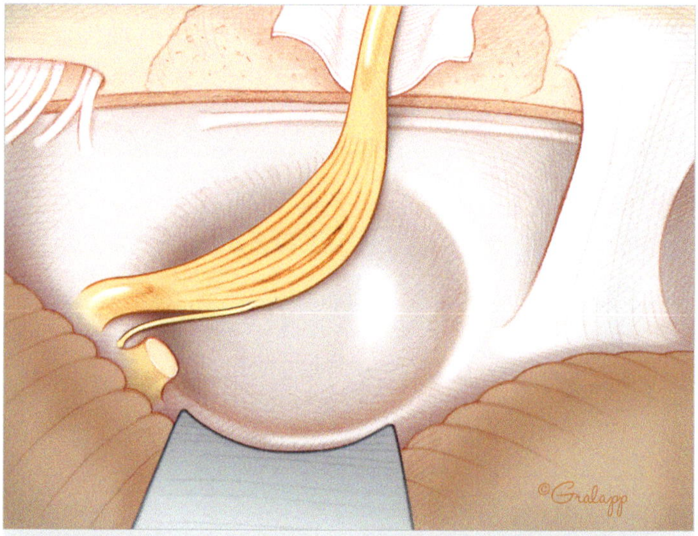

Fig. 9.13 Variability exists in the distance before the nervus intermedius joins the main facial nerve trunk.

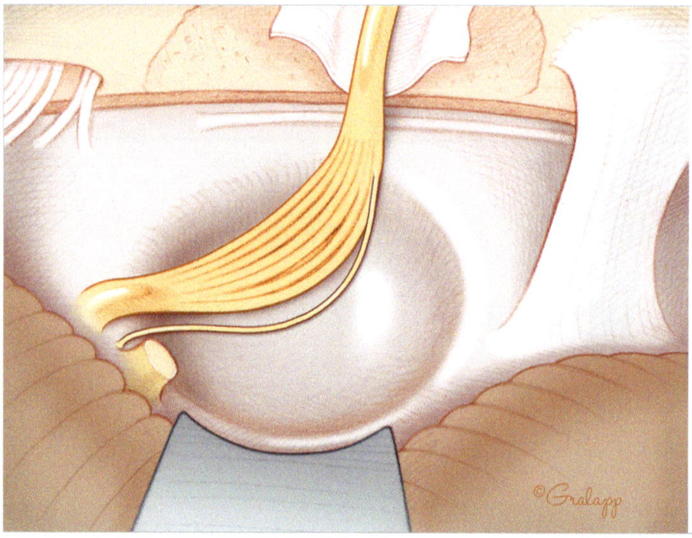

Fig. 9.14 Variability exists in the distance before the nervus intermedius joins the main facial nerve trunk.

9.3 Repair of the Facial Nerve

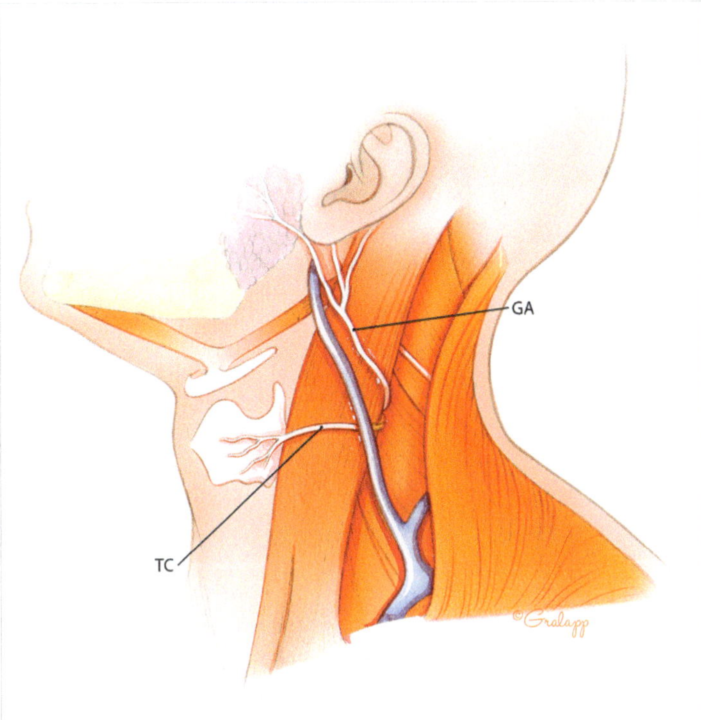

Fig. 9.15 Several nerves are available regionally for use in reconstructing the facial nerve. The greater auricular nerve is the most frequent nerve utilized for interposition grafting of the facial nerve. It is favored due to its proximity to the operative field, excellent size match, and minimal donor deficit. The transverse cervical nerve is another sensory branch suitable for use in facial nerve reconstruction. GA, greater auricular nerve; TC, transverse cervical nerve.

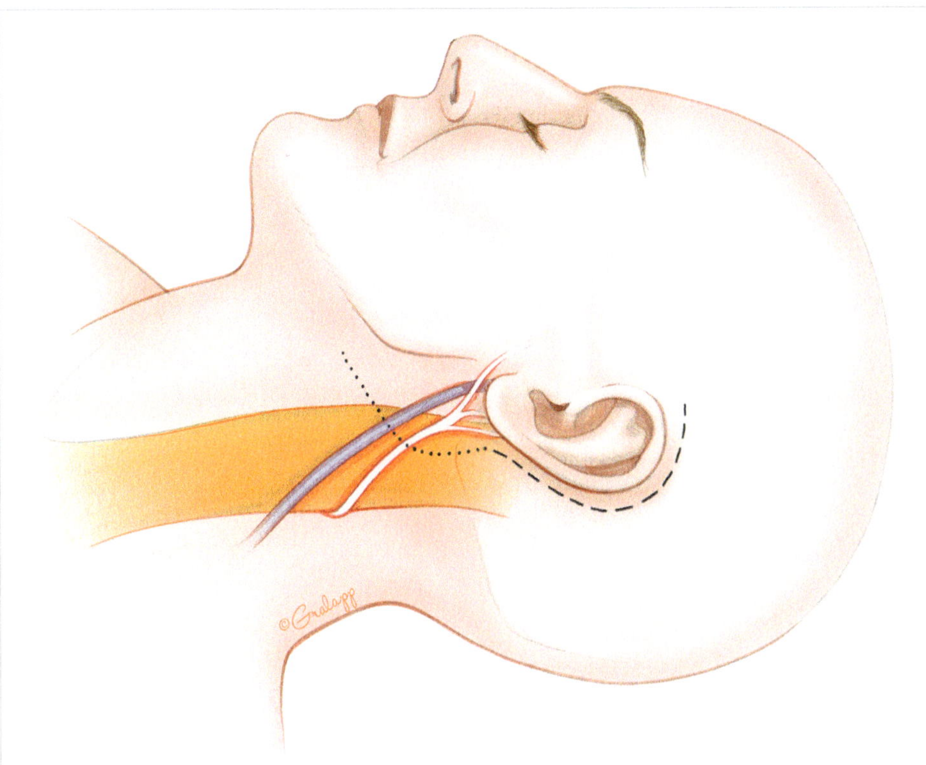

Fig. 9.16 To expose the greater auricular nerve, a postauricular incision is carried inferiorly into the upper neck. The incision can usually be placed in a natural skin crease, thus creating only a subtle scar.

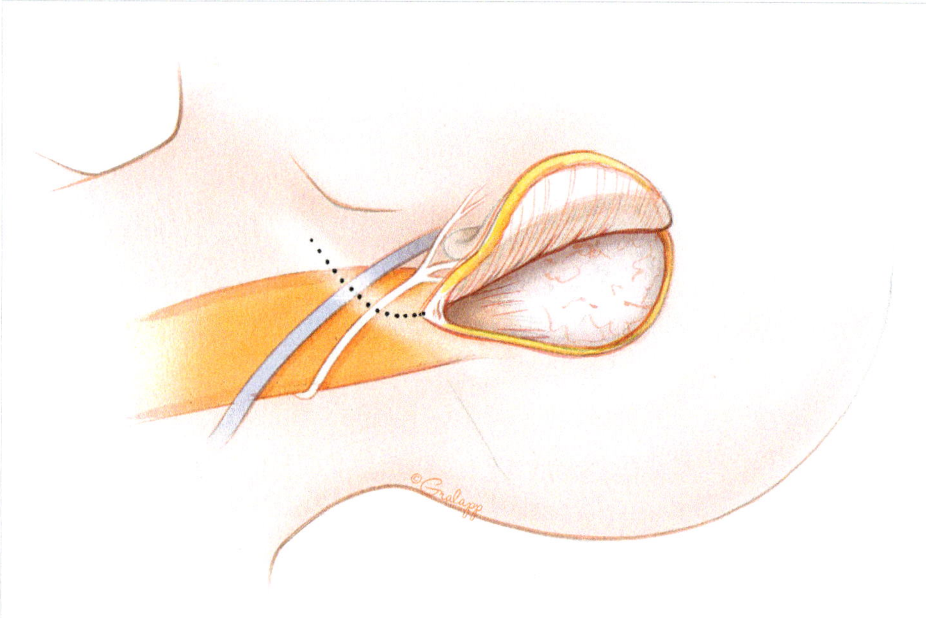

Fig. 9.17 After completing the intratemporal portion of the procedure, the incision is extended into the upper neck.

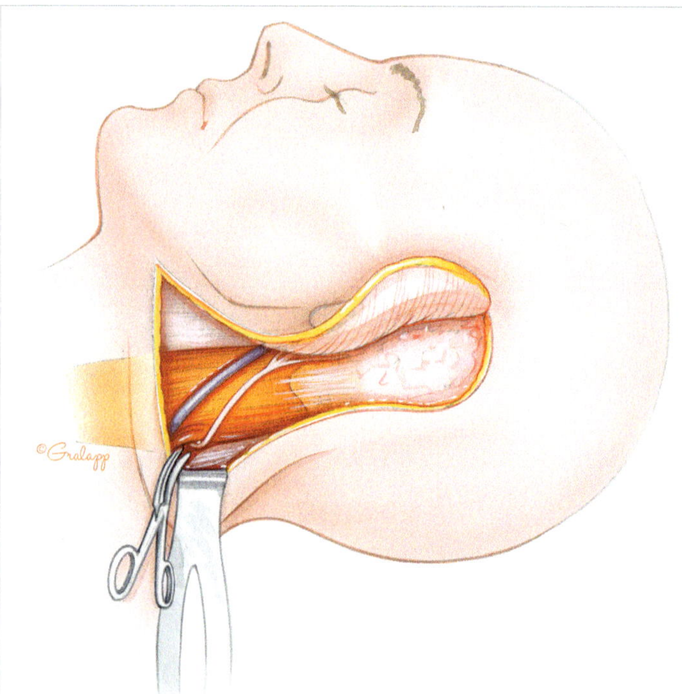

Fig. 9.18 The greater auricular nerve parallels the external jugular vein and courses superior to it across the surface of the sternomastoid muscle. To obtain a long segment of the nerve, it can be taken from its branch point under the pinna back to its exit from the spine.

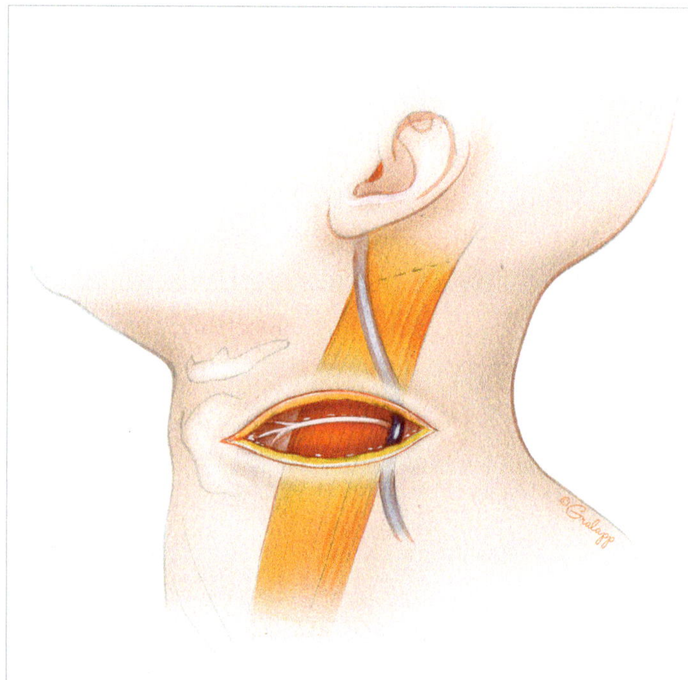

Fig. 9.19 The transverse cervical nerve is another sensory branch well suited for engrafting the facial nerve. It is particularly useful in malignant lesions of the temporal bone and parotid region which require resection of the greater auricular nerve with the tumor specimen.

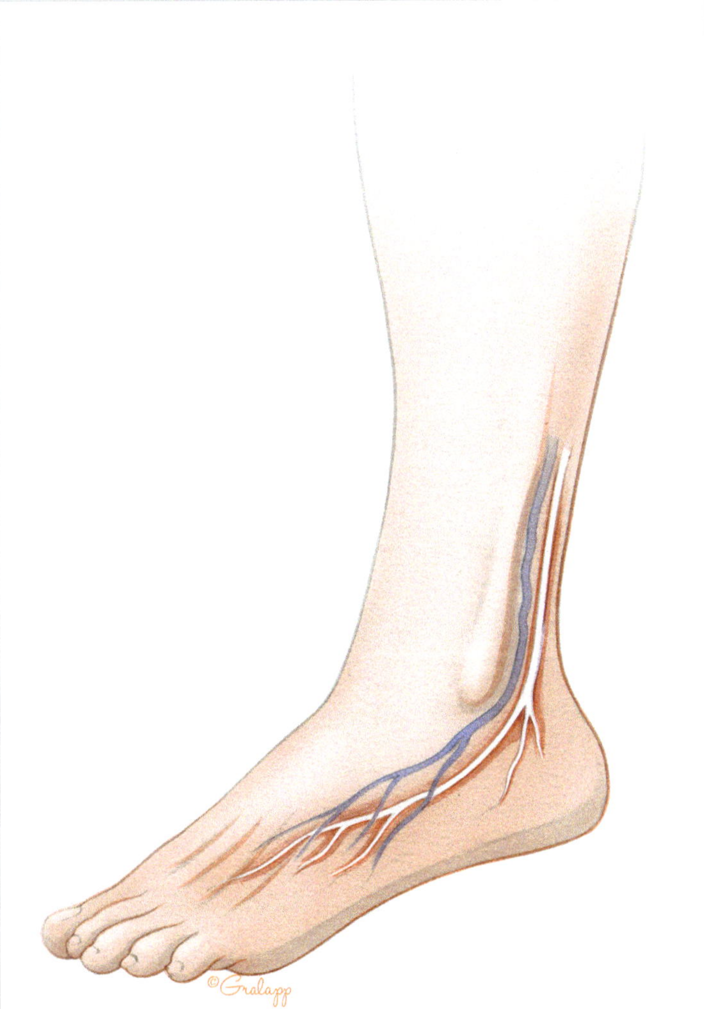

Fig. 9.20 When an unusually long nerve graft is required, the sural nerve can be harvested from the leg. This nerve courses behind the lateral malleolus in proximity to the lesser saphenous vein. The donor deficit consists of anesthesia of the heel region. The sural nerve is usually larger in diameter than the facial nerve. This makes it particularly suitable for defects which span the pes anserinus and require a branched graft.

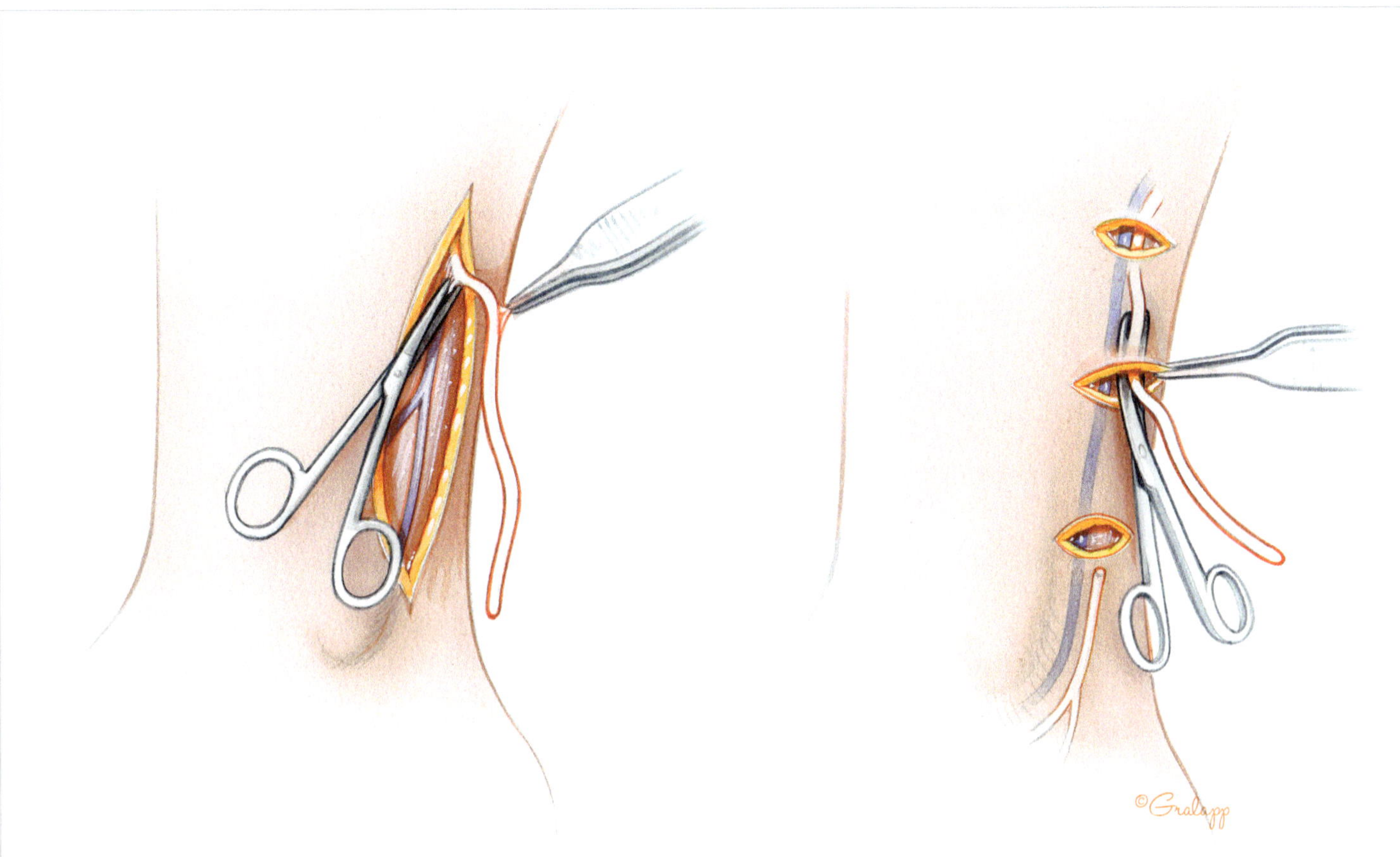

Fig. 9.21 The sural nerve can be harvested either through a longitudinal incision or a series of short stair-stepped transverse incisions.

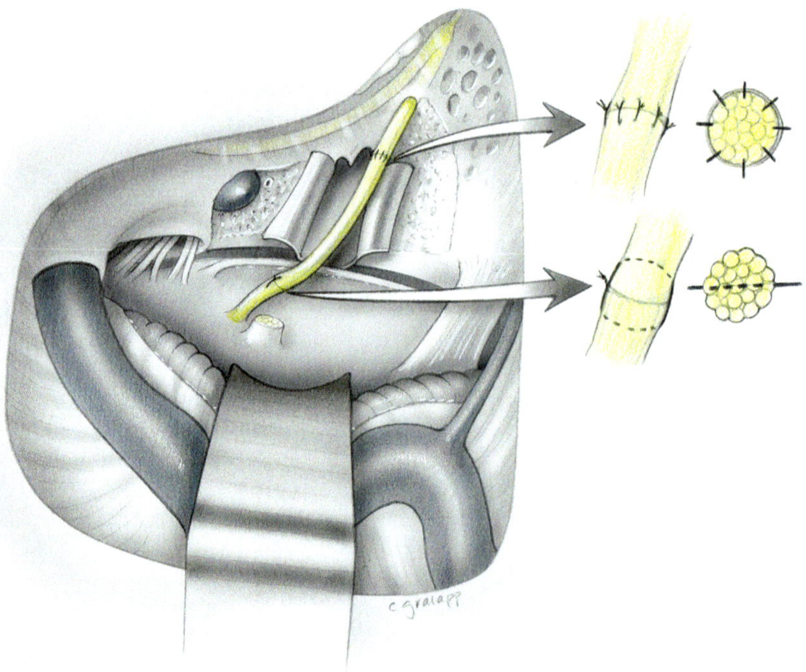

Fig. 9.22 Translabyrinthine view of a facial nerve transection near its pontine root entry zone with the defect extending to past the entry of the fallopian canal, which has been drilled open. The distal anastomosis is performed with epineural 9–0 sutures. As the intracranial nerve lacks an epineurium, a single central suture reapproximates the ends, often reinforced with a wrapping of fascia or other membrane.

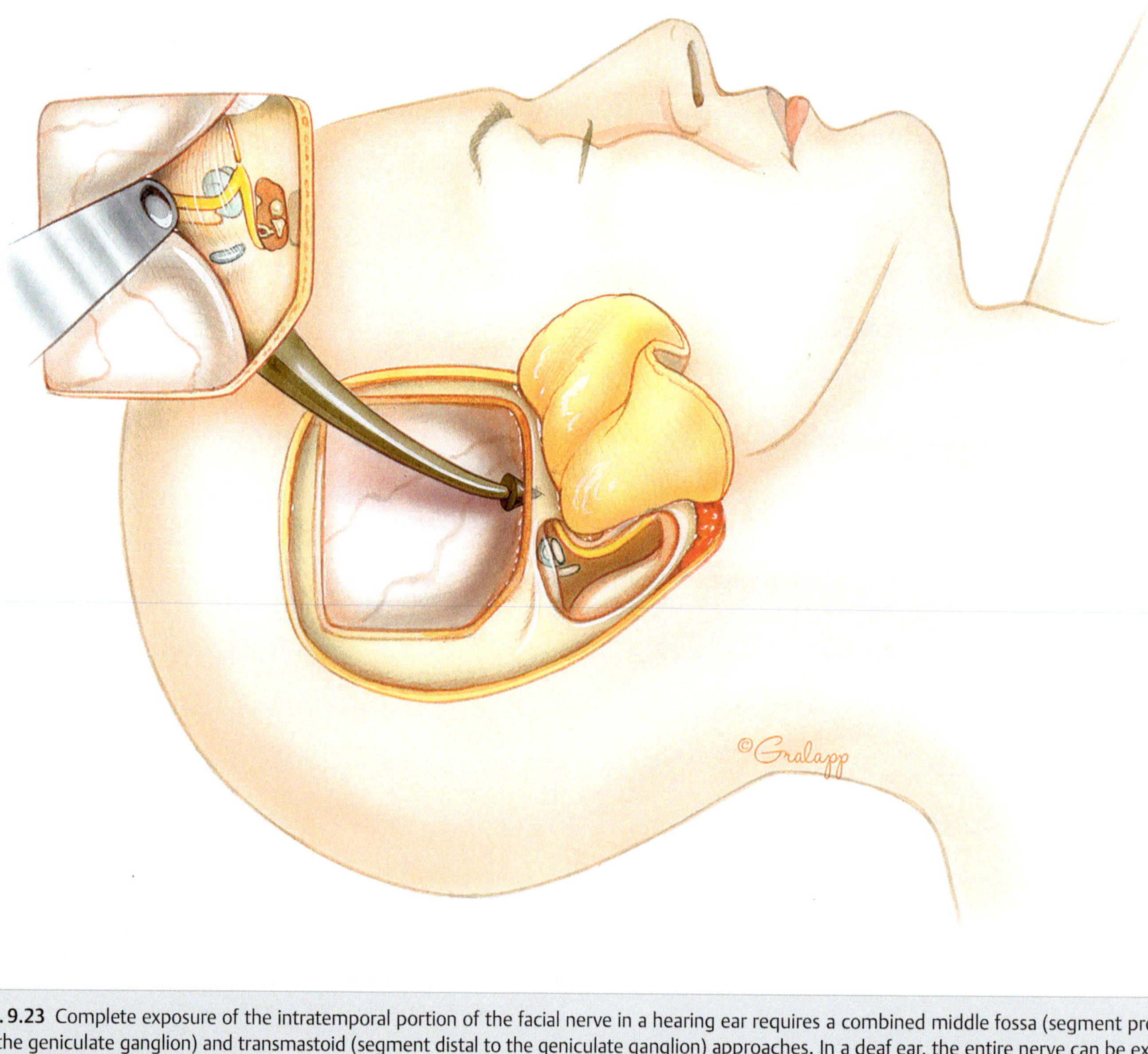

Fig. 9.23 Complete exposure of the intratemporal portion of the facial nerve in a hearing ear requires a combined middle fossa (segment proximal to the geniculate ganglion) and transmastoid (segment distal to the geniculate ganglion) approaches. In a deaf ear, the entire nerve can be exposed via a translabyrinthine approach.

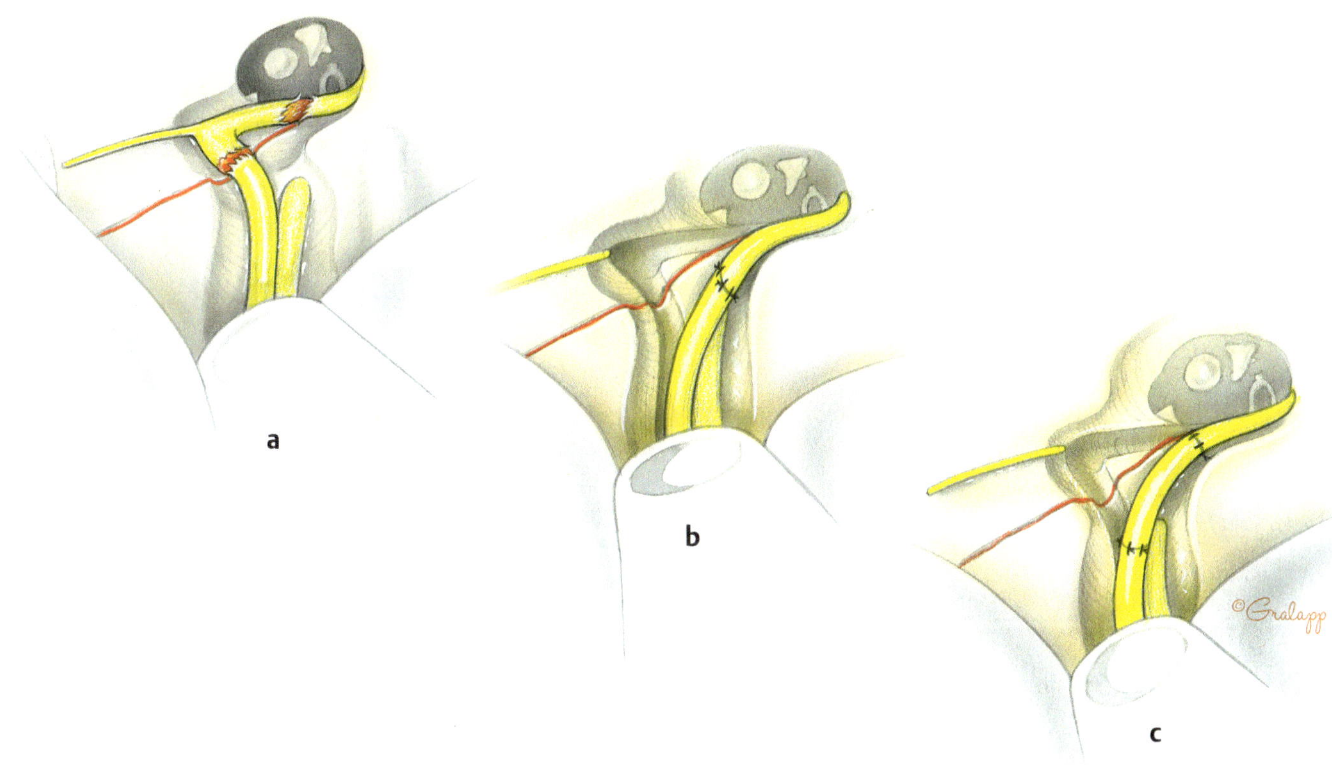

Fig. 9.24 Transection injury to the geniculate ganglion in transverse temporal bone fracture (A) can sometimes be repaired directly by rerouting the nerve across the base of the geniculate triangle (B). This has the advantage of a single anastomosis. In more extensive injury, an interposition nerve graft is needed (C).

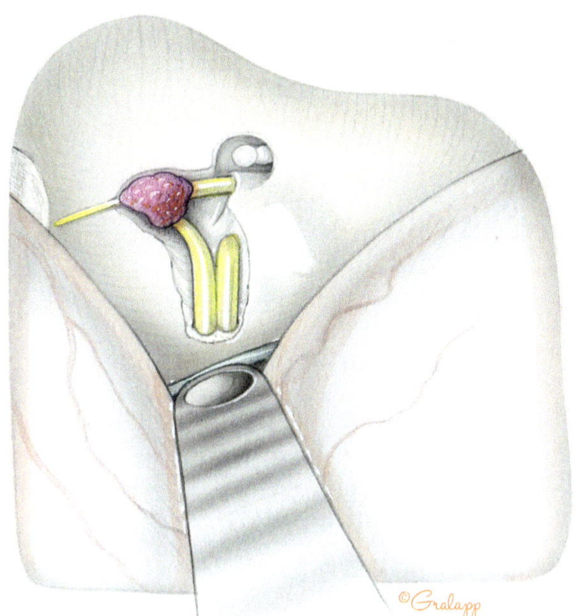

Fig. 9.25 The geniculate ganglion is a frequent site for destructive lesions of the facial nerve. Most common among these are temporal bone fracture and tumors such as hemangioma, schwannoma, and meningioma. In this middle fossa view, a hemangioma has resulted in focal destruction of the geniculate segment of the facial nerve.

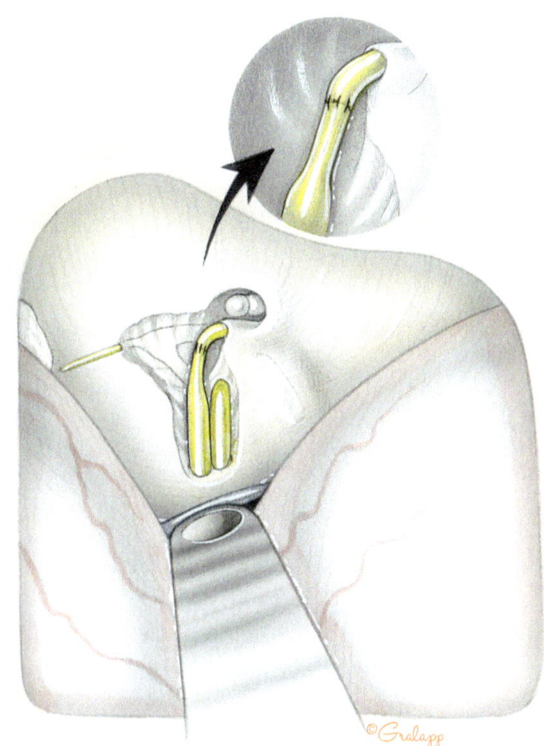

Fig. 9.26 Repair of the facial nerve by rerouting across the base of the geniculate triangle. The repair couples the labyrinthine and upper horizontal segments. It should be noted that while the native nerve can be preserved in many geniculate hemangiomas, schwannomas almost always necessitate resection and grafting.

9.4 Hypoglossal–Facial Anastomosis for Facial Reanimation

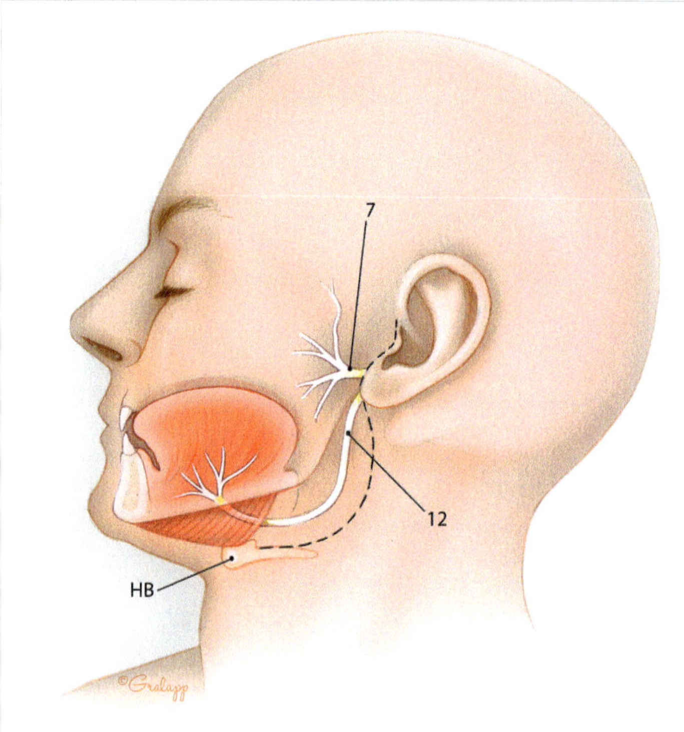

Fig. 9.27 Hypoglossal–facial anastomosis is performed through a preauricular incision (*dashed line*) which is carried into the upper neck approximately 2 cm beneath the mandible. 7, facial nerve; 12, hypoglossal nerve; HB, hyoid bone.

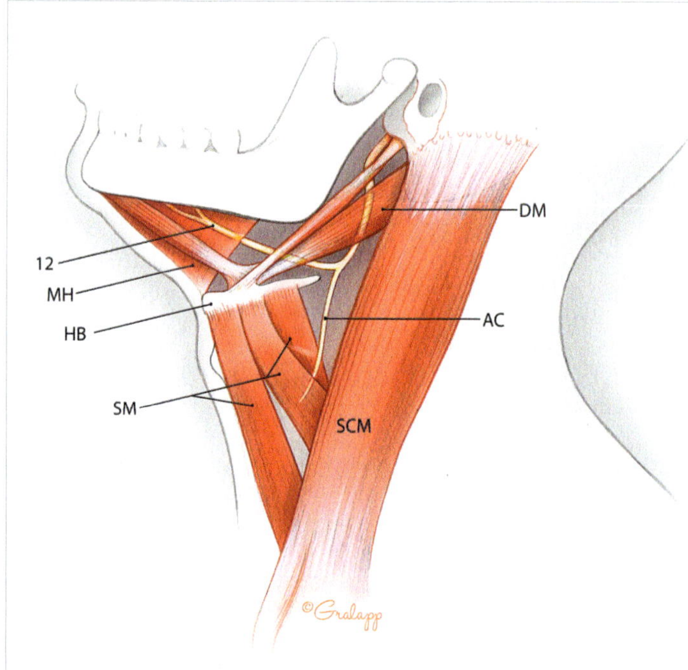

Fig. 9.28 The important landmarks in the surgical anatomy of the hypoglossal nerve include its close relationship to the medial surface of the posterior belly of the digastric muscle in the floor of the submandibular triangle. The ansa cervicalis, which innervates the strap muscles, branches off of the main nerve trunk posteriorly. 12, hypoglossal nerve; MH, mylohyoid muscle; HB, hyoid bone; SM, strap muscles; SM, styloid muscles; DM, digastric muscle; AC, ansa cervicalis; SCM, sternocleidomastoid muscle.

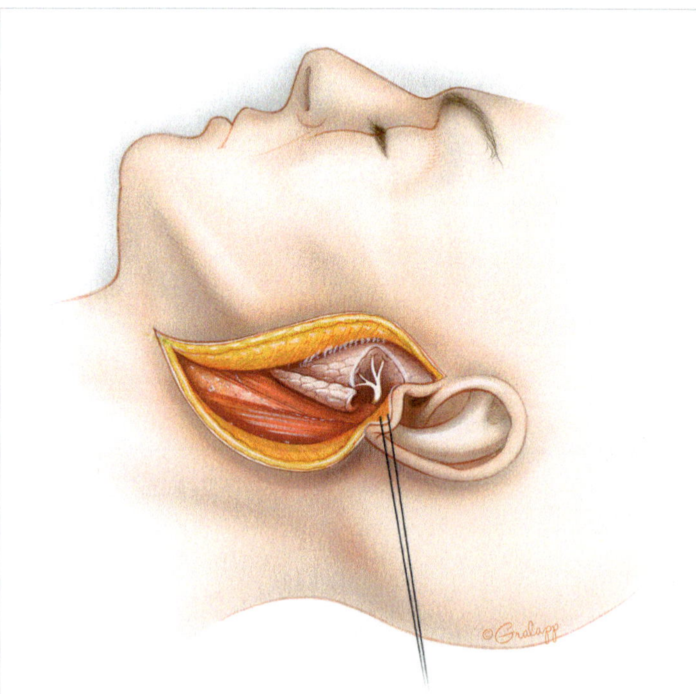

Fig. 9.29 In the initial stages of hypoglossal facial anastomosis procedure, the facial nerve is dissected from its exit from the stylomastoid foramen to the pes anserinus. Note that an extensive cheek flap, as utilized in parotidectomy, is unnecessary.

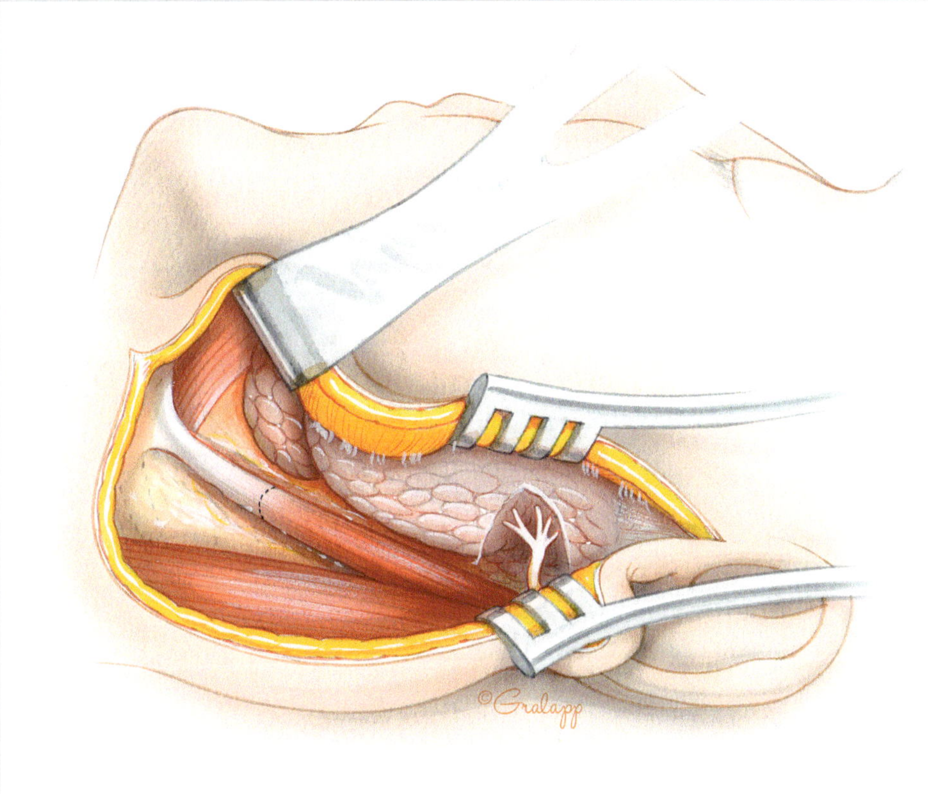

Fig. 9.30 After dissecting out the posterior belly of the digastric muscle, it is divided (*dashed line*) to provide unhindered exposure of the submandibular triangle. This muscle can also be left intact and retracted, but this is unusually more cumbersome than division and subsequent repair.

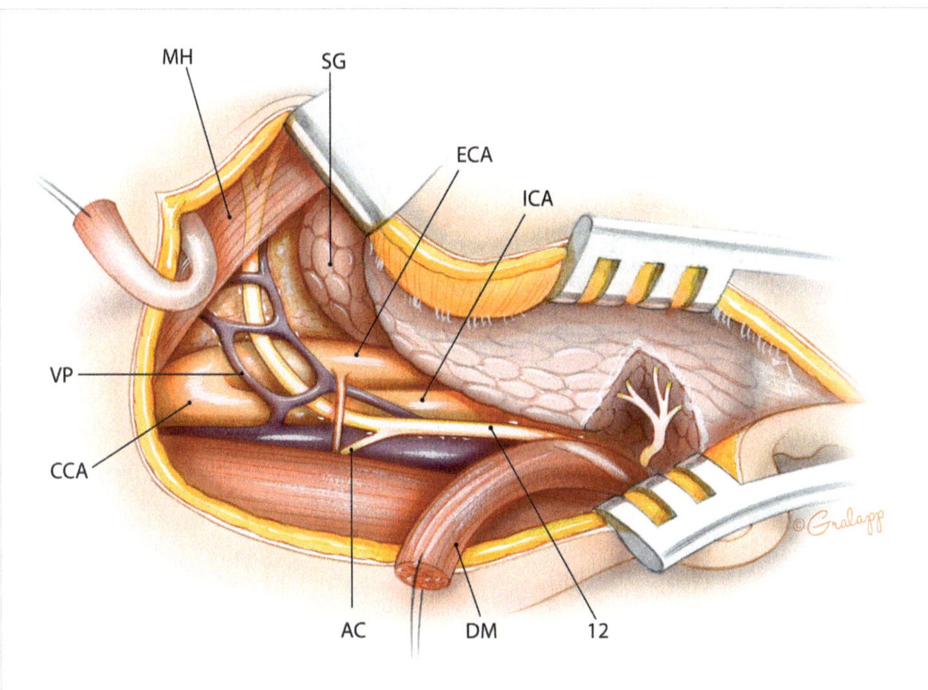

Fig. 9.31 In this surgical view, the contents of the submandibular triangle and upper neck have been rendered visible to demonstrate their relation to the hypoglossal nerve. Note the interconnecting network of veins typically parallel and cross over the hypoglossal nerve. As it enters the tongue, deep to the mylohyoid muscle, the hypoglossal nerve divides into its terminal branches. CCA, common carotid artery; VP, venous plexus of the submandibular triangle; A, ansa cervicalis; ECA, external carotid artery; DM, digastric muscle; 12, hypoglossal nerve; MH, mylohyoid muscle; SG, submandibular gland; ICA, internal carotid artery.

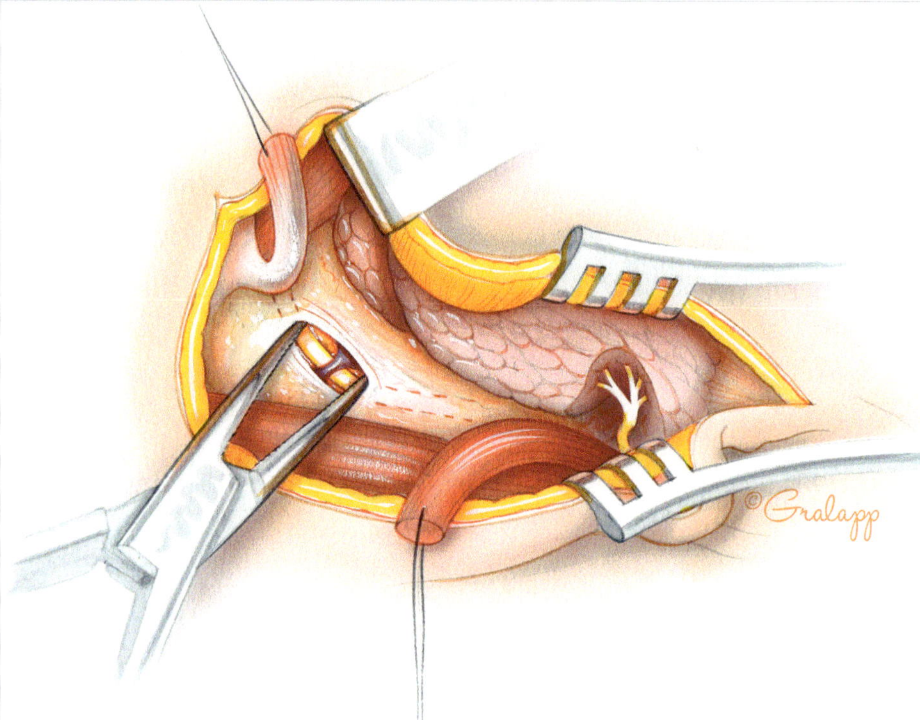

Fig. 9.32 The fascia of the submandibular triangle is opened deep to the course of the posterior belly of the digastric muscle. The tissues are dissected in a direction parallel to the course of the hypoglossal nerve. The veins which lie adjacent to the nerve often must be ligated.

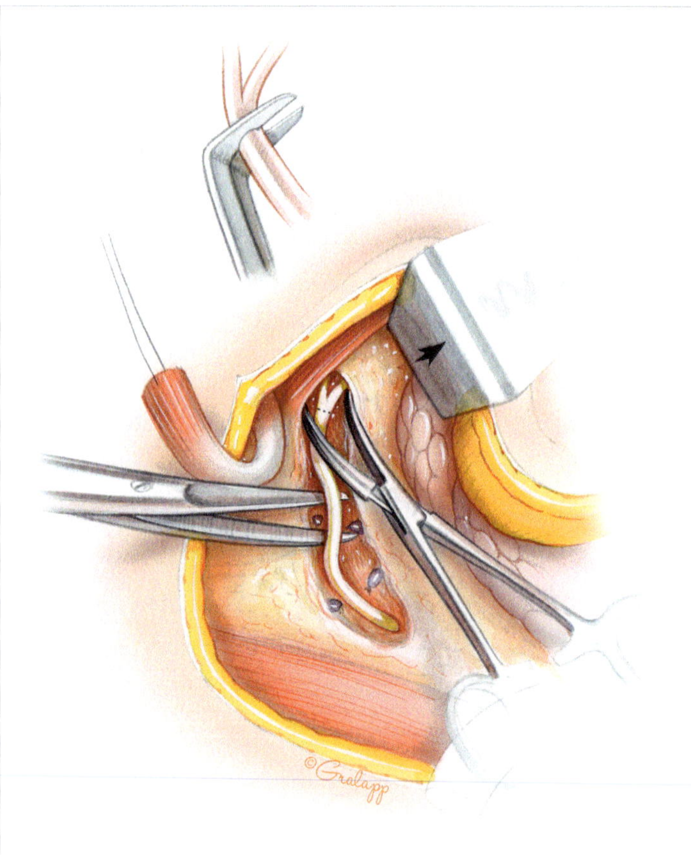

Fig. 9.33 To mobilize the nerve, it must be freed of all attachments, including those binding down its deep surface. The nerve is divided distally just proximal to its branch point within the tongue. Taking the nerve this far distally ensures that sufficient length will reach the transected facial nerve. Adequate exposure of the hypoglossal nerve's entry into the tongue requires vigorous retraction of the free margin of the mylohyoid muscle. Right angled scissors (e.g., upper lateral cartilage scissors) are helpful in accomplishing nerve division in the narrow field.

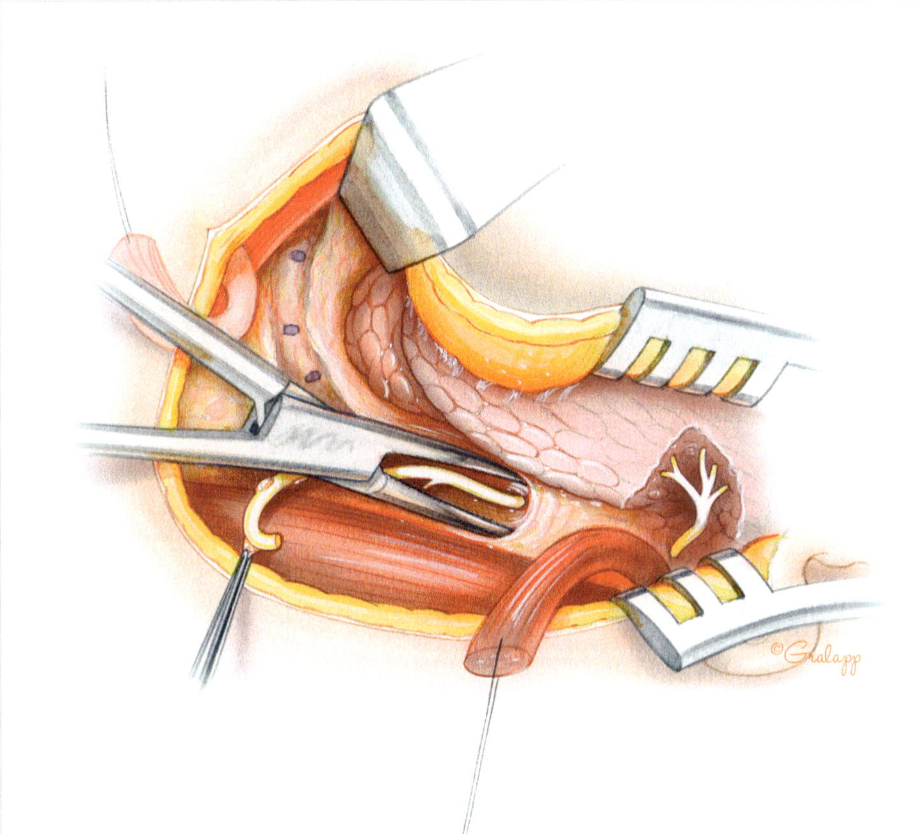

Fig. 9.34 The hypoglossal nerve is then dissected in the retrograde direction toward its exit from the cranial base. The ansa cervicalis is divided as is the small artery which usually crosses the nerve just superior to this point. In order to obtain a favorable angle of rotation for tension-free anastomosis, the nerve must be mobilized fairly high in the neck. It is helpful to leave small tags of connective tissue on the nerve, as depicted here, to serve as handles while manipulating the nerve.

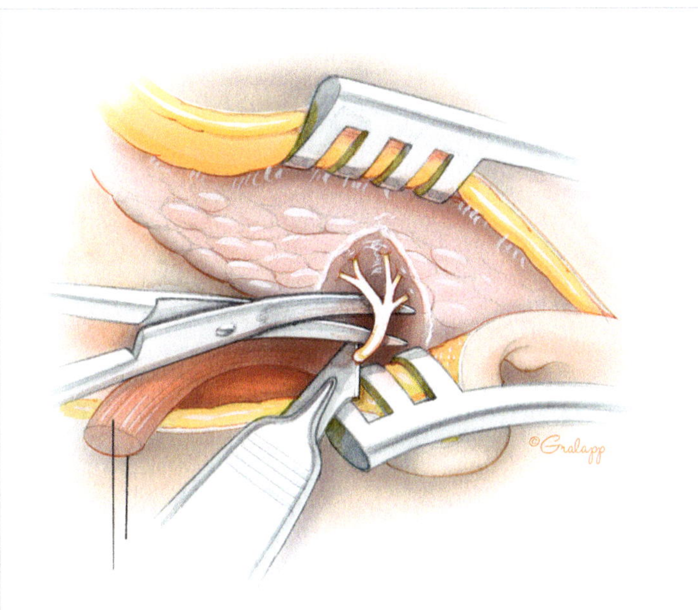

Fig. 9.35 The facial nerve is transected with a no. 11 blade just outside of the stylomastoid foramen. To permit its rotation inferiorly to meet the transposed hypoglossal nerve, the undersurface of the pes anserinus and the main nerve trunk are dissected free.

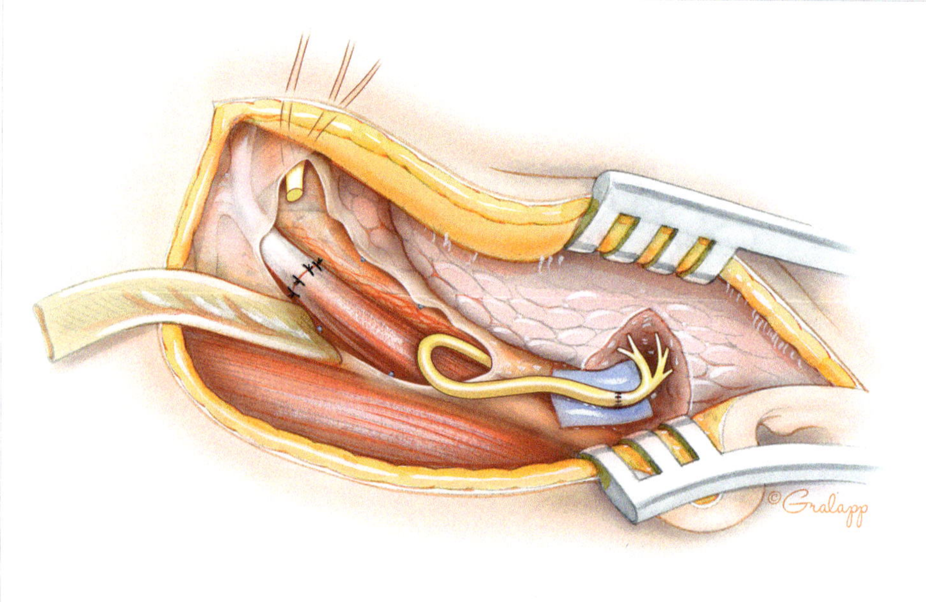

Fig. 9.36 The nerves are then anastomosed over a microsurgical background consisting of a colored piece of plastic sheet. Prior to anastomosis, the cut ends of the nerves are examined microscopically and freshened with sharp microscissors as required. Approximately six interrupted epineurial sutures are used.

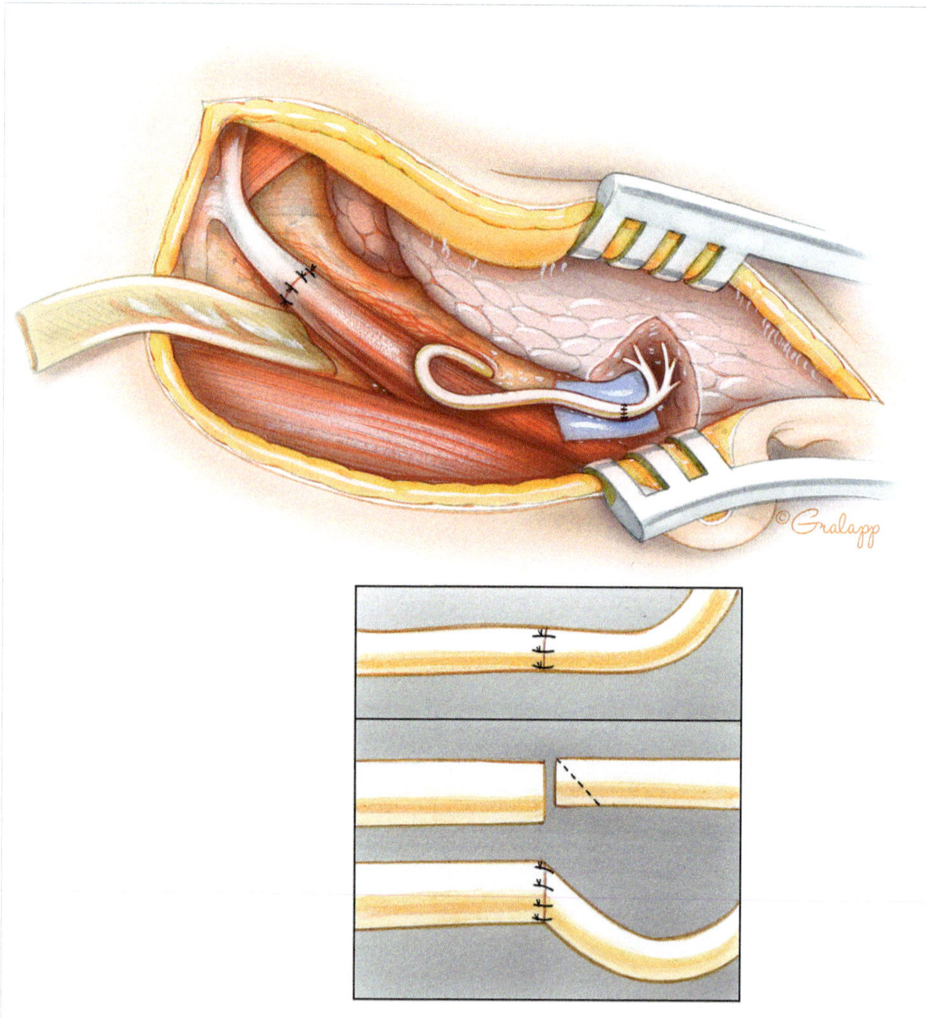

Fig. 9.37 When a size mismatch is present, the smaller nerve is beveled to allow precise coaptation of the epineurial sheaths.

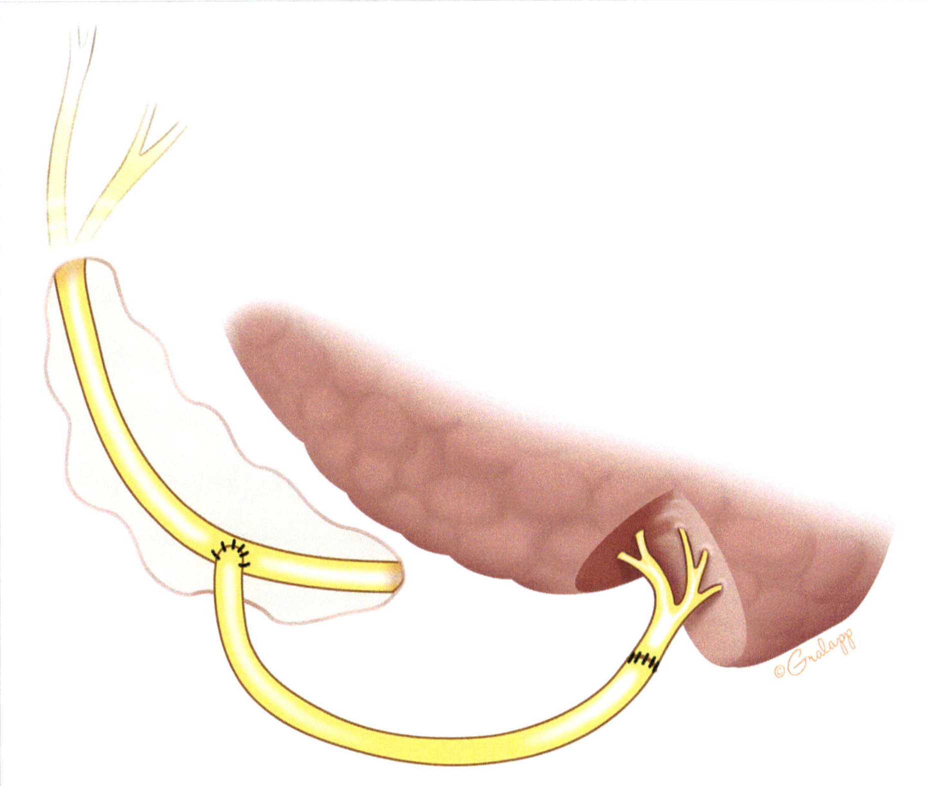

Fig. 9.38 An alternative technique is a jump graft connecting the hypoglossal and facial nerve.

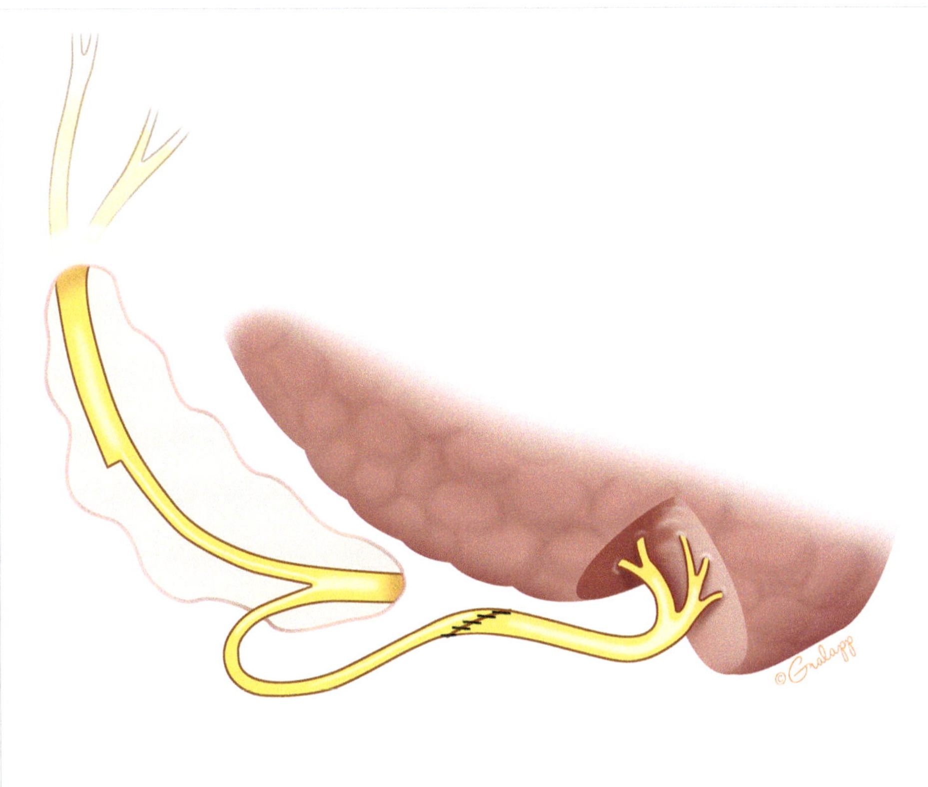

Fig. 9.39 In an effort to preserve tongue movement, some have advocated splitting the hypoglossal nerve.

9.5 Hypoglossal–Trigeminal–Facial Anastomosis

Jon-Paul Pepper

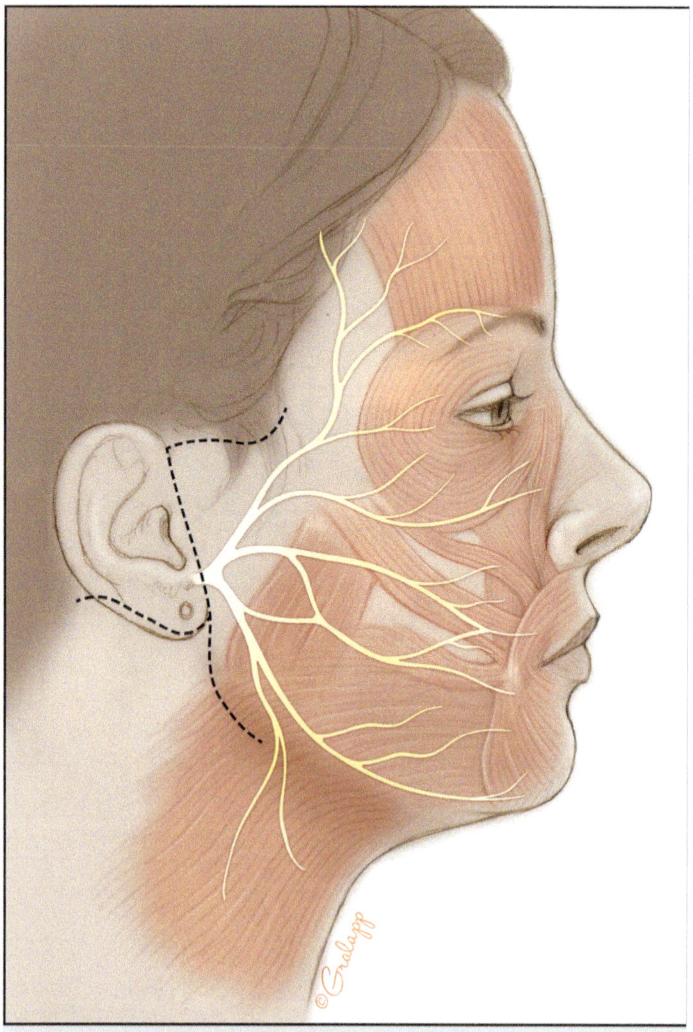

Fig. 9.40 The anatomy of the facial nerve is shown as it travels toward target muscles in the face. Also shown are typical facial incisions for combined hypoglossal-to-facial nerve and masseteric-to-facial nerve transfer procedures for facial reanimation in cases of chronic facial paralysis.

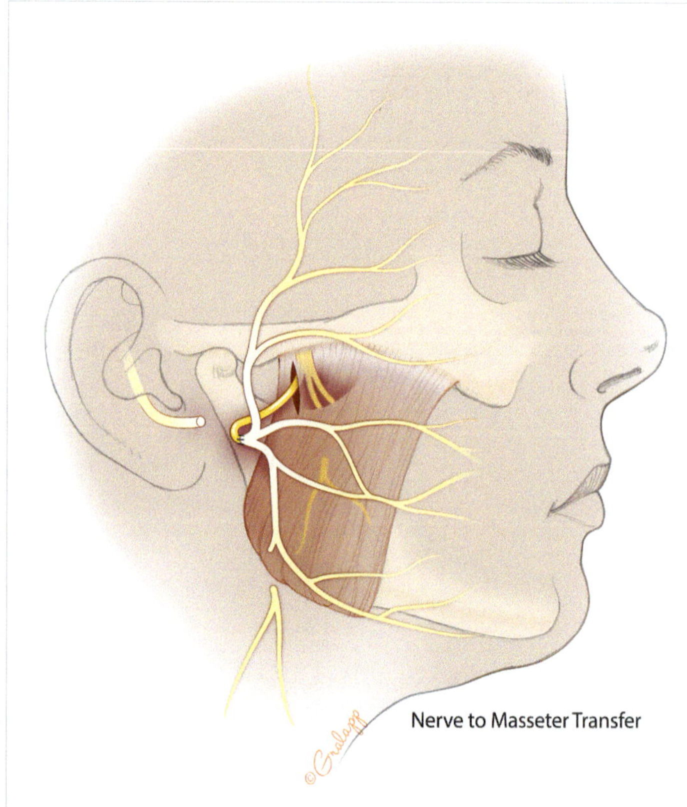

Fig. 9.41 Masseteric nerve transfer: the masseteric nerve courses through the sigmoid notch and into the fibers of the masseter muscle. It may be cut at its distal extent, and used as a source of nerve input for a chronically paralyzed facial nerve. The facial nerve may be cut near the stylomastoid foramen, and transposed to the nerve to masseter for coaptation.

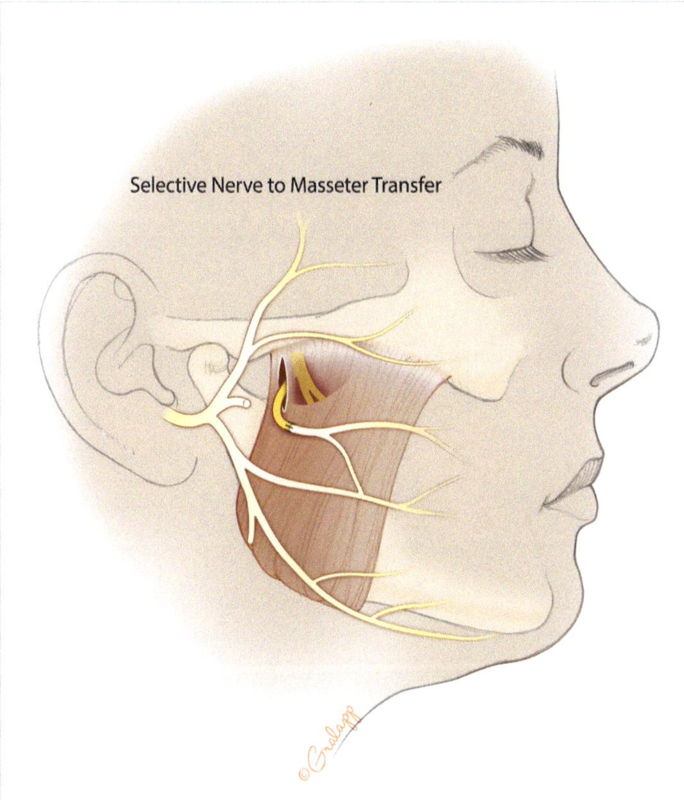

Fig. 9.42 Selective masseteric nerve transfer: the nerve to masseter may be used in selective fashion to resupply only a paralyzed buccal branch of the facial nerve for smile reanimation. This may be useful in cases where additional regeneration through the other branches of the facial nerve is expected. Alternatively, this is useful in combination with a hypoglossal nerve transfer.

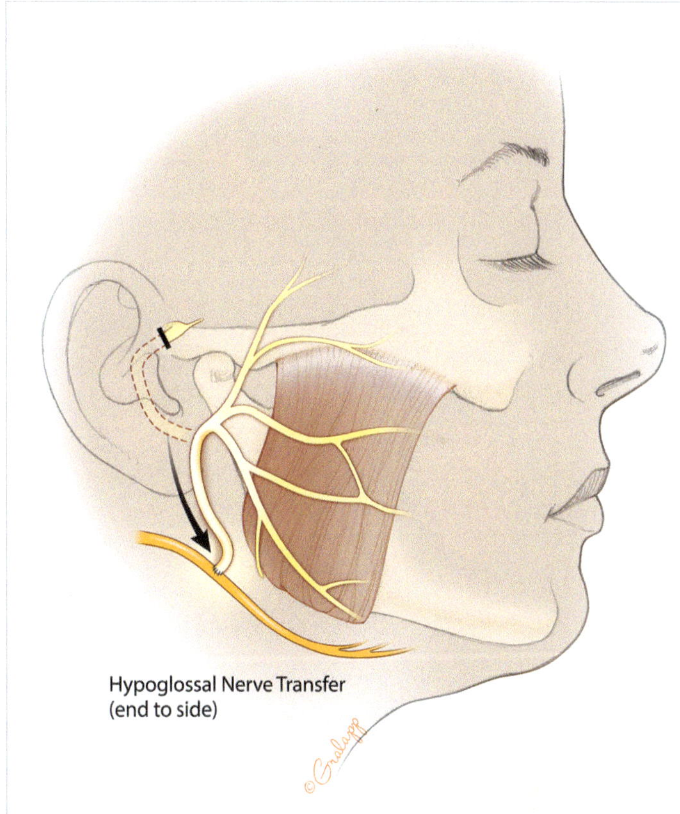

Fig. 9.43 Another alternative is to perform end-to-side facial hypoglossal anastomosis by mobilizing the facial nerve from the second genu (*solid line*). It is transected and freed from soft-tissue attachments near the stylomastoid foramen, then transposed toward the hypoglossal nerve. Approximately 50% of the hypoglossal nerve is spared in a partial neurotomy, thereby preventing hemiatrophy of the tongue.

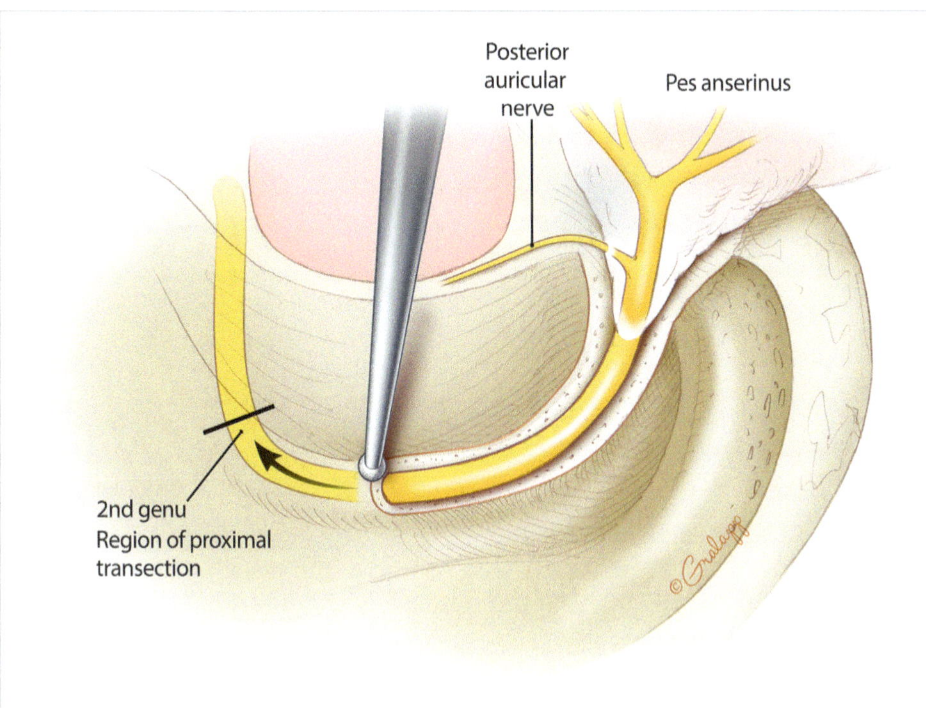

Fig. 9.44 Skeletonization of the facial nerve in the mastoid up to the level of the second genu.

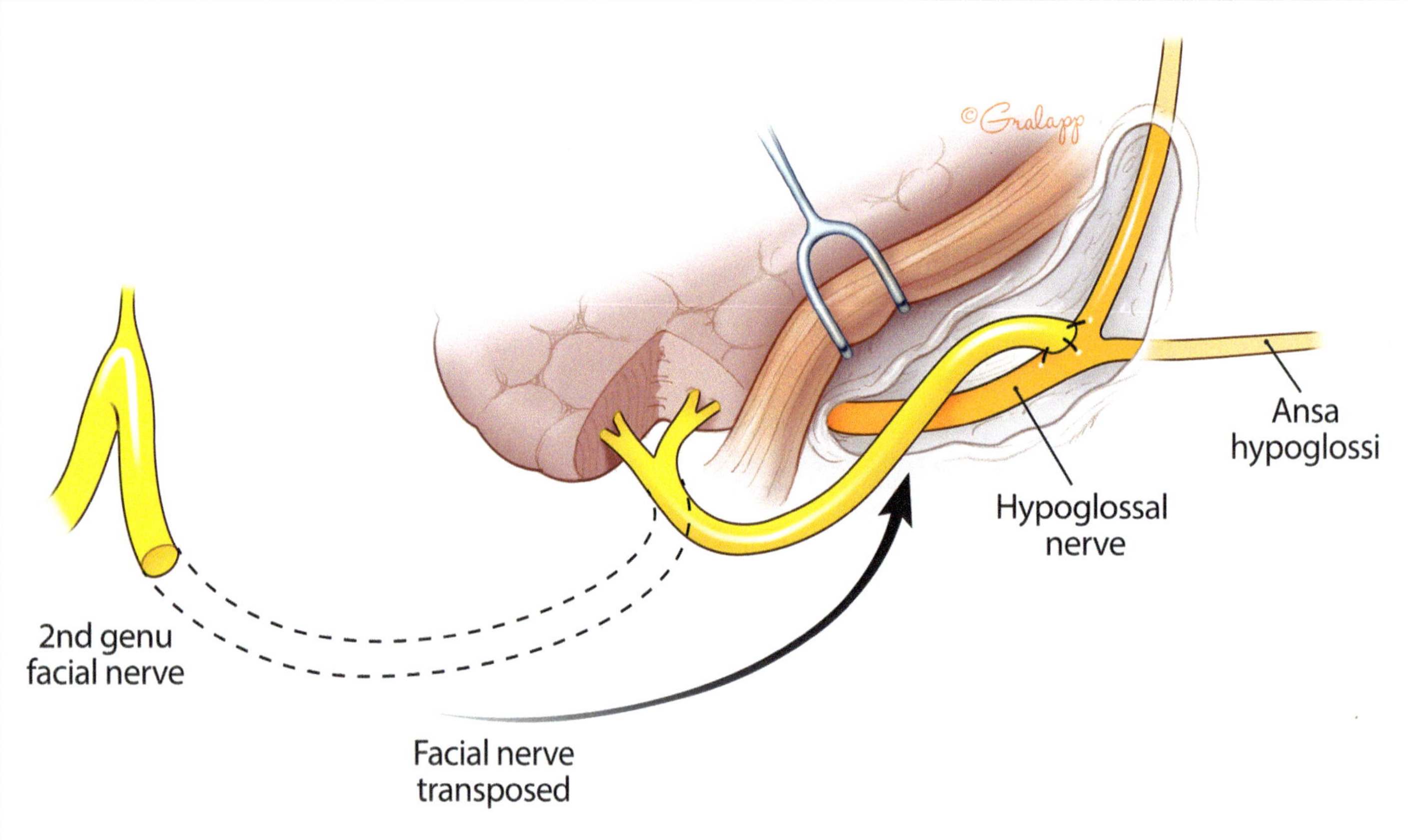

Fig. 9.45 The descending portion of the facial nerve from the mastoid is swung down for an end-to-side anastomosis with the hypoglossal nerve.

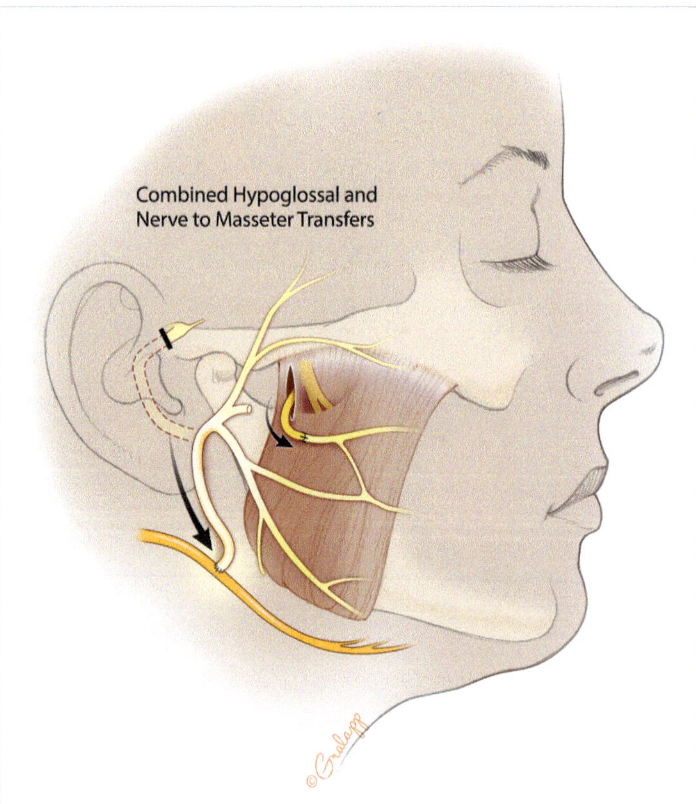

Fig. 9.46 Combined masseteric nerve and hypoglossal nerve transfers for facial reanimation: the end-to-side facial-to-hypoglossal nerve transfer may be combined with a selective nerve to masseter transfer in a single operation, thereby restoring facial tone (via hypoglossal nerve) and smile (via nerve to masseter).

9.6 Gracilis Microvascular Facial Reanimation

Jon-Paul Pepper

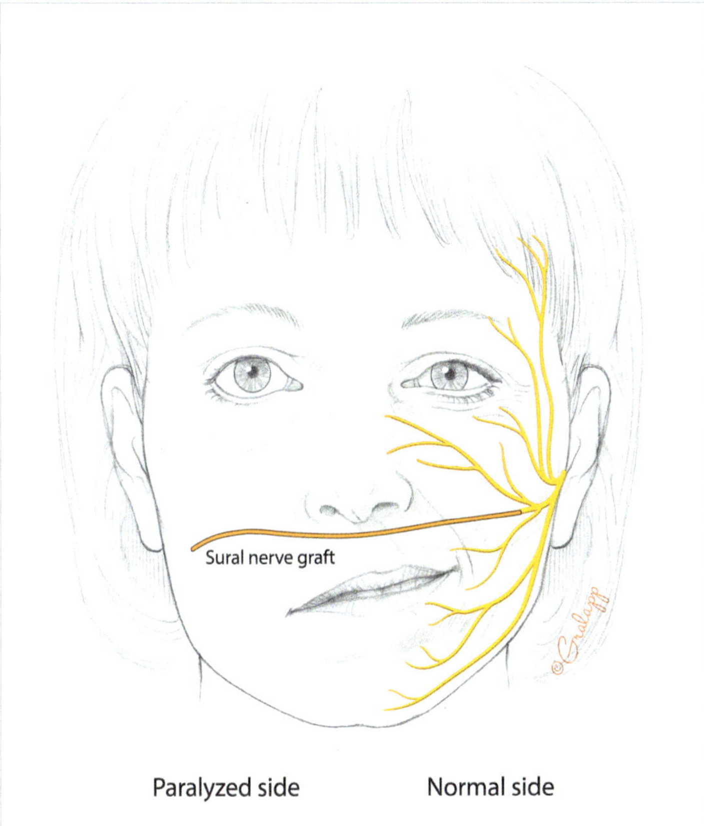

Fig. 9.47 For some cases of chronic facial paralysis, a long nerve graft may be harvested from the leg (not shown) and connected to a donor nerve branch on the nonparalyzed side of the face. The graft is then tunneled underneath the skin to the contralateral side. At a second surgery, this nerve graft may be connected to the gracilis muscle transplanted from the inner thigh region in order to reestablish movement of the corner of the mouth.

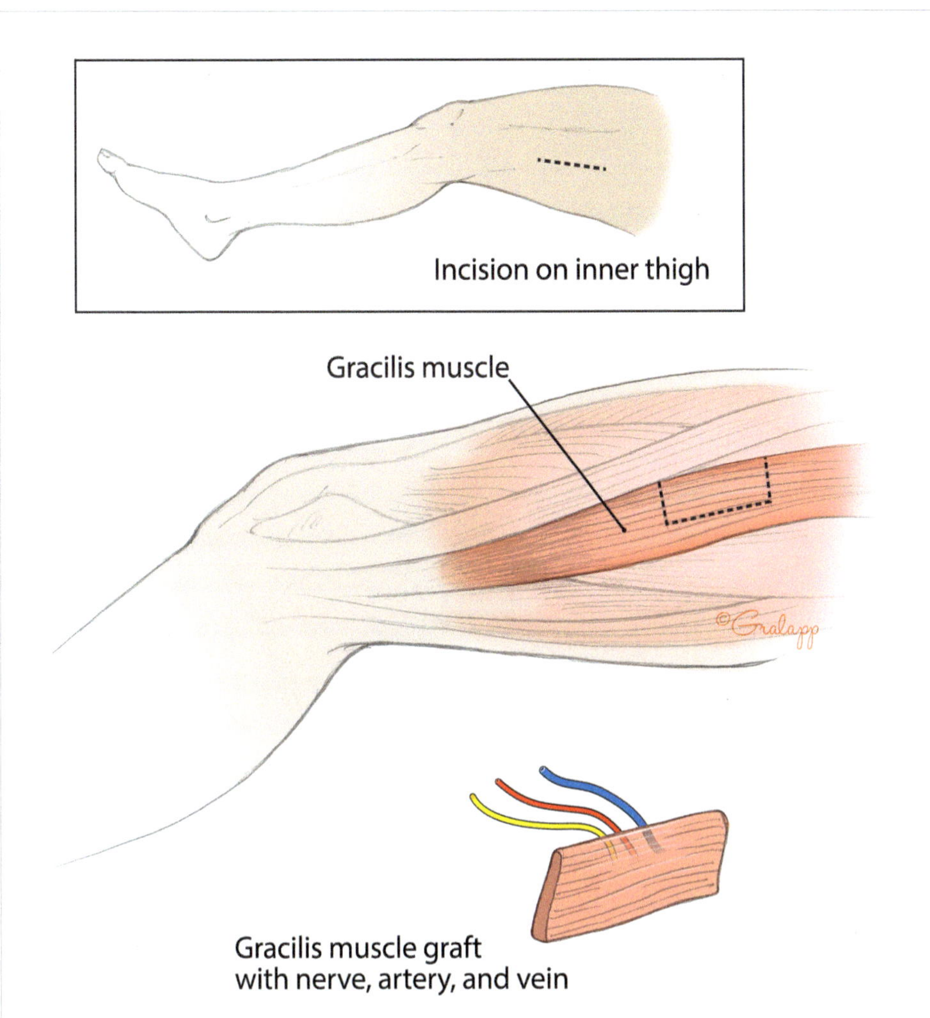

Fig. 9.48 Gracilis muscle harvest: the gracilis muscle free tissue transfer is harvested from the inner thigh region, with its accompanying nerve, artery, and vein. This muscle can then be transplanted to the paralyzed side of the face in order to reestablish movement of the corner of the mouth (smile).

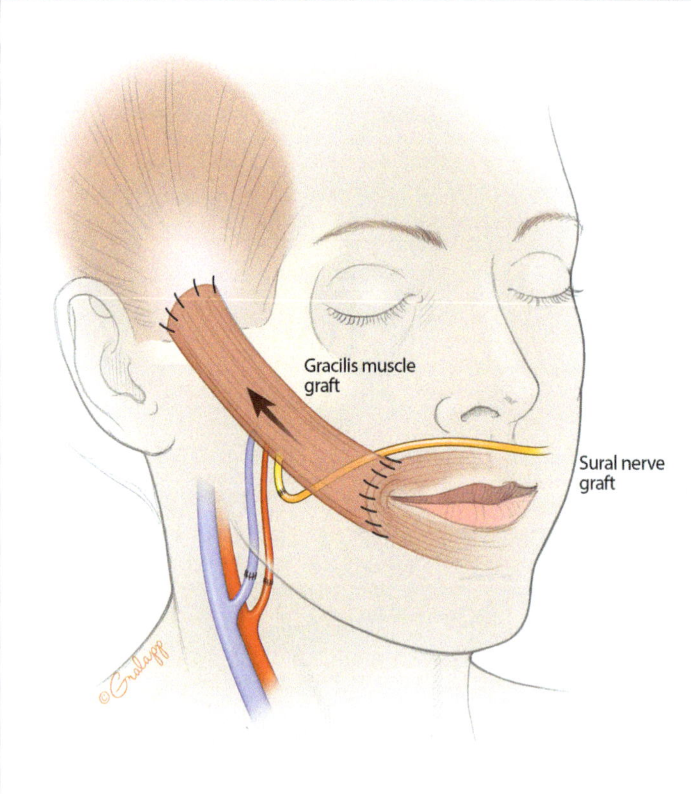

Fig. 9.49 Gracilis free tissue transfer for facial paralysis: the gracilis muscle free tissue transfer is connected to a new nerve and vascular supply in the face, to permit movement of the paralyzed side of the face. The gracilis muscle may be "powered" by the contralateral side of the face via a long graft, or by the nerve to masseter on the ipsilateral side (not shown).

9.7 Static and Dynamic Slings for Facial Reanimation

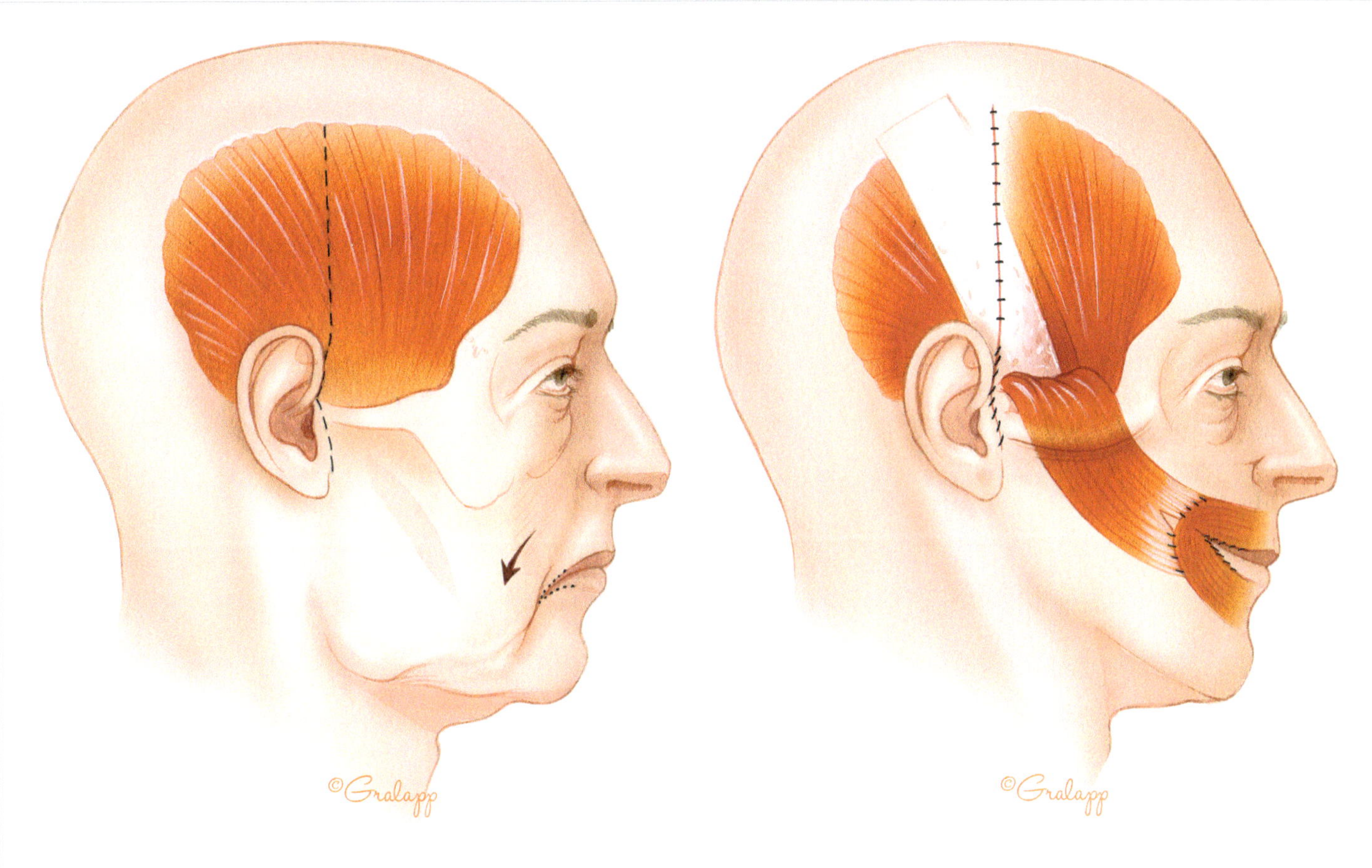

Fig. 9.50 In long-standing facial paralysis which is not suitable for a reinnervation procedure, a strip of temporalis muscle can be used to elevate the corner of the mouth. This so-called dynamic sling permits some degree of volitional elevation of the corner of the mouth. Two incisions (*dashed lines*) are required: preauricular–temporal and oral commissure. The muscle strip is tunneled under the cheek and then split before attachment to the musculofascial plane of the upper and lower lips. Overcorrection is wise, as some loosening inevitably occurs in the early postoperative period. A cosmetic donor deformity results from the decrease in temporal bulk coupled with a bulge over the zygomatic arch due to the folded muscle pedicle. This hollowed temple appearance can be compensated for by placement of a prosthetic disc (e.g., Silastic) in the temporal fossa or with fat grafting.

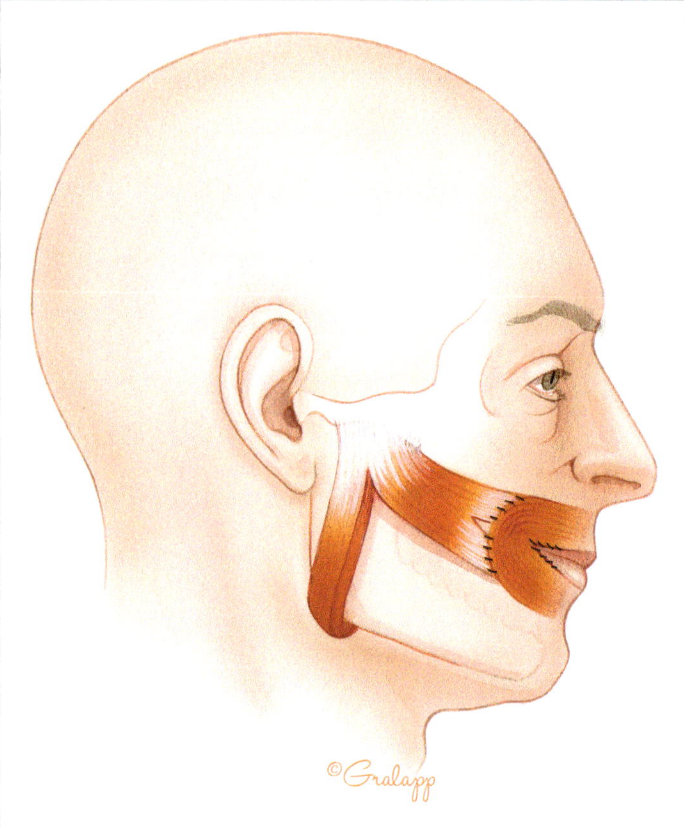

Fig. 9.51 A limited reanimation of the oral commissure can also be accomplished by its suspension with the anterior fibers of the masseter muscle. This technique is carried out via an intraoral approach.

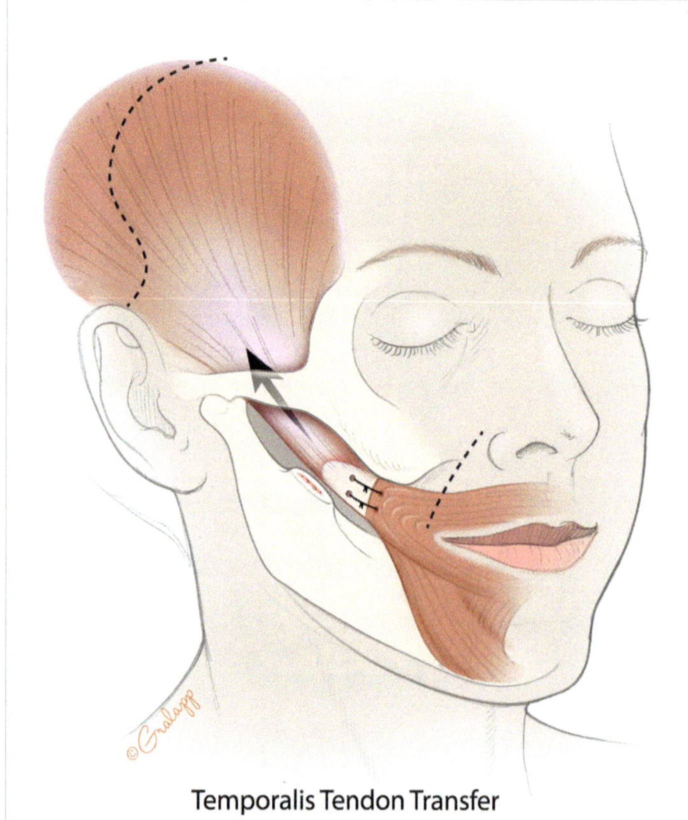

Fig. 9.52 Temporalis tendon transfer: the insertion of the temporalis tendon is identified at the medial aspect of the coronoid process of the mandible. An osteotomy is made to divide the coronoid with its fibrous attachments from the temporalis muscle and its associated tendon. This tendon–muscle complex is then advanced to the oral commissure for resuspension. Undue tension should be avoided, and this can be facilitated by release of the temporalis muscle from its fossa followed by resuspension with the correct length–tension relationship.

10 Vestibular Surgery

Robert K. Jackler

10.1 Introduction to Vestibular Surgery

The vast majority of vertiginous disorders are best managed medically. Since intratympanic therapy (e.g., dexamethasone, gentamycin) demonstrated efficacy in refractory cases of endolymphatic hydrops (Ménière's disease), surgery for vestibular disease has become less commonly done today than it was 20 years ago. Surgical removal of the semicircular canals (labyrinthectomy) remains useful in end-stage disease in a deaf ear. The remaining role for endolymphatic sac surgery (decompression or shunting) and selective vestibular nerve section is controversial, but these procedures are seldom undertaken today in most centers. The same is true for perilymphatic fistula repair: an entity viewed with much skepticism by most otologists and saved for rare instances of severe barotraumatic injury (e.g., scuba diving, rapid airplane decompression) or penetrating injury resulting in acute vertigo and hearing loss. While it is not widely practiced, semicircular canal occlusion and selective singular neurectomy are still occasionally performed for refractory positioning vertigo.

The most common surgical procedure practiced today for vestibular dysfunction is superior semicircular canal dehiscence repair first described in 1998 by Minor. Options for approach to the repair are middle fossa extradural craniotomy and the transmastoid approach. In cases of extensive middle fossa floor erosion with tegmen dehiscence, sometimes accompanied by encephalocele and/or cerebrospinal fluid leak, middle fossa approach is preferable. Management of the fistula may be either via re-covering or plugging the dehiscent canal. The author prefers a middle fossa repair with a thick layer of hydroxyapatite bone cement backed up by transmastoid plugging should symptoms be inadequately controlled.

Further Reading

1. Alarcón AV, Hidalgo LO, Arévalo RJ, Diaz MP. Labyrinthectomy and vestibular neurectomy for intractable vertiginous symptoms. Int Arch Otorhinolaryngol 2017;21(2):184–190 PubMed
2. Banakis Hartl RM, Cass SP. Effectiveness of transmastoid plugging for semicircular canal dehiscence syndrome. Otolaryngol Head Neck Surg 2018;158(3):534–540 PubMed
3. Bojrab DI II, LaRouere MJ, Bojrab DI, et al. Endolymphatic sac decompression with intra-sac dexamethasone injection in Menière's disease. Otol Neurotol 2018;39(5):616–621 PubMed
4. Carr SD, Rutka JA. Vestibular outcomes in bilateral posterior semicircular canal occlusion for refractory benign positional vertigo. Otol Neurotol 2018;39(8):1031–1036 PubMed
5. Corvera Behar G, García de la Cruz MA. Surgical treatment for recurrent benign paroxysmal positional vertigo. Int Arch Otorhinolaryngol 2017;21(2):191–194 PubMed
6. Diaz RC, LaRouere MJ, Bojrab DI, Zappia JJ, Sargent EW, Shaia WT. Quality-of-life assessment of Ménière's disease patients after surgical labyrinthectomy. Otol Neurotol 2007;28(1):74–86 PubMed
7. Handzel O, Brenner-Ullman A, Cavel O, et al. Clinical implications of the association between temporal bone tegmen defects and superior semicircular canal dehiscence. Otol Neurotol 2018;39(6):797–802 PubMed
8. Hornibrook J. Perilymph fistula: fifty years of controversy. ISRN Otolaryngol 2012;2012:281248 PubMed
9. Minor LB, Solomon D, Zinreich JS, Zee DS. Sound- and/or pressure-induced vertigo due to bone dehiscence of the superior semicircular canal. Arch Otolaryngol Head Neck Surg 1998;124(3):249–258 PubMed
10. Morvan JB, Gempp E, Rivière D, Louge P, Vallee N, Verdalle P. Perilymphatic fistula after underwater diving: a series of 11 cases. Diving Hyperb Med 2016;46(2):72–75 PubMed
11. Nguyen T, Lagman C, Sheppard JP, et al. Middle cranial fossa approach for the repair of superior semicircular canal dehiscence is associated with greater symptom resolution compared to transmastoid approach. Acta Neurochir (Wien) 2018;160(6):1219–1224 PubMed
12. Patnaik U, Srivastava A, Sikka K, Thakar A. Surgery for vertigo: 10-year audit from a contemporary vertigo clinic. J Laryngol Otol 2015;129(12):1182–1187 PubMed
13. Rodgers B, Lin J, Staecker H. Transmastoid resurfacing versus middle fossa plugging for repair of superior canal dehiscence: comparison of techniques from a retrospective cohort. World J Otorhinolaryngol Head Neck Surg 2016;2(3):161–167 PubMed
14. Sharon JD, Trevino C, Schubert MC, Carey JP. Treatment of Menière's disease. Curr Treat Options Neurol 2015;17(4):341–357 PubMed
15. Volkenstein S, Dazert S. Recent surgical options for vestibular vertigo. GMS Curr Top Otorhinolaryngol Head Neck Surg 2017;16:Doc01 PubMed

10.2 Endolymphatic Sac Surgery

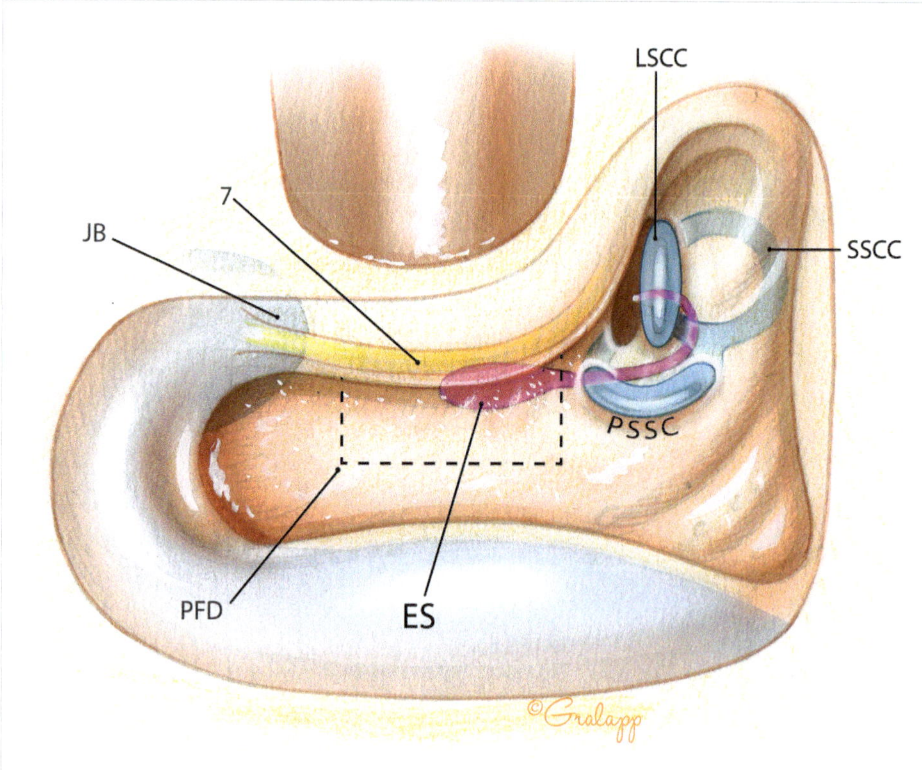

Fig. 10.1 In preparation for exposure of the endolymphatic sac, an intact canal wall mastoidectomy is performed. In contrast to many drawings which appear in otologic texts, the sac does not reside on the posterior fossa dura superficially in the mastoid. Instead it is positioned rather medially and sits inferior to the labyrinth. Surgical exposure of the sac is carried out through a roughly rectangular window (*dashed line*) which, when pneumatized, is known as the retrofacial air cell tract. This is bounded anteriorly by the mastoid segment of the facial nerve, posteriorly by the posterior fossa dura, superiorly by the posterior semicircular canal, and inferiorly by the jugular bulb. ES, endolymphatic sac; JB, jugular bulb; PFD, posterior fossa dura; 7, facial nerve; PSCC, posterior semicircular canal; LSCC, lateral semicircular canal; SSCC, superior semicircular canal.

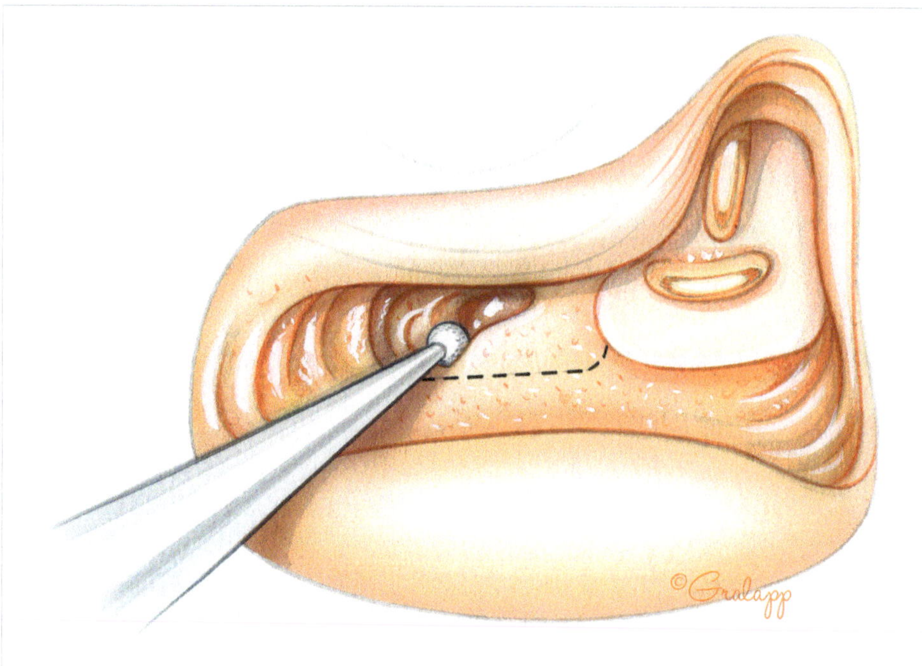

Fig. 10.2 A patch of posterior fossa dura is bared beneath the inferior margin of the posterior semicircular canal. It is usually not necessary to skeletonize this canal in order to gain adequate exposure. When an extensive retrofacial cell tract exists, the pneumatized cells can be safely and rapidly removed en route to the sac. The lower margin of the otic capsule can usually be appreciated by its denser nature, its more yellow color, and its fine pattern of superficial blood vessels.

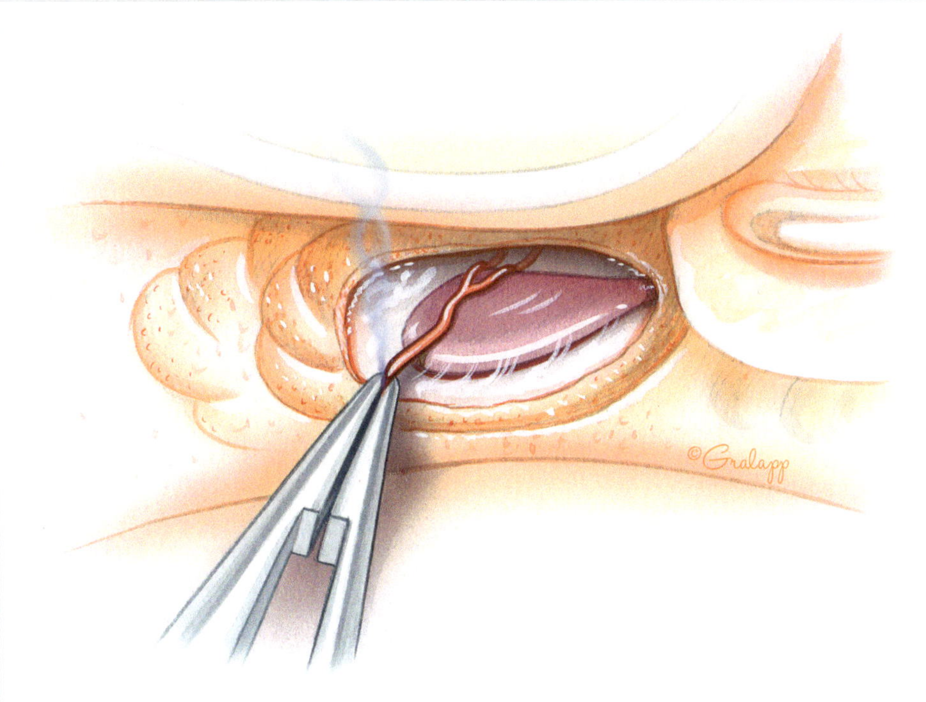

Fig. 10.3 The goal of sac decompression is not merely to identify its edge, but rather to remove bone completely from its lateral surface along with 1 to 2 mm of surrounding dura. Care must be taken to avoid injury to the endolymphatic aqueduct where it penetrates the otic capsule superiorly. While the entire sac is accessible in the great majority of cases, in a few percent it may lie either predominantly or even completely deep to the posterior semicircular canal. A small vessel typically traverses the apex of the sac. It is often injured during bone removal and must be controlled with either bipolar cautery or an absorbable gelatin sponge pledget.

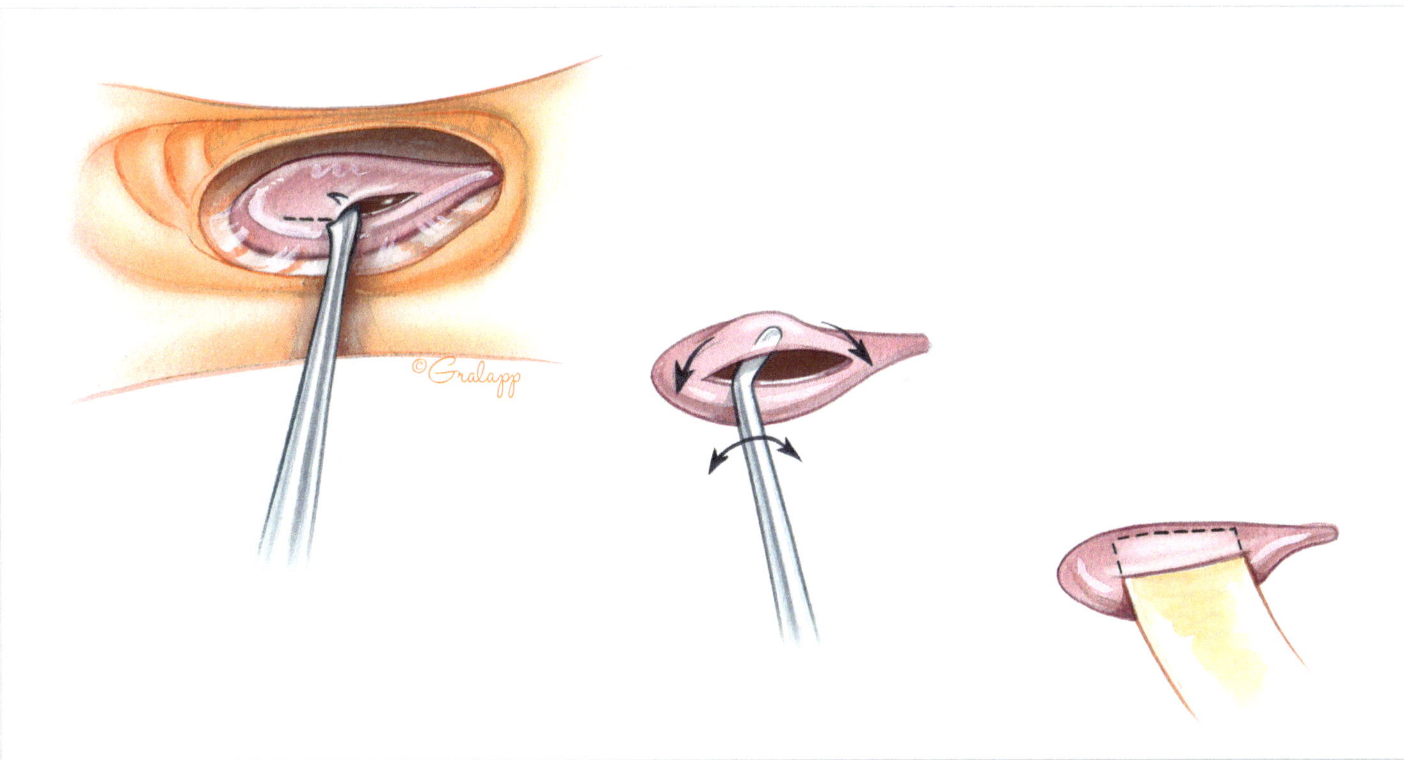

Fig. 10.4 Once the sac has been exposed, several options are available. In the simplest, the sac can be left alone in its "decompressed" state. Some surgeons inject a long-acting corticosteroid into the sac wall and between the leaves of the surrounding dura. Others open the lumen of the sac and create a shunt into either the mastoid or subarachnoid space, the latter being seldom practiced. Placement of a tube through the back wall of the sac into cerebrospinal fluid has been largely abandoned in recent years. In mastoid shunting, the lateral wall of the sac is opened with a sharp knife. While many surgeons use a Beaver blade for this maneuver, a disposable myringotomy knife or even a fine hook works well and is more economical. The endolymphatic sac does not possess a single large lumen, but is rather a network of channels partitioned by a fine reticular meshwork. These can be broken up by sweeping the lumen with a 3-mm blunt hook. A mastoid shunt can be created by inserting a thin (0.05-mm) sheet of silicon rubber as depicted in the illustration. Some surgeons advocate that the Silastic sheeting be rolled into a tube to help separate the leaves of the sac, although this can be somewhat tricky to insert. A few surgeons even insert a modified glaucoma valve, although there is little to commend about this strategy. It should be pointed out that there is much controversy concerning the efficacy of endolymphatic sac surgery, with many otologic surgeons turning away from it in recent years. While its role in the management of Meniere's disease remains the subject of much debate, it is quite clear that results do not depend on how the sac is handled (decompression, shunting, etc.).

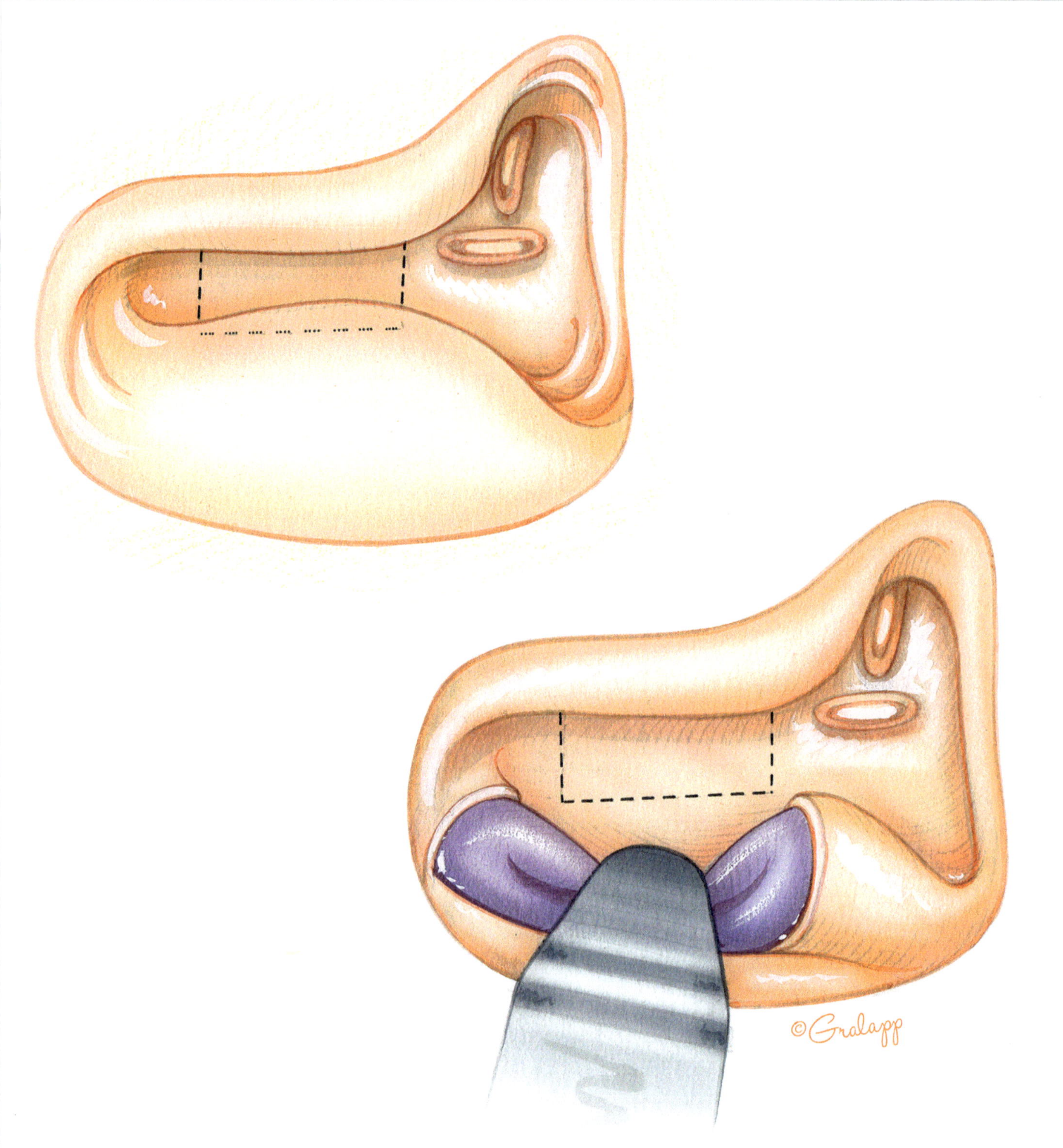

Fig. 10.5 When the sigmoid sinus is anteriorly placed, it can obstruct visualization of the retrofacial cell tract (*dashed lines*). In extreme cases, the sinus may even contact the posterior aspect of the ear canal. To accommodate for the anatomical variation of an anteriorly placed sigmoid sinus, bone is removed from the vessel's surface with a diamond burr and it is gently retracted. This maneuver provides ample access to the region of the endolymphatic sac.

10.3 Labyrinthectomy

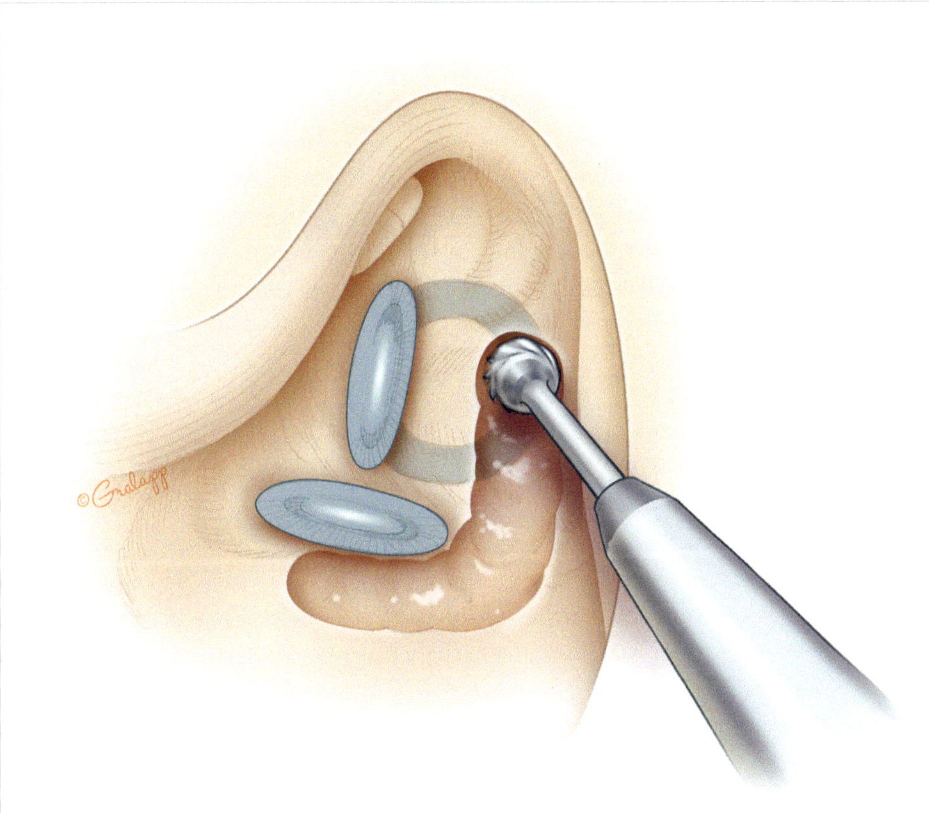

Fig. 10.6 Labyrinthectomy may be effective in alleviating medically refractory vestibular symptoms in an ear with no useful hearing. The goal is not to merely open the labyrinth, but to remove all five inner ear neuroepithelial elements (three semicircular canal ampullae and two otolithic organs: utricle and saccule). The procedure commences with drilling troughs parallel to the middle and posterior fossa dural plates with a cutting burr. This enables drilling toward the facial nerve with greater stability by using the side of the burr to cut through the hard otic capsule bone rather than the tip which is less controllable.

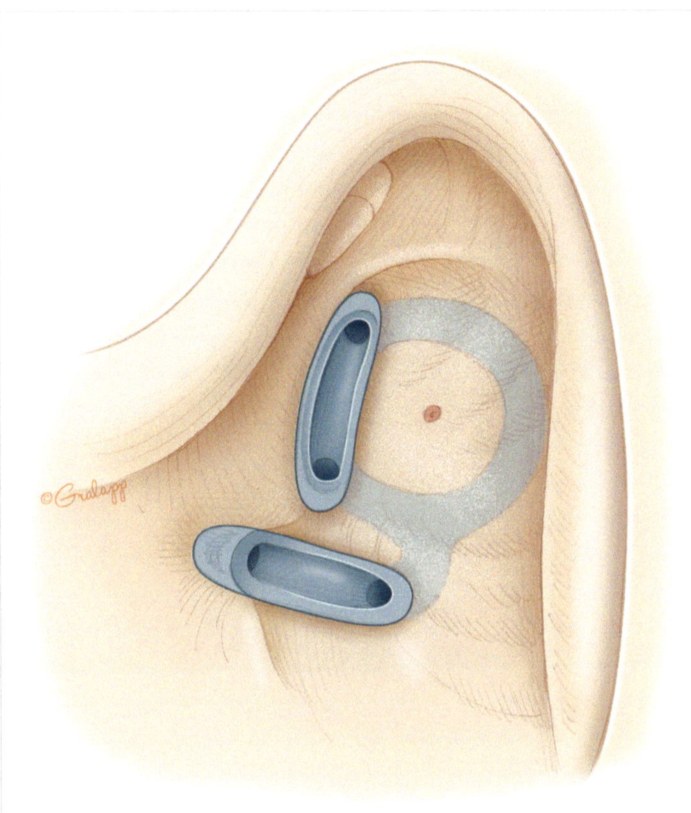

Fig. 10.7 Entry into the lateral canal and posterior canal.

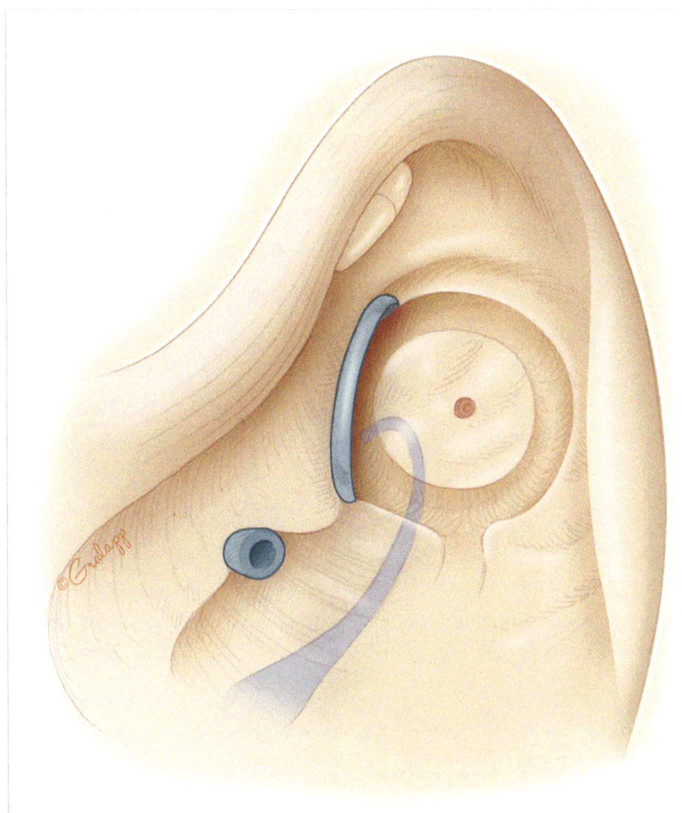

Fig. 10.8 The facial nerve lies immediately inferior to the full length of the lateral semicircular canal and is closely associated with the inferior end of the posterior semicircular canal. Note the endolymphatic sac and its duct in its J-shaped course to the vestibule passing in proximity to the common crus of the posterior and superior semicircular canals.

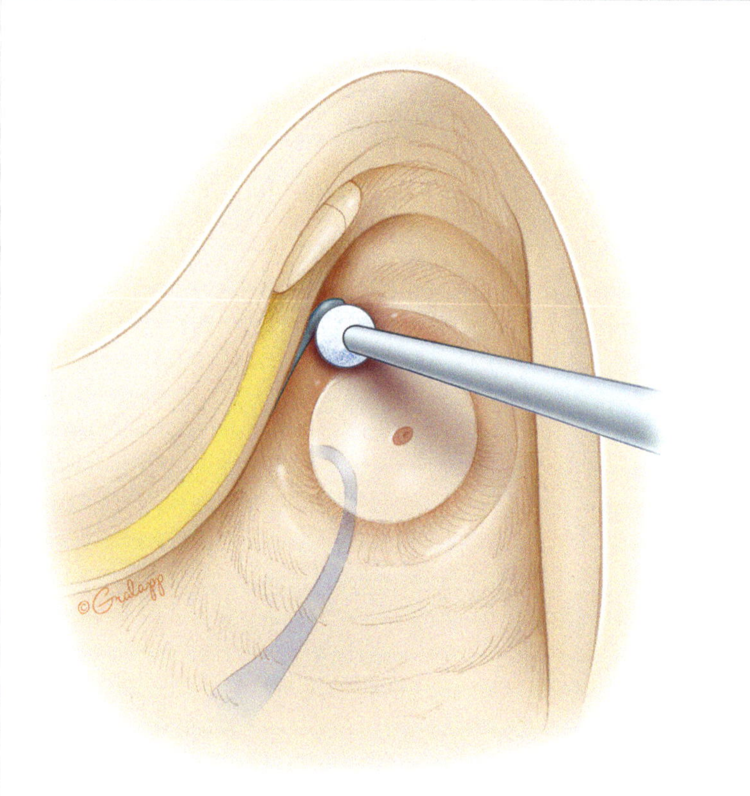

Fig. 10.9 Using a diamond burr and copious irrigation, the last portions of the lateral and posterior semicircular canals are removed. The remnant of the superior semicircular canal lies deep with the arcuate artery in the center of its loop.

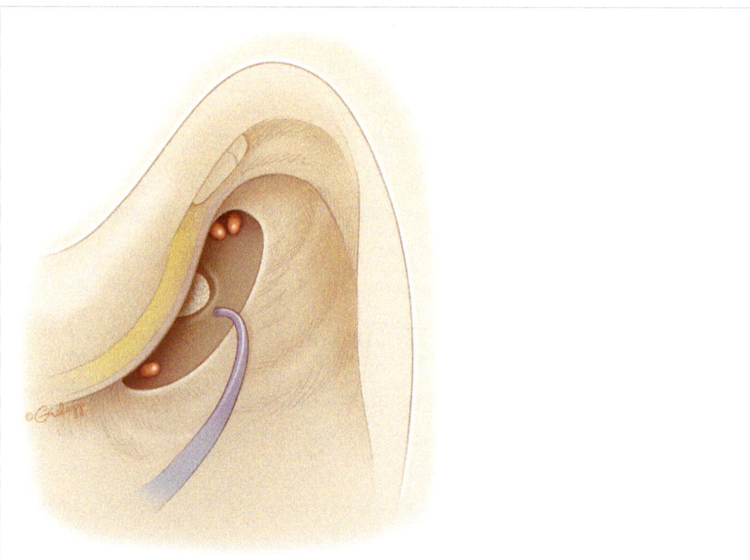

Fig. 10.10 Exposure of the vestibule of the inner ear which reveals the ampullae of the superior, lateral, and posterior semicircular canals.

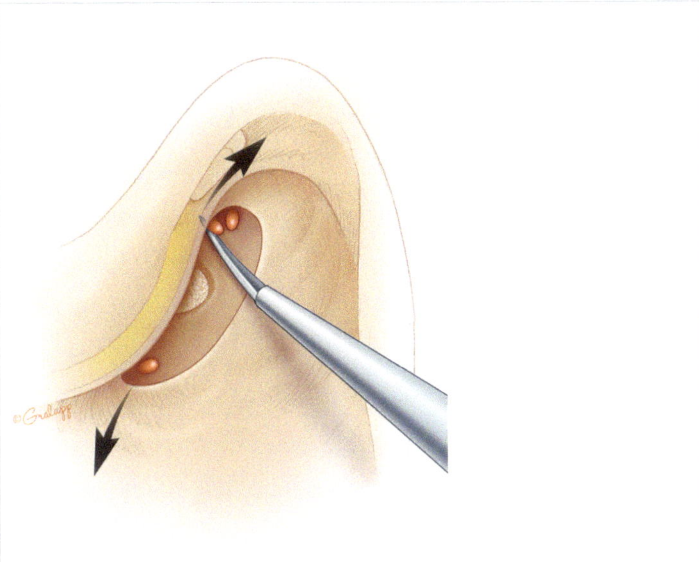

Fig. 10.11 Removal of the lateral and superior ampullae (above right) and posterior ampulla (below left).

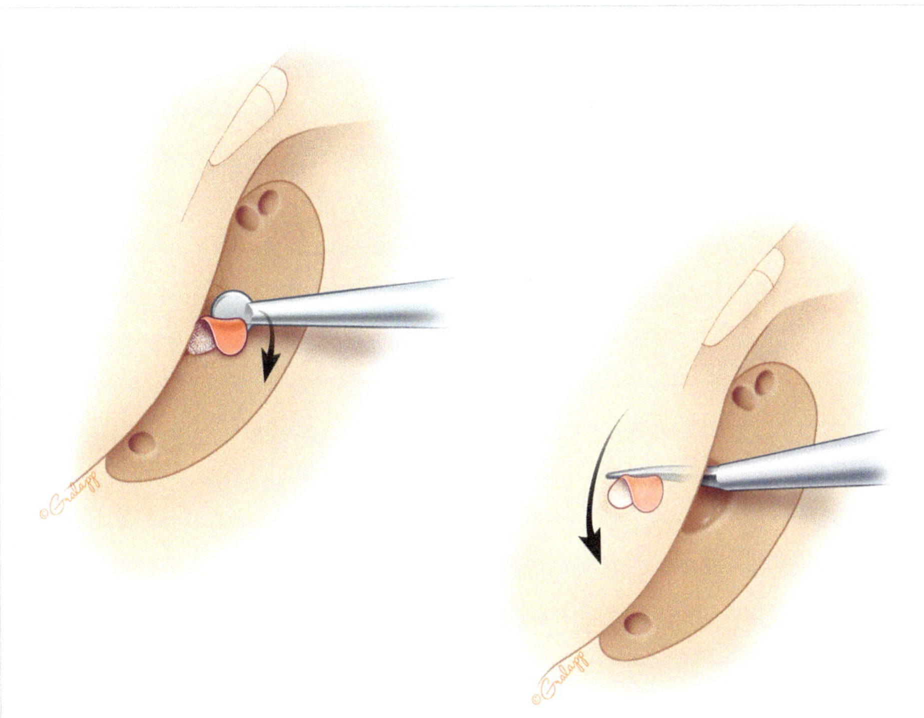

Fig. 10.12 Removal of the utricle from the elliptical recess is done under direct vision. Removal of the saccule requires a blind sweep using a long hook.

10.4 Superior Semicircular Canal Dehiscence

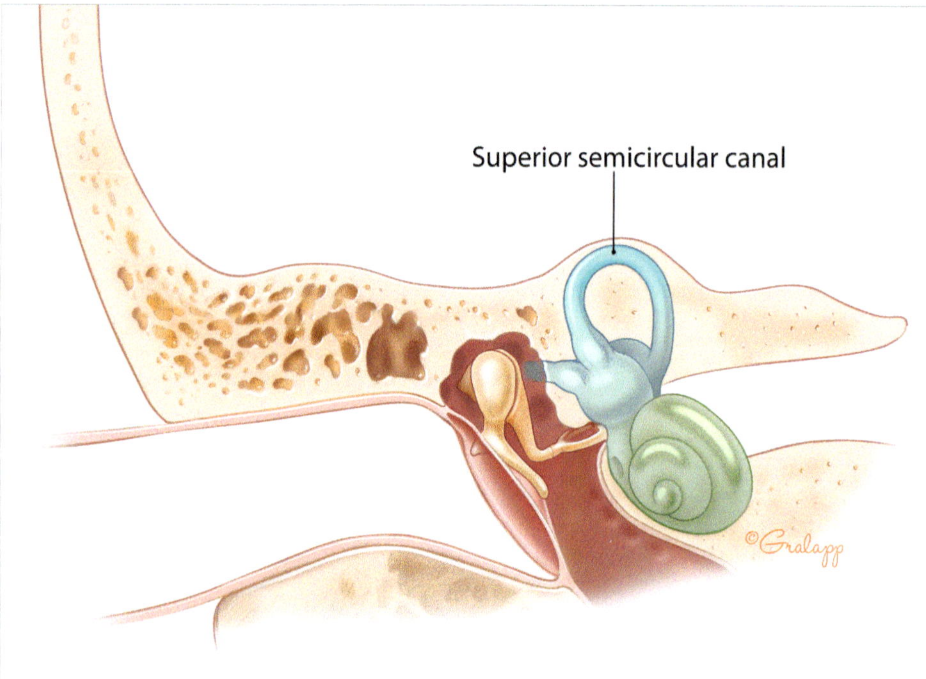

Fig. 10.13 Coronal view of the temporal bone depicting a normal superior semicircular canal.

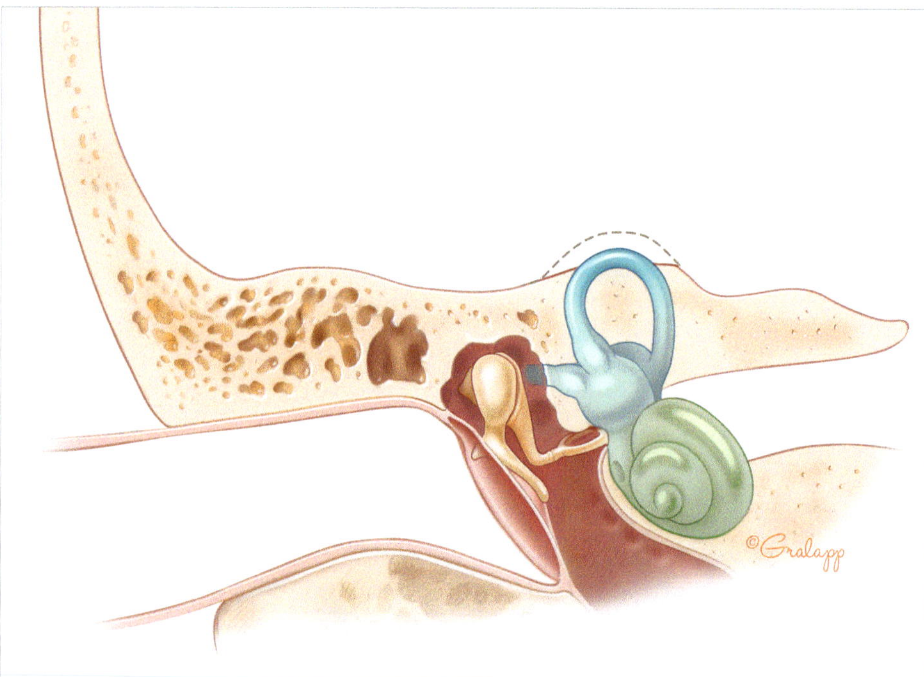

Fig. 10.14 Isolated superior semicircular canal dehiscence.

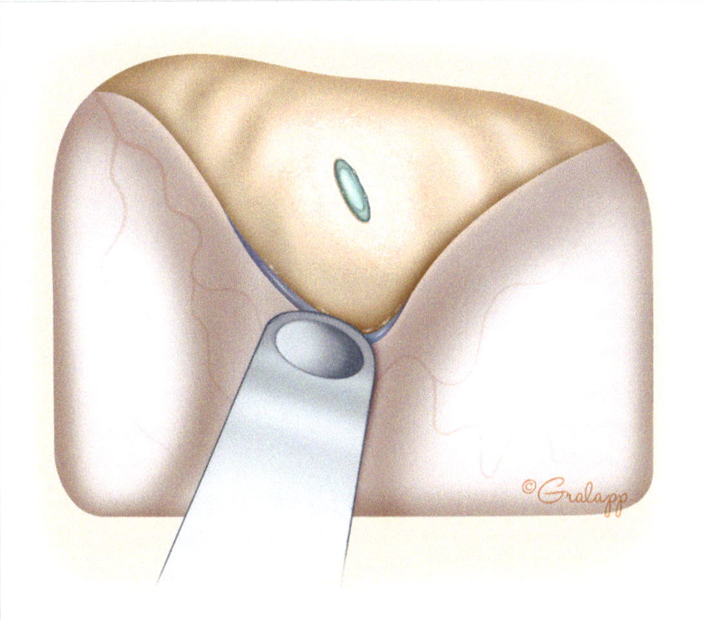

Fig. 10.15 Superior semicircular canal dehiscence on the temporal floor viewed via middle fossa craniotomy.

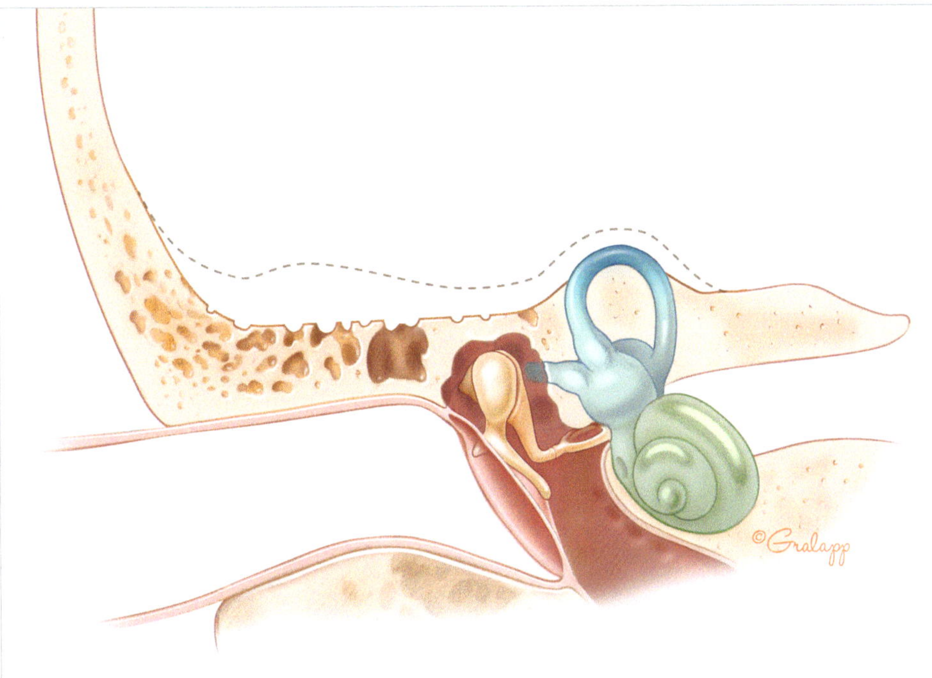

Fig. 10.16 Superior semicircular canal dehiscence often occurs together with diffuse resorption of the temporal floor. The tegmen mastoideum and tympani are often extensively eroded. In some cases, a meningoencephalocele may exist.

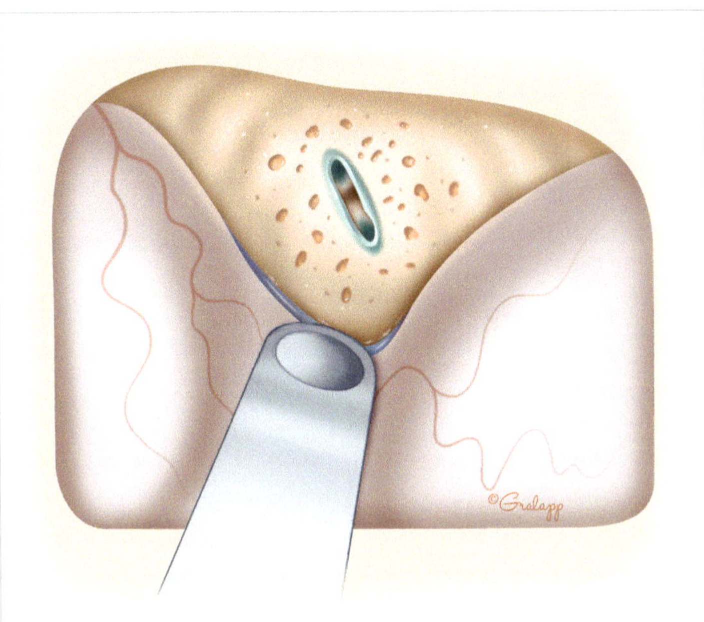

Fig. 10.17 Superior semicircular canal dehiscence often occurs as part of a diffuse resorption of the temporal floor (as seen via middle fossa craniotomy).

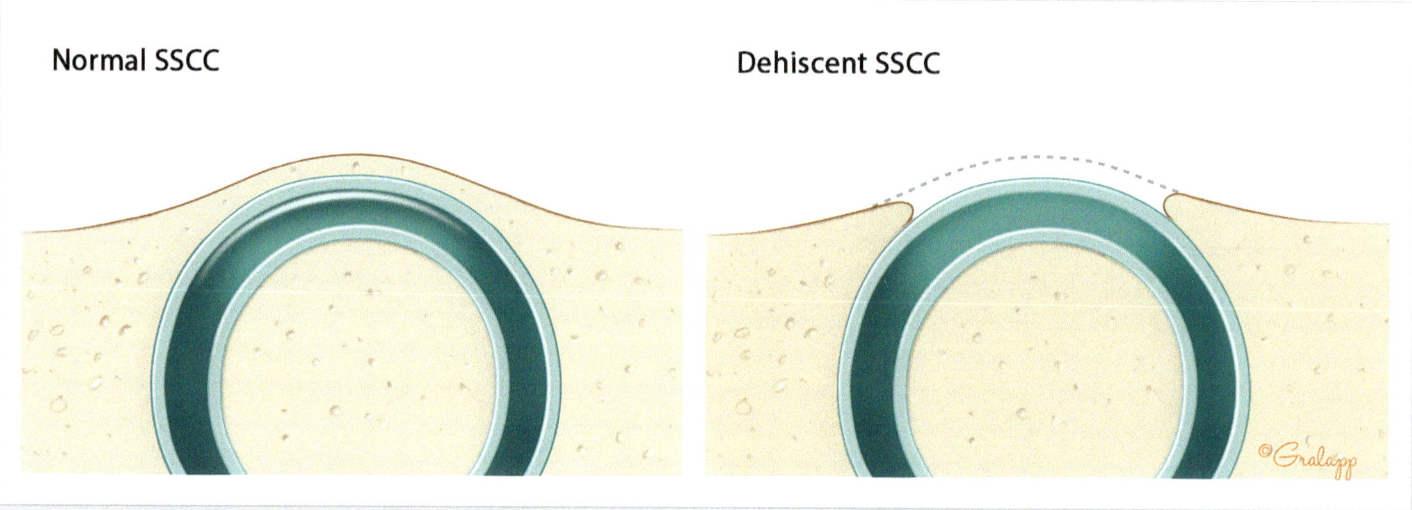

Fig. 10.18 Schematic coronal view of superior semicircular canal dehiscence showing absent bone but intact membranous labyrinth.

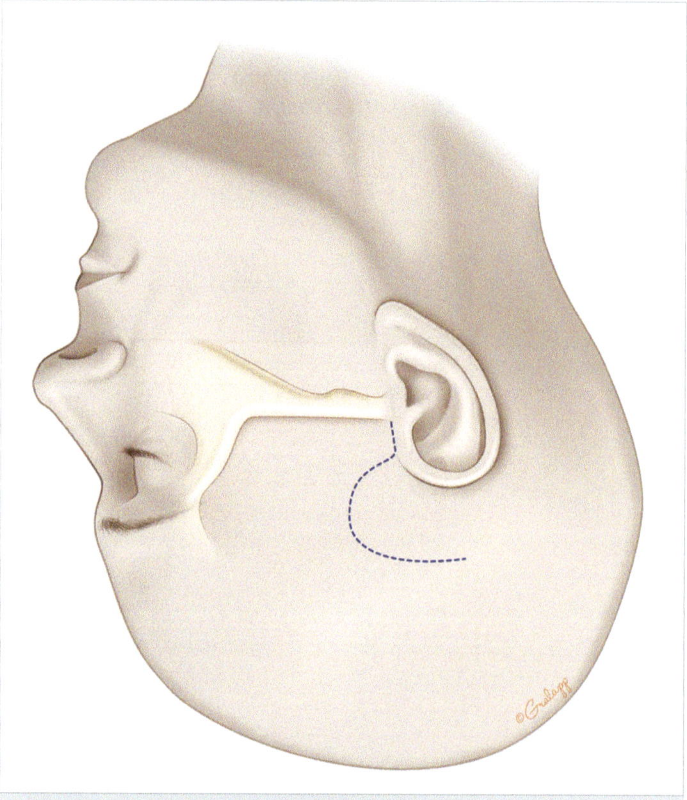

Fig. 10.19 Incision used for the small middle fossa craniotomy needed in superior semicircular canal dehiscence repair. Only a racing stripe of shaving is needed.

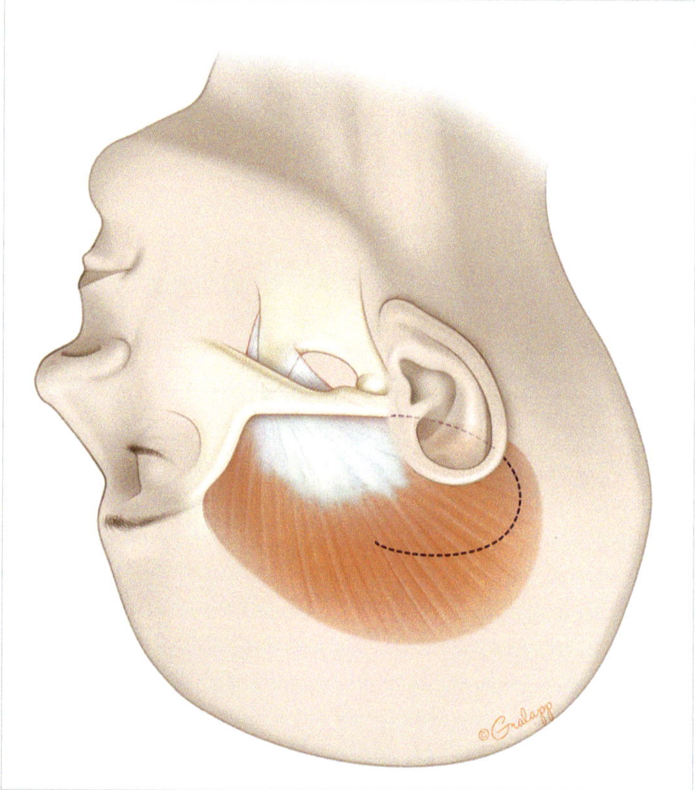

Fig. 10.20 A flap of temporalis muscle is developed opposite to the skin flap. The temporalis muscle is thinner posteriorly.

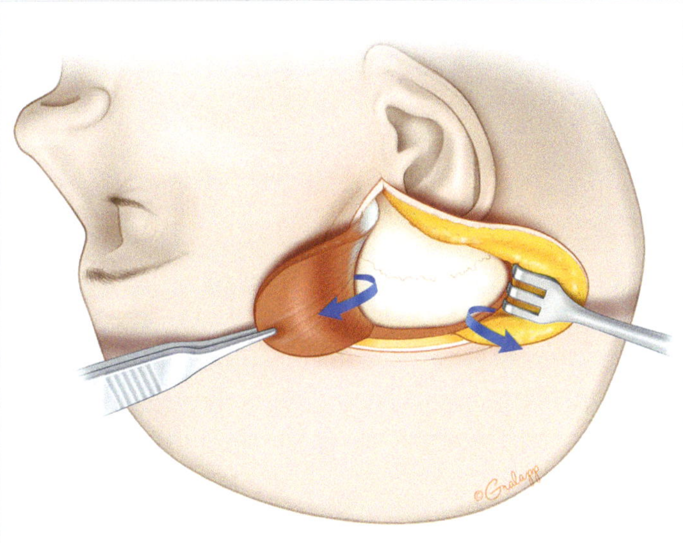

Fig. 10.21 The skin and muscle flaps are developed in opposite directions.

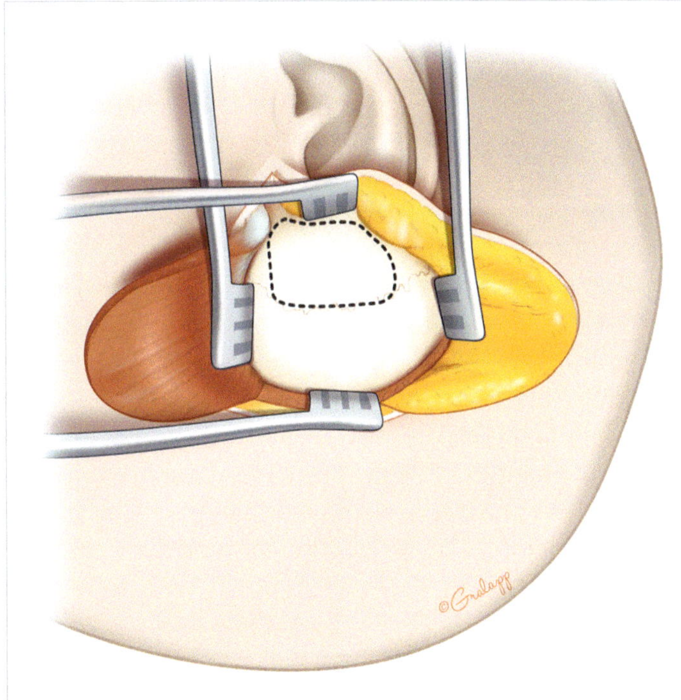

Fig. 10.22 Note that the craniotomy is centered over the mastoid, more posteriorly than in middle fossa approaches to the internal auditory canal.

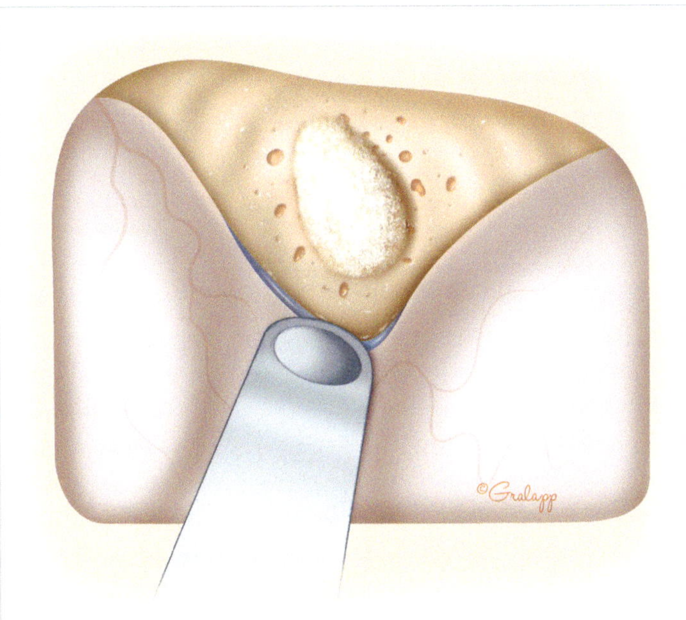

Fig. 10.23 In the resurfacing method, autologous bone paté (optional) may be placed over the canal fistula.

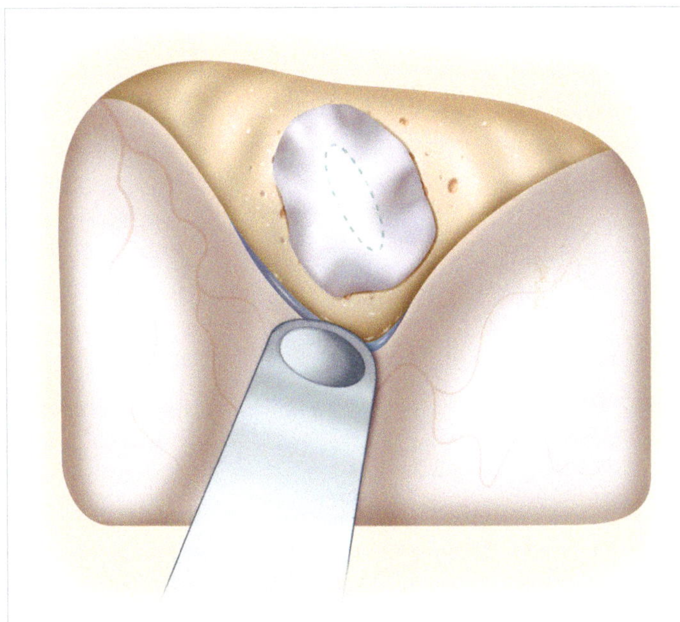

Fig. 10.24 Temporalis fascia is placed over the fistula.

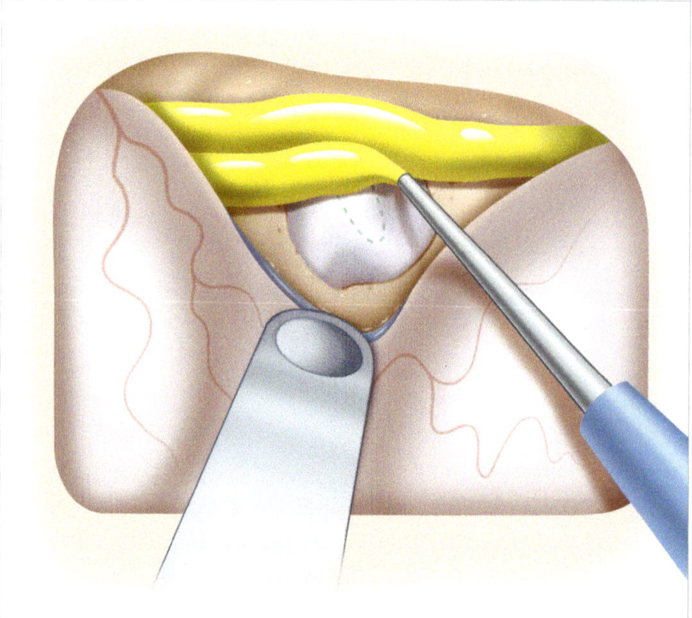

Fig. 10.25 Hydroxyapatite cement (e.g., Stryker HydroSet) is placed in its gel form. This product does not generate heat while setting.

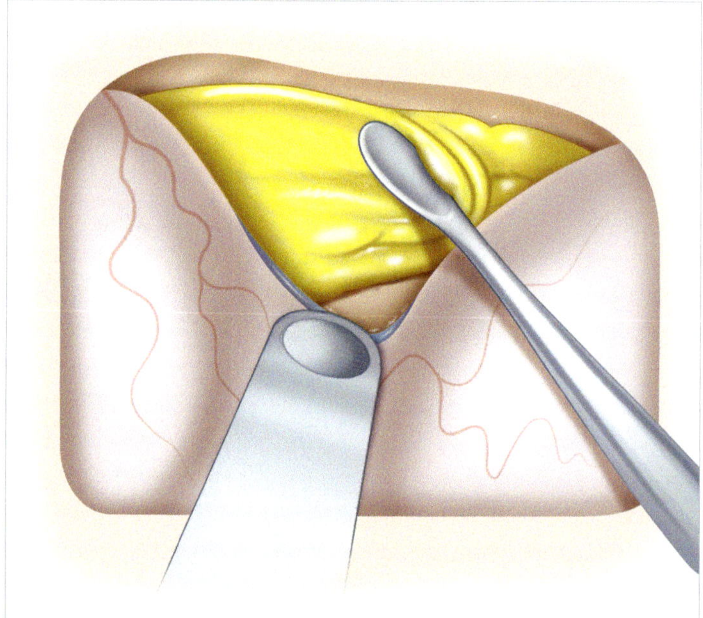

Fig. 10.26 The hydroxyapatite cement is smoothed to cover the fistula as well as reinforce the entire temporal floor.

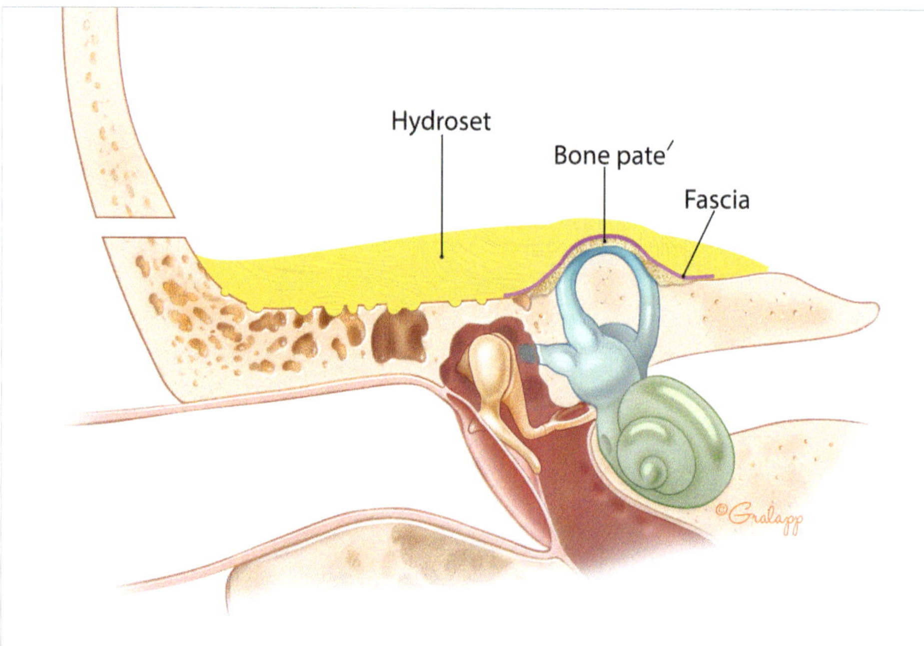

Fig. 10.27 Coronal view of completed resurfacing repair of a superior semicircular canal fistula.

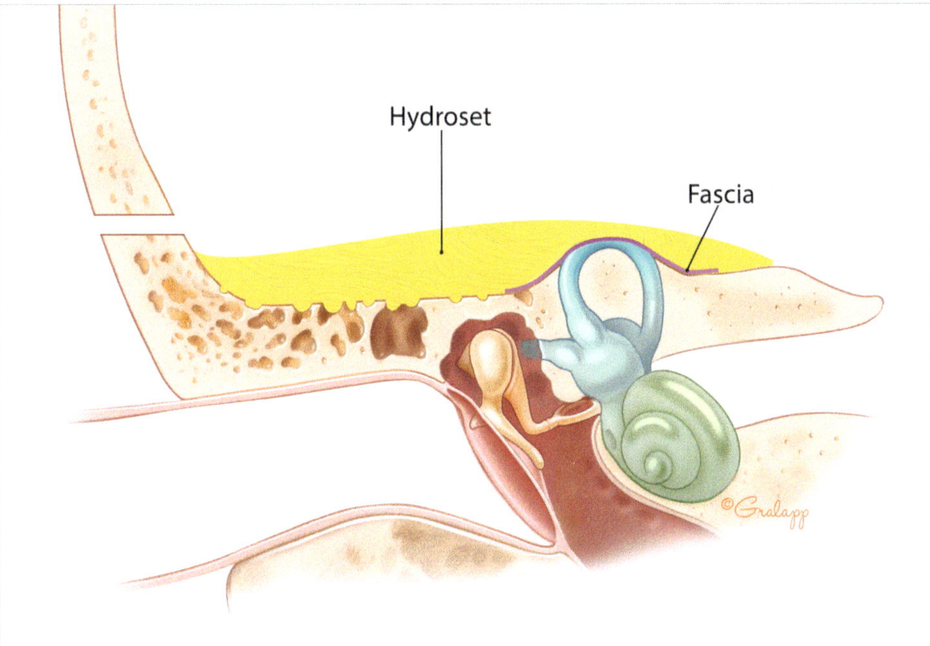

Fig. 10.28 Coronal view of completed resurfacing repair of a superior semicircular canal fistula.

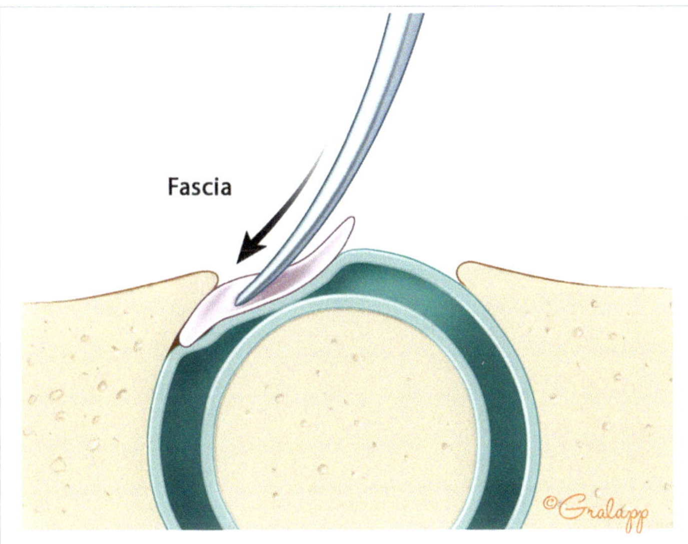

Fig. 10.29 The plugging method commences with inserting fascia in both limbs of the superior semicircular canal. Note that the membranous labyrinth is compressed.

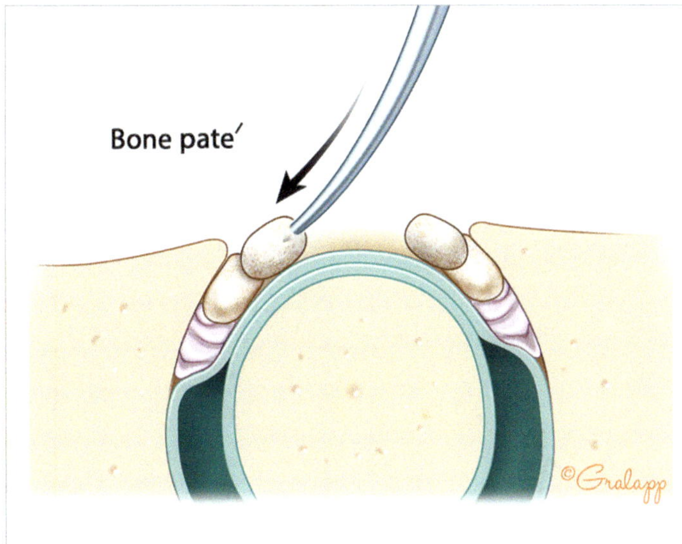

Fig. 10.30 Bone paté is placed to fill the canal.

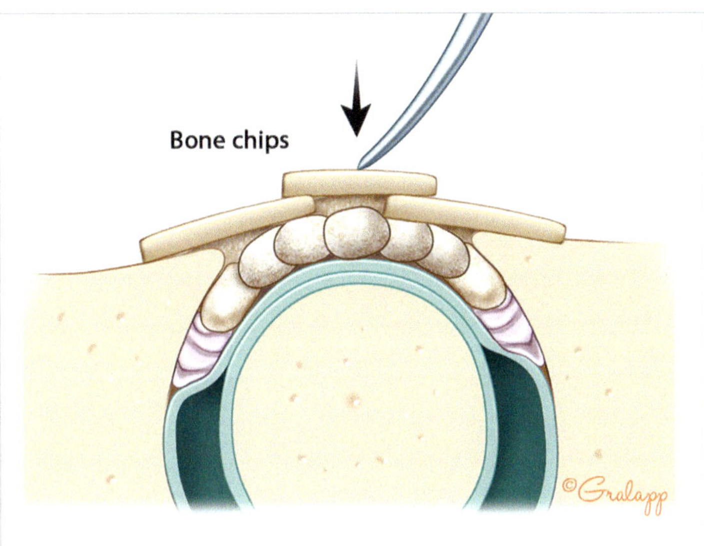

Fig. 10.31 Bone chips cover the site of the fistula.

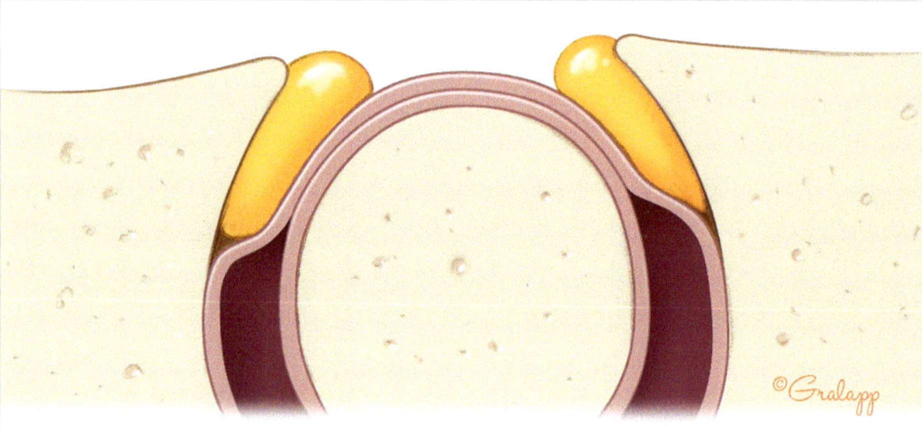

Fig. 10.32 Bone wax is an alternative means of plugging a dehiscent semicircular canal.

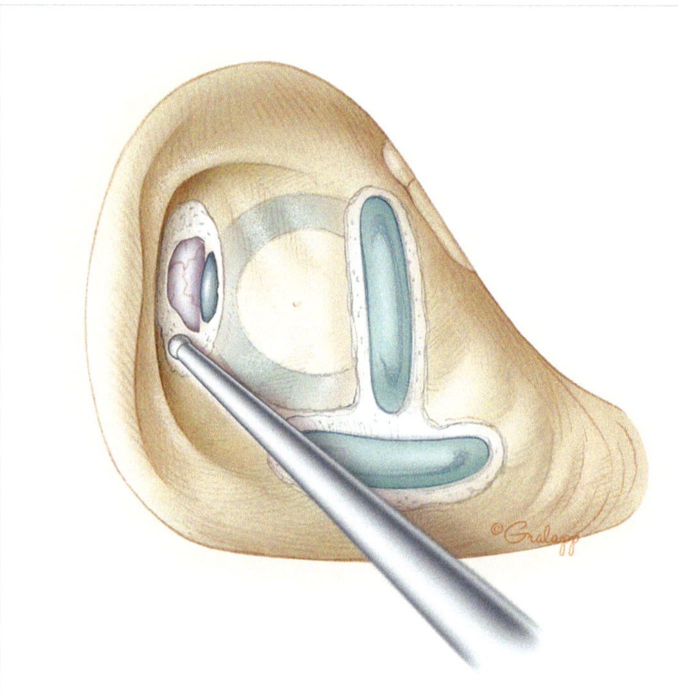

Fig. 10.33 Transmastoid approach to superior semicircular canal plugging showing identification of the dehiscence. The transmastoid approach has the advantage of being a more minor procedure than the middle fossa approach. However, it does not allow repair and/or reinforcement of the eroded roof of the middle ear and mastoid so common with superior semicircular dehiscence.

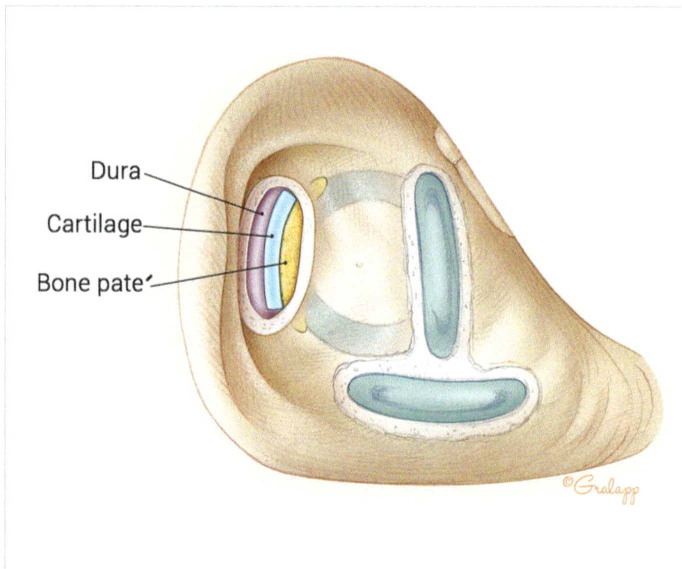

Fig. 10.34 Transmastoid dehiscence repair with cartilage and bone paté.

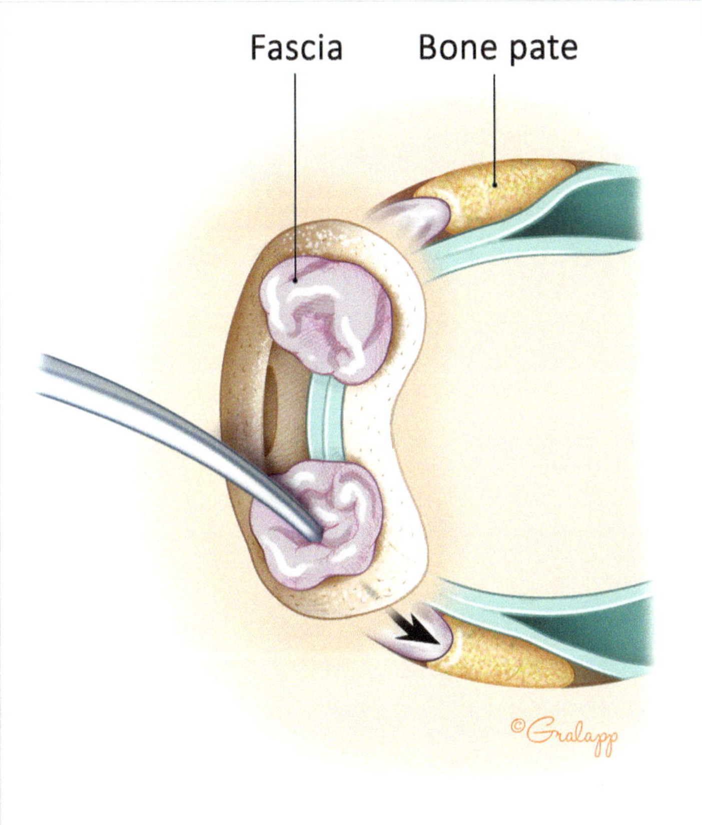

Fig. 10.35 Transmastoid superior canal plugging using bone paté and fascia.

11 Cochlear Implants

Nikolas H. Blevins and Jennifer Alyono

11.1 Introduction to Cochlear Implants

Cochlear implantation remains one of modern medicine's greatest innovations, having restored hearing to hundreds of thousands of individuals around the world. Refinements of implant technology and associated surgical techniques have improved outcomes, thereby allowing consideration of this treatment for new populations of children and adults. The wide adoption of hearing preservation techniques has demonstrated the benefits of retaining any residual cochlear function. Current meticulous surgical approaches are based on a solid appreciation of cochlear anatomy and how it relates to surrounding otologic structures.

The basic approach to implantation is similar regardless of the device used, despite a variety of manufacturers and electrode array configurations (with more being certain in the future). A limited postauricular incision provides the ability to place the receiver–stimulator behind and above the pinna. A mastoidectomy with facial recess provides access to the middle ear, through which the basal turn of the cochlea can be accessed via either the round window or a cochleostomy. It is now routine for implant surgeons to treat the inner ear with the care expected during stapedectomy. Electrode arrays have become thinner and less traumatic, requiring additional patience and precision for optimal placement.

Numerous surgical challenges can alter the course of implantation, including congenital malformations, spinal fluid leaks, and obstruction from fibrosis or ossification. Such challenges can be successfully met with appropriate alterations in surgical technique. As the field of cochlear implantation continues to evolve, new devices will bring both new opportunities and challenges. It is highly likely that an appreciation for cochlear anatomy and minimally invasive methods to access the inner ear will be increasingly vital to the success of the next generation of hearing restoration technology.

Further Reading

1. Coelho DH, Roland JT Jr. Implanting obstructed and malformed cochleae. Otolaryngol Clin North Am 2012;45(1): 91–110 PubMed
2. Franz BK, Clark GM, Bloom DM. Surgical anatomy of the round window with special reference to cochlear implantation. J Laryngol Otol 1987;101(2):97–102 PubMed
3. Mangus B, Rivas A, Tsai BS, Haynes DS, Roland JT Jr. Surgical techniques in cochlear implants. Otolaryngol Clin North Am 2012;45(1):69–80 PubMed
4. Millar DA, Hillman TA, Shelton C. Implantation of the ossified cochlea: management with the split electrode array. Laryngoscope 2005;115(12):2155–2160 PubMed
5. Niparko JK. Cochlear Implants Principles and Practice. Philadelphia, PA: Wolters Kluwer; 2012
6. Pakdaman MN, Herrmann BS, Curtin HD, Van Beek-King J, Lee DJ. Cochlear implantation in children with anomalous cochleovestibular anatomy: a systematic review. Otolaryngol Head Neck Surg 2012;146(2):180–190 PubMed
7. Santa Maria PL, Gluth MB, Yuan Y, Atlas MD, Blevins NH. Hearing preservation surgery for cochlear implantation: a meta-analysis. Otol Neurotol 2014;35(10):e256–e269 PubMed
8. Singla A, Sahni D, Gupta AK, Aggarwal A, Gupta T. Surgical anatomy of the basal turn of the human cochlea as pertaining to cochlear implantation. Otol Neurotol 2015;36(2):323–328 PubMed
9. Tóth M, Alpár A, Bodon G, Moser G, Patonay L. Surgical anatomy of the cochlea for cochlear implantation. Ann Anat 2006;188(4):363–370 PubMed
10. Waltzman SB, Roland JT Jr. Cochlear Implants, 3rd ed. New York, NY: Thieme; 2014
11. Wang L, Zhang D. Surgical methods and postoperative results of cochlear implantation in 79 cases of ossified cochlea. Acta Otolaryngol 2014;134(12):1219–1224 PubMed
12. Wanna GB, Noble JH, Carlson ML, et al. Impact of electrode design and surgical approach on scalar location and cochlear implant outcomes. Laryngoscope 2014;124(Suppl 6):S1–S7 PubMed
13. Wasson JD, Briggs RJ. Contemporary surgical issues in paediatric cochlear implantation. Int J Audiol 2016;55(55, Suppl 2): S77–S87 PubMed
14. Wootten CT, Backous DD, Haynes DS. Management of cerebrospinal fluid leakage from cochleostomy during cochlear implant surgery. Laryngoscope 2006;116(11):2055–2059 PubMed

11.2 Cochlear Implant Surgery

Nikolas H. Blevins and Jennifer Alyono

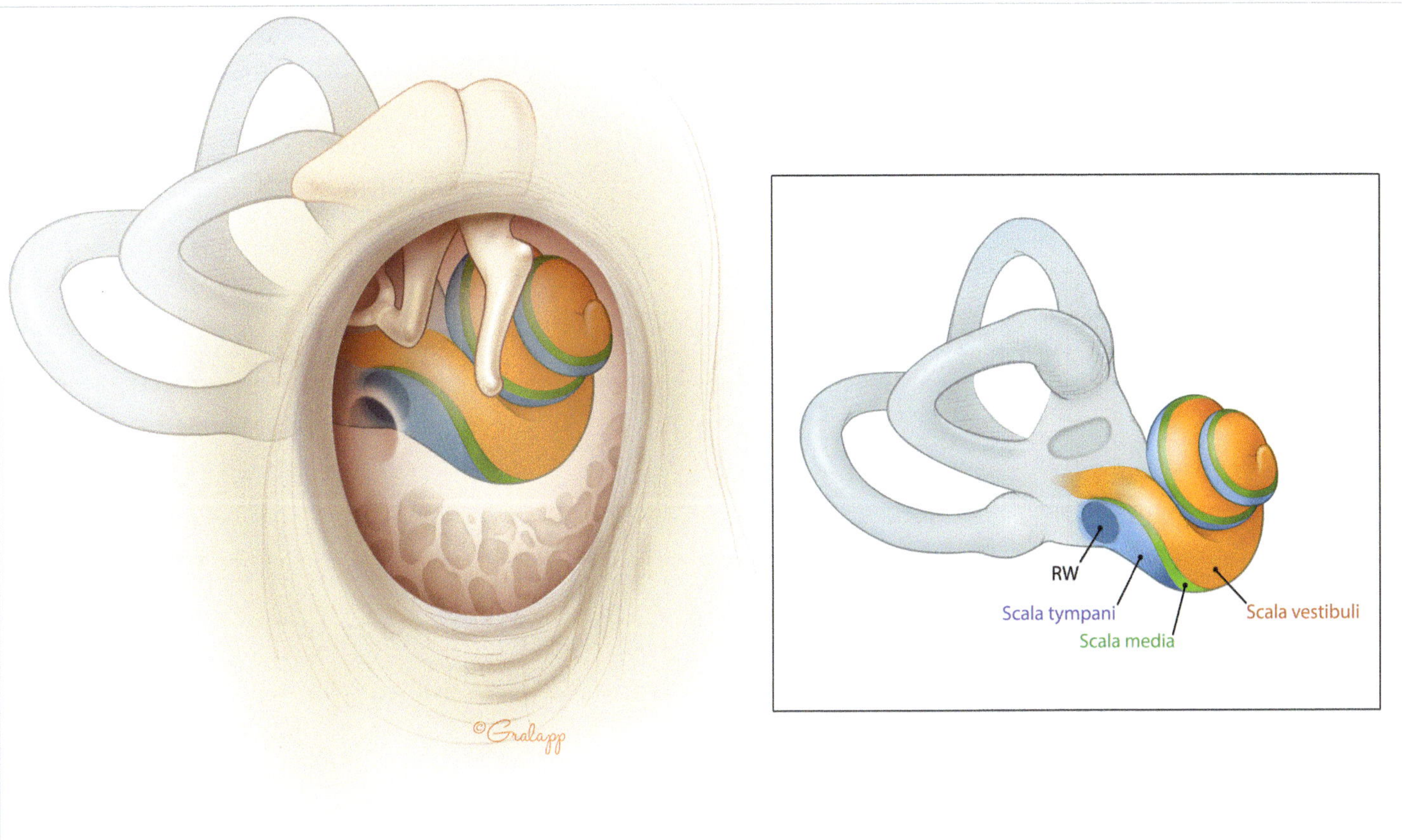

Fig. 11.1 Anatomical view of the inner ear scalae in relation to the ear canal, ossicles, and tympanic cavity. Note the extension of the basal turn of the cochlea inferior to the round window, and the hook of the scala media as it approaches the vestibule. The goal of cochlear implantation is atraumatic placement of the electrode array into the scala tympani. Whether this is performed through the round window or cochleostomy, a solid grasp of the location and interrelationships of the scalae is needed to avoid additional cochlear injury and potential reduction in performance. RW, round window.

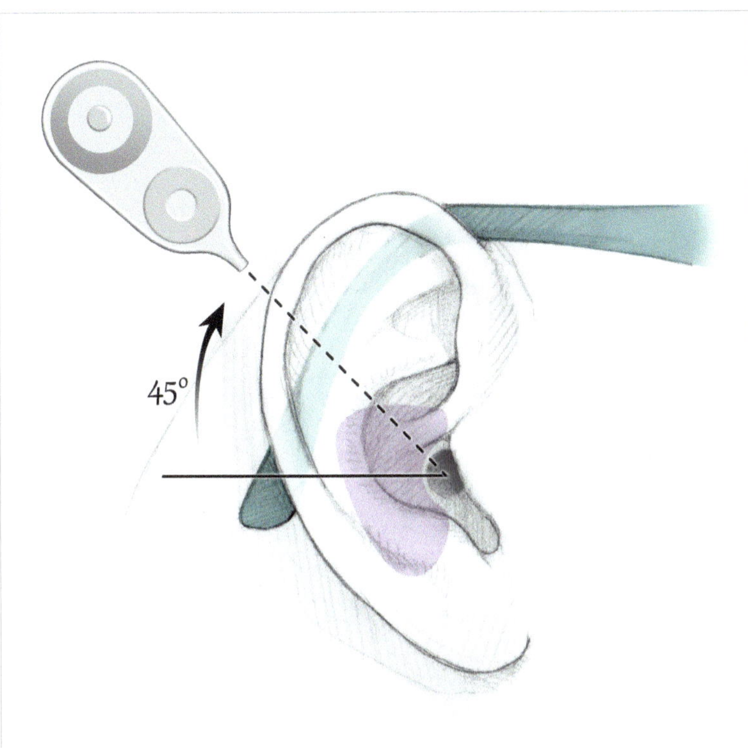

Fig. 11.2 Planning the placement of the receiver–stimulator should allow sufficient room between the pinna and the headpiece to enable the comfortable use of a behind-the-ear processor and eyeglasses. Approximately 3 to 4 cm should be left between the ear canal and the anterior edge of the device, which then provides additional distance to the magnet and headpiece. The device is angled up at about 45 degrees from the linea temporalis, which places it behind the bulk of the temporalis muscle.

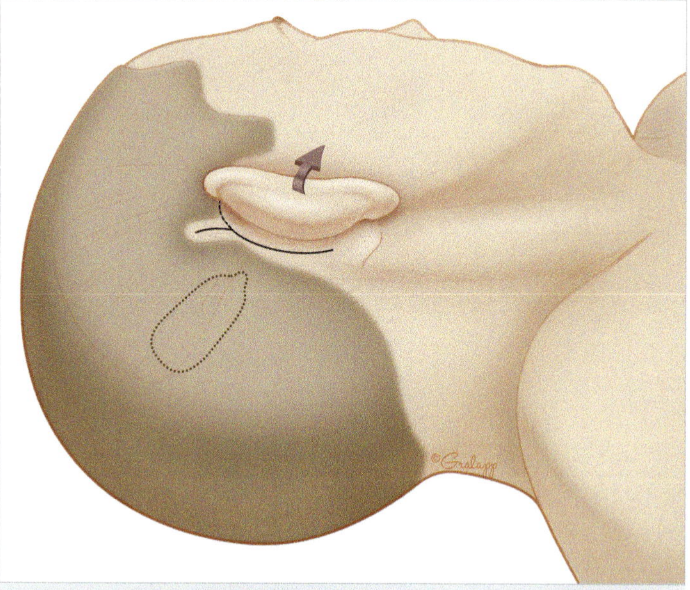

Fig. 11.3 A postauricular incision is most commonly used for cochlear implantation. The superior aspect of the incision can be continued anteriorly or extended superiorly. This modification can provide additional ease of exposure for creating a well to seat the receiver–stimulator. Minimal or no shaving of hair is required if drapes are secured sufficiently to adjacent skin. Sufficient space (at least 1.5 cm) between the incision and the anterior aspect of the implant should be allowed to minimize the chance of device extrusion through the incision.

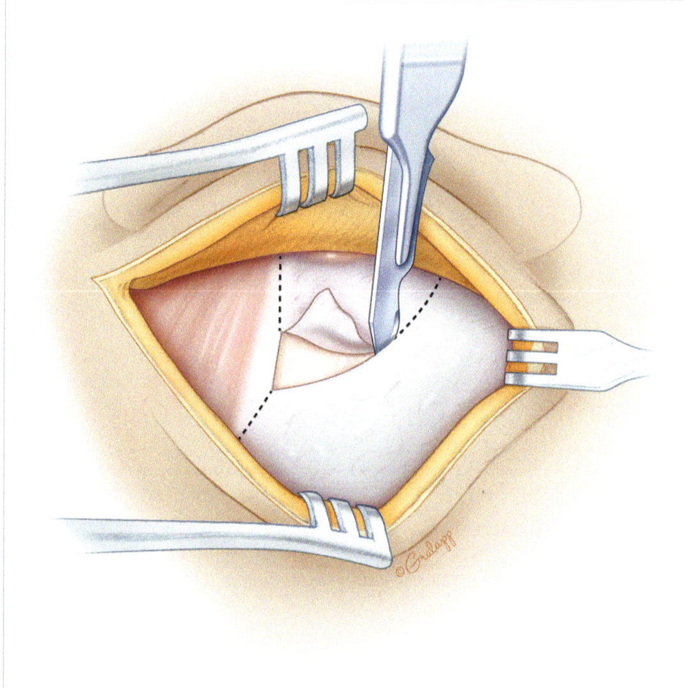

Fig. 11.4 The skin incision is carried down to the level of the temporalis fascia and mastoid periosteum. Minimizing anterior dissection along the temporalis muscle can reduce postoperative facial edema. A separate anteriorly based periosteal flap is created, which can be closed over the mastoidectomy and device at the conclusion of the procedure. Avoiding electrocautery for this step minimizes tissue shrinkage and facilitates closure. In small children where the flap is quite thin, the periosteum and muscle can be left attached to the skin. An extension of the periosteal incision posteriorly, curving up along the linea temporalis, allows for retraction of the temporalis muscle superiorly. This can help when creating the soft-tissue pocket for the receiver–stimulator.

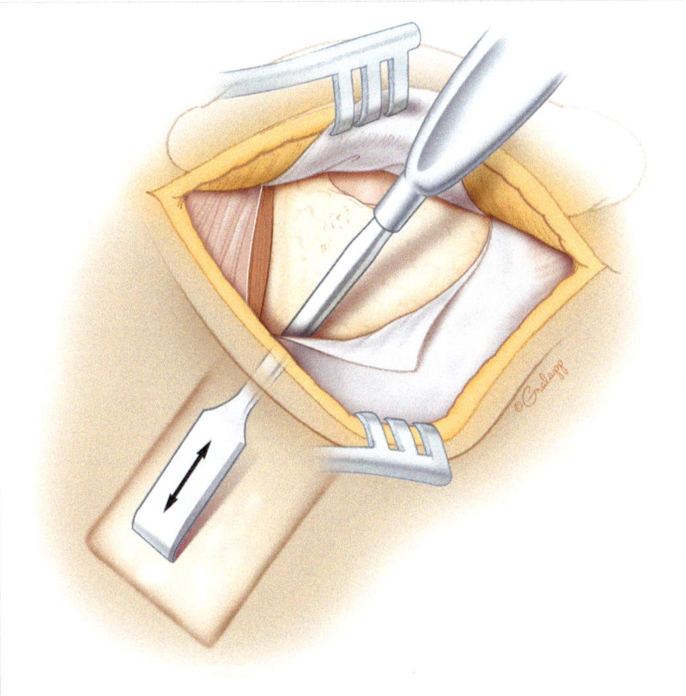

Fig. 11.5 A subperiosteal pocket is created to accept the receiver–stimulator. A device-specific template is used to gauge the size of the pocket, and to mark the location of a bony well to recess and stabilize the electronics case. The pocket should be kept just large enough to comfortably accept the template without the need for excessive force or bending. Using a periosteal elevator to make multiple parallel passes will create a rectangular pocket, and reduce the risk of excessive movement or migration. Care must be taken during this elevation in very young children or those with developmental abnormalities, since the cortical bone over dura may be quite thin or even dehiscent.

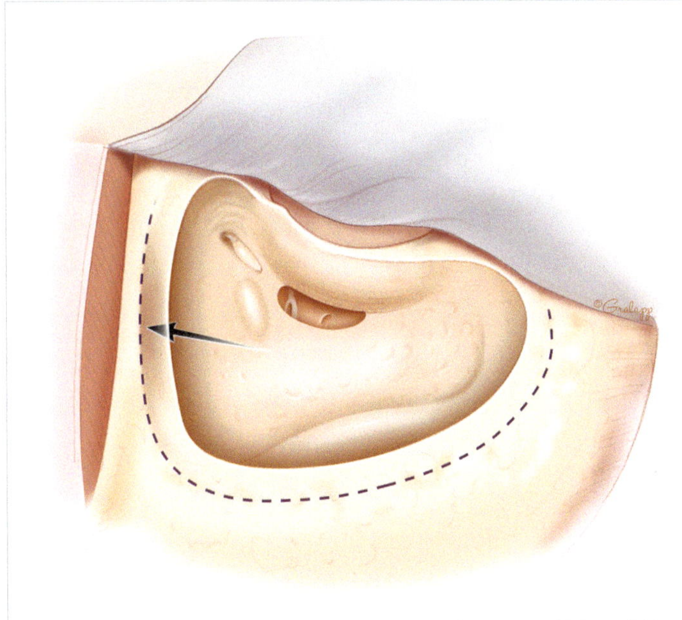

Fig. 11.6 Mastoidectomy is then performed. Unlike the conventional technique for chronic otitis media, the surrounding cortex is not "saucerized." Instead, bony overhangs are left superiorly, posteriorly, and inferiorly to help retain the coiled electrode lead. The creation of such overhangs should not be performed at the expense of safety. By carefully controlling the angle of view, the surgeon can ensure that the burr is always seen, even while creating the overhang. Most cochlear implant recipients have normally developed and aerated mastoids. Some air cells can be left intact provided that adequate exposure to completely open the facial recess is provided. The facial recess is then performed as described elsewhere. Adequate middle ear exposure through the facial recess is critical for array insertion. The facial nerve is identified through thin bone, as is the chorda tympani. The removal of bone anterior to the facial nerve will enable optimal view of the round window niche. Exposure of the incudostapedial joint and stapedial tendon can provide valuable landmarks. The incudal buttress is left intact.

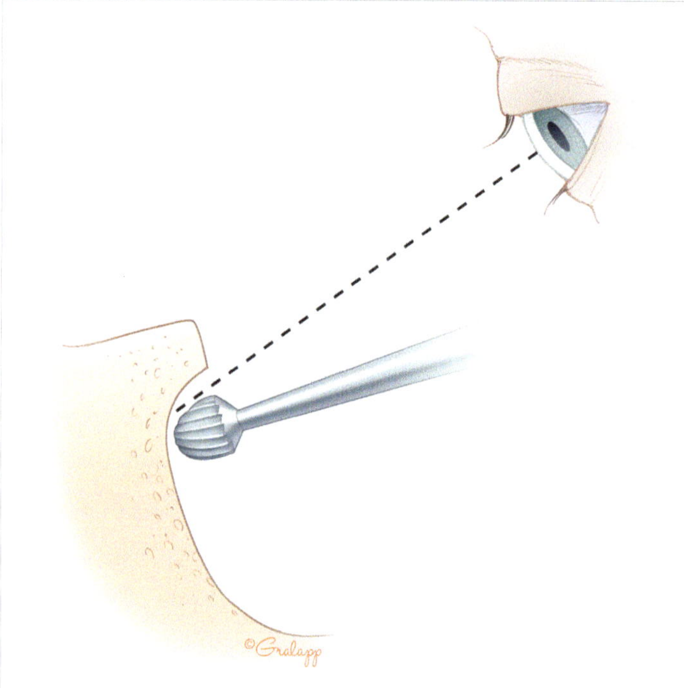

Fig. 11.7 Depiction of the importance of adjusting the surgical angle of view while leaving cortical overhangs during mastoidectomy. By moving the microscope appropriately, the surgeon can maintain continuous line-of-sight with the burr, ensuring that no structures are inadvertently injured.

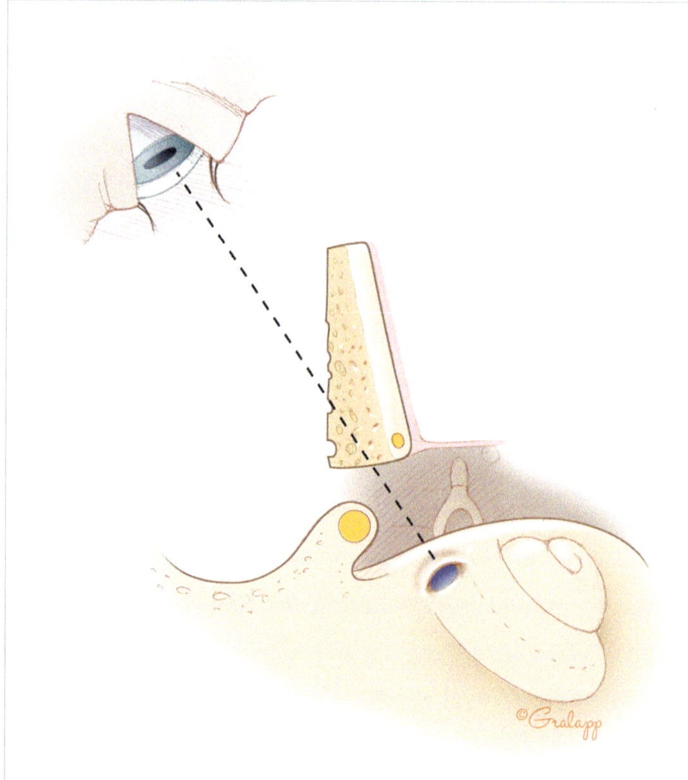

Fig. 11.8 It is critical that the posterior external canal wall be adequately thinned to provide optimal exposure of the round window. The canal moves anteriorly as it extends medially, and following its contour to maintain uniform thickness is essential. Incomplete canal wall thinning will prevent identification of the chorda tympani, and leave the facial recess significantly smaller than it should be. Similarly, the persistence of medial canal bone can prevent sufficient exposure of the bone anterior to the facial nerve, and prevent the identification of the round window niche.

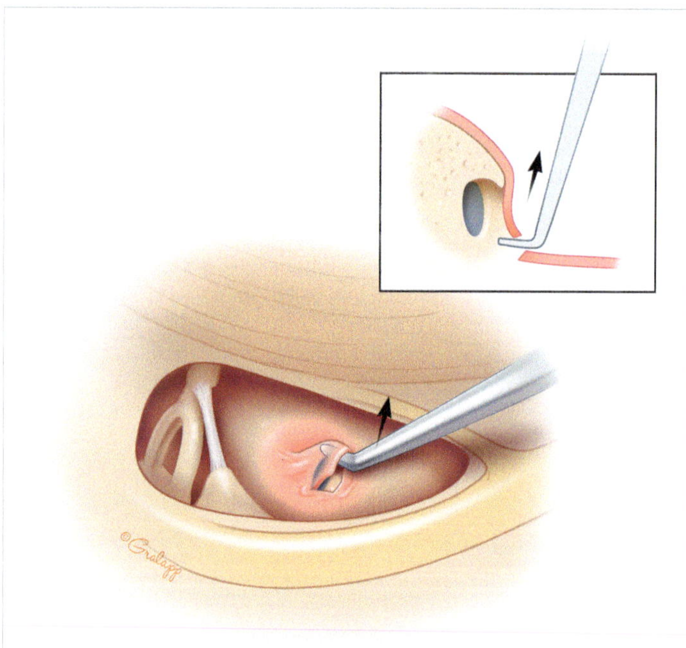

Fig. 11.9 The round window niche is often covered by a layer of mucosa, sometimes referred to as the "round window niche membrane." This membrane can be differentiated from the true round window membrane by its location at the opening of the niche and its more pink color in comparison to the bluish round window membrane. When encountered, this mucosa can be gently dissected away from the underlying niche and round window membrane with a small right-angled hook.

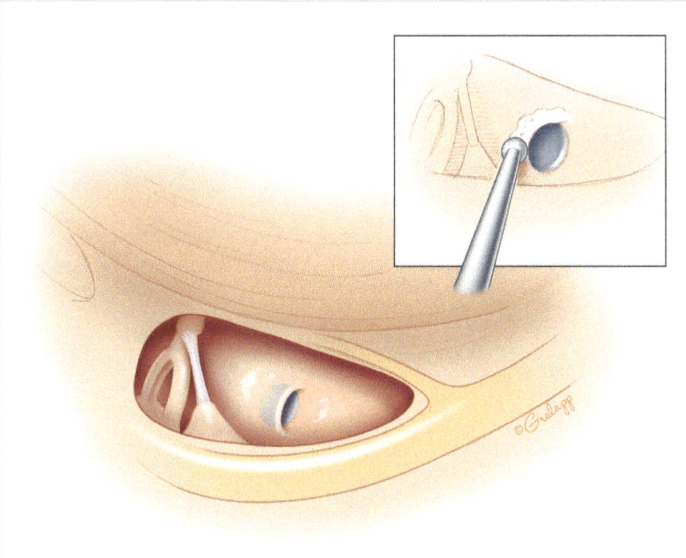

Fig. 11.10 Once the round window niche is identified and cleared of overlying mucosa, the round window membrane can be exposed. The round window membrane is usually bluish in appearance, and has a distinctive white-gray annular ligament at its periphery. Adequate exposure of the round window membrane is essential for optimal electrode placement. The membrane is usually covered to a variable extent by the bone of the round window overhang. A 1-mm diamond burr at low speed can be used to safely remove the overhang while preserving the integrity of the underlying membrane. An adequate view of the anterior margin of the membrane is most important given the optimal trajectory of planned electrode array insertion. Small pieces of gelatin foam sponges with 1:1,000 epinephrine can be used to achieve hemostasis at this point. The avoidance of bone dust or blood is needed to prevent their introduction to the inner ear during array placement. Steroids and hyaluronic acid lubricant can be introduced to the niche at this point if desired.

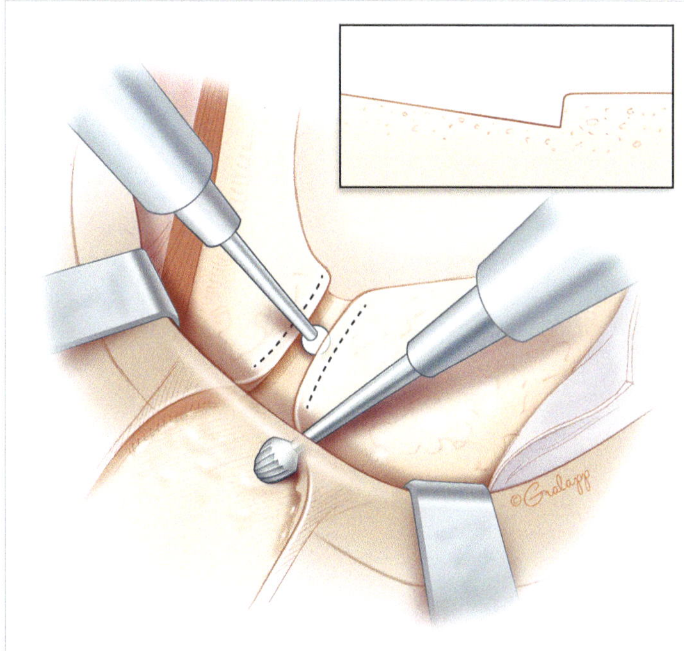

Fig. 11.11 A shallow well can be drilled to accept the electronics casing of the receiver–stimulator snugly. Device-specific templates are used to ensure the correct location and orientation of this well. Bone removal is performed under the posterior skin flap, and adequate retraction and adjustment of the surgeon's angle of view is needed to perform this in a safe manner. Initial bone removal can be performed with a large cutting burr, with a smaller cutting or diamond burr being used to create a sharp ledge anteriorly to prevent migration of the device over time. A smaller burr is used to drill a trough from the well to the mastoid cavity. Overhangs can be left to help hold the electrode lead securely. Many surgeons have completely dispensed with drilling such a well. The creation of a secure soft-tissue pocket alone is sufficient to prevent migration. This is a particular consideration in young children with thin bone. In these cases, avoiding the creation of a well may reduce the risk of intracranial complications. A small piece of muscle and fascia can be harvested from the posterior aspect of the incision for later use in closure. This is then an opportunity to achieve hemostasis fully before opening the device onto the operative field.

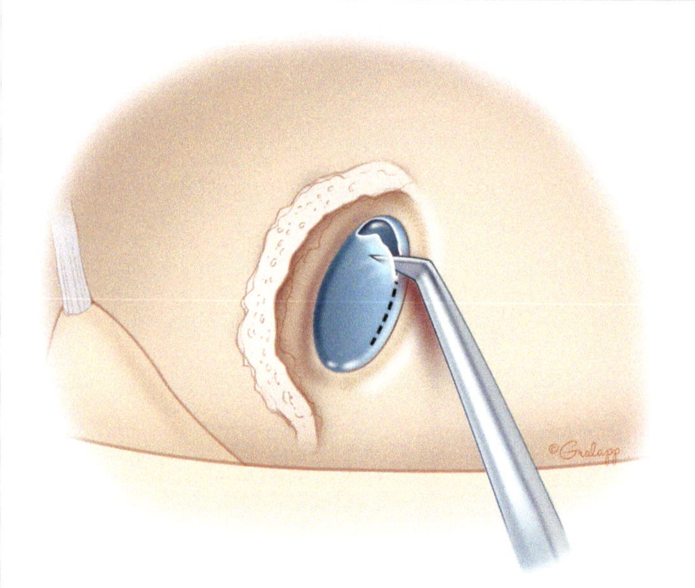

Fig. 11.12 The middle ear and mastoid are irrigated to remove any blood or bone dust. The device is then opened, inspected, and placed in the pocket. The anterior margin of the round window membrane is incised with a sharp pick or needle. There is more room anteriorly between the round window membrane and the underlying basilar membrane. Also, an anterior incision encourages the optimal direction of array insertion. When a sufficient amount of membrane has been incised, the opening will be visible without the need for tissue excision or flap creation. Similar to stapedectomy, the surgeon should avoid suctioning directly over the incision to maintain the perilymph within the scala. The application of additional topical steroids and hyaluronic acid may be beneficial at this step.

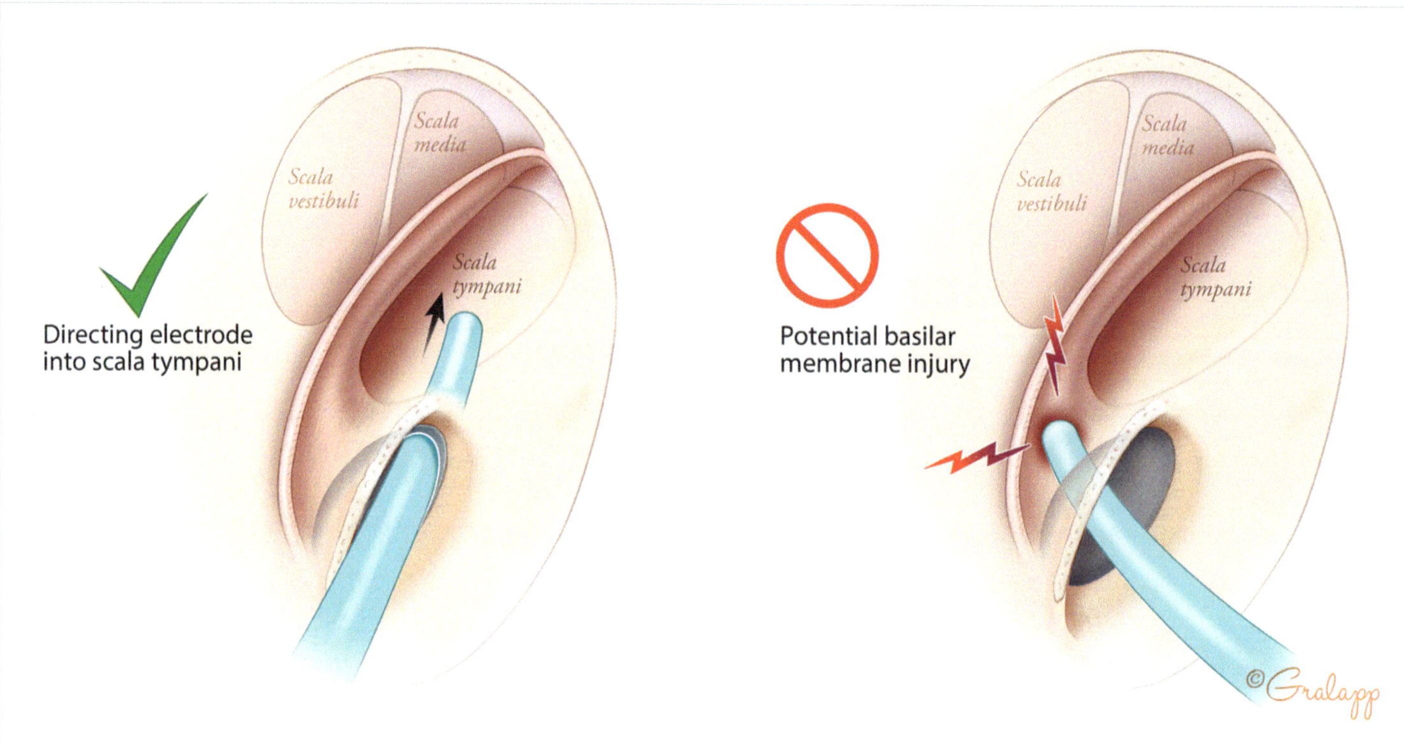

Fig. 11.13 The electrode array is threaded into the scala tympani through the anterior incision in the round window membrane. Note that an anterior trajectory of insertion will guide the array into the basal turn and minimize the risk of direct trauma to the basilar membrane (left panel). A superiorly directed trajectory (right panel) of insertion may cause the array to impact and damage the basilar membrane. Such a direction may result from the suboptimal exposure of the round window membrane from incomplete drilling of the niche overhang, or from incising the round window membrane too far posterior.

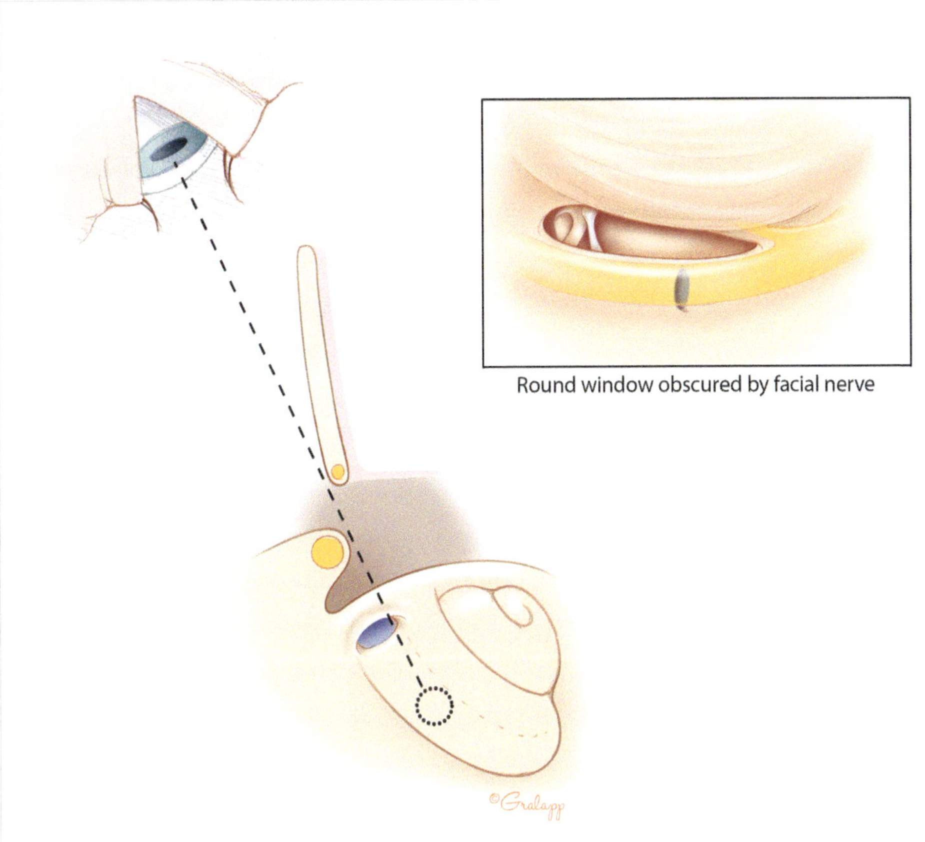

Fig. 11.14 In some cases, the surgeon's view of the round window may be obstructed by the facial nerve despite optimal drilling. In such cases, the surgeon will usually still have a view anterior and inferior to the round window along the inferior side of the promontory, where a cochleostomy can be created. Identification of this region may be facilitated if there is even a slight view of the anterior margin of the niche.

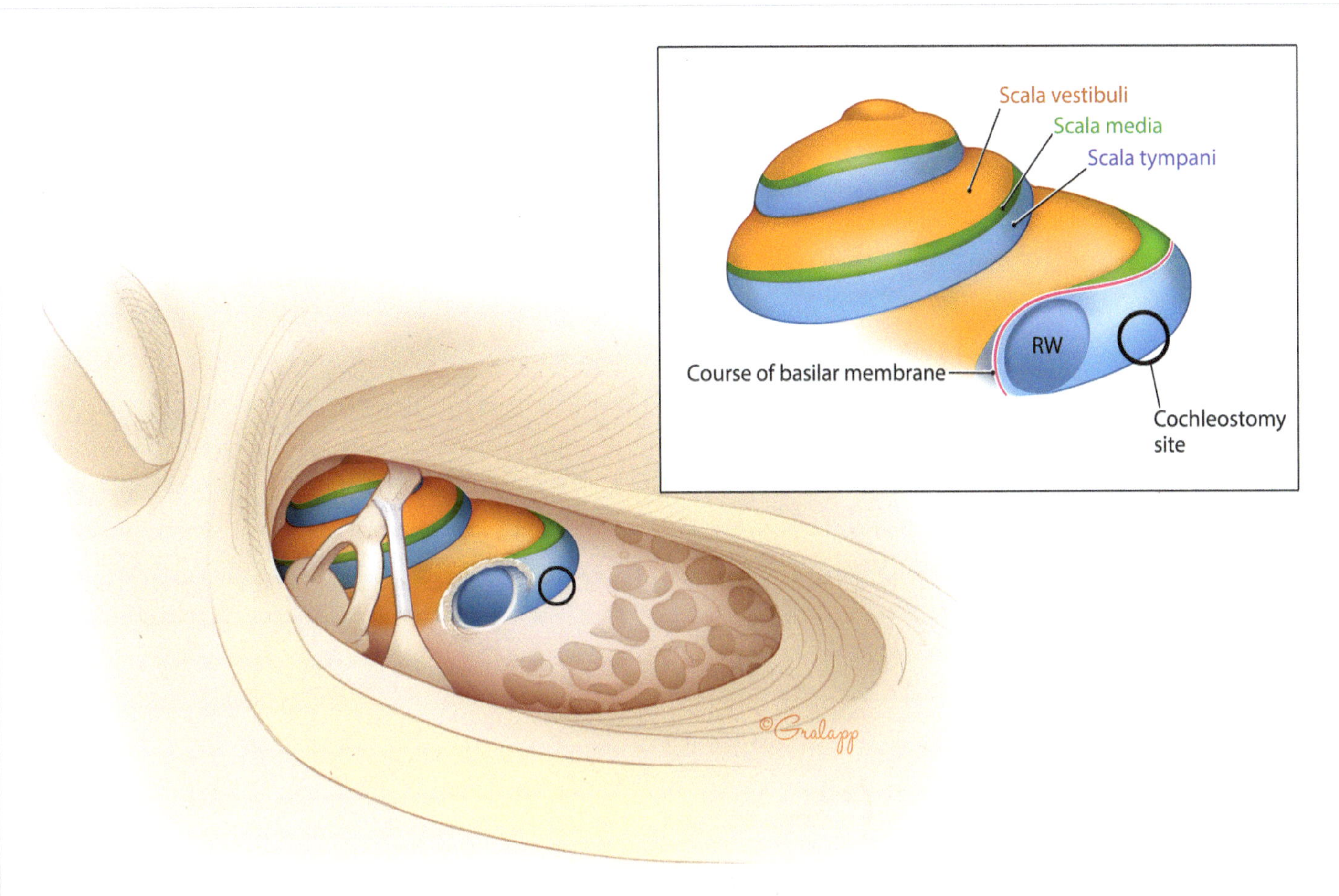

Fig. 11.15 The optimal placement of a cochleostomy is anterior and inferior to the round window. Such placement ensures that drilling will occur into the scala tympani, and away from the spiral ligament and basilar membrane. Such an inferior cochleostomy also provides a straight path to the first turn of the cochlea, and allows insertion of the electrode array with minimal force or curvature. RW, round window.

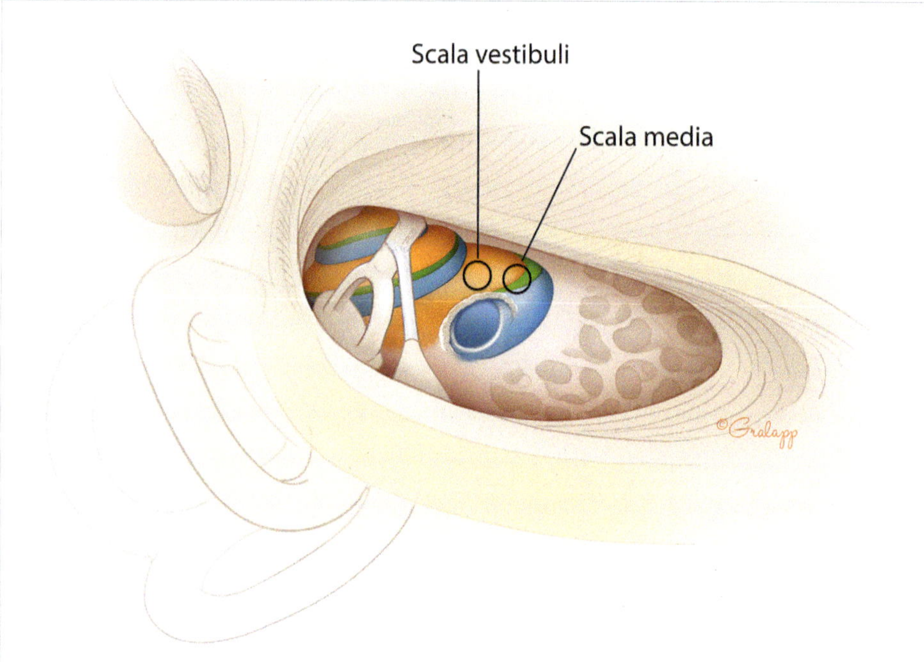

Fig. 11.16 Suboptimal cochleostomy locations. Placement of a cochleostomy just anterior to the round window risks direct damage to the basilar membrane, spiral ligament, and enters into the scala media. Similarly, placement of a cochleostomy superior to the round window will enter the scala vestibuli. Both of these approaches are to be avoided if possible to minimize the risk of trauma and ensure that the array remains within the scala tympani. Intentionally drilling in these areas or extending a scala tympani cochleostomy into the other scala may be needed if there is fibrosis or ossification obstructing the lumen of the scala tympani.

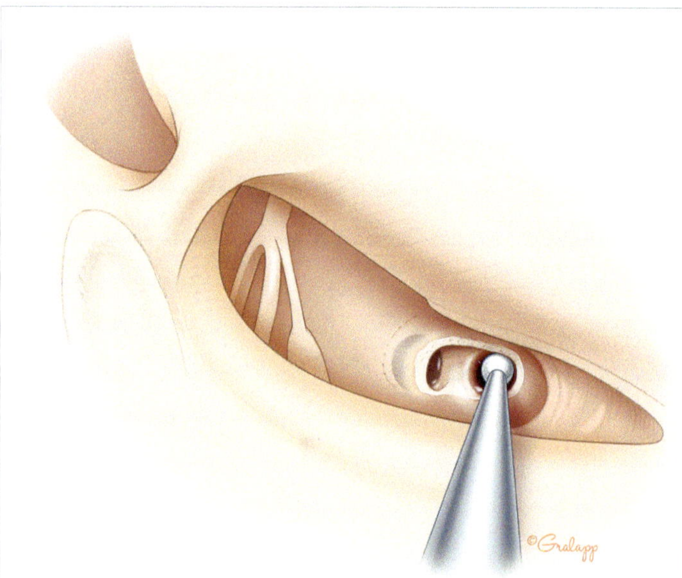

Fig. 11.17 A small diamond burr is used at low speed to drill a cochleostomy. The direction of bone removal should be in the anterior–superior direction for optimal cochleostomy. Drilling directly anterior risks moving tangential to the inferior portion of the basal turn. Care should be taken to attempt to identify and preserve the endosteum over a wide area. The endosteum can then be entered with a sharp hook. Avoid drilling directly into the inner ear to minimize trauma. Such an approach minimizes the risk of damage to the basilar membrane (*dashed line*) and remaining neural elements.

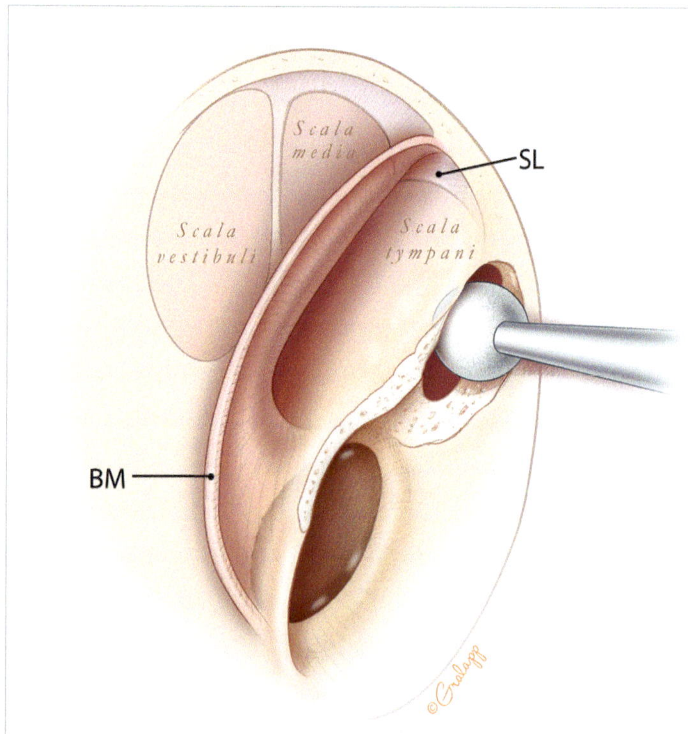

Fig. 11.18 Schematic depiction of a cochleostomy into the inferior aspect of the scala tympani. This minimizes cochlear injury by avoiding both the basilar membrane (BM) and the spiral ligament (SL). The trajectory of drilling should be aimed somewhat superiorly to enter the scala and avoid drilling tangentially past the inferior aspect of the basal turn.

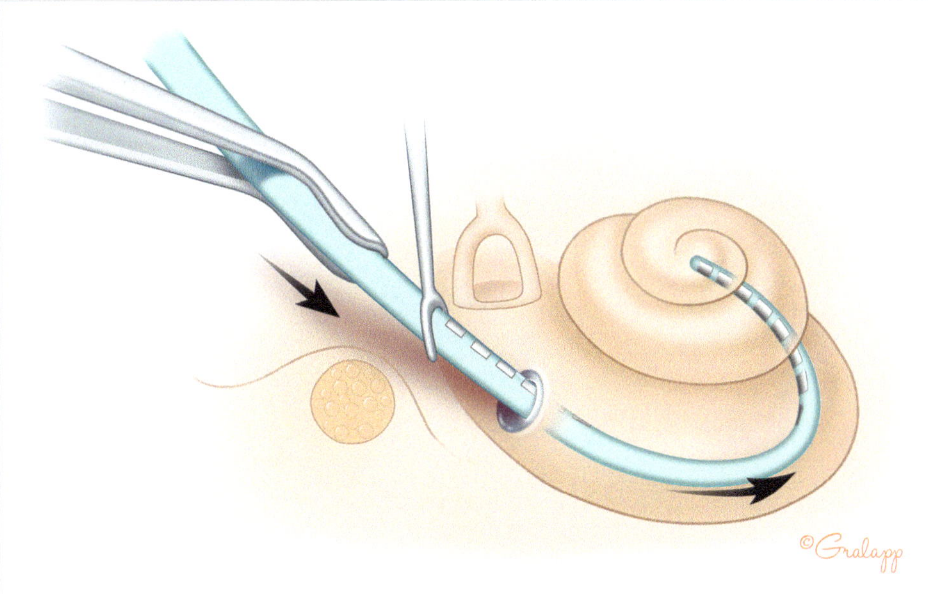

Fig. 11.19 The electrode array is gently inserted into the inner ear. A similar approach is used whether through the round window or a cochleostomy. The array is directed anteriorly in the direction of the basal turn. A combination of forceps and "claw" guides can enable a slow and steady insertion. Many surgeons advocate a slow insertion (over 1 minute in duration). This may decrease trauma to cochlear tissues by allowing the equilibration of perilymphatic pressures changes from the volume of the array. Similarly, slow insertion speeds may reduce trauma from friction to the anti-modiolar wall.

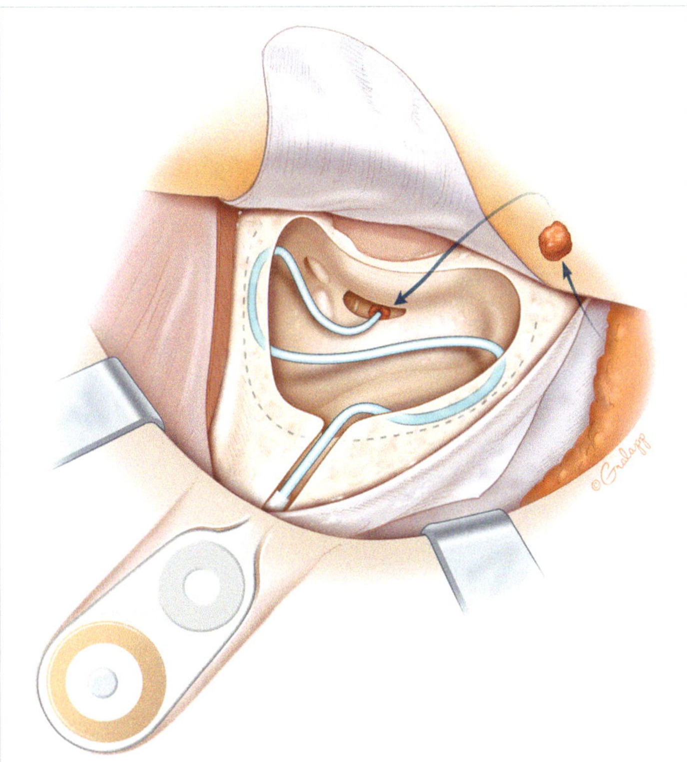

Fig. 11.20 Following complete insertion, the electrode array can be surrounded by small pieces of muscle and fascia obtained from the posterior incision. In the absence of a spinal fluid leak, it is not necessary to pack these pieces into the inner ear itself. Such tissue can help stabilize the array and reduce the risk of displacement. This may also reseal the inner ear, lessening the potential for a perilymphatic leak and the risk of bacterial spread from the middle ear to the perilymph. The facial recess can be similarly closed with muscle to further stabilize the array and its lead. Care should be taken to avoid packing these tissues against the ossicles to maintain the conductive mechanism for any remaining acoustic hearing postoperatively. The electrode lead is coiled into the mastoid cavity. The bony overhangs left during drilling will often help hold the loops in place.

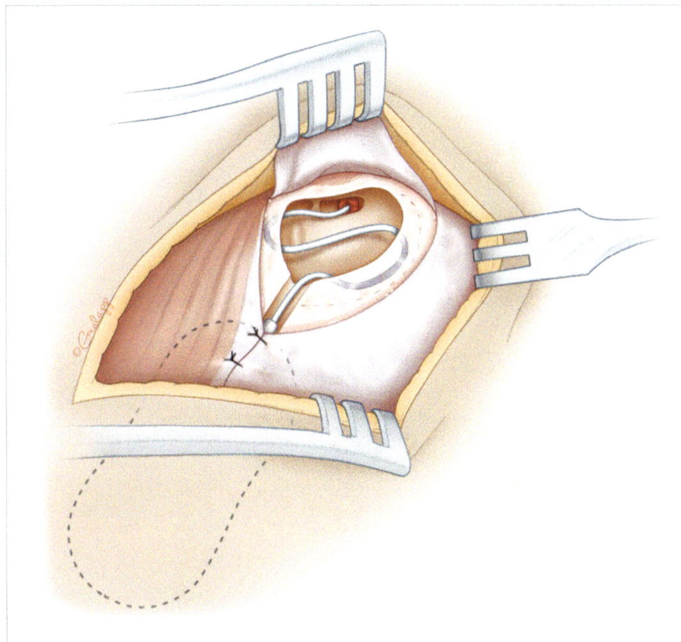

Fig. 11.21 The periosteal incision is closed tightly over the anterior portion of the receiver–stimulator. These sutures help anchor the device in the pocket and secure it in the bony recess if one was created.

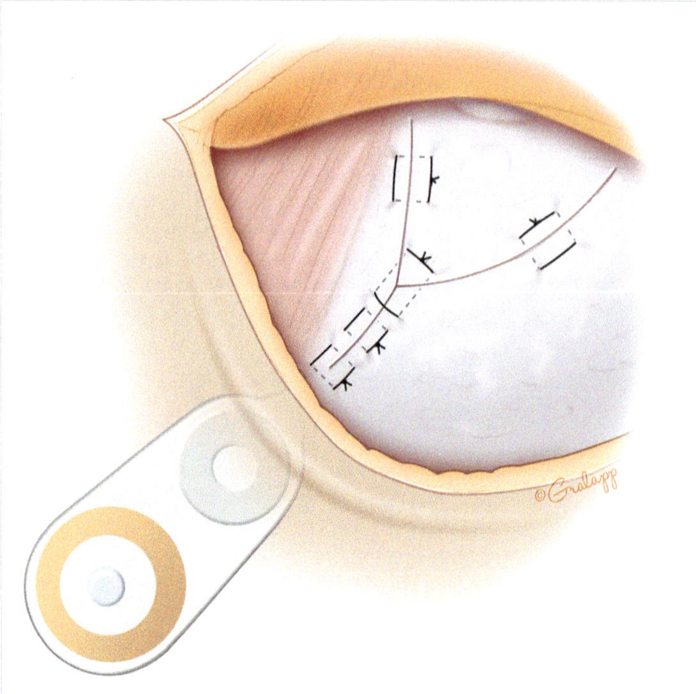

Fig. 11.22 The anteriorly based periosteal flap is closed over the mastoid cavity, providing separation between the device and the skin incision. The skin is then closed and a mastoid pressure dressing applied for 24 hours.

11.3 Cochlear Implant Surgical Variations

Nikolas H. Blevins and Jennifer Alyono

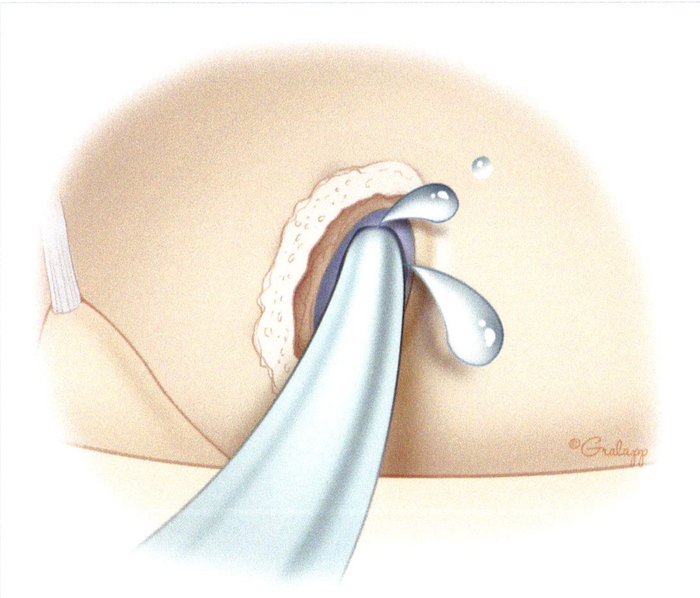

Fig. 11.23 Entering the inner ear may precipitate a spinal fluid leak. This may either be brisk ("gusher") or slow ("oozer"). In the case of a slow leak, the flow of spinal fluid may be controlled with the full insertion of the electrode array and placement of surrounding tissue as described above. In more brisk leaks, as is commonly seen in congenitally malformed inner ears, additional packing may be required to control the leak.

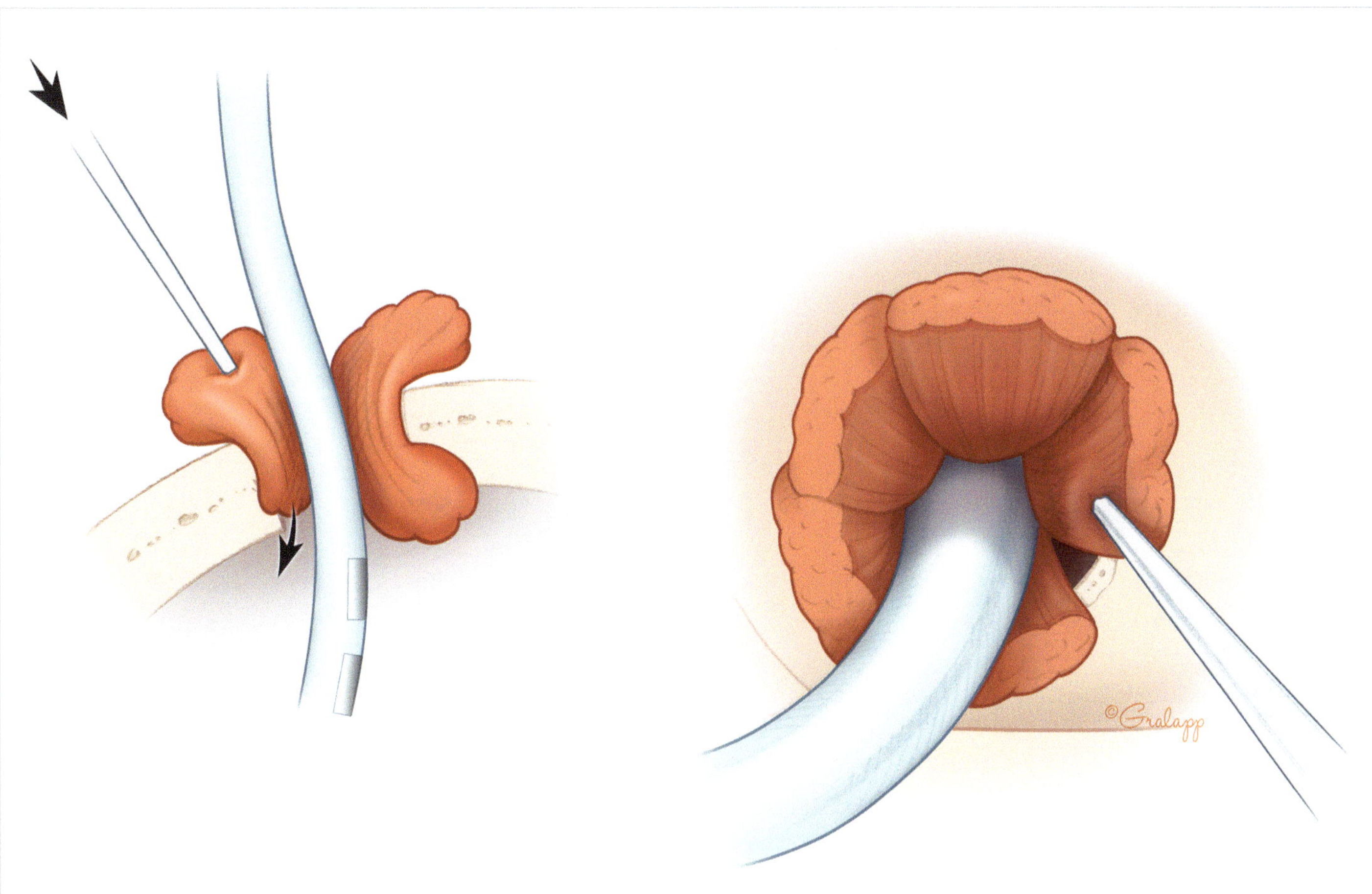

Fig. 11.24 In the case of a brisk spinal fluid leak, as may be seen from a common cavity malformation, the surgeon may elect to open the cochleostomy slightly larger, thereby affording the opportunity to pack muscle tightly between the array and the bone of the otic capsule circumferentially. Fibrin glue can also assist in creating a seal. This will be sufficient in most cases, although consideration can be given to formally oversewing the ear canal and obliterating the Eustachian tube to provide definitive closure.

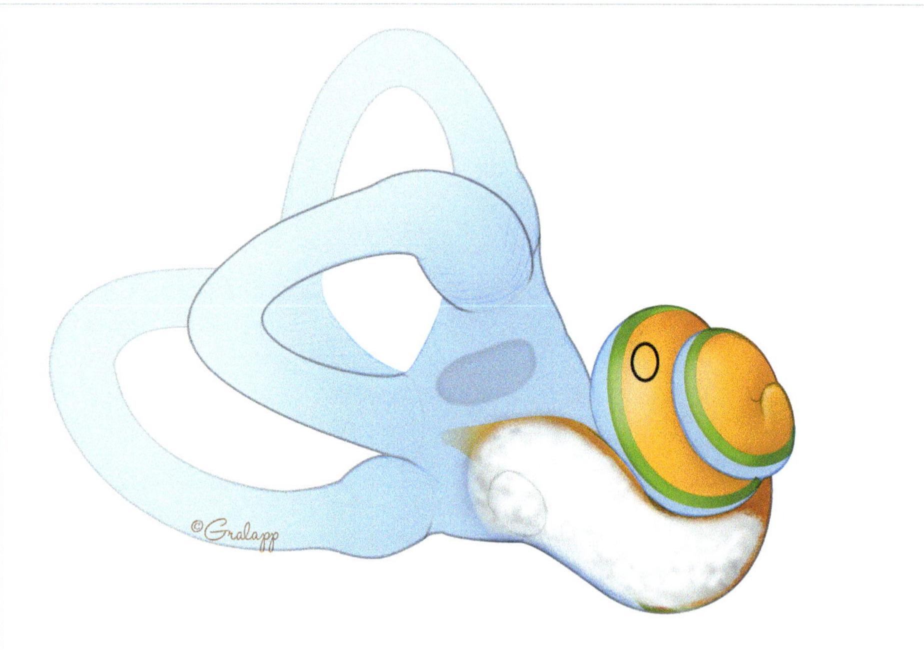

Fig. 11.25 In the case of ossification or fibrosis, the basal turn is often the most affected portion of cochlea. In such cases, the round window niche may be replaced by fibrotic tissue and "chalky" new bone.

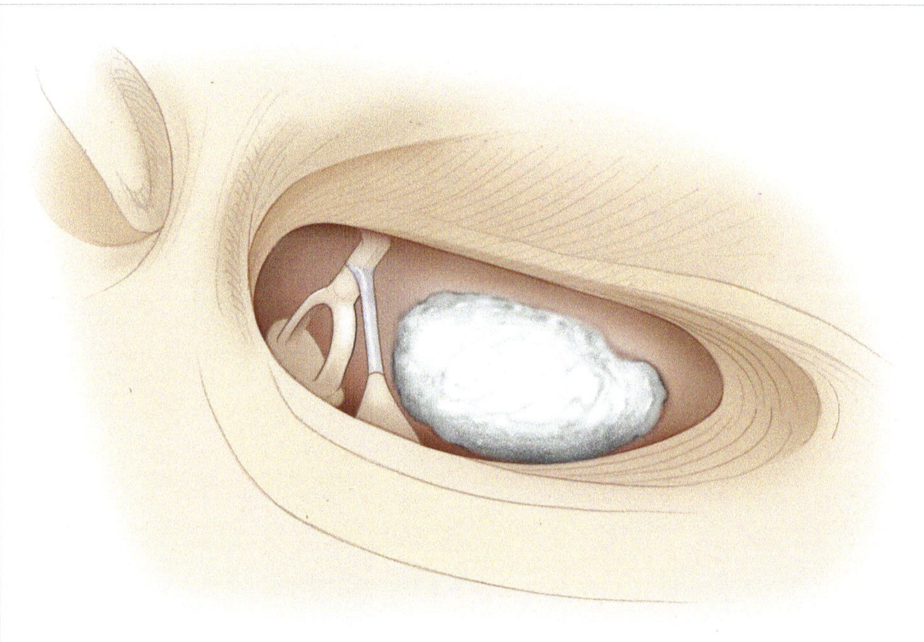

Fig. 11.26 Most ossification relevant to cochlear implantation lies within the cochlear lumen, but occasionally it extends into the middle ear and obscures the round window. This illustration depicts a plaque of dystrophic calcification obscuring the round window.

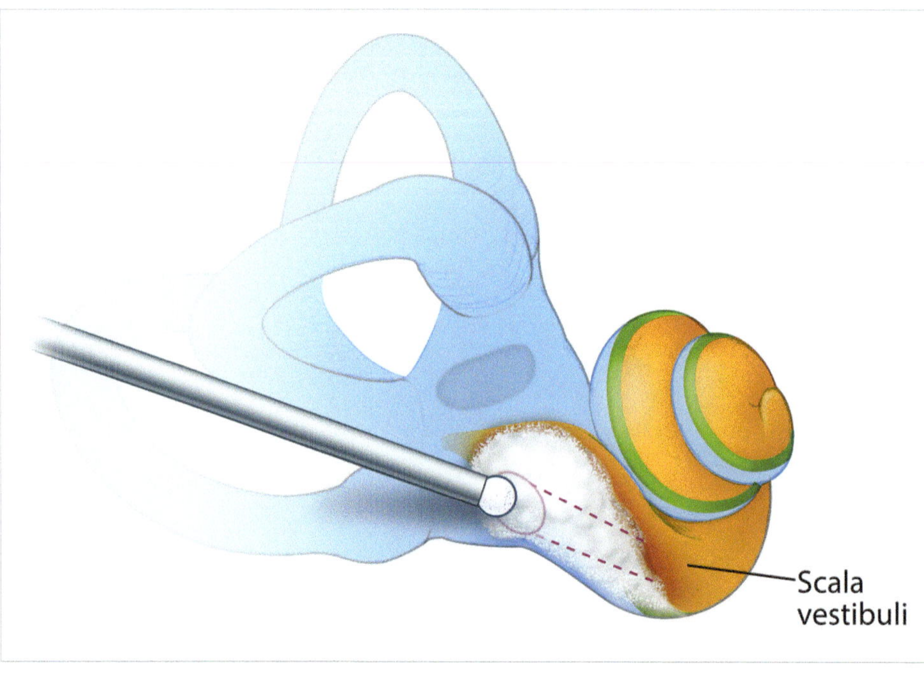

Fig. 11.27 Drilling anterior, and following the abnormal bone along the path expected for the basal turn, may eventually lead to an opening in the more anterior aspect of the cochlea. This may enable a complete insertion of a conventional array into the cochlea. Often the scala vestibuli is relatively less affected than the scala tympani, providing a path for insertion. A combination of preoperative high-resolution CT and MRI sequences optimized to show intracochlear fluids can be invaluable in planning for such cases.

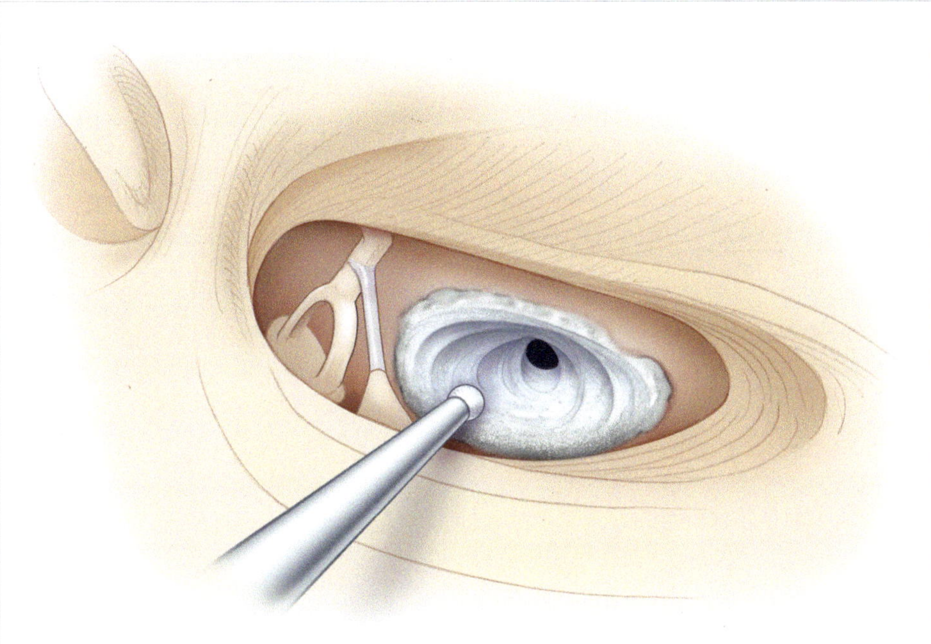

Fig. 11.28 Drilling anteriorly through calcification of the basal turn to reach an open scala vestibuli.

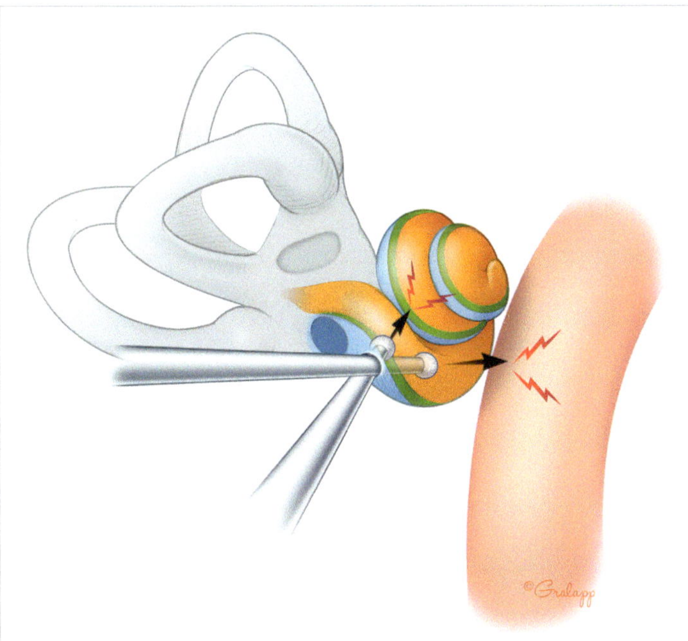

Fig. 11.29 Maintaining orientation within an abnormal cochlea can be challenging, whether the distorted anatomy is from fibrosis, ossification, or congenital malformation. The surgeon must maintain orientation using whatever landmarks are present. Removal of bone too superior can risk entering the modiolus, thereby injuring neural tissues and creating an iatrogenic spinal fluid leak. Similarly, drilling too far anteriorly risks injury to the genu of the intratemporal carotid.

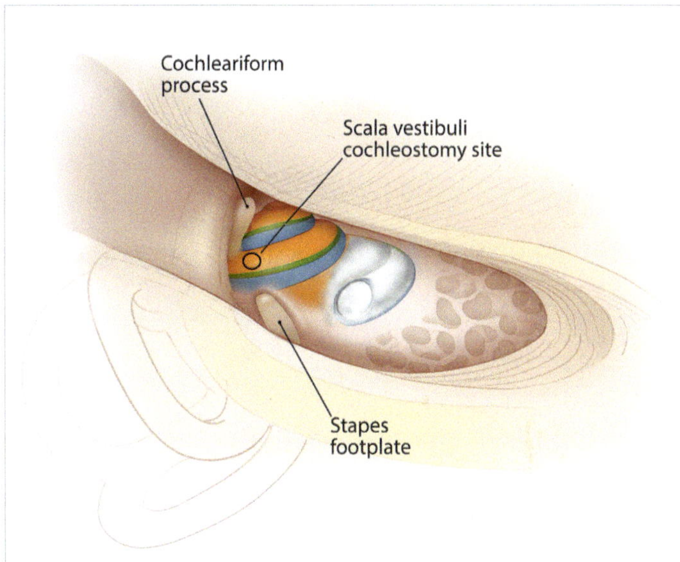

Fig. 11.30 A mid-turn cochleostomy can be performed, though the facial recess after the incus, incudal buttress, and stapes superstructure are removed. Drilling can then be performed in the area between the anterior oval window and the base of the cochleariform process. Although this will usually enter into the scala vestibuli, any lumen can be used if this approach is needed.

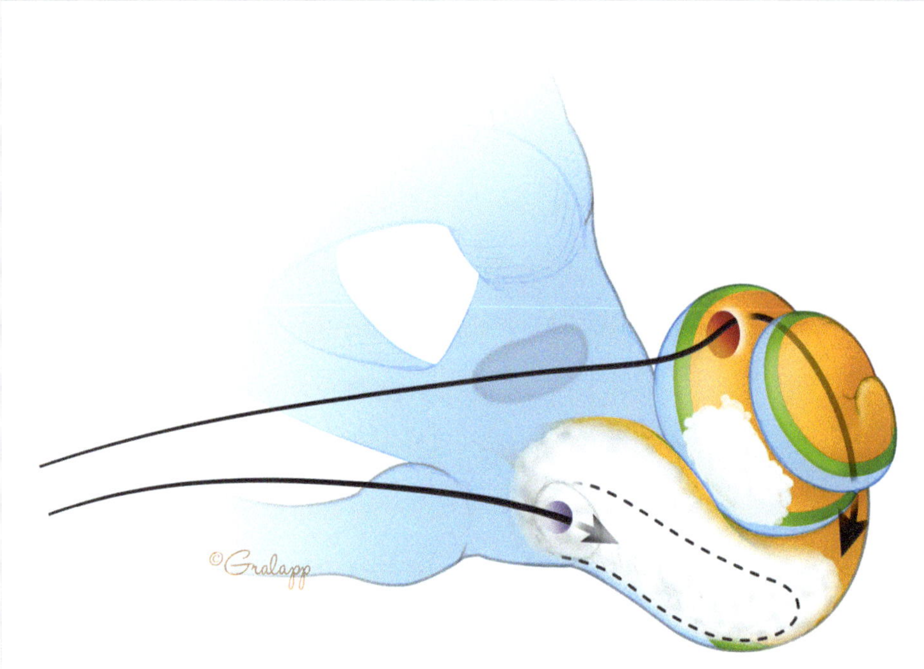

Fig. 11.31 Upon creation of a mid-turn cochleostomy, a split array can be placed. One array is placed as far as possible into the basal turn. The other array can be threaded into the mid-turn in an antegrade fashion if possible. A retrograde insertion (as shown) can also be considered if that provides for a greater number of intracochlear electrodes.

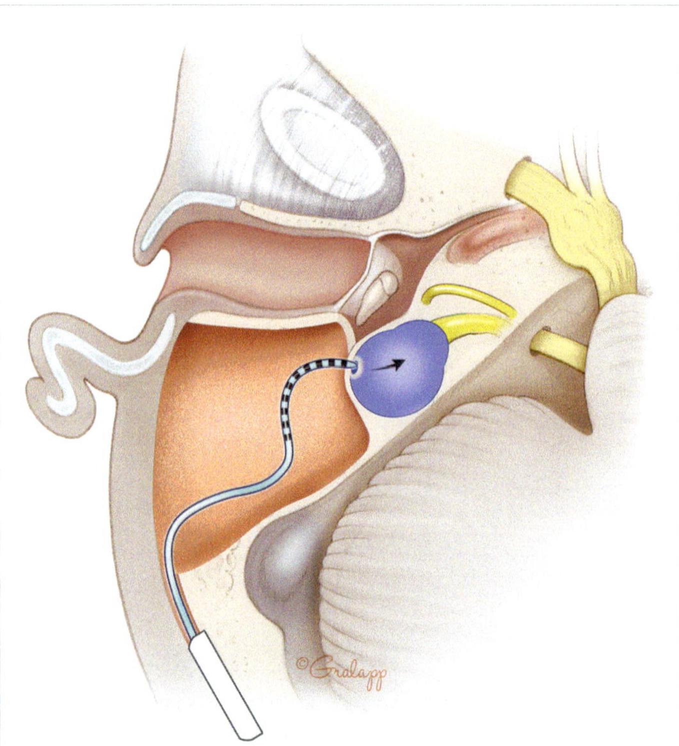

Fig. 11.32 Cochlear implantation of a malformed inner ear presents special challenges. Because the spiral geometry of the cochlea may be altered (e.g., incomplete partition) or absent (e.g., common cavity), the relationship between the electrodes and the auditory nerve may be altered. In addition, because the cochlear modiolus may be malformed, a connection between the perilymph and cerebrospinal fluid may exist at the lateral terminus of the internal auditory canal.

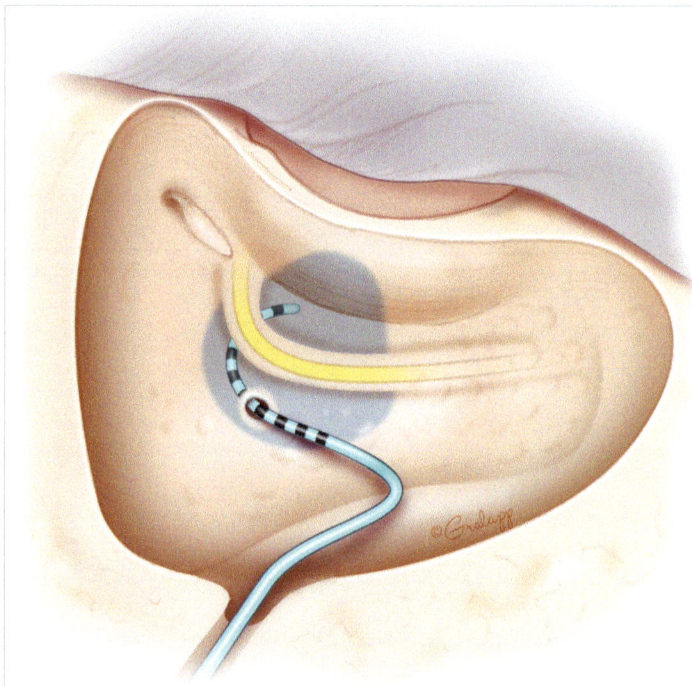

Fig. 11.33 In cases of common cavity malformation, cochleostomy can be performed posterior to the facial nerve. Drilling of the facial recess, while also allowing access to the cavity, is typically unnecessary. A more posterior cochleostomy also allows for better access in case packing of a CSF leak is required.

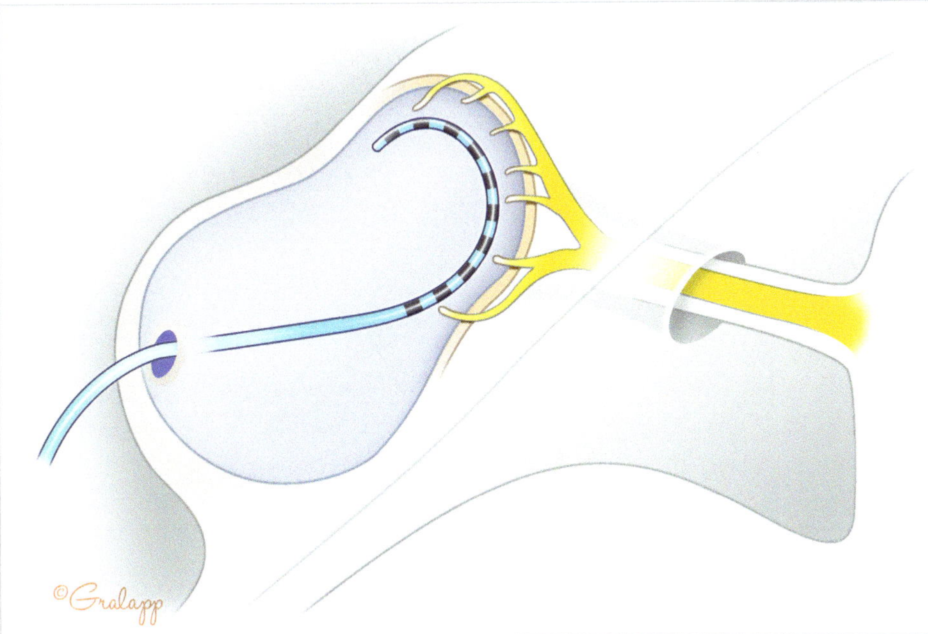

Fig. 11.34 A straight electrode advances along the periphery of the cavity in proximity to the auditory dendrites and ganglia.

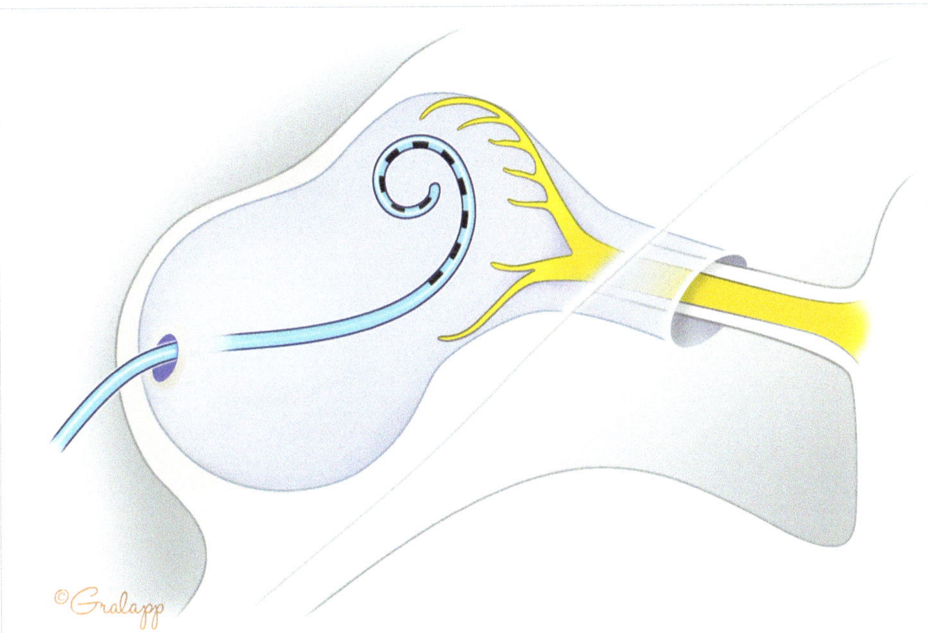

Fig. 11.35 A coiled electrode may position more centrally in the deformed inner ear, more remote form the neural elements.

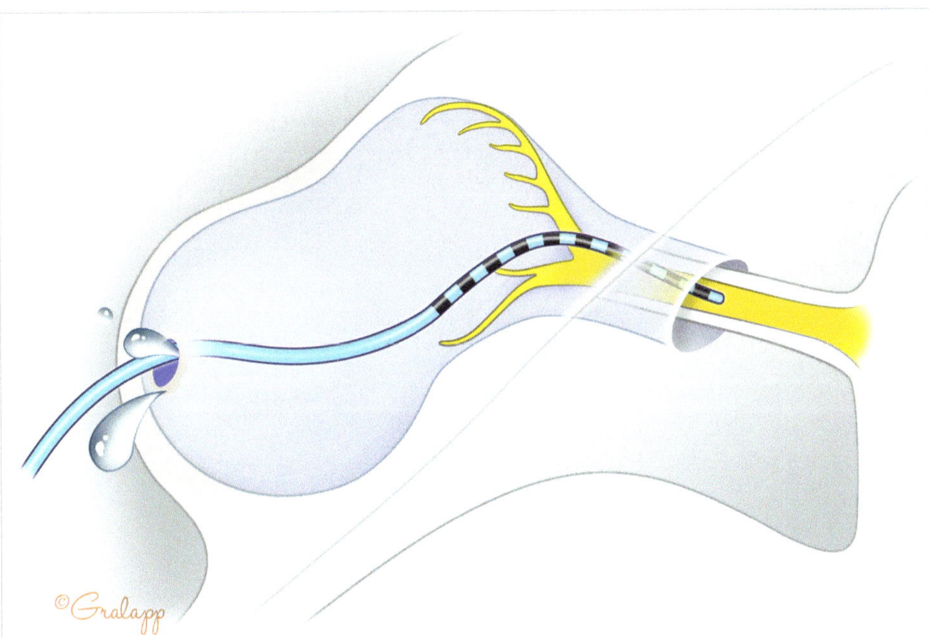

Fig. 11.36 In severe inner ear malformation, it is common to have poor partitioning between the deformed inner ear and cerebrospinal fluid (CSF) space at lateral extremity of the internal auditory canal. This can result in brisk CSF leakage. In addition, a straight electrode is prone to penetrate the internal auditory canal. It is prudent to obtain an intraoperative X-ray to ensure proper placement.

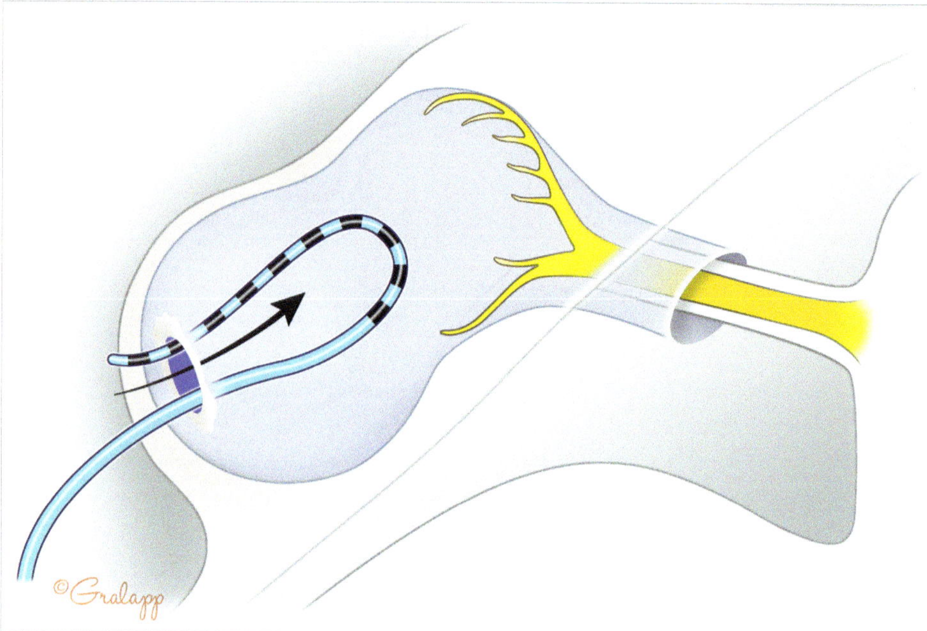

Fig. 11.37 One technique to exert a degree of control over electrode placement in a deformed inner ear lacking internal architecture is inserting a loop via a slot-shaped bony opening.

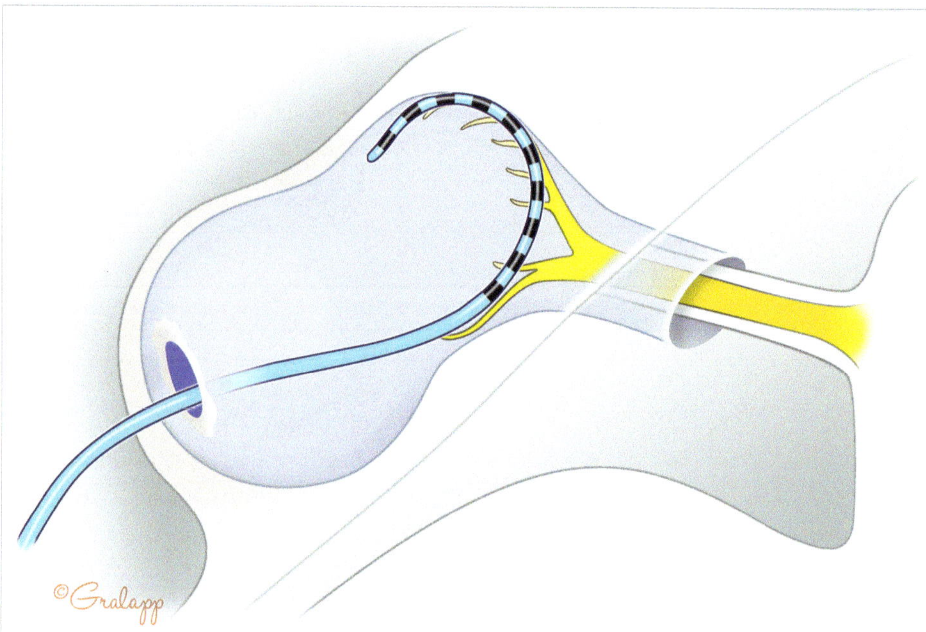

Fig. 11.38 The loop deploys peripherally in proximity to neural elements. This technique reduces the risk of the electrode penetrating the internal auditory canal.

12 Temporal Bone Fractures, Encephaloceles, and Cerebrospinal Fluid Leaks

Robert K. Jackler

12.1 Introduction

Most fractures of the temporal bone result from blunt trauma. Longitudinal fractures usually result from a temporal or parietal blow and usually do not disrupt the otic capsule (cochlea and semicircular canals). They often disrupt the ossicular chain, especially the incudostapedial joint, which is usually repaired on a delayed basis. Transverse fractures generally require a more severe degree of trauma, typically to the occiput, and are often accompanied by intracranial injury. Transverse fractures frequently traverse the otic capsule resulting in deafness.

In most cases, traumatic cerebrospinal fluid (CSF) leak stops spontaneously without need for surgical intervention. In severe injuries, persistent leak may necessitate operative repair, most often reconstruction of the temporal floor. Facial paralysis associated with temporal bone fracture has a good prognosis when the fallopian canal is not severely disrupted. In cases of delayed paralysis, most experts favor expectant management. In immediate-onset facial paralysis associated with fallopian canal disruption, surgical exploration with decompression and/or repair may be indicated.

CSF leak via the ear may be spontaneous, follow trauma, or arise as a complication of skull base surgery. Most postoperative and posttraumatic CSF leaks are treated conservatively initially with surgical repair reserved for persistent cases or when meningitis has occurred. Spontaneous CSF leaks most often arise from deficiencies in the tegmen mastoideum or tympani and are more common in obese individuals. Often, there is widespread thinning of the cranial base and underlying hydrocephalus should be suspected. CSF leak may occur via the inner ear when congenital malformation connects the perilymphatic space with the cerebellopontine angle cistern, most often via the internal auditory canal.

Most encephaloceles of the temporal bone are spontaneous and may be accompanied by CSF leak. Superior semicircular canal dehiscence may accompany spontaneous encephalocele. Encephaloceles are sometimes encountered following mastoidectomy in which the tegmen has been disrupted or following temporal bone trauma. Generally, middle fossa encephaloceles are best repaired from above via an extradural middle fossa craniotomy approach with repair of both the dura and bony defect. The herniated brain from the floor of the temporal lobe may be repositioned intracranially before repair, but the hernia is most often devitalized and should be resected.

Further Reading

1. Bhindi A, Carpineta L, Al Qassabi B, et al. Hearing loss in pediatric temporal bone fractures: evaluating two radiographic classification systems as prognosticators. Int J Pediatr Otorhinolaryngol 2018;109:158–163 PubMed
2. Diaz RC, Cervenka B, Brodie HA. Treatment of temporal bone fractures. J Neurol Surg B Skull Base 2016;77(5):419–429 PubMed
3. Eddelman DB, Munich S, Kochanski RB, et al. Repair of temporal bone defects via the middle cranial fossa approach: treatment of 2 pathologies with 1 operation. Neurosurgery 2018 PubMed
4. Gioacchini FM, Cassandro E, Alicandri-Ciufelli M, et al. Surgical outcomes in the treatment of temporal bone cerebrospinal fluid leak: a systematic review. Auris Nasus Larynx 2018;45 (5):903–910 PubMed
5. Gonen L, Handzel O, Shimony N, Fliss DM, Margalit N. Surgical management of spontaneous cerebrospinal fluid leakage through temporal bone defects–case series and review of the literature. Neurosurg Rev 2016;39(1):141–150, discussion 150 PubMed
6. Grinblat G, Dandinarasaiah M, Prasad SC, et al. Temporal bone meningo-encephalic-herniation: etiological categorization and surgical strategy. Otol Neurotol 2018;39(3):320–332 PubMed
7. Jeevan DS, Ormond DR, Kim AH, et al. Cerebrospinal fluid leaks and encephaloceles of temporal bone origin: nuances to diagnosis and management. World Neurosurg 2015;83 (4):560–566 PubMed
8. Kutz JW Jr, Johnson AK, Wick CC. Surgical management of spontaneous cerebrospinal fistulas and encephaloceles of the temporal bone. Laryngoscope 2018;128(9):2170–2177 PubMed
9. Rereddy SK, Mattox DE. Spontaneous defects between the mastoid and posterior cranial fossa. Acta Otolaryngol 2016;136(4):340–343 PubMed
10. Yetiser S, Hidir Y, Birkent H, Satar B, Durmaz A. Traumatic ossicular dislocations: etiology and management. Am J Otolaryngol 2008;29(1):31–36 PubMed

12.2 Temporal Bone Fractures

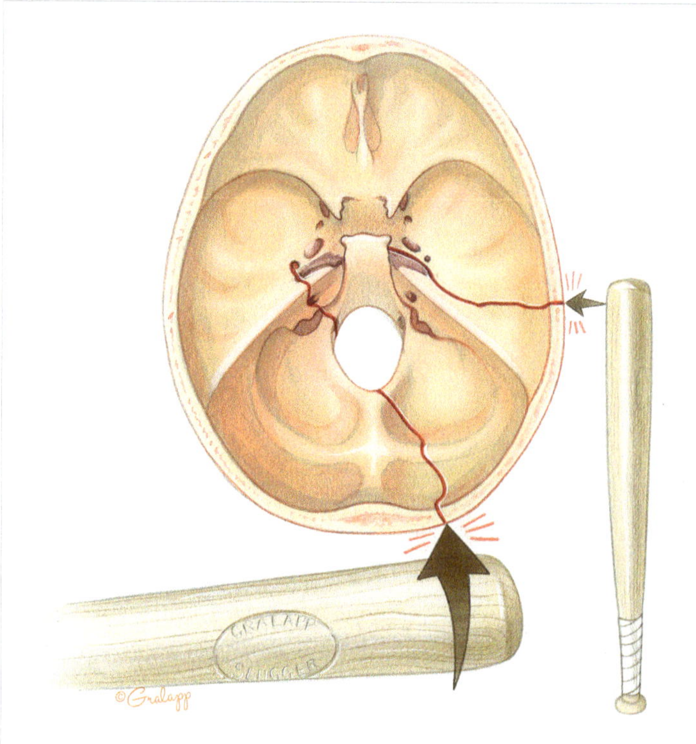

Fig. 12.1 Fractures through the petrous pyramid may result from either posterior or lateral blows to the head. The skull base fractures more easily when struck from the side, on the thin temporal squamosa, than posteriorly on the thick occipital bone. Fractures resulting from temporal blows tend to propagate medially along a course parallel to the long axis of the petrous pyramid and thus are termed "longitudinal." Strong occipital blows characteristically produce a fracture which disrupts the foramen magnum ring and then propagates anteriorly across the petrous pyramid at right angles to its long axis. These are termed "transverse fractures." Longitudinal fractures tend to be associated with conductive hearing loss due to hemotympanum and ossicular disruption. Transverse fractures tend to break the otic capsule and result in permanent sensory hearing loss and acute vertigo. Either can produce facial nerve injury or cerebrospinal fluid leakage.

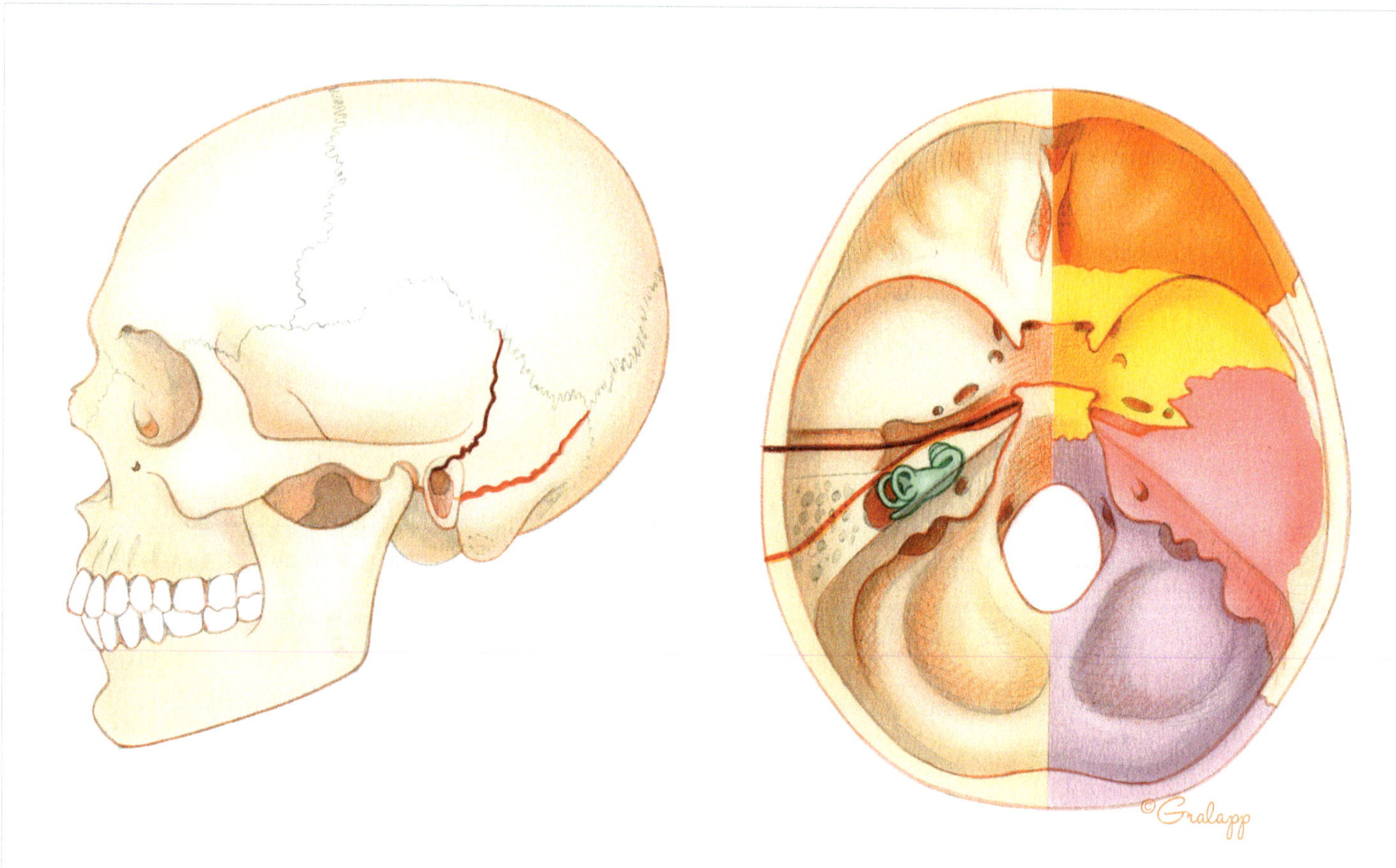

Fig. 12.2 In longitudinal temporal bone fractures, the break originates through cortical areas of weakness such as through the external auditory canal anteriorly, or through the mastoid air cells posteriorly. Fractures originating through the external canal will usually present with bloody otorrhea, a torn tympanic membrane, and a bony canal step-off. Those originating more posterior will have an intact tympanic membrane, hemotympanum, and a Battle's sign due to blood seeping from the mastoid emissary vein. Regardless of their origin, the fractures generally pass through the middle ear space to be deflected anteriorly by the otic capsule to the foramen lacerum. The inner ear and fallopian canal are usually spared.

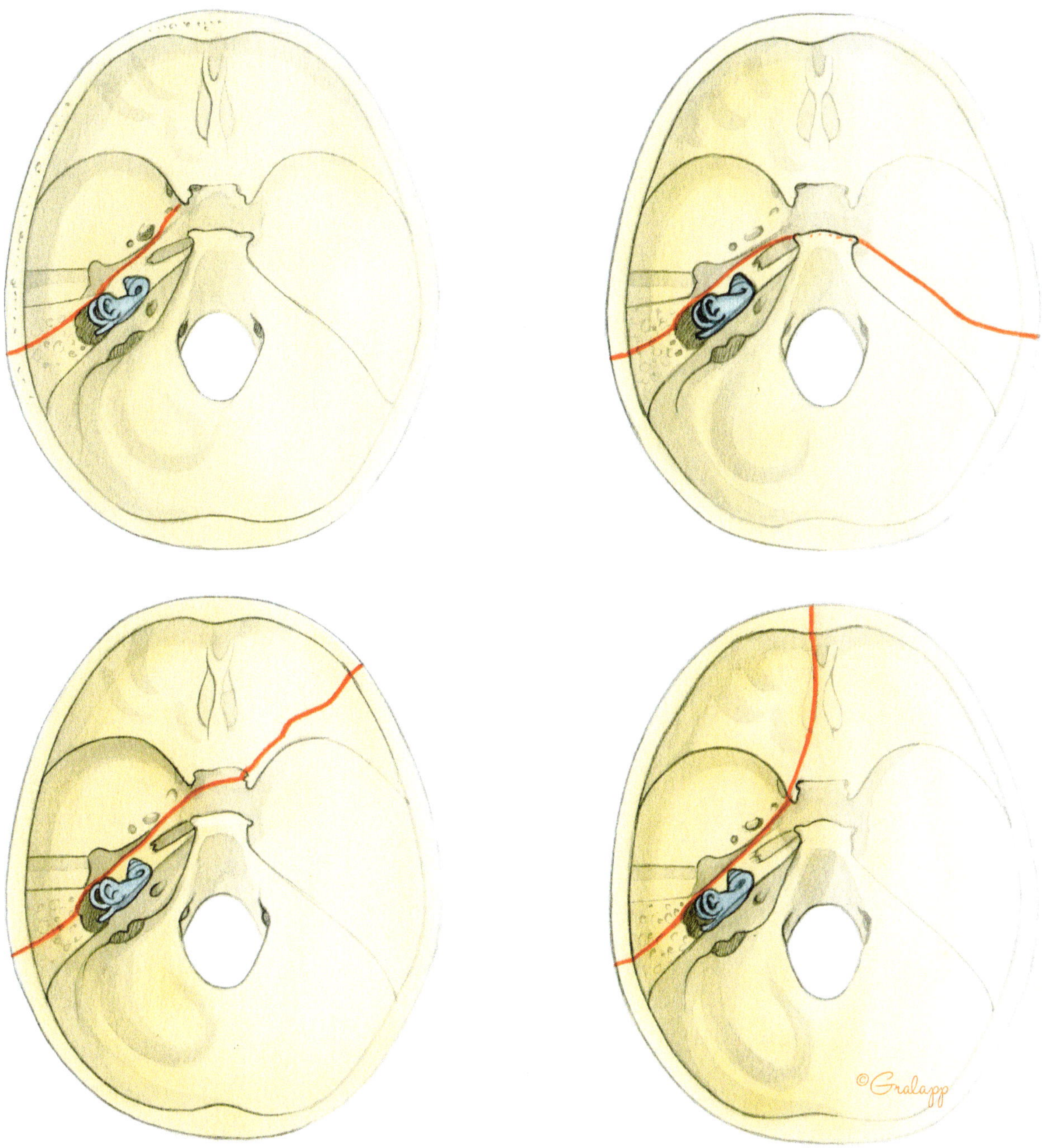

Fig. 12.3 Possible courses of longitudinal temporal bone fractures: the majority of fractures will terminate in the floor of the middle fossa, or in the sphenoid bone (*top left*). Approximately one-third will extend across the midline to be continuous with a contralateral temporal bone fracture (*top right*). A minority of fractures will extend anteriorly to exit the cranium through the anterior fossa floor laterally (*bottom left*), or at the midline through the cribriform plate (*bottom right*).

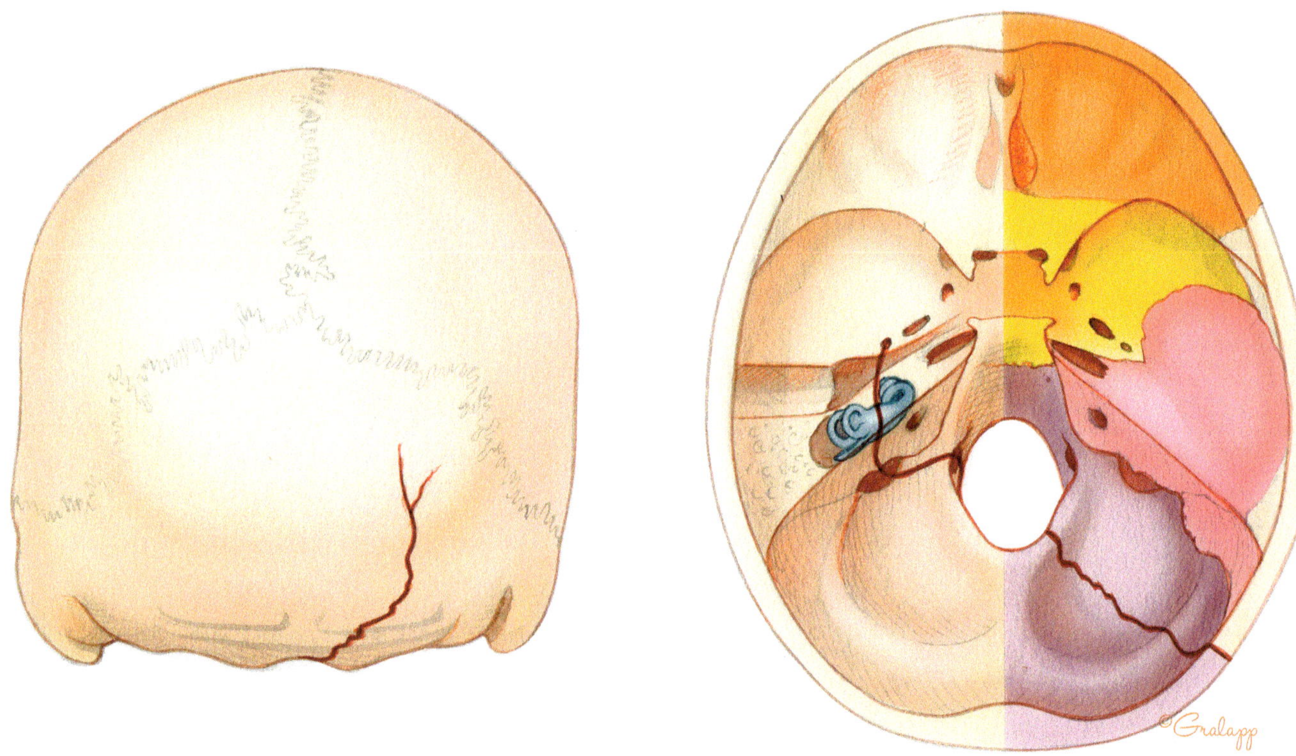

Fig. 12.4 In transverse temporal bone fractures, the cortical origin of the fracture is generally in the occipital bone, where it extends to the foramen magnum. The fracture then traverses the petrous pyramid perpendicular to its long axis, passing from the foramen magnum to the floor of the middle fossa. The otic capsule is usually fractured, resulting in complete loss of inner ear function and often facial nerve injury.

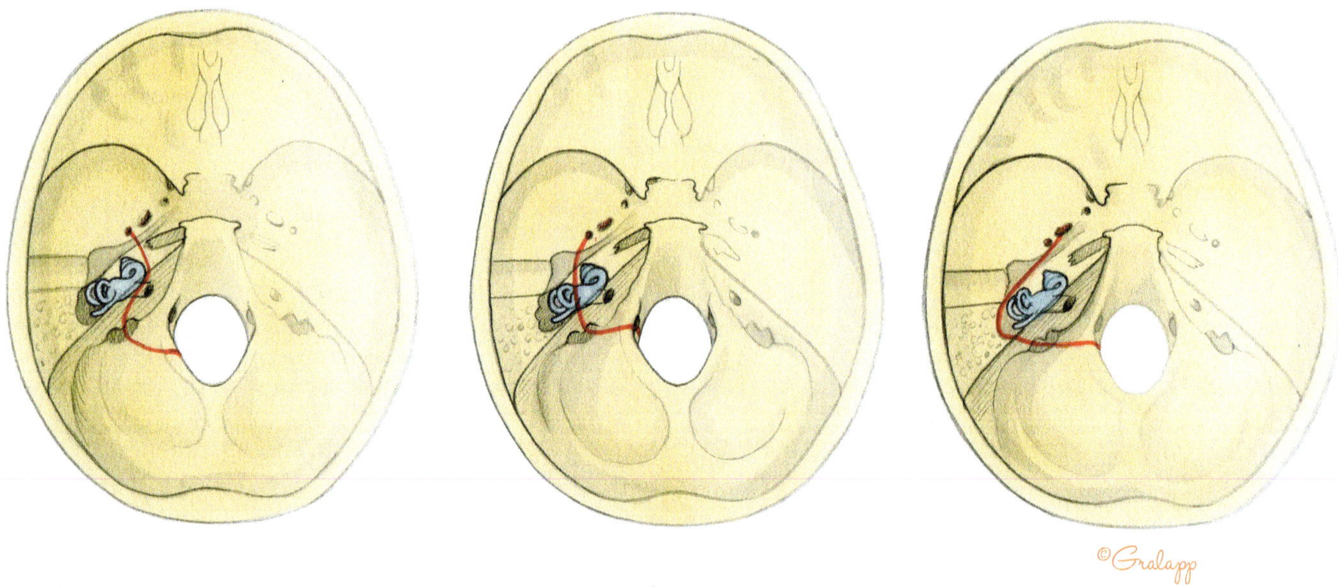

Fig. 12.5 Possible courses of transverse temporal bone fractures: In its course from the foramen magnum to the floor of the middle fossa, the transverse fracture may pass either lateral to, through or medial to, the otic capsule. The most common path is directly through the otic capsule, thereby disrupting the inner ear (*center*). In the rare case where the fracture spares the otic capsule by passing medial to it (*left*), the facial and vestibulocochlear nerves are at risk as the fracture traverses the internal auditory canal. Also rare, the fracture may spare the otic capsule by passing lateral to it through the middle ear (*right*).

12.3 Encephaloceles

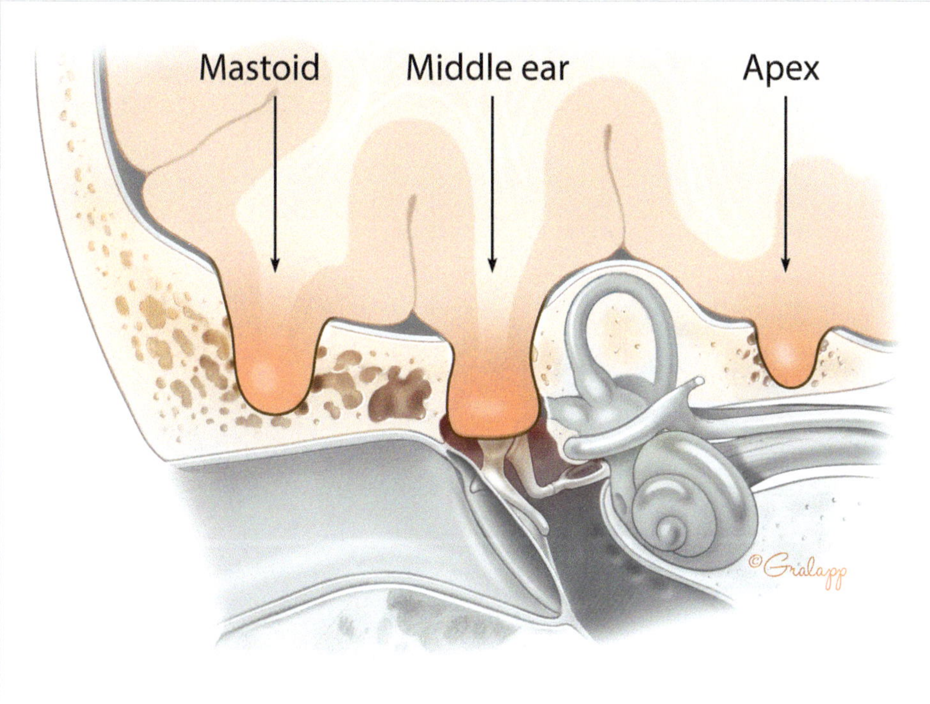

Fig. 12.6 Encephaloceles of the temporal bone most commonly occur through the floor of the middle cranial fossa. These may penetrate the roof of the mastoid, middle ear, or petrous apex. Most frequently, they are traumatic in origin arising either due to cranial base fracture or following iatrogenic injury sustained during mastoid surgery. Spontaneous meningoceles and encephaloceles also occur, presumably due to prominent arachnoid granulations which penetrate the eggshell thin tegmen mastoideum or tympani. Chronically increased intracranial pressure may play a role in such cases.

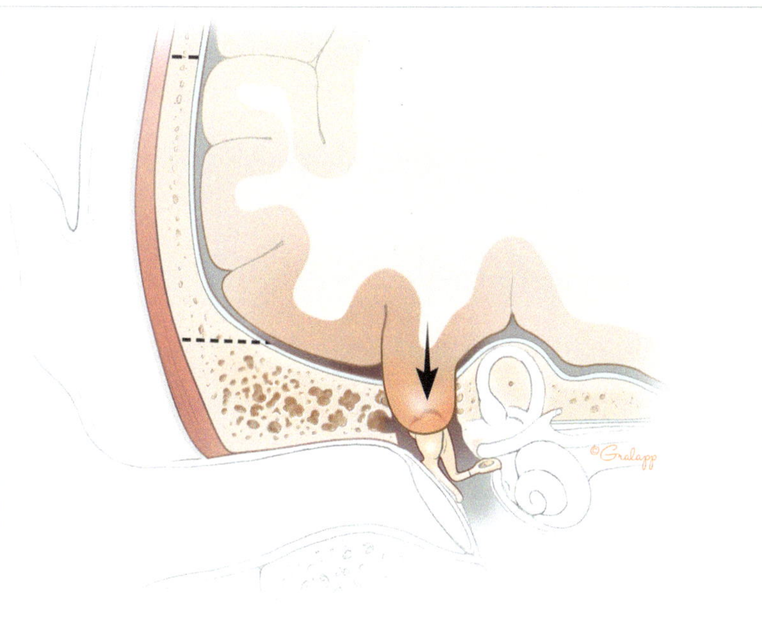

Fig. 12.7 Encephaloceles of the temporal bone with a small brain hernia impinging upon the ossicular chain resulting in conductive hearing loss. This may occur with either intact dura or a dural defect in which case brain may be visible behind the tympanic membrane. *Dashed lines* show bone cuts for middle fossa extradural repair of the dehiscent tegmen.

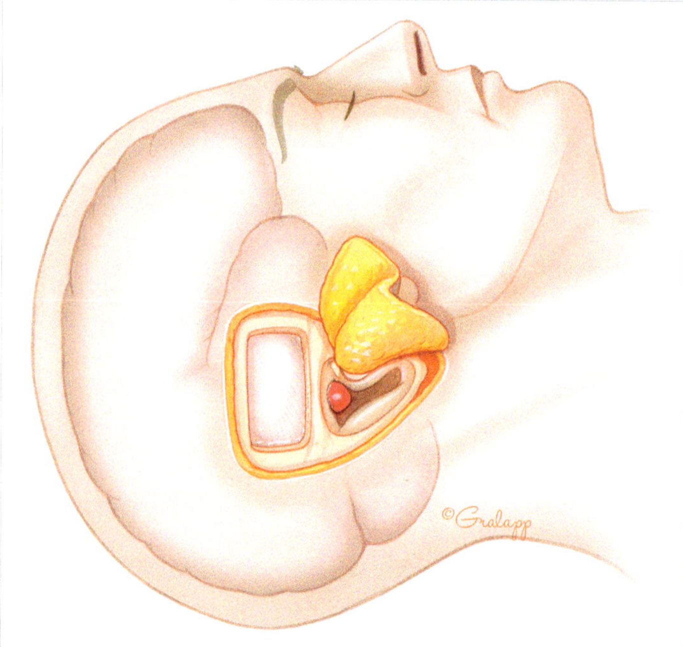

Fig. 12.8 Operative view of a meningoencephalocele herniating into the mastoid via the tegmen. A small middle fossa craniotomy has been performed to gain access to the temporal floor from above.

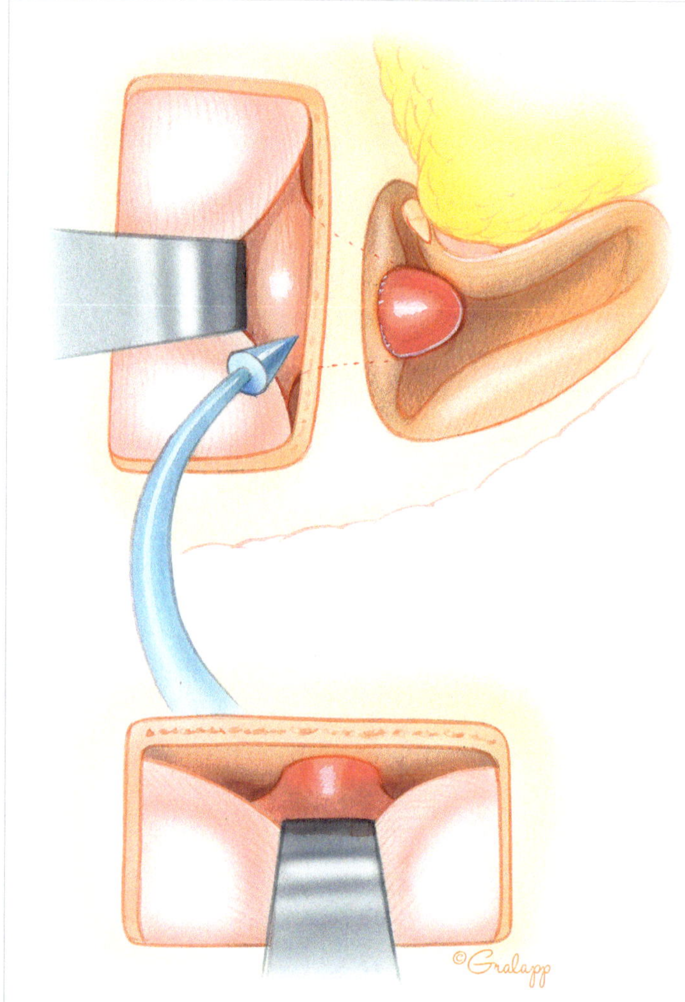

Fig. 12.9 Extradural retraction of the temporal lobe brings into view the base of the hernia.

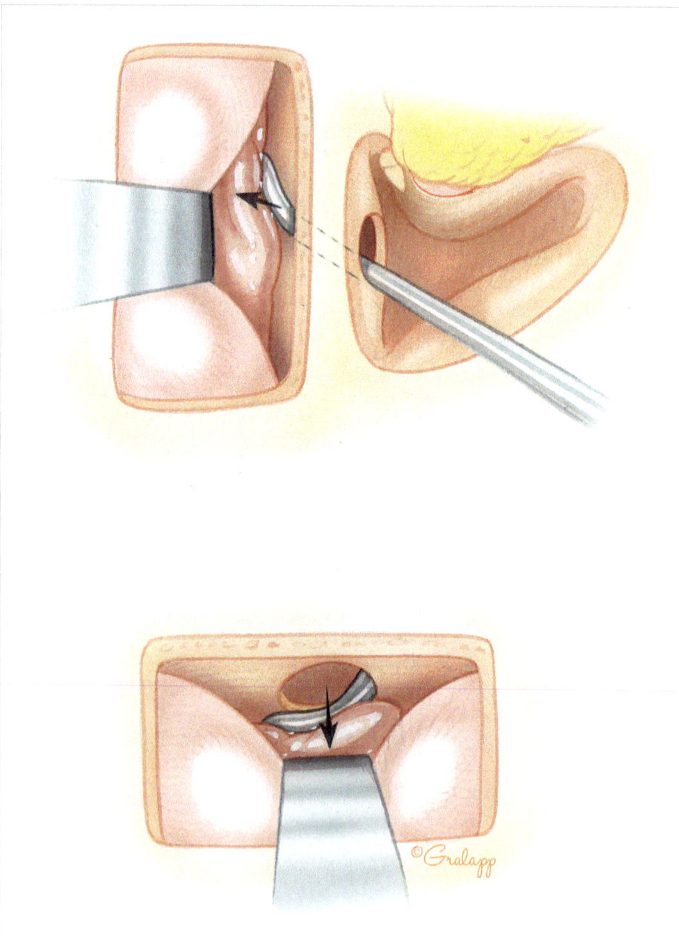

Fig. 12.10 When the brain is not necrotic, an attempt should be made to reduce the hernia back into the temporal fossa.

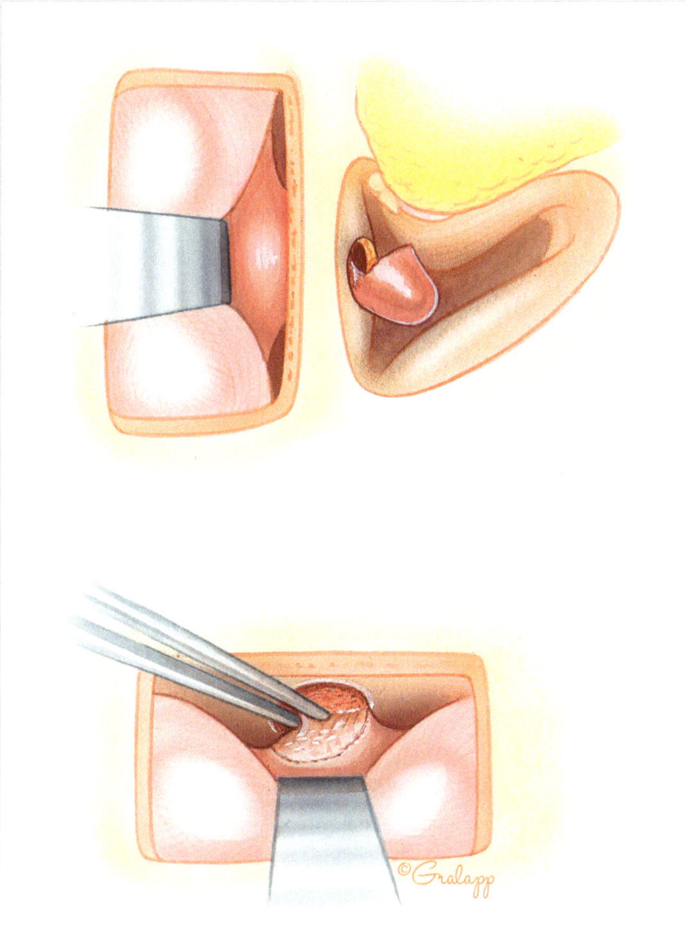

Fig. 12.11 When the brain hernia is necrotic or cannot be reduced, it should be amputated at the level of the cranial base.

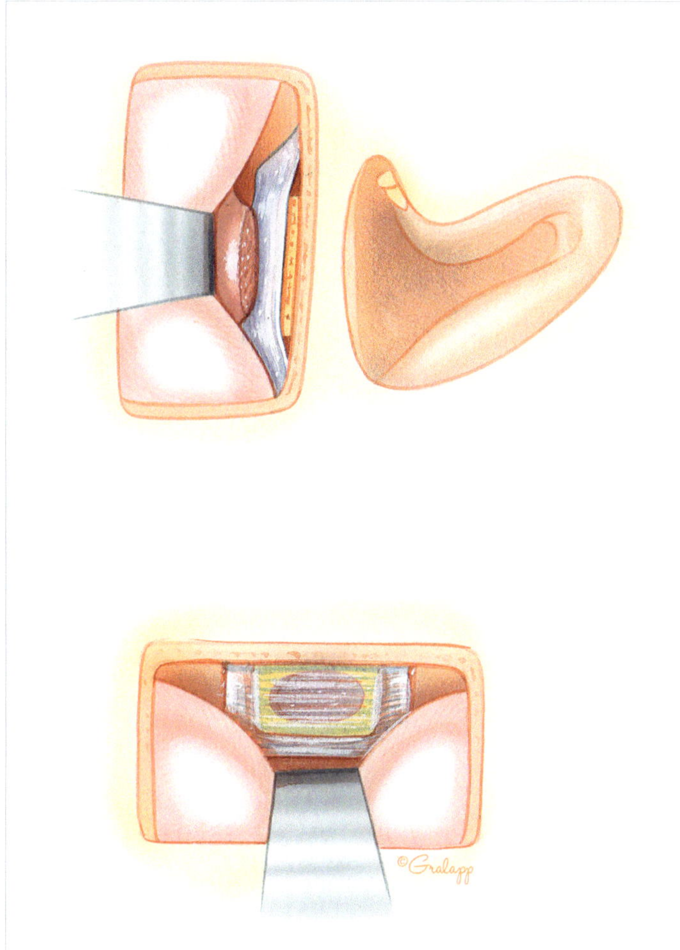

Fig. 12.12 Narrow deficiencies in the temporal floor can be repaired with a soft-tissue graft alone, but a supplemental osseous layer is desirable. Wider defects should be bridged by a bone graft, as depicted here, in addition to a connective tissue sheet.

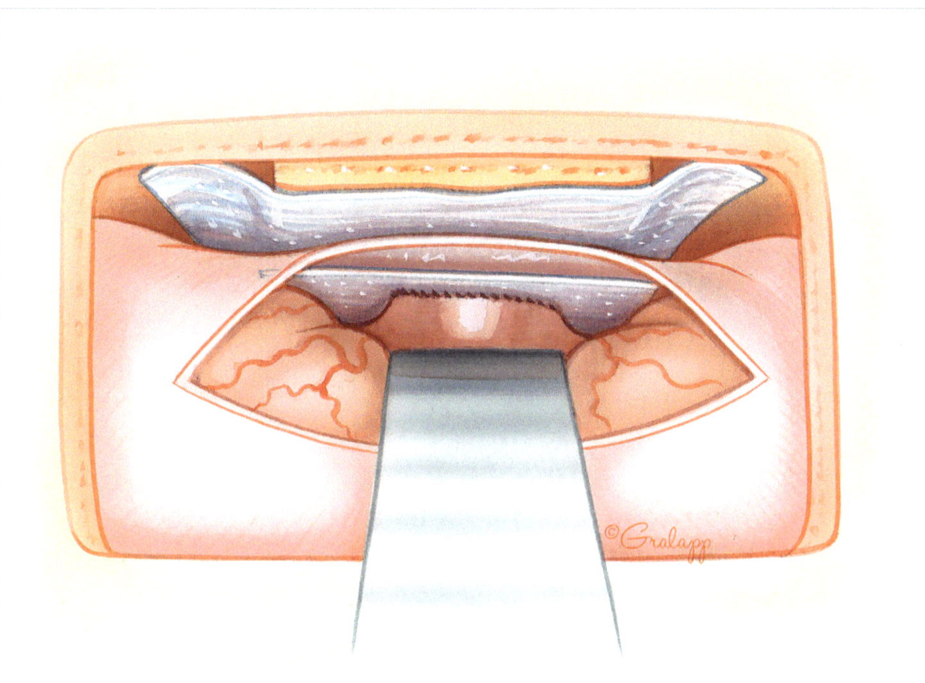

Fig. 12.13 When the dural defect is large, placing a supplemental fascia graft intradurally is desirable. The advantage of an intradural graft is that the weight of the brain helps to coapt the graft with the surrounding dura.

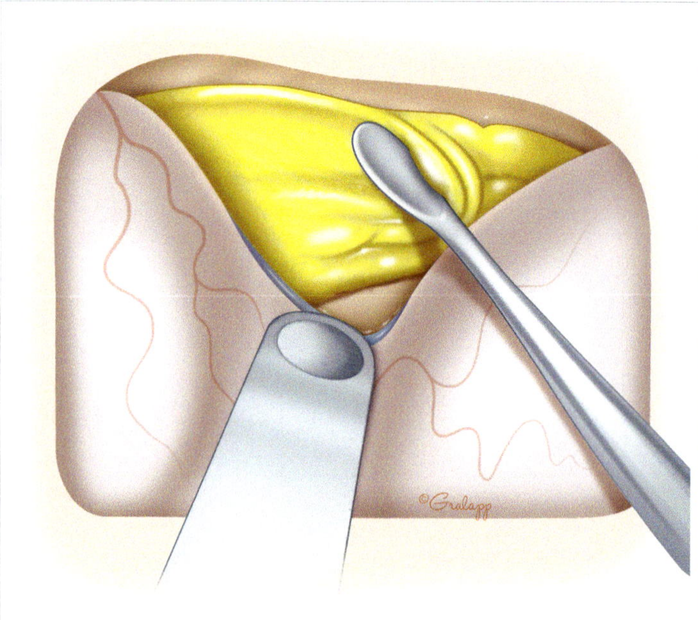

Fig. 12.14 The author's preferred method is to use fascia followed by hydroxyapatite cement smoothed to cover the cranial base defect as well to reinforce the entire temporal floor to deter recurrence.

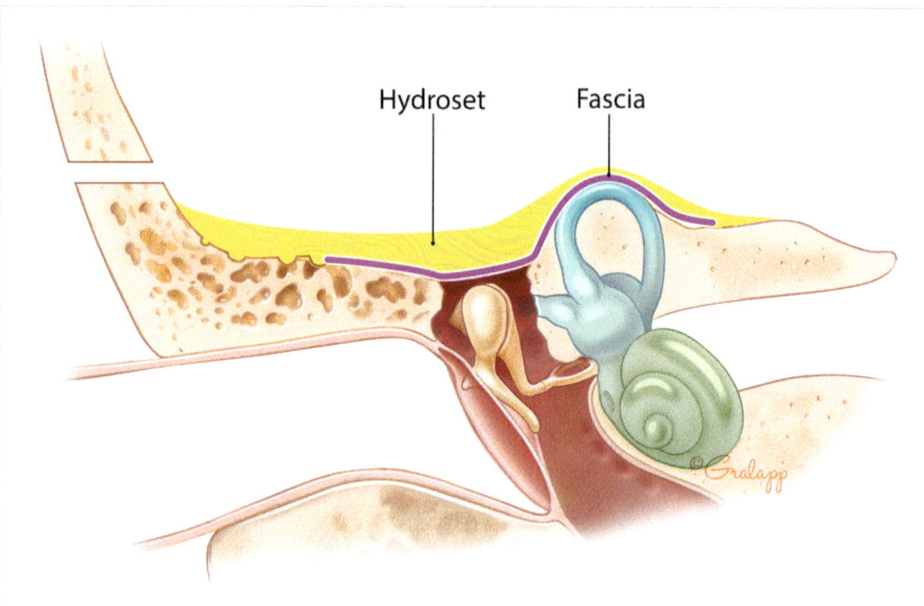

Fig. 12.15 Overview of a repaired temporal floor defect which is best accomplished with a multilayer closure including fascia, bone (either split calvarial or artificial hydroxyapatite as shown here), and sometimes muscle. Fascia is placed both over the bony defect with a second layer placed over the dural defect.

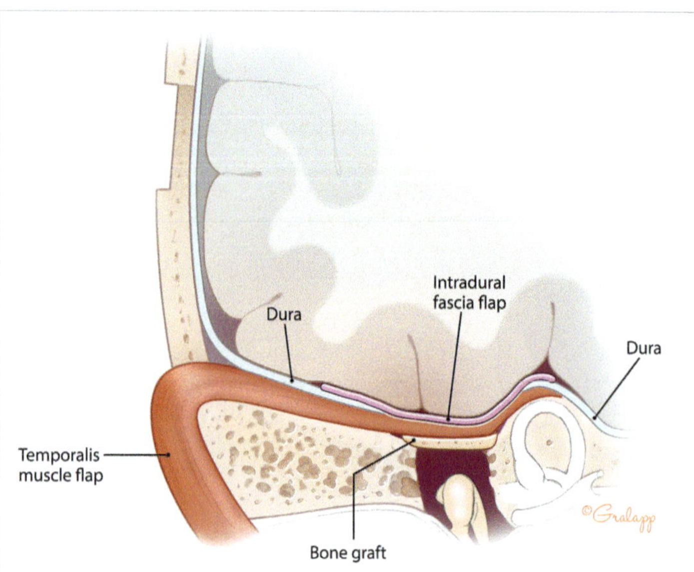

Fig. 12.16 The temporal craniotomy flap has been split with a reciprocating saw to provide a bone graft to cover the widely diastatic gap over the middle ear. A temporalis muscle rotation flap has been used to reinforce the closure. Dural repair may be intradural, as shown here, or extradural.

12.4 Cerebrospinal Fluid Leaks

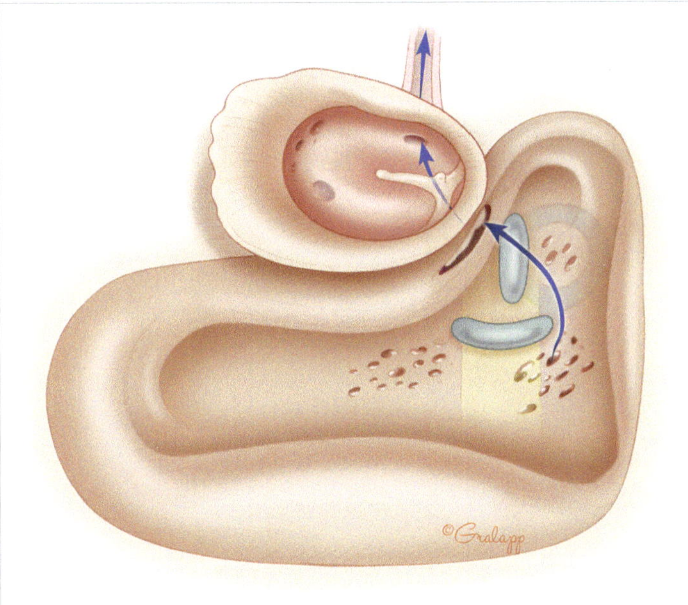

Fig. 12.17 Multiple pathways exist for CSF leakage through the ear. Most common are traumatic and spontaneous leaks that occur via the middle fossa floor (tegmen tympani and mastoideum). Following skull base tumor surgery, the leakage from the posterior fossa flows via perilabyrinthine tracts as shown in the illustration above. Finally, leak may flow though the inner ear, especially when congenitally malformed, or following cochlear implant surgery. (see 11.2 Cochlear Implant Surgical Variations)

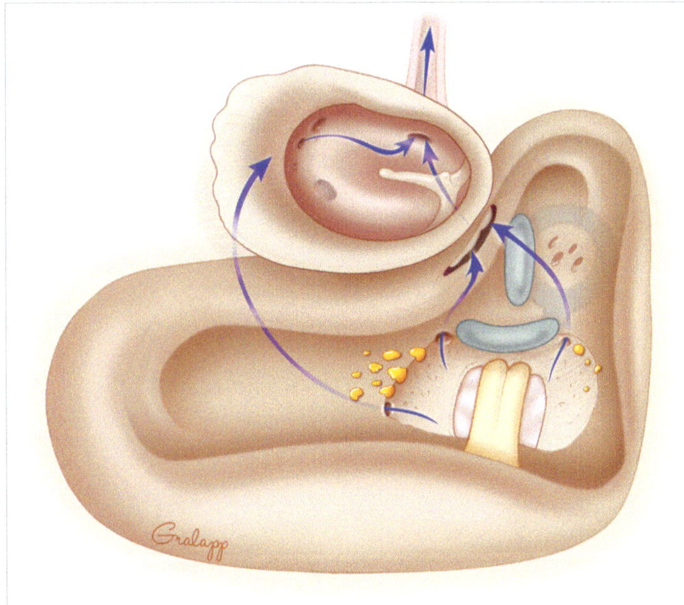

Fig. 12.18 Following a retrosigmoid approach to acoustic neuroma, air cell tracts around the internal auditory canal have been opened. CSF may reach the Eustachian tube via the aditus (common route) or via a direct infralabyrinthine–infracochlear route to the hypotympanum.

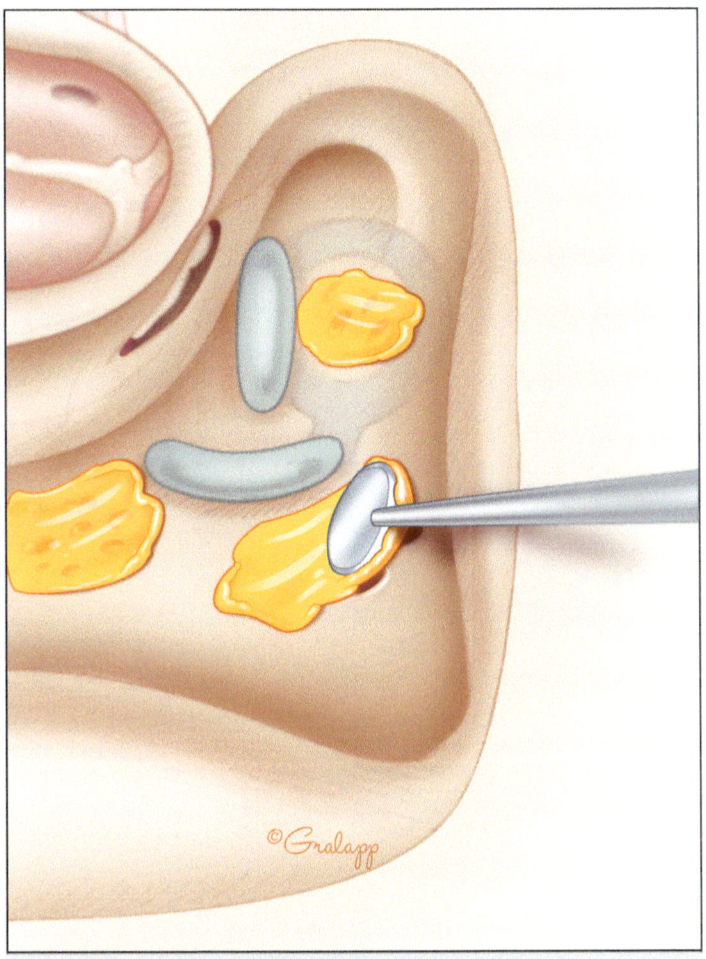

Fig. 12.19 In a hearing ear, the perilabyrinthine cell tract can be meticulously sealed with bone wax.

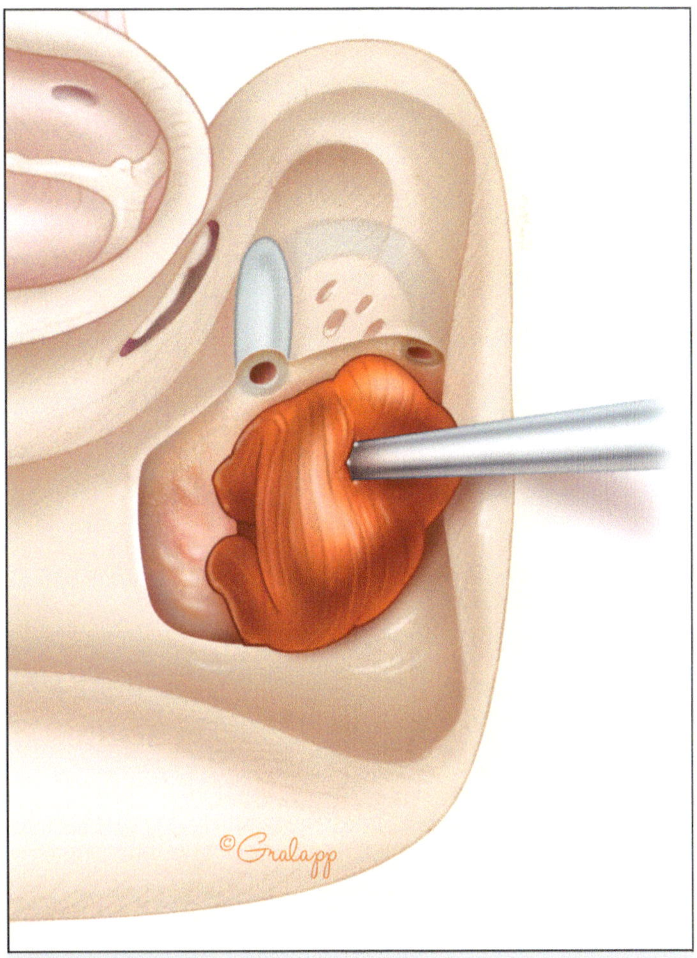

Fig. 12.20 In a nonhearing ear, the labyrinth can be resected to enable a combination of fascia and muscle to directly seal the dural opening.

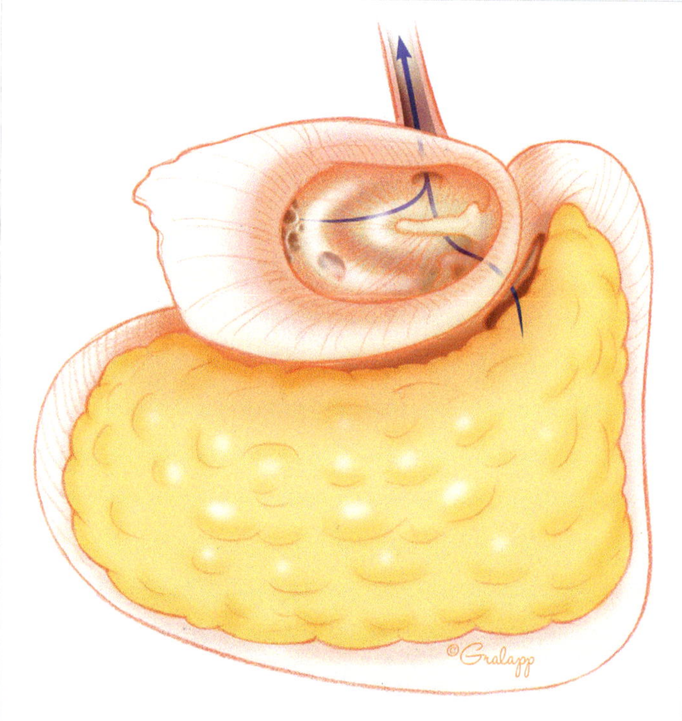

Fig. 12.21 Management of CSF otorhinorrhea illustrated by leakage occurring after a translabyrinthine approach to acoustic neuroma. In this case, CSF traverses the fat graft in the petrous defect to pass through the aditus to the middle ear and then via the Eustachian tube to the nasopharynx (*arrow*).

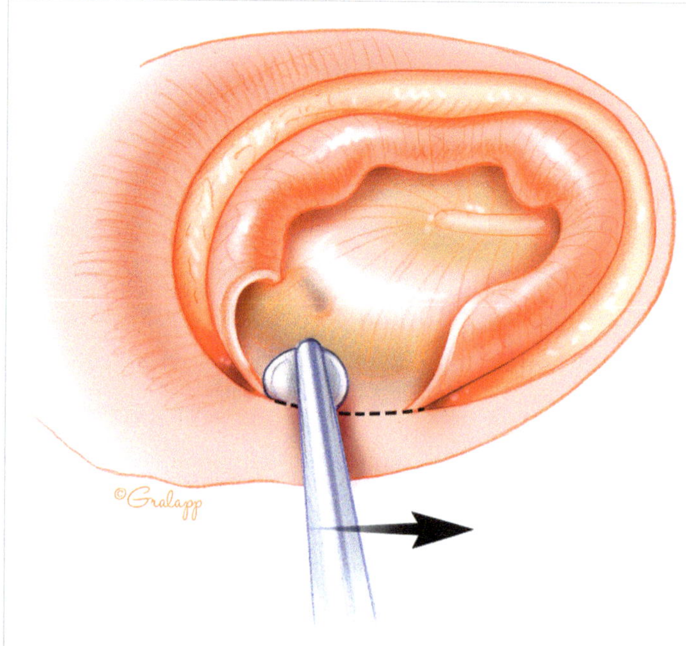

Fig. 12.22 The first stage in obliteration of the middle ear and closure of the Eustachian tube begins with removal of the skin of the external auditory canal. This is important to perform thoroughly to avoid creation of an iatrogenic cholesteatoma.

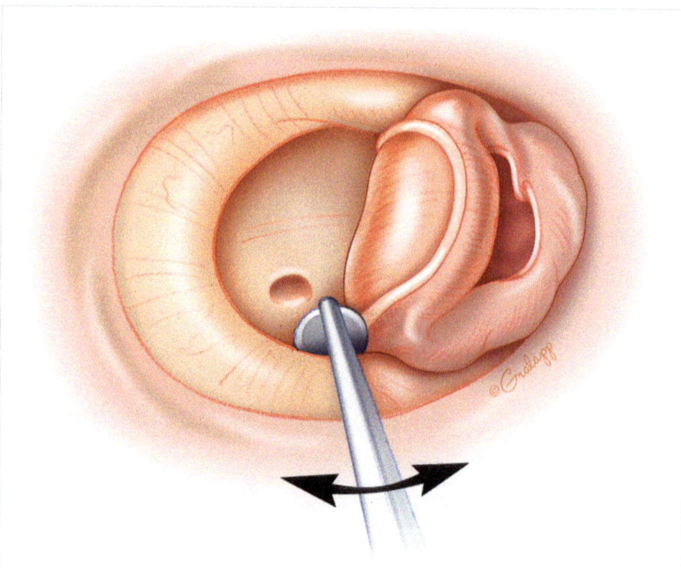

Fig. 12.23 Dissection of the tympanic annulus from its sulcus.

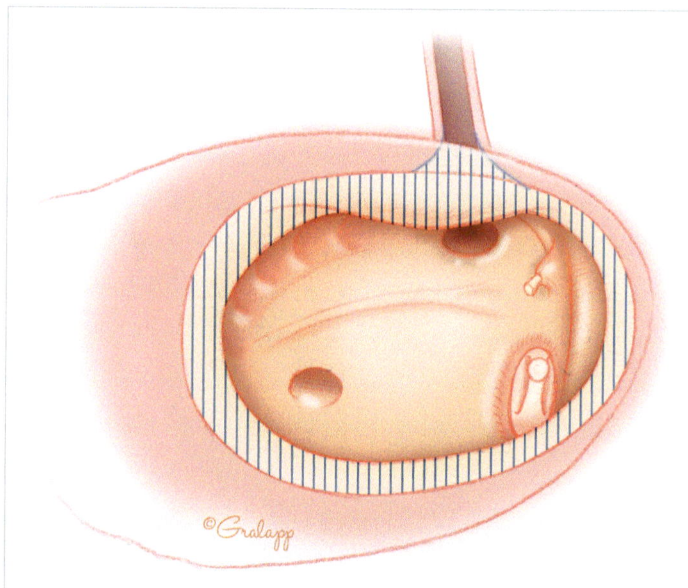

Fig. 12.24 To ensure removal of all squamous remnants, the annular sulcus is drilled away. Note that the bone overlying the Eustachian tube infundibulum must be widely excavated.

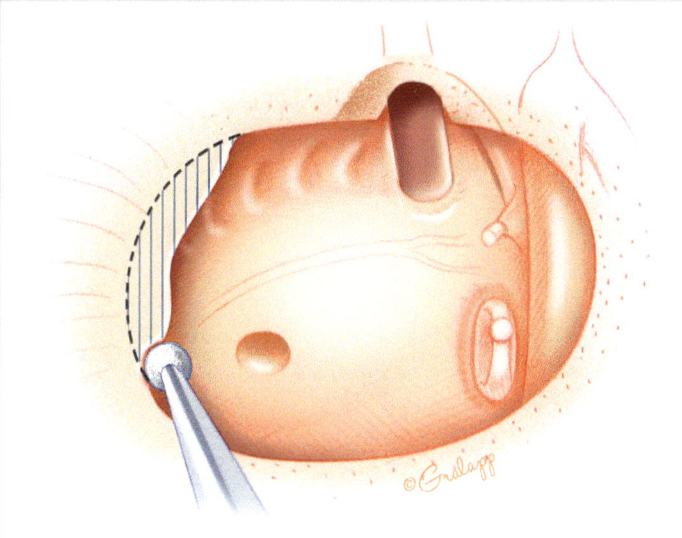

Fig. 12.25 The orifice of the Eustachian tube has been exposed.

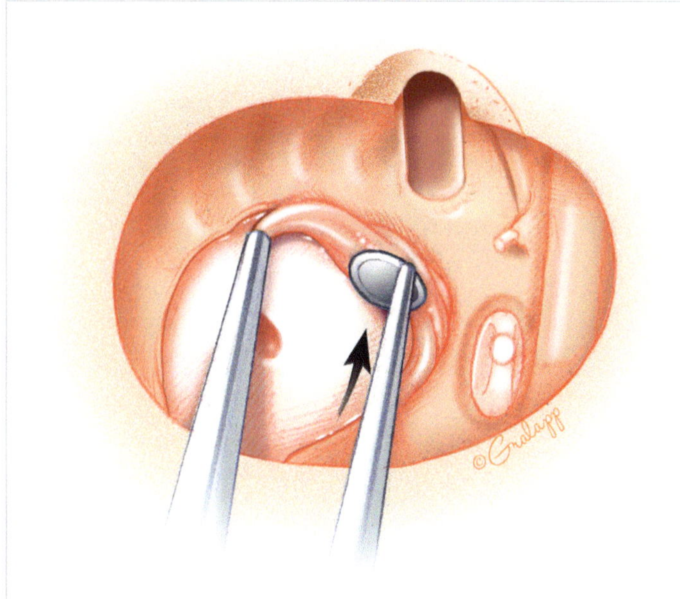

Fig. 12.26 To reduce the likelihood of mucocele formation, mucosa from the middle ear is removed.

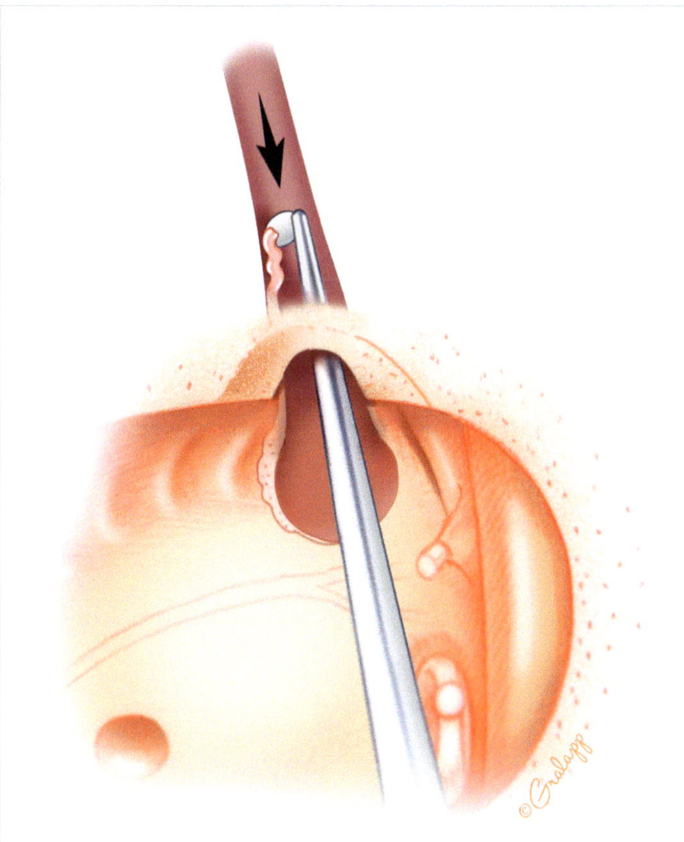

Fig. 12.27 Mucosa is scraped from the Eustachian tube. As the party wall with the carotid artery can be dehiscent, this should be done without excessive vigor.

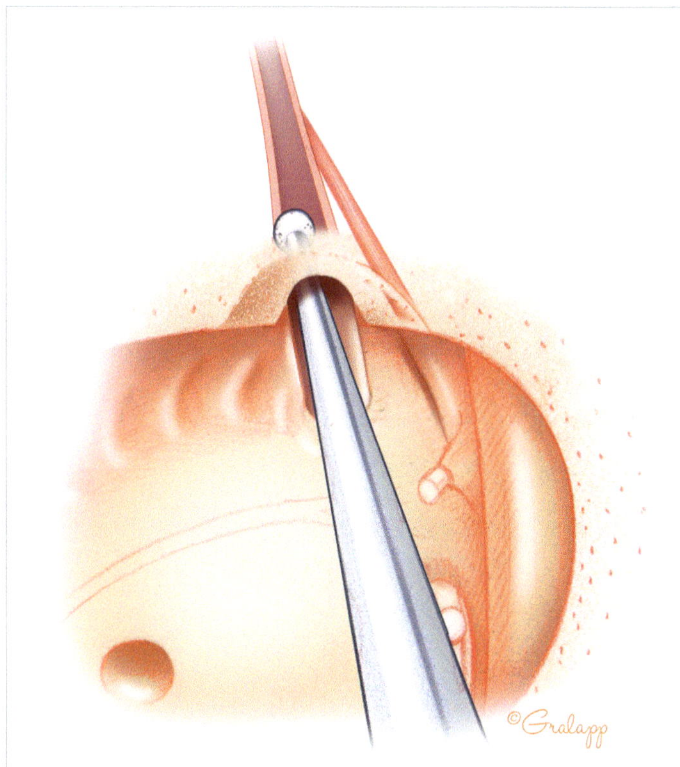

Fig. 12.28 Using a diamond burr, the middle ear orifice of the Eustachian tube is funneled.

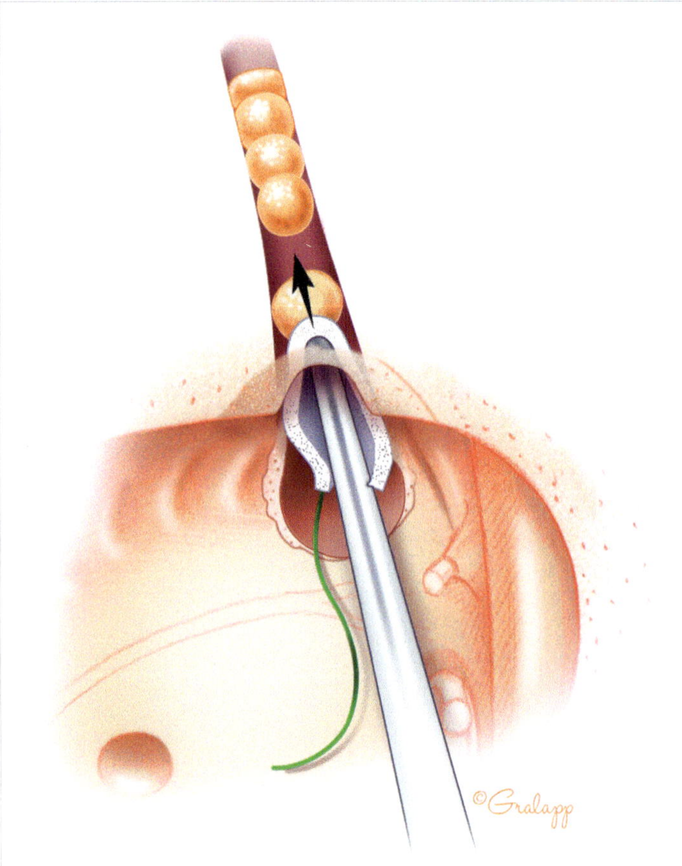

Fig. 12.29 The Eustachian tube is obliterated with bone wax. A series of small "peas" of bone wax are impacted sequentially with a ¼ inch cottonoid pledget.

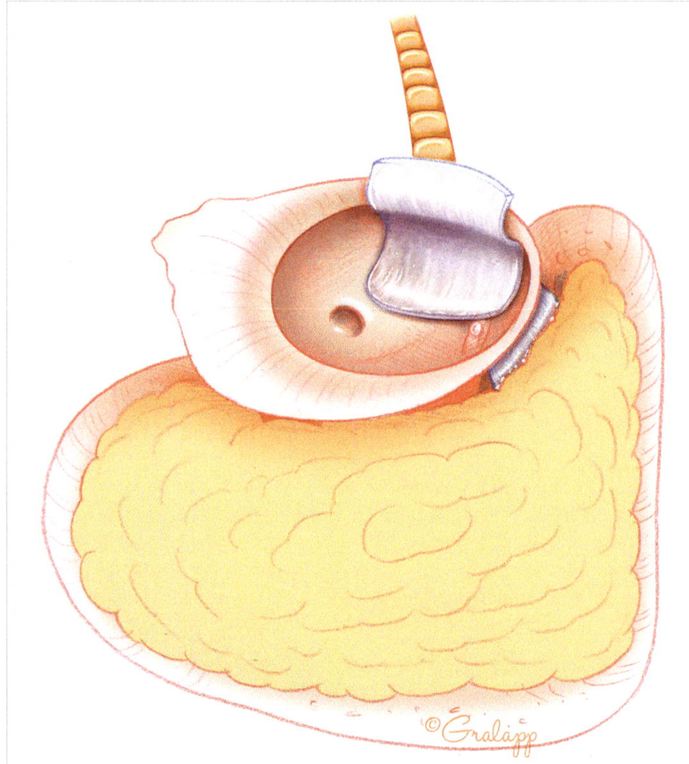

Fig. 12.30 After scraping excess wax from the Eustachian tube orifice, temporalis fascia is placed over the orifice and over the aditus.

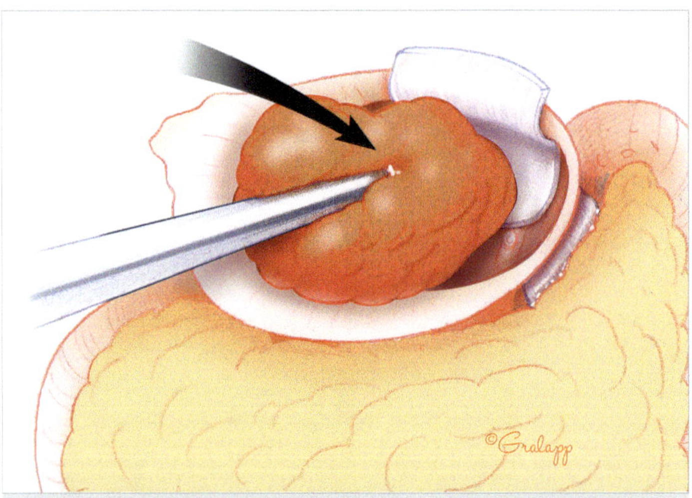

Fig. 12.31 A free graft of temporalis muscle is mortised into the medial ear canal to obliterate the middle ear cavity and hold the fascia in place over the Eustachian tube orifice.

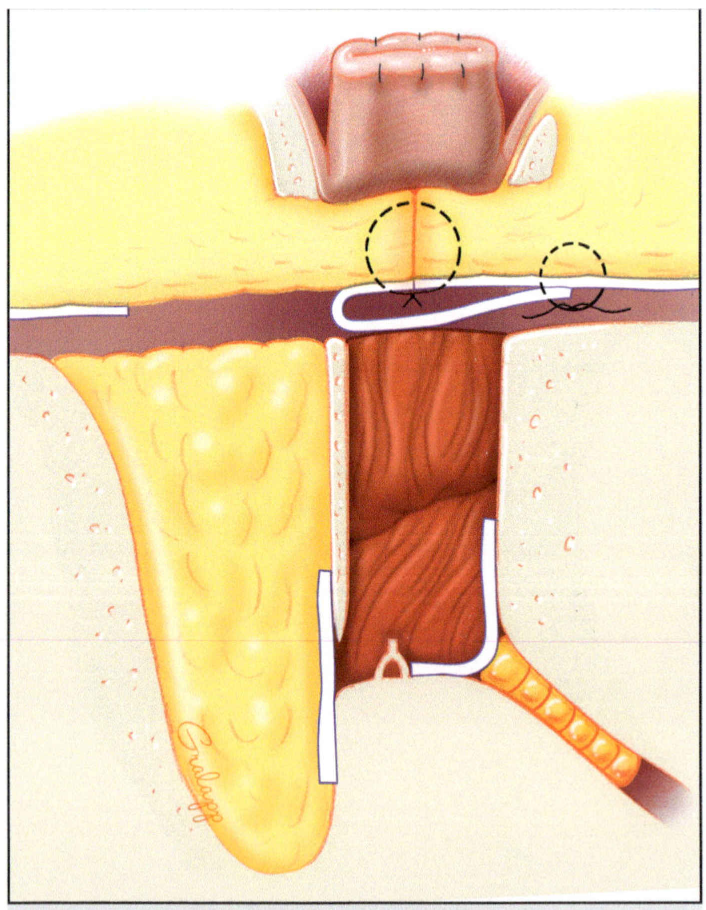

Fig. 12.32 Completed temporal bone obliteration for CSF leak. The technique for ear canal closure to withstand CSF pressure is illustrated in the next section.

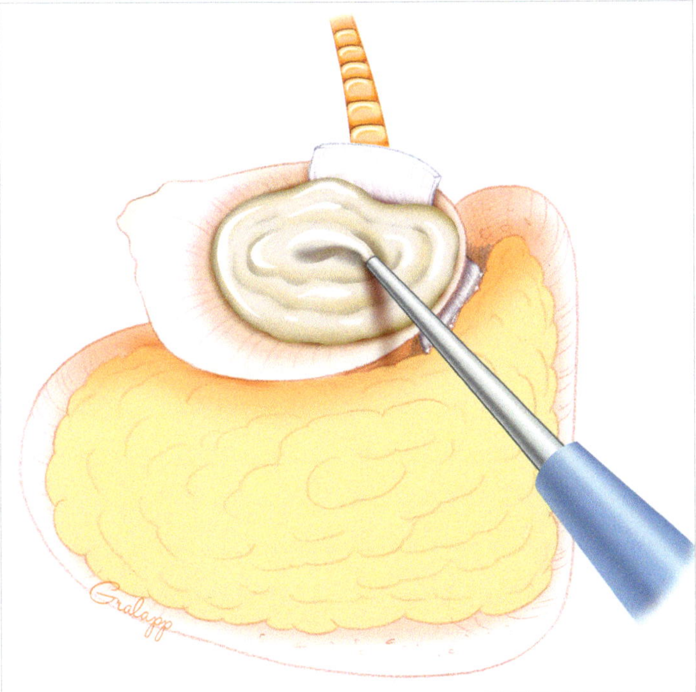

Fig. 12.33 Hydroxyapatite is an alternative means of filling the middle ear and bony ear canal.

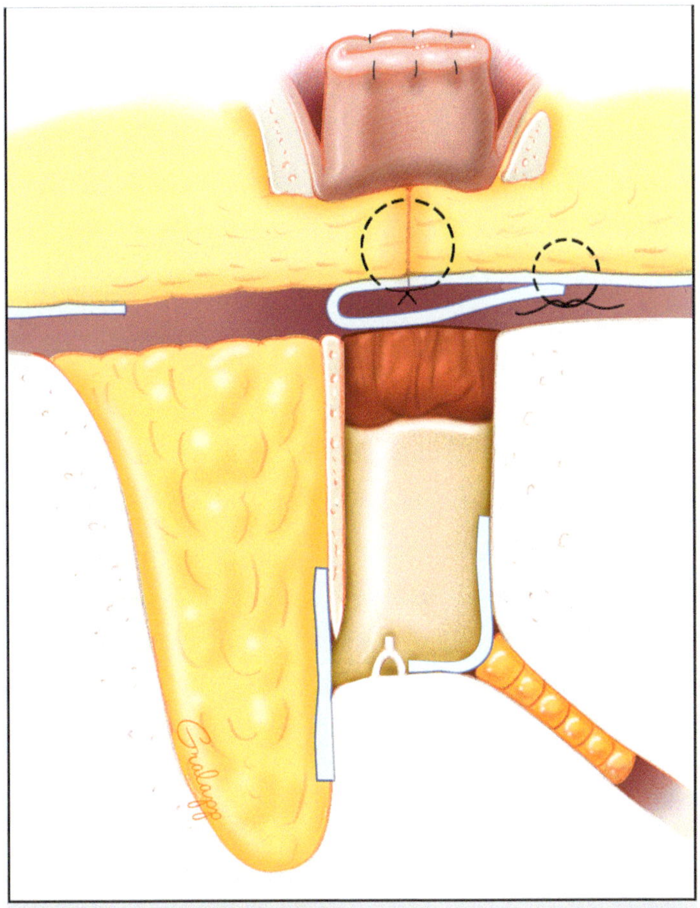

Fig. 12.34 Schematic showing use of hydroxyapatite to obliterate the middle ear and osseous ear canal.

12.5 Ear Canal Closure

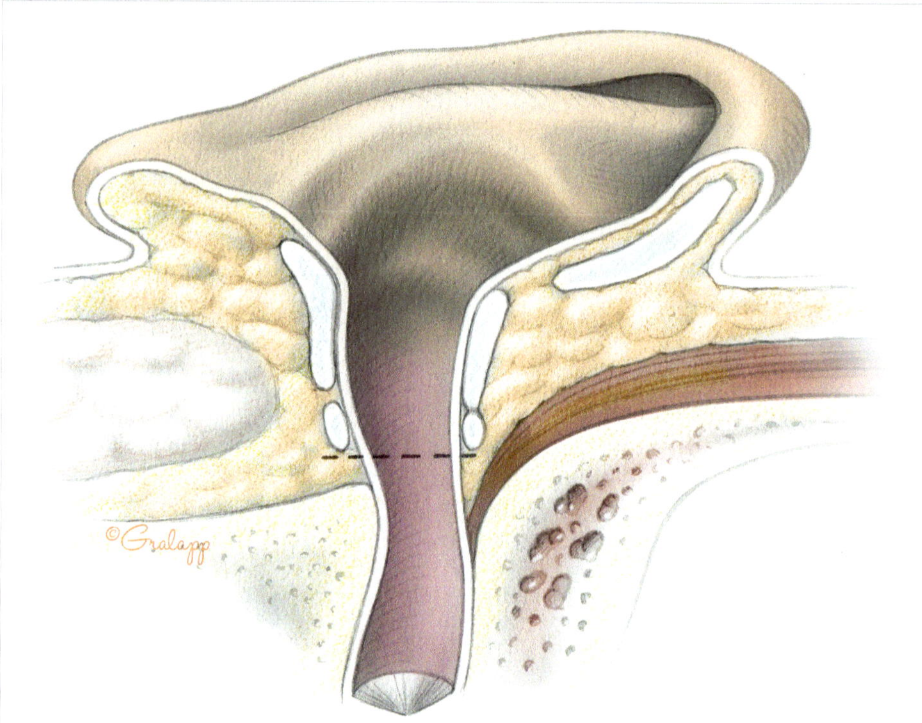

Fig. 12.35 The goal of ear canal closure during skull base surgery is to create a sealed cavity into which an adipose tissue graft or muscle flap can be placed. Prior to obliterating the surgical defect, all skin and as much mucous membrane as possible must be removed from the defect. When the dura has been violated, it is essential that the closure be watertight to avoid CSF leakage. This requires a multiple layer closure and meticulous technique. It is usually done in the early stages of the procedure, although it can be accomplished at any convenient stage. The ear canal is initially transected at the level of the bony cartilaginous junction as depicted here. For the technique of meatal closure employed in temporal bone resection for carcinoma of the ear canal, see 13.2 Lateral Temporal Bone Resection.

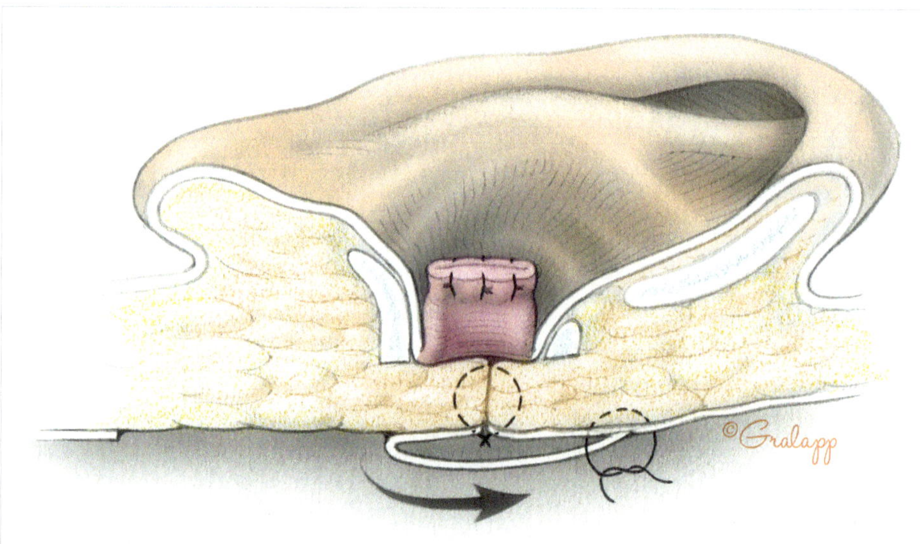

Fig. 12.36 Completed meatal closure involves three layers: the everted meatal skin, the intervening fibrous tissue, and an inner periosteal-fascial flap. Of the three, the middle layer is often least substantial.

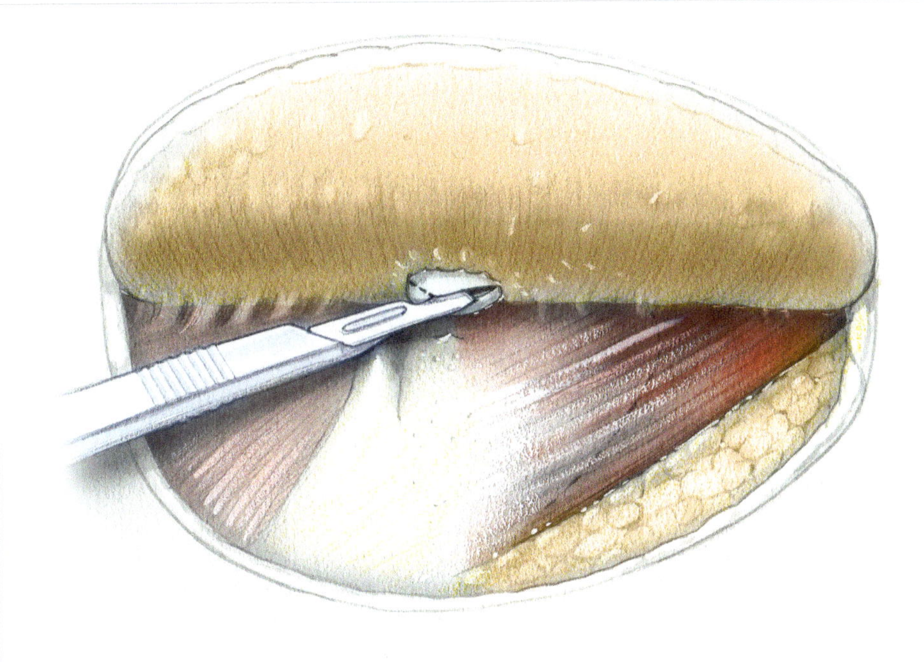

Fig. 12.37 The posterior aspect of the ear canal is transected sharply at the bony cartilaginous junction. As the canal possesses numerous small vessels, it is helpful to apply a line of bipolar cautery to the external (periosteal) surface before making this incision.

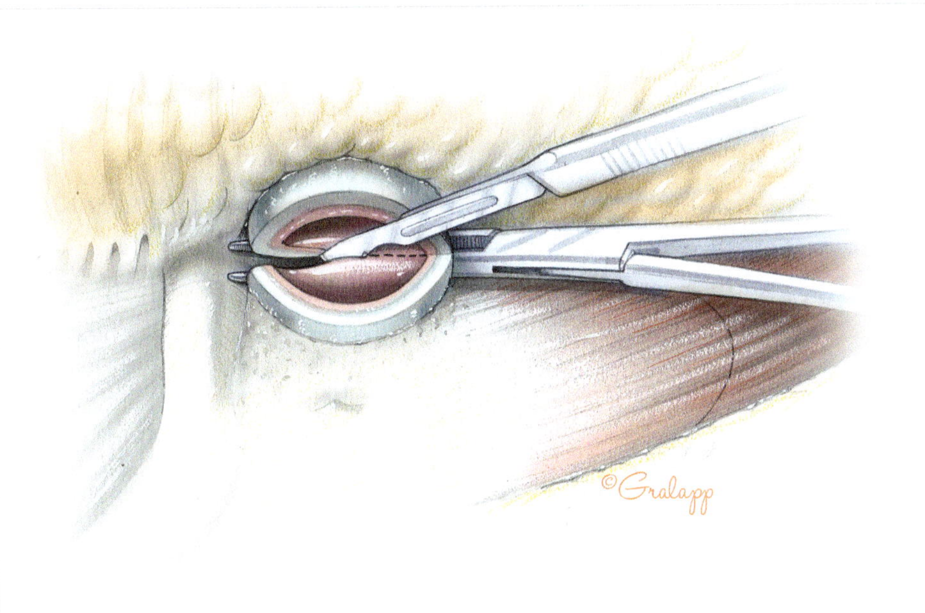

Fig. 12.38 Prior to transection of the anterior aspect of the cartilaginous ear canal, a clamp is insinuated between it and the parotid fascia. This maneuver reduces the likelihood of bothersome bleeding from the parotid gland, and thus speeds the procedure.

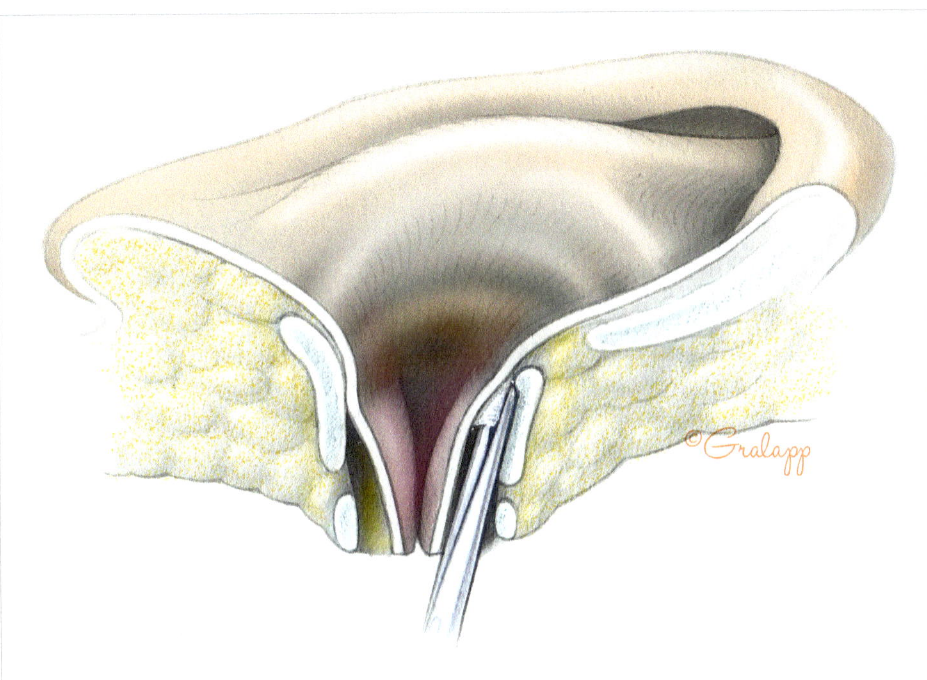

Fig. 12.39 The skin of the lateral portion of the ear canal is dissected from its underlying cartilage in retrograde fashion. When approaching the lateral margin of this elevation, care must be taken to avoid buttonholing the flap. This is unlikely to occur anteriorly as the tragus is long and broad and there is no need to dissect all the way to its free edge. Posteriorly, however, the canal skin abruptly drapes over the conchal margin where it is vulnerable. Keeping a finger in the meatus while dissecting from the postauricular side provides useful tactile feedback as to the remaining length of mobilization required.

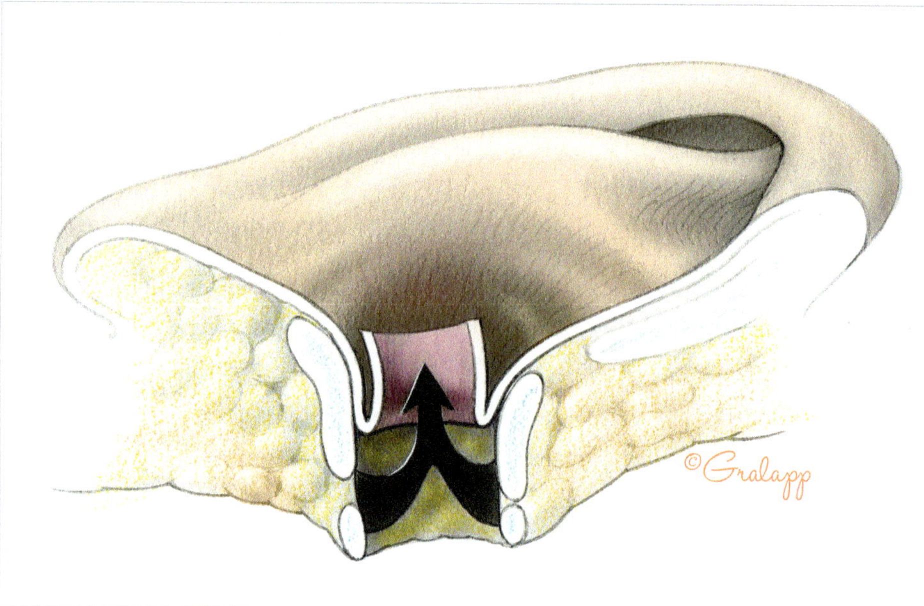

Fig. 12.40 The skin of the lateral portion of the ear canal is dissected from its underlying cartilage in retrograde fashion. When approaching the lateral margin of this elevation, care must be taken to avoid buttonholing the flap. This is unlikely to occur anteriorly as the tragus is long and broad and there is no need to dissect all the way to its free edge. Posteriorly, however, the canal skin abruptly drapes over the conchal margin where it is vulnerable. Keeping a finger in the meatus while dissecting from the postauricular side provides useful tactile feedback as to the remaining length of mobilization required.

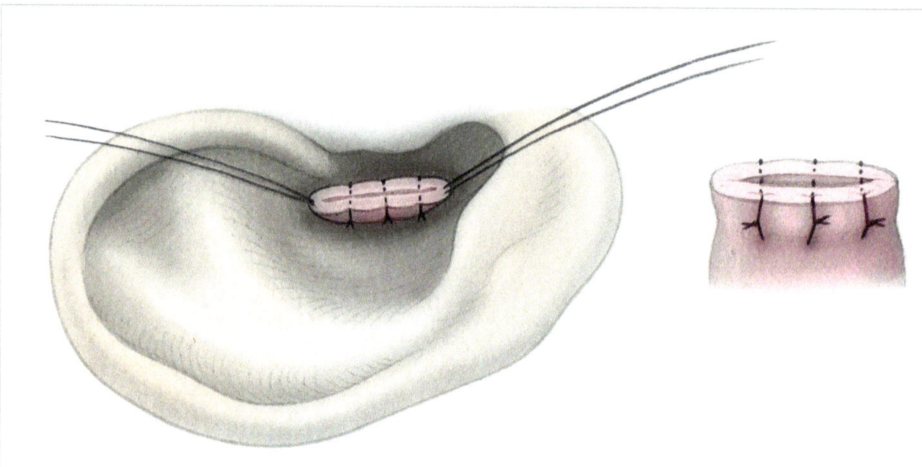

Fig. 12.41 While being stabilized with the traction sutures, a series of interrupted vertical mattress sutures are used to seal the meatus. The lower pass of these sutures is placed rather far down the skin cuff to help coapt the long sleeve of subcutaneous tissue. Once these sutures have been placed, the everted canal remains in place and the traction sutures can be removed or tied to serve as a subcutaneous closure at the extremity of the suture line.

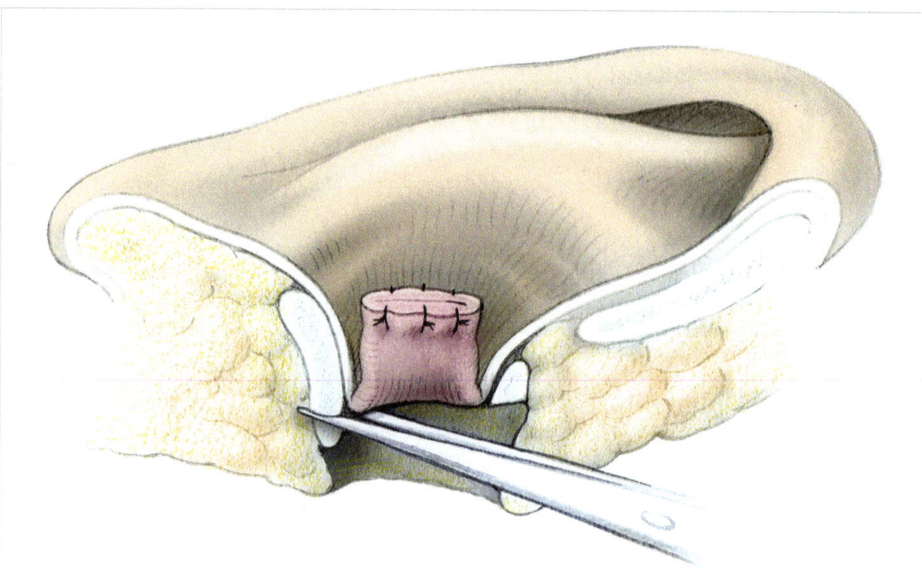

Fig. 12.42 Working from the postauricular side, the canal cartilage is removed or scored to break its spring. This facilitates coaptation of the submeatal soft tissues to serve as a second closure layer.

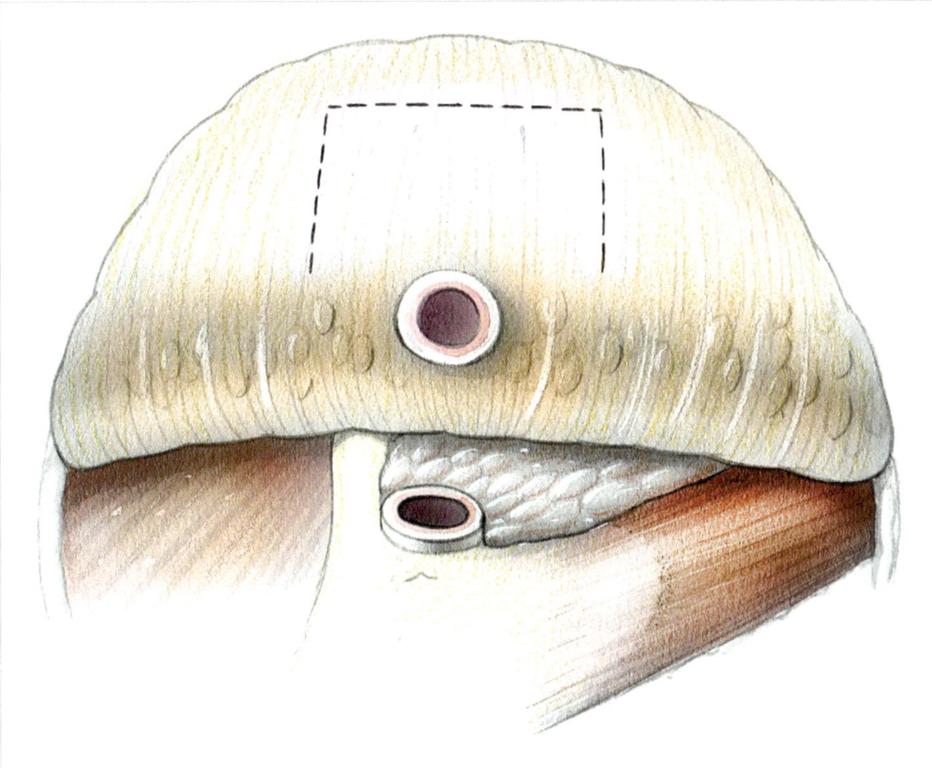

Fig. 12.43 A third layer of closure is developed from the pericranium and fascia of the undersurface of the flap. This can be designed in a number of ways (e.g., anteriorly based, inferiorly based) according to the nature of the tissue available.

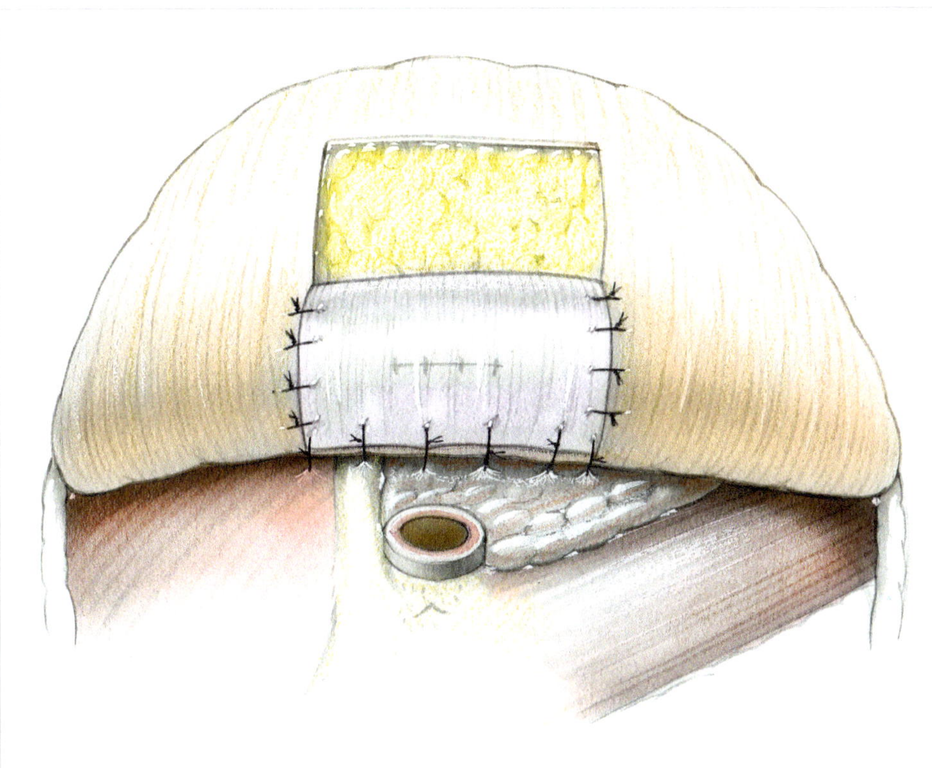

Fig. 12.44 The suture line anterior to the ear canal is anchored in the parotid fascia. As this layer has little strength, this line of sutures is laid in as a row and then tied gently by hand. During the rest of the procedure (tumor exposure and resection), care must be taken with the positioning of retractors so as not to disrupt this inner surface of the meatal closure.

13 Temporal Bone Resection

Robert K. Jackler

13.1 Introduction to Temporal Bone Resection

Resection of part of, or all of, the temporal bone is most commonly performed for squamous cell carcinoma arising from the ear canal or middle ear. Unlike similar tumors of the pinna, which arise from sun exposure, these tumors most often occur in the setting of chronic inflammation. These lesions have a tendency to penetrate the cranial base and can become lethal. With aggressive surgical resection followed by radiation, high rates of cure can be realized.

Tumors limited to the ear canal and adjacent structures are managed by lateral temporal bone resection with *en bloc* removal of the ear canal. When extension warrants, the parotid, temporomandibular joint, infratemporal fossa contents, and neck nodes may need to be removed as well. The so-called total temporal bone resection is a misnomer. A true total resection of the temporal bone would require sacrifice of the carotid, jugular bulb, and cranial nerves VII, IX, X, and XI—a morbidity that is seldom justifiable. When a squamous cell malignancy has invaded the medial wall of the middle ear, most ear surgeons remove the lateral segment *en bloc* and then drill away the medial temporal bone and petrous apex, removing the inner ear, and skeletonizing the great vessels.

Some surgeons leave resection cavities open following temporal bone resection arguing that it may heal as an open mastoidectomy cavity and thus may help preserve healing. As the cochlea will receive a full therapeutic dose of radiation (approximately 70 Gy), long-term preservation of auditory function is unlikely. Importantly, leaving the cavity open delays healing and thus the onset of radiation therapy. It also creates exposed bone in the mastoid and middle ear and greatly increases the risk of osteoradionecrosis. To accelerate healing, it is preferable to swing in a vascularized muscle flap such as suturing a split temporalis muscle flap to the sternocleidomastoid muscle.

Further Reading

1. Allanson BM, Low TH, Clark JR, Gupta R. Squamous cell carcinoma of the external auditory canal and temporal bone: an update. Head Neck Pathol 2018;12(3):407–418 PubMed
2. Beyea JA, Moberly AC. Squamous cell carcinoma of the temporal bone. Otolaryngol Clin North Am 2015;48(2):281–292 PubMed
3. Chen J, Lin F, Liu Z, Yu Y, Wang Y. Pedicled temporalis muscle flap stuffing after a lateral temporal bone resection for treating mastoid osteoradionecrosis. Otolaryngol Head Neck Surg 2017;156(4):622–626 PubMed
4. Komune N, Komune S, Morishita T, Rhoton AL Jr. Microsurgical anatomy of subtotal temporal bone resection en bloc with the parotid gland and temporomandibular joint. Neurosurgery 2014;10(Suppl 2):334–356, discussion 356 PubMed
5. Kutz JW Jr, Mitchell D, Isaacson B, et al. En bloc resection of the temporal bone and temporomandibular joint for advanced temporal bone carcinoma. Otolaryngol Head Neck Surg 2015;152(3):571–573 PubMed
6. Lassig AA, Spector ME, Soliman S, El-Kashlan HK. Squamous cell carcinoma involving the temporal bone: lateral temporal bone resection as primary intervention. Otol Neurotol 2013;34(1):141–150 PubMed
7. Sinha S, Dedmon MM, Naunheim MR, Fuller JC, Gray ST, Lin DT. Update on surgical outcomes of lateral temporal bone resection for ear and temporal bone malignancies. J Neurol Surg B Skull Base 2017;78(1):37–42 PubMed
8. Yuhan BT, Nguyen BK, Svider PF, et al. Osteoradionecrosis of the temporal bone: an evidence-based approach. Otol Neurotol 2018;39(9):1172–1183 PubMed

13.2 Lateral Temporal Bone Resection

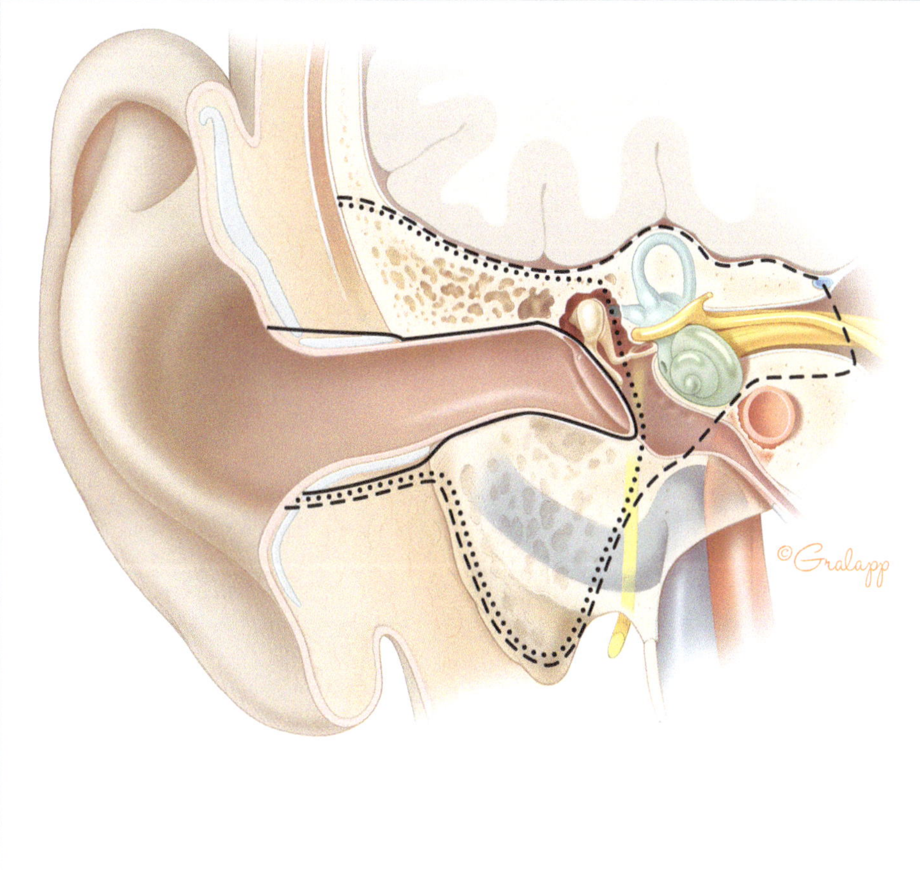

Fig. 13.1 Temporal bone resection for malignancy encompasses three related procedures of progressively increasing depth: sleeve resection of the external auditory canal (*solid line*), lateral temporal bone resection (*dotted line*), and total temporal bone resection (*dashed line*). The illustration depicts these procedures in the coronal view. Most of these resections are performed for squamous cell carcinoma arising from the external auditory canal. It is generally acknowledged that sleeve resection is an insufficient therapy for malignant disease. In the lateral temporal bone resection, the ear canal is removed *en bloc* with the tympanic membrane and lateral ossicles. A parotidectomy and/or neck dissection often supplements the temporal bone specimen. In total temporal bone resection, creation of an *en bloc* specimen is difficult and probably unnecessary. It requires an extensive dissection of the intrapetrous carotid artery, a measure usually of little benefit in deeply invasive squamous cell carcinoma. Most contemporary otologists perform the so-called total temporal bone resection by first carrying out a lateral temporal bone resection and then removing the medial petrous bone piecemeal with a drill. This procedure is indicated for deep extension which penetrates beyond the medial wall of the middle ear and/or mastoid.

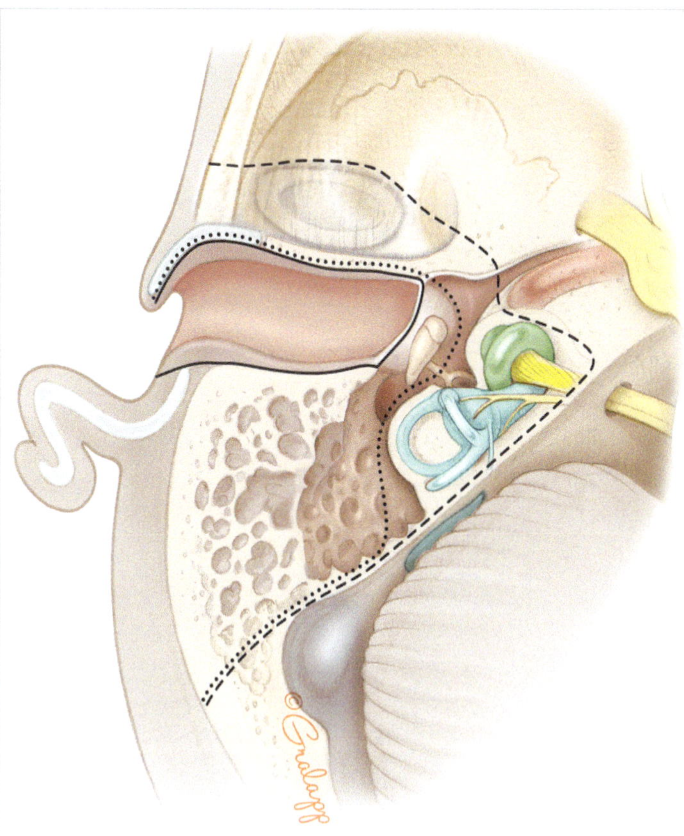

Fig. 13.2 Axial view of the three types of temporal bone resection for malignancy: sleeve resection of the external auditory canal (*solid line*), lateral temporal bone resection (*dotted line*), total temporal bone resection (*dashed line*).

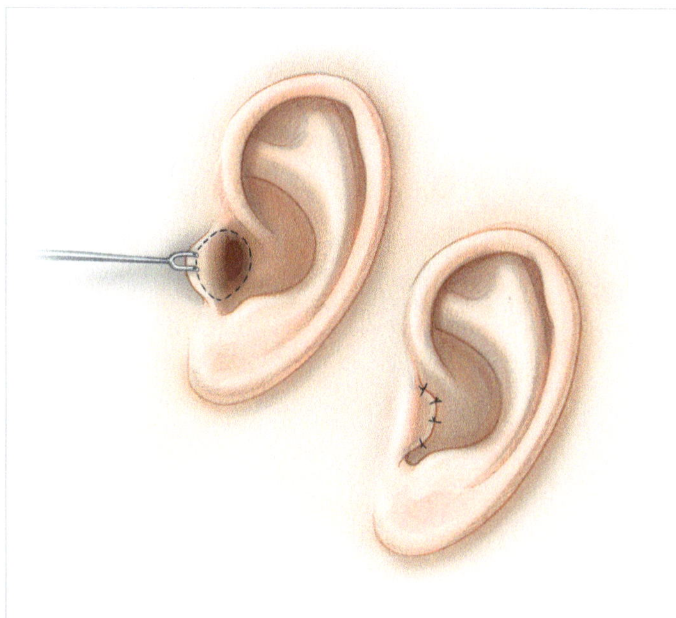

Fig. 13.3 At the beginning of the temporal bone resection for ear canal malignancy, the ear canal is transected and the meatus sutured closed. The lateral margin is sent for frozen section. Note that the technique employed is different from that used during skull base surgery (see 12.5 Ear Canal Closure). Simply sewing the tragal skin to the conchal margin permits resection of the skin of the entire ear canal. To break the spring of the conchal cartilage, it is crosshatched with a scalpel.

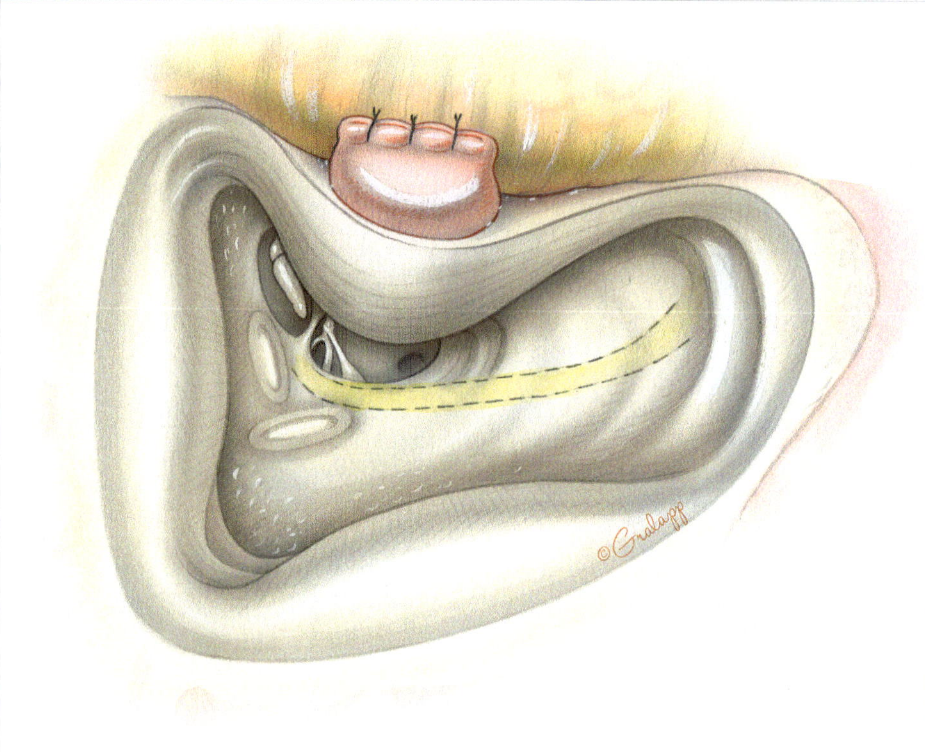

Fig. 13.4 After transection of the cartilaginous canal just medial to the meatus, a ring of skin and cartilage is harvested from the specimen side and sent for frozen section analysis. If tumor is seen in the specimen (uncommon), then further resection of the meatus and pinna is performed as necessary. To discourage spillage of tumor cells, the meatus is sewn shut. An intact canal wall mastoidectomy is then performed with opening of the facial recess (for technique, see 7.5 Facial Recess Approach). FR, facial recess.

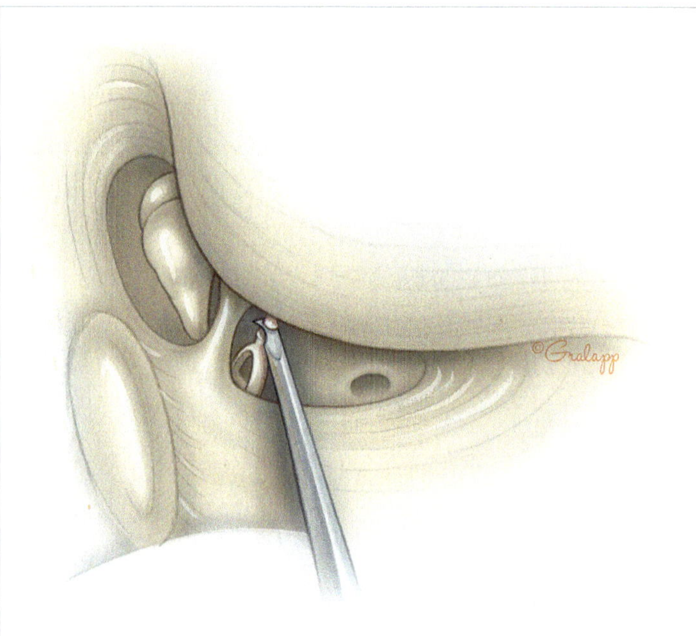

Fig. 13.5 Working via the facial recess, the incudostapedial joint is severed sharply. A disposable myringotomy knife is a convenient tool for accomplishing this maneuver.

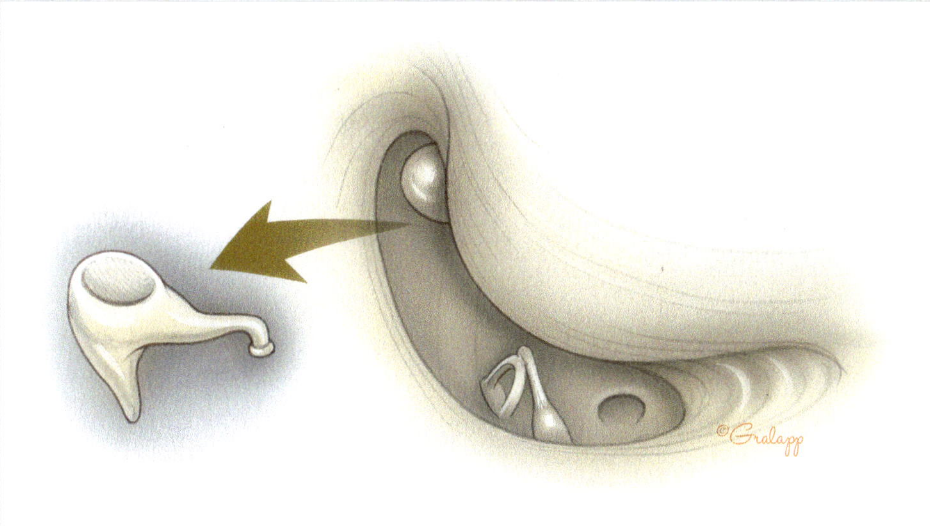

Fig. 13.6 The bone bridge separating the epitympanum from the facial recess is then drilled away and the incus is removed. The tensor tympani muscle also needs to be transected (not shown here).

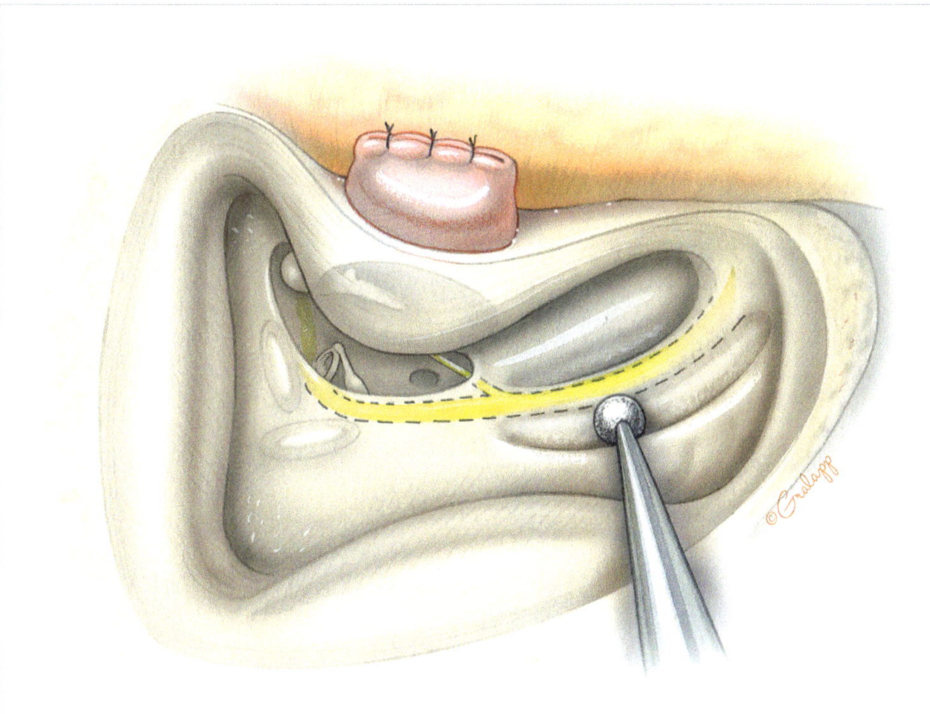

Fig. 13.7 The descending portion of the fallopian canal is then skeletonized, leaving a thin bony covering. Identification of the position of the facial nerve is important for the next step during which the facial recess opening is then extended inferiorly into the hypotympanum.

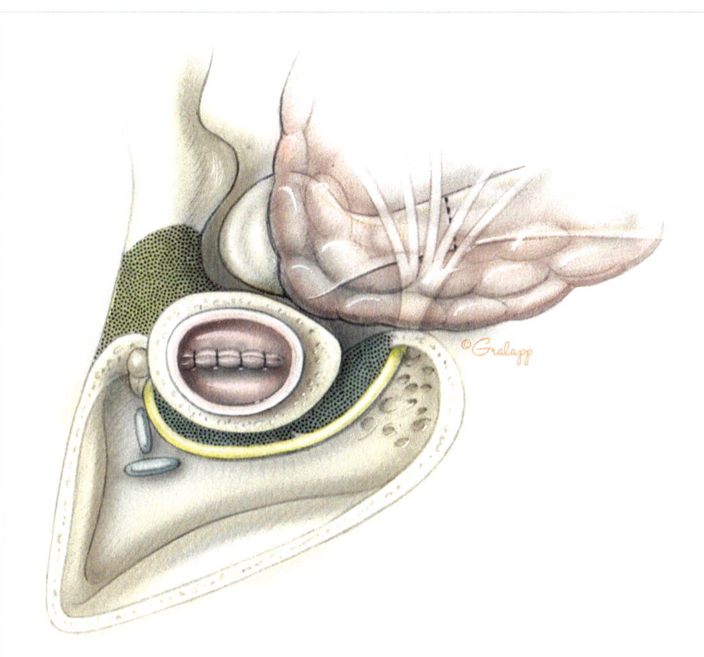

Fig. 13.8 To isolate the ear canal as an *en bloc* specimen, bone must be removed from 360 degrees around the canal (*green stippled area*). An extended facial recess approach is connected to the posterior and inferior aspects of the middle ear. The anterior wall of the mastoid is removed between the inferior margin of the osseous ear canal and the stylomastoid foramen. Superiorly, the root of the zygoma and the posterior aspect of the glenoid fossa are removed (*yellow stippled area*).

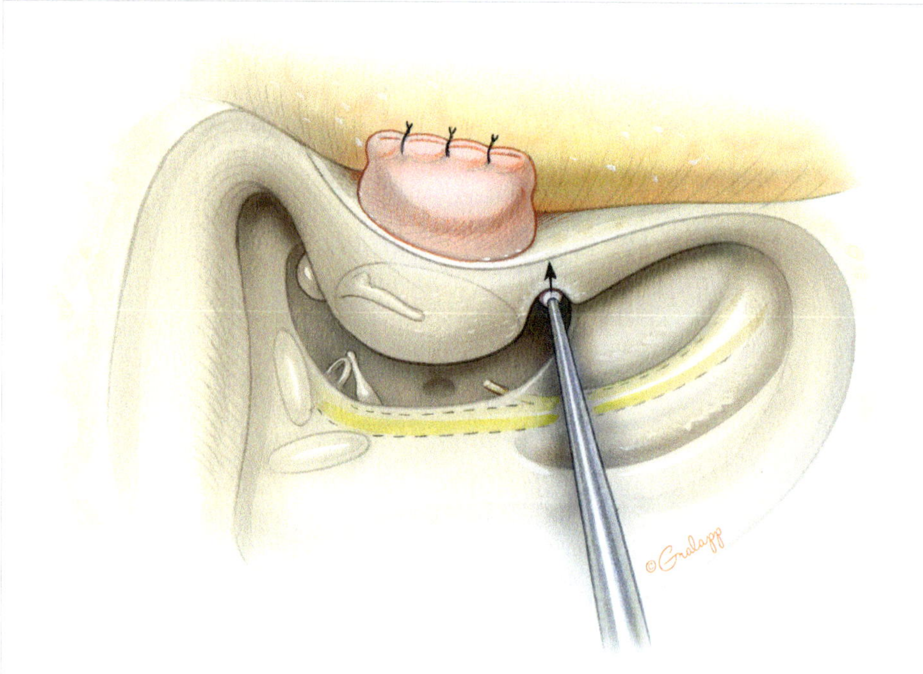

Fig. 13.9 While connecting the facial recess into the hypotympanum, the chorda tympani nerve is sharply transected. Care must be taken while working in this narrow interval to avoid injury to the descending facial nerve with the shaft of the drill. A cut is then made parallel to the bony ear canal through the front face of the mastoid.

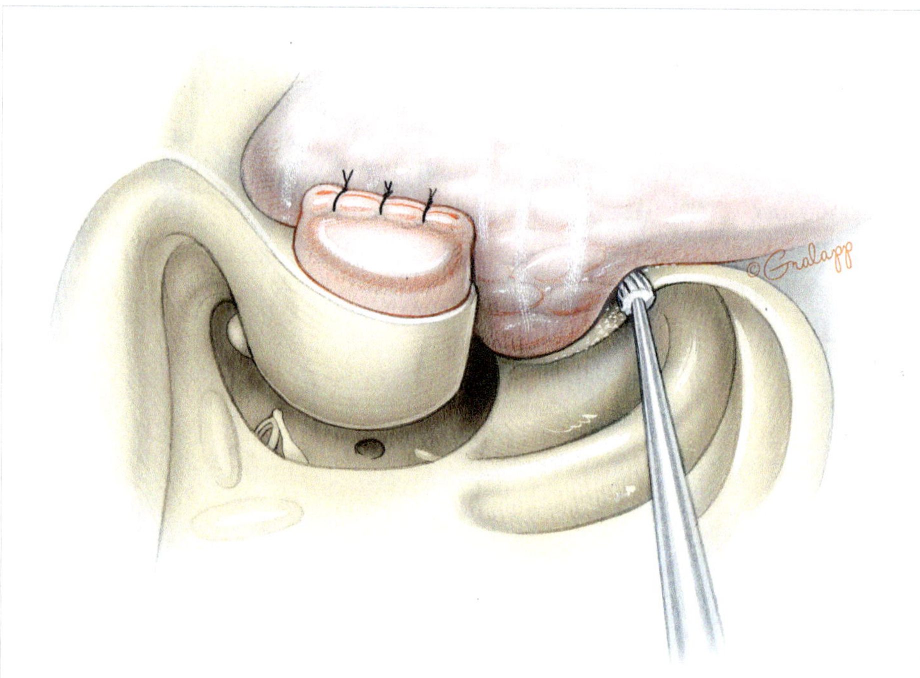

Fig. 13.10 The remainder of the anterior face of the mastoid is removed down to the level of the stylomastoid foramen.

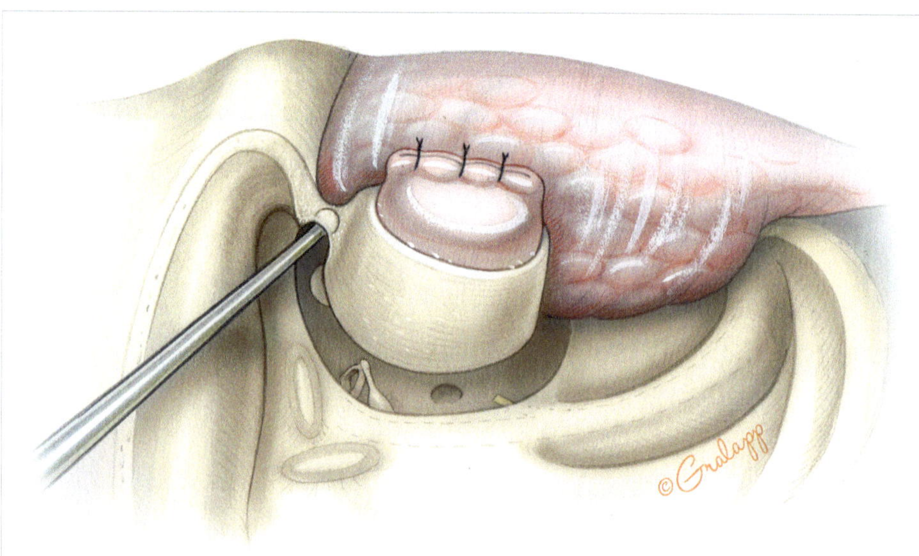

Fig. 13.11 Working between the floor of the middle cranial fossa and the roof of the ear canal, the root of the zygoma is drilled away. It is necessary to continue drilling until the anterior epitympanum has been opened into the glenoid fossa.

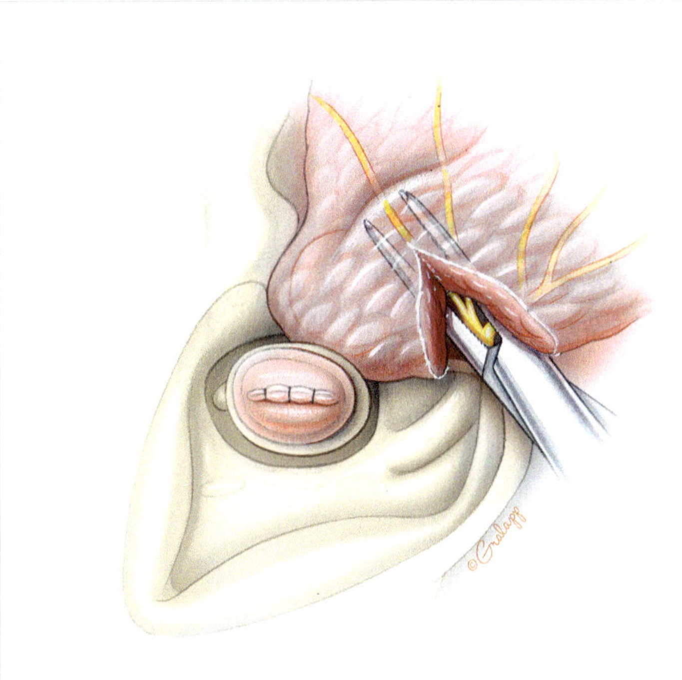

Fig. 13.12 When the anterior aspect of the ear canal is involved by tumor, it is often appropriate to remove a cuff of tissue anteriorly. This includes part or all of the parotid gland and the tissue which resides between the ear canal and mandibular condyle. Parotidectomy is commenced by identification of the facial nerve as it exits the stylomastoid foramen. In the absence of gross tumor involvement of the parotid region, then only the portion of the gland which abuts the ear canal needs to be removed. In such cases, only the part of the parotid which lies posterior to the upper branch of the facial nerve must be included with the specimen.

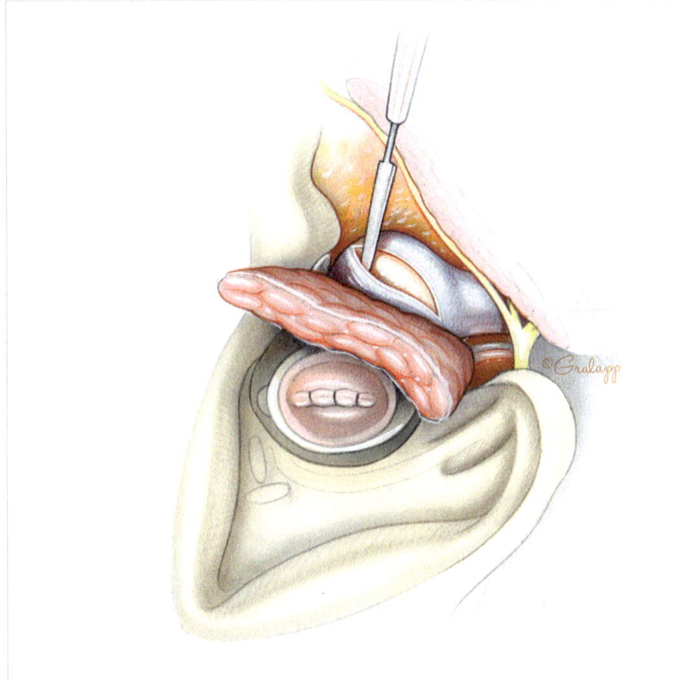

Fig. 13.13 Once the parotid has been reflected posteriorly, the mandibular condyle is addressed. There are three options for handling the condyle: taking only its capsule, partial resection, and complete resection. When leaving the condyle in situ, an incision is made in its capsule with cutting electrocautery.

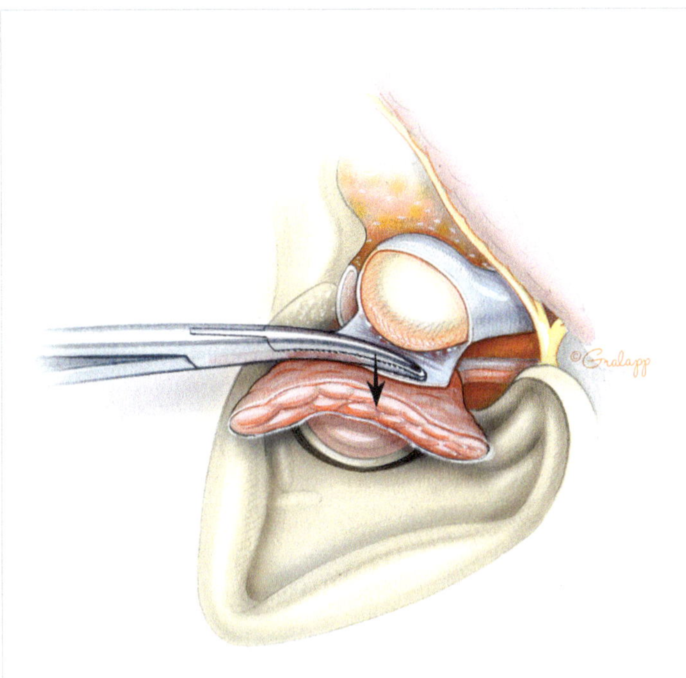

Fig. 13.14 The capsule is then dissected off the condylar head.

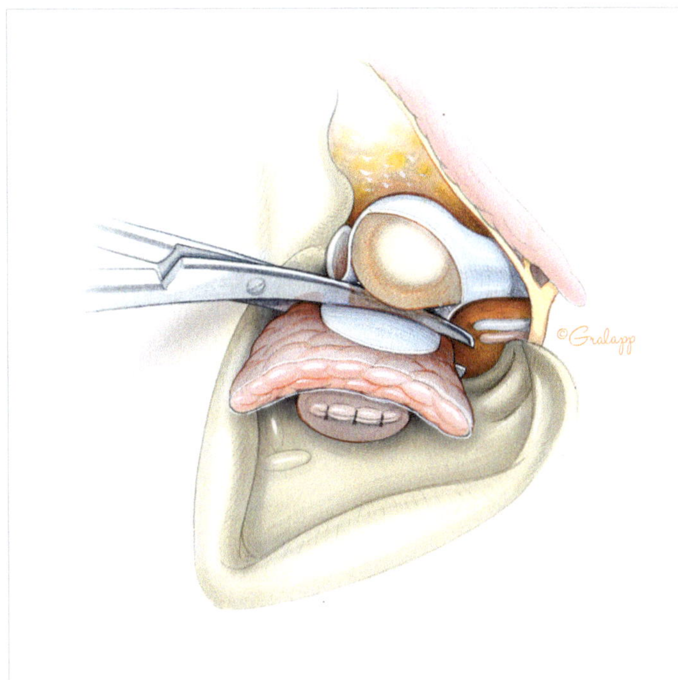

Fig. 13.15 The leathery condylar capsule is transected on the deep side with Mayo scissors. The superficial temporal artery and vein need to be controlled at this point.

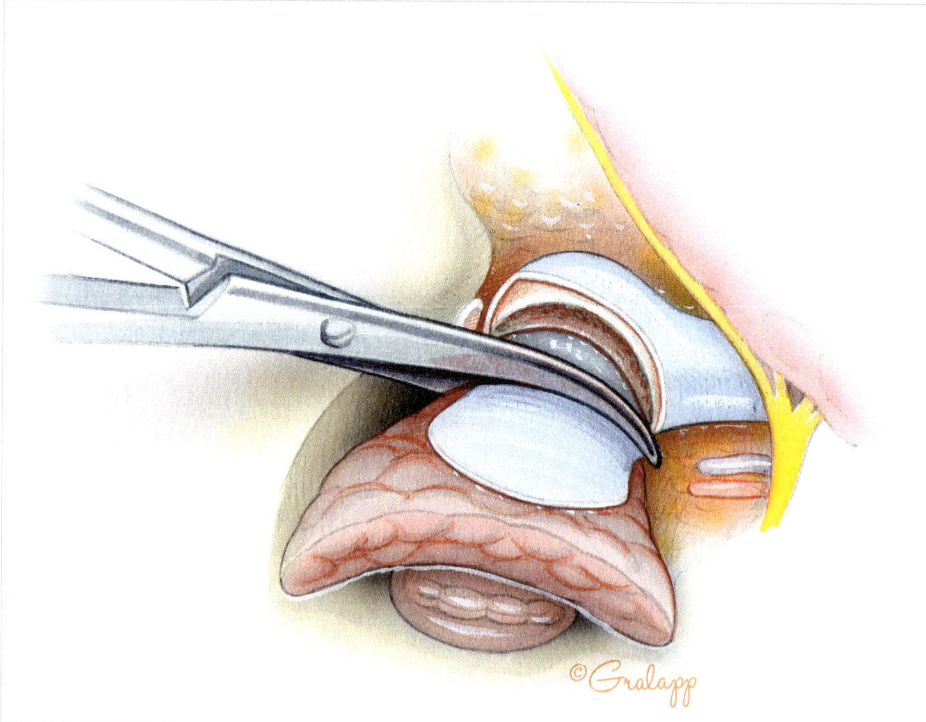

Fig. 13.16 Partial condylectomy can be accomplished with a drill, leaving intact a portion of the articular face of the joint. This maneuver facilitates removal of a wider cuff of soft tissue anterior to the deep portion of the ear canal. Complete condylectomy is accomplished by treading a Gigli saw around the condylar neck. While isolating the condylar neck, care must be taken to avoid injury to the internal maxillary artery.

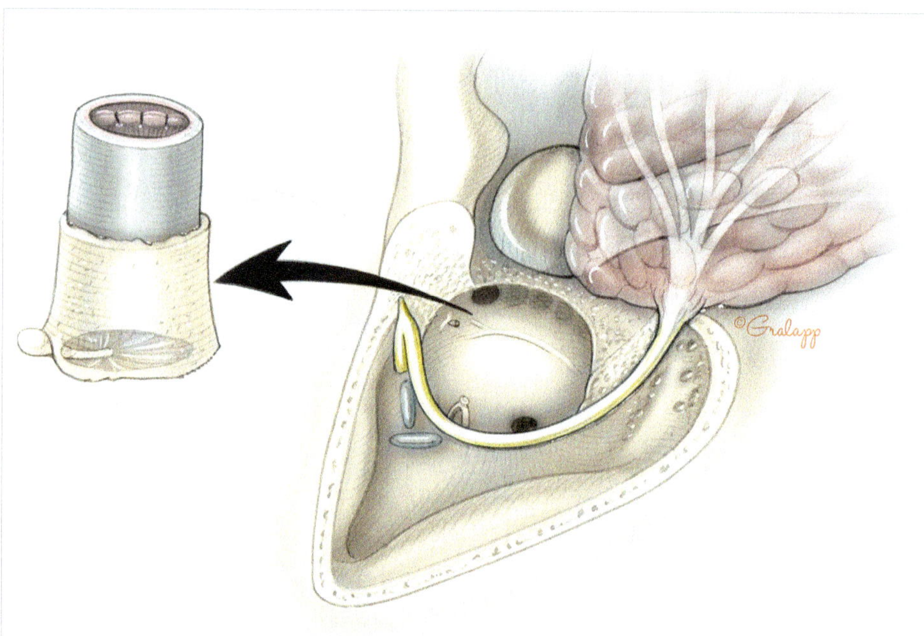

Fig. 13.17 The specimen in a lateral temporal bone resection includes both the cartilaginous and osseous ear canal as well as the tympanic membrane with malleus attached.

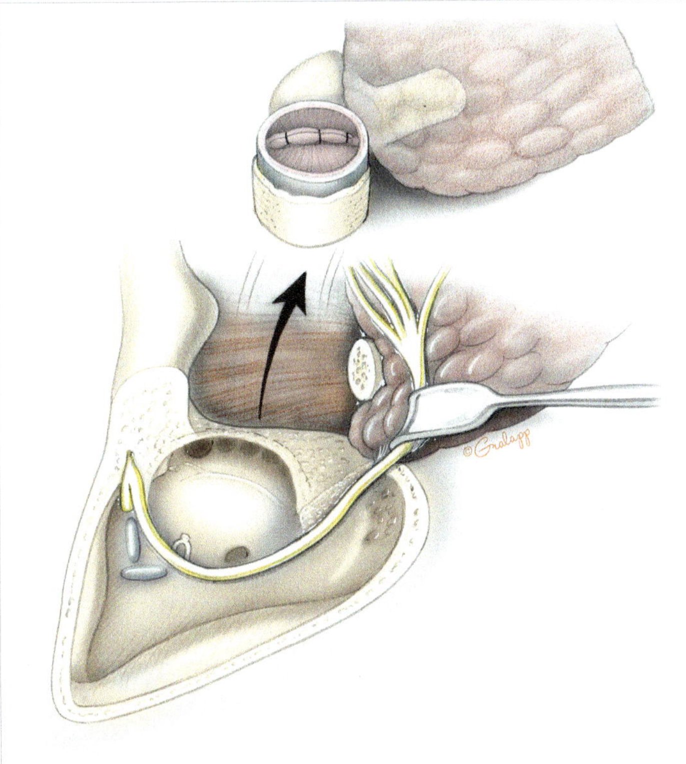

Fig. 13.18 Lateral temporal bone resection may include a resection of the parotid and condylar head in continuity with the ear canal.

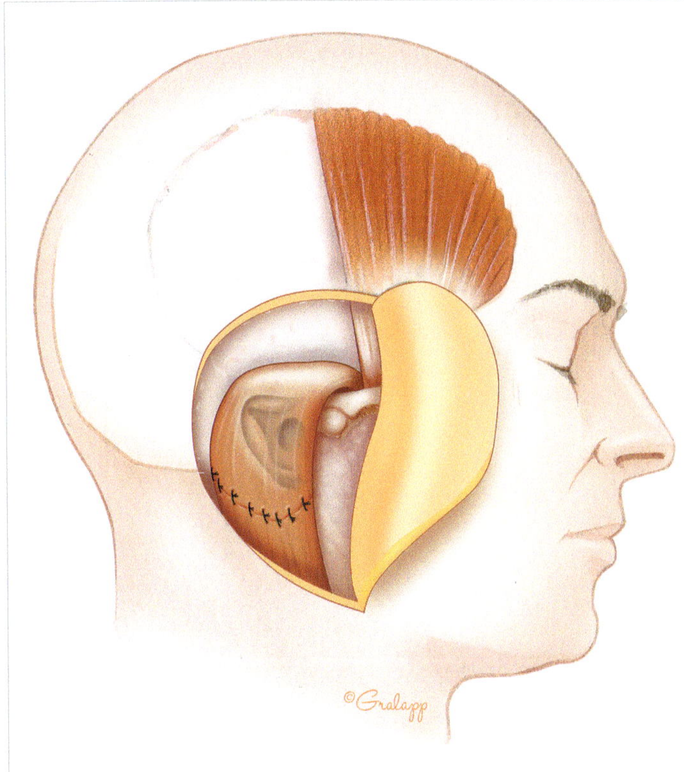

Fig. 13.19 To foster rapid healing in preparation for radiotherapy, the posterior half of the temporalis muscle can be rotated as a flap. Securing the flap to the sternocleidomastoid muscle is a very effective means of setting the flap into position. Leaving the cavity open predisposes to the development of osteoradionecrosis. Hearing is unlikely to be rehabilitated in an ear that is to be subjected to radiation at the level of 60 to 70 Gy.

13.3 Extended Temporal Bone Resection

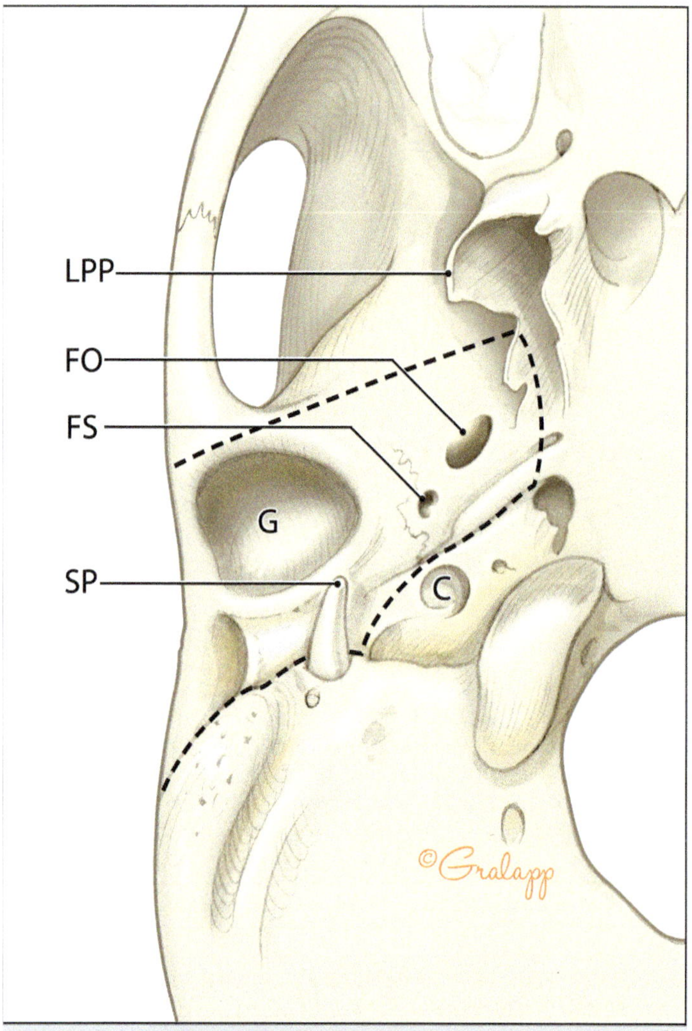

Fig. 13.20 Osseous anatomy of the lateral skull base as seen from below illustrating the resection limits of the infratemporal fossa extension of temporal bone resection (*dotted line*). LPP, lateral pterygoid process; FO, foramen ovale; FS, foramen spinosum; G, glenoid fossa; SP, styloid process; C, carotid canal.

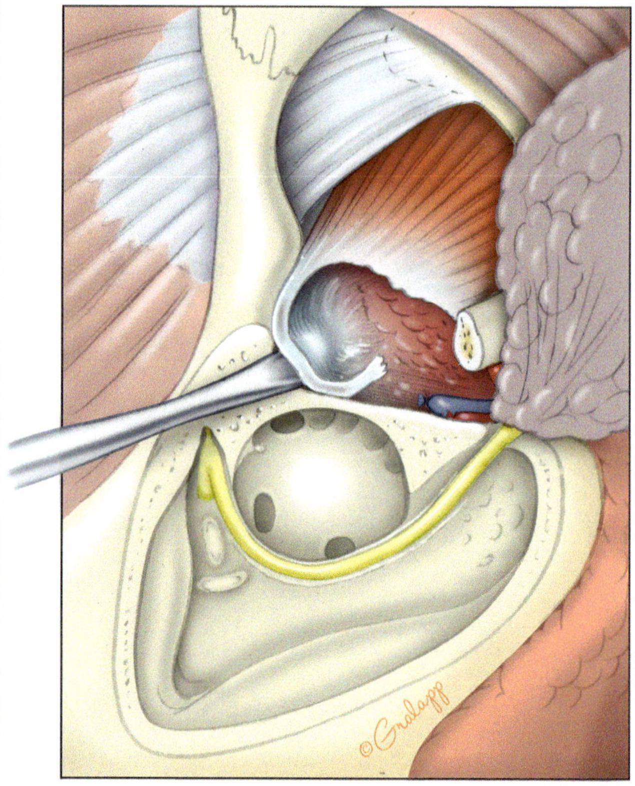

Fig. 13.21 Following removal of the *en bloc* lateral temporal bone specimen including resection of the mandibular condyle, the TMJ capsule is dissected off of the glenoid fossa. TM, temporalis muscle; LP, lateral pterygoid muscle.

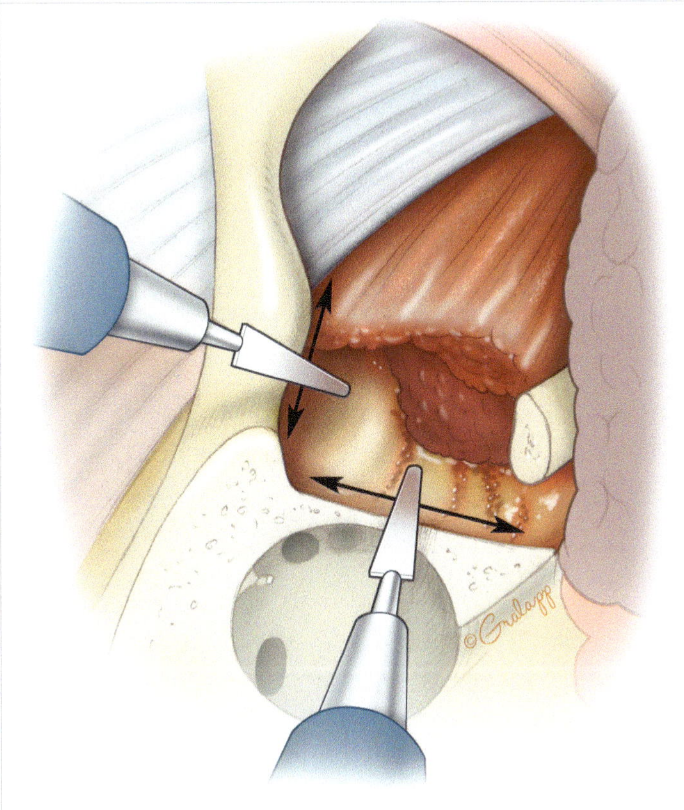

Fig. 13.22 Ear canal squamous cell carcinoma which has penetrated anteriorly beyond the confines of the ear canal may spread medially along the anterior face of the temporal bone. Electrocautery can be used to dissect muscles and ligaments from the anterior surface of the temporal bone and temporal floor.

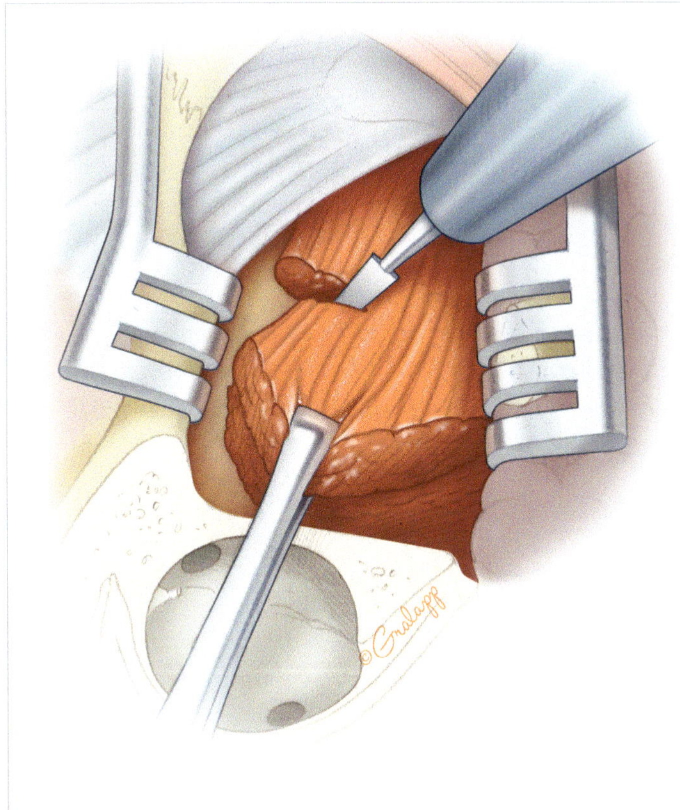

Fig. 13.23 The pterygoid muscle mass is sequentially resected.

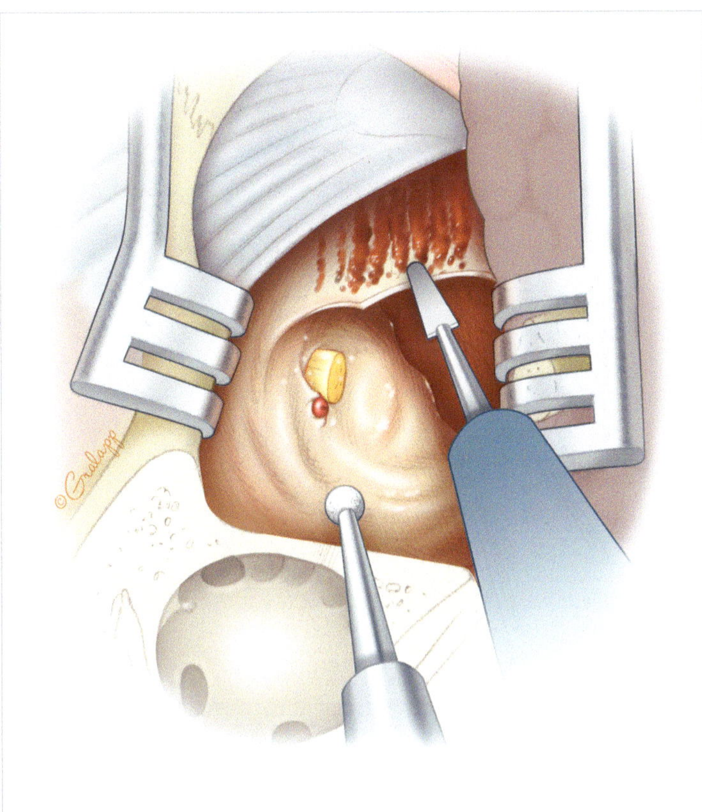

Fig. 13.24 Resection of pterygoid muscle is completed to the level of the lateral pterygoid plate. A diamond burr is used to excavate a bony margin on the anterior surface of the petrous bone. The middle meningeal artery and third division of the trigeminal nerve lie transected where they traverse the middle fossa floor.

14 Petrous Apex

Robert K. Jackler

14.1 Introduction to the Petrous Apex

The petrous apex is the medial portion of the petrous ridge situated between the inner ear and the clivus. In its base lies foramen lacerum traversed by the internal carotid artery. Above lies Meckel's cave and the fifth nerve as well as the sixth nerve in Dorello's canal. In most patients, the petrous apex is filled with marrow with, at most, a small amount of pneumatization. In less than 10% of adults, the petrous apex is extensively pneumatized. A word to clarify the nomenclature of petrous apex surgical approaches is needed. The term "*petrous apicectomy*" which implies removal of the petrous apex is often inappropriately used to describe drainage procedures which more accurately should be referred to as "*petrous apicotomy*."

The most common petrous apex lesion is fluid in a well-pneumatized petrous apex which is confined to the air cell tracts without osseous erosion. This entity should almost always be followed medically as one would for a maxillary antral inclusion cyst. The most common surgical petrous apex lesion is cholesterol granuloma, an expansile, destructive lesion driven by persistent blood seepage into mucosal spaces from adjacent richly vascularized bone marrow. Eroding laterally, cholesterol granulomas may invade the inner ear with resultant hearing loss and vertigo. Eroding superiorly, they cause diplopia due to pressure on the abducens nerve in Dorello's canal and facial sensory disturbance due to pressure on the fifth nerve due to erosion of the floor of Meckel's cave. The surgical treatment of petrous apex cholesterol granuloma is by establishing a drainage tract into the middle ear. The hypotympanic, infracochlear route is most direct when the anatomy is favorable. An alternative route, which is deeper, narrower, and more technically challenging, is the infralabyrinthine pathway between the posterior semicircular canal, descending facial nerve, and jugular bulb. When the anatomy is favorable, transsphenoidal drainage may also be feasible. When drainage laterally into the middle ear or medially into the sphenoid is not anatomically feasible, or drainage procedures have failed to adequately alleviate symptoms, resection of the granuloma via an extradural middle fossa craniotomy may be considered. In this procedure, care must be taken to avoid injury to the carotid artery, as its bony wall is often eroded.

Two forms of infection may involve the petrous apex. Most common in the antibiotic era is otogenic skull base osteomyelitis. This aggressive infection is most often caused by pseudomonas in elderly diabetics or fungus (e.g., *Aspergillus fumigatus*) in immunocompromised patients. Skull base osteomyelitis propagates through marrow rather than air cells. It is generally a nonsurgical disease except when sequestration has occurred or when tissue is needed to establish the causative organism. Petrous apicitis, by contrast, is infection within the air cells of a pneumatized apex. Apical infection may cause a syndrome of ear pain and discharge, diplopia, and retro-orbital pain often referred to eponymically as Gradenigo's syndrome. Drainage of apicitis is via petrous apicotomy which may be conducted via numerous pathways including those above, below, or through (e.g., traversing the superior semicircular canal loop) the labyrinth or beneath the cochlea. The general rule is to *"follow the pus"* preferably using small curettes, which better respect the integrity of the otic capsule than high-speed drills.

The most common primary tumor of the petrous apex is chondrosarcoma arising from foramen lacerum at the petroclival junction. Secondary tumors include metastases, especially involving prostate and breast cancers. Arachnoid cyst descending from Meckel's cave is an uncommon petrous apex lesion.

Further Reading

1. Chole RA. Petrous apicitis: surgical anatomy. Ann Otol Rhinol Laryngol 1985;94(3):251–257 PubMed
2. Cristobal R, Oghalai JS. Peripetrosal arachnoid cysts. Curr Opin Otolaryngol Head Neck Surg 2007;15(5):323–329 PubMed
3. Dhanasekar G, Jones NS. Endoscopic trans-sphenoidal removal of cholesterol granuloma of the petrous apex: case report and literature review. J Laryngol Otol 2011;125 (2):169–172 PubMed
4. Fournier HD, Mercier P, Roche PH. Surgical anatomy of the petrous apex and petroclival region. Adv Tech Stand Neurosurg 2007;32:91–146 PubMed
5. Isaacson B. Cholesterol granuloma and other petrous apex lesions. Otolaryngol Clin North Am 2015;48(2):361–373 PubMed
6. Jackler RK, Cho M. A new theory to explain the genesis of petrous apex cholesterol granuloma. Otol Neurotol 2003;24 (1):96–106, discussion 106 PubMed
7. Lee DH, Kim MJ, Lee S, Choi H. Anatomical factors influencing pneumatization of the petrous apex. Clin Exp Otorhinolaryngol 2015;8(4):339–344 PubMed
8. Sanna M, Dispenza F, Mathur N, De Stefano A, De Donato G. Otoneurological management of petrous apex cholesterol granuloma. Am J Otolaryngol 2009;30(6):407–414 PubMed
9. Shoman N, Donaldson AM, Ksiazek J, Pensak ML, Zimmer LA. First stage in predicative measure for transnasal transsphenoidal approach to petrous apex cholesterol granuloma. Laryngoscope 2013;123(3):581–583 PubMed
10. Sweeney AD, Osetinsky LM, Carlson ML, et al. The natural history and management of petrous apex cholesterol granulomas. Otol Neurotol 2015;36(10):1714–1719 PubMed
11. Taklalsingh N, Falcone F, Velayudhan V. Gradenigo's syndrome in a patient with chronic suppurative otitis media, petrous apicitis, and meningitis. Am J Case Rep 2017;18:1039–1043 PubMed
12. Wick CC, Hansen AR, Kutz JW Jr, Isaacson B. Endoscopic infracochlear approach for drainage of petrous apex cholesterol granulomas: a case series. Otol Neurotol 2017;38(6):876–881 PubMed

14.2 Petrous Apicotomy

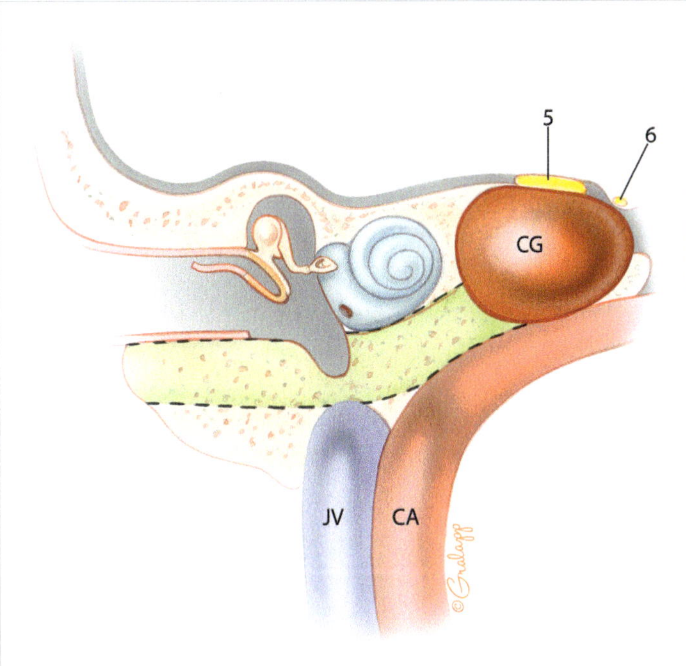

Fig. 14.1 The petrous apex is the medial portion of the petrous bone that lies between the inner ear and the clivus. Petrous "apicectomy" is the term commonly applied to a procedure which reaches the apical portion of the petrous bone by skirting around the inner ear. It is inherently a drainage procedure which creates only a relatively small entry into the apical region. Thus, the commonly used term petrous "apicectomy" is a misnomer when used in this context. Petrous *apicotomy* would actually be a more accurate description for the procedure. Petrous apicotomy is primarily indicated for drainage of cholesterol granuloma and purulent infections. Fundamentally, there are two routes used to reach the petrous apex: those which pass near the labyrinth and those which skirt the cochlea. In recent years, the hypotympanic–subcochlear route depicted here has become the most popular. The bone removed during this procedure is depicted in this schematic coronal illustration as the color green. Note the relationship of the apical cholesterol granuloma to the fifth and sixth nerves. This explains the frequent occurrence of deep ear and retro-orbital pain as well as diplopia in these lesions. JV, jugular vein; CA, carotid artery; CG, cholesterol granuloma; 5, trigeminal nerve; 6, abducens nerve.

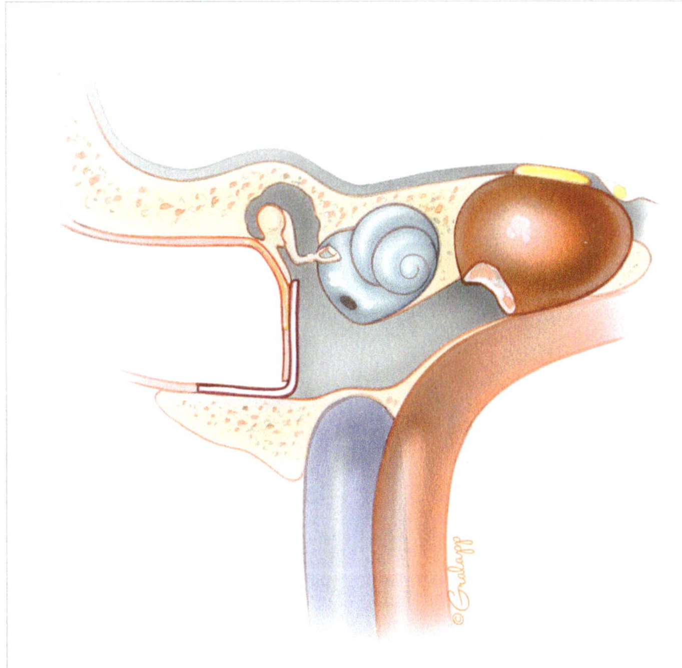

Fig. 14.2 Coronal schematic view of the bone removed during the hypotympanic-subcochlear approach to the petrous apex. Note that the floor of the ear canal and hypotympanum has been removed to the level of the jugular bulb. Superiorly, the opening is bounded by the cochlea. More medially, the opening courses over the genu of the carotid artery. As shown here, the hypotympanic defect is enclosed with a fascia graft, resulting in a larger than normal tympanic membrane.

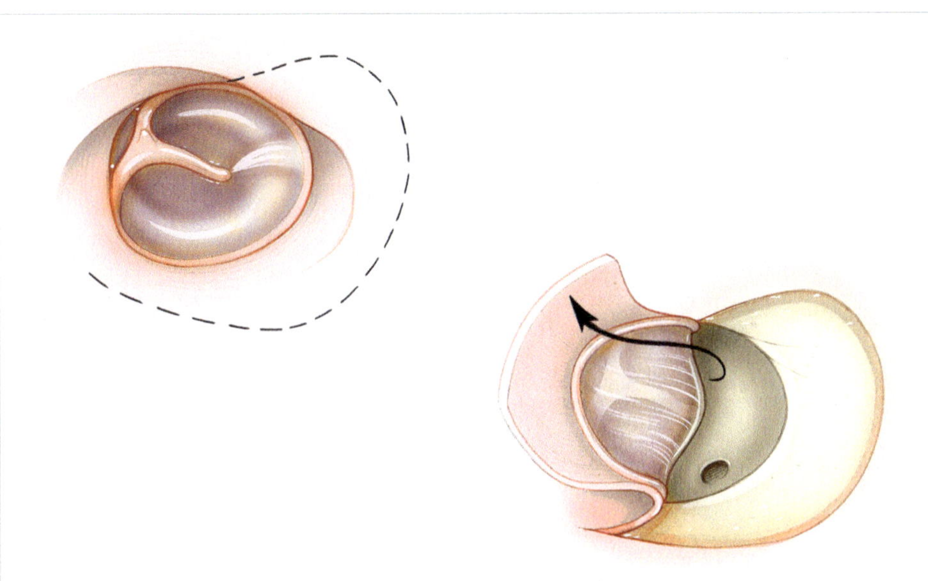

Fig. 14.3 The superiorly based tympanomeatal flap employed in the subcochlear approach to the petrous apex is designed to provide wide exposure of the hypotympanic region.

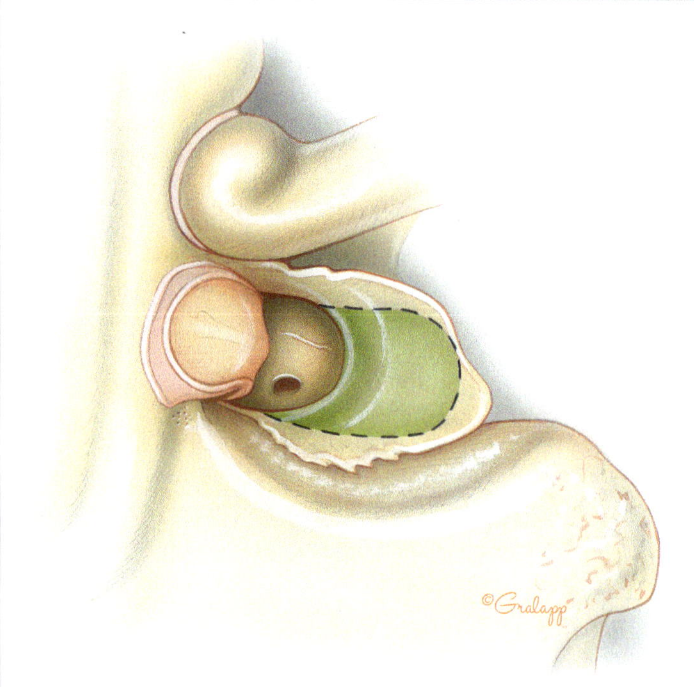

Fig. 14.4 The tympanic bone showing the bone removed (*green*) on route to the petrous apex.

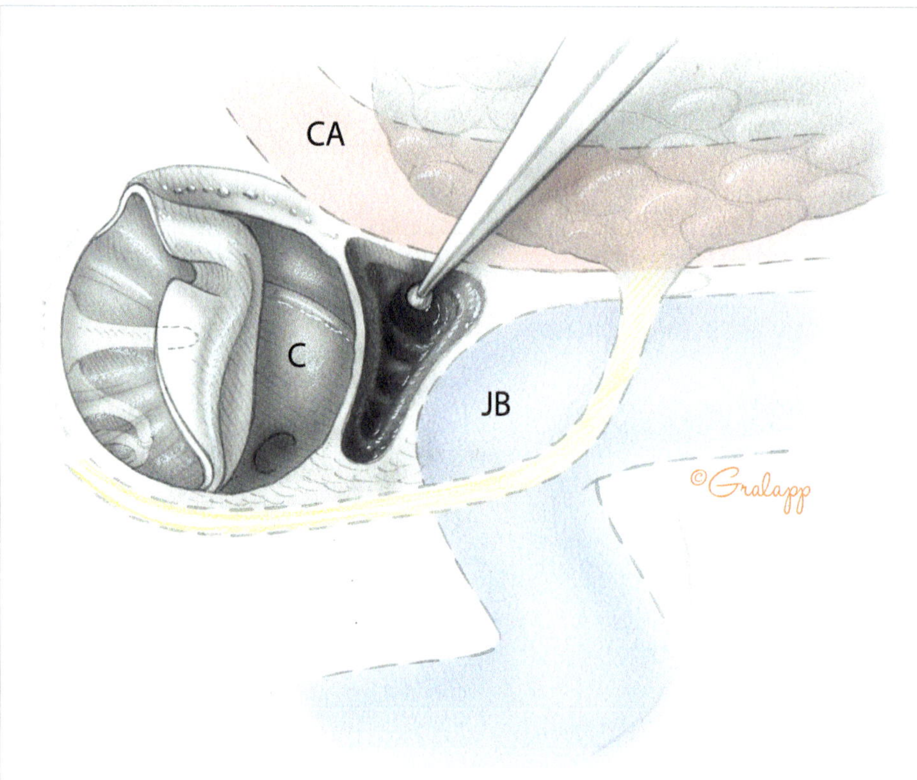

Fig. 14.5 In the subcochlear approach, the petrous apex, bone is excavated from the triangle bounded by the cochlea (C) superiorly, the jugular bulb (JB) posteriorly, and the carotid artery (CA) anteriorly.

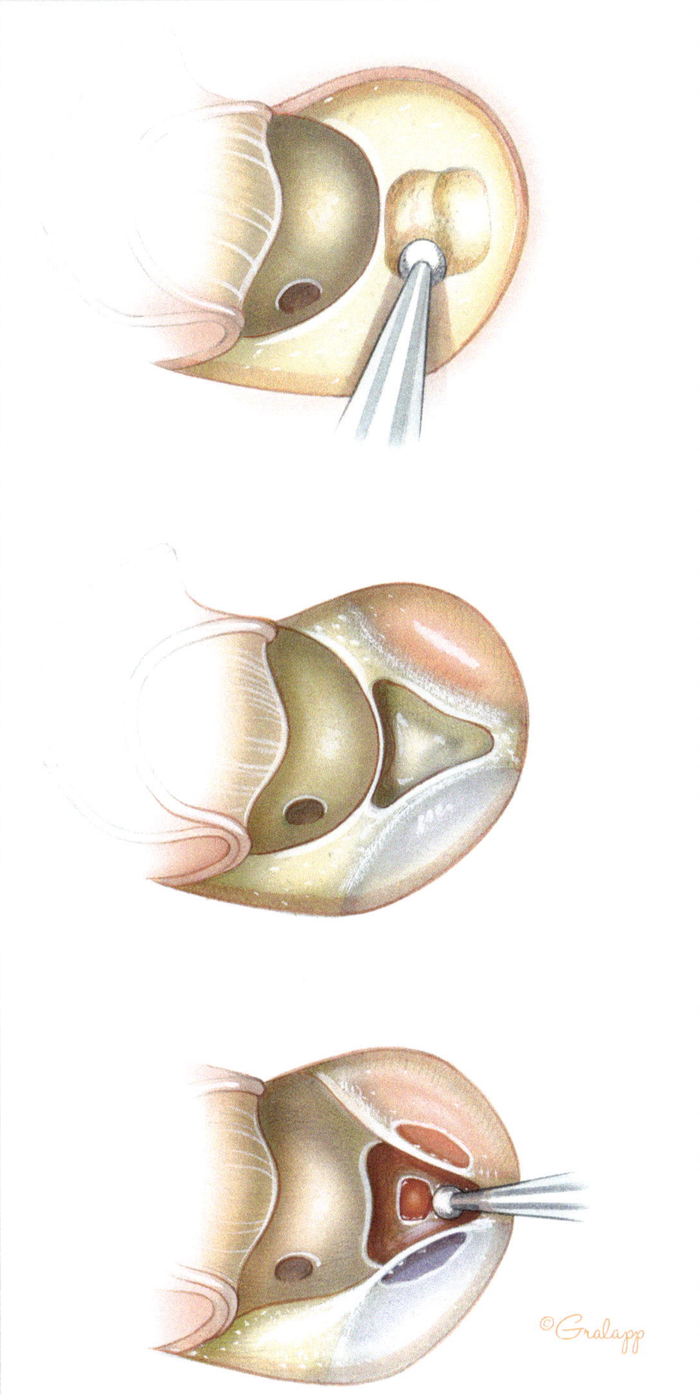

Fig. 14.6 Bony removal is commenced in the hypotympanic region. For orientation, it is usually best to identify the walls of both the jugular and carotid. This can be safely accomplished working gently with a diamond burr. The wall of the cholesterol granuloma is often fairly robust and may need to be opened sharply. When in doubt, aspiration with a needle may help confirm the identity of the cyst wall prior to its incision. Image guidance could also be helpful in verifying cyst location. The window created into the cyst should be as large as possible. To evacuate as much cyst contents as possible, the cyst cavity should be copiously lavaged with bacitracin saline through a plastic tube (e.g., no. 14 Angiocath). The passageway to the apex is usually sufficiently large to remain open by itself. When the connection is fairly small, a rolled sheet of thin silicon rubber (0.005 inch) is placed through the opening to discourage the formation of webs. A rolled sheet is better than a length of catheter, as it expands and accommodates to the maximal diameter of the opening. A fraction of surgically created apex drainage tracts close over time.

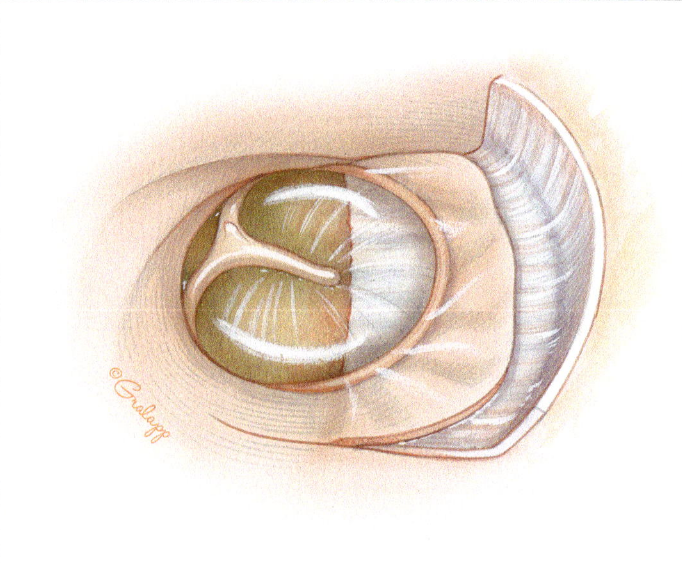

Fig. 14.7 After drainage of the cyst, the infracochlear opening remains open and is marsupialized into the tympanic cavity. As the tympanomeatal flap is now too short to cover the hypotympanic defect, it is augmented with a temporalis fascia graft. Once healing has taken place, the otoscopic appearance is of an enlarged tympanic membrane.

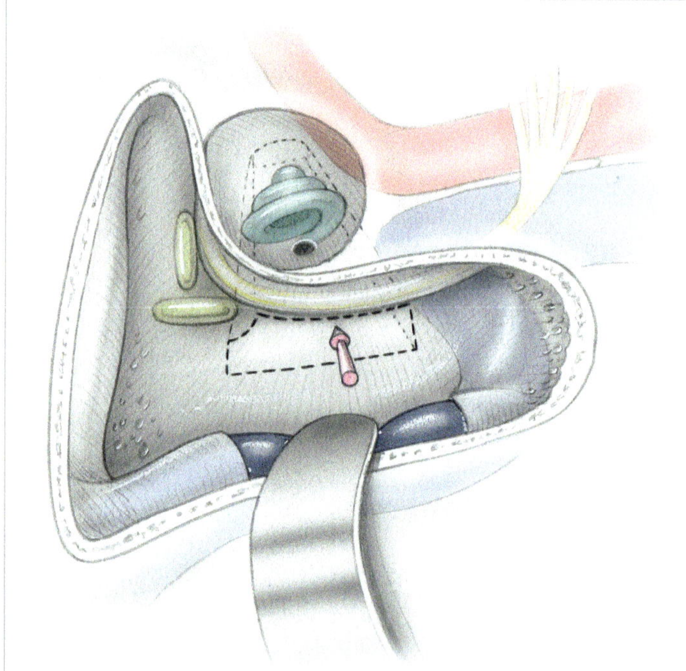

Fig. 14.8 The infralabyrinthine approach is an alternative route to the petrous apex for the drainage of cholesterol granuloma or infectious petrous apicitis. The opening enters via a rectangular space bounded superiorly by the posterior semicircular canal, inferiorly by the jugular bulb, posteriorly by the posterior fossa dura, and anteriorly by the descending facial nerve. The amount of room available via this exposure can be estimated from preoperative CT scans. As the main portion of the petrous apex lies anterior to the cochlea, this pathway is deep and narrow. To obtain a favorable angle for tunneling deep to the facial nerve, the sigmoid sinus can be decompressed and posteriorly displaced as depicted here. In contrast to cholesterol granuloma surgery, apical drainage for chronic otitis media may follow a variety of perilabyrinthine routes. The time-tested dictums are to use hand instruments (e.g., curettes) which better respect otic capsule bone and to identify diseased tracts by following the cholesteatoma and/or pus.

14.3 Petrous Apicectomy

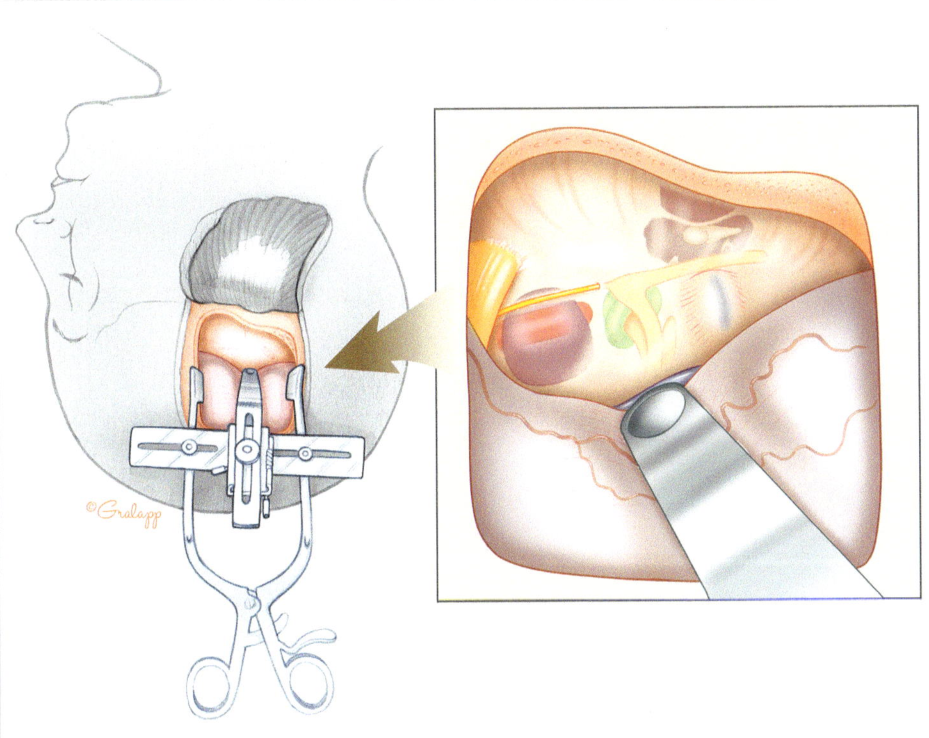

Fig. 14.9 The middle fossa approach may be used for exposure of apical petrous lesions. Examples include tumors such as chondrosarcoma and for the resection of cystic lesions. Cholesterol granuloma of the petrous apex may require resection when they are recurrent or when no lateral (subcochlear or infralabyrinthine) or medial (transsphenoidal) drainage route exists.

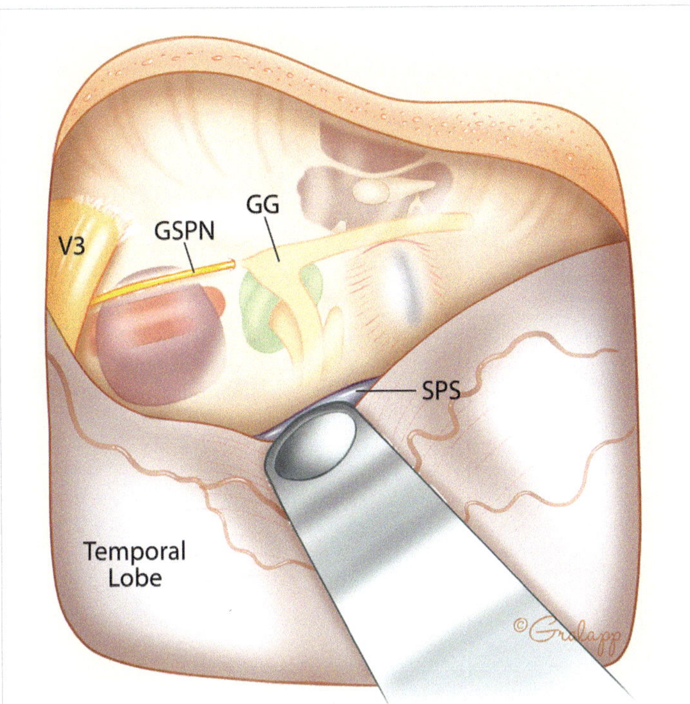

Fig. 14.10 Anatomical detail of the middle fossa floor in relation to a petrous apex cholesterol granuloma. Note that the retractor is engaged at the crest of the petrous pyramid in the groove of the superior petrosal sinus. As with all subtemporal approaches, venous bleeding from the anterior aspect of the floor almost invariably needs to be controlled with packing. GG, geniculate ganglion; V3, third division of the trigeminal nerve at the foramen ovale; GSPN, greater superficial petrosal nerve; SPS, superior petrosal sinus.

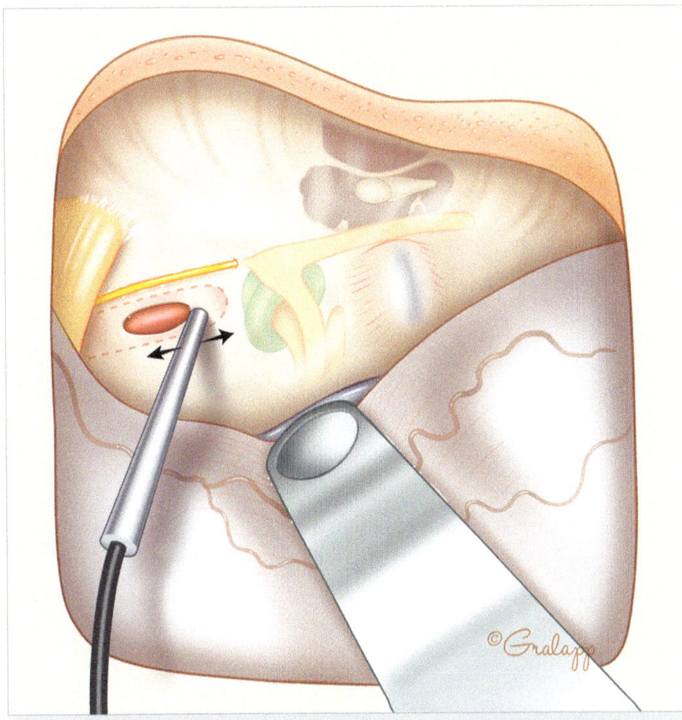

Fig. 14.11 The intrapetrous carotid artery may be congenitally dehiscent on the middle fossa floor or may have been eroded by disease. A Doppler probe may be useful in identifying the carotid before making an incision in the roof of the cholesterol granuloma.

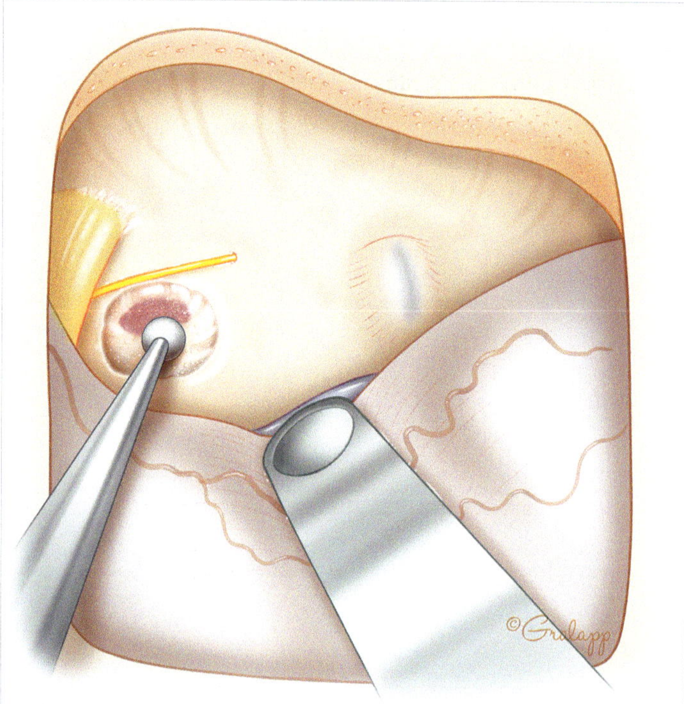

Fig. 14.12 A diamond burr is used to expose the roof of the cyst.

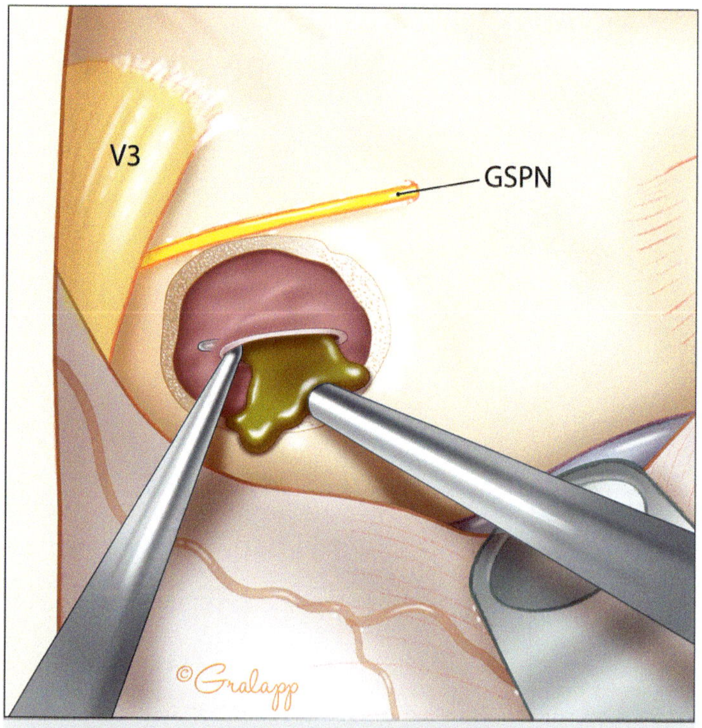

Fig. 14.13 The roof of the cholesterol granuloma is incised with release of its contents. GSPN, greater superficial petrosal nerve; V3, the third division of the trigeminal nerve entering foramen ovale.

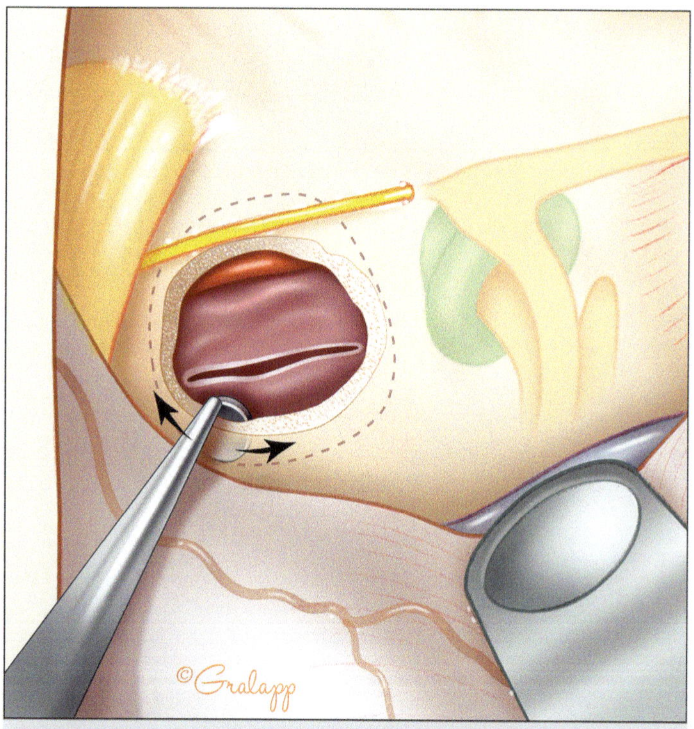

Fig. 14.14 The wall of the cholesterol granuloma is dissected from its bony cavity.

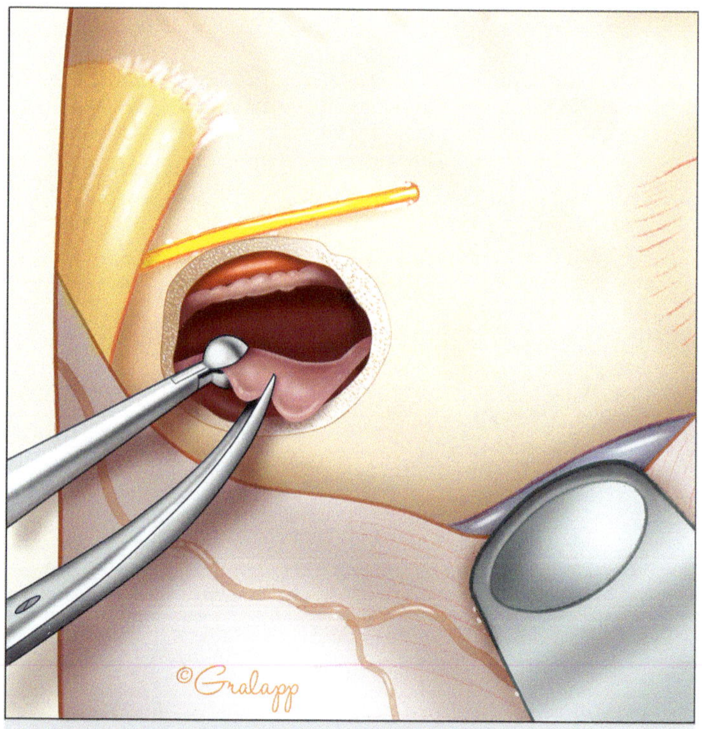

Fig. 14.15 The liberated cyst wall is excised.

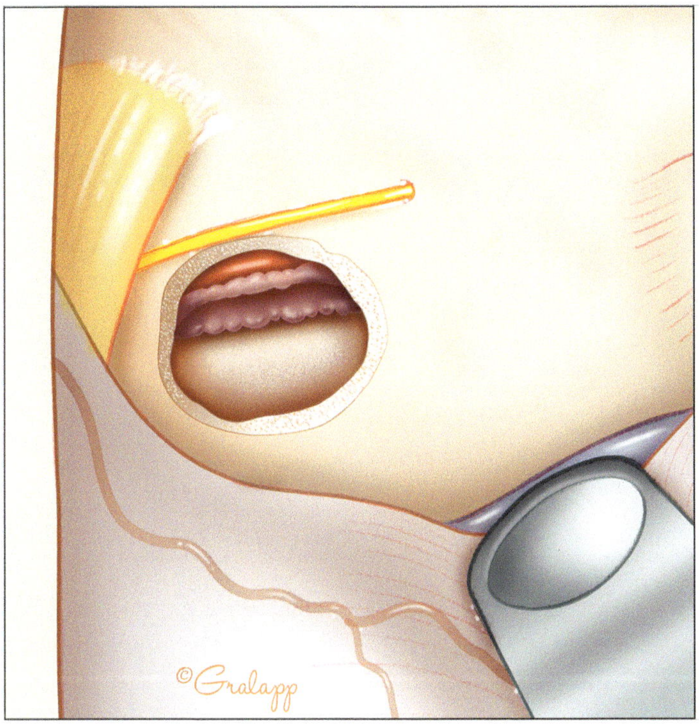

Fig. 14.16 If the cyst membrane is adherent to a dehiscent vessel wall, a portion of the cyst capsule is left on the carotid artery to avoid possible vascular injury with resultant stroke.

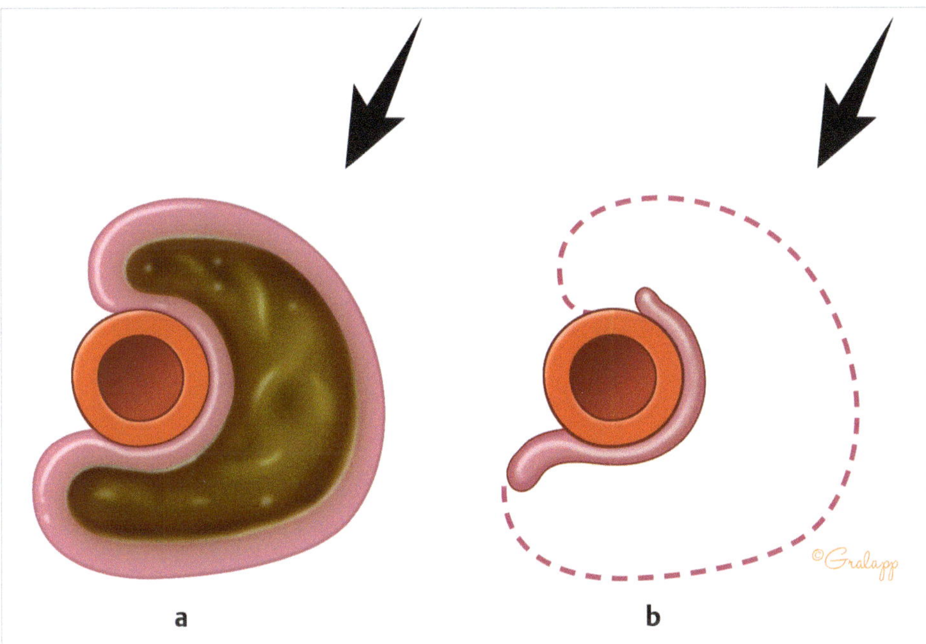

Fig. 14.17 Sagittal schematic illustration of the relationship between a petrous apex cholesterol granuloma and the intrapetrous carotid (**a**). When the cyst wall adheres to the carotid wall, it may be wisest to leave the adherent portion (**b**). The arrow represents the surgeon's point of view.

14.4 Transsphenoidal Approach to Petrous Apex

Peter H. Hwang

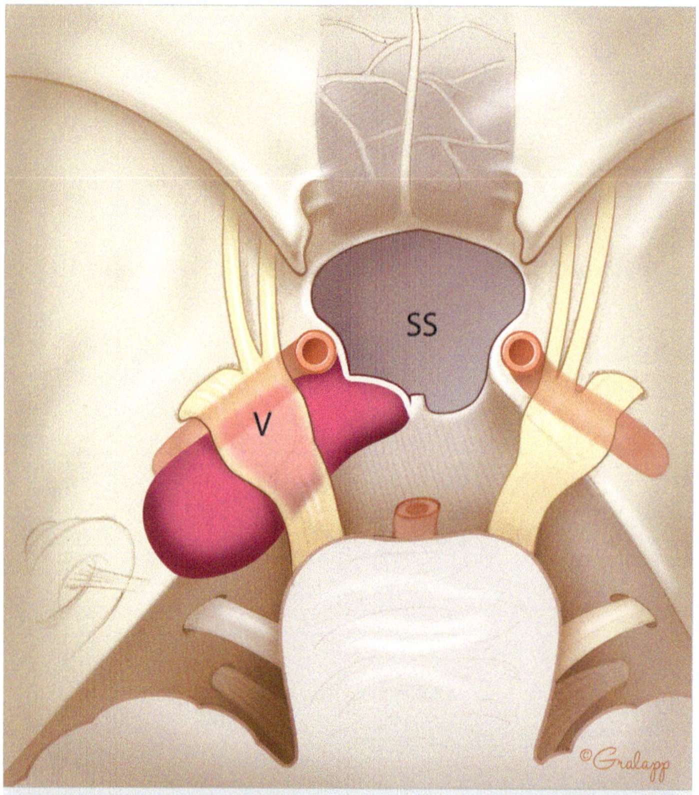

Fig. 14.18 Petrous apex cholesterol granuloma, axial view. This lesion, which extends medial to the carotid artery, has a favorable anatomy for drainage into the sphenoid sinus. V, trigeminal nerve; SS, sphenoid sinus with the intersinus septum removed.

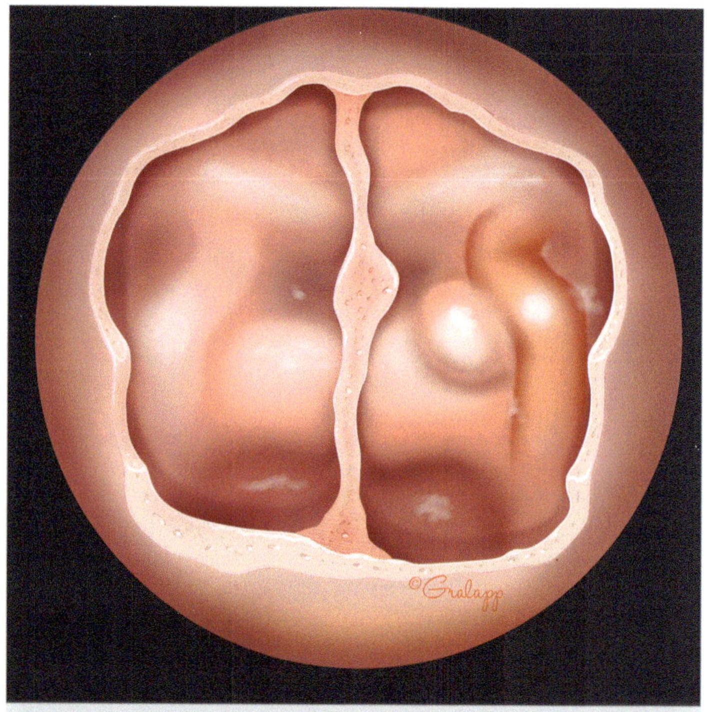

Fig. 14.19 The cholesterol granuloma makes a bulge in the posterolateral wall of the sphenoid sinus just medial to the carotid artery.

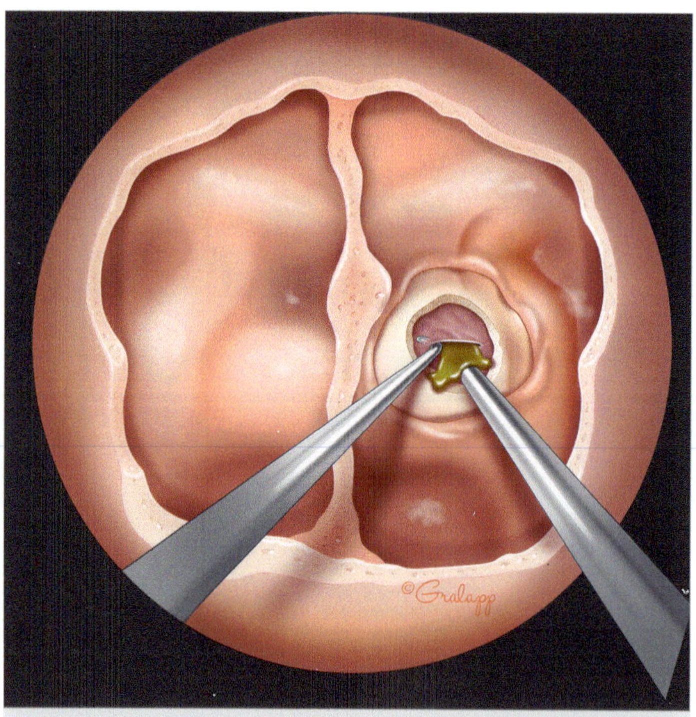

Fig. 14.20 The cyst is marsupialized into the sphenoid sinus.

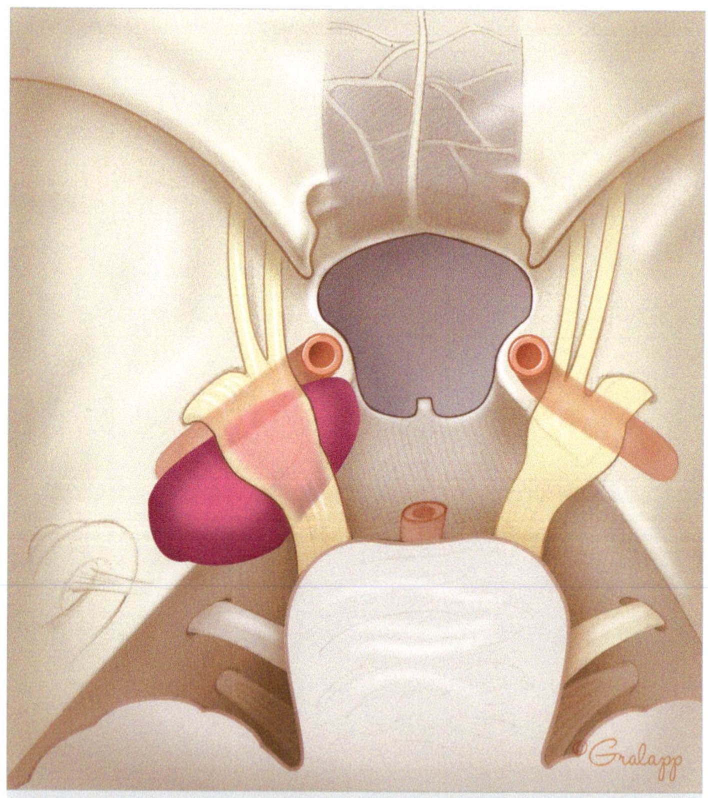

Fig. 14.21 Petrous apex cholesterol granuloma, axial view. This lesion, which extends to the medial edge of the carotid artery, is accessible for drainage into the sphenoid sinus.

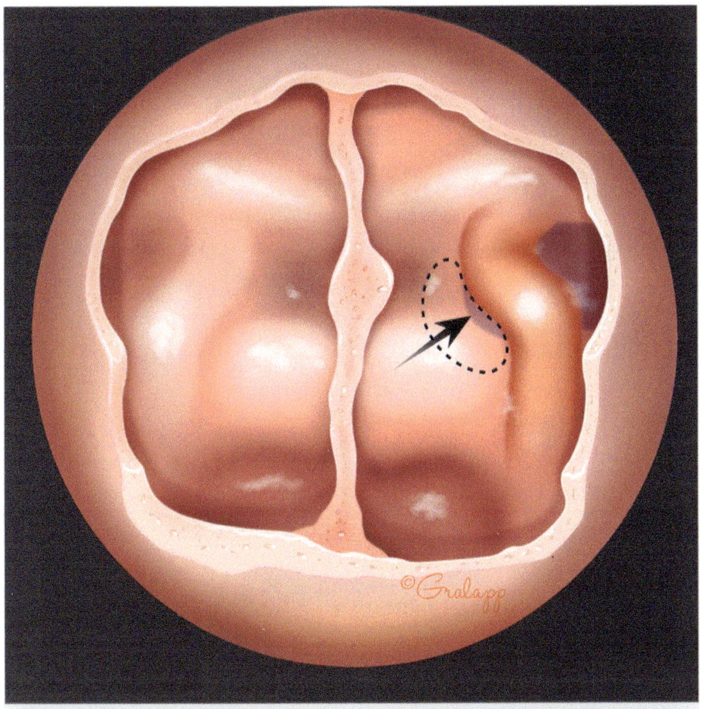

Fig. 14.22 Aspect of the posterolateral wall of the sphenoid sinus to be opened (*dotted lines*) to create the pathway needed to gain access to the cyst.

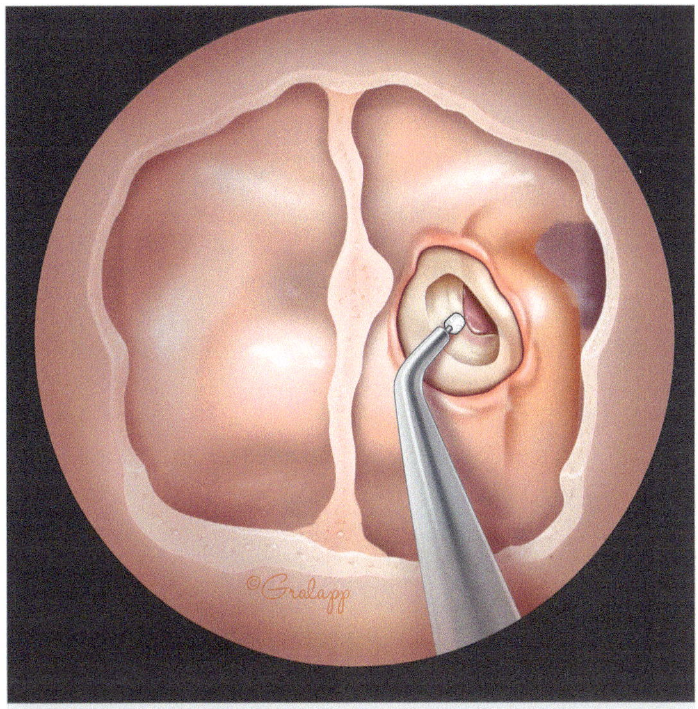

Fig. 14.23 Removal of bone with an angled drill.

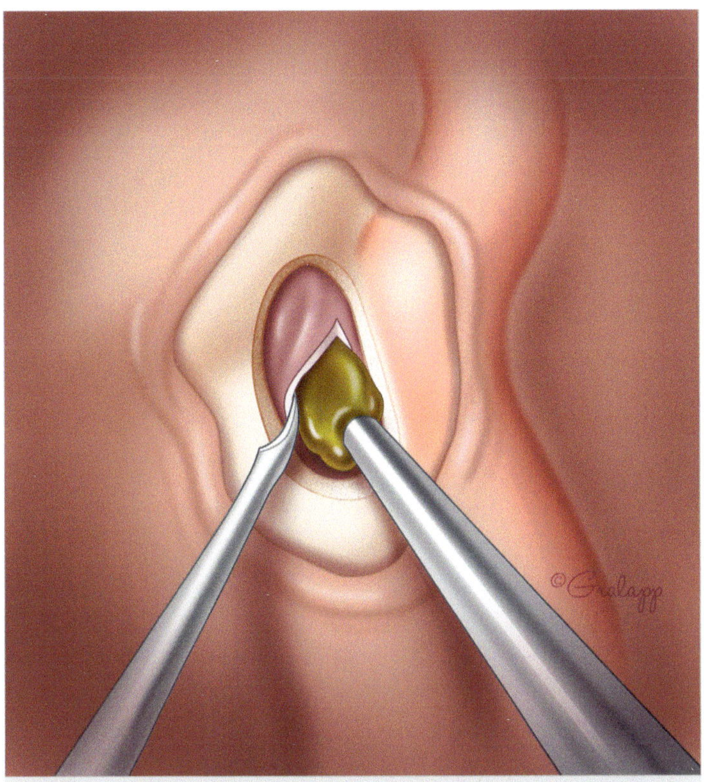

Fig. 14.24 Incision of the cyst wall and evacuation of its contents. To avoid possible stenosis of the drainage portal, the widest possible marsupialization should be created.

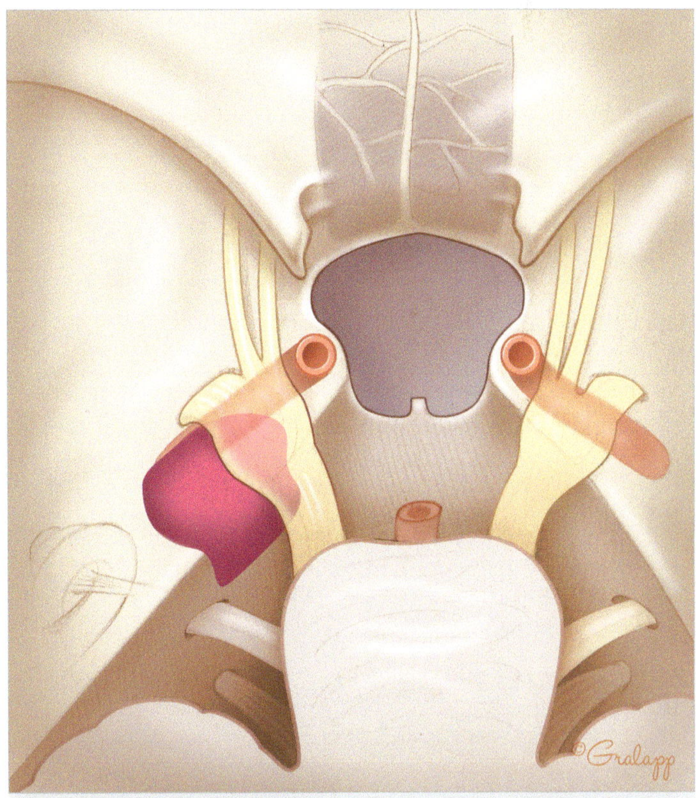

Fig. 14.25 Petrous apex cholesterol granuloma, axial view. This lesion, which is situated well lateral to the medial edge of the carotid artery, is not easily accessible for drainage into the sphenoid sinus.

15 Pulsatile Tinnitus

Robert K. Jackler

15.1 Introduction to Pulsatile Tinnitus

Pulsatile tinnitus may have many sources. Most commonly it occurs in conductive hearing loss, especially middle ear effusion, due to reduced external hearing and augmented vascular pulsations conducted through the fluid. Persistent and troubling pulsatile tinnitus is most often not due to ear disease but rather the ear picking up uncommonly noisy blood flow in adjacent vascular structures. The most common cause is turbulent flow in the sigmoid sinus. This may be due to irregularities in the vessel's wall caused by arachnoid granulations, mural thrombus, or diverticulum. Pulsatile tinnitus typically emanates from the dominant sigmoid sinus, most commonly on the right side. While the characteristic of the pulsation simulates the pitch of arterial flow, it is due to the high pressures in the brain's primary venous outflow conduit. Characteristically compression of the jugular vein in the neck either transiently muffles or eliminates the pulsation that, in turn, is augmented when the compression is released. On examination, pulsatile tinnitus may be subjective (only heard by the patient) or objective (audible to the examiner via a stethoscope). Audible pulsatile tinnitus is most often due to arteriovenous fistula.

Imaging such as CT or MR angiography is important to evaluate for dural arteriovenous fistula which is usually treated endovascularly. In evaluation of pulsatile tinnitus, the author prefers a combination of CT temporal bone (to identify sinus wall dehiscence, high jugular bulb, anomalous carotid artery, superior semicircular canal dehiscence, or glomus tumor) combined with CT angiography imaging both arterial (AV fistula) and venous (intraluminal sigmoid irregularities) anatomies. Ophthalmological examination for papilledema and visual field defect is often indicated to evaluate for pseudotumor cerebri. Treatment of troublesome pulsatile tinnitus of venous origin involves creation of a sound baffle in the mastoid and/or hypotympanum. Ligation of the jugular vein in the neck or packing of the jugular bulb is contraindicated due to the risk of triggering intracranial venous insufficiency. Endovascular procedures, including stenting, are alternative options especially for the obliteration of arteriovenous fistulae.

Further Reading

1. Ahsan SF, Seidman M, Yaremchuk K. What is the best imaging modality in evaluating patients with unilateral pulsatile tinnitus? Laryngoscope 2015;125(2):284–285 PubMed
2. DeHart AN, Shaia WT, Coelho DH. Hydroxyapatite cement resurfacing the dehiscent jugular bulb: novel treatment for pulsatile tinnitus. Laryngoscope 2018;128(5):1186–1190 PubMed
3. Lansley JA, Tucker W, Eriksen MR, Riordan-Eva P, Connor SEJ. Sigmoid sinus diverticulum, dehiscence, and venous sinus stenosis: potential causes of pulsatile tinnitus in patients with idiopathic intracranial hypertension? AJNR Am J Neuroradiol 2017;38(9):1783–1788 PubMed
4. Pegge SAH, Steens SCA, Kunst HPM, Meijer FJA. Pulsatile tinnitus: differential diagnosis and radiological work-up. Curr Radiol Rep 2017;5(1):5 PubMed
5. Reardon MA, Raghavan P. Venous abnormalities leading to tinnitus: imaging evaluation. Neuroimaging Clin N Am 2016;26(2):237–245 PubMed
6. Serulle Y, Miller TR, Gandhi D. Dural arteriovenous fistulae: imaging and management. Neuroimaging Clin N Am 2016;26(2):247–258 PubMed
7. Sismanis A. Pulsatile tinnitus: contemporary assessment and management. Curr Opin Otolaryngol Head Neck Surg 2011;19(5):348–357 PubMed
8. Song JJ, Kim YJ, Kim SY, et al. Sinus wall resurfacing for patients with temporal bone venous sinus diverticulum and ipsilateral pulsatile tinnitus. Neurosurgery 2015;77(5):709–717, discussion 717 PubMed
9. Trivelato FP, Araújo JF, Dos Santos Silva R, Rezende MT, Ulhôa AC, Castro GD. Endovascular treatment of pulsatile tinnitus associated with transverse sigmoid sinus aneurysms and jugular bulb anomalies. Interv Neuroradiol 2015;21(4):548–551 PubMed
10. Wang AC, Nelson AN, Pino C, Svider PF, Hong RS, Chan E. Management of sigmoid sinus associated pulsatile tinnitus: a systematic review of the literature. Otol Neurotol 2017;38(10):1390–1396 PubMed
11. Yeo WX, Xu SH, Tan TY, Low YM, Yuen HW. Surgical management of pulsatile tinnitus secondary to jugular bulb or sigmoid sinus diverticulum with review of literature. Am J Otolaryngol 2018;39(2):247–252 PubMed

15.2 Pulsatile Tinnitus of Dural Sinus Origin

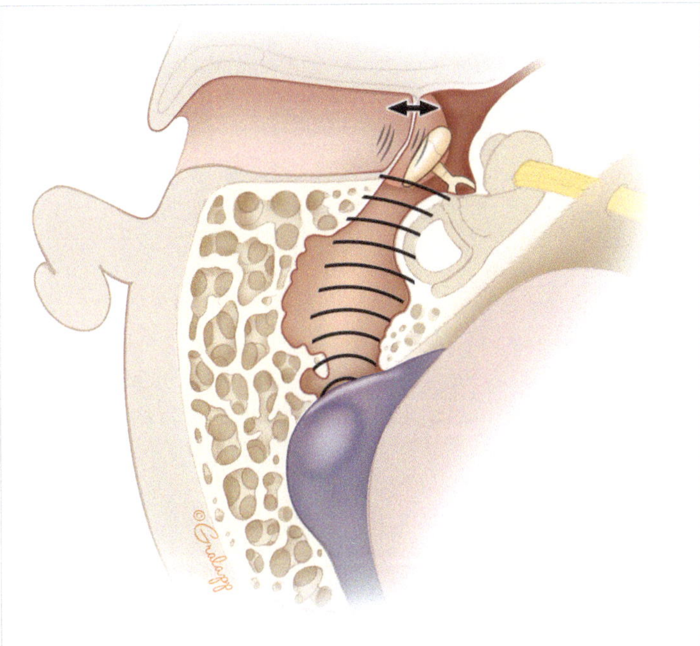

Fig. 15.1 Flow in the venous sinuses is rapid and under high pressure. When the bony covering of the sigmoid sinus is dehiscent, sound generated may pass via the mastoid air cells to the tympanum with it and can vibrate the tympano-ossicular chain resulting in pulsatile tinnitus. This is the most common cause of troubling pulsatile tinnitus.

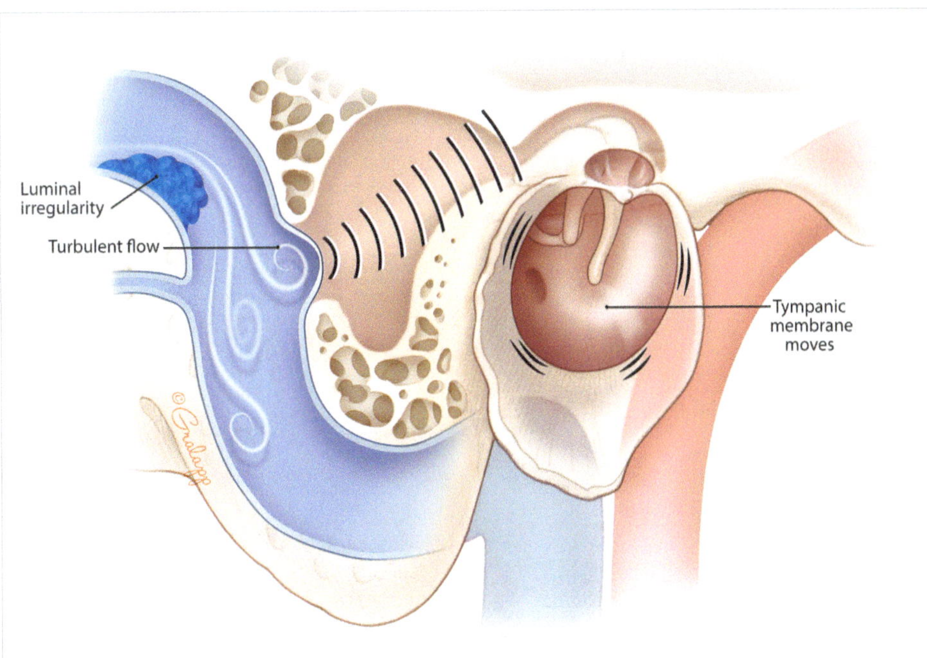

Fig. 15.2 Smooth flow within the sinus generates little noise. Turbulent flow augments the audibility of venous sounds. In many cases, prominent arachnoid granulations impinge upon the lumen in proximity to the transverse–sigmoid sinus junction.

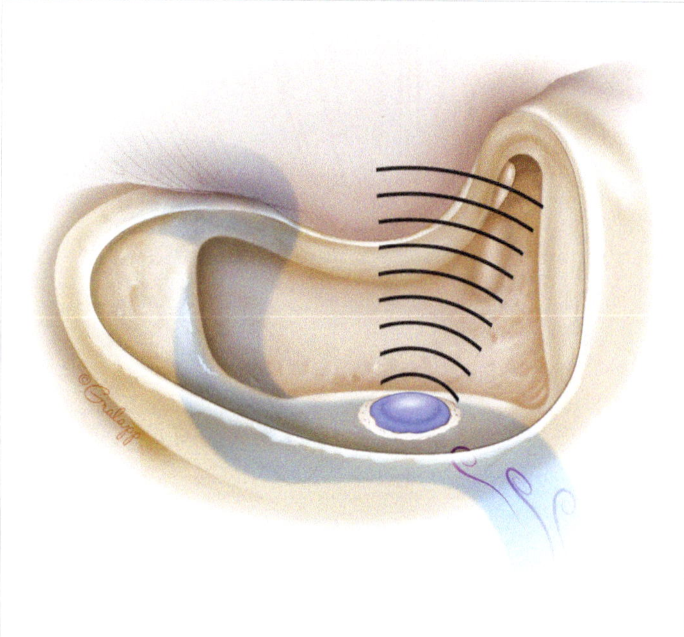

Fig. 15.3 Mastoidectomy exposing the dehiscent segment of the sigmoid sinus. Care is taken not to disturb the intact sigmoid bone covering and to avoid enlarging the dehiscence.

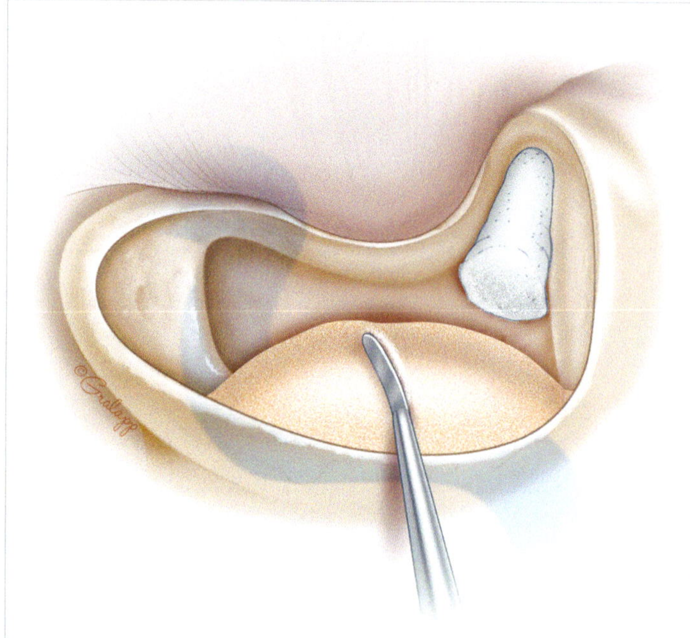

Fig. 15.4 Covering of the dehiscent sinus with a thick coating of hydroxyapatite cement to create a sound baffle. This has proved highly effective in abating pulsatile tinnitus in properly selected patients. Note the temporary placement of absorbable gelatin sponge in the aditus-ad-antrum to protect the ossicles from coming in contact with the cement.

15.3 Pulsatile Tinnitus of Carotid and Jugular Bulb Origin

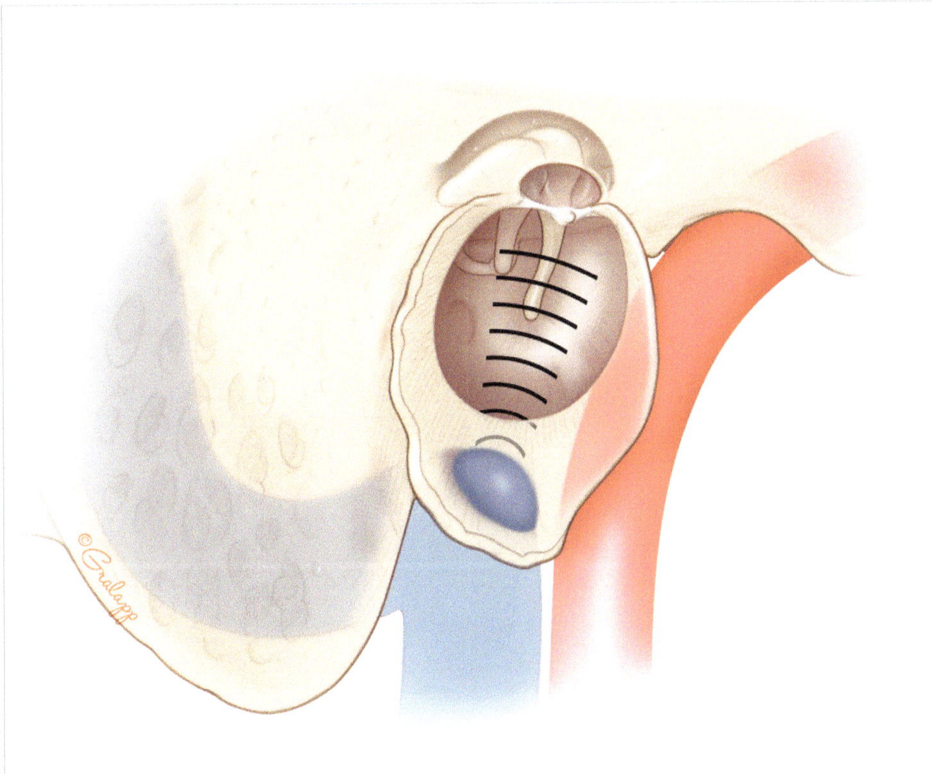

Fig. 15.5 Dehiscent carotid artery into the hypotympanum may result in pulsatile tinnitus.

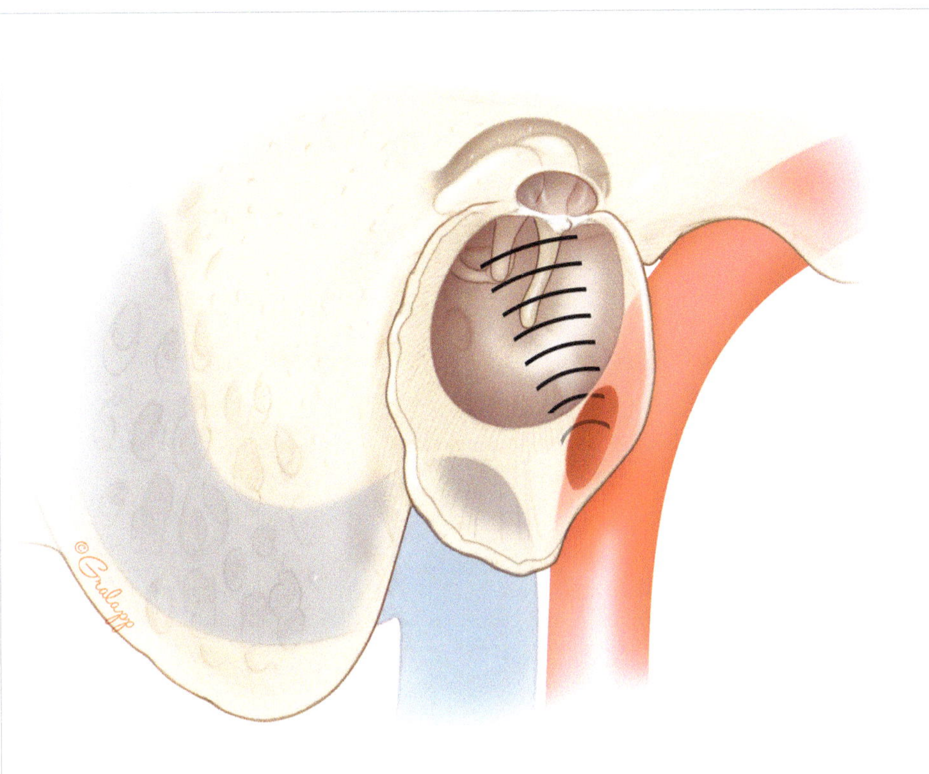

Fig. 15.6 Dehiscent jugular bulb into the hypotympanum may result in pulsatile tinnitus.

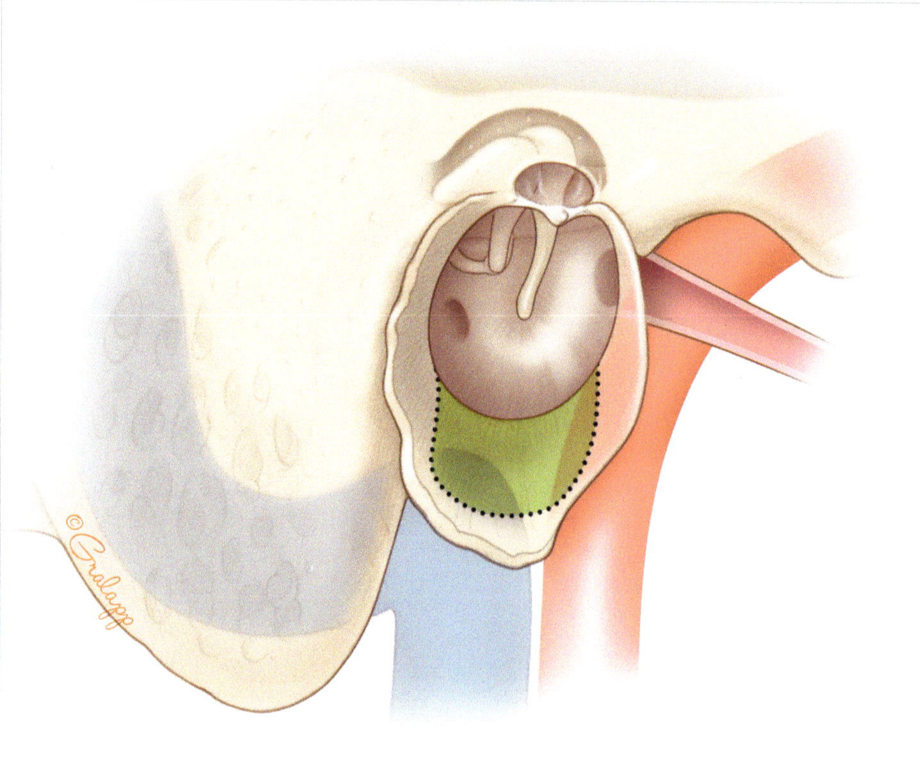

Fig. 15.7 Hypotympanic approach for exposure of the great vessels. This procedure is done postauricularly with lowering of the floor of the osseous ear canal in preparation.

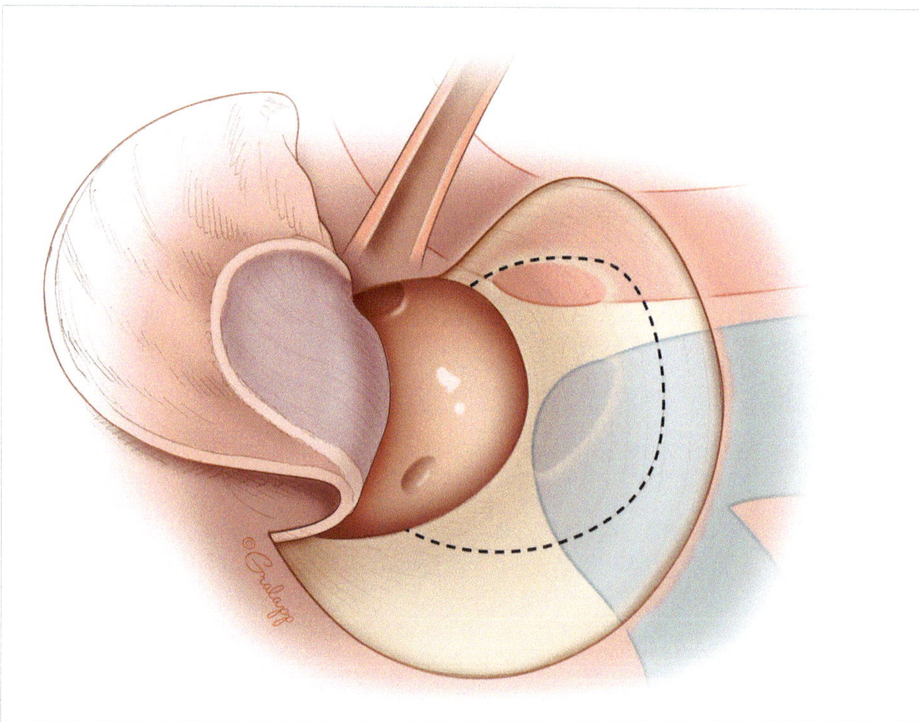

Fig. 15.8 A superiorly based tympanomeatal flap is elevated.

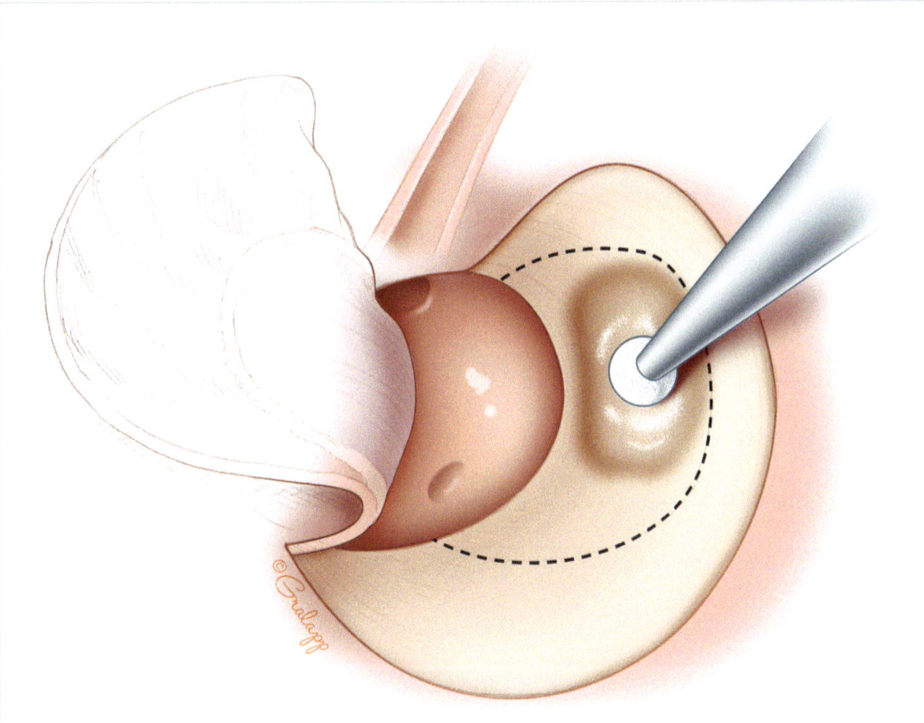

Fig. 15.9 The hypotympanum is drilled open.

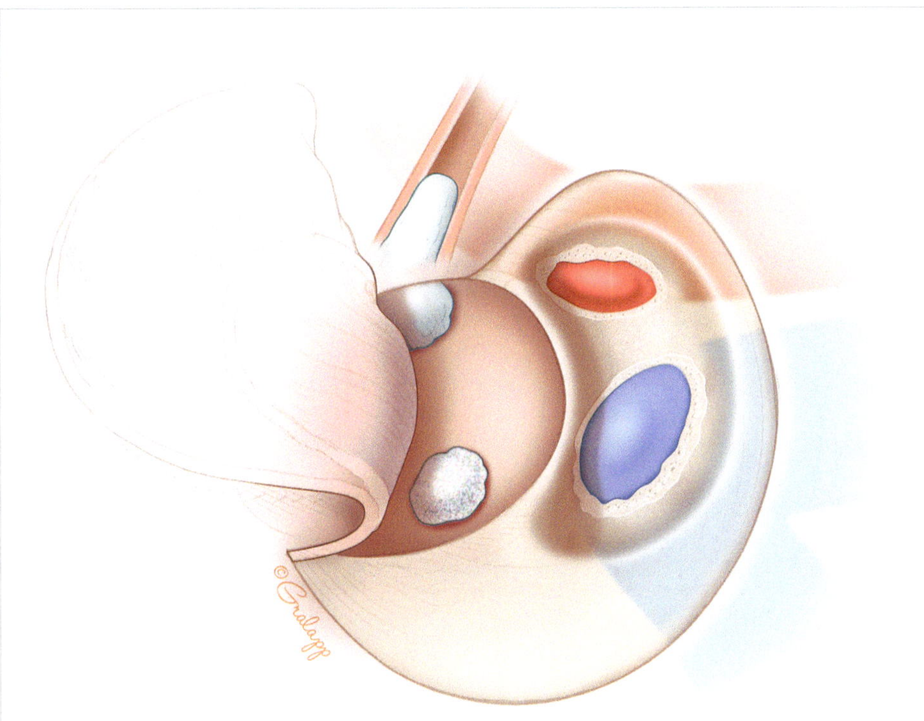

Fig. 15.10 Exposure of the carotid artery and jugular bulb in the hypotympanum.

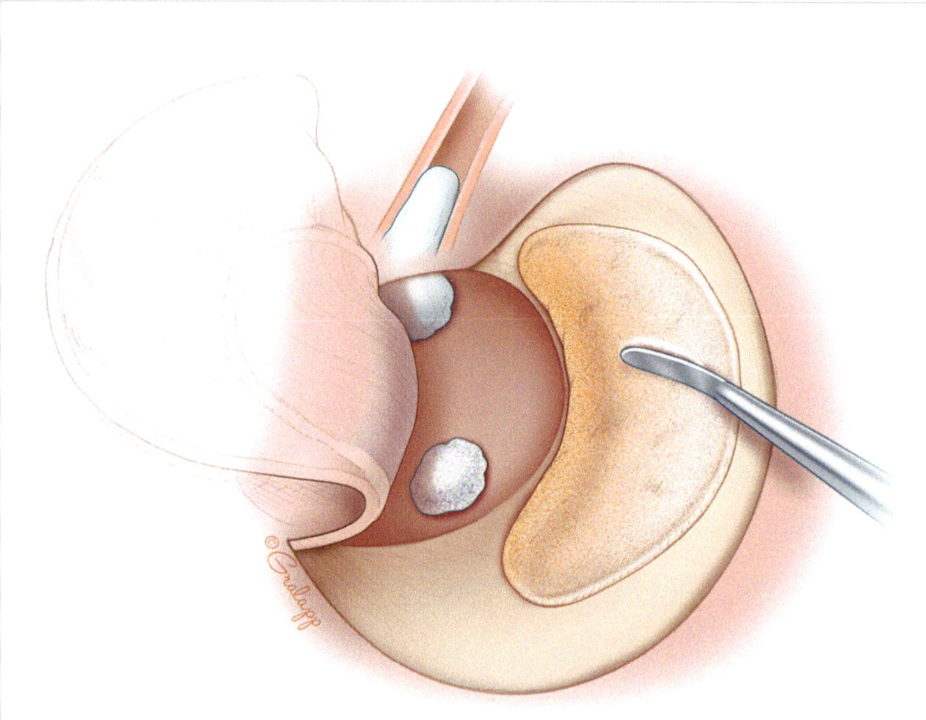

Fig. 15.11 Covering of the carotid artery and jugular bulb with hydroxyapatite cement to create a sound baffle. Temporary absorbable gelatin sponge packing is placed in the round window and a small Merocel pack is placed in the Eustachian tube orifice to protect them.

16 Appendix: Educational Handouts for Patients

Robert K. Jackler

At the Stanford Ear Institute, we employ a series of handouts to help explain ear disease and planned surgeries to patients and their families. We include these compilations in this book so that otologists around the world can adopt them for use with their own patients.

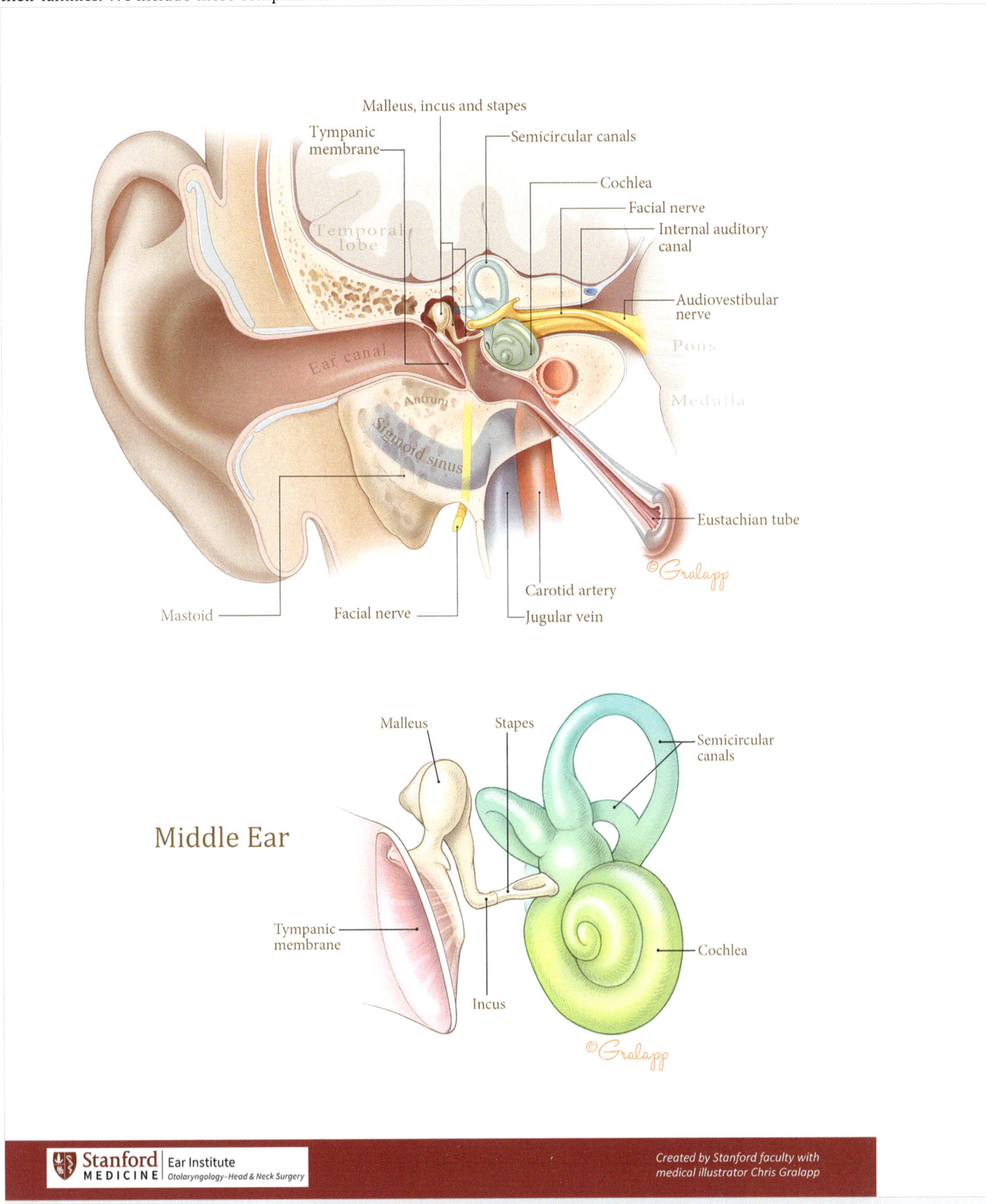

Fig. 16.1 Anatomy of the ear.

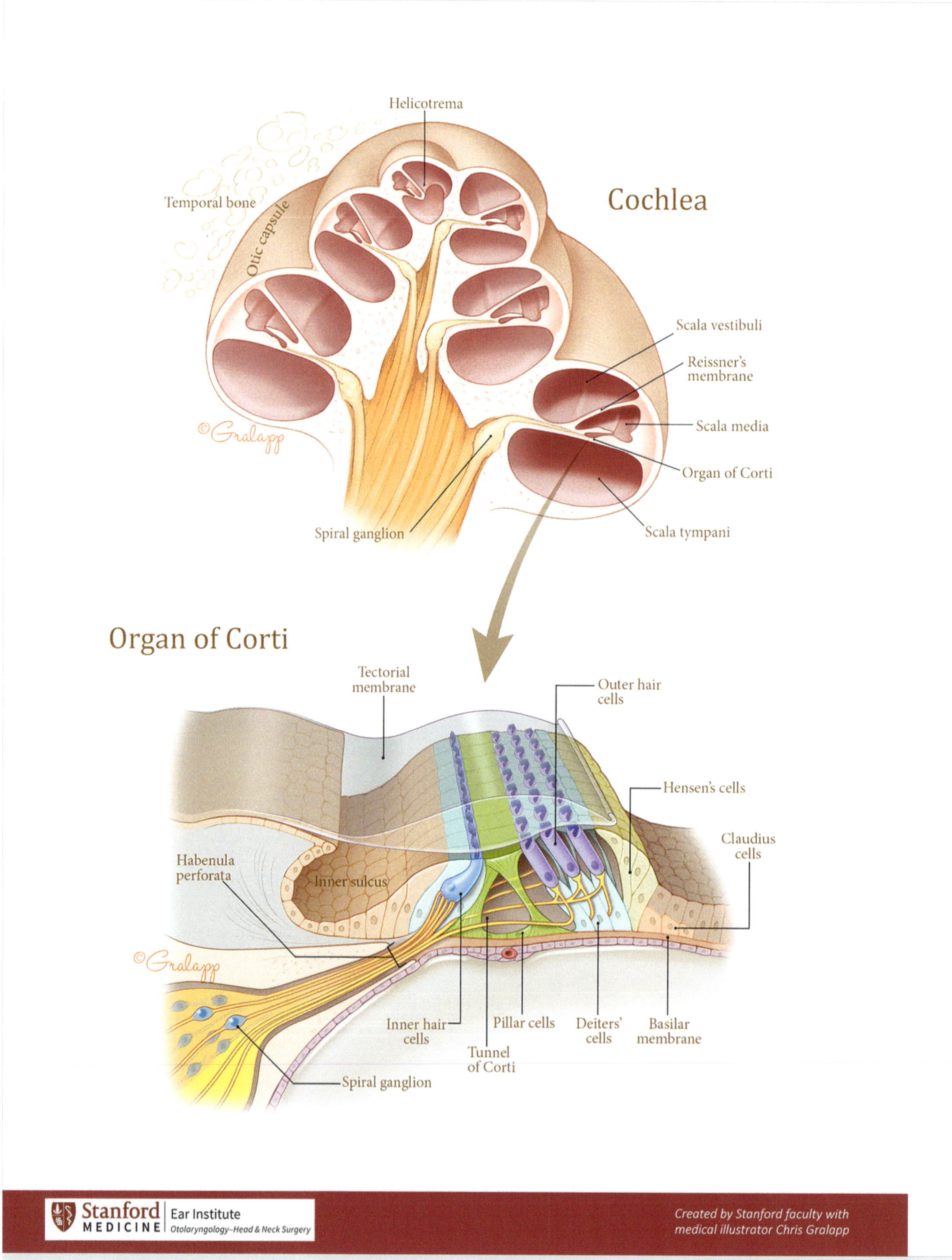

Fig. 16.2 Anatomy of hearing.

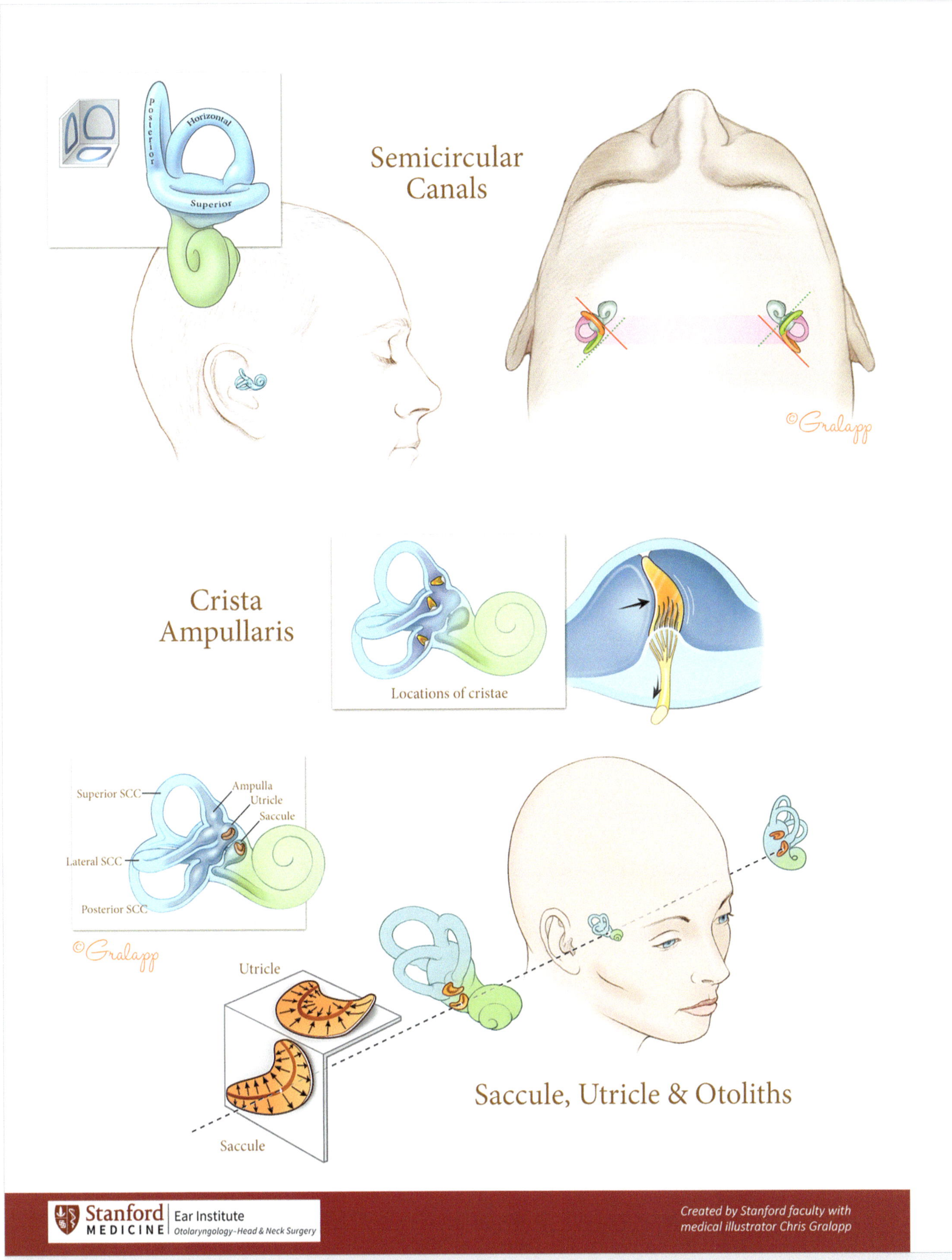

Fig. 16.3 Anatomy of balance.

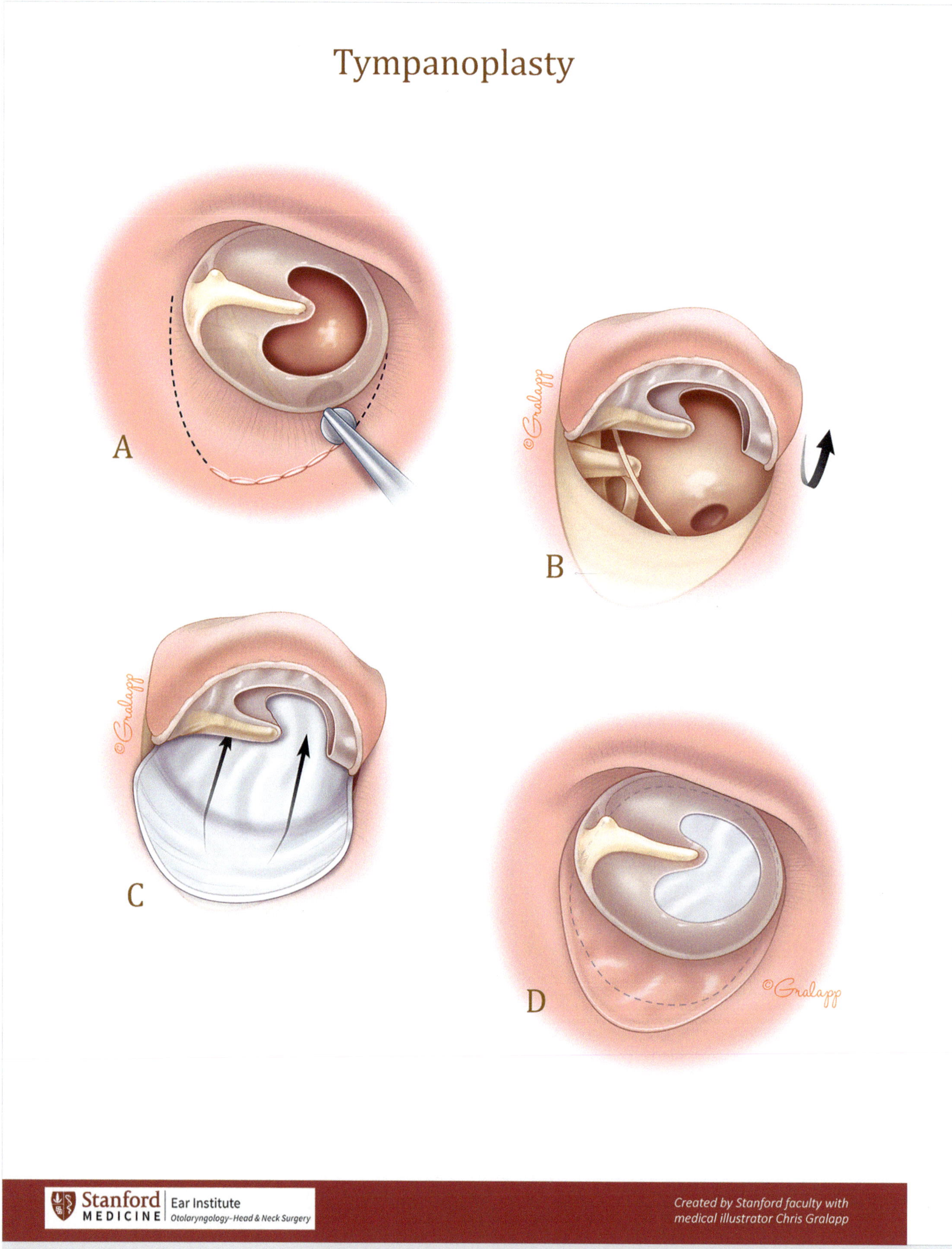

Fig. 16.4 Tympanoplasty.

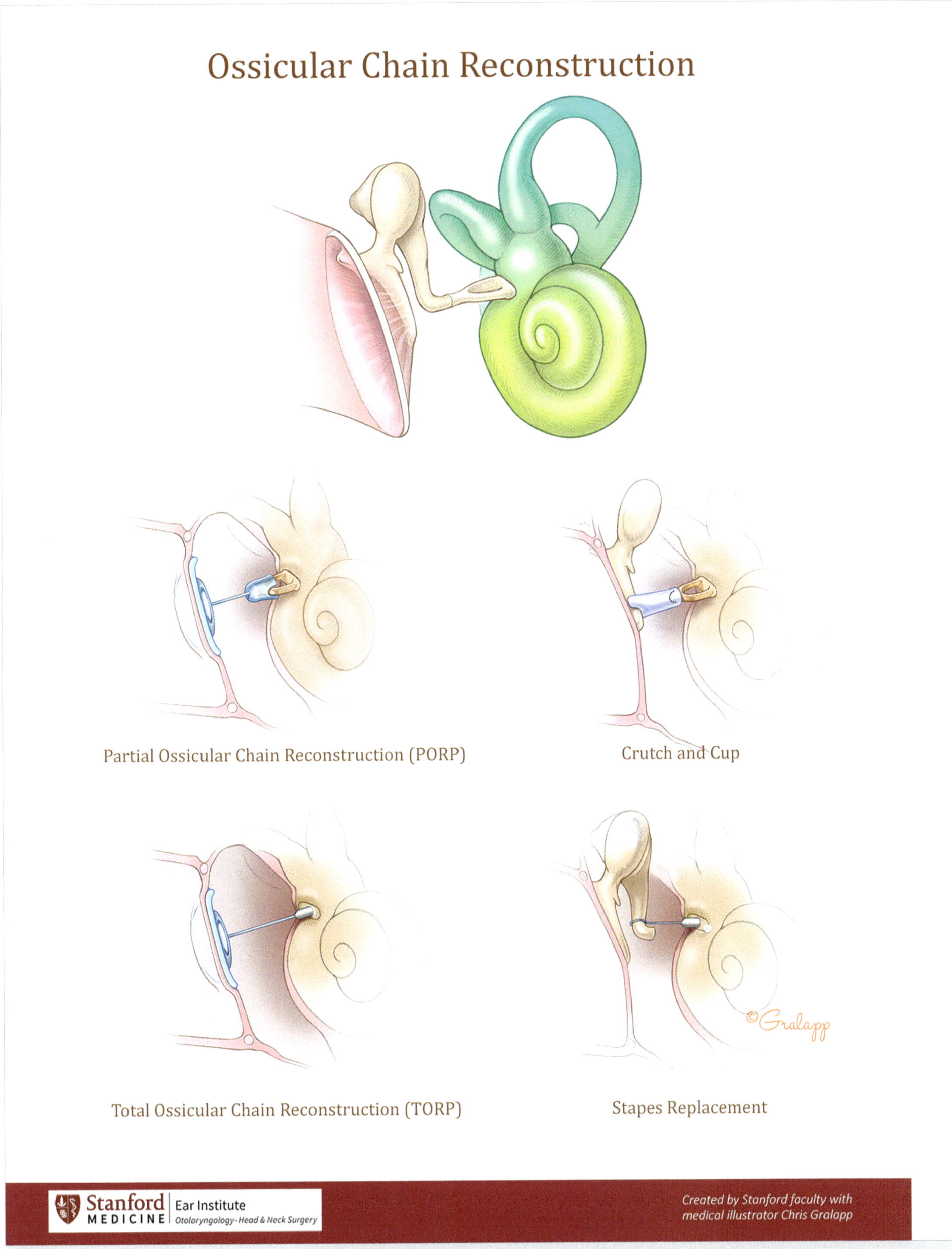

Fig. 16.5 Ossicular chair reconstruction.

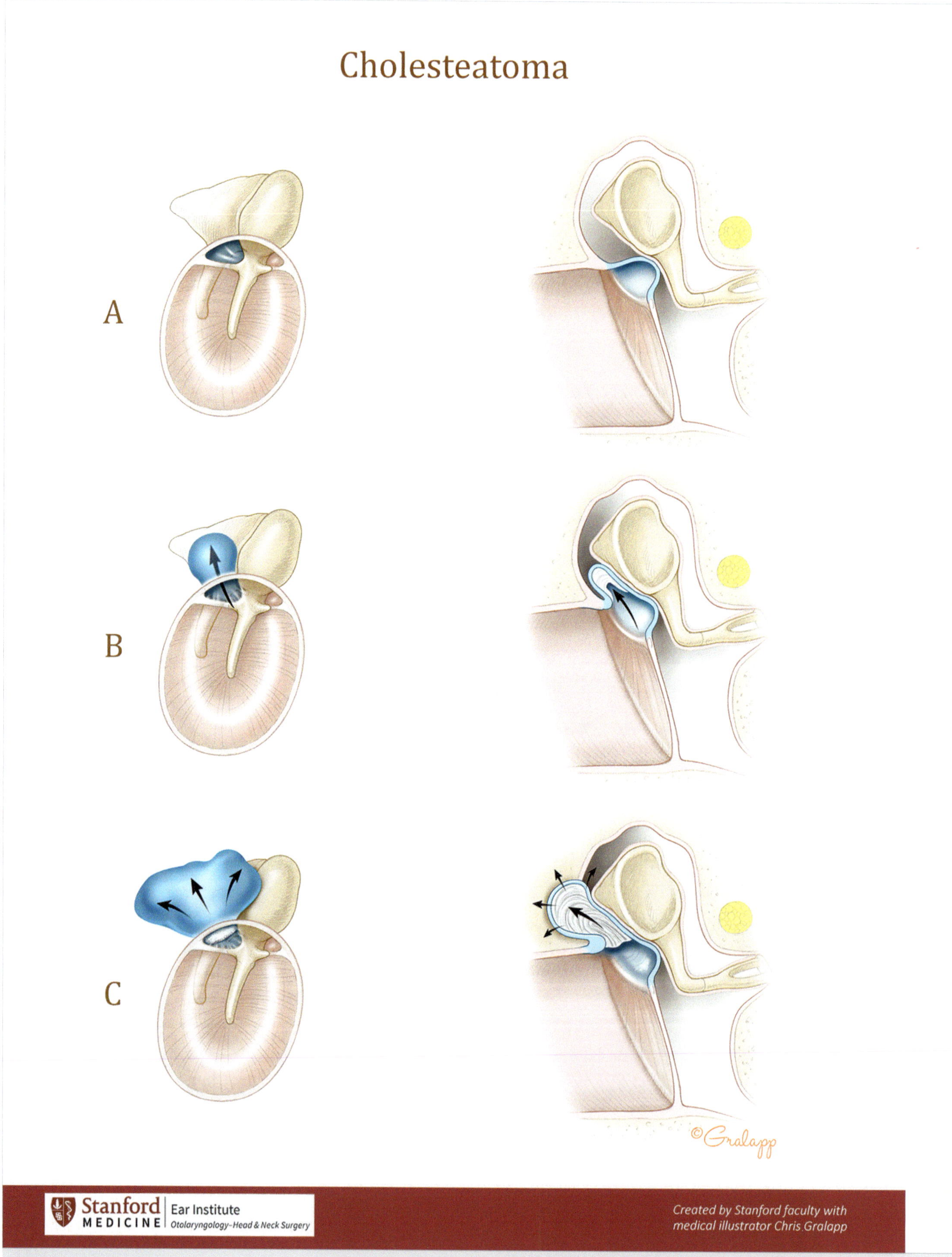

Fig. 16.6 Cholesteatoma.

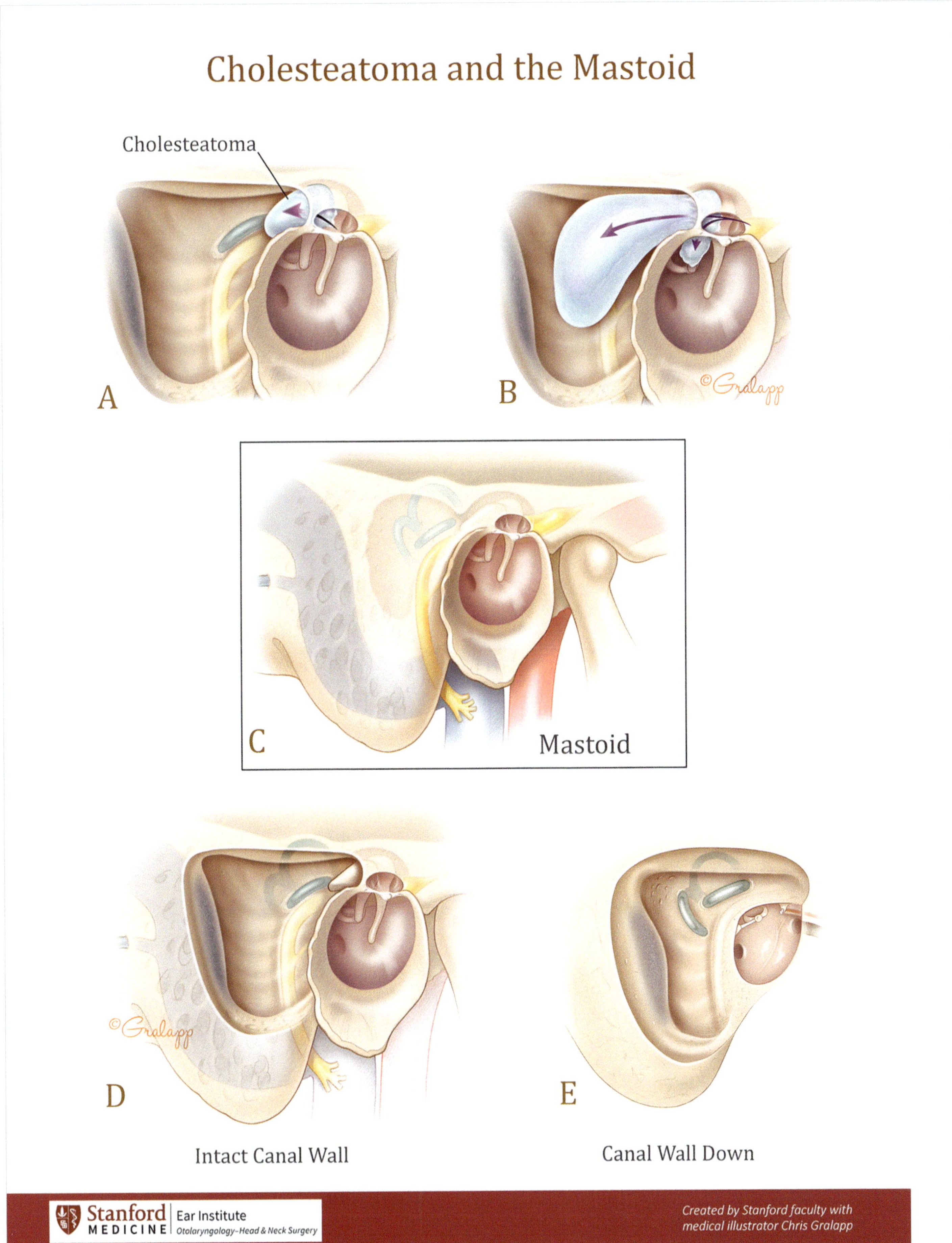

Fig. 16.7 Cholesteatoma and mastoidectomy.

Otosclerosis & Stapes Surgery

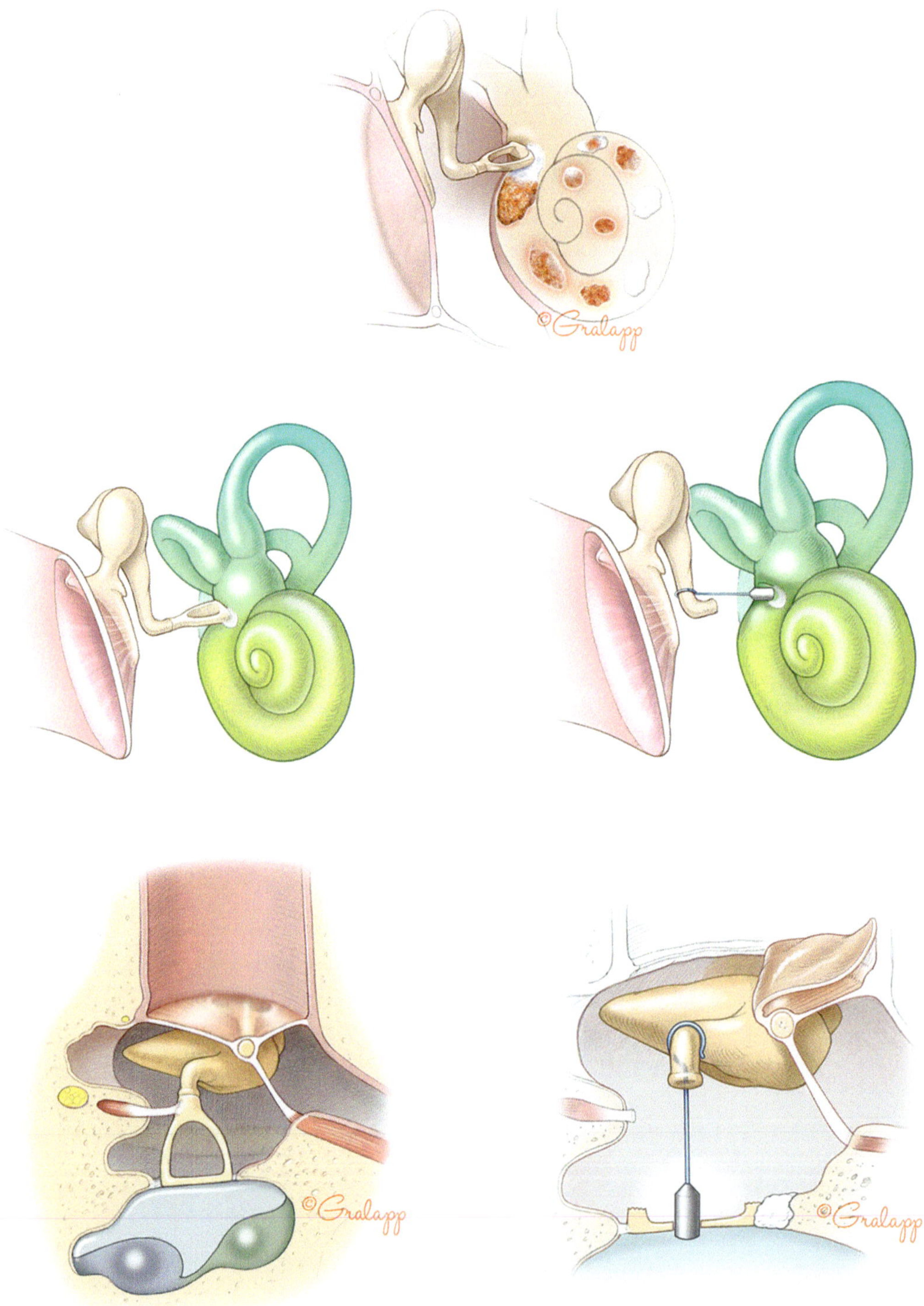

Stanford MEDICINE | Ear Institute
Otolaryngology-Head & Neck Surgery

Created by Stanford faculty with medical illustrator Chris Gralapp

Fig. 16.8 Otosclerosis and stapes surgery.

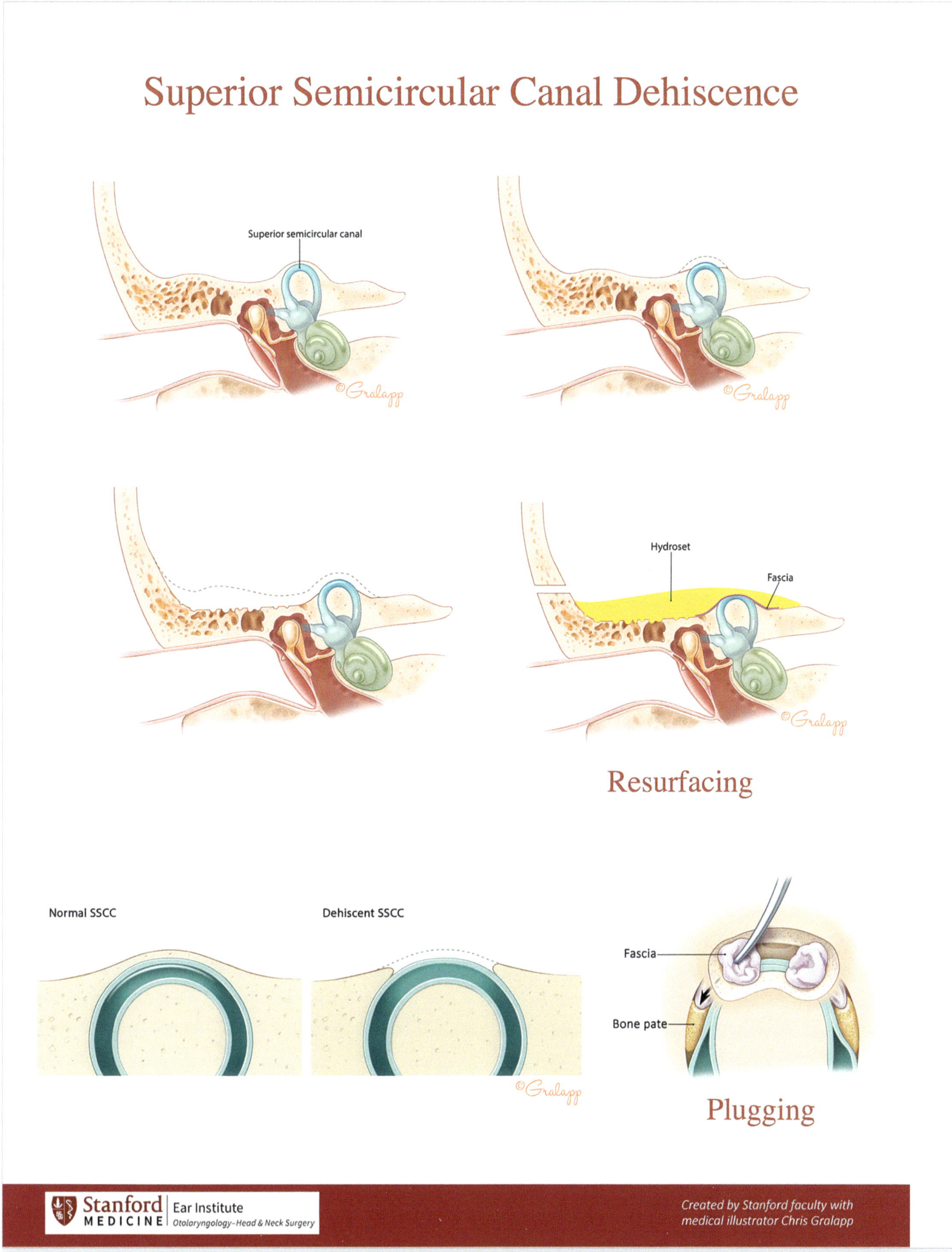

Fig. 16.9 Superior semicircular canal dehiscence.

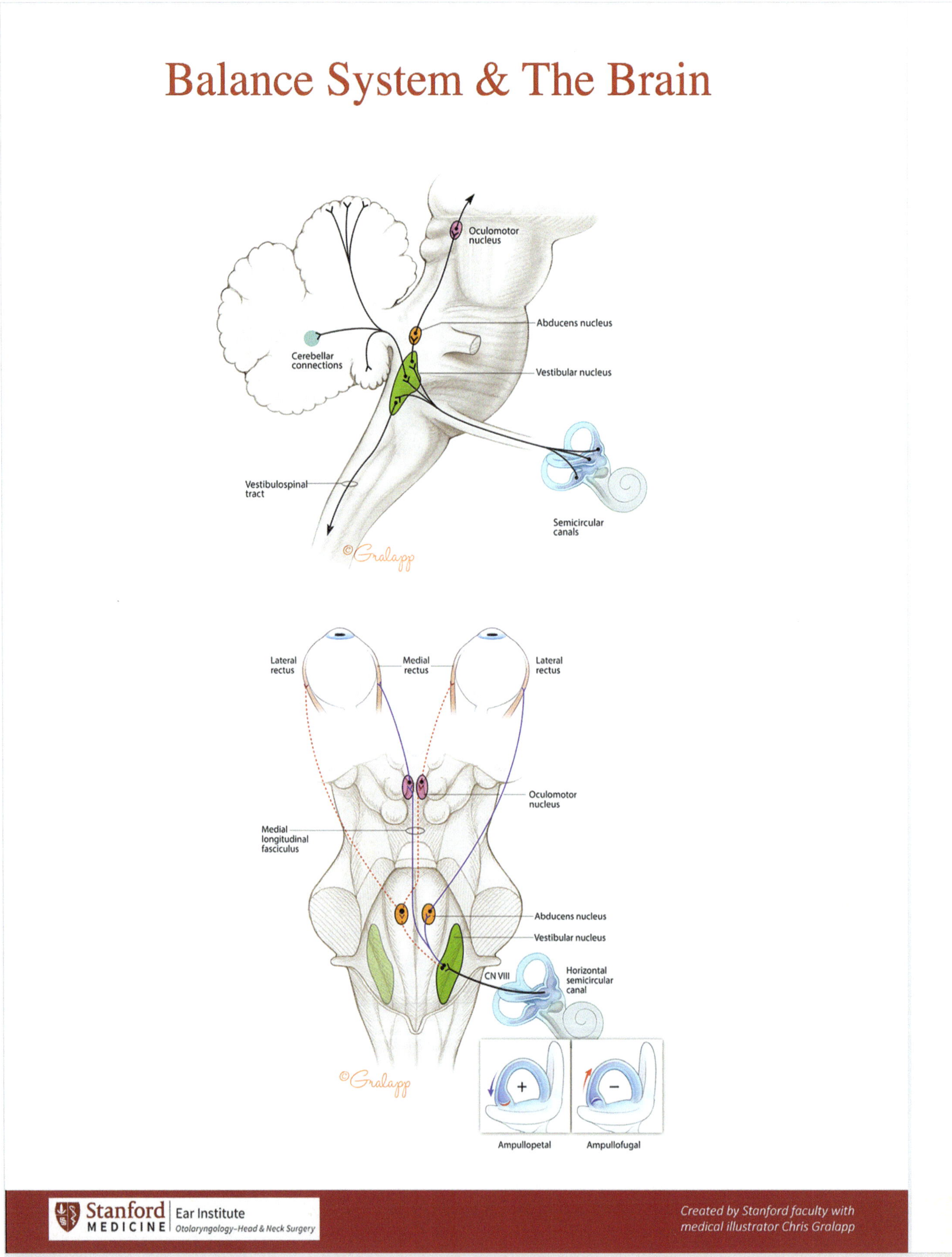

Fig. 16.10 Balance system and the brain.

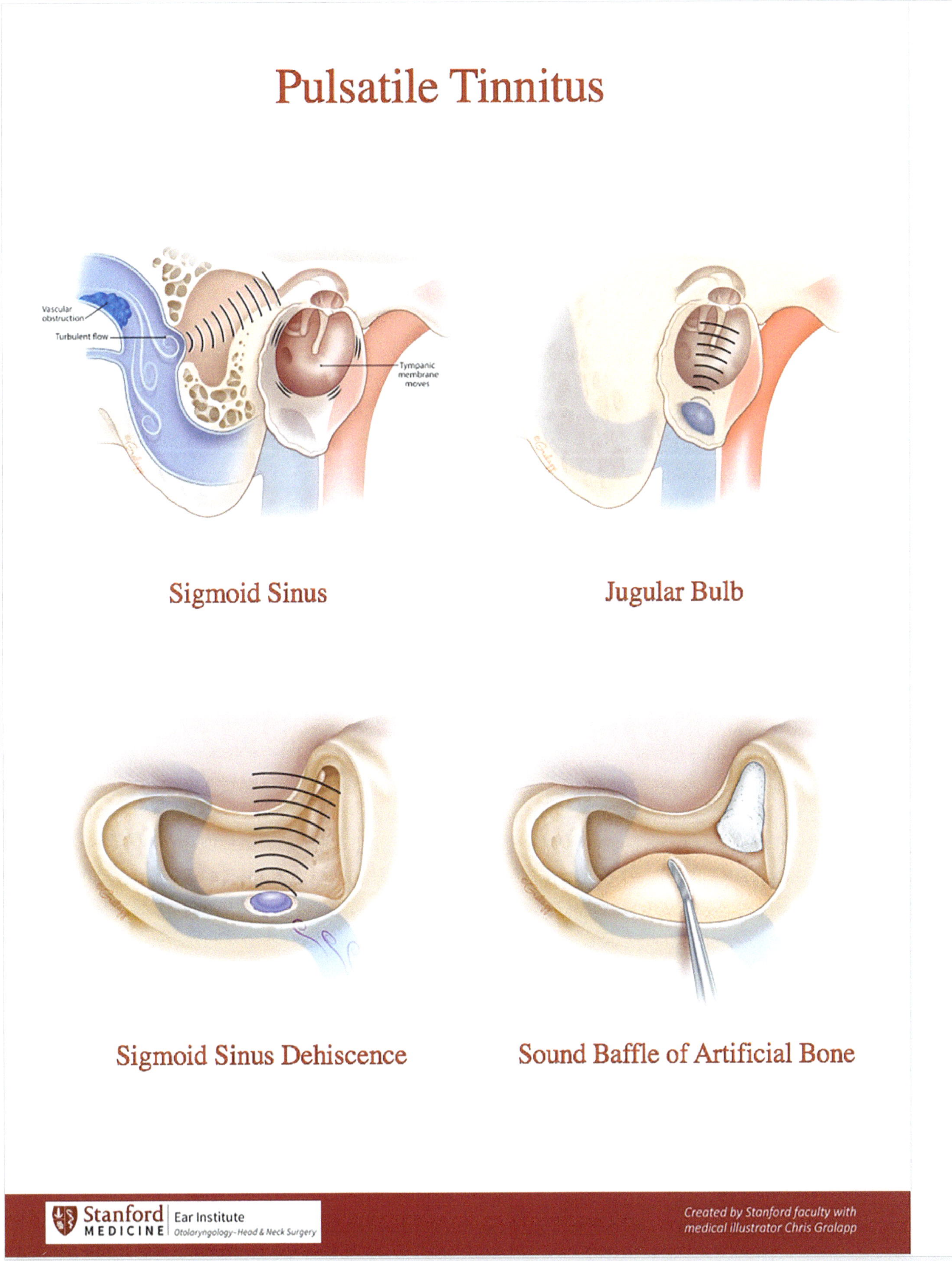

Fig. 16.11 Pulsatile tinnitus.

Index

A

B

C

R

S

T